Atlas of
Essential
Orthopaedic Procedures

Atlas of Essential Orthopaedic Procedures

Edited by

Evan Flatow, MD
Chairman
Department of Orthopaedics
Mount Sinai School of Medicine
New York, New York

Alexis Chiang Colvin, MD
Assistant Professor
Department of Orthopaedics
Mount Sinai School of Medicine
New York, New York

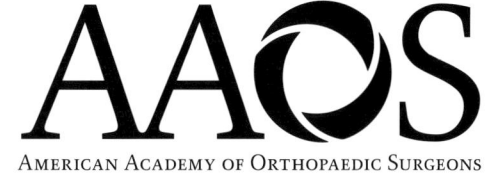

American Academy of Orthopaedic Surgeons

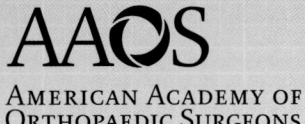

American Academy of Orthopaedic Surgeons Board of Directors, 2013-2014

Joshua J. Jacobs, MD
President

Frederick M. Azar, MD
First Vice-President

David Teuscher
Second Vice-President

John R. Tongue, MD
Past President

Andrew N. Pollak, MD
Treasurer

Annunziato Amendola, MD

William J. Best

Joseph A. Bosco III, MD

Matthew B. Dobbs, MD

Wilford K. Gibson, MD

David Mansfield, MD

John J. McGraw, MD

Todd A. Milbrandt, MD

Steven D.K. Ross, MD

David C. Templeman, MD

Karen L. Hackett, FACHE, CAE
(ex officio)

Staff

Constance M. Filling, *Chief Education Officer*

Hans Koelsch, PhD, *Director, Department of Publications*

Jane Baque, *Senior Manager, Publications Websites*

Laurie Braun, *Managing Editor*

Juliet Orellana, *Copy Editor*

Mary Steermann Bishop, *Senior Manager, Production and Content Management*

Courtney Astle, *Editorial Production Manager*

Abram Fassler, *Publishing Systems Manager*

Suzanne O'Reilly, *Graphic Designer*

Susan Morritz Baim, *Production Coordinator*

Karen Danca, *Permissions Coordinator*

Charlie Baldwin, *Production Database Associate*

Hollie Muir, *Production Database Associate*

Emily Nickel, *Page Production Assistant*

Michelle Bruno, *Editorial Coordinator*

Rachel Winokur, *Publications Assistant*

Brian Moore, *Manager, Electronic Media Programs*

The material presented in the **Atlas of Essential Orthopaedic Procedures** has been made available by the American Academy of Orthopaedic Surgeons for educational purposes only. This material is not intended to present the only, or necessarily best, methods or procedures for the medical situations discussed, but rather is intended to represent an approach, view, statement, or opinion of the author(s) or producer(s), which may be helpful to others who face similar situations.

Some drugs or medical devices demonstrated in Academy courses or described in Academy print or electronic publications have not been cleared by the Food and Drug Administration (FDA) or have been cleared for specific uses only. The FDA has stated that it is the responsibility of the physician to determine the FDA clearance status of each drug or device he or she wishes to use in clinical practice.

Furthermore, any statements about commercial products are solely the opinion(s) of the author(s) and do not represent an Academy endorsement or evaluation of these products. These statements may not be used in advertising or for any commercial purpose.

All rights reserved. No part of this publication may be reproduced, stored in a retrieval system, or transmitted, in any form, or by any means, electronic, mechanical, photocopying, recording, or otherwise, without prior written permission from the publisher.

ISBN 978-0-89203-634-9

Library of Congress Control Number: 2013933777

Printed in the USA

Published 2013 by the
American Academy of Orthopaedic Surgeons
6300 North River Road
Rosemont, IL 60018

Copyright 2013
by the American Academy of Orthopaedic Surgeons

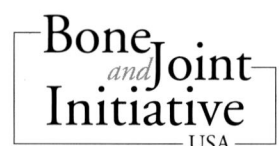

Acknowledgments

Editorial Board
Atlas of Essential Orthopaedic Procedures

Editors

Evan Flatow, MD
Chairman
Department of Orthopaedics
Mount Sinai School of Medicine
New York, New York

Alexis Chiang Colvin, MD
Assistant Professor
Department of Orthopaedics
Mount Sinai School of Medicine
New York, New York

Section Editors

Eben A. Carroll, MD *(Trauma)*
Assistant Professor
Department of Orthopaedic Surgery
Wake Forest University
Winston-Salem, North Carolina

Henry G. Chambers, MD *(Pediatrics)*
Professor of Clinical Orthopaedic Surgery
Department of Orthopaedic Surgery
University of California, San Diego
San Diego, California

Alexis Chiang Colvin, MD *(Sports Medicine)*
Assistant Professor
Department of Orthopaedics
Mount Sinai School of Medicine
New York, New York

Edward Diao, MD *(Hand and Wrist)*
Professor Emeritus
Chief of Hand Surgery
University of California, San Francisco
California Pacific Medical Center
San Francisco, California

Christopher D. Harner, MD *(Sports Medicine)*
Professor
Chief of Sports Medicine
Department of Orthopaedic Surgery
University of Pittsburgh Medical Center for Sports Medicine
Pittsburgh, Pennsylvania

Andrew C. Hecht, MD *(Spine)*
Chief, Spine Surgery
Assistant Professor, Orthopaedics and Neurosurgery
Mount Sinai Medical Center
New York, New York

William Macaulay, MD *(Adult Reconstruction)*
Chief, Division of Adult Reconstruction of the Hip and Knee
Department of Orthopaedics
Columbia University Medical Center
New York, New York

Michael Pinzur, MD *(Foot and Ankle)*
Professor of Orthopaedic Surgery
Department of Orthopaedic Surgery
Loyola University Health System
Maywood, Illinois

John W. Sperling, MD, MBA *(Shoulder and Elbow)*
Consultant
Department of Orthopedic Surgery
Mayo Clinic
Rochester, Minnesota

Lawrence X. Webb, MD *(Trauma)*
Chairman
Georgia Orthopaedic Trauma Institute
Medical Center of Central Georgia
Macon, Georgia

Contributors

Nicholas A. Abidi, MD
Director
Department of Orthopaedic Surgery
Santa Cruz Orthopaedic Institute, Inc.
Capitola, California

Julie E. Adams, MD, MS
Assistant Professor
Department of Orthopaedic Surgery
University of Minnesota
Minneapolis, Minnesota

John Akins, MD
Orthopaedic Surgeon
Department of Orthopaedic Surgery
Mountain View Specialty Clinic
Mountain View, Arkansas

David W. Altchek, MD
Co-chief, Sports Medicine and Shoulder Service
Sports Medicine and Shoulder Services
Hospital for Special Surgery
New York, New York

Annunziato Amendola, MD
Professor
Department of Orthopaedic Surgery and Rehabilitation
University of Iowa Hospitals and Clinics
Iowa City, Iowa

Howard An, MD
Professor and Director of Spine Surgery
Department of Orthopaedics
Rush University Medical Center
Chicago, Illinois

Robert A. Arciero, MD
Professor of Orthopaedics
Department of Orthopaedics
University of Connecticut Health Center
Farmington, Connecticut

Bernard R. Bach, Jr, MD
The Claude N. Lambert, MD – Helen Susan Thomson
 Professor of Orthopaedic Surgery
Director, Division of Sports Medicine
Director, Sports Medicine Fellowship
Rush University Medical Center
Chicago, Illinois

Semon Bader, MD
Walnut Creek, California

Geoffrey S. Baer, MD, PhD
Assistant Professor
Department of Orthopedics and Rehabilitation
Division of Sports Medicine
University of Wisconsin
Madison, Wisconsin

Sarvottam Bajaj, BE
Midwest Orthopaedics at Rush
Rush University Medical Center
Chicago, Illinois

Champ L. Baker III, MD
Staff Physician
The Hughston Clinic
Columbus, Georgia

Champ L. Baker, Jr, MD
The Hughston Clinic
Columbus, Georgia

Kelley Banagan, MD
Assistant Professor, Spine Surgery
Department of Orthopaedics
University of Maryland
Baltimore, Maryland

Alireza Behboudi, DO
Orthopedic Surgeon
Department of Orthopedic Surgery
East Texas Medical Center
Tyler, Texas

Stephen Benirschke, MD
Department of Orthopaedics and Sports Medicine
Harborview Medical Center
Seattle, Washington

Gregory C. Berlet, MD
Attending Physician
Department of Orthopedic Foot and Ankle Surgery
Orthopedic Foot & Ankle Center
Columbus, Ohio

Louis U. Bigliani, MD
Professor and Chairman
Department of Orthopaedics
Columbia University Medical Center
New York, New York

Randy Bindra, MD
Orthopaedic Surgeon
Department of Orthopaedic Surgery
Loyola University Medical Center
Maywood, Illinois

Michael V. Birman, MD
Hand and Microvascular Surgery Fellow
Department of Orthopaedic Surgery
Columbia University Medical Center
New York, New York

Scott D. Boden, MD
Director
The Emory Spine Center
Emory University School of Medicine
Atlanta, Georgia

Davide Edoardo Bonasia, MD
Orthopaedic Surgeon
I Clinica Ortopedica, AO CTO Hospital
University of Torino
Torino, Italy

Christopher M. Bono, MD
Associate Professor of Orthopaedic Surgery
Harvard Medical School
Chief, Orthopaedic Spine Service
Brigham and Women's Hospital
Boston, Massachusetts

Robert B. Bourne, MD, FRCSC
Professor of Surgery
Division of Orthopaedic Surgery
Western University
London, Ontario, Canada

Karl F. Bowman, Jr, MD
Fellow, Sports Medicine
Center for Sports Medicine
Department of Orthopaedic Surgery
University of Pittsburgh
Pittsburgh, Pennsylvania

James P. Bradley, MD
Clinical Professor
Burke & Bradley Orthopedics
University of Pittsburgh Medical Center
Pittsburgh, Pennsylvania

Jaycen Brown, BS
Clinical Manager
Stanley Graves MDPC
Phoenix, Arizona

LCDR Brandon Bryant, MD, USN
Assistant Professor of Orthopaedic Surgery
Department of Orthopaedic Surgery and Sports Medicine
Portsmouth Naval Medical Center
Portsmouth, Virginia

James B. Carr, MD
(deceased)
Roanoke, Virginia

Eben A. Carroll, MD
Assistant Professor
Department of Orthopaedic Surgery
Wake Forest University
Winston-Salem, North Carolina

Cordelia Carter, MD
Assistant Professor
Department of Orthopaedics and Rehabilitation
Yale University
New Haven, Connecticut

Danielle Casagrande, MD
Orthopaedic Resident
Department of Orthopaedics
University of Texas Medical Branch
Galveston, Texas

Thomas D. Cha, MD, MBA
Spine Surgeon
Department of Orthopaedic Surgery
Massachusetts General Hospital
Boston, Massachusetts

Peter Chalmers, MD
Resident
Department of Orthopaedic Surgery
Rush University Medical Center
Chicago, Illinois

Henry G. Chambers, MD
Professor of Clinical Orthopaedic Surgery
Department of Orthopaedic Surgery
University of California, San Diego
San Diego, California

Paul D. Choi, MD
Assistant Professor of Clinical Orthopaedics
Department of Orthopaedic Surgery
Children's Hospital Los Angeles
University of Southern California
Los Angeles, California

Loretta Chou, MD
Professor
Department of Orthopaedic Surgery
Stanford University
Stanford, California

Michael P. Clare, MD
Director of Foot and Ankle Fellowship Education
Florida Orthopaedic Institute
Tampa, Florida

J. Chris Coetzee, MD, FRCSC
Twin Cities Orthopedics
Edina, Minnesota

Brian J. Cole, MD, MBA
Professor, Section Head
Department of Orthopaedics, Anatomy and Cell Biology
Cartilage Restoration Center
Rush University Medical Center
Chicago, Illinois

Alexis Chiang Colvin, MD
Assistant Professor
Department of Orthopaedics
Mount Sinai School of Medicine
New York, New York

Andrew J. Cosgarea, MD
Professor and Director of Sports Medicine
Department of Orthopaedic Surgery
Johns Hopkins University
Baltimore, Maryland

Michael J. Coughlin, MD
Chief, Coughlin Foot and Ankle Clinic
Department of Orthopaedic Surgery
Saint Alphonsus Regional Medical Center
Boise, Idaho

Jonathan R. Danoff, MD
Postdoctoral Residency Fellow
Department of Orthopaedic Surgery
New York Presbyterian/Columbia University Medical Center
New York, New York

Michael R. Dayton, MD
Assistant Professor
Department of Orthopaedics
University of Colorado Denver
Aurora, Colorado

Samuel M. Davis, MD
Assistant Professor
Department of Orthopaedic Surgery
Emory University
Atlanta, Georgia

Thomas M. DeBerardino, MD
Associate Professor
Department of Orthopaedic Surgery
University of Connecticut Health Center
Farmington, Connecticut

Gregory K. Deirmengian, MD
Assistant Professor of Orthopaedic Surgery
Rothman Institute
Thomas Jefferson Medical School
Philadelphia, Pennsylvania

Edward Diao, MD
Professor Emeritus
Chief of Hand Surgery
University of California, San Francisco
California Pacific Medical Center
San Francisco, California

Gregory S. DiFelice, MD
Orthopaedic Surgeon
Department of Orthopaedic Surgery
Hospital for Special Surgery
New York, New York

Joshua S. Dines, MD
Orthopedic Surgeon
Sports Medicine and Shoulder Service
Hospital for Special Surgery
New York, New York

Henry J. Dolch, DO
Orthopaedic Trauma Surgeon
Orthopaedic Trauma Group
Charleston Area Medical Center
Charleston, West Virginia

James C. Dreese, MD
Assistant Professor
Department of Orthopaedics
University of Maryland
Baltimore, Maryland

Thomas R. Duquin, MD
Assistant Professor
Department of Orthopaedic Surgery
State University of New York, University at Buffalo
Buffalo, New York

Mark E. Easley, MD
Associate Professor
Department of Orthopaedic Surgery
Duke University Medical Center
Durham, North Carolina

T. Bradley Edwards, MD
Attending Shoulder Surgeon
Fondren Orthopedic Group
Texas Orthopedic Hospital
Houston, Texas

John J. Elias, PhD
Senior Research Scientist
Calhoun Research Laboratory
Akron General Medical Center
Akron, Ohio

Jesse James F. Exaltacion, MD
Fellow, Adult Reconstructive Surgery
Center for Orthopaedic Surgery
The Methodist Hospital
Houston, Texas

COL James R. Ficke, MD
Chairman
Department of Orthopaedics and Rehabilitation
San Antonio Military Medical Center
Fort Sam Houston, Texas

Larry D. Field, MD
Director
Upper Extremity Service
Mississippi Sports Medicine and Orthopaedic Center
Jackson, Mississippi

Steven J. Fineberg, MD
Research Coordinator
Department of Orthopaedic Surgery
Rush University Medical Center
Chicago, Illinois

Jennifer FitzPatrick, MD
Orthopedic Surgeon
Department of Orthopedics
University of Colorado
Aurora, Colorado

John C.P. Floyd, MD
Associate Professor
Mercer University School of Medicine
Associate Director
Georgia Orthopaedic Trauma Institute
Macon, Georgia

John M. Flynn, MD
Associate Chief
Professor of Orthopaedic Surgery
University of Pennsylvania School of Medicine
Department of Pediatric Orthopaedics
The Children's Hospital of Philadelphia
Philadelphia, Pennsylvania

Brett A. Freedman, MD
Chief, Spine and Neurosurgery Service
Department of Orthopaedics and Rehabilitation
Landstuhl Regional Medical Center
Landstuhl, Germany

Carol Frey, MD
Orthopaedic Surgeon
Assistant Professor
Clinical Orthopaedic Surgery
University of California, Los Angeles
Los Angeles, California

Freddie H. Fu, MD
David Silver Professor and Chairman
Department of Orthopaedic Surgery
University of Pittsburgh
Pittsburgh, Pennsylvania

Bethany Gallagher, MD
Assistant Professor
Department of Orthopaedics
Vanderbilt University
Nashville, Tennessee

Lauren E. Geaney, MD
Orthopaedic Resident
Department of Orthopaedic Surgery
University of Connecticut
Farmington, Connecticut

William B. Geissler, MD
Professor and Chief
Division of Hand and Upper Extremity Surgery
Department of Orthopaedic Surgery
University of Mississippi Medical Center
Jackson, Mississippi

Jeffrey A. Geller, MD
Associate Professor of Orthopaedic Surgery
Department of Orthopaedic Surgery
New York-Presbyterian Hospital/Columbia University
New York, New York

Neil Ghodadra, MD
Department of Orthopedic Surgery and Sports Medicine
Southern California Orthopedic Institute
Van Nuys, California

Filippos S. Giannoulis, MD
Orthopaedic Surgeon
Hand, Upper Extremity, and Microsurgery Department
Athens UAT Hospital
Athens, Greece

Thomas V. Giel III, MD
Orthopaedic Surgeon
Division of Sports Medicine
OrthoMemphis
Memphis, Tennessee

Hilton Phillip Gottschalk, MD
Pediatric Orthopaedic Surgeon
Central Texas Pediatric Orthopedics
Dell Children's Hospital
Austin, Texas

James A. Goulet, MD
Professor
Department of Orthopaedic Surgery
University of Michigan
Ann Arbor, Michigan

Stanley C. Graves, MD
Director
Stanley Graves MD PC
Phoenix, Arizona

Steven B. Haas, MD
Chief, Knee Service
Hospital for Special Surgery
New York, New York

Mark E. Hake, MD
Resident
Department of Orthopaedic Surgery
University of Michigan
Ann Arbor, Michigan

Jason J. Halvorson, MD
Chief Resident
Department of Orthopaedic Surgery
Wake Forest University School of Medicine
Winston-Salem, North Carolina

Christopher D. Harner, MD
Professor
Chief of Sports Medicine
Department of Orthopaedic Surgery
University of Pittsburgh Medical Center for Sports Medicine
Pittsburgh, Pennsylvania

Andrew C. Hecht, MD
Chief, Spine Surgery
Assistant Professor, Orthopaedics and Neurosurgery
Mount Sinai Medical Center
New York, New York

John G. Heller, MD
Baur Professor of Orthopaedic Surgery
Department of Orthopaedic Surgery
Emory University School of Medicine
Atlanta, Georgia

Christopher B. Hirose, MD
Orthopaedic Surgeon
The Coughlin Clinic
Saint Alphonsus Regional Medical Center
Boise, Idaho

Reimer Hoffmann, MD
Consultant Hand Surgeon
HPC Oldenburg
Oldenburg, Germany

Donald W. Hohman, Jr, MD
Orthopaedic Resident
Department of Orthopaedic Surgery
State University of New York, University at Buffalo
Buffalo, New York

Harish Hosalkar, MD
Attending Orthopedic Surgeon
Department of Orthopedics
Rady Children's Hospital
San Diego, California

Jonathan A. Hoskins, MD
Research Associate
Department of Orthopaedic Surgery
Rush University Medical Center
Chicago, Illinois

William J. Hozack, MD
Professor of Orthopaedic Surgery
Rothman Institute
Thomas Jefferson Medical School
Philadelphia, Pennsylvania

Stephanie Hsu, MD
Fellow
Center for Shoulder, Elbow, and Sports Medicine
Columbia University
New York, New York

Stephen J. Incavo, MD
Section Head, Adult Reconstructive Surgery
Department of Orthopaedics
The Methodist Hospital
Houston, Texas

Peter Johnston, MD
Southern Maryland Orthopaedics and Sports Medicine
Leonardtown, Maryland

Clifford B. Jones, MD, FACS
Clinical Professor
Michigan State University College of Human Medicine
Orthopaedic Associates of Michigan
Grand Rapids, Michigan

Jesse B. Jupiter, MD
Hansjorg Wyss AO Professor
Department of Orthopaedic Surgery
Massachusetts General Hospital
Boston, Massachusetts

Jay V. Kalawadia, MD
Resident Physician
Department of Orthopaedic Surgery
Northwestern University
Chicago, Illinois

Daniel G. Kang, MD
Orthopaedic Surgery Resident
Department of Orthopaedic Surgery and Rehabilitation
Walter Reed National Military Medical Center
Bethesda, Maryland

Christopher A. Keen, MD
Fellow
Department of Orthopaedic Surgery and Rehabilitation
University of Mississippi Health Care
Jackson, Mississippi

James F. Kellam, BSc, MD, FRCSC, FACS, FRCSI
Director of Orthopaedic Trauma Program
Department of Orthopaedic Surgery
Carolinas Medical Center
Charlotte, North Carolina

Stephen Kim, MD
Attending Physician
Resurgens Orthopaedics
Kennestone Hospital
Marietta, Georgia

Mininder S. Kocher, MD, MPH
Associate Director
Division of Sports Medicine
Boston Children's Hospital
Boston, Massachusetts

Patricia Kramer, PhD
Research Associate Professor
Department of Anthropology
University of Washington
Seattle, Washington

Jonathan H. Lee, MD
Assistant Professor, Clinical Orthopaedic Surgery
Department of Orthopaedics
Columbia University Medical Center
New York, New York

Ronald A. Lehman, Jr, MD
Chief, Pediatric and Adult Spine
Associate Professor of Surgery
Walter Reed National Medical Center
Bethesda, Maryland

Thomas P. Lehman, PT, MD
Associate Professor
Department of Orthopedic Surgery
University of Oklahoma Health Sciences Center
Oklahoma City, Oklahoma

Lawrence G. Lenke, MD
Jerome J. Gilden Distinguished Professor of Orthopaedic Surgery
Chief of Spine Surgery
Department of Orthopaedic Surgery
Washington University School of Medicine
Saint Louis, Missouri

Albert Lin, MD
Assistant Professor
Department of Orthopaedics
Division of Sports Medicine
University of Pittsburgh Medical Center
Pittsburgh, Pennsylvania

Sheldon S. Lin, MD
Associate Professor
Department of Orthopaedics
University of Medicine & Dentistry of New Jersey
New Jersey Medical School
Newark, New Jersey

© 2013 American Academy of Orthopaedic Surgeons

Randall T. Loder, MD
Department of Orthopaedic Surgery
Riley Children's Hospital
Indianapolis, Indiana

John D. Lubahn, MD
Hand, Microsurgery, and Reconstructive Orthopaedics, LLP
Erie, Pennsylvania

Steven C. Ludwig, MD
Associate Professor and Chief of Spine Surgery
Department of Orthopaedics
University of Maryland
Baltimore, Maryland

Jeffrey Macalena, MD
Assistant Professor
Department of Orthopaedic Surgery
University of Minnesota
Minneapolis, Minnesota

William Macaulay, MD
Chief, Division of Adult Reconstruction of the Hip and Knee
Department of Orthopaedics
Columbia University Medical Center
New York, New York

Tahir Mahmud, BSc(Hons), MBBS, MRCS(Eng), FRCS(Tr & Orth)
Fellow, Adult Lower Limb Reconstruction
Division of Orthopaedic Surgery
London Health Sciences Centre
University Hospital
London, Ontario, Canada

Richard C. Mather III, MD
Assistant Professor
Department of Orthopaedic Surgery
Duke University Medical Center
Durham, North Carolina

Kristofer S. Matullo, MD
Head of Hand Surgery
Orthopaedic Surgical Specialists
St. Luke's University Hospital
Bethlehem, Pennsylvania

Augustus D. Mazzocca, MS, MD
Associate Professor of Orthopaedic Surgery
Director of Resident Education
Department of Orthopaedics
University of Connecticut
Farmington, Connecticut

Michael David McKee, MD, FRCSC
Professor of Surgery
Department of Surgery
Division of Orthopaedics
St. Michael's Hospital
University of Toronto
Toronto, Ontario, Canada

Siddhant K. Mehta, MD
Postdoctoral Research Fellow
Department of Orthopaedic Surgery and Rehabilitation
University of Mississippi Medical Center
Jackson, Mississippi

Anna N. Miller, MD
Assistant Professor
Department of Orthopaedic Surgery
Wake Forest School of Medicine
Winston-Salem, North Carolina

Bradley Moatz, MD
Resident Physician
Department of Orthopaedics
Union Memorial Hospital
Baltimore, Maryland

Scott J. Mubarak, MD
Department of Orthopedics
Pediatric Orthopedic and Scoliosis Center
Rady Children's Hospital
University of California, San Diego
San Diego, California

Daniel J. Nagle, MD
Clinical Professor
Department of Orthopaedic Surgery
Feinberg School of Medicine
Northwestern University
Chicago, Illinois

Blaise Alexander Nemeth, MD, MS
Associate Professor, Clinical Health Science
Department of Orthopedics and Rehabilitation
University of Wisconsin School of Medicine and Public Health
Madison, Wisconsin

Gregory P. Nicholson, MD
Associate Professor
Department of Orthopaedic Surgery
Rush University Medical Center
Chicago, Illinois

Kenneth Noonan, MD
Associate Professor
Department of Pediatric Orthopedics
University of Wisconsin Health
Madison, Wisconsin

Thomas Obermeyer, MD
Fellow, Shoulder and Elbow Surgery
Department of Orthopaedic Surgery
Mount Sinai Medical Center
New York, New York

Matthew Oglesby, BA
Research Coordinator
Department of Orthopaedic Surgery
Rush University Medical Center
Chicago, Illinois

Nirav K. Pandya, MD
Attending Orthopaedic Surgeon
Department of Pediatric Orthopaedics
Children's Hospital and Research Center Oakland
University of California, San Francisco
Oakland, California

Wayne Paprosky, MD
Professor
Department of Orthopaedic Surgery
Adult Joint Reconstruction
Rush University Medical Center
Chicago, Illinois

Andrew Park, MD
Department of Orthopedic Surgery
Methodist Hospital for Surgery
Addison, Texas

Richard D. Parker, MD
Professor and Chairman
Department of Orthopaedics
Cleveland Clinic Foundation
Cleveland, Ohio

Bradford Parsons, MD
Assistant Professor of Orthopaedic Surgery
Department of Orthopaedic Surgery
Mount Sinai School of Medicine
New York, New York

Chirag S. Patel, MD
Resident
Department of Orthopaedic Surgery
Stanford University
Redwood City, California

Neeraj M. Patel, MD, MPH, MBS
Benjamin Fox Orthopaedic Research Fellow
Division of Orthopaedic Surgery
Children's Hospital of Philadelphia
Philadelphia, Pennsylvania

Steven L. Peterson, MD, DVM
Staff Hand Surgeon
Operative Care Division
Portland Veterans Administration Medical Center
Portland, Oregon

Terrence M. Philbin, DO
Attending Physician
Department of Orthopedic Surgery
Orthopedic Foot and Ankle Center
Columbus, Ohio

Maya Pring, MD
Associate Professor
Department of Orthopaedic Surgery
University of California, San Diego
San Diego, California

Sheeraz Qureshi, MD
Orthopaedic Spine Surgeon
Department of Orthopaedics
Mount Sinai Hospital
New York, New York

Steven M. Raikin, MD
Director, Foot and Ankle Service
Professor, Orthopaedic Surgery
Rothman Institute
Philadelphia, Pennsylvania

Matthew L. Ramsey, MD
Professor and Vice Chairman
Department of Orthopaedic Surgery
Rothman Institute
Thomas Jefferson University
Philadelphia, Pennsylvania

Anil S. Ranawat, MD
Orthopaedic Surgeon
Department of Sports Medicine and Joint Preservation
Hospital for Special Surgery
New York, New York

Ghazi Rayan, MD
Clinical Professor
Department of Orthopedics
Oklahoma University
Oklahoma City, Oklahoma

Brett Rebal, BA
Research Fellow
Medical Student
Department of Orthopaedics
Columbia University Medical Center
New York, New York

Keith R. Reinhardt, MD
Fellow
Department of Orthopedic Surgery
Harvard Brigham and Women's Hospital
Boston, Massachusetts

K. Daniel Riew, MD
Mildred B. Simon Distinguished Professor
Department of Orthopaedic Surgery
Washington University School of Medicine
St. Louis, Missouri

David Ring, MD, PhD
Director of Research
Orthopaedic Hand and Upper Extremity Service
Massachusetts General Hospital
Boston, Massachusetts

Pascal Rippstein, MD
Medical Director/Chief Department of Foot and Ankle
Schulthess Clinic
Zurich, Switzerland

Mark William Rodosky, MD
Chief, Division of Shoulder Surgery
Department of Orthopaedic Sports Medicine
University of Pittsburgh
Pittsburgh, Pennsylvania

Arnaldo I. Rodríguez Santiago, MD
Shoulder/Elbow Surgeon
Department of Orthopedic Surgery
HIMA San Pablo Caguas
Caguas, Puerto Rico

© 2013 American Academy of Orthopaedic Surgeons

Anthony A. Romeo, MD
Professor, Division of Orthopaedics
Director, Section of Shoulder and Elbow Surgery
Team Physician, Chicago White Sox
Department of Orthopaedic Surgery
Division of Sports Medicine
Rush University Medical Center
Chicago, Illinois

Melvin P. Rosenwasser, MD
Robert E. Carroll Professor of Orthopaedic Surgery
Department of Orthopaedic Surgery
Columbia University
New York, New York

Roberto Rossi, MD
Professor
Department of Orthopaedics
University of Turin
Turin, Italy

Michael J. Salata, MD
Director, Joint Preservation and Cartilage Restoration Center
Department of Orthopaedic Surgery
University Hospitals of Cleveland
Cleveland, Ohio

Paul M. Saluan, MD
Director, Pediatric and Adolescent Sports Medicine
Department of Orthopaedic Surgery
Cleveland Clinic Sports Health
Cleveland, Ohio

Felix H. Savoie III, MD
Professor
Department of Orthopaedic Surgery
Tulane University
New Orleans, Louisiana

Andrew J. Schoenfeld, MD
Assistant Professor
Department of Orthopaedic Surgery
Texas Tech University Health Sciences Center
El Paso, Texas

Patrick Schottel, MD
Resident
Department of Orthopaedic Surgery
Hospital for Special Surgery
New York, New York

William C. Schroer, MD
Research Director
St. Louis Joint Replacement Institute
SSM DePaul Health Center
St. Louis, Missouri

Alexandra Schwartz, MD
Professor
Department of Orthopaedic Surgery
University of California, San Diego
San Diego, California

Laura E. Scordino, MD
Orthopaedic Surgery Resident
Department of Orthopaedic Surgery
University of Connecticut
Farmington, Connecticut

Giles R. Scuderi, MD
Vice President, Orthopaedic Service Line
Department of Orthopaedics
North Shore Long Island Jewish Health System
Long Island, New York

Scott Scuderi, BS
Research Assistant
Insall Scott Kelly Institute for Orthopaedics and Sports Medicine
New York, New York

Ari D. Seidenstein, MD
Orthopaedic Surgeon
Hartzband Center for Hip and Knee Replacement, LLC
Hackensack University Medical Center/Holy Name Medical Center
Paramus, New Jersey

Christopher L. Sherman, DO, MS
Department of Orthopaedic Surgery
Riverside County Regional Medical Center
Moreno Valley, California

Seth L. Sherman, MD
Assistant Professor
Department of Orthopaedic Surgery
University of Missouri
Columbia, Missouri

Alexander Y. Shin, MD
Professor of Orthopedic Surgery
Department of Orthopedics
Mayo Clinic
Rochester, Minnesota

Benjamin J. Shore, MD, FRCSC
Instructor in Orthopaedic Surgery
Department of Orthopaedic Surgery
Boston Children's Hospital
Harvard Medical School
Boston, Massachusetts

Peter Silvero, MD
Orthopaedic Surgeon
Associates in Orthopaedic Surgery
Jordan Valley Medical Center
Salt Lake City, Utah

Micah Sinclair, MD
Hand Surgery Fellow
Department of Orthopaedics
University of Utah
Salt Lake City, Utah

Kern Singh, MD
Assistant Professor
Department of Orthopaedic Surgery
Rush University Medical Center
Chicago, Illinois

Ernest L. Sink, MD
Associate Professor
Department of Pediatric Orthopaedic Surgery
Hospital for Special Surgery
New York, New York

David L. Skaggs, MD
Professor and Chief of Orthopaedic Surgery
Children's Orthopaedic Center
Children's Hospital Los Angeles
Los Angeles, California

Nicholas R. Slenker, MD
Orthopaedic Resident
Rothman Institute
Thomas Jefferson University Hospital
Philadelphia, Pennsylvania

Dean G. Sotereanos, MD
Professor
Hand and Upper Extremity Surgery
Allegheny General Hospital
Pittsburgh, Pennsylvania

Scott Sporer, MD, MS
Associate Professor
Department of Orthopaedic Surgery
Rush University Medical Center
Chicago, Illinois

Scott P. Steinmann, MD
Professor of Orthopedic Surgery
Mayo Clinic
Rochester, Minnesota

MAJ Daniel J. Stinner, MD
Chief Resident, Orthopaedic Surgery
Department of Orthopaedics and Rehabilitation
San Antonio Military Medical Center
Fort Sam Houston, Texas

Eric J. Strauss, MD
Assistant Professor
Department of Orthopaedic Surgery
New York University Hospital for Joint Diseases
New York, New York

John M. Tabit, DO
Orthopaedic Traumatologist
The Orthopaedic Trauma Group
Charleston Area Medical Center
Charleston, West Virginia

Miho J. Tanaka, MD
Director, Women's Sports Medicine Initiative
Regeneration Orthopedics
Chesterfield, Missouri

Oliver O. Tannous, MD
Resident
Department of Orthopaedics
University of Maryland Medical Center
Baltimore, Maryland

Nikhil A. Thakur, MD
Assistant Professor
Department of Orthopaedics
State University of New York Upstate Medical University
Syracuse, New York

Matthew M. Tomaino, MD, MBA
Tomaino Orthopaedic Care
Rochester, New York

Michael E. Torchia, MD
Consultant
Department of Orthopedic Surgery
Mayo Clinic
Rochester, Minnesota

P. Justin Tortolani, MD
Director, Spine Education and Research
Department of Orthopaedic Surgery
Medstar Union Memorial Hospital
Baltimore, Maryland

Carola van Eck, MD, PhD
Orthopaedic Surgery Resident
Department of Orthopaedic Surgery
University of Pittsburgh Medical Center
Pittsburgh, Pennsylvania

Thomas F. Varecka, MD
Assistant Professor
University of Minnesota
Department of Orthopaedic Surgery
Hennepin County Medical Center
Minneapolis, Minnesota

Aaron I. Venouziou, MD
Fellow
Division of Upper Extremity Surgery
Allegheny General Hospital
Pittsburgh, Pennsylvania

Armando F. Vidal, MD
Assistant Professor
Sports Medicine and Shoulder Service
University of Colorado School of Medicine
Denver, Colorado

Dharmesh Vyas, MD
Assistant Professor
Department of Orthopaedic Surgery
University of Pittsburgh Medical Center
Pittsburgh, Pennsylvania

Emily A. Wagstrom, MD
Resident Physician
Department of Orthopaedics
University of Iowa
Iowa City, Iowa

Eric Wall, MD
Professor
Department of Pediatric Orthopaedic Surgery
Cincinnati Children's Hospital Medical Center
Cincinnati, Ohio

Arthur K. Walling, MD
Foot and Ankle Surgery Fellowship Director
Florida Orthopaedic Institute
Tampa, Florida

Lawrence X. Webb, MD
Chairman
Georgia Orthopaedic Trauma Institute
Medical Center of Central Georgia
Macon, Georgia

Robin West, MD
Orthopaedic Surgeon
Associate Professor
University of Pittsburgh Medical Center
Pittsburgh, Pennsylvania

Matthew J. White, MD
Orthopaedic Surgeon
Physicians' Clinic of Iowa
Cedar Rapids, Iowa

Neil J. White, MD, FRCSC
Hand Surgeon
Orthopaedic Trauma Surgeon
Department of Orthopaedics
University of Calgary
Calgary, Alberta, Canada

Kevin W. Wilson, MD
Orthopaedic Surgery Resident
Department of Orthopaedics and Rehabilitation
Walter Reed National Military Medical Center
Bethesda, Maryland

Michael A. Wirth, MD
Professor and Charles A. Rockwood, Jr, MD, Chair
Department of Orthopaedics
University of Texas Health Science Center
San Antonio, Texas

Bryan Witt, DO
Orthopaedic Surgery Resident
Department of Orthopaedic Surgery
Doctors Hospital
Columbus, Ohio

Brian R. Wolf, MD, MS
Congdon Professor of Orthopaedic Surgery
Department of Orthopaedics and Rehabilitation
University of Iowa
Iowa City, Iowa

Adam B. Yanke, MD
Resident
Department of Orthopaedic Surgery
Rush University
Chicago, Illinois

Vamshi Yelavarthi, BA
Medical Student
Boston University School of Medicine
Boston, Massachusetts

Dedication

To our families, for their love and support; to our teachers, for their wisdom; and to our patients, from whom we learned the value of our craft.

Preface

Orthopaedic surgeons face an ever-growing body of information to be mastered, yet the demands on their time have never been greater. The *Atlas of Essential Orthopaedic Procedures* has been developed by the American Academy of Orthopaedic Surgeons (AAOS) to provide a concise yet comprehensive multimedia resource for the busy orthopaedic surgeon. Every specialty is represented, and each of the 107 procedures has been selected thoughtfully by experts in each specialty. The authors are surgeons who are recognized leaders in their field. The management of each condition is detailed in an easy-to-access format that begins with patient selection, takes the reader through a detailed, step-by-step description of the author's procedure, and includes the author's surgical pearls. The 70 surgical videos complement the chapters and enhance the learning experience.

The *Atlas of Essential Orthopaedic Procedures* is a highly visual, technique-oriented reference. The chapters are heavily illustrated with radiographs, intraoperative photographs, and line drawings. They contain few citations because the emphasis is on conveying the practical techniques of expert surgeons rather than on reviewing the literature. We expect this publication to be a one-stop destination for the surgeon who is confronted with a multitude of conditions requiring knowledge of these essential surgical techniques.

The *Atlas of Essential Orthopaedic Procedures* would not have been possible without the support of the AAOS and the efforts of numerous individuals. First, the authors are owed a debt of gratitude for providing the outstanding text, illustrations, and video that are certain to make this publication a standard reference for the orthopaedic surgeon. Second, we are grateful to the section editors for their outstanding work in reviewing the text and video. These busy surgeons have devoted many hours to this project over the course of several years, in addition to the many other demands on their time. Our gratitude goes to the following, listed in alphabetical order: Eben A. Carroll, MD (*Trauma*); Henry G. Chambers, MD (*Pediatrics*); Edward Diao, MD (*Hand and Wrist*); Christopher D. Harner, MD (*Sports Medicine*); Andrew C. Hecht, MD (*Spine*); William Macaulay, MD (*Adult Reconstruction*); Michael Pinzur, MD (*Foot and Ankle*); John W. Sperling, MD, MBA (*Shoulder and Elbow*); and Lawrence X. Webb, MD (*Trauma*). Also, we would be remiss if we failed to acknowledge the loss to the orthopaedic community with the passing of one of our authors, Dr. James Carr, who was a renowned orthopaedic surgeon and educator.

Finally, we thank the members of the AAOS Publications and Electronic Media departments who were instrumental in the production of this groundbreaking multimedia reference. The project had the good fortune of benefiting from the leadership of two Directors of Publications: Marilyn Fox, PhD, whose vision and support made this possible and whose tenure ended recently; and Hans Koelsch, PhD, her able successor. Jane Baque, Senior Manager, Publications Websites; Laurie Braun, Managing Editor, Textbooks; Rachel Winokur, Publications Assistant; and Brian Moore, Manager, Electronic Media Programs, are all to be commended for their extraordinary efforts in organizing and editing the text and video. In addition, the AAOS Production Department deserves recognition for their talent and professionalism in ensuring that the presentation of a tremendously complex art program comprising many hundreds of graphic elements was completed to high quality standards.

We hope you agree that these efforts have resulted in a publication that will improve patient care and should be a vital part of every orthopaedic surgeon's library.

Evan Flatow, MD
Alexis Chiang Colvin, MD
Editors

Table of Contents

Section 1: Sports Medicine
Section Editors: Christopher D. Harner, MD; Alexis Chiang Colvin, MD

1. Arthroscopic Repair of Partial-Thickness Rotator Cuff Tears 3
   Matthew J. White, MD; Geoffrey S. Baer, MD, PhD

2. Arthroscopic and Open Bankart Repair 9
   LCDR Brandon Bryant, MD, USN; James P. Bradley, MD

3. Arthroscopic Superior Labrum Anterior-to-Posterior Repair 17
   James C. Dreese, MD; Danielle Casagrande, MD

4. Biceps Tenotomy and Tenodesis.. 25
   Peter Chalmers, MD; Seth L. Sherman, MD; Neil Ghodadra, MD;
   Richard C. Mather III, MD; Anthony A. Romeo, MD

5. Anatomic Acromioclavicular Joint Reconstruction.. 31
   Albert Lin, MD; Mark William Rodosky, MD

6. Open Reduction and Internal Fixation of Clavicle Fractures.. 35
   Laura E. Scordino, MD; Thomas M. DeBerardino, MD

7. Open Treatment of Medial and Lateral Epicondylitis.. 39
   Champ L. Baker III, MD; John Akins, MD; Champ L. Baker, Jr, MD

8. Distal Biceps Repair 43
   Lauren E. Geaney, MD; Robert A. Arciero, MD; Anthony A. Romeo, MD;
   Augustus D. Mazzocca, MS, MD

9. Ulnar Collateral Ligament Reconstruction... 49
   Joshua S. Dines, MD; David W. Altchek, MD

10. Arthroscopic Management of Femoroacetabular Impingement.. 55
    Alexis Chiang Colvin, MD

11. Meniscectomy 59
    Semon Bader, MD; Paul M. Saluan, MD; Richard D. Parker, MD

12. Meniscal Repair 67
    Karl F. Bowman, Jr, MD; Christopher D. Harner, MD

13. Medial Meniscal Root Repair 73
    Dharmesh Vyas, MD; Christopher D. Harner, MD

14. Microfracture... 79
    Armando F. Vidal, MD; Jennifer FitzPatrick, MD

15. Surgical Treatment of Osteochondritis Dissecans Lesions.. 85
    Sarvottam Bajaj, BE; Michael J. Salata, MD; Brian J. Cole, MD, MBA

16. Anterior Cruciate Ligament Reconstruction: Single-Bundle Transtibial Technique........................ 95
    Eric J. Strauss, MD; Adam B. Yanke, MD; Bernard R. Bach, Jr, MD

17. Anterior Cruciate Ligament Reconstruction: Two-Tunnel Technique 103
    Dharmesh Vyas, MD; Christopher D. Harner, MD

18. Anatomic Anterior Cruciate Ligament Double-Bundle Reconstruction 109
    Jeffrey Macalena, MD; Carola van Eck, MD, PhD; Freddie H. Fu, MD

19. Pediatric Anterior Cruciate Ligament Reconstruction 117
    Davide Edoardo Bonasia, MD; Roberto Rossi, MD; Brian R. Wolf, MD, MS;
    Annunziato Amendola, MD

20. Medial Patellofemoral Ligament Reconstruction for Recurrent Patellar Instability 125
    Andrew J. Cosgarea, MD; Miho J. Tanaka, MD; John J. Elias, PhD

21. Realignment for Patellofemoral Arthritis 131
    Albert Lin, MD; Robin West, MD

© 2013 American Academy of Orthopaedic Surgeons

22 Surgical Treatment of Traumatic Quadriceps and Patellar Tendon Injuries of the Knee................... 137
Patrick Schottel, MD; Keith R. Reinhardt, MD; Gregory S. DiFelice, MD;
Anil S. Ranawat, MD

Section 2: Shoulder and Elbow
Section Editor: John W. Sperling, MD, MBA

23 Arthroscopic Subacromial Decompression and Distal Clavicle Resection 149
Albert Lin, MD; Mark William Rodosky, MD

24 Arthroscopic Management of Frozen Shoulder... 153
Peter N. Chalmers, MD; Seth L. Sherman, MD; Neil Ghodadra, MD;
Gregory P. Nicholson, MD

25 Arthroscopic Rotator Cuff Repair 159
Thomas R. Duquin, MD; Donald W. Hohman, Jr, MD

26 Percutaneous Pinning of Proximal Humerus Fractures... 169
Bradford O. Parsons, MD

27 Fixation of Proximal Humerus Fractures.. 175
Michael E. Torchia, MD; Thomas S. Obermeyer, MD

28 Hemiarthroplasty for Proximal Humerus Fractures.. 183
Arnaldo I. Rodriguez-Santiago, MD; T. Bradley Edwards, MD

29 Total Shoulder Arthroplasty for Osteoarthritis 191
Stephanie H. Hsu, MD; Louis U. Bigliani, MD

30 Reverse Total Shoulder Arthroplasty for Rotator Cuff Arthropathy 197
Peter Silvero, MD; Michael A. Wirth, MD

31 Arthroscopy of the Elbow.. 203
Thomas V. Giel III, MD; Larry D. Field, MD; Felix H. Savoie III, MD

32 Open Treatment of Radial Head Fractures and Olecranon Fractures............................. 211
Julie E. Adams, MD, MS; Scott P. Steinmann, MD

33 Open Reduction and Internal Fixation of Distal Humerus Fractures.............................. 219
Michael David McKee, MD, FRCSC

34 Total Elbow Arthroplasty 225
Peter Johnston, MD; Matthew L. Ramsey, MD

Section 3: Hand and Wrist
Section Editor: Edward Diao, MD

35 Carpal Tunnel Release.. 235
Edward Diao, MD

36 Surgical Treatment of Cubital Tunnel Syndrome.. 241
Reimer Hoffmann, MD; John D. Lubahn, MD

37 First Dorsal Extensor Compartment Release 247
Aaron I. Venouziou, MD; Filippos S. Giannoulis, MD; Dean G. Sotereanos, MD

38 Trigger Finger Release.. 253
Randy Bindra, MD; Micah Sinclair, MD

39 Open Reduction and Internal Fixation of the Distal Radius With a Volar Locking Plate 259
Jesse B. Jupiter, MD; David Ring, MD, PhD

40 External Fixation of Distal Radius Fractures 263
Michael V. Birman, MD; Jonathan R. Danoff, MD; Neil J. White, MD;
Melvin P. Rosenwasser, MD

41 Open Reduction and Internal Fixation of Scaphoid Fractures 269
Kristofer S. Matullo, MD; Alexander Y. Shin, MD

42 Open Reduction and Internal Fixation of Phalangeal Fractures 275
William B. Geissler, MD

| 43 | Surgical Fixation of Metacarpal Fractures | 281 |

William B. Geissler, MD; Christopher A. Keen, MD

| 44 | Excision of Ganglion Cysts of the Wrist and Hand | 287 |

Daniel J. Nagle, MD; Jay V. Kalawadia, MD

| 45 | Surgical Excision of Digital Mucous Cysts | 293 |

Matthew M. Tomaino, MD, MBA

| 46 | Surgical Treatment of Basal Joint Arthritis of the Thumb | 295 |

Edward Diao, MD

| 47 | Partial Palmar Fasciectomy for Dupuytren Disease | 305 |

Thomas P. Lehman, PT, MD; Steven L. Peterson, MD, DVM; Ghazi Rayan, MD

Section 4: Adult Reconstruction
Section Editor: William Macaulay, MD

| 48 | Hip Arthroplasty via Small-Incision Enhanced Posterior Soft-Tissue Repair | 313 |

Jonathan H. Lee, MD; William Macaulay, MD; Brett Rebal, BA

| 49 | Hip Arthroplasty via a Direct Lateral Approach | 319 |

Tahir Mahmud, BSc (Hons), MBBS, FRCS (Tr & Orth); Robert B. Bourne, MD, FRCSC

| 50 | Direct Anterior Approach for Hip Arthroplasty | 325 |

Gregory K. Deirmengian, MD; William J. Hozack, MD

| 51 | Revision Total Hip Arthroplasty via Extended Trochanteric Osteotomy | 333 |

Scott M. Sporer, MD, MS; Wayne G. Paprosky, MD, FACS

| 52 | Total Knee Arthroplasty via the Medial Parapatellar Approach | 341 |

Stephen J. Incavo, MD; Michael R. Dayton, MD; Jesse James F. Exaltacion, MD

| 53 | Total Knee Arthroplasty via Small-Incision Midvastus Approach | 345 |

Steven B. Haas, MD, MPH; Stephen Kim, MD

| 54 | Total Knee Arthroplasty via the Mini-Subvastus Approach | 351 |

William C. Schroer, MD

| 55 | Revision Total Knee Arthroplasty via Quadriceps Snip | 359 |

Ari Seidenstein, MD; Scott Scuderi, BS; Giles R. Scuderi, MD

| 56 | Revision Total Knee Arthroplasty via Tibial Tubercle Osteotomy | 363 |

Jeffrey A. Geller, MD

Section 5: Trauma
Section Editors: Lawrence X. Webb, MD; Eben A. Carroll, MD

| 57 | General Principles of Surgical Débridement | 369 |

Lawrence X. Webb, MD; Henry J. Dolch, DO

| 58 | Fasciotomy for Compartment Syndrome of the Leg | 371 |

Lawrence X. Webb, MD; Alireza Behboudi, DO

| 59 | Open Reduction and Internal Fixation of Forearm Fractures | 375 |

Thomas F. Varecka, MD

| 60 | Open Reduction and Internal Fixation of Posterior Wall Acetabular Fractures | 385 |

Lawrence X. Webb, MD

| 61 | Open Reduction and Internal Fixation of Femoral Neck Fractures | 393 |

Lawrence X. Webb, MD; John C.P. Floyd, MD

| 62 | Intertrochanteric Fracture Fixation Using a Sliding Hip Screw or Cephalomedullary Nail | 401 |

Alexandra K. Schwartz, MD; Christopher L. Sherman, DO, MS

| 63 | Intramedullary Nailing of Diaphyseal Femur Fractures | 407 |

Anna N. Miller, MD

| 64 | Surgical Fixation of Fractures of the Distal Femur | 413 |

James F. Kellam, BSc, MD, FRCSC, FACS, FRCSI

65 Open Reduction and Internal Fixation of Tibial Plateau Fractures................................... 421
    James A. Goulet, MD; Mark E. Hake, MD

66 Tibial Diaphyseal Intramedullary Nailing 429
    Clifford B. Jones, MD, FACS

67 Open Reduction and Internal Fixation of the Tibial Plafond..................................... 437
    Stephen K. Benirschke, MD; Patricia Kramer, PhD

68 Surgical Treatment of Ankle Fractures 443
    Eben A. Carroll, MD; Jason J. Halvorson, MD

69 Surgical Management of Fractures of the Talus... 451
    John M. Tabit, DO; Lawrence X. Webb, MD

70 Open Reduction and Internal Fixation of Calcaneal Fractures 459
    Michael P. Clare, MD

71 Open Reduction and Internal Fixation of Fracture-Dislocations of the Tarsometatarsal Joint.............. 467
    Terrence M. Philbin, DO; Gregory C. Berlet, MD

72 Open Reduction and Internal Fixation of Proximal Fifth Metatarsal Fractures 473
    Mark E. Easley, MD

Section 6: Foot and Ankle
Section Editor: Michael Pinzur, MD

73 Ankle Arthroscopy: Diagnostics, Débridement, and Removal of Loose Bodies....................... 485
    Carol Frey, MD

74 Arthroscopic Treatment of Osteochondral Lesions of the Talus 491
    Steven M. Raikin, MD; Nicholas R. Slenker, MD

75 Augmented Lateral Ankle Ligament Reconstruction for Persistent Ankle Instability 499
    Nicholas A. Abidi, MD

76 Achilles Tendon Rupture Repair 505
    Stanley C. Graves, MD; Jaycen Brown, BS

77 Tibiotalar Arthrodesis 509
    Siddhant K. Mehta, MD; Nicholas A. Abidi, MD; Sheldon S. Lin, MD

78 Subtalar Arthrodesis 515
    James B. Carr, MD

79 Arthrodesis of the Tarsometatarsal Joint... 519
    J. Chris Coetzee, MD, FRCSC; Pascal Rippstein, MD

80 Surgical Treatment of Navicular Stress Fractures 527
    Bethany Gallagher, MD; Arthur K. Walling, MD

81 Arthrodesis of the Hallux Metatarsophalangeal Joint 531
    Chirag S. Patel, MD; Loretta Chou, MD

82 Proximal and Distal First Metatarsal Osteotomies for Hallux Valgus 535
    Christopher B. Hirose, MD; Michael J. Coughlin, MD

83 Chronic Exertional Compartment Syndrome and Release 541
    Emily A. Wagstrom, MD; Annunziato Amendola, MD; Brian R. Wolf, MD, MS

84 Transtibial Amputation 545
    COL James R. Ficke, MD; MAJ Daniel J. Stinner, MD

85 Midfoot Amputations 551
    Terrence M. Philbin, DO; Bryan Witt, DO

Section 7: Spine
Section Editor: Andrew C. Hecht, MD

- 86 Anterior Cervical Diskectomy and Fusion 559
  Howard S. An, MD; Thomas D. Cha, MD, MBA

- 87 Anterior Cervical Corpectomy and Fusion/Instrumentation 563
  Daniel G. Kang, MD; Ronald A. Lehman, Jr, MD; K. Daniel Riew, MD

- 88 Posterior Cervical Foraminotomy 575
  Kern Singh, MD; Steven J. Fineberg, MD; Matthew Oglesby, BA; Jonathan A. Hoskins, MD; Vamshi Yelavarthi, BA

- 89 Posterior Cervical Laminectomy and Fusion 579
  Sheeraz A. Qureshi, MD, MBA; Andrew C. Hecht, MD

- 90 Cervical Laminoplasty 585
  Nikhil A. Thakur, MD; Brett A. Freedman, MD; John G. Heller, MD

- 91 Placement of Thoracic Pedicle Screws 591
  Kevin W. Wilson, MD; Ronald A. Lehman, Jr, MD; Lawrence G. Lenke, MD

- 92 Lumbar Microdiskectomy 601
  Bradley Moatz, MD; P. Justin Tortolani, MD

- 93 Lumbar Laminectomy 607
  Samuel M. Davis, MD; Scott D. Boden, MD

- 94 Instrumented Lumbar Fusion 611
  Andrew J. Schoenfeld, MD; Christopher M. Bono, MD

- 95 Transforaminal Lumbar Interbody Fusion 617
  Oliver O. Tannous, MD; Kelley Banagan, MD; Steven C. Ludwig, MD

- 96 Anterior Lumbar Interbody Fusion 625
  Andrew Park, MD

Section 8: Pediatrics
Section Editor: Henry G. Chambers, MD

- 97 Closed and Open Reduction of Supracondylar Humerus Fractures 633
  David L. Skaggs, MD; Paul D. Choi, MD; Cordelia Carter, MD

- 98 Reduction and Fixation of Lateral Condyle Fractures of the Distal Humerus 641
  Neeraj M. Patel, MD, MPH, MBS; John M. Flynn, MD

- 99 Intramedullary Fixation of Radial and Ulnar Shaft Fractures in Skeletally Immature Patients 647
  Maya E. Pring, MD; Hilton P. Gottschalk, MD; Henry G. Chambers, MD

- 100 Incision and Drainage of the Septic Hip 653
  Benjamin J. Shore, MD, FRCSC; Mininder S. Kocher, MD, MPH

- 101 Percutaneous in Situ Fixation of Slipped Capital Femoral Epiphysis 657
  Randall T. Loder, MD

- 102 Fixation of Pediatric Femur Fractures 663
  Ernest L. Sink, MD

- 103 Femoral Derotation Osteotomy in Adolescents and Young Adults 673
  Harish S. Hosalkar, MD

- 104 Surgical Reduction and Fixation of Tibial Spine Fractures in Children 677
  Eric Wall, MD

- 105 Treatment of Clubfoot Using the Ponseti Method 683
  Blaise Alexander Nemeth, MD, MS; Kenneth J. Noonan, MD

- 106 Treatment of Tarsal Coalitions 689
  Scott J. Mubarak, MD

- 107 Lower Extremity Surgery in Children With Cerebral Palsy 695
  Nirav K. Pandya, MD; Henry G. Chambers, MD

Sports Medicine

Section Editors
Christopher D. Harner, MD
Alexis Chiang Colvin, MD

1. **Arthroscopic Repair of Partial-Thickness Rotator Cuff Tears** 3
   Matthew J. White, MD; Geoffrey S. Baer, MD, PhD

2. **Arthroscopic and Open Bankart Repair** 9
   LCDR Brandon Bryant, MD, USN; James P. Bradley, MD

3. **Arthroscopic Superior Labrum Anterior-to-Posterior Repair** 17
   James C. Dreese, MD; Danielle Casagrande, MD

4. **Biceps Tenotomy and Tenodesis** 25
   *Peter Chalmers, MD; Seth L. Sherman, MD; Neil Ghodadra, MD;
   Richard C. Mather III, MD; Anthony A. Romeo, MD*

5. **Anatomic Acromioclavicular Joint Reconstruction** 31
   Albert Lin, MD; Mark William Rodosky, MD

6. **Open Reduction and Internal Fixation of Clavicle Fractures** 35
   Laura E. Scordino, MD; Thomas M. DeBerardino, MD

7. **Open Treatment of Medial and Lateral Epicondylitis** 39
   Champ L. Baker III, MD; John Akins, MD; Champ L. Baker, Jr, MD

8. **Distal Biceps Repair** 43
   *Lauren E. Geaney, MD; Robert A. Arciero, MD;
   Anthony A. Romeo, MD; Augustus D. Mazzocca, MS, MD*

9. **Ulnar Collateral Ligament Reconstruction** 49
   Joshua S. Dines, MD; David W. Altchek, MD

10. **Arthroscopic Management of Femoroacetabular Impingement** 55
    Alexis Chiang Colvin, MD

11   Meniscectomy **59**
Semon Bader, MD; Paul M. Saluan, MD; Richard D. Parker, MD

12   Meniscal Repair **67**
Karl F. Bowman, Jr, MD; Christopher D. Harner, MD

13   Medial Meniscal Root Repair **73**
Dharmesh Vyas, MD; Christopher D. Harner, MD

14   Microfracture **79**
Armando F. Vidal, MD; Jennifer FitzPatrick, MD

15   Surgical Treatment of Osteochondritis Dissecans Lesions **85**
Sarvottam Bajaj, BE; Michael J. Salata, MD; Brian J. Cole, MD, MBA

**16   Anterior Cruciate Ligament Reconstruction: Single-Bundle
        Transtibial Technique** **95**
Eric J. Strauss, MD; Adam B. Yanke, MD; Bernard R. Bach, Jr, MD

17   Anterior Cruciate Ligament Reconstruction: Two-Tunnel Technique ... **103**
Dharmesh Vyas, MD; Christopher D. Harner, MD

**18   Anatomic Anterior Cruciate Ligament Double-Bundle
        Reconstruction** **109**
Jeffrey Macalena, MD; Carola van Eck, MD, PhD; Freddie H. Fu, MD

19   Pediatric Anterior Cruciate Ligament Reconstruction **117**
*Davide Edoardo Bonasia, MD; Roberto Rossi, MD;
Brian R. Wolf, MD, MS; Annunziato Amendola, MD*

**20   Medial Patellofemoral Ligament Reconstruction for
        Recurrent Patellar Instability** **125**
Andrew J. Cosgarea, MD; Miho J. Tanaka, MD; John J. Elias, PhD

21   Realignment for Patellofemoral Arthritis **131**
Albert Lin, MD; Robin West, MD

**22   Surgical Treatment of Traumatic Quadriceps and Patellar Tendon
        Injuries of the Knee** **137**
*Patrick Schottel, MD; Keith R. Reinhardt, MD;
Gregory S. DiFelice, MD; Anil S. Ranawat, MD*

Chapter 1
Arthroscopic Repair of Partial-Thickness Rotator Cuff Tears

Matthew J. White, MD   Geoffrey S. Baer, MD, PhD

Patient Selection

Rotator cuff surgery is one of the more common procedures performed by orthopaedic surgeons. As knowledge of the anatomy and function of the rotator cuff improves, more sophisticated methods have been developed to repair this musculotendinous construct. Partial-thickness articular-surface rotator cuff repair and transosseous-equivalent repair represent two techniques that expand the treatment options for rotator cuff damage.

Indications

The indications for partial-thickness articular-surface rotator cuff repair and transosseous-equivalent repair are similar. The patient should have documented clinical findings in the presence of radiographically confirmed rotator cuff injury and should have undergone a concerted attempt at nonsurgical modalities such as rest, activity modification, medication, and physical therapy. Failure of nonsurgical treatment necessitates further treatment in the form of open or arthroscopic surgery. Subsequent decisions are based on the intraoperative findings. Fukuda et al[1] demonstrated that partial-thickness rotator cuff tears have a poor healing capacity, which may limit the success of nonsurgical treatment. These tears also have a tendency to progress when treated with acromioplasty alone.[2] On the other hand, results of repair for these tears have been excellent, especially in the young patient.[3] Acute full-thickness tears of the rotator cuff should be managed surgically. For both full- and partial-thickness chronic tears, nonsurgical treatment should be used initially. In patients who report continued pain despite these nonsurgical measures, some authors recommend surgical repair of the tear regardless of size.[4]

Contraindications

Contraindications to the surgical repair of rotator cuff tears are limited to patients in poor medical health and patients who cannot perform the necessary postoperative rehabilitation.

Preoperative Imaging

Each patient should have a shoulder series of plain radiographs. At our institution, we obtain AP, Neer AP, outlet, and axillary views of the affected shoulder. These views will demonstrate possible fracture, bony abnormality, acromion type, or, in some cases, humeral subluxation/escape. If suspicion exists about a full- or partial-thickness rotator cuff tear, advanced imaging can be ordered, the most common of which is MRI (**Figure 1, A** and **B**). Magnetic resonance arthrography (MRA) is an additional option. In a recent meta-analysis, MRA showed excellent diagnostic capabilities for both full- and partial-thickness rotator cuff tears.[5] One of the newer modalities for detecting shoulder pathology is ultrasonography (**Figure 1, C**). Vlychou et al[6] found ultrasonography to be almost equally as effective as MRI in detecting rotator cuff tears. Ultrasonography is a less expensive alternative to MRI for the diagnosis of rotator cuff tears, but it is also highly operator-dependent and slightly less sensitive. In addition, ultrasonography may not be available to all surgeons. Ultrasonography has the advantage of potentially being done at the same time as the office visit and can provide dynamic imaging.

Procedure

Room Setup/Patient Positioning

We prefer to perform shoulder arthroscopy with the patient in the lateral decubitus position. A standard arthroscopic pump is used for fluid control, and an arm holder is positioned at the distal portion of the operating table to keep the arm in approximately 20° of forward flexion and 20° to 40° of abduction with the assistance of a 5- to 10-lb weight.

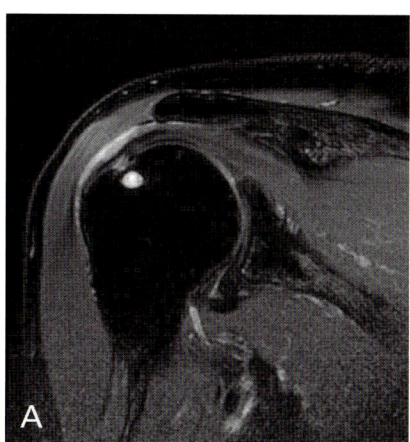
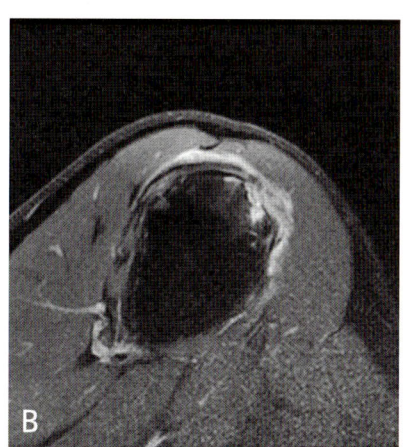
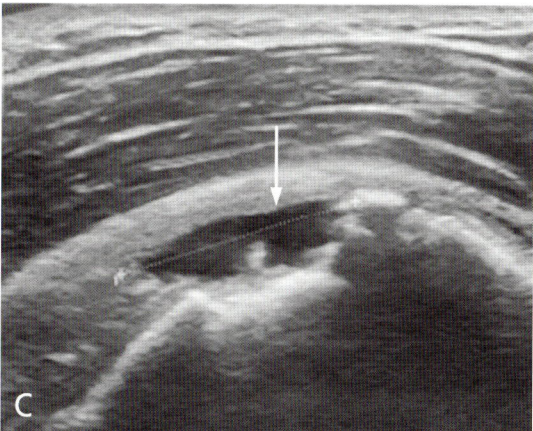

Figure 1 Partial-thickness articular-surface rotator cuff tears. **A,** Coronal T2-weighted MRI demonstrates a partial-thickness articular-surface supraspinatus tear. **B,** Sagittal T2-weighted MRI shows a tear. **C,** Longitudinal ultrasound image demonstrates a partial-thickness supraspinatus tear.

Dr. Baer or an immediate family member serves as a board member, owner, officer, or committee member of the Big Ten Fellowship Society. Neither Dr. White nor any immediate family member has received anything of value from or owns stock in a commercial company or institution related directly or indirectly to the subject of this chapter.

© 2013 American Academy of Orthopaedic Surgeons

Section 1: Sports Medicine

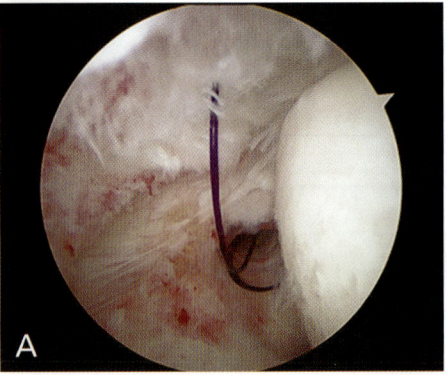
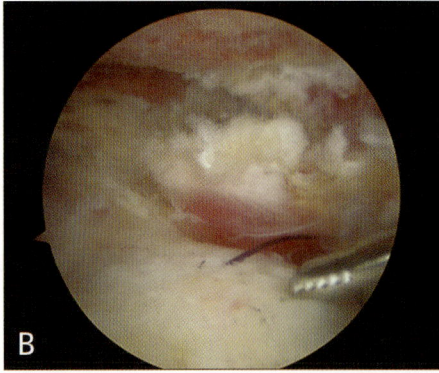

Figure 2 Arthroscopic views demonstrate technique for locating a rotator cuff tear. **A**, Monofilament suture is placed into the glenohumeral joint percutaneously to locate a partial-thickness rotator cuff tear. **B**, The monofilament suture indicates the location of the tear. A standard shaver is used to perform a bursectomy.

Table 1 Ellman Classification of Partial-Thickness Rotator Cuff Tears

Location	Grade (Depth of Lesion)
A (articular surface)	1 (<3 mm deep)
B (bursal surface)	2 (3–6 mm deep)
C (interstitial)	3 (>6 mm deep)

Special Instruments/Equipment

Instruments typically needed include a burr or curet for footprint decortications, an arthroscopic shaver, an array of graspers, a spinal needle, variously sized arthroscopic cannulas, a knot pusher, and arthroscopic scissors. Also needed is a suture punch for antegrade suture passing, a looped tissue penetrator for retrograde suture passing, or a suture lasso device for antegrade or retrograde passing.

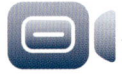 **Video 1.1** Repair of Partial Thickness Rotator Cuff Tears. Richard Angelo, MD (15 min)

Surgical Technique

Diagnostic Arthroscopy

The bony landmarks should be marked before incision because this provides a visible layout for portal positioning. We typically use the standard posterior and anterior portals as well as combinations of anterolateral and lateral portals and, occasionally, a Neviaser portal. The posterior portal is established first, approximately 1 cm medial and 2 cm inferior to the posterolateral corner of the acromion, in the "soft spot." Once this viewing portal is established, we place an anterior portal through the rotator interval using an outside-in technique with a spinal needle and standard arthroscopic cannula. We then perform a systematic glenohumeral inspection to examine for other shoulder pathology. Once this inspection is performed, we turn our attention to the articular aspect of the rotator cuff.

Certainly, large full-thickness rotator cuff tears are much easier to see. When inspecting the cuff from the articular surface, the surgeon can rotate the arm so that the entire undersurface of the cuff can be seen from anterior to posterior. In addition, the arthroscope can be switched to the anterior portal for a different viewing perspective. A 70° arthroscope also may be used to allow further visualization, especially for far anterior or far posterior tears. In the case of a partial-thickness articular-surface tear, taking the arm out of traction and increasing abduction and/or rotation often helps with visualization of the tear. Gentle débridement of frayed tissue with a shaver may make it easier to see the edges of intact tendon. If the margins of a tear can be appreciated, then a probe of known size can be used to estimate the depth of the tear and guide treatment. At this point, it is best to evaluate the nature of the tissue on the bursal side of the rotator cuff. A spinal needle can be placed percutaneously through the cuff pathology and then monofilament suture passed through and retrieved through the anterior portal in the glenohumeral joint (**Figure 2**). This makes it easier to locate the affected portion of cuff from the subacromial side. At this point, the arthroscope and instruments are transitioned to the subacromial space, where a thorough bursectomy is performed, making sure to get as far lateral as possible. The lateral portal provides an excellent working position for a shaver or radiofrequency wand. Subacromial decompression should be performed only if acromial pathology is noted. Without the bursa obstructing the view, the rotator cuff can be inspected further. A full-thickness tear will be quite apparent, and the repair can begin. If a partial-thickness tear is present, the surgeon can identify the monofilament suture that was previously placed. The bursal side of the cuff is inspected. If this tissue is intact, then the tear is treated as a partial-thickness articular-surface tear.

Repair of Partial-Thickness Articular-Surface Tears

For partial-thickness articular-surface rotator cuff tears, our treatment is guided by the Ellman classification system[7] (**Table 1**). A partial-thickness articular-surface tear less than 3 mm deep is considered an A1 tear and can be treated with débridement alone. A full-radius shaver works well for débriding degenerative and frayed tissue without damaging intact tendon. If the tear is between 3 and 6 mm (<50%), then treatment options include simple débridement or intratendon repair. An intratendon repair can be a favorable way of using intact tissue to the surgeon's advantage because it provides a road map for cuff placement and decreases the amount of tissue that must heal. Our technique for intratendon repair, described below, has been described previously by other surgeons.[8]

Viewing through the arthroscope in the posterior portal in the glenohumeral joint, we place a spinal needle just lateral to the edge of the acromion in a transtendinous fashion to locate the position for the suture anchors, which will be placed at the medial margin of the rotator cuff footprint at an angle of approximately 45°. This may be easier to achieve with the arm in slight adduction. Once the position is determined, the footprint is prepared with a shaver or burr, and a dual-loaded suture anchor is placed transtendinously into the footprint. Another suture anchor can be placed if the

© 2013 American Academy of Orthopaedic Surgeons

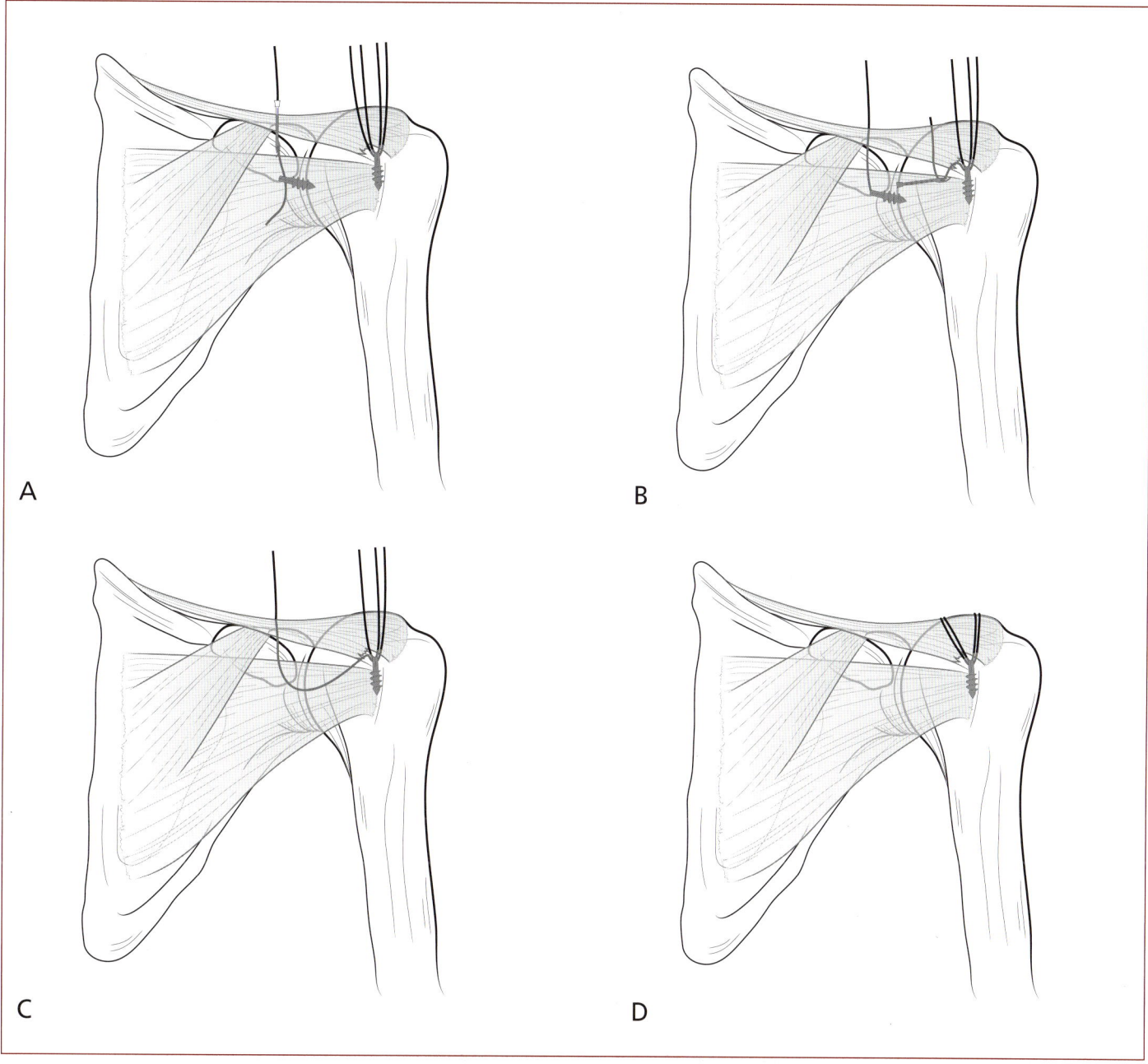

Figure 3 Illustrations show arthroscopic repair of a partial-thickness articular-surface tear. **A,** A shuttle relay is passed through the spinal needle and retrieved through the anterior portal. **B,** One end of the suture also is retrieved through the anterior portal. **C,** One end of the suture is engaged in the eyelet of the shuttle relay and then pulled back out of the healthy portion of the partially torn tendon. **D,** A complete repair of a partial-thickness articular-side rotator cuff tear is shown.

anterior-posterior dimension of the tear is large. Suture passing then begins. Different techniques can be used, depending on the amount of delamination present. Extensive delamination lends itself to the use of an instrument such as a suture lasso from within the glenohumeral joint. The 90° suture lasso allows the surgeon to pierce the lower lamina of cuff tissue from the anterior portal in the direction of the anchor. The suture then is passed out the anterior portal and tied down on top of the lamina. Visualization can be difficult using this technique, so it is best used in the presence of true delamination. If extensive delamination is not present, using a combination of shuttle relays from the subacromial space may be easier (**Figure 3**). This can be done by placing a spinal needle just off the acromion into the healthy portion of the tendon. A monofilament suture relay then is passed into the joint to retrieve one limb of suture. This suture is pulled out the anterolateral subacromial portal. This step is repeated in different portions of the healthy tendon until all four sutures have been retrieved subacromially and demonstrate a tissue bridge of at least 5 mm. The matching sutures then are tied down on top of the rotator cuff using a sliding knot followed by alternating half hitches. As each suture is tied down, it should be inspected from both the subacromial space and the glenohumeral joint.

Repair of Large Articular-Surface Tears Using the Transosseous-Equivalent Technique

If the partial-thickness tear is larger than 6 mm (>50%), the tissue often is not amenable to intratendon repair, and débridement alone almost ensures further propagation.[9] We prefer to complete these tears to a full-thickness depth and then perform our standard rotator cuff repair. The easiest way to complete the tear is from the subacromial side; this can be done using the monofilament location suture discussed earlier. A standard shaver can be used to débride the tissue until the greater tuberosity is seen and the full dimension of the tear is noted. At this point, several repair options are available, including single-row, double-row, and double-row transosseous-equivalent techniques, depending on the appearance of the tear. The transosseous-equivalent repair technique is discussed here.

Transosseous-equivalent repair has been shown to be an excellent option for treatment of full-thickness rotator cuff tears, with demonstrated success at least equivalent to that of single-row repairs as well as other types of double-row fixation.[10,11] The transosseous-equivalent technique has been shown to restore as much of the anatomic footprint as possible and increase the surface area for healing.[12] Of all the repair techniques, transosseous-equivalent repair achieves the highest contact pressure between tendon and tuberosity.[13] This may prevent spot welding as the only form of healing and may impact long-term outcomes. Repair integrity at 1 year evaluated by MRI has been quite good.[14]

After the portals are established and a thorough glenohumeral inspection has been performed, demonstrating a near–full-thickness tear, a marking suture is placed through the tear and the focus shifts to the subacromial space. A full bursectomy is performed. A subacromial decompression is performed only if the patient has noted acromial pathology. Once the bursectomy has been performed, the rotator cuff should be examined carefully to evaluate for any bursal-side cuff pathology. The lateral viewing portal can provide better visualization to define the tear. Alternatively, a 70° arthroscope can be used for a different view. Establishing an anterior subacromial portal as well as a second lateral portal directly in line with the tear can help with visualization of the tear as well as suture management. With a deep partial-thickness tear, we probe the tear and, in cases in which the tear is almost full thickness, we complete the tear with an arthroscopic shaver, débriding the degenerative edges to the tear. Once the degenerative tissue has been débrided, the footprint is prepared, using a curet or high-speed burr to decorticate the tuberosity back to bleeding bone. The surgeon must take care to only decorticate and not burr away significant portions of the greater tuberosity. The use of a radiofrequency electrode is avoided here because it could cause thermal necrosis on the healing surface. Typically, one or two suture anchors are placed percutaneously along the medial margin of the footprint at an angle of less than 45° (the deadman's angle). If the surgeon prefers not to use percutaneous placement, the anterolateral portal can be used for placement. Taking the patient's arm out of abduction can help facilitate this. We always use double-loaded suture anchors for transosseous-equivalent repair to increase configuration options and provide a backup suture if one is unloaded inadvertently.

Many options exist for passing suture for the rotator cuff repair. Suture lassos and looped tissue penetrators are useful options for retrograde passing; other devices can be used to pass suture in an antegrade fashion. Suture lassos come in a variety of angles that can make it easier to navigate difficult corners or viewing angles. Looped tissue penetrators may require a Neviaser portal. Antegrade passers eliminate the need for suture relay and can be used through standard portals. All techniques should result in a horizontal mattress configuration for matching sutures. The initial suture passes should be placed medial enough to ensure the lateral edge reaches all the way to the greater tuberosity.

Regardless of the type of suture-passing device used, good suture management is critical to success. We prefer to pass all of the sutures first, working anterior to posterior and parking the sutures out of the anterior or accessory lateral cannula. Once all the sutures are passed, we begin tying down the medial-row sutures from posterior to anterior, parking the sutures out of the accessory lateral portal. All knots are tied down with an adequate tissue bridge, using a sliding knot followed by a series of alternating half hitches. Sutures should not be cut at this point. The tied sutures should be parked opposite the remaining untied sutures. Once all of the knots for the medial row have been tied, we then check the rotator cuff configuration and the remaining footprint. Once the medial-row sutures have been tied down, we choose the pairs of sutures that lie best over the lateral aspect of the cuff for final fixation. The surgeon must take care to avoid any obvious "dog ear" configuration of the tissue. Once we determine which pairs of sutures will be used for lateral-row fixation, we take one of the sutures from each pair and thread it through the lateral-row anchor. We typically use a medium size knotless anchor for the lateral-row anchor; four No. 2 sutures can typically be placed through this style of anchor. We then locate a position off the lateral aspect of the greater tuberosity for placement of the anterior lateral anchor. The same process is repeated with the second suture from each pair passed through a second lateral anchor that is placed at the posterolateral aspect of the tear. This creates a crossed pattern of sutures (**Figure 4**). If the tear is quite large, we adjust the configuration accordingly and may place three or four medial anchors converging into two lateral anchors (**Figure 5**). The arm can be taken out of abduction during these steps to eliminate any concern about overtensioning. The final view should demonstrate a tension-free, well-approximated cuff repair, with the lateral edge compressed to the greater tuberosity. We confirm the repair in the glenohumeral joint as well as in the subacromial space. The portal sites are closed, and an abduction sling is placed.

Treatment of Bursal-Side Tears
Bursal-side partial-thickness tears typically are categorized as superficial or deep tears. Most superficial tears are treated with simple débridement. These tears often are associated with concomitant bursal pathology—a subacromial or acromioclavicular joint spurring—that requires appropriate treatment. We treat deep bursal-side tears similarly to deep articular-side tears by first probing the tear to get a sense of the amount of intact tissue that remains. When the tissue is felt to be very thin, we complete the tear with an arthroscopic shaver and repair the tear, depending on its size, as described previously for large tears.

Complications
Complications that can occur following rotator cuff repair typically include but are not limited to continued pain, retear, motion difficulty or stiffness, and loss of strength. When pain continues following surgical repair, attention should be paid to possible failed decompression or concomitant pathology that was not addressed (eg, biceps tendinopathy, labral pathology, acromioclavicular joint spurs, degenerative joint disease). Diagnostic injections can help determine whether failed decompression, biceps-generated pain, or acromioclavicular joint pathology is responsible. Retearing can occur

even in patients who have demonstrated symptomatic relief of their initial tear.[15] This can be related to tissue quality as well as initial tear size. If pain continues and a retear is demonstrated, revision should be considered if the tissue is in reasonable condition. Stiffness can result when a patient lacks commitment to the rehabilitation protocol. Alternatively, stiffness may be the result of an inflammatory response such as adhesive capsulitis; this can be helped with anti-inflammatory medication or injection. Individually directed rehabilitation protocols also can be of assistance. If all of these measures fail, arthroscopic capsular release can be effective.

Postoperative Care and Rehabilitation

Patients are supported in an abduction sling for 4 to 6 weeks depending on the tissue quality and the size of the tear. The first 2 weeks are dedicated to gentle Codman exercises. At 2 weeks, we begin passive range-of-motion exercises in formal physical therapy and at home with a stick-and-pulley system. Generally, at 6 weeks, active range-of-motion exercises are initiated. Return to activity occurs when the patient has good motion and is pain free. Full return to higher impact activities such as manual labor or overhead activities usually is delayed until 6 to 12 months postoperatively.

Pearls

- A patient who has pain with resisted rotator cuff testing but demonstrates normal strength could have a partial-thickness rotator cuff tear. If MRI is the modality of choice in the surgeon's practice, MRA should be considered to increase the specificity for identification of the partial-thickness tear.
- We generally fix any tear greater than 6 mm or greater than 50% of the thickness of the tendon. The easiest way to determine the size of the tear is with a calibrated probe or shaver of known size.
- Suture management probably is the most important aspect of rotator cuff surgery. Keeping sutures "docked" or "parked" away from the set the surgeon is working with makes visualization much easier and limits the chance of crossing the sutures, especially when using a transosseous-equivalent technique.
- To make it easier to locate the partial-thickness tear on the subacromial side, a spinal needle can be placed percutaneously through the tear. Then, a monofilament suture can be passed through the needle and parked out of the anterior glenohumeral portal. The location of the partial-thickness tear is indicated by the monofilament suture position when viewed from the subacromial side.
- A thorough bursectomy enhances visualization and minimizes the possibility of getting the sutures snagged in the tissue. In addition, it affords full identification of the tear, which facilitates surgical planning.

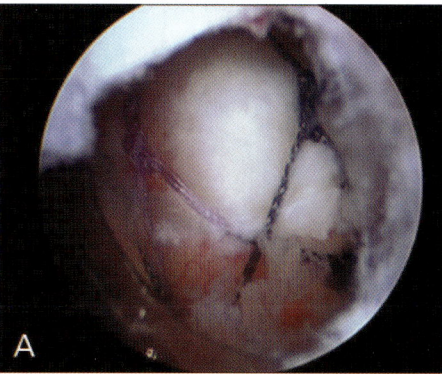 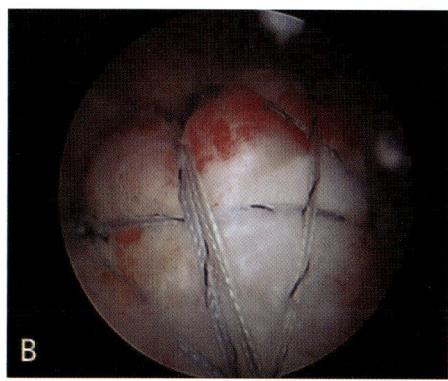

Figure 4 Arthroscopic views show completed rotator cuff repair. **A,** The final crossed pattern of sutures for transosseous-equivalent repair of the rotator cuff using two medial and two lateral anchors. **B,** The suture configuration for a larger tear requiring three medial anchors and two lateral anchors.

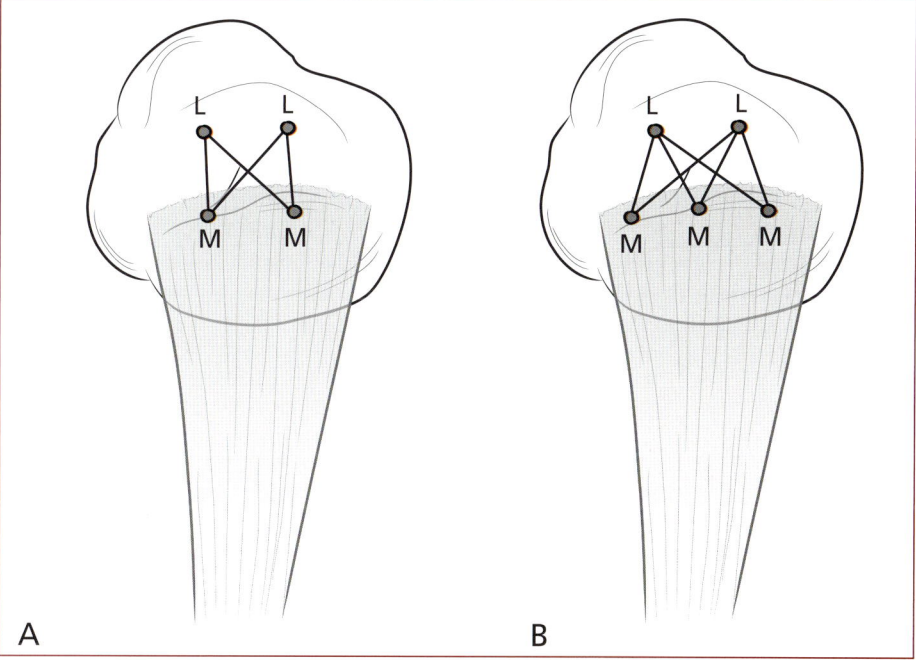

Figure 5 Illustrations show suture configuration possibilities for transosseous-equivalent rotator cuff repair. **A,** Two medial-row pairs of sutures are tied down with sliding/locking knots. Then, one suture from each suture stack is brought to a lateral anchor placed at the anterolateral aspect of the tear, and the second suture from each suture stack is passed to a second lateral anchor at the posterolateral aspect of the tear. **B,** In large tears requiring three pairs of medial sutures, one suture from each knot stack may be brought out to either an anterolateral or posterolateral anchor, creating the transosseous-equivalent repair with compression of the cuff tissue over the footprint. L = lateral anchor, M = medial knot stack.

References

1. Fukuda H, Hamada K, Nakajima T, Yamada N, Tomonaga A, Goto M: Partial-thickness tears of the rotator cuff: A clinicopathological review based on 66 surgically verified cases. *Int Orthop* 1996;20(4):257-265.
2. Kartus J, Kartus C, Rostgård-Christensen L, Sernert N, Read J, Perko M: Long-term clinical and ultrasound evaluation after arthroscopic acromioplasty in patients with partial rotator cuff tears. *Arthroscopy* 2006;22(1):44-49.
3. Kamath G, Galatz LM, Keener JD, Teefey S, Middleton W, Yamaguchi K: Tendon

integrity and functional outcome after arthroscopic repair of high-grade partial-thickness supraspinatus tears. *J Bone Joint Surg Am* 2009;91(5):1055-1062.

4. Lähteenmäki HE, Hiltunen A, Virolainen P, Nelimarkka O: Repair of full-thickness rotator cuff tears is recommended regardless of tear size and age: A retrospective study of 218 patients. *J Shoulder Elbow Surg* 2007;16(5):586-590.

5. de Jesus JO, Parker L, Frangos AJ, Nazarian LN: Accuracy of MRI, MR arthrography, and ultrasound in the diagnosis of rotator cuff tears: A meta-analysis. *AJR Am J Roentgenol* 2009;192(6):1701-1707.

6. Vlychou M, Dailiana Z, Fotiadou A, Papanagiotou M, Fezoulidis IV, Malizos KN: Symptomatic partial rotator cuff tears: Diagnostic performance of ultrasound and magnetic resonance imaging with surgical correlation. *Acta Radiol* 2009;50(1):101-105.

7. Ellman H: Diagnosis and treatment of incomplete rotator cuff tears. *Clin Orthop Relat Res* 1990;254:64-74.

8. Ide J, Maeda S, Takagi K: Arthroscopic transtendon repair of partial-thickness articular-side tears of the rotator cuff: Anatomical and clinical study. *Am J Sports Med* 2005;33(11):1672-1679.

9. Strauss EJ, Salata MJ, Kercher J, et al: Multimedia article: The arthroscopic management of partial-thickness rotator cuff tears. A systematic review of the literature. *Arthroscopy* 2011;27(4):568-580.

10. Nho SJ, Slabaugh MA, Seroyer ST, et al: Does the literature support double-row suture anchor fixation for arthroscopic rotator cuff repair? A systematic review comparing double-row and single-row suture anchor configuration. *Arthroscopy* 2009;25(11):1319-1328.

11. Toussaint B, Schnaser E, Bosley J, Lefebvre Y, Gobezie R: Early structural and functional outcomes for arthroscopic double-row transosseous-equivalent rotator cuff repair. *Am J Sports Med* 2011;39(6):1217-1225.

12. Park MC, Tibone JE, ElAttrache NS, Ahmad CS, Jun BJ, Lee TQ: Part II: Biomechanical assessment for a footprint-restoring transosseous-equivalent rotator cuff repair technique compared with a double-row repair technique. *J Shoulder Elbow Surg* 2007;16(4):469-476.

13. Mazzocca AD, Bollier MJ, Ciminiello AM, et al: Biomechanical evaluation of arthroscopic rotator cuff repairs over time. *Arthroscopy* 2010;26(5):592-599.

14. Frank JB, ElAttrache NS, Dines JS, Blackburn A, Crues J, Tibone JE: Repair site integrity after arthroscopic transosseous-equivalent suture-bridge rotator cuff repair. *Am J Sports Med* 2008;36(8):1496-1503.

15. Galatz LM, Ball CM, Teefey SA, Middleton WD, Yamaguchi K: The outcome and repair integrity of completely arthroscopically repaired large and massive rotator cuff tears. *J Bone Joint Surg Am* 2004;86(2):219-224.

Video Reference

1.1 Angelo R: Repair of partial thickness rotator cuff tears, in Burkhart SS, Savoie FH, eds: *Arthroscopic Surgical Techniques: Rotator Cuff Repair*. Rosemont, IL, American Academy of Orthopaedic Surgeons, 2009.

Chapter 2
Arthroscopic and Open Bankart Repair

LCDR Brandon Bryant, MD, USN   *James P. Bradley, MD*

Patient Selection
Indications
Patients who present with a history of a traumatic shoulder dislocation should undergo a comprehensive history and a physical examination of both shoulders. Overhead and contact athletes with documented anteroinferior glenohumeral instability should be considered for either arthroscopic or open Bankart repair.[1] Older and recreational athletes without engaging Hill-Sachs lesions or large (> 25%) bony Bankart lesions should be initially considered for a supervised physical therapy program.[2,3] In patients who have recurrent dislocation events or those with persistent symptoms despite initial nonsurgical management, we recommend surgical intervention. Arthroscopic Bankart repair has emerged as an equivalent treatment method for successful stabilization compared with the previous gold standard of open repair techniques.[4-7]

Contraindications
The decision whether to pursue an arthroscopic repair versus an open repair is often one of surgeon preference, although certain conditions exist under which open techniques are preferred. The presence of significant glenoid bone loss (>25%), an engaging Hill-Sachs lesion, glenohumeral capsulolabral attenuation (congenital or as a result of previous thermal use or failed instability surgery), connective tissue disorders, and concomitant subscapularis tears or humeral avulsions of the glenohumeral ligament (HAGL lesions) are considered contraindications to performing an arthroscopic Bankart repair.[3,8] Patients with chronic recurrent instability after surgical or nonsurgical treatment represent a relative contraindication; the decision to proceed with arthroscopic repair should be based on imaging and tissue quality during diagnostic arthroscopy.[2,3,8,9]

Preoperative Imaging
Preoperative radiographs are needed to assess the position of the humeral head with respect to the glenoid and the presence and size of any associated Hill-Sachs or bony glenoid defects, and to rule out any associated fractures, such as of the greater tuberosity. We routinely obtain true AP, axillary lateral, and scapular Y views. Additional views, such as the apical oblique, West Point, and Didiee, can be obtained to further define bony glenoid defects; the Stryker notch and true AP in internal rotation views can better assess Hill-Sachs defects.[9,10]

MRI, with or without gadolinium arthrography, is routinely obtained preoperatively to assess the capsule, labrum, rotator cuff, cartilage, and bony anatomy (**Figure 1**). When significant bone defects are observed on either plain radiographs or MRI, a three-dimensional CT scan can be obtained. This modality allows for the subtraction of the humeral head with direct measurement of the glenoid face, in addition to accurate sizing of humeral head defects.[3,9]

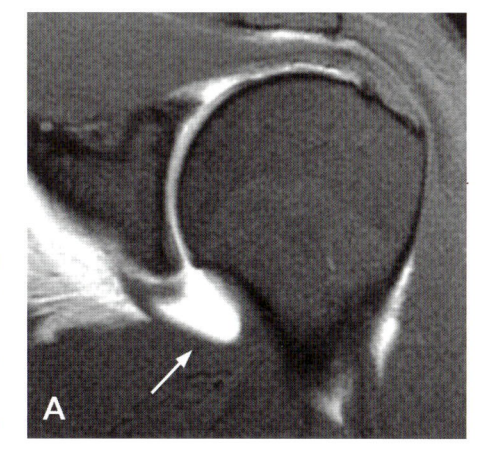

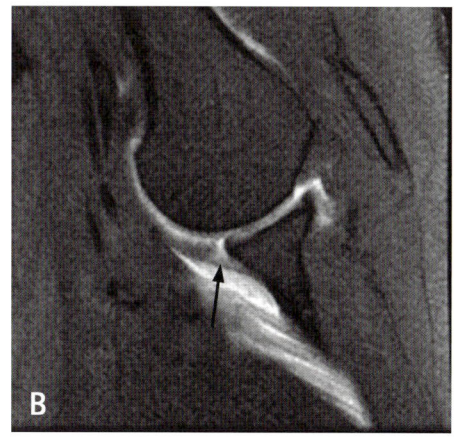

Figure 1 Preoperative T2-weighted magnetic resonance arthrograms of the shoulder of a patient with an anteroinferior labral tear, or Bankart lesion (arrows). **A,** Coronal image. **B,** Abduction external rotation image.

Procedure
Room Setup/Patient Positioning
We routinely perform a diagnostic shoulder arthroscopy on all patients with anterior instability to determine, based on the findings of the arthroscopy and in conjunction with preoperative history and imaging, whether open or arthroscopic repair is needed. We prefer to use the standard lateral decubitus position for shoulder arthroscopy, although the beach-chair position can also be effectively used. We use a vacuum beanbag to hold the patient in the lateral decubitus position. It is important to protect the axillary nerve with a gel pad and to place pillows between the legs and beneath the contralateral leg to protect the peroneal nerve (**Figure 2**).

If it is determined that an open repair will be performed, the patient is taken out of lateral arm traction and placed back into the supine position. The surgical arm is placed on an arm board, and folded surgical towels are placed beneath the scapula directly posterior. The patient is moved to the surgical-side edge of the

---

Dr. Bradley or an immediate family member has received royalties from Arthrex; has received research or institutional support from Arthrex; and serves as a board member, owner, officer, or committee member of the American Orthopaedic Society for Sports Medicine. Neither Dr. Bryant nor any immediate family member has received anything of value from or owns stock in a commercial company or institution related directly or indirectly to the subject of this chapter.

Section 1: Sports Medicine

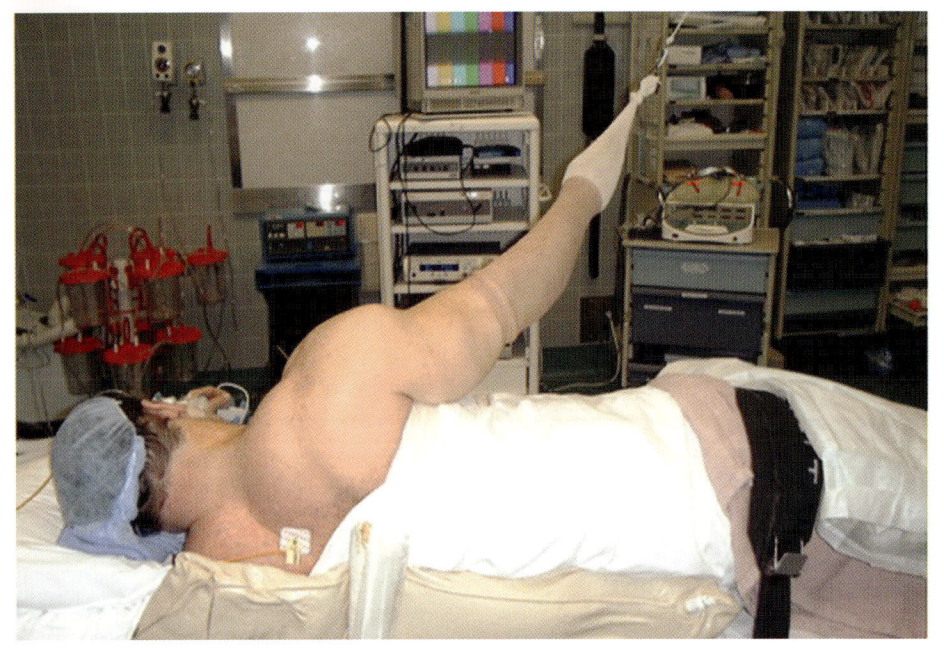

Figure 2 Photograph shows lateral decubitus positioning for shoulder arthroscopy. A beanbag and an axillary roll are used, and pillows are placed underneath and between the legs, padding all prominences.

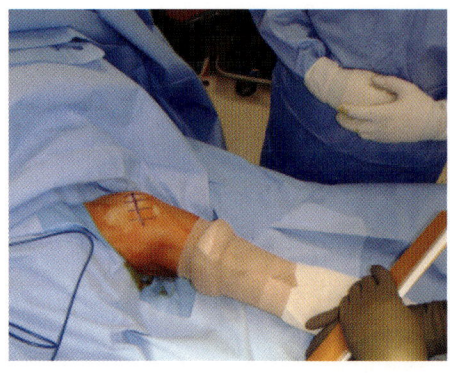

Figure 3 Photograph shows a patient positioned supine for open anterior Bankart repair, with the surgical arm prepared and draped free on an arm board.

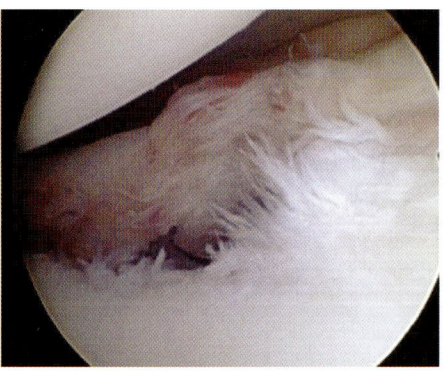

Figure 4 A Bankart lesion in a left shoulder as viewed through an arthroscope in the posterior portal.

table to facilitate improved visualization and room for the procedure. The arm is draped free to the level of the shoulder to facilitate full positioning control throughout the procedure (**Figure 3**).

Special Instruments/Equipment/Implants

Successful arthroscopic Bankart repair can be performed using standard shoulder arthroscopy equipment. The particular equipment used is dependent on surgeon preference. Many different cannulas, anchors, and soft-tissue suture-passing devices have been developed, any of which can be used to perform successful repair. Success is related more to surgical technique than to the specific devices used. We prefer to use curved suture-shuttling devices for exchange suture passing from the anchors through soft tissue, and we routinely use 2.4- or 2.0-mm biocomposite bone anchors that are preloaded with a single No. 2 high-strength braided nonabsorbable suture.

During open Bankart repair, adequate visualization is paramount. A three-pronged pitchfork glenoid retractor; a long, narrow right-angle retractor; Richardson retractors; and a humeral head depressor/retractor are all used throughout the procedure to maintain critical visualization.

Surgical Technique
Arthroscopic Bankart Repair

Following the induction of general anesthesia, an evaluation under anesthesia of both the affected and the unaffected shoulder is performed with the patient supine. The patient is then placed into the lateral decubitus position as described previously. A foam arm traction sleeve is placed on the surgical arm and secured with self-adherent wrap. Lateral traction is then applied using 5 to 10 pounds, depending on patient size, in approximately 20° of forward flexion and 20° to 30° of abduction. After a sterile local preparation and using an 18-gauge spinal needle, the posterior portal is infiltrated with 1% lidocaine with epinephrine (1:100,000); then the needle is advanced into the glenohumeral joint, and a total of 50 mL is instilled. Many authors believe that this step decreases overall bleeding, allowing lower arthroscopic pump pressures to be used. The pump is typically maintained at 40 to 60 mm Hg throughout the case.

The shoulder and the upper arm are then prepared and draped in standard fashion. The posterior portal is established, the arthroscope is introduced, and a comprehensive diagnostic arthroscopy is performed (**Figure 4**). If none of the contraindicating factors described previously are present, arthroscopic Bankart repair is performed. If contraindications to arthroscopic repair are present, preparations are made for an open repair: The posterior portal is closed and covered with a local impermeable sterile dressing, and the patient is transferred to the supine position as described previously.

A standard anterior portal is established, and a clear 8.25-mm cannula is placed. The anterior portal is positioned slightly lateral in the interval, just at the superior margin of the subscapularis, which allows for proper placement of the anteroinferior glenoid anchors. A third (anterosuperior) portal is then established, high in the rotator interval. A smaller 5.75-mm clear cannula is placed here, decreasing overcrowding of the interval. The anterosuperior portal will eventually be used for the arthroscope, whereas the standard anterior and posterior portals will be used as working portals.

Preparation of the labrum is performed next. This is considered a critical aspect of this procedure and should not be trivialized. An arthroscopic elevator is used via the anterior portal to mobilize the labrum (**Figure 5, A**). This is done carefully within the tear cleft, between the labrum and glenoid bone, ensuring that the sharp elevator does not iatrogenically create a radial split in the labral tissue. The labrum may be scarred in a nonanatomic position along the medial glenoid neck and must be elevated to allow for later anatomic repair. Although ALPSA (an-

Chapter 2: Arthroscopic and Open Bankart Repair

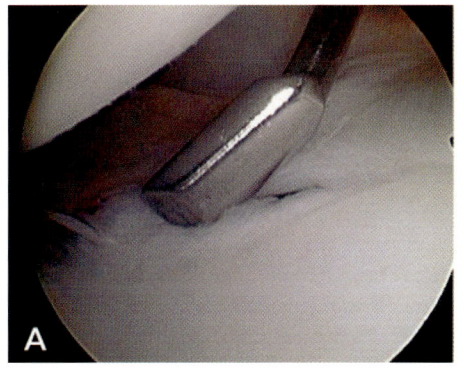

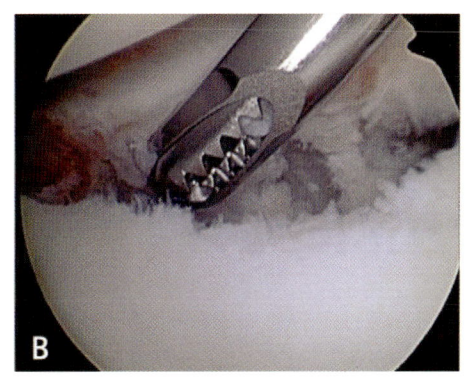

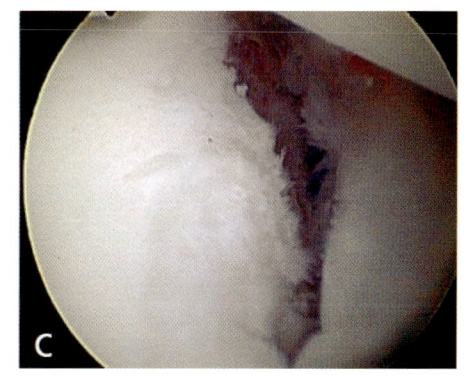

Figure 5 Arthroscopic views show labrum preparation for arthroscopic Bankart lesion repair. **A,** An arthroscopic elevator device is used to mobilize the labral tear in the interval between the glenoid rim and the anteroinferior labrum. **B,** An arthroscopic shaver is used to prepare the glenoid rim and the labrum for repair. **C,** View of the anterior glenoid from the anterosuperior portal following labrum mobilization and glenoid preparation. Note the roughened glenoid rim and bleeding tissues.

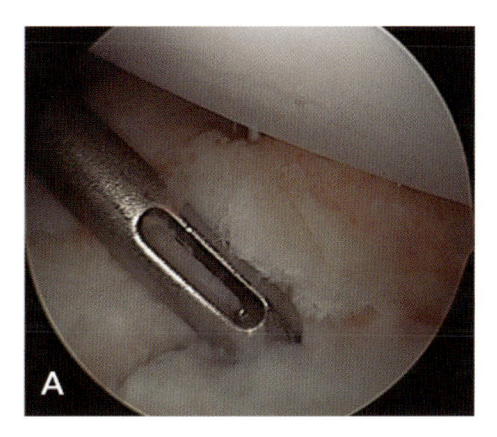

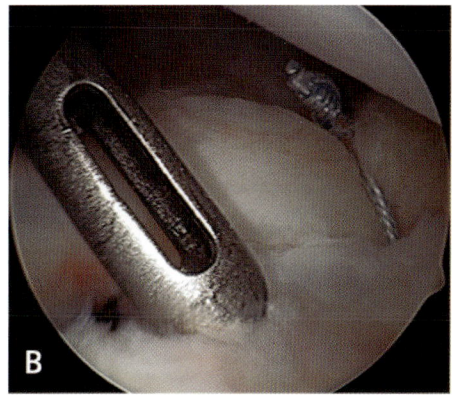

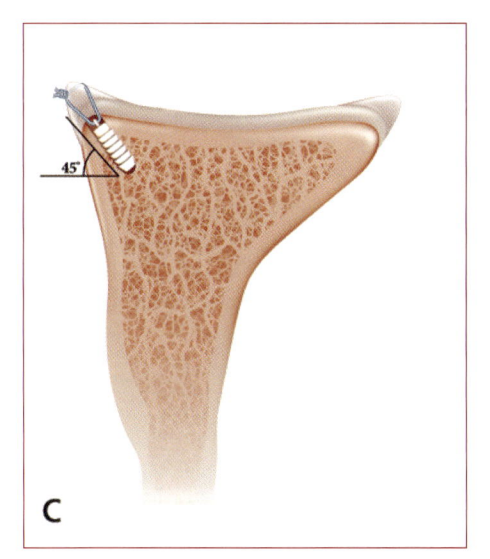

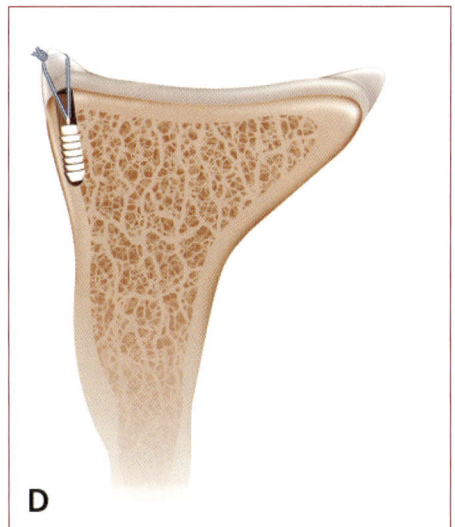

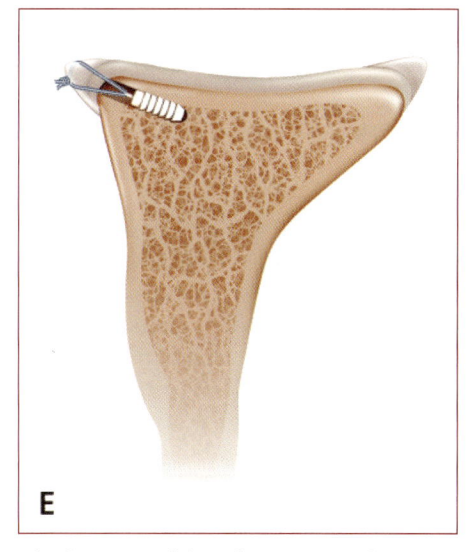

Figure 6 Anchor placement for arthroscopic Bankart repair. **A,** Arthroscopic view shows anchor guide placement of the inferiormost anchor at the 6-o'clock position. **B,** Arthroscopic view shows placement of the second anchor at the 5-o'clock position. Note that the sutures for the first anchor are secured and the suture tails are cut. **C,** Illustration shows the proper angle of anchor placement, 45° from the glenoid face. The correct entry location, approximately 2 mm onto the glenoid face from the edge of the rim, is also illustrated. Illustrations show improper anchor placement, with the anchor placed too perpendicular to the glenoid and buried too far into the glenoid (**D**) and the anchor placed too parallel to the glenoid and buried too far into the glenoid (**E**).

terior labral periosteal sleeve avulsion) lesions are less common, they should be evaluated for and elevated if present. Next, the glenoid rim is prepared for anchor placement. A 4.0-mm shaver or burr is used along the glenoid rim to roughen the surface, creating a bleeding bed of bone (**Figure 5, B** and **C**). It is imperative not to remove glenoid bone during this step, creating iatrogenic glenoid bone deficiency.

Anchors are then placed through the standard anterior portal, beginning inferiorly on the glenoid near the 6-o'clock position (**Figure 6, A**). Occasionally, this inferior anchor is placed via a percutaneously placed 5-o'clock portal to avoid a significantly oblique trajectory, which can result in missing adequate glenoid bone for purchase. (All clockface positions described in this chapter are for a right shoulder.) Proper anchor placement is imperative; it should allow for anatomic restoration of the glenolabral concavity. Anchors are placed on the anterior rim of the glenoid, roughly 2 mm from the anterior edge and at a 45° angle to the

© 2013 American Academy of Orthopaedic Surgeons

Section 1: Sports Medicine

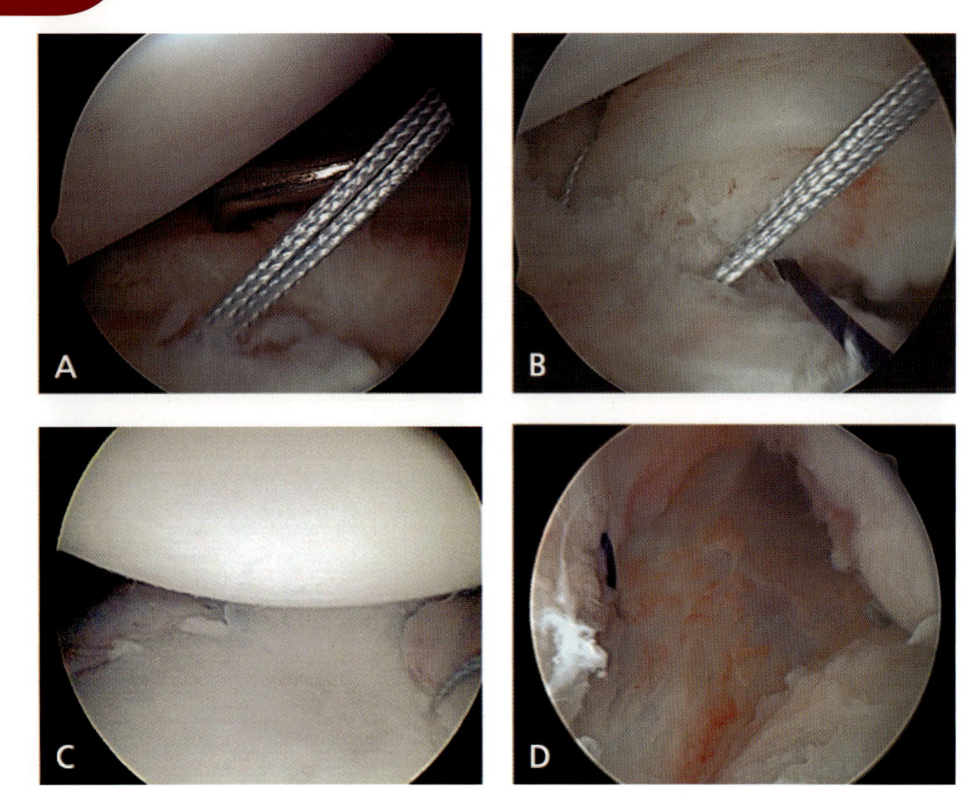

Figure 7 Arthroscopic views show anchor suturing and closure for arthroscopic Bankart repair. **A,** A suture-passing device penetrates the tissue roughly 1 cm from the glenoid edge (at the level of the placed anchor) and passes under the torn anterior labrum. **B,** Passage of a No. 0 absorbable synthetic monofilament suture for shuttling of one of the suture limbs from the placed anchor. **C,** Completed Bankart repair. Note the rolled labral edge or bumper and the centering of the humeral head on the glenoid after placement of knots and half-hitches. **D,** Closure of the posterior capsular rent (portal) using a No. 0 absorbable synthetic monofilament suture and a locking sliding knot.

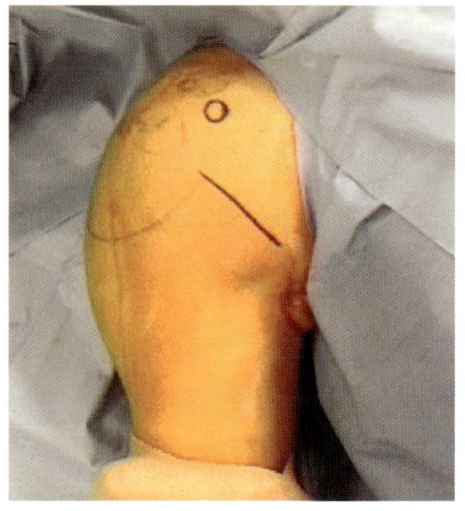

Figure 8 Photograph shows location of the anterior shoulder incision for an open Bankart repair in a right shoulder, within the natural axillary crease and the Langer lines.

glenoid surface, ensuring that the repair is not in a medialized position (**Figure 6, B** through **E**). At least three anchors are placed, roughly 6 to 7 mm apart, marching up the anterior glenoid rim, until the entire Bankart lesion is repaired. Care must be taken to avoid closing a sublabral hole, or foramen, or a Buford complex. Following the placement of each anchor, one limb of suture from the anchor is passed through the capsulolabral tissue using a retrograde technique. Numerous commercially available suture-passing devices can be used to effectively perform this portion of the procedure. The suture passer is used to grab the capsulolabral tissue approximately 1 cm off the glenoid edge, inferior to the placed anchor, advancing the tissue in a south-to-north manner. This ultimately brings the torn inferior tissue superiorly to the point of fixation (anchor), resuspending the capsuloligamentous complex that often will have fallen inferomedially (**Figure 7, A** and **B**). Sutures are then tied in sequential order using a locking, sliding knot, seated away from the glenoid face, and backed up with three half-hitches (**Figure 7, C**). The final result is a rolled labral edge or bumper and centering of the humeral head on the glenoid.

Once all the anchors have been placed and secured, a straight punch is used via the posterior portal in the bare area of the humeral head to allow for a small vascular infusion that provides valuable marrow elements and growth factors for tissue-healing. The capsular rent caused by the posterior portal is then closed using a simple No. 0 absorbable synthetic monofilament suture (**Figure 7, D**). All portal incisions are then closed with 2-0 nylon suture using an inverted figure-of-8 technique. Postoperative dressings are applied, and the patient is placed in a sling with an abduction pillow and an ice pack over the dressing.

Open Bankart Repair

With the patient positioned supine as described previously, the entire arm and shoulder girdle are prepared and draped with the arm free. A standard deltopectoral incision is used, with the skin incision beginning 1 cm lateral to the tip of the coracoid and extending distally to the axillary crease (**Figure 8**). The subcutaneous tissues are undermined, and the deltopectoral interval is identified with localization of the cephalic vein. The cephalic vein is retracted laterally with the deltoid and is preserved whenever possible. Blunt dissection is then performed deep to the deltoid muscle, allowing for exposure of the deeper clavipectoral fascia. This fascia is then incised along its lateral border, followed by blunt dissection beneath the conjoined tendon; the acromial branch of the thoracoacromial artery is often encountered lateral to the coracoid in this interval and should be ligated. The conjoined tendon is then retracted medially using a long, narrow right-angle retractor. This medial retraction needs only to be slight, as the nearby musculocutaneous nerve can be injured with heavy retraction.

The subscapularis tendon is then visualized with the shoulder externally rotated to 65°, and its upper and lower borders are identified, including the location of the biceps tendon and the lesser tuberosity. We perform a subscapularis split approach as described by Kim and Jobe,[2] which we believe allows for earlier range of motion, negating the need for tendon healing back to the lesser tuberosity (as required with subscapularis elevation off its insertion), and presents less overall risk to this important structure. The subscapularis is incised in line with its fibers between the upper two thirds and lower one third of the tendon. Care is taken not to penetrate too deeply, avoiding capsular incision and arthrotomy. This horizontal subscapularis incision is taken from its lateral border, medially to the musculotendinous junction. A periosteal (key) elevator is used to separate the more superficial subscapularis tissue from the underlying anterior capsule (Figure 9). This is performed beginning medially, where there is more anatomic separation of these structures, facilitating the identification of this interval. Separation of the subscapularis and the anterior capsule is performed laterally in the same manner. Multiple No. 2 braided traction sutures are placed on both the upper and lower subscapularis limbs, to facilitate traction and identification later.

Self-retaining Gelpi retractors are then positioned between the two subscapularis limbs, followed by placement of a three-pronged pitchfork retractor on the anterior glenoid neck. This retractor is an important tool and provides adequate visualization of the anterior glenoid rim during the course of the Bankart repair.

The anterior capsule is then incised from lateral to medial, roughly parallel to the subscapularis split and toward the 3-o'clock position of the glenoid. This incision should be made just superior to the capsular thickening, which represents the anterior band of the inferior glenohumeral ligament. Care is taken not to cut into the anterior labrum. Multiple No. 2 braided traction sutures are placed on both the superior and the inferior limbs of the capsule. These traction sutures are purposely passed at the level of the glenoid in the medial-to-lateral direction, which will serve as a marker preventing overtightening later during the repair. A humeral head retractor is then positioned carefully between the humeral head and the posterior glenoid, allowing for improved visualization of the anterior glenoid rim (Figure 10).

The anterior labrum is then inspected for a Bankart lesion. The Bankart tear and the anterior labrum are then dissected free from the anterior glenoid and mobilized. The anterior glenoid rim is prepared using both a small curet and a burr, to freshen the area for repair (to create a bleeding bed). As with the arthroscopic technique, care must be taken not to remove significant anterior glenoid bone, thus creating a glenoid bone deficiency state. Bone anchors preloaded with needles on heavy nonabsorbable sutures are then sequentially placed along the anterior glenoid rim at the 5:30, 4-o'clock, and 3-o'clock positions (Figure 11). Beginning with the most inferiorly placed anchor, the sutures are passed beneath the labrum and through the inferior limb of the capsule. Each suture limb from each anchor is passed in

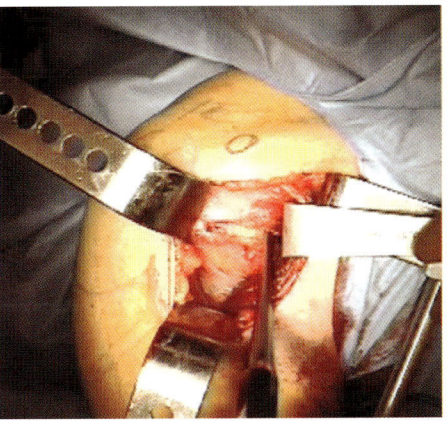

Figure 9 Intraoperative photograph shows a subscapularis split approach for an open Bankart repair in a right shoulder. The subscapularis tendon is split using electrocautery longitudinally, in line with its fibers, without penetrating the anterior capsule.

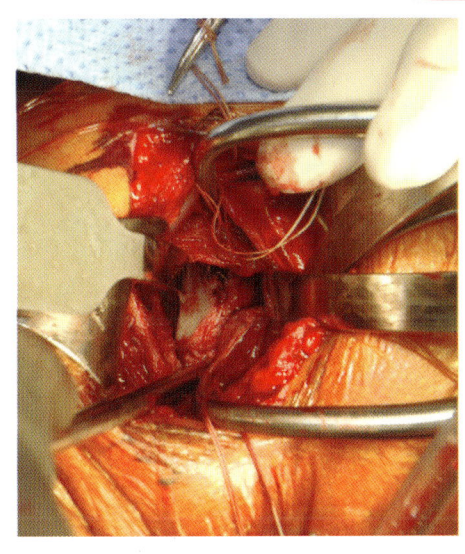

Figure 10 Intraoperative photograph shows visualization of an anterior Bankart lesion and the glenoid in a right shoulder.

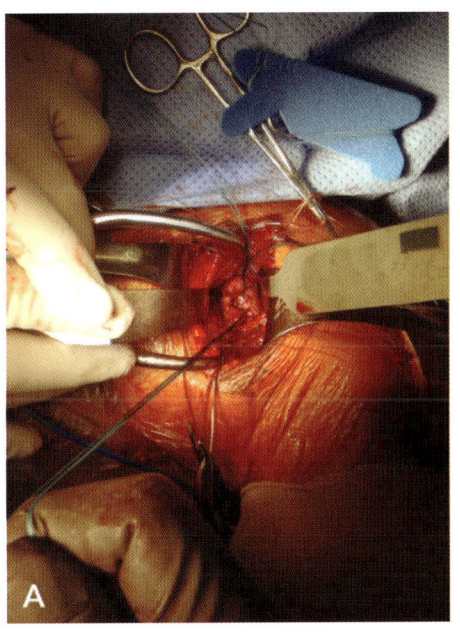

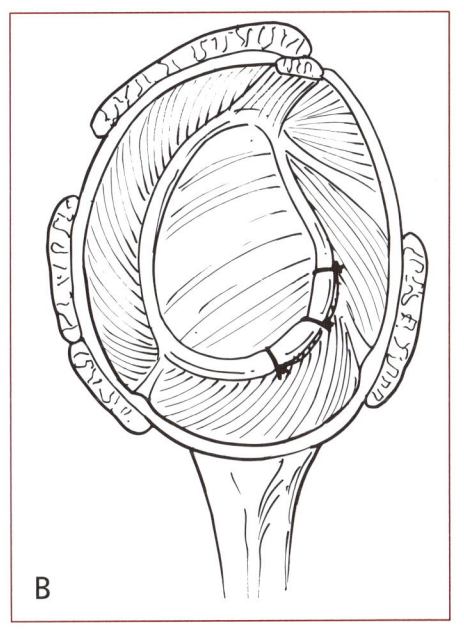

Figure 11 Anchor placement in open Bankart repair. **A,** Intraoperative photograph shows suture anchors placed along the anteroinferior glenoid margin. **B,** Illustration shows anchor placement with respect to the glenoid face. Anchors are placed roughly at the 5:30, 4-o'clock, and 3-o'clock positions (in a right shoulder) for most Bankart tear patterns. More extensive tears may require placement of additional anchors posteroinferiorly.

this manner, creating a horizontal mattress suture configuration (Figure 12, A). Sutures are passed while pulling the traction sutures on the inferior capsular limb in a superior direction, which allows for a superior shift of tissue. It is important to pass these sutures through the capsule at the level of the glenoid in the medial-lateral plane. Passing the sutures lateral to the glenoid will result in overtightening of the anterior capsule, with resultant loss of external rotation. The sutures from the middle (4-o'clock) anchor are passed in the same manner. The sutures from the superior (3-o'clock) anchor are passed through the superior limb of the capsule, using the traction sutures to pull inferiorly during needle passage (Figure 12, B).

The sutures from the middle anchor are then also passed through the superior capsular limb, which will result in overlapping of the two limbs. This is performed with the arm in roughly 65° of abduction. The arm is taken through gentle external and internal rotation, assessing the amount of capsular tightening and ensuring that enough external rotation is present and not overly constrained. Once all sutures have been passed, they

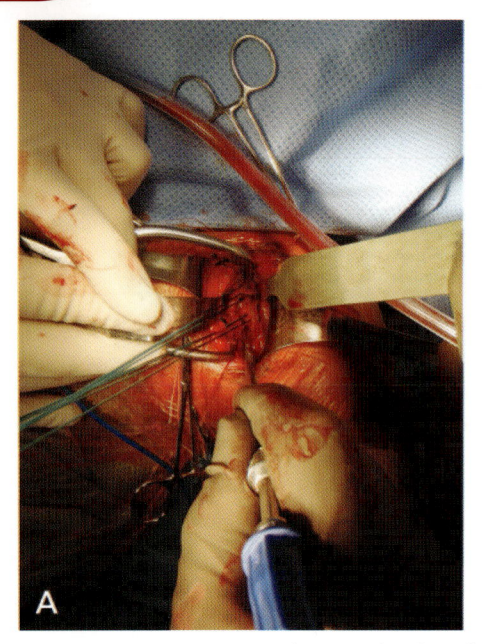

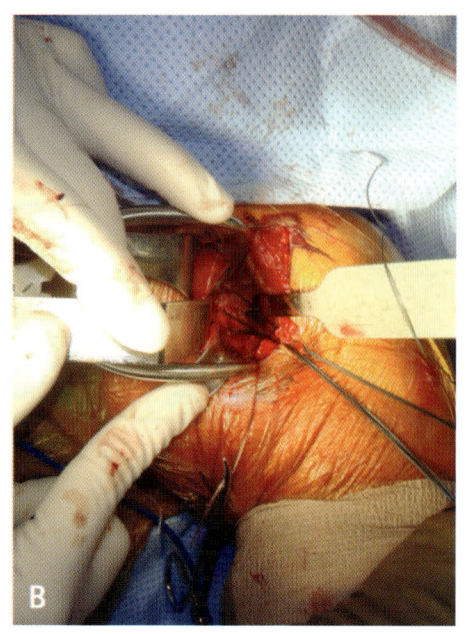

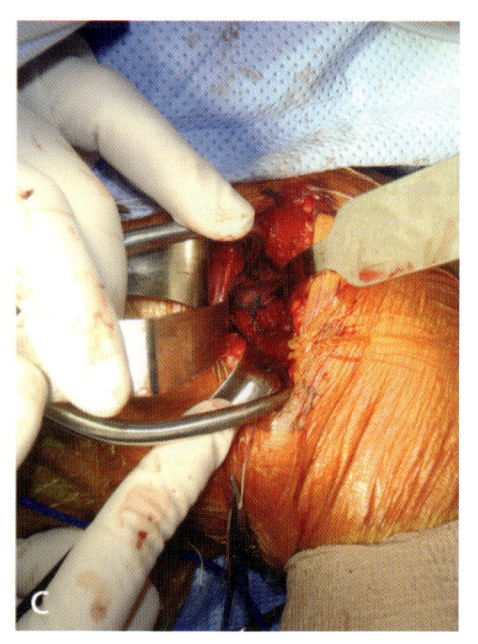

Figure 12 Intraoperative photographs show final steps in an open Bankart repair. **A,** Both suture limbs are passed through the anteroinferior labrum in a horizontal mattress fashion. **B,** Superior and inferior anterior capsular leaflets are repaired, shifting the inferior leaflet superiorly. **C,** The repaired anterior capsule.

are sequentially tied, beginning inferiorly. The suture tails are then cut. At this stage, the capsule and labrum have been repaired back to the glenoid rim and the capsule overlapped at its medial side (**Figure 12, C**). The glenohumeral joint is then copiously irrigated, and the humeral head retractor is removed. This completes the Bankart repair portion of the procedure. Irrigation and closure are then performed.

The subscapularis is closed using interrupted inverted No. 0 absorbable sutures in a side-to-side fashion. The deltopectoral interval is not closed with sutures, although it can be loosely reapproximated with No. 2-0 absorbable sutures according to the surgeon's preference. Subcutaneous tissues are reapproximated with No. 2-0 absorbable sutures, and the skin is closed with a running subcuticular absorbable suture. Adhesive skin strips are applied superficially, and a sterile dressing is applied. The arm is placed in a sling, with an abduction pillow and an ice pack over the dressing.

Complications

Complications for both arthroscopic and open Bankart repair can be separated into two categories: intraoperative and postoperative. A thorough understanding of shoulder anatomy and careful surgical technique are imperative to avoid these complications. Nerve injury, vascular injury, hardware failure, chondrolysis, and over- or undertensioning of the capsulolabral complex have been known to occur.[11,12]

The axillary and musculocutaneous nerves in particular are at risk during this procedure. The axillary nerve has been shown to lie approximately 10 to 15 mm beneath the inferior capsule.[12] Overzealous plication of the inferior capsule can result in injury to this nerve. The musculocutaneous nerve lies 5 to 8 cm inferior to the coracoid and is most at risk during the open approach, with excessive medial retraction of the conjoined tendon.[12] Nerve injury to the brachial plexus can also occur and is thought to result from excessive arm traction and increased cervical flexion or extension during the procedure.[12] During positioning, neutral cervical alignment should be confirmed and continually checked by the anesthesiologist throughout the case.

The use of suture anchors or other devices is not without the potential for iatrogenic injury. Anchors that are placed proud (not below the articular margin) or not firmly seated within the bone can cause abrasive cartilage wear or become loose bodies. Surgical technique is crucial with both anchor placement and the tying of arthroscopic knots. Knots that are not tied securely with good technique can result in a failed repair.

Chondrolysis has been shown to occur with the use of postoperative intra-articularly placed pain pumps, particularly those using bupivacaine.[12] Chondrolysis has also been seen in the absence of pain pump use; its exact mechanism is not currently completely understood. The use of intra-articular pain pumps following shoulder surgery should be avoided.

Over- or undertensioning of the capsule and labral repair can lead to either stiffness or continued laxity, respectively.

Postoperative complications, including stiffness, infection, and persistent pain, can occur. Some degree of stiffness, particularly in external rotation, is to be expected with either open or arthroscopic Bankart repair. Excessive overtightening of the anteroinferior capsule can result in significant external rotation losses and may increase the contact pressures within the glenohumeral joint.[11,12] These increased pressures can further lead to accelerated degenerative arthritic breakdown of the joint. Infection following open or arthroscopic Bankart surgery is rare; it is seen in up to 6% of open cases and less than 1% of arthroscopic procedures.[12] The most common causative organism with shoulder cases is *Propionibacterium acnes*. With any suspected infection, appropriate cultures should be obtained and the laboratory should be asked to specifically look for *P acnes*, because this requires special culture techniques and longer result times. In all cases of infection, antibiotics should begin immediately after the culture has been obtained and should be tailored to the organism grown. Persistent postoperative pain can be difficult to manage. A thorough examination should always be performed, with adjunctive imaging tests as indicated to aid in diagnosis. Nonsurgical management is the rule of thumb unless the specific etiology is found and can be addressed surgically.

Postoperative Care and Rehabilitation

Patients undergoing both open and arthroscopic Bankart repair are initially placed in an abduction pillow sling that is to be worn full time for 6 weeks. Patients are encouraged to perform elbow and wrist motion exercises immediately. Passive shoulder abduction in the scapular plane and active internal and external shoulder rotation with the arm adducted at the side (elbow flexed at 90°) are also started immediately. External rotation is limited to 10° for the first 2 weeks and 20° from weeks 2 to 4. Formal physical therapy is commenced at 4 weeks, with progressive range-of-motion and isometric periscapular exercises. The goal by week 12 is the restoration of motion in forward flexion, internal rotation, abduction, and approximately 50% external rotation comparable to the contralateral shoulder. From 3 to 6 months postoperatively, progressive strengthening, plyometrics, and sport-specific exercises are started. For contact athletes, the goal is return to play at 6 months.

Pearls

- The surgeon must be familiar with the indications for and contraindications to arthroscopic Bankart repair; open repair should be used when indicated.
- During arthroscopic Bankart repair, two anterior portals should be used—one in the standard position above the subscapularis tendon and one in a superior portion of the rotator interval—to prevent overcrowding.
- During arthroscopic Bankart repair, occasionally a percutaneous anchor can be placed to allow for access to the most inferior aspects of the glenoid and to prevent oblique trajectories for suture tying.
- Preparation of the labrum and stimulation of a bleeding osseous glenoid bed is a critical step in Bankart repair and should be carefully performed to prevent iatrogenic injury to the labrum and the glenoid bone stock.
- Anchors should be placed from inferior to superior and tied while being placed to facilitate proper tensioning.
- During the approach for open Bankart repair, the subscapularis should be separated from the underlying capsule to facilitate capsuloligamentous repair during suture repair.
- With open Bankart repair, the arm should be held in 65° of abduction during final capsular repair.

References

1. Mazzocca AD, Brown FM Jr, Carreira DS, Hayden J, Romeo AA: Arthroscopic anterior shoulder stabilization of collision and contact athletes. *Am J Sports Med* 2005;33(1):52-60.
2. Kim D, Jobe F: Open anterior instability repair, in ElAttrache N, ed: *Surgical Techniques in Sports Medicine*, ed 1. Philadelphia, PA, Lippincott Williams & Wilkins, 2007, pp 3-10.
3. Burkhart S, Klein J: Arthroscopic bankart repair, in ElAttrache N, ed: *Surgical Techniques in Sports Medicine*, ed 1. Philadelphia, PA, Lippincott Williams & Wilkins, 2007, pp 11-16.
4. Bottoni CR, Smith EL, Berkowitz MJ, Towle RB, Moore JH: Arthroscopic versus open shoulder stabilization for recurrent anterior instability: A prospective randomized clinical trial. *Am J Sports Med* 2006;34(11):1730-1737.
5. Carreira DS, Mazzocca AD, Oryhon J, Brown FM, Hayden JK, Romeo AA: A prospective outcome evaluation of arthroscopic Bankart repairs: Minimum 2-year follow-up. *Am J Sports Med* 2006;34(5):771-777.
6. Owens BD, DeBerardino TM, Nelson BJ, et al: Long-term follow-up of acute arthroscopic Bankart repair for initial anterior shoulder dislocations in young athletes. *Am J Sports Med* 2009;37(4):669-673.
7. Robinson CM, Howes J, Murdoch H, Will E, Graham C: Functional outcome and risk of recurrent instability after primary traumatic anterior shoulder dislocation in young patients. *J Bone Joint Surg Am* 2006;88(11):2326-2336.
8. Boselli KJ, Cody EA, Bigliani LU: Open capsular shift: There still is a role! *Orthop Clin North Am* 2010;41(3):427-436.
9. Provencher MT, Ghodadra N, Romeo AA: Arthroscopic management of anterior instability: Pearls, pitfalls, and lessons learned. *Orthop Clin North Am* 2010;41(3):325-337.
10. Matsen FA III, Chebli C, Lippitt S; American Academy of Orthopaedic Surgeons: Principles for the evaluation and management of shoulder instability. *J Bone Joint Surg Am* 2006;88(3):648-659.
11. Boone JL, Arciero RA: Management of failed instability surgery: How to get it right the next time. *Orthop Clin North Am* 2010;41(3):367-379.
12. Kang RW, Frank RM, Nho SJ, et al: Complications associated with anterior shoulder instability repair. *Arthroscopy* 2009;25(8):909-920.

Chapter 3
Arthroscopic Superior Labrum Anterior-to-Posterior Repair

James C. Dreese, MD   Danielle Casagrande, MD

Introduction

Superior labrum anterior-to-posterior (SLAP) tears have become increasingly recognized with the improved diagnostic capability of arthroscopy and advanced imaging modalities. First described in a group of throwing athletes by Andrews et al[1] in 1985, SLAP tears were further classified by Snyder et al[2] in 1990. Common to all SLAP tears is detachment of the superior labrum, with or without involvement of the biceps anchor.

Classification

The original Snyder classification system remains the most widely recognized; it describes four types of SLAP lesions (**Figure 1**). Type I lesions involve fraying on the inner margin of the superior labrum and local degeneration. The superior labrum and biceps anchor remain attached and stable. These lesions are believed to result from age-related degenerative changes and are common in the middle-aged and elderly. Type I lesions are thought to be largely asymptomatic. The type II lesion is the most common type of SLAP tear requiring repair. Type II lesions are characterized by detachment of the superior labrum and biceps tendon anchor from the superior glenoid rim. Abnormal mobility of the superior labrum and biceps anchor is present, resulting in an unstable lesion. Numerous authors have described successful repair of type II SLAP lesions.[3-24] In 1998, Morgan et al[3] further classified type II SLAP tears into three subvariants. The anterior variant and posterior variant represent isolated anterior and posterior detachments, respectively, of the superior labrum and biceps complex; the posterior subtype is most common in throwing athletes. The anterior and posterior variant represents a combined detachment of the anterior and posterior labrum and biceps complex. Type III SLAP lesions demonstrate a buckle-handle tear of the superior labrum with an intact biceps anchor. When the mobile fragment is large, it may displace into the glenohumeral joint, resulting in mechanical symptoms and pain. Type IV SLAP lesions involve a bucket-handle tear with extension of the labral tear into the biceps tendon. Typically, a portion of the biceps attachment to the superior glenoid remains intact despite the unstable torn portion.

In 1995, Maffet et al[6] described three additional SLAP variants with injury patterns involving both the superior labrum–biceps anchor complex and labrum. A type V SLAP lesion describes a type II lesion with anterior extension involving the anteroinferior labrum. Type VI lesions are characterized by an unstable anterior or posterior flap of the superior labrum in conjunction with a type II lesion. Type VII lesions are type II lesions with a separation of the biceps attachment extending into the middle glenohumeral ligament, rendering it incompetent. Powell et al[7] described three additional SLAP variants: type VIII is a type II lesion with posterior labral extension, type IX is a type II lesion with a circumferential labral tear, and type X is a type II lesion with a posteroinferior labral tear.

Clinical Diagnosis

Clinical diagnosis of SLAP tears can be difficult. The superior labrum injury often occurs in conjunction with other shoulder pathology, such as an anterior/posterior labral tear and rotator cuff tears. The most common presenting symptom

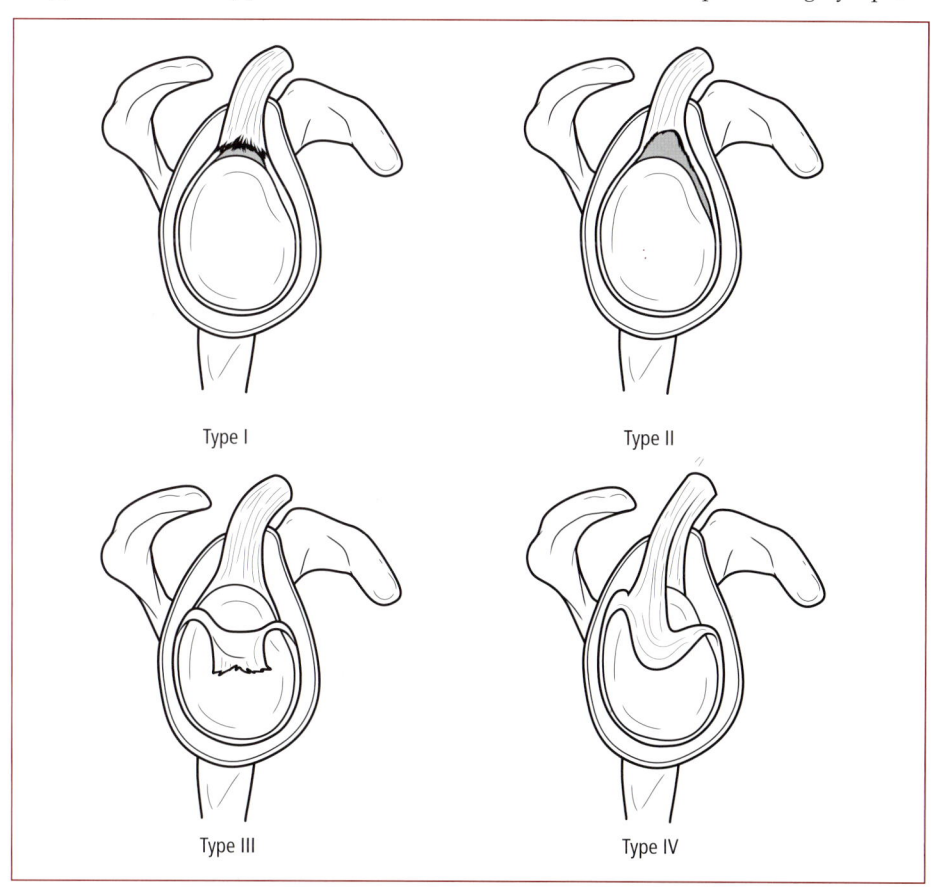

Figure 1 Illustration shows the Snyder classification of superior labrum anterior-to-posterior (SLAP) tears. Type I: Local degeneration and fraying on the inner margin of the superior labrum are seen. Type II: The superior labrum and biceps tendon anchor are detached from the superior glenoid rim. Type III: A bucket-handle tear of the superior labrum is present; the biceps anchor is intact. Type IV: The bucket-handle tear extends into the biceps tendon.

Dr. Dreese or an immediate family member is a member of a speakers' bureau or has made paid presentations on behalf of Cayenne Medical and serves as a paid consultant to or is an employee of Cayenne Medical. Neither Dr. Casagrande nor any immediate family member has received anything of value from or owns stock in a commercial company or institution related directly or indirectly to the subject of this chapter.

is pain, which may be described as sharp or aching and may be anterior or posterior in location. No single examination finding has been proven to be both highly sensitive and specific for SLAP tears.[8]

Suspicion of SLAP pathology is based on injury mechanism, physical examination, and radiographic evaluation. Nonsurgical treatment includes rest from aggravating activities, nonsteroidal anti-inflammatory drugs, posterior capsule stretching, and strengthening of the rotator cuff and scapular stabilizers. An intra-articular injection may give patients temporary pain relief and confirm the glenohumeral joint as the source of discomfort.

Patient Selection
Indications
Indications for surgical treatment are variable. In general, if a 3-month trial of nonsurgical measures fails to alleviate the patient's symptoms, consideration of arthroscopy is warranted. Arthroscopy remains the gold standard in the diagnosis and treatment of SLAP lesions. Arthroscopic identification of normal superior labrum–biceps complex variants is crucial to avoid unnecessary repair and potential resultant complications. In most instances, type I SLAP tears are considered a normal finding that does not require treatment. Type II lesions should be repaired when the physical examination is consistent and arthroscopy does not reveal another explanation for the patient's pain. Repair of type II SLAP tears has evolved in the past 20 years. Techniques involving the use of arthroscopic tacks, staples, and suture anchors have been described with varying success.[3-5,9] Careful evaluation of all pathologies should be considered in determining the etiology of the pain and the most effective treatment. Although outcomes following repair of type II SLAP tears with suture anchors in young, active patients generally have been good, repair of incidental degenerative SLAP tears in older patients with concomitant shoulder pathology such as rotator cuff tears should be avoided.[4] A randomized controlled trial in patients older than 50 years with both rotator cuff and labral pathology revealed better clinical results with combined rotator cuff repair and biceps tenotomy than with rotator cuff repair and SLAP repair.[10] Biceps tenodesis may be a more effective treatment than SLAP repair for type II tears in patients older than 40 years.[11] Pathologic findings with a stable biceps anchor (type III and some type IV lesions) often can be treated adequately with débridement of the unstable fragment alone. When resecting the unstable bucket-handle fragment, care must be taken to not destabilize the middle glenohumeral ligament. Type IV lesions may be treated with repair, biceps tenodesis, or biceps tenotomy. Young patients with minimal involvement of the biceps anchor are good candidates for débridement of the unstable fragment alone or direct suture anchor repair. As with type II tears, active patients with a partial-thickness tear of the biceps tendon greater than 25%, chronic atrophic changes of the tendon, subluxation of the tendon from the bicipital groove, or tendon atrophy such that the tendon is less than 75% its normal width may benefit from biceps tenodesis.[12] Low-demand patients with extensive partial-thickness tearing, evidence of subluxation, or both are candidates for biceps tenotomy. Type V through type X SLAP tears are a combination of superior labral injuries and disruption of the capsule and labrum. Treatment is directed at anatomic restoration of the labral and ligamentous attachments. As with type IV lesions, SLAP repair, biceps tenodesis, and biceps tenotomy may be appropriate depending on the patient's age and the arthroscopic findings.

Contraindications
Contraindications to the surgical management of SLAP lesions may be absolute or relative. Absolute contraindications include the presence of active infection and medical comorbidities—the risks of which outweigh the potential benefits of repair. The presence of a normal superior labral anatomic variant such as a sublabral foramen or Buford complex rather than a SLAP tear also is an absolute contraindication. Relative contraindications include older patients with concomitant findings that explain their disability, such as rotator cuff tears. Adhesive capsulitis should be managed nonsurgically initially, despite findings of a possible SLAP tear. Evidence of extensive tearing of the long head of the biceps, biceps subluxation, and extensive degenerative tearing of the long head of the biceps all are relative contraindications to SLAP repair and are better suited for tenodesis or tenotomy. Determination of the best treatment for each patient is made based on the preoperative symptoms, age of the patient, and surgical findings. Preoperative consultation with the patient regarding possible treatments is necessary to establish better understanding and expectations of treatment alternatives and expected outcomes.

Preoperative Imaging
Diagnostic imaging begins with standard shoulder radiographs: glenoid AP, acromioclavicular AP, scapular Y, and axillary views. Plain radiographs rule out other potential sources of shoulder pain such as degenerative arthritis of the glenohumeral and acromioclavicular joints.

MRI is the study of choice in evaluating SLAP pathology, rotator cuff injuries, and labral pathology. The presence of a paralabral cyst within the spinoglenoid notch is highly suggestive of a SLAP tear. Understanding normal anatomic variation in the superior labrum–biceps complex is critical to the identification of pathologic SLAP tears. An arthroscopic study of 546 patients revealed a 3.3% incidence of a sublabral foramen, an 8.6% incidence of a sublabral foramen with a cord-like middle glenohumeral ligament, and a 1.5% incidence of an absent anterosuperior labrum with a cord-like middle glenohumeral ligament (Buford complex).[13] Conventional MRI has been reported to be 84% to 98% sensitive and 63% to 91% specific in the detection of SLAP tears.[14,15]

Magnetic resonance arthrography (MRA) includes an intra-articular contrast injection in conjunction with MRI. If adequate distension of the joint is achieved, extravasation of contrast into or underneath the superior labrum–biceps complex is highly suggestive of SLAP pathology. Although debate exists about whether MRA or high-resolution MRI is more effective in diagnosing SLAP tears, MRA is undeniably more effective than low-resolution MRI in making the diagnosis. Both coronal and axial images are particularly helpful in making the diagnosis using multiplanar MRI. A distinction between normal superior labrum–biceps complex variants and findings of SLAP tears must be made.

Procedure
Surgical Considerations
Recent research has drawn attention to the technique of SLAP repair. Current techniques generally involve placement of one or more suture anchors into the glenoid to secure the superior labrum–biceps complex. In doing so, it is imperative that a proper angle of insertion be used to avoid injury to the articular cartilage, penetration through the glenoid

neck, or both. Morgan et al[3] reported the importance of portal placement in directing suture anchors into the glenoid at an angle of approximately 45°. Conventional arthroscopy most often uses one or two anterior cannulas within the rotator interval. Other authors have described using a small drill sleeve through the posterior portion of the rotator interval, just anterior to the supraspinatus, as an alternative when placing suture anchors posterior to the biceps anchor.[5,16,17] Several published studies have suggested that posterosuperior suture anchors placed via various portals during SLAP repair may penetrate through the glenoid rim and potentially endanger the suprascapular nerve.[18-20]

We recently investigated the risk of injury to the suprascapular nerve when using anterior versus anterolateral arthroscopic cannulas for suture anchor placement during SLAP repair (R Morgan, R Henn, J Dreese, unpublished data presented at the AAOS annual meeting, 2013). Ten matched cadaveric pairs were randomized to SLAP repair via anterior versus anterolateral portals. Suture anchors were placed in the 10-, 11-, and 1-o'clock positions in the right shoulder (2-, 1-, and 11-o'clock positions in the left shoulder). Following placement of the suture anchors, the suprascapular nerve was dissected and the glenoid rim was exposed to determine whether glenoid rim perforation occurred. All far posterior suture anchors (10 o'clock in the right shoulder; 2 o'clock in the left shoulder) perforated through the glenoid rim, whether placed through an anterior or anterolateral portal. Far posterior anchors placed through the anterolateral portal were, on average, located just 2 mm from the suprascapular nerve, whereas anchors placed through an anterior portal were on average 8 mm from the suprascapular nerve. Posterosuperior anchors (11 o'clock in the right shoulder; 1 o'clock in the left shoulder) showed an 80% rate of glenoid perforation when placed through an anterolateral portal and 60% when placed through a rotator interval portal.

A portal medial to the acromion and posterior to the distal clavicle directly above the glenoid has been described.[21] The resulting approach is oriented less than 45° from vertical, potentially damaging the articular cartilage of the superior glenoid. It has been suggested that placing posterosuperior suture anchors during SLAP repair is best achieved from a starting point along the posterolateral acromion. Morgan et al[3] described a trans–rotator cuff portal for placement of suture anchors into the posterosuperior glenoid during SLAP repair. The authors placed the portal 1 cm lateral and 1 cm anterior to the posterolateral corner of the acromion; this portal was named the port of Wilmington. Several authors have reported excellent results in repairing SLAP lesions via a trans–rotator cuff portal.[3,4,22] This technique provides an adequate angle of insertion into the glenoid, but it carries the risk of injury to the tendinous insertion of the rotator cuff. A recent study reported on a series of six patients who sustained tendinous detachment of the supraspinatus, infraspinatus, or both as a result of arthroscopic portal placement during SLAP repair via a trans–rotator cuff approach.[23] The authors concluded that a trans–rotator cuff portal should be placed percutaneously without the use of a cannula and medial to the musculotendinous junction with the assistance of spinal needle localization.

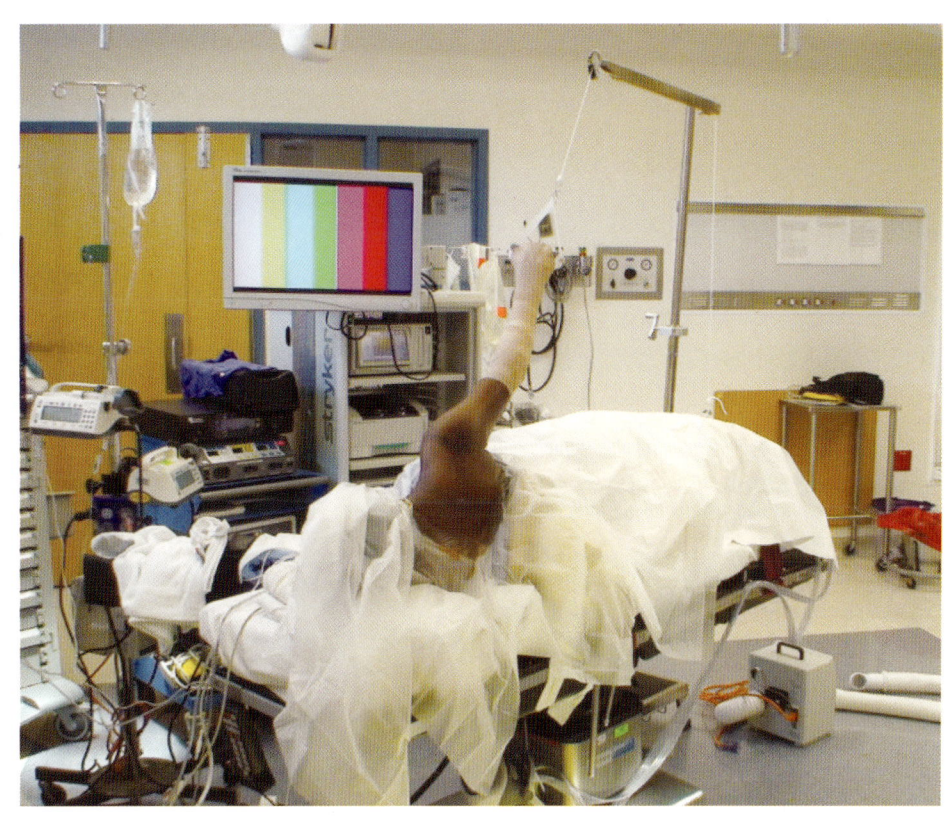

Figure 2 Photograph shows a patient in the lateral decubitus position.

Room Setup/Patient Positioning

Surgical treatment of SLAP tears can be performed under regional anesthesia with intravenous sedation and with the patient in the modified beach-chair or lateral decubitus position. Both positions provide adequate visualization and access to the superior labrum–biceps complex. An examination under anesthesia is performed to ensure full passive range of motion (ROM) and identify patterns of instability. Comparison with the contralateral shoulder must be made to distinguish laxity from pathologic instability. If the patient is positioned in the modified beach-chair position with the extremity prepared in sterile fashion and with the use of an arm holder. If the lateral decubitus position (**Figure 2**) is used, the patient lies on the contralateral side on a well-padded beanbag. Careful attention is paid to padding the contralateral knee to prevent peroneal nerve injury. The involved extremity is placed into a pulley system with 5 to 10 lb of traction, 30° to 45° of abduction, and 10° to 20° of forward elevation. Sterile draping must allow access to the sternum anteriorly and the medial border of the scapula posteriorly. The bony landmarks of the shoulder (acromion, clavicle, acromioclavicular joint, coracoid process) are demarcated with an indelible ink marker (**Figure 3**). In particular, careful attention is paid to correctly localize the coracoid process to avoid injury to the neurovascular structures.

Special Instruments/Equipment/Implants

Typically, arthroscopy is performed with a 30° arthroscope, but it also may be performed with a 70° arthroscope if the need

Section 1: Sports Medicine

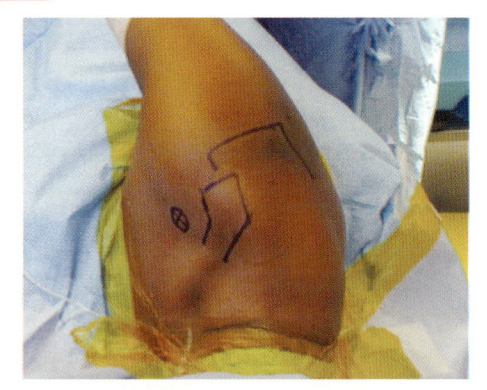

Figure 3 Photograph shows bony landmark demarcation on the right shoulder of a patient in the lateral decubitus position. The coracoid process is indicated with an encircled X.

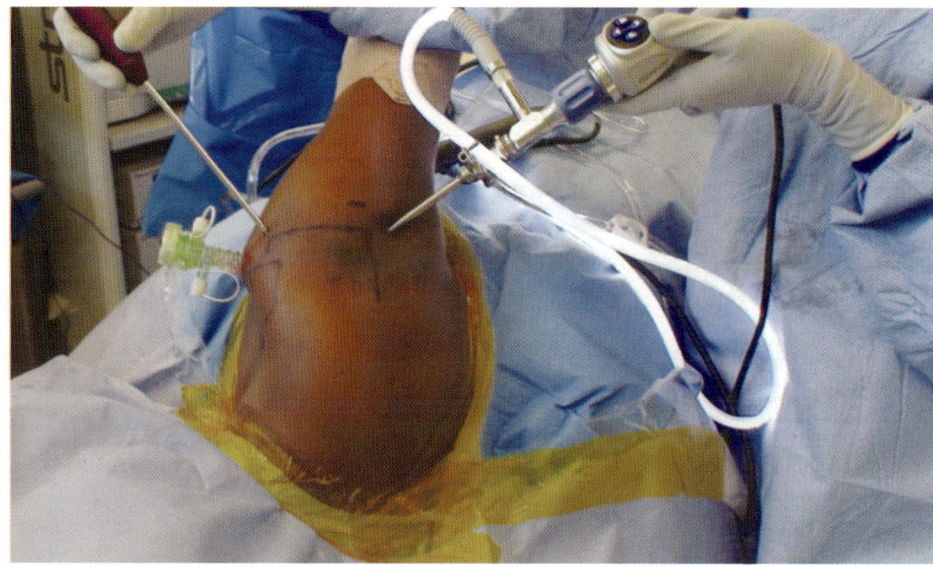

Figure 4 Photograph shows the placement of the drill sleeve through a rotator interval approach.

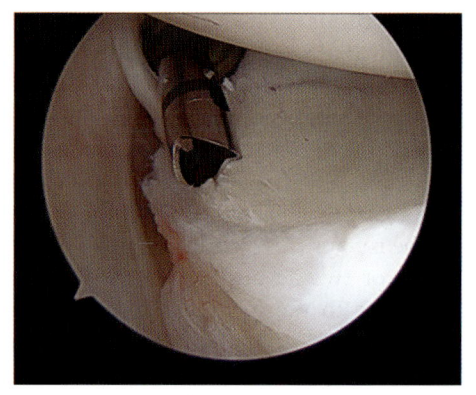

Figure 5 Arthroscopic view demonstrates the tangential approach to the posterosuperior glenoid when passing the drill sleeve through an anterosuperior portal. This has been shown to significantly increase the risk of glenoid rim perforation and may potentially place the suprascapular nerve at risk of injury.

arises. Repair typically uses one, two, or three 7-mm clear cannulas to allow transport of the arthroscopic instrumentation. Instruments may include a probe, an elevator and/or rasp, a shaver and/or burr, a drill, a cannulated drill sleeve, suture anchor(s), a suture-passing device, a looped suture grasper, a knot pusher, and a suture cutter.

Surgical Technique
Diagnostic Arthroscopy
Diagnostic arthroscopy is undertaken through a posterior viewing portal. With the patient in the beach-chair position, this portal is made just distal and medial to the posterolateral corner of the acromion. With the patient in the lateral decubitus position, this portal is made just distal and lateral to the posterolateral corner of the acromion. The appropriate placement can be determined by rotating the shoulder and palpating the soft spot of the glenohumeral joint.

A 7-mm clear cannula is established high in the rotator interval (**Figure 4**). This is safely localized with the assistance of a spinal needle, switching stick, and cannulated trocar. Careful attention is paid to placing the cannula lateral to the coracoid process to avoid neurovascular injury.

A comprehensive examination of the glenohumeral joint is undertaken. The articular surfaces of the humeral head and glenoid are inspected to rule out degenerative change, glenoid rim deficiency (bony Bankart injury), and impaction injuries to the humeral head (Hill-Sachs deformity). The superior labrum–biceps anchor is evaluated for injury. The superior labrum is probed for evidence of a SLAP tear, and the long head of the biceps (both the intra-articular and intertubercular segments) is evaluated for intrasubstance tearing or degeneration, dynamic versus fixed subluxation, synovitis, and injury to the biceps pulley. The subscapularis insertion on the lesser tuberosity is inspected closely for evidence of tearing, which has been reported widely in conjunction with biceps tendon tearing and instability. The rotator interval, particularly the middle and superior glenohumeral ligaments, is evaluated for injury. The anteroinferior and posteroinferior labrum, anterior and posterior bands of the inferior glenohumeral ligaments or capsule, and axillary pouch are inspected for evidence of injury. The articular side of the supraspinatus and infraspinatus is examined for injury. The anatomic findings are compared to normal anatomic variants such as the Buford complex and sublabral foramen.

Cannula Placement
If a confirmed SLAP lesion is identified, a second cannula may be established low in the rotator interval just above the subscapularis tendon to assist in suture management. This 5- or 7-mm clear cannula is placed over a cannulated trocar, similar to the first clear cannula. This cannula functions as a second working portal and facilitates suture management.

The type of SLAP tear is determined. Unstable superior labrum–biceps complex fragments are débrided with an oscillating shaver. For SLAP tears with an unstable superior labrum–biceps complex (type II and types V through X), the superior labrum is mobilized gently, and soft tissue is débrided from the glenoid rim with a shaver to create a bleeding surface and facilitate healing. As discussed previously, placement of suture anchors posterior to the long head of the biceps insertion through an anterosuperior portal or rotator interval portal may lead to a tangential approach to the glenoid, potentially causing penetration through the posterior glenoid rim and endangering the suprascapular nerve. **Figure 4** depicts the positioning of a rotator interval approach. **Figure 5** reveals the tangential approach to the posterosuperior glenoid through an anterosuperior portal.

Suture Anchor Placement
The port of Wilmington is localized with the assistance of a spinal needle (**Figure 6, A**). The posterolateral corner of the acromion is palpated. A spinal needle is passed from a point 1 cm anterior and

© 2013 American Academy of Orthopaedic Surgeons

Chapter 3: Arthroscopic Superior Labrum Anterior-to-Posterior Repair

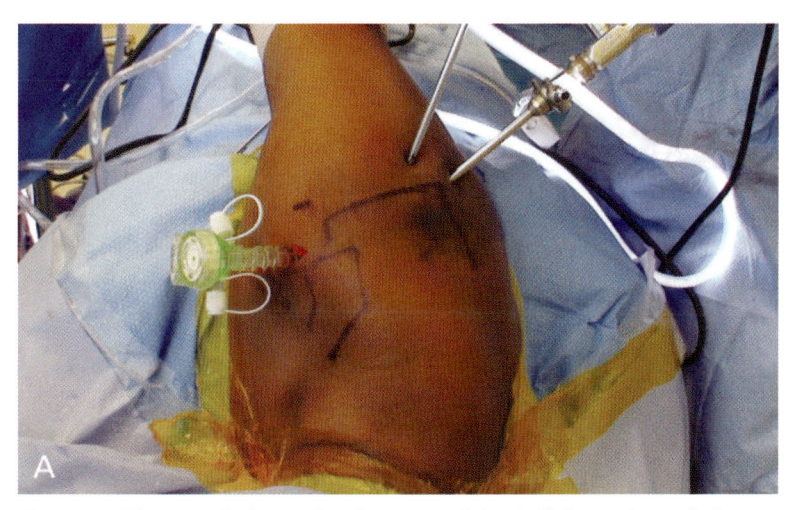

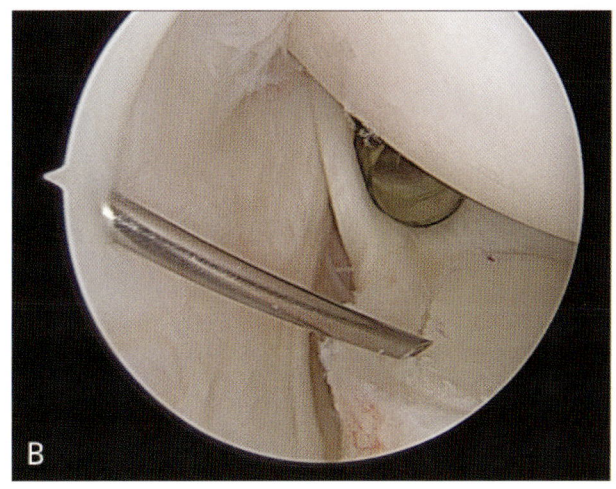

Figure 6 Photograph shows the placement of the drill sleeve through the port of Wilmington (**A**). Arthroscopic view shows the approach to the posterosuperior glenoid using spinal needle passage through the port of Wilmington (**B**).

lateral to this landmark, directed at the superior labrum–biceps anchor. The spinal needle is visualized to ensure passage medial to the tendinous insertion of the supraspinatus and infraspinatus tendons, as shown in **Figure 6, B**. The spinal needle is removed, and a 3-mm drill sleeve with a sharp trocar is placed through the musculotendinous junction of the rotator cuff.

One or two suture anchors are placed posterior to the biceps anchor through the port of Wilmington. The number of anchors depends on the posterior extension of the SLAP tear. When placement of multiple posterior suture anchors is necessary, the suture anchors are placed through a 3-mm drill sleeve with a single pass through the musculotendinous junction of the rotator cuff. Sutures are retrieved through the anteroinferior cannula when applicable; alternatively, they may be retrieved through a single anterosuperior portal. The anterosuperior cannula is advanced over the superior labrum–biceps complex. A suture passer is advanced through the anterosuperior portal and passed through the superior labrum at the far posterior position. The suture passer and the superior most suture in the far posterior suture anchor are grasped through the anteroinferior cannula. The suture is advanced through the suture passer, and the two free limbs are advanced out the anterosuperior cannula as the suture passer is withdrawn. The inferior suture from the far posterior suture anchor is retrieved through the anterosuperior cannula. The anterosuperior cannula is advanced to the base of the superior labrum–biceps anchor to prevent excessive tension and displacement during the arthroscopic knot-tying. We use a sliding, locking knot configuration with two alternating half hitches, followed by switching of the post and then tying a third half hitch. The anterosuperior cannula is maintained at the base along the superior base of the superior labrum–biceps anchor. The suture passer is advanced through the anterosuperior cannula through the superior labrum along the posterior border of the long head of the biceps. The suture passer and the superior suture of the posterosuperior suture anchor are retrieved through the anteroinferior cannula. The free end of the suture is advanced through the suture passer, and the suture passer is advanced through the anterosuperior cannula. The inferior suture of the posterosuperior suture anchor is retrieved through the anterosuperior cannula. Standard knot-tying technique is used to secure the posterosuperior anchor along the posterior border of the superior labrum–biceps complex.

After the suture anchor(s) posterior to the biceps anchor have been placed and secured, an anterosuperior suture anchor is placed just anterior to the biceps anchor. This anchor is placed at the 1-o'clock position in the right shoulder; in most patients, this anchor may be placed safely through an anterosuperior or rotator interval portal. Arthroscopic evaluation of the approach to the glenoid afforded by each portal is critical in the safe placement of suture anchors. The sutures are shuttled out the inferior portal in the rotator interval. A suture passer is used to shuttle the more superior suture in the anterosuperior anchor behind the superior labrum at the 1-o'clock position. Care is taken to not overconstrain the middle and superior glenohumeral ligaments. Standard knot-tying technique is used to secure the knot at the repair site.

Repair of concomitant anterior and posterior labral tears is performed. Our preference is to first perform anterior labral repair/capsulorrhaphy, when indicated, followed by superior labrum–biceps complex repair and then posterior labral repair/capsulorrhaphy. The rationale for this order is that, particularly with the patient in the lateral decubitus position, visualization and exposure of the anteroinferior glenoid and labrum are more difficult following a posterior labral repair/capsulorrhaphy, but the posterior labrum is accessed easily following anterior and superior labral repair. **Figure 7** summarizes the stepwise arthroscopic technique for suture anchor repair of a type II SLAP tear.

Alternative Repair Techniques and Considerations

Multiple alternatives to the technique described previously have been described. Bioabsorbable tacks are no longer used because of the frequency of associated synovitis, implant failure, and recurrent instability.[24,25] Knotless anchors may be used in place of standard suture anchors. Although knotless anchors may offer technical advantages, research suggests they may be more prone to early gap formation at the repair site. Biomechanical cadaver studies have shown higher comparative load–to–2-mm gapping in the knotless constructs, but similar overall load to failure in both constructs.[26,27] The clinical effect of this difference in vivo is not yet well established.

Controversy exists regarding the optimal suture configuration and orientation of suture anchors in repairing the

© 2013 American Academy of Orthopaedic Surgeons

Section 1: Sports Medicine

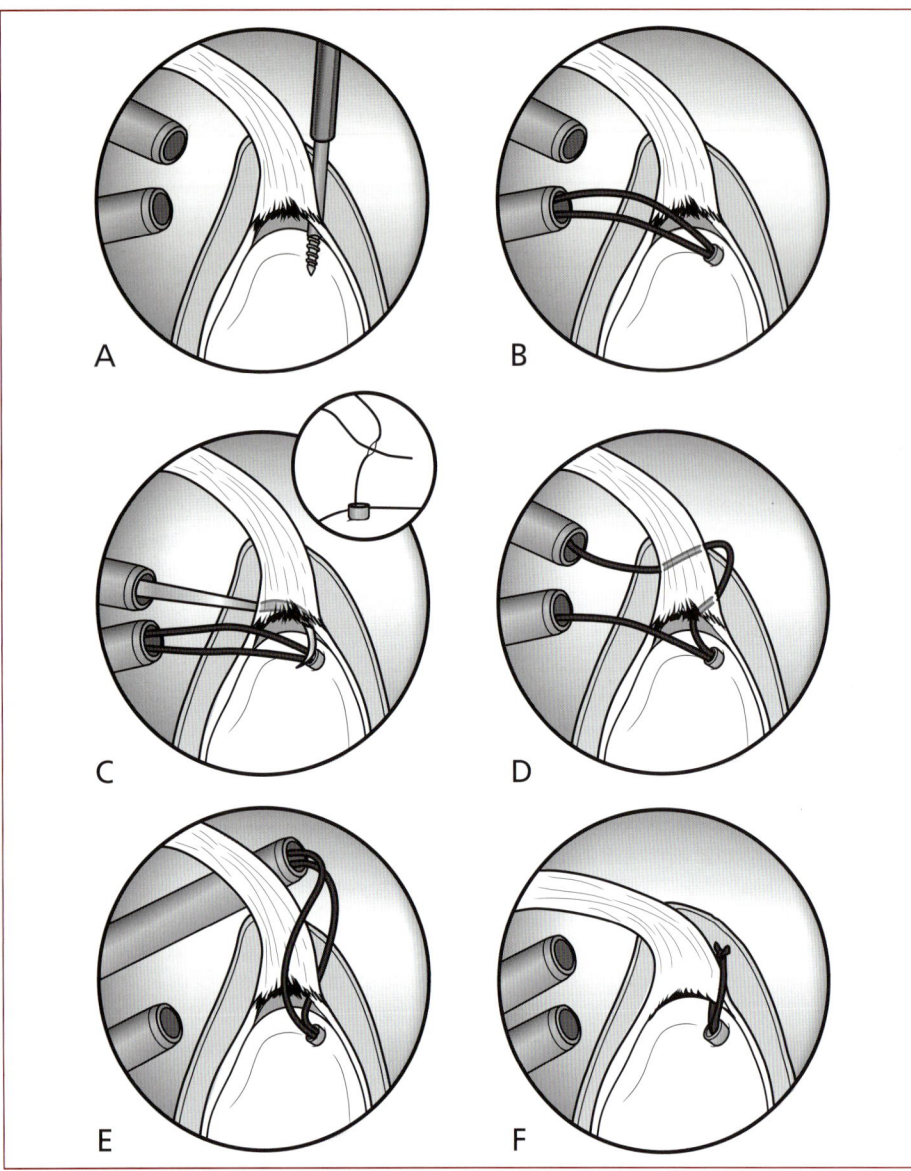

Figure 7 Illustrations demonstrate the arthroscopic suture anchor technique for the repair of type II SLAP tears. **A,** Suture anchor insertion is directed at a 45° angle to the glenoid rim to limit the risk of articular cartilage injury. **B,** The suture limbs are retrieved through the anteroinferior portal. **C,** A wire suture passer then is passed under the torn superior labrum and retrieved through the anteroinferior portal. **D,** The medial suture limb of the suture anchor is fed through the wire suture loop. The suture loop is advanced under the superior labrum and retrieved through the anterosuperior cannula. **E,** A standard arthroscopic knot-tying technique is used to secure the repair. **F,** The completed SLAP repair.

superior labrum. Suture configurations include a simple suture technique (only one suture passed through the labrum) and horizontal mattress construct (both sutures passed through the labrum). Although one biomechanical study showed a potential load-to-failure advantage with the horizontal mattress configuration around the biceps anchor,[28] another showed a simple suture construct to be more secure.[29] Debate also exists regarding the need for a suture anchor anterior to the biceps anchor. Variable biomechanical results have been published regarding the optimal orientation of suture anchors, with one study concluding that placement of a suture anchor anterior to the biceps anchor does not improve biomechanical properties.[30]

Complications

Complications from SLAP repair surgery can result from poor management preoperatively, intraoperatively, or postoperatively, or a combination of all three. Preoperatively, it is important to correlate the patient's signs and symptoms with the recognized pathology. Although tests for SLAP tears all have high sensitivity, the specificity of the same tests lags far behind in most studies. As a result, the rate of false-positives is quite high. Typical clinically symptomatic SLAP lesions occur in individuals younger than 40 years who are active or have sustained a traumatic injury. Repetitive throwing athletes may not recall a traumatic event. Patients older than 40 years may have degenerative changes of the superior labrum that may be mistaken for a symptomatic SLAP tear. Painful lesions of the superior labrum also may occur and require treatment for resolution of symptoms. The misguided repair of a degenerative superior labrum leads to persistence of the unaddressed pathology (eg, rotator cuff tear, degenerative arthritis) and increased risk of postoperative adhesive capsulitis. Awareness of the patient's age, mechanism of injury, and anatomic findings are thus important in surgical decision making.

Intraoperative complications may result from an error in technique or an error in judgment. Appropriate access to the glenoid for the placement of suture anchors depends on accurate cannula placement. Access to the superior glenoid requires a high portal placement to allow a descending course for the arthroscopic drill and suture anchor. Otherwise, the drill and suture anchor may not be contained within the superior glenoid, placing the suprascapular nerve at risk and potentially compromising the biomechanical integrity of the anchor. A suture anchor placed anterior to the biceps anchor may risk overconstraining the middle and superior glenohumeral ligaments, leading to an increased risk of adhesive capsulitis and loss of external rotation with the arm at the side. Creation of a large defect through the musculotendinous junction of the rotator cuff, which may occur during placement of a large cannula, may be a source of persistent shoulder pain. Neurovascular injury may result from cannula placement medial to the coracoid process.

Errors in judgment can take several forms. A normal superior labrum variant can be easily mistaken for a SLAP tear. A meniscoid labrum must be distinguished from a SLAP tear by the lack of tearing and inflammatory tissue underneath the superior labrum and the presence of articular cartilage underneath the loose labrum. Care must be taken to recognize other normal anatomic variants to avoid repairing a sublabral foramen or misinterpreting a cord-like middle glenohumeral ligament (Buford complex). Errors in judgment also may involve selecting a treatment with a high likelihood of failure. Repair of a badly degenerated or torn superior labrum or an unstable long head

Table 1 Range-of-Motion Goals Following SLAP Repair

Weeks	Forward Flexion	External Rotation
0-2	90°	10°
2-4	120°	30°
4-6	140°	45°
6-8	160°	60°
8-10	Full[a]	Full[a]

[a]Preferably within 5° of the contralateral side.
SLAP = superior labrum anterior-to-posterior.

of the biceps or repair in patients older than 40 years has been shown to have a high rate of failure. Better results with biceps tenodesis or tenotomy versus labral repair have been shown in these patient populations.[11] Subpectoral biceps tenodesis has been shown to be highly effective and avoids the risk of persistent discomfort sometimes seen in a more proximal bicipital groove tenodesis.[31]

Potential postoperative shoulder complications include shoulder stiffness, infection, and persistent pain. Patients must be cautioned not to remain in a sling too long, and the importance of early ROM should be emphasized.

Postoperative Care and Rehabilitation

Stage 1 (0 to 4 Weeks)

Patients younger than 25 years begin physical therapy at 1 week postoperatively. Those older than 25 years start physical therapy within 3 to 4 days postoperatively. Patients typically visit physical therapy 2 or 3 times per week.

The patient is placed in a shoulder sling in the operating room. The sling may be removed for dressing and hygiene but should be worn for 3 to 4 weeks. If the patient is having trouble regaining ROM or notably stiff at the 1-week postoperative visit, the sling may be removed earlier at the surgeon's discretion. A home program including wand exercises and an overhead pulley is instituted when range of motion does not progress per protocol.

The sling may be removed for tabletop activities within pain tolerance, such as eating, tooth brushing, writing, and occasional keyboard use. The sling also may be removed for exercises, showering, and dressing.

Exercises include elbow ROM, squeezing a tennis ball for grip, cocontraction of the biceps/triceps at 0°, 30°, 60°, 90°, and 120°, pendulum exercises, passive ROM from 0° to 120° of forward elevation in the scapular plane, and external rotation to 30° with the arm at the side.

Stage 2 (4 to 12 Weeks)

Patients have 1 or 2 physical therapy visits per week. The frequency may be increased if ROM is lagging behind.

Range of Motion

ROM goals are outlined in **Table 1**. The patient goes through active and passive ROM for all shoulder motions, limiting external rotation to 45° until 4 to 6 weeks postoperatively. Full external rotation is allowed by 10 to 12 weeks.

Pearls

- MRA should be considered for the evaluation of a shoulder when a strong suspicion for a SLAP lesion exists.
- The surgeon should look for pathologies other than SLAP lesions in patients older than 40 years, particularly in patients with no history of traumatic injury.
- Degenerative SLAP tears in patients older than 40 years are good candidates for biceps tenodesis or tenolysis rather than SLAP repair.
- Controversy exists regarding the role of superior labral repair in conjunction with biceps tenodesis or tenolysis in patients with unstable superior labral lesions in the setting of degenerative SLAP tears.
- Types I, III, and IV SLAP lesions have a stable biceps anchor and often can be treated nonsurgically or with simple débridement of the torn biceps tendon.
- Type II and types V through X SLAP tears are unstable lesions that benefit from restoration of the labral attachment.
- In type IV lesions, when less than 30% of the biceps tendon is involved, débridement of the labral tear and its extension into the biceps is warranted. When more than 30% of the biceps tendon is involved, the treatment typically is biceps tenodesis and labral repair in younger patients or labral débridement and biceps tenotomy versus tenodesis in older patients.
- The surgeon should not repair normal anatomic variants such as a sublabral foramen, a meniscoid labrum, or a Buford complex.
- Placement of arthroscopic cannulas through the rotator cuff should be avoided. If a trans–rotator cuff portal is used, precise placement of a 3-mm drill sleeve with a sharp trocar through the musculotendinous junction can be used to limit the risk of injury to the tendinous insertion which may result in disability. Localization of the approach with a spinal needle facilitates efficient placement of the drill sleeve and limits traumatic injury to the rotator cuff musculature.
- Postoperatively, early ROM may help limit the risk of adhesive capsulitis.

References

1. Andrews JR, Carson WG Jr, McLeod WD: Glenoid labrum tears related to the long head of the biceps. *Am J Sports Med* 1985;13(5):337-341.
2. Snyder SJ, Karzel RP, Del Pizzo W, Ferkel RD, Friedman MJ: SLAP lesions of the shoulder. *Arthroscopy* 1990;6(4):274-279.
3. Morgan CD, Burkhart SS, Palmeri M, Gillespie M: Type II SLAP lesions: Three subtypes and their relationships to superior instability and rotator cuff tears. *Arthroscopy* 1998;14(6):553-565.
4. Ide J, Maeda S, Takagi K: Sports activity after arthroscopic superior labral repair using suture anchors in overhead-throwing athletes. *Am J Sports Med* 2005;33(4):507-514.
5. Cohen DB, Coleman S, Drakos MC, et al: Outcomes of isolated type II SLAP lesions treated with arthroscopic fixation using a bioabsorbable tack. *Arthroscopy* 2006;22(2):136-142.
6. Maffet MW, Gartsman GM, Moseley B: Superior labrum-biceps tendon complex lesions of the shoulder. *Am J Sports Med* 1995;23(1):93-98.
7. Powell SE, Nord KD, Ryu RK: The diagnosis, classification, and treatment of SLAP lesions. *Oper Tech Sports Med* 2004;12:99-110.
8. Parentis MA, Glousman RE, Mohr KS, Yocum LA: An evaluation of the provocative tests for superior labral anterior posterior lesions. *Am J Sports Med* 2006;34(2):265-268.

9. Rhee YG, Lee DH, Lim CT: Unstable isolated SLAP lesion: Clinical presentation and outcome of arthroscopic fixation. *Arthroscopy* 2005;21(9):1099.

10. Franceschi F, Longo UG, Ruzzini L, Rizzello G, Maffulli N, Denaro V: No advantages in repairing a type II superior labrum anterior and posterior (SLAP) lesion when associated with rotator cuff repair in patients over age 50: A randomized controlled trial. *Am J Sports Med* 2008;36(2):247-253.

11. Boileau P, Parratte S, Chuinard C, Roussanne Y, Shia D, Bicknell R: Arthroscopic treatment of isolated type II SLAP lesions: Biceps tenodesis as an alternative to reinsertion. *Am J Sports Med* 2009;37(5):929-936.

12. Sethi N, Wright R, Yamaguchi K: Disorders of the long head of the biceps tendon. *J Shoulder Elbow Surg* 1999;8(6):644-654.

13. Rao AG, Kim TK, Chronopoulos E, McFarland EG: Anatomical variants in the anterosuperior aspect of the glenoid labrum: A statistical analysis of seventy-three cases. *J Bone Joint Surg Am* 2003;85(4):653-659.

14. Connell DA, Potter HG, Wickiewicz TL, Altchek DW, Warren RF: Noncontrast magnetic resonance imaging of superior labral lesions: 102 cases confirmed at arthroscopic surgery. *Am J Sports Med* 1999;27(2):208-213.

15. Tung GA, Entzian D, Green A, Brody JM: High-field and low-field MR imaging of superior glenoid labral tears and associated tendon injuries. *AJR Am J Roentgenol* 2000;174(4):1107-1114.

16. Gartsman GM, Hammerman SM: Superior labrum, anterior and posterior lesions: When and how to treat them. *Clin Sports Med* 2000;19(1):115-124.

17. Samani JE, Marston SB, Buss DD: Arthroscopic stabilization of type II SLAP lesions using an absorbable tack. *Arthroscopy* 2001;17(1):19-24.

18. Koh KH, Park WH, Lim TK, Yoo JC: Medial perforation of the glenoid neck following SLAP repair places the suprascapular nerve at risk: A cadaveric study. *J Shoulder Elbow Surg* 2011;20(2):245-250.

19. Yoo JC, Lee YS, Ahn JH, Park JH, Kang HJ, Koh KH: Isolated suprascapular nerve injury below the spinoglenoid notch after SLAP repair. *J Shoulder Elbow Surg* 2009;18(4):e27-e29.

20. Gumina S, Albino P, Giaracuni M, Vestri A, Ripani M, Postacchini F: The safe zone for avoiding suprascapular nerve injury during shoulder arthroscopy: An anatomical study on 500 dry scapulae. *J Shoulder Elbow Surg* 2011;20(8):1317-1322.

21. Yamaguchi K, Bindra R: Disorders of the biceps tendon, in Iannotti JP, Williams GR Jr, eds: *Disorders of the Shoulder.* Philadelphia, PA, Lippincott Williams & Williams, 1999, pp 187-188.

22. O'Brien SJ, Allen AA, Coleman SH, Drakos MC: The trans-rotator cuff approach to SLAP lesions: Technical aspects for repair and a clinical follow-up of 31 patients at a minimum of 2 years. *Arthroscopy* 2002;18(4):372-377.

23. Stephenson DR, Hurt JH, Mair SD: Rotator cuff injury as a complication of portal placement for superior labrum anterior-posterior repair. *J Shoulder Elbow Surg* 2012;21(10):1316-1321.

24. Sassmannshausen G, Sukay M, Mair SD: Broken or dislodged poly-L-lactic acid bioabsorbable tacks in patients after SLAP lesion surgery. *Arthroscopy* 2006;22(6):615-619.

25. Freehill MQ, Harms DJ, Huber SM, Atlihan D, Buss DD: Poly-L-lactic acid tack synovitis after arthroscopic stabilization of the shoulder. *Am J Sports Med* 2003;31(5):643-647.

26. Nho SJ, Frank RM, Van Thiel GS, et al: A biomechanical analysis of anterior Bankart repair using suture anchors. *Am J Sports Med* 2010;38(7):1405-1412.

27. Sileo MJ, Lee SJ, Kremenic IJ, et al: Biomechanical comparison of a knotless suture anchor with standard suture anchor in the repair of type II SLAP tears. *Arthroscopy* 2009;25(4):348-354.

28. Domb BG, Ehteshami JR, Shindle MK, et al: Biomechanical comparison of 3 suture anchor configurations for repair of type II SLAP lesions. *Arthroscopy* 2007;23(2):135-140.

29. Yoo JC, Ahn JH, Lee SH, et al: A biomechanical comparison of repair techniques in posterior type II superior labral anterior and posterior (SLAP) lesions. *J Shoulder Elbow Surg* 2008;17(1):144-149.

30. Morgan RJ, Kuremsky MA, Peindl RD, Fleischli JE: A biomechanical comparison of two suture anchor configurations for the repair of type II SLAP lesions subjected to a peel-back mechanism of failure. *Arthroscopy* 2008;24(4):383-388.

31. Mazzocca AD, Cote MP, Arciero CL, Romeo AA, Arciero RA: Clinical outcomes after subpectoral biceps tenodesis with an interference screw. *Am J Sports Med* 2008;36(10):1922-1929

Chapter 4
Biceps Tenotomy and Tenodesis

Peter Chalmers, MD   Seth L. Sherman, MD   Neil Ghodadra, MD
Richard C. Mather III, MD   Anthony A. Romeo, MD

Patient Selection

The long head of the biceps tendon (LHBT) runs a unique anatomic course through the anterior shoulder, ascending proximally through the intertubercular groove before turning 30° medially and posteriorly, where a "pulley" composed of the coracohumeral ligament, the superior glenohumeral ligament, the supraspinatus tendon, and the subscapularis tendon supports the LHBT.[1] The LHBT then travels intra-articularly but extrasynovially through the glenohumeral joint and inserts onto the supraglenoid tubercle and/or superior labrum.[2] LHBT pathology can occur at several locations through its anatomic course: in the intertubercular groove, within the glenohumeral joint, and at its attachment site. Depending on the location, the etiology of this tendinopathy may be osteophytes within the intertubercular groove, microtrauma from repetitive overhead activities, acromial morphology, internal impingement, ischemia, tendon instability, or trauma.[3] Tendinitis and tendinosis commonly occur in association with subacromial impingement, rotator cuff pathology, tears of the anterior capsuloligamentous complex, labral tears, glenohumeral instability, and acromioclavicular arthrosis.[2] Acutely, the tendon may be swollen and hemorrhagic, but with chronic friction and traction the tendon can become thinned, frayed, and atrophied, which can lead to tendon rupture, commonly with subsequent pain relief.[4] The functional consequences of this rupture are unclear. The importance of the LHBT in shoulder function has been debated in the literature, with some authors arguing that contraction of the LHBT plays no role in shoulder motion[5] or stability and others arguing that the LHBT acts as an important humeral head depressor.[2]

The LHBT is among the primary pain-generating structures of the anterior shoulder. Because LHBT tendinosis rarely occurs in isolation, however, determining whether a patient's pain is due in part to LHBT pathology can be challenging.[3] The history should elicit a full description of the location of the pain, the shoulder positions and movements that exacerbate this pain (typically overhand or underhand throwing, lifting, or extending the arm), and the patient's occupation and sporting activities. Patients may or may not give a history of a specific traumatic event. Classically, LHBT pain begins in the anterior shoulder and radiates distally into the biceps muscle belly. Snapping, grinding, or popping symptoms may be described. Physical examination should include a standard shoulder evaluation, including inspection, palpation, and range of motion; a complete neurovascular examination; and a battery of provocative maneuvers to test for subacromial impingement, rotator cuff tears, instability, and acromioclavicular pathology.

Indications

The indications for biceps tenotomy and tenodesis are similar. They include lesions involving more than 25% to 50% of the tendon; type II or IV superior labral anterior-to-position (SLAP) tears in older, less active patients;[6] bicipital tendon instability; failed SLAP repairs; and anterior shoulder pain that is attributable to LHBT pathology and is unresponsive to nonsurgical management.[2,7] Once LHBT pathology has been identified, nonsurgical management should be attempted. Initial nonsurgical treatment includes rest, ice, oral anti-inflammatory medications, range-of-motion exercises, stretching, physical therapy, iontophoresis, phonophoresis, and glenohumeral or subacromial corticosteroid injections. In addition, the LHBT sheath can be selectively injected, although injection into the substance of the tendon should be avoided. The effect of LHBT sheath injection upon the risk of subsequent rupture is unknown, and patients should be counseled regarding this potential risk before injection. Failed tenodesis may indicate for tenotomy and vice versa.[7]

Contraindications

Few contraindications to arthroscopic biceps tenodesis exist. One relative contraindication is pseudoparalysis of the shoulder.[6]

Preoperative Imaging

Imaging is used along with the patient's history and physical examination to support the diagnosis of LHBT pathology. Radiographs obtained to evaluate for LHBT pathology should include AP, lateral, and axillary views of the shoulder, as well as a scapular outlet view to examine acromial pathology. The intertubercular groove can be visualized in profile by placing the cassette at the apex of the externally rotated shoulder with the x-ray beam collinear with the humeral shaft.

Traditionally, arthrography also was used to diagnose LHBT pathology. Ultrasonography also has been used and is sensitive and specific, but the technician-dependent nature of the results limits widespread application.[2] MRI has largely supplanted these methods. Findings associated with LHBT pathology include ovalization of the tendon (which is normally kidney bean–shaped), increased intrasubstance signal intensity on T2-weighted images, and tendon dislocation from the intertubercular groove.[2] Magnetic resonance arthrography further increases the sensitivity and specificity

---

Dr. Mather or an immediate family member serves as an unpaid consultant to Pivot Medical and has received research or institutional support from Forest Pharmaceuticals. Dr. Romeo or an immediate family member has received royalties from Arthrex; is a member of a speakers' bureau or has made paid presentations on behalf of Arthrex, DJ Orthopaedics, and the Joint Restoration Foundation; serves as a paid consultant to or is an employee of Arthrex; has received research or institutional support from Arthrex and DJ Orthopaedics; has received nonincome support (such as equipment or services), commercially derived honoraria, or other non–research-related funding (such as paid travel) from Arthrex and DJ Orthopaedics; and serves as a board member, owner, officer, or committee member of the American Orthopaedic Society for Sports Medicine, the American Shoulder and Elbow Surgeons, and the Arthroscopy Association of North America. None of the following authors or any immediate family member has received anything of value from or owns stock in a commercial company or institution related directly or indirectly to the subject of this chapter: Dr. Chalmers, Dr. Sherman, and Dr. Ghodadra.

of this modality for evaluation of LHBT pathology.[2] In addition, it offers excellent delineation of associated shoulder injuries.

The gold standard diagnostic test is shoulder arthroscopy. Any patient undergoing shoulder arthroscopy should undergo a full evaluation of the biceps tendon. LHBT pathology is commonly discovered incidentally during glenohumeral arthroscopies performed for other indications, and the surgeon should be prepared to intervene if indicated.[8]

Procedure
Surgical Decision Making
Debate exists within the literature about whether tenotomy or tenodesis provides better outcomes.[9,10] Among proponents of tenodesis, additional debate exists regarding whether proximal or subpectoral tenodesis is preferable,[2,3,7,11-15] whether to perform osseous or soft-tissue tenodesis,[2,3,12,13,15] and which method of fixation to use.[2,3,12-15] The most appropriate procedure, approach, and fixation method likely depends on the individual patient.[2,3,7,11-15]

Both tenotomy and tenodesis have been used with success.[9] Tenotomy is simpler to perform, but it is associated with several potential complications of unclear clinical significance. First, clinical examiners commonly note a postoperative "Popeye" deformity in up to 70% of patients; however, several series have noted that patients were unbothered by the changed cosmetic appearance of their arm.[6,9] Older patients and patients with arms with excess adipose tissue are less likely to be bothered by this deformity. Secondly, because the LHBT acts as an elbow flexor and supinator, weakness could ensue from tenotomy. In one series of 54 patients who underwent unilateral LHBT tenotomy, the maximum number of elbow flexion repetitions with a 10-lb weight was 32.3 and 34.2 repetitions in operated and nonoperated arms, respectively.[10] A difference of this magnitude is likely to be clinically significant only for younger, more active patients. Finally, tenotomy destroys the anatomic length-tension relationship of the muscle; thus, unopposed biceps contraction could result in muscle cramping and atrophy. In a recent systematic review, Frost et al[9] were unable to find any discernable clinical difference between the procedures and recommended tenotomy for reasons of ease, speed, thrift, and simplicity of postoperative management. Because tenodesis avoids potential complications, it may be preferable for active or young (<50 years) patients. Conversely, tenotomy may be preferable in older patients, less active patients, and patients unwilling or unable to participate in postoperative therapy or adhere to postoperative restrictions.[10]

One alternate procedure that has been described for isolated LHBT instability is repair of the surrounding soft tissues that form a pulley for the tendon—specifically the subscapularis tendon, the supraspinatus tendon, the coracohumeral ligament, and the superior glenohumeral ligament. Although repair is theoretically superior because it allows LHBT preservation, outcomes have been disappointing. Repairs have led to LHBT rupture in 25% of cases, with 33% of the tendons not ruptured exhibiting a positive Speed test.[1] In addition to the risk of rupture and an inability to address the pathology in question, these repairs risk overtightening the structures of the rotator interval and causing a loss of external rotation. We therefore prefer to perform tenotomy or tenodesis.

Several methods of tenodesis have been described. Tenodesis can be performed at the proximal end of the intertubercular groove through an arthroscopic approach[15] or under the inferior edge of the pectoralis major insertion through an open approach.[13] Although the arthroscopic approach prevents the need for an additional incision, it leaves several centimeters of LHBT within the intertubercular groove. This residual tendon can continue to produce anterior shoulder pain or may subsequently rupture because of osteophytes impinging upon the tendon in the groove. Also, the arthroscopic approach is more technically challenging and obscures re-creation of the length-tension relationship of the tendon. In addition, the bulk of the tenodesis at the proximal end of the intertubercular groove could contribute to subacromial impingement postoperatively. Furthermore, proximal tenodesis places the repair within the inflamed zone. In recent series of 188 tenodeses, a significantly higher failure rate was reported for the proximal (12%) over the distal (2.7%) procedure.[11] We therefore prefer the subpectoral approach, although both approaches are reasonable, and some patients may prefer to avoid the additional axillary incision of a subpectoral tenodesis.

Soft-tissue tenodesis and tenodesis to bone have both been described. Soft-tissue tenodesis places shear stress on the structures sutured to the tendon, which can include the coracohumeral ligament, the superior glenohumeral ligament, and the supraspinatus and subscapularis tendons. This technique also may predispose to scar tissue and adhesion formation within the subacromial and subpectoral spaces, may increase the severity of subacromial impingement by increasing superior muscular pull on the humerus, allows recurrent subluxation within the groove, and may not reconstruct the anatomy of the LHBT. Osseous tenodesis may be performed using a bone tunnel, a keyhole, a suture anchor, or an interference screw.[13] Biomechanical studies have demonstrated interference screw fixation to have the least displacement after cycling and the highest ultimate load to failure.[12] This method also provides the smoothest tendon-bone transition and intramedullary placement of the tendon to aid healing. We therefore prefer osseous subpectoral tenodesis with interference screw fixation. Both subpectoral and proximal osseous tenodesis techniques are described here.

Room Setup/Patient Positioning
LHBT tenodesis should commence with a standard diagnostic glenohumeral arthroscopy, which begins with administration of a scalene block and standard preoperative intravenous antibiotics. Because it provides easy access to the axilla for subpectoral tenodesis, the beach-chair position is preferable to the lateral decubitus position. An articulated arm holder is attached to the operating table and covered with a sterile drape to facilitate joint positioning.

Surgical Technique
The acromion, distal clavicle, and coracoid are marked. The joint is entered posteriorly with an 18-gauge spinal needle 2 cm medial and inferior to the posterolateral corner of the acromion, aiming toward the coracoid. A stab wound is made and a blunt obturator is introduced into the joint, aiming toward the labral attachment of the long head of the biceps. The arthroscope is then introduced. The LHBT should first be examined with no fluid pressure, or "dry." Pressurization of the arthroscopic fluid can compress the LHBT peritendinous vessels, obscuring the "lipstick" lesion.[13] An anteromedial portal is then introduced using the outside-in technique, inserting a spinal needle lateral to the tip of the coracoid. Once the needle is visualized, a stab wound is made in the

skin and a 7-mm smooth cannula is introduced into the joint.

A probe is inserted through the anterior cannula. The LHBT is pulled into the joint to examine the portion of the tendon that normally lies within the intertubercular groove, which is commonly inflamed or otherwise abnormal.[13] This also allows the surgeon to assess the mobility of the tendon. The tendon should be displaced medially and laterally to assess for instability and occult coracohumeral and superior glenohumeral ligament injuries. The peel-back test should be performed, in which the humerus is abducted and externally rotated while the LHBT insertion is observed for SLAP tears. The active compression test should also be performed, in which the arm is placed in 90° of flexion, full elbow extension, and 15° of internal rotation. If the biceps anchor and tendon move medial and inferior and become entrapped with these movements, the test is considered positive for LHBT instability. A standard diagnostic arthroscopy can then be performed. Other procedures being done concomitantly, such as rotator cuff repair, should be performed before tenotomy or tenodesis.

If the surgeon elects for subpectoral tenodesis, the LHBT is released from the supraglenoid tubercle with electrocautery, an arthroscopic shaver, a thermal ablative device, or arthroscopic scissors.

If the surgeon elects for arthroscopic proximal tenodesis, several additional steps should be performed before tendon release. The tendon must first be transfixed with a spinal needle at the entrance to the intertubercular groove. Suture is then passed to mark the tenodesis site. An additional anterolateral portal 3 cm from the anterior acromion and 3 cm lateral to the anteromedial portal is made. The arthroscope is inserted through this anterolateral portal. The groove is then identified medial to the lateral edge of the greater tuberosity. The groove is opened with electrocautery and the tendon is removed from the groove, which is further cleared of soft tissue. The guidewire is then drilled into the center of the groove, perpendicular to the humerus and parallel to the lateral border of the acromion, 1 cm distal to the superior aspect of the groove. This guidewire is then overdrilled with an 8-mm cannulated acorn reamer to 25 mm. The tunnel created is then chamfered using a shaver or burr to facilitate tendon seating. The suture previously placed through the tendon is then passed through the tenodesis screwdriver loaded with an 8 × 25-mm screw. The screwdriver is used to seat the tendon into the tunnel, and the screw is advanced next to the tendon until flush. Whether the tendon is tied depends on the surgeon's preference for improved fixation versus the possibly increased risk of subacromial impingement. Tendon tension can be assessed with a probe.

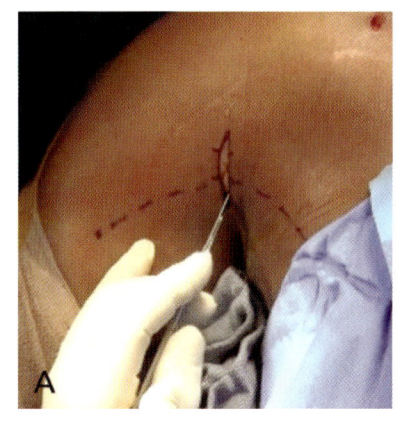

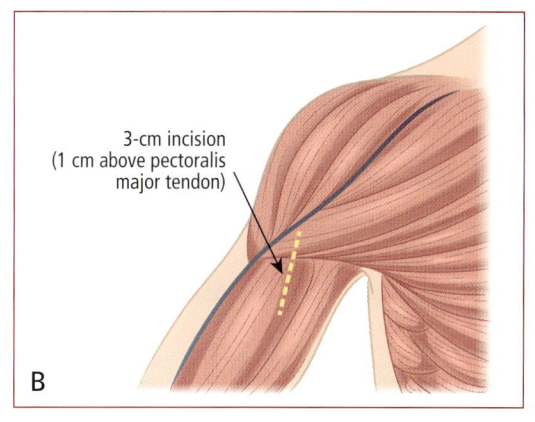

Figure 1 Intraoperative photograph (**A**) and illustration (**B**) show the incision for subpectoral biceps tenodesis. A 3-cm longitudinal incision is made, with its proximal edge 1 cm superior to the inferior edge of the pectoralis major insertion.

If the surgeon elects for subpectoral tenodesis, attention is turned to the axilla and preparation is made for an open procedure after arthroscopic tenotomy. The patient is reclined an additional 30° from the beach-chair position. Internal rotation and abduction brings the insertion of the pectoralis major into tension, allowing identification of the inferior edge. A 3-cm longitudinal incision is marked, with the proximal edge beginning 1 cm superior to the inferior edge of the pectoralis major insertion (**Figure 1**). This incision can be placed within the axilla for cosmesis if the surgeon is intimately familiar with the anatomy. The subcutaneous tissues are injected with bupivacaine and epinephrine to improve postoperative pain control and minimize intraoperative hemorrhage. The skin and subcuticular tissues are incised with a scalpel. Electrocautery should be used to minimize bleeding and maximize visualization. A Gelpi or Weitlaner self-retaining retractor can also improve visualization.

After the subcutaneous adipose tissue has been cleared, the medial-lateral orientation of the fibers of the pectoralis major should be seen. If these structures cannot be visualized, the dissection may be too lateral. If the cephalic vein is visible, the dissection is both too lateral and too proximal. Blunt finger dissection at the inferior edge of these fibers should identify the coracobrachialis and the LHBT, which is palpable on the anteromedial surface of the humerus. The fascia overlying the coracobrachialis and LHBT should be incised from proximal to distal. A pointed Hohmann retractor can be placed on the humerus to retract the pectoralis tendon proximally and laterally. A blunt Chandler retractor can be used to retract the coracobrachialis and short head of the biceps medially; such retraction should be performed gently to avoid musculocutaneous nerve injury.

A right-angle clamp can then be used to retrieve the tendon out of the groove and deliver it from the wound (**Figure 2, A**). The tendon should be resected such that 20 to 25 mm of tendon remains proximal to the musculotendinous junction. A stout large-caliber suture is then used to place a Krackow whip-stitch into the proximal 15 mm of tendon. These measurements help to ensure proper tensioning of the LHBT once it is tenodesed.

A 2-cm × 1-cm patch of periosteum within the groove roughly 1 cm proximal to the inferior edge of the pectoralis major insertion is reflected. A guidewire is then drilled into this prepared bed. This guidewire should be placed in the center of the groove at the intersection of the middle and distal thirds of the groove. An 8-mm cannulated acorn reamer is then used to make a 15-mm-deep tunnel over the guidewire. Care should be taken not to violate the posterior cortex. The field should be irrigated to remove any osseous fragments. One limb of the suture should then be threaded through the tenodesis screwdriver loaded with an 8 × 15-mm polyetheretherketone tenodesis screw (**Figure 2, B**). The driver is used to push the tendon to the deepest aspect of the tunnel, and the tenodesis screw is then advanced next to the tendon into the tunnel until flush

© 2013 American Academy of Orthopaedic Surgeons

Section 1: Sports Medicine

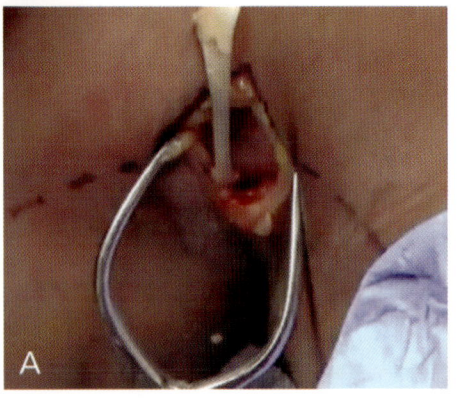

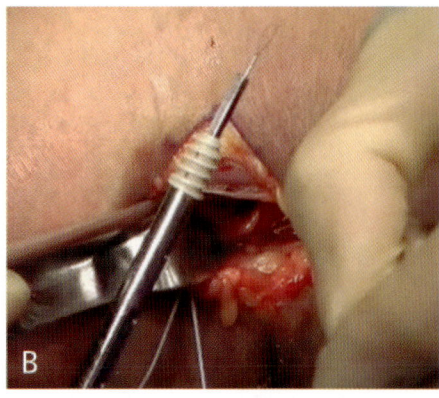

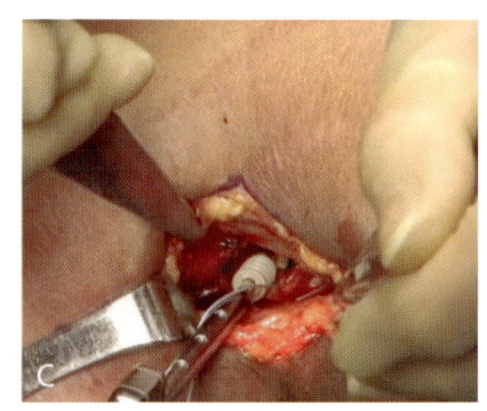

Figure 2 Intraoperative photographs show biceps tenodesis. **A,** The proximal cut edge of the tendon is delivered out of the wound. **B,** A tenodesis screw is loaded onto the driver. Note that one limb of the suture fixating the tendon must then be loaded onto the screwdriver. **C,** The tendon is pushed into the deepest aspect of the tunnel, and the tenodesis screw is advanced over the tendon.

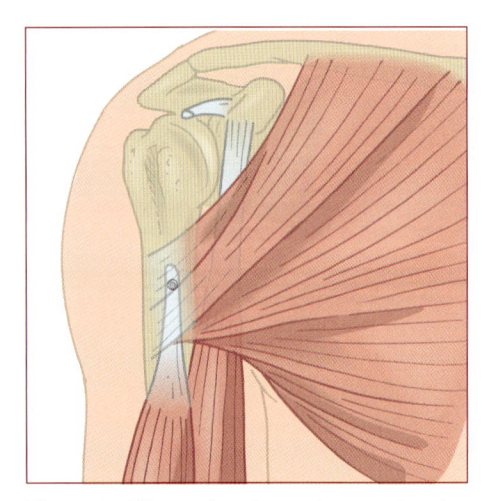

Figure 3 Illustration shows the completed subpectoral tenodesis. After fixation, the musculotendinous junction rests at its native anatomic position under the pectoralis major tendon.

(**Figure 2, C**). The two ends of the stout large-caliber suture can then be tied and cut (**Figure 3**). After further irrigation, the wound is closed per the surgeon's preference. We use 2-0 absorbable monofilament suture for subcuticular closure with Dermabond (Ethicon) to reduce bacterial contamination from the adjacent axilla.

Tenotomy
If the surgeon elects for tenotomy, the setup, patient positioning, and approach are the same as that for tenodesis. The LHBT is also released as described for tenodesis, but once the tendon has been confirmed to retract from the intra-articular space, the procedure is complete. Because the tendon is commonly hypertrophied and entrapped within the joint, further tendon resection may be necessary to cause the tendon to retract. Retraction is necessary because free-floating tendon may otherwise cause symptoms within the joint.

Complications
Loss of range of motion, hematoma, seroma, infection, irritation from hardware, axillary nerve injury, musculocutaneous nerve injury, brachial artery injury, axillary artery injury, heterotopic ossification, and proximal humeral fracture are all theoretically possible following LHBT tenotomy or tenodesis. In a recent series of 353 subpectoral tenodeses performed at our institution and followed for an average of 2.3 years, only 7 complications were observed (2%). Two patients reported persistent bicipital pain; in another two, fixation failed and the "Popeye" deformity developed; and the following developed in one patient each: a deep infection that required irrigation and débridement; reflex sympathetic dystrophy that required stellate ganglion block; and musculoskeletal neurapraxia that spontaneously resolved.[14] Although many authors have worried that tenotomy or tenodesis could lead to proximal humeral migration and rapid progression of rotator cuff arthropathy given the potential role of the LHBT as a humeral head depressor, numerous studies have failed to validate these concerns.[6]

Postoperative Care and Rehabilitation
Postoperative limitations secondary to any concomitant procedures performed typically supersede any management required by biceps tenotomy or tenodesis. Postoperative treatment is generally similar to that applied after acromioplasty. A sling is worn for 3 to 4 weeks. During the initial 6 weeks, the patient progresses to full passive and active range of motion. The patient is advised against active flexion and supination of the surgical arm until 6 weeks postoperatively to protect the tenodesis. Patients are typically able to resume a lightened work schedule at 3 to 4 weeks, depending on their occupation.

Pearls
- Although identification of LHBT pathology on history and physical examination can be difficult, the reliable response of appropriately indicated patients to tenodesis rewards careful patient selection.
- Patients with LHBT instability should be carefully evaluated for other lesions. Because of the anatomic arrangement of the pulley, tendon subluxation is inevitably associated with concomitant pathology.
- LHBT tendinosis is commonly associated with other injuries and should be examined for in patients with subacromial impingement, rotator cuff pathology, tears of the anterior capsuloligamentous complex, labral tears, glenohumeral instability, and acromioclavicular arthrosis.
- Although tenotomy and tenodesis outcomes may be similar, each procedure can provide maximum benefit to different patient populations. In younger, more active patients, tenodesis may prevent complications potentially associated with tenotomy; in older, less active, and obese patients, tenotomy may provide equivalent outcomes with decreased surgical time, expense, and difficulty.
- Subpectoral tenodesis has several advantages over arthroscopic proximal tenodesis and should be considered in the appropriate patient.
- Interference screw fixation provides biomechanically superior fixation.

References

1. Walch G, Nove-Josserand L, Levigne C, Renaud E: Tears of the supraspinatus tendon associated with "hidden" lesions of the rotator interval. *J Shoulder Elbow Surg* 1994;3(6):353-360.
2. Provencher MT, LeClere LE, Romeo AA: Subpectoral biceps tenodesis. *Sports Med Arthrosc* 2008;16(3):170-176.
3. Mazzocca AD, Cote MP, Arciero CL, Romeo AA, Arciero RA: Clinical outcomes after subpectoral biceps tenodesis with an interference screw. *Am J Sports Med* 2008;36(10):1922-1929.
4. Nho SJ, Frank RM, Reiff SN, Verma NN, Romeo AA: Arthroscopic repair of anterosuperior rotator cuff tears combined with open biceps tenodesis. *Arthroscopy* 2010;26(12):1667-1674.
5. Yamaguchi K, Riew KD, Galatz LM, Syme JA, Neviaser RJ: Biceps activity during shoulder motion: An electromyographic analysis. *Clin Orthop Relat Res* 1997;336:122-129.
6. Boileau P, Baqué F, Valerio L, Ahrens P, Chuinard C, Trojani C: Isolated arthroscopic biceps tenotomy or tenodesis improves symptoms in patients with massive irreparable rotator cuff tears. *J Bone Joint Surg Am* 2007;89(4):747-757.
7. Heckman DS, Creighton RA, Romeo AA: Management of failed biceps tenodesis or tenotomy: Causation and treatment. *Sports Med Arthrosc* 2010;18(3):173-180.
8. Gill HS, El Rassi G, Bahk MS, Castillo RC, McFarland EG: Physical examination for partial tears of the biceps tendon. *Am J Sports Med* 2007;35(8):1334-1340.
9. Frost A, Zafar MS, Maffulli N: Tenotomy versus tenodesis in the management of pathologic lesions of the tendon of the long head of the biceps brachii. *Am J Sports Med* 2009;37(4):828-833.
10. Kelly AM, Drakos MC, Fealy S, Taylor SA, O'Brien SJ: Arthroscopic release of the long head of the biceps tendon: Functional outcome and clinical results. *Am J Sports Med* 2005;33(2):208-213.
11. Friedman DJ, Dunn JC, Higgins LD, Warner JJ: Proximal biceps tendon: Injuries and management. *Sports Med Arthrosc* 2008;16(3):162-169.
12. Mazzocca AD, Bicos J, Santangelo S, Romeo AA, Arciero RA: The biomechanical evaluation of four fixation techniques for proximal biceps tenodesis. *Arthroscopy* 2005;21(11):1296-1306.
13. Mazzocca AD, Rios CG, Romeo AA, Arciero RA: Subpectoral biceps tenodesis with interference screw fixation. *Arthroscopy* 2005;21(7):896.
14. Nho SJ, Reiff SN, Verma NN, Slabaugh MA, Mazzocca AD, Romeo AA: Complications associated with subpectoral biceps tenodesis: Low rates of incidence following surgery. *J Shoulder Elbow Surg* 2010;19(5):764-768.
15. Romeo AA, Mazzocca AD, Tauro JC: Arthroscopic biceps tenodesis. *Arthroscopy* 2004;20(2):206-213.

Chapter 5
Anatomic Acromioclavicular Joint Reconstruction

Albert Lin, MD   Mark William Rodosky, MD

Patient Selection

Acromioclavicular (AC) joint injuries are common injuries that account for as many as half of all athletic shoulder injuries.[1] The most frequent mechanism of AC joint separation is a direct fall onto an adducted shoulder. The forces transmitted often result in inferior and medial displacement of the acromion while the clavicle remains stabilized to the bony thorax through the sternoclavicular joint.[2] Patients may present with local swelling, apparent deformity with prominence of the distal clavicle, pain over the AC joint, and accentuation of pain with cross-body adduction or abduction. The stability of an AC joint separation on physical examination may also be assessed, with the ability to reduce depending on the acuity of the injury and the severity of soft-tissue injuries. In higher-energy injuries, associated injuries to the clavicle, scapula, proximal humerus, and neurovascular structures such as the brachial plexus should be assessed. AC joint separations are often classified by the Rockwood classification scheme (**Table 1**), which usually dictates the treatment options. Type I injuries, where there is no appreciable deformity of the AC joint, and type II injuries, where there may be disruption of the AC joint capsule but not of the coracoclavicular ligaments and thus no vertical instability, are almost uniformly treated nonsurgically.

Indications for surgical treatment include type IV, V, and VI AC joint separations; these represent higher-energy mechanisms of injury and associated soft-tissue disruption. These injuries are not reducible on physical examination, with type IV AC joint separations representing posterior displacement of the clavicle through the trapezius; type V injuries representing detachment of the deltoid, trapezius, and fascia or the dynamic stabilizers of the AC joint from the clavicle; and type VI injuries representing a rare entity in which the clavicle is inferiorly displaced under the coracoid in the setting of high-energy trauma with associated fractures of the shoulder girdle and brachial plexus.

The decision regarding nonsurgical versus surgical treatment of type III injuries is controversial.[3-6] Type III injuries represent injuries to both the AC joint capsule and the coracoclavicular ligaments, resulting in horizontal and vertical instability, and are manually reducible on physical examination. There is no consensus in the literature regarding surgical versus nonsurgical treatment.[3-6] Surgical treatment for a type III injury can usually be reserved for patients who have persistent pain and instability after a trial of conservative therapy of at least 3 months. A relative indication for acute stabilization of a type III injury may be a sport or job that places a high demand on the shoulder.[1]

Contraindications to AC joint stabilization or reconstruction include type I and II injuries, coracoid fracture, clavicle fracture, glenohumeral arthritis, and patients who lack the ability to comply with postoperative rehabilitation protocols.

Several procedures exist to stabilize the AC joint. The authors' preferred method is open anatomic AC joint reconstruction using hamstring autograft or allograft because biomechanical testing has demonstrated this to be the strongest construct that most closely approximates the native AC joint.[7]

Preoperative Imaging
Radiography

Standard radiographs are crucial for diagnosing and classifying AC joint injuries. Routine shoulder radiographs should include true AP and axillary lateral views. The axillary lateral view can be invaluable in distinguishing a type IV injury (**Figure 1, A**).[1] To assess the AC joint, a Zanca view (10° to 15° cephalic tilt) with the patient upright and the injured arm

Table 1 Rockwood Classification of Acromioclavicular Joint Injuries

Type	AC Ligaments	CC Ligaments	Deltopectoral Fascia	Radiographic CC Distance Increase	Radiographic AC Appearance	AC Joint Reducible?
I	Sprained	Intact	Intact	Normal (1.1 to 1.3 cm)	Normal	N/A
II	Disrupted	Sprained	Intact	<25%	Widened	Yes
III	Disrupted	Disrupted	Disrupted	25% to 100%	Widened	Yes
IV	Disrupted	Disrupted	Disrupted	Increased	Posterior clavicle displacement	No
V	Disrupted	Disrupted	Disrupted	100% to 300%	N/A	No
VI	Disrupted	Intact	Disrupted	Decreased	N/A	No

AC = acromioclavicular, CC = coracoclavicular, N/A = not applicable.

Adapted from Simovitch R, Sanders B, Ozbaydar M, Lavery K, Warner JJ: Acromioclavicular joint injuries: Diagnosis and management. *J Am Acad Orthop Surg* 2009;17(4):207-219.

Neither of the following authors nor any immediate family member has received anything of value from or owns stock in a commercial company or institution related directly or indirectly to the subject of this chapter: Dr. Lin and Dr. Rodosky.

Section 1: Sports Medicine

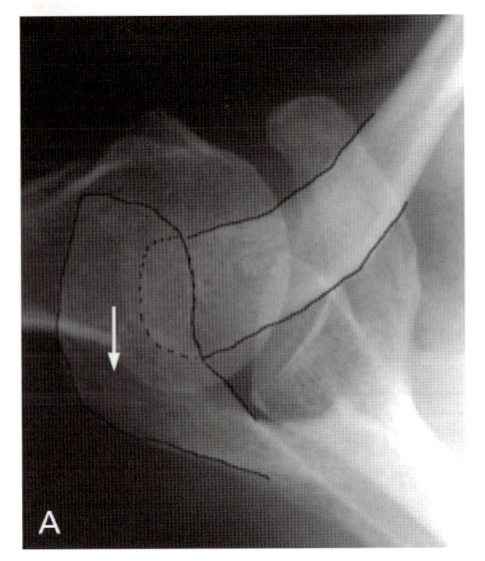

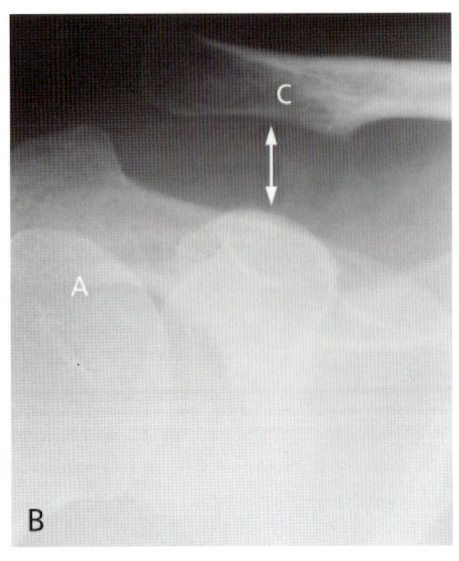

Figure 1 Axillary lateral (**A**) and Zanca view (**B**) radiographs demonstrate increased coracoclavicular interspace distance (double-headed arrow in **B**) and posterior displacement of the clavicle (posteriorly directed arrow in **A**), distinguishing this injury as a type IV acromioclavicular joint separation. The acromion (A) and clavicle (C) are outlined in **A**. (Reproduced from Simovitch R, Sanders B, Ozbaydar M, Lavery K, Warner JJ: Acromioclavicular joint injuries: Diagnosis and management. *J Am Acad Orthop Surg* 2009;17[4]:207-219.)

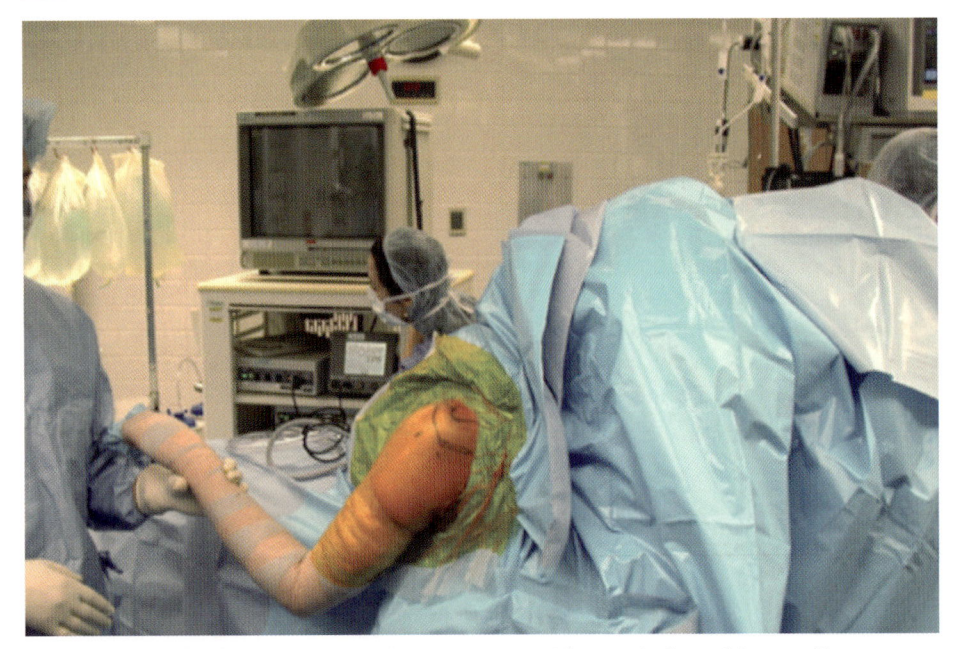

Figure 2 Photograph shows beach-chair positioning. The arm is draped free to allow for manipulation and manual reduction. (Reproduced from Mostofi A, Rios C, Tennent T, Arciero R, Mazzocca A: Acromioclavicular joint injuries. *Orthopaedic Knowledge Online Journal* 2008;6[4]:SHO020.)

unsupported should be obtained (**Figure 1, B**).[1] The uninjured extremity should be assessed, if possible on the same film, to allow comparison of AC joint asymmetry and coracoclavicular distance. Although not routinely taken, a Stryker notch view can be obtained if a coracoid fracture is suspected and not adequately visualized on the other films.[1]

Computed Tomography
CT scans are not usually obtained in isolated AC joint injuries. However, a CT scan can be helpful if there are suspected associated injuries such as sternoclavicular joint disruption, a physeal fracture in adolescent patients or patients with open physes, scapular fractures, glenoid fractures, distal clavicle fractures, and proximal humeral fractures.

Procedure
Room Setup/Patient Positioning
The patient is placed in about 60° of elevation either on a standard operating table or in a beach-chair configuration[5] (**Figure 2**). The head is supported with foam and tilted away from the surgical site to allow for maximal exposure. A bump is placed under the medial scapular edge to elevate the coracoid anteriorly.[5] The preparation area is wide, extending to at least the midline of the chest and superiorly to the midline of the chin and neck to expose the sternoclavicular joint if necessary and the posterior clavicle for visualization of the shoulder girdle. The preparation area is also wide in case there is an unforeseen complication to the underlying subclavian vessels, the brachial plexus, or the lung. The arm should be draped free to allow manipulation and reduction. All bony prominences elsewhere are well padded and protected.

Special Instruments/Equipment
The following equipment should be available for this procedure:
- Gelpi retractors
- Needle-tip Bovie electrocautery
- Small periosteal elevator
- No. 2 nonabsorbable suture, such as Ethibond (Ethicon)
- Cannulated reamer set
- Low-profile, malleable guidewire
- Threaded guide pins for cannulated reamers
- Reduction clamps
- Mini C-arm for imaging
- Graft-harvesting station (if hamstring autograft is obtained)
- Suture-passing devices, such as a Hewson or curved suture-passing device

Surgical Technique
Exposure
A saber-cut incision is used. The incision is usually 3 to 3.5 cm medial to the AC joint, proceeding along the Langer's line and curving medially toward the coracoid[5] (**Figure 3**). A well-placed incision will allow visualization of both the AC joint laterally and the coracoid medially. Once through the skin, superficial bleeding is controlled. Using a needle-tip Bovie, the incision is performed through the subcutaneous layer to the level of the deltotrapezial fascia in line with the skin incision. Large full-thickness skin flaps are then elevated on either side at the level of the fascia to improve visualization. It is essential that the flaps are full thickness to prevent loss of vascularity of the skin. The deltotrapezial fascia is then incised off the clavicle in a medial-to-lateral direction, creating anterior and posterior flaps. This will serve to "skeletonize" the

Chapter 5: Anatomic Acromioclavicular Joint Reconstruction

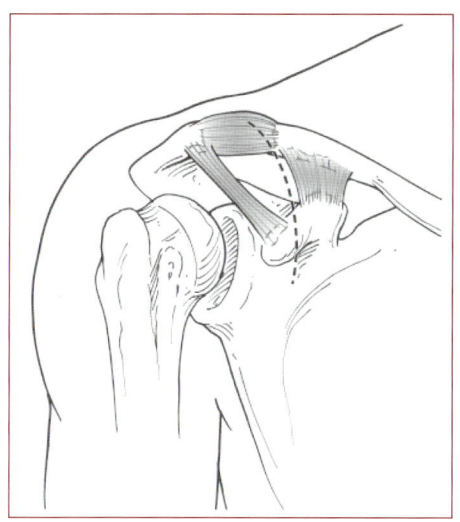

Figure 3 Illustration shows the saber-cut skin incision (dashed line) used for acromioclavicular (AC) joint reconstruction. The incision must be lateral enough to allow exposure of the AC joint and extend medial enough to allow access and exposure of the coracoid.

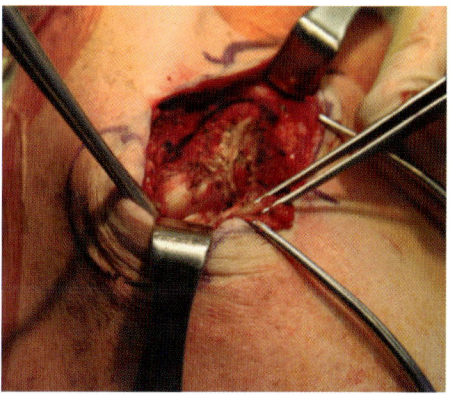

Figure 4 Intraoperative photograph shows the elevation of full-thickness deltotrapezial fascial flaps to skeletonize the clavicle; the flaps are preserved for later closure. (Reproduced from Mostofi A, Rios C, Tennent T, Arciero R, Mazzocca A: Acromioclavicular joint injuries. *Orthopaedic Knowledge Online Journal* 2008;6[4]:SHO020.)

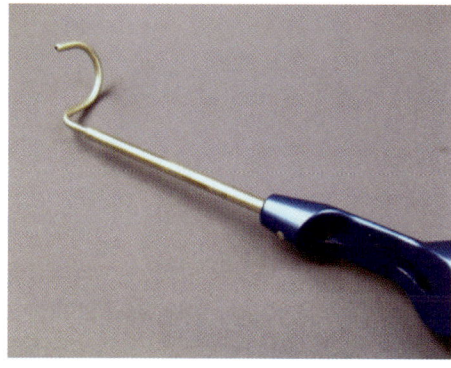

Figure 5 Photograph depicts one of many suture-passing devices that can be used to loop the graft and nonabsorbable suture around and underneath the coracoid. (Reproduced from Mostofi A, Rios C, Tennent T, Arciero R, Mazzocca A: Acromioclavicular joint injuries. *Orthopaedic Knowledge Online Journal* 2008;6[4]:SHO020.)

clavicle. Once full-thickness flaps are initially created with the Bovie, a small periosteal elevator can then be used to more safely complete the skeletonization of the clavicle. It is critical that the periosteal/fascial flaps be kept full thickness to allow for appropriate closure of the fascia[5] (**Figure 4**).

Trial Reduction

Once the AC joint is fully exposed, a trial reduction is attempted by pushing upward on the elbow, which serves to reduce the scapulothoracic complex toward the anatomically positioned distal clavicle. Interposing soft tissue on the distal clavicle may prevent reduction and must be completely cleared to allow for appropriate reduction. An initial reduction can be confirmed with a mini C-arm.

Preparation of the Allograft

On a separate table, a gracilis autograft or a tibialis allograft is prepared. The two free ends are whipstitched, and excess tissue at the free ends is removed to facilitate easier passage through the bone tunnels.

Graft Passage

Next, attention is turned toward the coracoid. Ideally, the coracoid has been well exposed both medially and laterally during the initial approach and can be palpated with confidence to allow passage of a curved suture-passing device[5] (**Figure 5**) or a large right-angle clamp. The curved suture passer is placed in a medial-to-lateral direction under the coracoid to avoid injury to the neurovascular bundle. Then a looped wire is placed in the suture passer medial to lateral, and this wire is used to shuttle the graft and nonabsorbable suture around and underneath the coracoid.

Tunnel Drilling for Conoid and Trapezoid Reconstruction

Next, attention is directed toward the clavicle for bone tunnel placement and reconstruction of the conoid and trapezoid ligaments. A threaded cannulated guide pin is placed posteromedially on the clavicle about 4.5 cm away from the AC joint for the conoid reconstruction, and another pin is placed 3 cm from the AC joint more centered on the clavicle and in parallel fashion to the previously placed pin for the trapezoid reconstruction[5] (**Figure 6**). A cannulated reamer is then used on power over the guide pins to create the bone tunnels. The size of the tunnel will depend on the measured size of the grafts; a smaller reamer can be used first with successive dilation to a larger-sized reamer if there is doubt about the size of the tunnel. Care must be taken in particular with reaming over the conoid pin to ensure that the posterior cortex of the clavicle is not breached.

Reconstruction of the AC Joint

Using a Hewson suture passer from superior to inferior, the free ends of the graft and nonabsorbable suture are crossed over each other and passed through the two bone tunnels to re-create the coracoclavicular ligaments[1,5] (**Figure 7**). Thus, the graft and suture are crossed over in

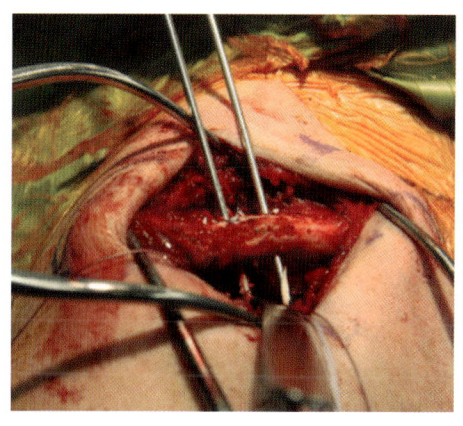

Figure 6 Intraoperative photograph shows two guide pins placed in parallel fashion. The conoid guide pin is placed approximately 4.5 cm from the acromioclavicular (AC) joint posteromedially on the clavicle. The trapezoid guide pin is placed about 3 cm from the AC joint lateral to the conoid guide pin and centered on the clavicle. (Reproduced from Mostofi A, Rios C, Tennent T, Arciero R, Mazzocca A: Acromioclavicular joint injuries. *Orthopaedic Knowledge Online Journal* 2008;6[4]:SHO020.)

a figure-of-8 fashion. An assistant then manually reduces the AC joint by placing upward pressure on the elbow. The AC joint should be overreduced because there is usually some displacement long term after reconstruction. The nonabsorbable suture is tied in place for augmentation and nonbiologic stabilization. While maintaining manual reduction, the graft is pulled back and forth and cycled several times to ensure that there is no displacement or migration once the graft is fixed in place. With maximal traction placed on the graft and the AC joint reduced, the two ends are then sutured onto each other in side-to-side fashion with

© 2013 American Academy of Orthopaedic Surgeons

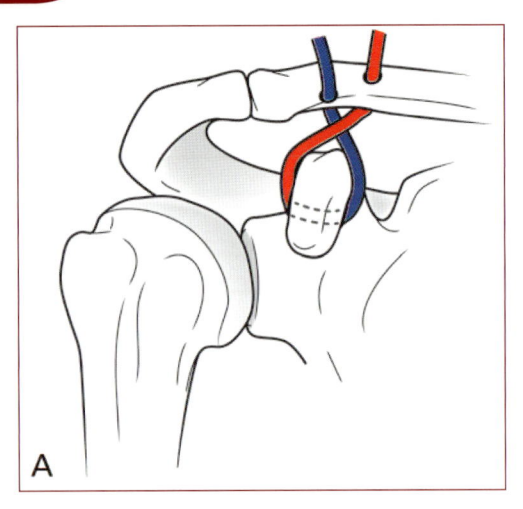

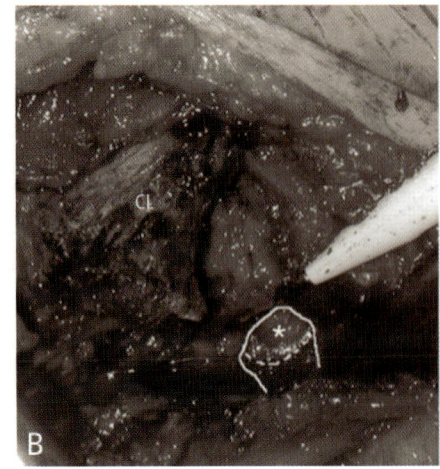

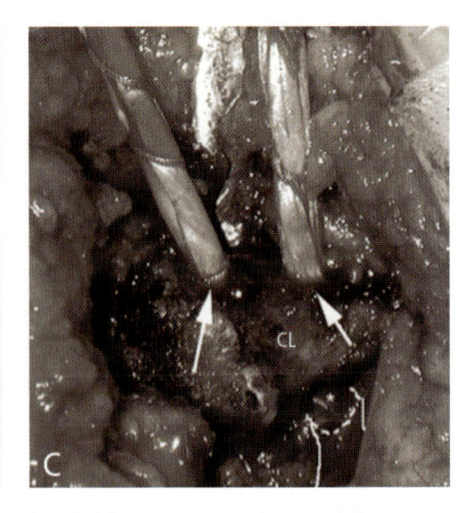

Figure 7 Reconstruction of the coracoclavicular ligaments. **A,** Illustration shows the graft and nonabsorbable suture passed around the coracoid and crossed as the free ends are brought through the conoid and trapezoid bone tunnels. **B,** Intraoperative photograph shows a suture passer being passed from medial to lateral around the coracoid tip (*) and used to retrieve the anterior tibialis allograft around the coracoid process. **C,** The graft ends are pulled through two bone tunnels (arrows) in the clavicle (CL) to approximate the pull of the conoid and trapezoid ligaments. (Panels **B** and **C** are reproduced from Simovitch R, Sanders B, Ozbaydar M, Lavery K, Warner JJ: Acromioclavicular joint injuries: Diagnosis and management. *J Am Acad Orthop Surg* 2009;17[4]:207-219.)

several figure-of-8 sutures with a heavy, absorbable suture such as a 0 or #1 Vicryl (Ethicon), completing the reconstruction.

Closure
The deltotrapezial fascia is closed using 0 Vicryl sutures, the deep dermal layer is closed using 2-0 or 3-0 Vicryl sutures, and the superficial skin is closed with a running 4-0 Monocryl suture (Ethicon).

Complications
Complications of anatomic AC joint reconstruction include early or late fracture of the coracoid process and the clavicle. Osteolysis of either the coracoid or clavicle may occur from the use of nonabsorbable nonbiologic fixation. Iatrogenic injury to the brachial plexus or axillary artery can occur with graft passage around the coracoid. Dissection that strays medially and inferiorly can injure the subclavian vessels and lung in very rare instances. Persistent pain, recurrent instability, loss of reduction, and persistent deformity are also complications of AC joint reconstruction.

Postoperative Care and Rehabilitation
The patient is kept in a simple sling for 2 weeks in a normal resting position. Pendulum exercises are initiated at 2 weeks and at 4 weeks the sling is discontinued, and arm use is allowed for light activities of daily living. At 8 weeks, formal physical therapy is initiated for active and passive range of motion. Light resistance is initiated at 3 months. Full return to labor or sports is initiated once full strength and range of motion are obtained, usually between 4 and 6 months.

Pearls
- A bump is placed under the medial scapular border for stabilization and anteriorization of the coracoid.
- The head should be tilted maximally away from the surgical field; this will facilitate drilling of the conoid tunnel.
- Full-thickness flaps of the deltotrapezial fascia are made when exposing the clavicle. This is critical for later closure.
- When passing the graft, the medial coracoid must be adequately exposed. Passage of the graft medial to lateral is recommended to avoid injury to the brachial plexus and axillary artery.
- The size of the reamer must be accounted for when placing the guide pins to avoid breaching the posterior or anterior cortex of the clavicle.
- Frayed edges at the whipstitched ends should be adequately débrided to facilitate easy graft passage through the bony tunnels.
- Use of heavy, ultra-high-strength nonabsorbable sutures for nonbiologic fixation should be avoided because this increases the risk of late osteolysis of either the coracoid or the clavicle.
- If there is doubt about the size of the bone tunnel, the surgeon should start with a smaller reamer and incrementally increase the reamer size.
- When fixing the graft in place, the joint should be overreduced because there is often some loss of reduction over time.
- The graft is cycled several times back and forth through the tunnels to ensure that there is no displacement or migration of the graft after it is fixed in place.

References
1. Simovitch R, Sanders B, Ozbaydar M, Lavery K, Warner JJ: Acromioclavicular joint injuries: Diagnosis and management. *J Am Acad Orthop Surg* 2009;17(4):207-219.
2. Rios CG, Arciero RA, Mazzocca AD: Anatomy of the clavicle and coracoid process for reconstruction of the coracoclavicular ligaments. *Am J Sports Med* 2007;35(5):811-817.
3. Bannister GC, Wallace WA, Stableforth PG, Hutson MA: The management of acute acromioclavicular dislocation: A randomised prospective controlled trial. *J Bone Joint Surg Br* 1989;71(5):848-850.
4. McFarland EG, Blivin SJ, Doehring CB, Curl LA, Silberstein C: Treatment of grade III acromioclavicular separations in professional throwing athletes: Results of a survey. *Am J Orthop (Belle Mead NJ)* 1997;26(11):771-774.
5. Mostofi A, Rios C, Tennent T, Arciero R, Mazzocca A: Acromioclavicular joint injuries. *Orthopaedic Knowledge Online.* 2011.
6. Phillips AM, Smart C, Groom AF: Acromioclavicular dislocation: Conservative or surgical therapy. *Clin Orthop Relat Res* 1998;353:10-17.
7. Mazzocca AD, Santangelo SA, Johnson ST, Rios CG, Dumonski ML, Arciero RA: A biomechanical evaluation of an anatomical coracoclavicular ligament reconstruction. *Am J Sports Med* 2006;34(2):236-246.

Chapter 6

Open Reduction and Internal Fixation of Clavicle Fractures

Laura E. Scordino, MD   Thomas M. DeBerardino, MD

Introduction

Clavicle fractures are common, accounting for 2.6% to 5.0% of adult fractures.[1-3] Historically, clavicle fractures were thought to heal with predictability while being managed almost exclusively nonsurgically. This treatment was based largely on two retrospective studies performed in the 1960s by Neer[4] and Rowe[5] that suggested that surgical treatment actually resulted in an increased number of nonunions and complications compared with nonsurgical treatment.

Today, with improved surgical techniques, growing evidence indicates that early surgical treatment may be beneficial in appropriately selected patients. In fact, in a recent prospective multicenter randomized clinical trial by the Canadian Orthopaedic Trauma Society, a comparison of nonsurgical treatment and plate fixation of midshaft clavicle fractures revealed that plate fixation resulted in significantly better radiographic outcomes; Constant scores; Disability of the Arm, Shoulder, and Hand (DASH) scores; functional outcomes; and cosmetic scores.[6]

Classification

Clavicle fractures are generally classified based on the location of the fracture within the clavicle as well as the degree of comminution and angulation. The classification devised by Allman[7] is commonly used; it categorizes clavicle fractures as proximal, midshaft, or distal. The location of the fracture within the clavicle and the degree of displacement, angulation, and comminution all play a role in determining treatment recommendations.[3,8,9]

Overall, fractures of the midshaft make up about 70% to 80% of all clavicle fractures, whereas those of the lateral or distal portion make up approximately 21% and medial-end fractures approximately 2% to 3%.[1,8-10] Midshaft fractures occur more commonly as a result of high energy and in a younger patient population and are more commonly displaced, whereas lateral and medial-end fractures occur more commonly in the elderly and are nondisplaced.[2,8,9]

Patient Selection
Indications

Overall surgical indications include open fractures, "floating shoulder," impending skin necrosis, associated neurovascular injuries, and multiply injured trauma patients.[3,8] More recently, studies have suggested that improved outcomes are associated with surgical fixation of fractures with shortening greater than 15 to 20 mm, with 100% displacement, or with comminution.[6]

Contraindications

Nonsurgical treatment is generally recommended for nondisplaced or minimally displaced fractures and in older, sicker patients who are either low demand or are medically unfit to undergo surgery. If nonsurgical treatment is pursued, a sling and a course of non–weight bearing is sufficient.[3,8]

Preoperative Imaging

Orthogonal views of the clavicle are the best means of evaluating the fracture. The fracture should be evaluated for location within the clavicle, displacement, comminution, angulation, and associated fractures to the scapula and the proximal humerus. Evaluation of an AP radiograph of the chest should include not only the clavicle fracture itself but also associated chest injury, including rib fractures, pneumothorax, or hemothorax.

Other views that can supplement the initial views include the apical oblique view (affected shoulder tilted 45° anterior and x-ray beam 20° cephalad), which may help diagnose minimally displaced fractures.[11] This view also can help in judging the adequacy of reduction in the operating room. The abduction lordotic view (x-ray beam angled 25° cephalad with shoulder abducted above 135°) is useful to evaluate healing after internal fixation.[12] Other radiographs that may be obtained include a stress view for a lateral clavicle fracture to evaluate for acromioclavicular joint separation and the integrity of the coracoclavicular ligaments.

In addition to radiographs, preoperative CT scans of the clavicle are being increasingly used. They are used particularly for evaluation of nonunions as well as medial-end fractures extending into the sternoclavicular joint.

Procedure
Room Setup/Patient Positioning

The surgical technique for midshaft clavicle fractures is described here. Many surgical procedures are available for clavicle fracture fixation, depending on surgeon preference and fracture characteristics.

Initially, the patient is placed supine or in a modified beach-chair position on a radiolucent operating table. Intraoperative fluoroscopy should be available. A bump can be placed under the medial portion of the scapula of the surgical shoulder. A pneumatically controlled arm positioner can be used to negate the weight of the arm and facilitate surgery (**Figure 1**). Before marking out the skin incision, palpation of the bony landmarks should be performed, including the soft triangle in the superolateral shoulder area bounded by the acromion laterally and the scapular spine posteriorly. Just anterior to this soft triangle is the acromioclavicular joint, and just anteromedial to this is the coracoid process. The clavicle should be palpated along its S-shaped curve medially to where it articulates with the sternum at the sternoclavicular joint. The location of the incision depends on the fixation technique used.

Surgical Technique
Plate Fixation

Plate fixation is the most commonly used technique for management of clavicle fractures. Contoured clavicle plates are

---

Dr. DeBerardino is a member of a speakers' bureau or has made paid presentations on behalf of Arthrex, Genzyme, and the Musculoskeletal Transplant Foundation; serves as a paid consultant to or is an employee of Arthrex; serves as an unpaid consultant to Advanced Biomedical Technologies; has stock or stock options held in Advanced Biomedical Technologies; and has received research or institutional support from Arthrex and the Musculoskeletal Transplant Foundation. Neither Dr. Scordino nor any immediate family member has received anything of value from or owns stock in a commercial company or institution related directly or indirectly to the subject of this chapter.

Section 1: Sports Medicine

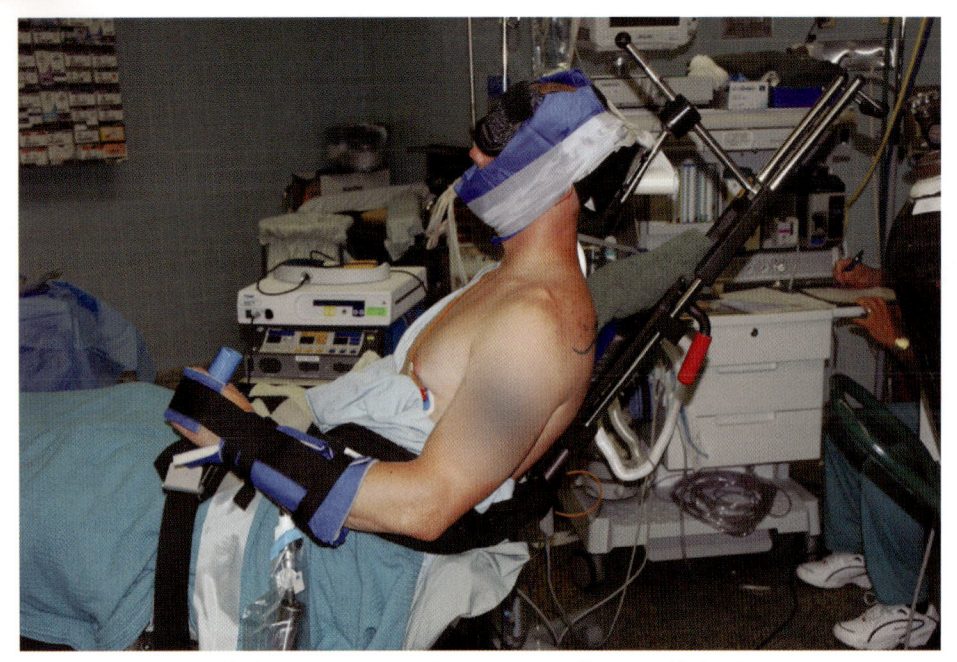

Figure 1 Photograph shows a patient with a pneumatically controlled arm positioner in place for left shoulder surgery.

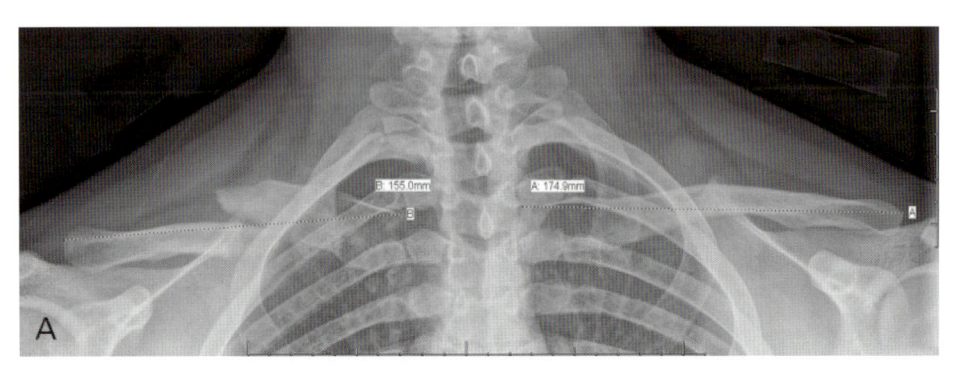

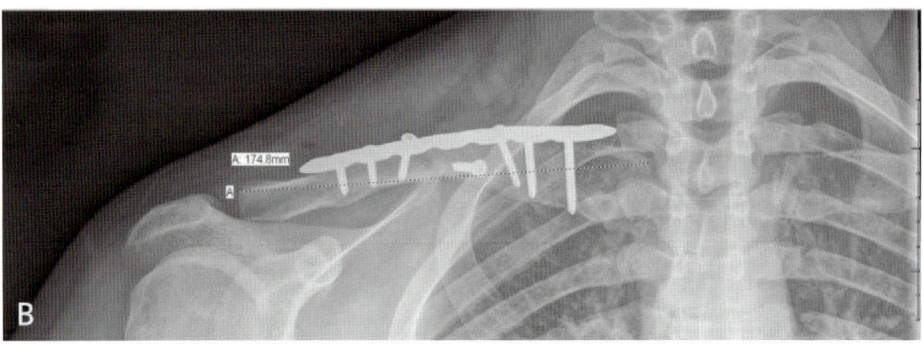

Figure 2 AP radiographs of a patient with a right midshaft clavicle fracture. **A,** Preoperative radiograph demonstrates 2 cm of shortening. **B,** Postoperative radiograph shows that clavicle length symmetric to the uninjured left side is restored with plate fixation. An interfragmentary screw and a contoured clavicle fracture plate were used.

available for superior plating of the midshaft (**Figure 2**); a different set of contoured plates is available for the lateral portion of the clavicle. Options for better contouring include trying a plate that is meant for the contralateral side or flipping the plates to use the medial side on the lateral side (for midshaft fractures only) and vice versa. Alternatively, a standard plate, such as a 3.5-mm limited-contact dynamic compression plate, can be bent to fit the clavicle of each individual patient.

The main ways of positioning the plate are superiorly or anteroinferiorly. The approaches are nearly identical, except that with anterior placement of the plate, the deltoid and pectoralis major must be extraperiosteally elevated. Advantages of the anteriorly placed plate include decreased hardware prominence and screws directed posteriorly instead of inferiorly, toward the traversing neurovascular structures.

We prefer a longitudinal incision made just inferior to and in line with the clavicle (**Figure 3**). The supraclavicular nerves are preserved as they cross perpendicular to the clavicle just deep to the level of the platysma (**Figure 4**). A 3.5-mm limited-contact dynamic compression plate or precontoured locking plate is applied to the clavicle with a minimum of three bicortical screws placed on either side of the fracture. A lag screw can be applied perpendicularly across the fracture fragment to generate compression and increase stability in a simple fracture pattern. For a comminuted fracture, a bridge plating technique can be used without fracture exposure, placing the plate over the top of the periosteum.[3,8,13]

Intramedullary Nailing

Intramedullary (IM) nailing is ideal for simple fractures of the middle third of the shaft that will have good cortical contact after fixation. IM nailing is not ideal for comminuted fractures, and this type of fixation does not resist torsional forces as well as plating does.[3] Proposed advantages are smaller skin incisions, less soft-tissue stripping compared to plate fixation, easier removal of hardware, and fewer potentially weak areas after hardware removal.[3]

The most commonly used technique uses a 2- to 3-cm incision over the fracture fragment. The platysma is dissected through, and the middle branches of the supraclavicular nerve are protected. The medial fracture fragment is elevated with a bone-reducing clamp and the canal is prepared, with care taken not to disrupt the medial cortex. The lateral fragment is then elevated, which can be aided by externally rotating the arm. The drill is advanced through the posterolateral cortex of the lateral fragment, with care taken to ensure that the exit point is not too superior, to avoid pin prominence). The clavicle pin is passed from the fracture site out the posterolateral cortex, and a small incision is made over the palpable tip.

After fracture reduction, the pin is driven in the opposite direction, into the medial fragment toward the anterior cortex. Two nuts are used on the lateral portion of the pin, both to provide compression against the lateral cortex of the clavicle and to provide a means to advance and remove the clavicle pin construct throughout fixation. Furthermore, the laterally placed nuts prevent medial

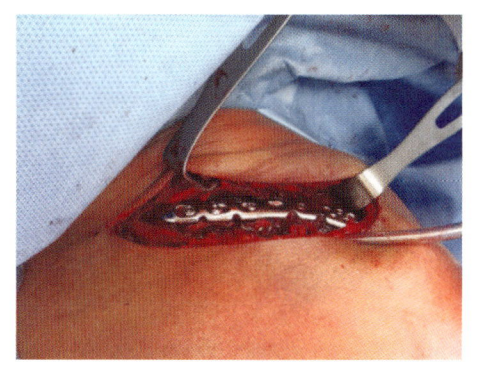

Figure 3 Intraoperative photograph shows the typical incision for a left midshaft clavicle fracture. A contoured clavicle plate and screws are used to maintain reduction.

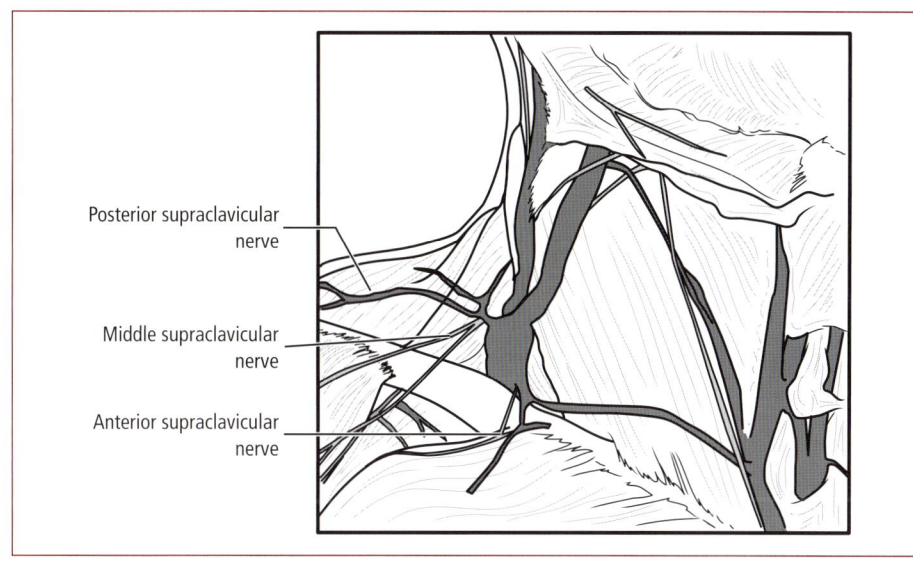

Figure 4 Illustration shows the anatomy of the supraclavicular nerves.

pin migration. The clavicle pin can be removed under general or local anesthetic in 10 to 12 weeks, after the fracture site has healed.[3,14]

Additional Considerations for Lateral Clavicle Fractures
Fixation of lateral clavicle fractures depends largely on patient selection as well as fracture characteristics. Often, lateral clavicle fractures are nondisplaced and occur in low-demand, elderly patients with poor bone quality. Lateral clavicle fractures can be managed nonsurgically; although the risk of nonunion is increased, this has been shown to have little effect on quality of life and is even associated with high patient satisfaction.[8] Fixation options include coracoclavicular screws, plate and hook-plate fixation, and the suture and sling technique.[8] Late intervention for acromioclavicular arthritis may include either arthroscopic or open distal clavicle resection.

Additional Considerations for Medial Clavicle Fractures
The mainstay of treatment for medial clavicle fractures is also largely nonsurgical because most are extra-articular and minimally displaced. Fracture displacement posteriorly and compression on the superior mediastinal structure clearly indicate a need for treatment. First, closed reduction is attempted; if this fails, open reduction and internal fixation is performed. Fixation with either suture or nonabsorbable wide fiber suture obviates the need to return to the operating room for removal of hardware and avoids the risk of metal hardware migration.

Complications
Complications of the surgical management of clavicle fractures include infection, nonunion, malunion, the need for hardware removal, neurologic complications, refracture, and osteoarthritis of the acromioclavicular joint.

Infection has been reported to occur in 0% to 18% of surgically treated clavicle fractures, with decreasing rates in more recent studies.[3,15]

Nonunions are often symptomatic in young patients, causing pain, decreased shoulder function, weakness, and a clicking sensation. At one time, nonunions were thought to occur with a frequency of less than 1% after nonsurgical management of clavicular fractures. A recent meta-analysis, however, reported that the nonunion rate for displaced midshaft clavicle fractures treated with plate fixation was 2.2% (10 of 460 patients) and with IM nail fixation was 2.0% (3 of 152 patients), whereas nonsurgical treatment resulted in a 15.1% (24 of 159 patients) nonunion rate.[16] Many of the included studies, though, were level III and IV evidence. Risk factors for nonunion include increasing age, female sex, fracture displacement, and comminution.[17]

Malunion occurs in almost every fracture that is treated nonsurgically; this is due to angulation (particularly anterior-posterior) and shortening.[3] Most malunions are asymptomatic, although some recent studies suggest that comminution, initial displacement greater than 15 to 20 mm, and increasing age are predictive of symptomatic malunions.[6]

Neurologic complications, with a prevalence ranging from 0.3% to greater than 20%, can occur as a result of the initial injury, with fracture compression of nerves; or as a late complication, such as if the brachial plexus or the subclavian vessels become encased within a hypertrophic callus.[5,6] This has been referred to as thoracic outlet syndrome and often is associated with ulnar nerve symptoms.[3,8]

Patients run the risk of refracturing the clavicle if they return to sports too soon or have risk factors such as alcohol abuse or epilepsy. Refracture is also a possibility after the removal of hardware. Refracture rates have been cited as ranging from 0% to 8%.[8,15]

Another late complication is posttraumatic osteoarthritis of the acromioclavicular joint, which often manifests as activity-related pain located anteriorly over the acromioclavicular joint; the pain can be reproduced with palpation or with cross-arm adduction. Posttraumatic osteoarthritis of the acromioclavicular joint is most commonly associated with intra-articular lateral clavicle fractures, although it can also occur with extra-articular fractures. Treatment includes distal clavicle excision (arthroscopic or open technique).[8]

The most dangerous intraoperative complication is injury to the subclavian artery or vein by drill penetration or during fracture immobilization.[3,8] If this rare complication occurs, repair by vascular or cardiothoracic surgeons may be indicated.

Postoperative Care and Rehabilitation
Postoperatively, patients remain in a sling for comfort for approximately 4 weeks. Range of motion at the wrist and elbow and active-assisted range of motion to 90° of forward flexion with the sling removed should be performed at least five times a day. Once radiographic and clinical healing has been achieved at approximately

6 weeks, resisted activity at the shoulder can be initiated. Often, return to sport is not suggested until 3 months postoperatively.

Pearls
- Landmarks should be drawn out, including the superior/inferior clavicle margins, the sternoclavicular joint, the acromioclavicular joint, and the planned incision.
- The patient should be in a modified beach-chair position.
- A bump placed under the medial portion of the scapula to be operated on helps with reduction.
- A pneumatically controlled arm positioner allows precise positioning of the arm, negates the weight of the arm, facilitates the surgery, and frees fellows and residents to assist with the operation rather than holding the limb during the case.
- Placing the incision inferior to the clavicle avoids hardware that lies directly under the skin.
- Fracture reduction is aided by reduction clamps.
- We prefer anterior-inferior plating, because it avoids hardware prominence, for patients who will carry heavy loads over their shoulders, such as firefighters.
- In addition to standard radiographs, an apical oblique view is helpful to evaluate fracture reduction.
- Nonabsorbable suture can be looped around small segmental fragments to bring them into apposition with the main fracture lines.

References

1. Postacchini F, Gumina S, De Santis P, Albo F: Epidemiology of clavicle fractures. *J Shoulder Elbow Surg* 2002;11(5):452-456.
2. Nordqvist A, Petersson C: The incidence of fractures of the clavicle. *Clin Orthop Relat Res* 1994;300:127-132.
3. Jeray KJ: Acute midshaft clavicular fracture. *J Am Acad Orthop Surg* 2007;15(4):239-248.
4. Neer CS II: Nonunion of the clavicle. *J Am Med Assoc* 1960;172:1006-1011.
5. Rowe CR: An atlas of anatomy and treatment of midclavicular fractures. *Clin Orthop Relat Res* 1968;58:29-42.
6. Canadian Orthopaedic Trauma Society: Nonoperative treatment compared with plate fixation of displaced midshaft clavicular fractures: A multicenter, randomized clinical trial. *J Bone Joint Surg Am* 2007;89(1):1-10.
7. Allman FL Jr: Fractures and ligamentous injuries of the clavicle and its articulation. *J Bone Joint Surg Am* 1967;49(4):774-784.
8. Khan LA, Bradnock TJ, Scott C, Robinson CM: Fractures of the clavicle. *J Bone Joint Surg Am* 2009;91(2):447-460.
9. Robinson CM: Fractures of the clavicle in the adult: Epidemiology and classification. *J Bone Joint Surg Br* 1998;80(3):476-484.
10. Stanley D, Trowbridge EA, Norris SH: The mechanism of clavicular fracture: A clinical and biomechanical analysis. *J Bone Joint Surg Br* 1988;70(3):461-464.
11. Weinberg B, Seife B, Alonso P: The apical oblique view of the clavicle: Its usefulness in neonatal and childhood trauma. *Skeletal Radiol* 1991;20(3):201-203.
12. Riemer BL, Butterfield SL, Daffner RH, O'Keeffe RM Jr: The abduction lordotic view of the clavicle: A new technique for radiographic visualization. *J Orthop Trauma* 1991;5(4):392-394.
13. Ring D, Jupiter J: Plate fixation of clavicle fractures, in Wiesel S, ed: *Operative Techniques in Orthopaedic Surgery*. Philadelphia, PA, Lippincott Williams & Wilkins, 2011, pp 3177-3179.
14. Tucker BS, Basamania C, Pepe MD: Intramedullary fixation of clavicle fractures, in Wiesel S, ed: *Operative Techniques in Orthopaedic Surgery*. Philadelphia, PA, Lippincott Williams & Wilkins, 2011, pp 3181-3190.
15. Böstman O, Manninen M, Pihlajamäki H: Complications of plate fixation in fresh displaced midclavicular fractures. *J Trauma* 1997;43(5):778-783.
16. Zlowodzki M, Zelle BA, Cole PA, Jeray K, McKee MD; Evidence-Based Orthopaedic Trauma Working Group: Treatment of acute midshaft clavicle fractures: Systematic review of 2144 fractures. *J Orthop Trauma* 2005;19(7):504-507.
17. Hill JM, McGuire MH, Crosby LA: Closed treatment of displaced middle-third fractures of the clavicle gives poor results. *J Bone Joint Surg Br* 1997;79(4):537-539.

Chapter 7
Open Treatment of Medial and Lateral Epicondylitis

Champ L. Baker III, MD   John Akins, MD   Champ L. Baker, Jr, MD

Patient Selection

Lateral and medial epicondylitis are common elbow conditions that cause pain, local tenderness, and limitations of activity. Most of these conditions can be managed successfully with nonsurgical treatment. Surgical intervention is reserved for patients with persistent symptoms and disability despite appropriate nonsurgical management of a minimum of 6 months' duration.

When considering surgical treatment of lateral epicondylitis, the surgeon should take care to differentiate this condition from other causes of lateral elbow pain, such as cervical radiculopathy, radial tunnel syndrome, posterolateral impingement, posterolateral rotatory instability, or radiocapitellar arthrosis, which require different treatment. For medial epicondylitis, the surgeon must examine the patient for associated ulnar neuritis and must consider other conditions causing medial elbow pain, such as attenuation of the ulnar collateral ligament with resultant instability or flexor pronator muscle ruptures.

Open, percutaneous, and, more recently, arthroscopic techniques have all been proven successful in the surgical management of recalcitrant epicondylitis.[1-8] This chapter presents open treatment of lateral and medial epicondylitis.

Preoperative Imaging

Lateral and medial epicondylitis are clinical diagnoses. However, imaging may provide additional information and may be useful to rule out other conditions. Plain radiographs can demonstrate calcifications about the epicondyle in approximately 20% of patients. MRI is useful to evaluate for intra-articular pathology, assess the collateral ligaments, and determine the extent of tearing of the extensor or flexor pronator origin.[9] Increased signal intensity on T2-weighted images may be seen in the extensor carpi radialis brevis (ECRB) tendon origin or the common flexor origin (**Figure 1**).

Procedure

Room Setup/Patient Positioning

The operating room setup is essentially the same for open treatment of lateral or medial epicondylitis. General anesthesia is preferred as long as patient comorbidities permit. Regional anesthesia can be used if needed but may not allow for an appropriate postoperative neurologic examination.

The patient is positioned supine on the operating table with the surgical arm placed on an arm board. A tourniquet is applied to the upper arm as high as possible. Standard sterile draping techniques are used. The hand and lower arm can be covered with a stockinette, although the entire upper extremity from fingertips to upper arm is prepped.

Special Instruments/Equipment/Implants

No special equipment or implants are required for the open treatment of lateral or medial epicondylitis. For surgeons who prefer to drill the epicondyle to stimulate a healing response, a 0.062-in Kirschner wire or a 5/64-in drill bit can be used.

Surgical Technique

Lateral Epicondylitis

The lateral epicondyle is palpated and outlined on the skin. An incision of approximately 4 cm is made anteromedial to the epicondyle (**Figure 2, A**). The subcutaneous tissues are divided to the level of the deep fascia overlying the extensor tendons. The interface between the extensor carpi radialis longus (ECRL) and the extensor digitorum communis (EDC) is identified. This interface is split superficially to a depth of 2 to 3 mm (**Figure 2, B**). The ECRL is then separated from the underlying ECRB by scalpel dissection and is retracted anteriorly. The

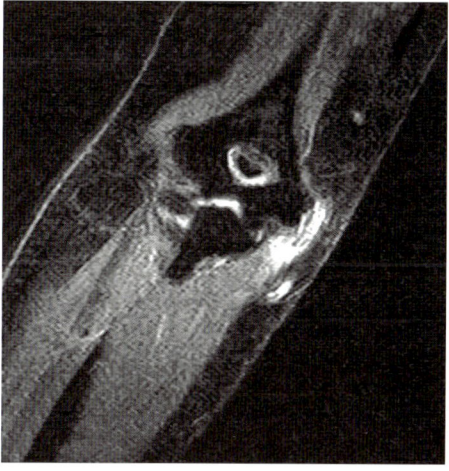

Figure 1 T2-weighted sagittal short-tau inversion recovery MRI of the elbow demonstrates medial epicondylitis. Note the increased signal intensity in the flexor pronator origin.

ECRB tendon origin is now readily visible. The pathologic angiofibroblastic tendinosis tissue is apparent by its dull, gray, friable appearance. All abnormal tissue is sharply excised en bloc with a scalpel (**Figure 2, C**). Using what is known as the Nirschl scratch test, the surgeon uses a scalpel to scrape away the remaining abnormal edematous tendinosis tissue, which peels off while leaving the healthy tendon intact.[4,5] A drill or rongeur is used on the lateral condyle to enhance the vascular supply (**Figure 2, D**). The ECRL and EDC aponeurosis is reapproximated with a running No. 1 absorbable suture (**Figure 2, E**). The subcutaneous tissues and skin are closed in a routine fashion. A well-padded posterior splint is applied with the elbow flexed to 90°.

Medial Epicondylitis

We prefer to use a modification of the technique of Vangsness and Jobe[1] to treat medial epicondylitis. First, the medial epicondyle, the olecranon, and the position of the ulnar nerve are outlined on the skin. A 4- to 5-cm incision is made, starting at the medial epicondyle and progressing distally (**Figure 3, A**). The subcutaneous tissues are divided to the level of the flexor pronator deep fascia, taking care to not injure the medial antebrachial cutaneous nerve (**Figure 3, B**). The portion of the common flexor origin encompassing the pronator teres (PT) and

---

Dr. Champ L. Baker III or an immediate family member has stock or stock options held in Arthrex. Dr. Champ L. Baker, Jr., or an immediate family member has received royalties from Arthrex; serves as an unpaid consultant to Arthrex and Smith & Nephew; and has stock or stock options held in Arthrex. Neither Dr. Atkins nor any immediate family member has received anything of value from or has stock or stock options held in a commercial company or institution related directly or indirectly to the subject of this chapter.

Section 1: Sports Medicine

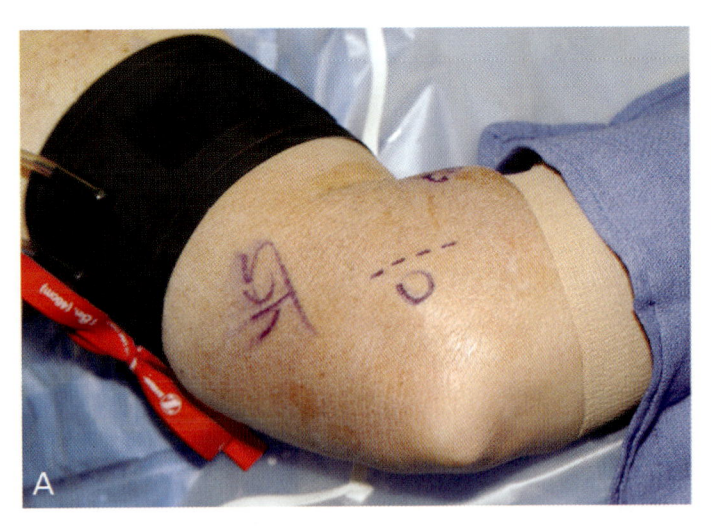

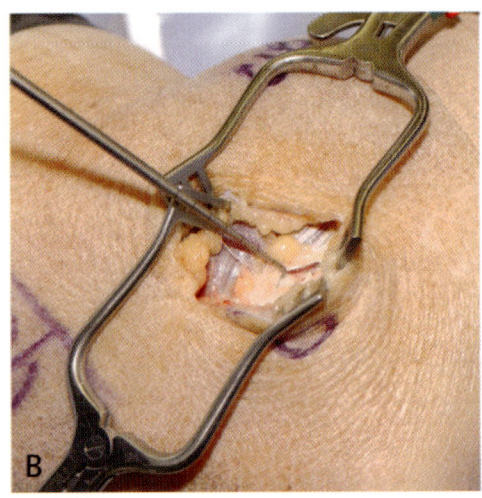

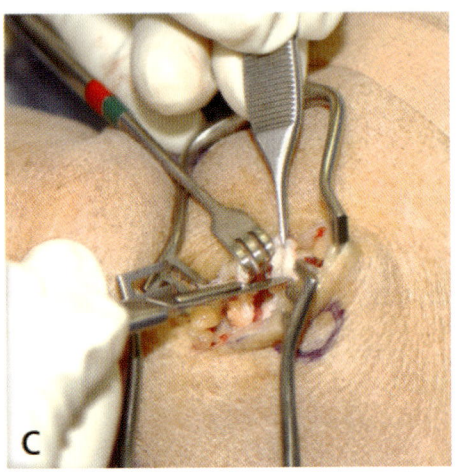

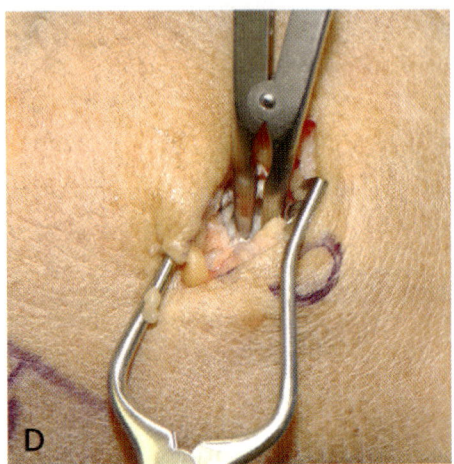

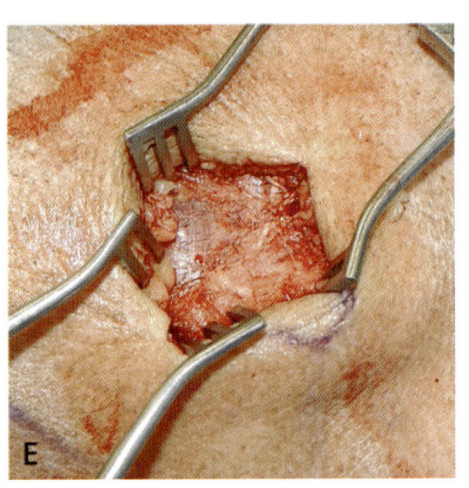

Figure 2 Intraoperative photographs demonstrate open treatment of lateral epicondylitis. **A,** The planned incision is marked anteromedial to the palpable and outlined lateral epicondyle. **B,** The interface between the anterior extensor carpi radialis longus (ECRL) and the more posterior extensor digitorum communis (EDC) is identified and superficially split. **C,** The pathologic extensor carpi radialis brevis tendinosis tissue is resected en bloc with a scalpel. **D,** A rongeur is used to roughen the lateral condyle to create a healing response. **E,** The ECRL/EDC aponeurosis is repaired with a running No. 1 absorbable suture (not visible in this photo). Débridement and closure of the extensor split is complete.

the flexor carpi radialis (FCR) is sharply detached from the medial epicondyle and reflected distally (**Figure 3, C** and **D**). It is important to leave a good cuff of tissue on the medial epicondyle for later flexor origin repair. The PT and the FCR are the most common sites of pathologic tendinosis tissue. Abnormal tissue is identified again by its characteristic dull, gray, edematous appearance.[6] Resection of the pathologic tissue is accomplished with sharp dissection and completed with the scalpel scratch test (**Figure 3, E**). The medial epicondyle is roughened with a rongeur to stimulate a healing response (**Figure 3, F**).

Management of the ulnar nerve during the procedure is based on the preoperative clinical evaluation. In patients with mild preoperative ulnar nerve symptoms, we prefer to perform an in situ ulnar nerve decompression (**Figure 3, G**). For patients with moderate or severe ulnar neuropathy or with evidence of a subluxating or dislocating ulnar nerve, we perform an anterior subcutaneous ulnar nerve transposition.

The flexor origin is securely repaired back to the medial epicondyle with several No. 1 absorbable sutures (**Figure 3, H**). The subcutaneous tissues and skin are closed in a routine fashion. A well-padded posterior splint is applied with the elbow flexed to 90°.

Complications

Following open treatment of lateral epicondylitis, the primary complication is persistent pain due to either inadequate resection of pathologic tendinosis tissue or an incorrect diagnosis by the physician. Excessive surgical dissection can cause iatrogenic injury to the lateral ulnar collateral ligament and can result in posterolateral rotatory instability of the elbow.

With open treatment of medial epicondylitis, a potential complication is injury to the medial antebrachial cutaneous nerve from the surgical approach, with resultant neuroma formation. Inadequate repair of the flexor pronator mass after tendinosis resection can result in postoperative weakness and pain. Injury to the underlying ulnar collateral ligament during resection of the flexor pronator pathoanatomy can result in iatrogenic valgus instability of the elbow. Failure to recognize and appropriately address the presence of concurrent preoperative ulnar nerve symptoms will lead to persistent ulnar neuropathy and a poorer outcome.

Postoperative Care and Rehabilitation

Similar postoperative protocols are followed for both lateral and medial epicondylitis. The splint is removed at approximately 1 week after surgery, and range-of-motion exercises for the elbow and wrist are instituted. Gentle strengthening exercises are begun around 4 to 6 weeks after surgery once full painless motion is obtained. A counterforce

Chapter 7: Open Treatment of Medial and Lateral Epicondylitis

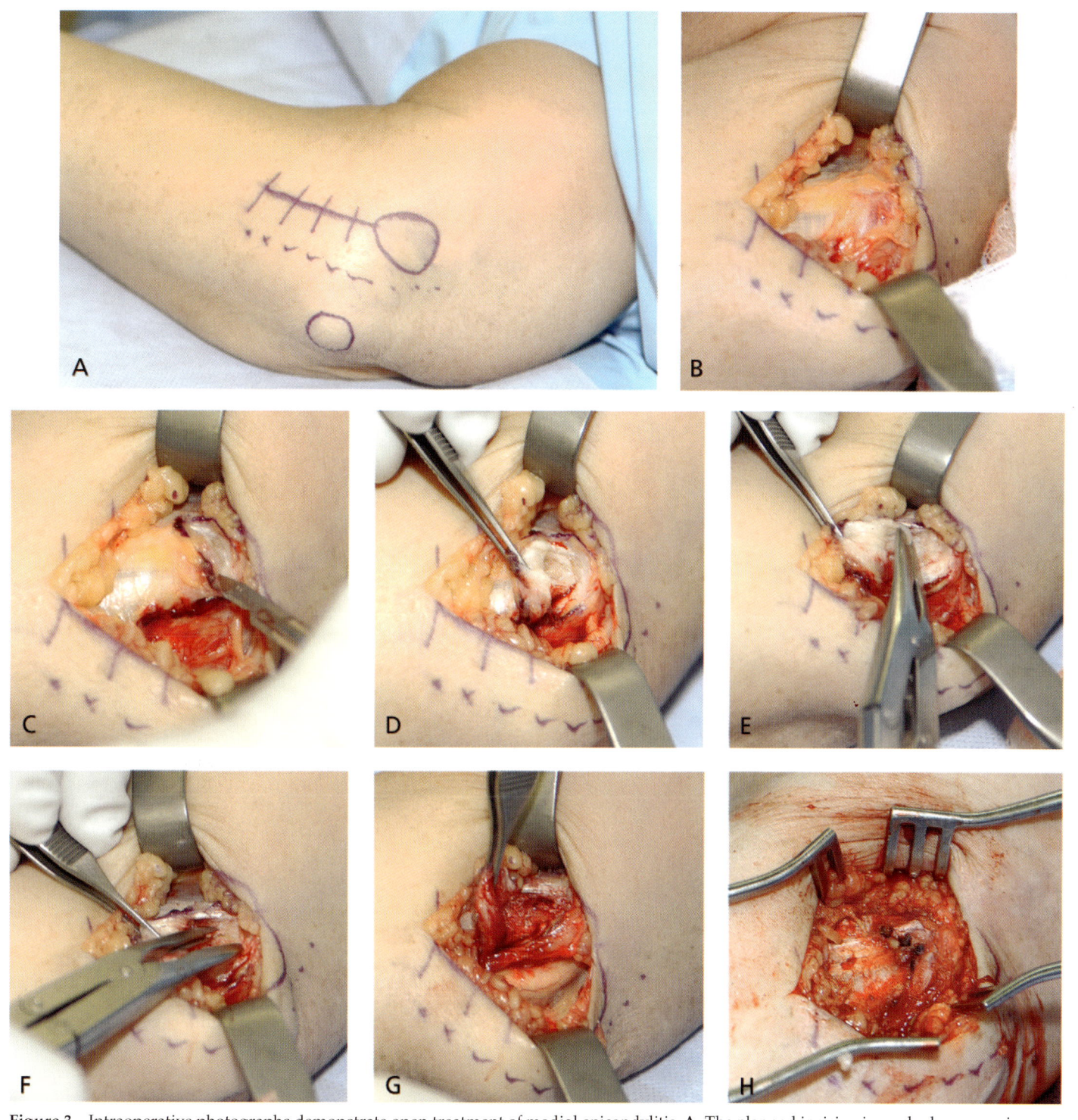

Figure 3 Intraoperative photographs demonstrate open treatment of medial epicondylitis. **A,** The planned incision is marked, progressing distally from the medial epicondyle. The medial epicondyle, the olecranon, and the position of the ulnar nerve are outlined on the skin. **B,** Dissection progresses through the subcutaneous tissues to the deep fascia of the flexor pronator mass. **C,** The planned area of detachment of the flexor pronator origin is outlined and scored with a scalpel. **D,** A portion of the flexor pronator origin is detached from the medial epicondyle and reflected distally. A good cuff of tissue remains proximally for later repair. **E,** The tendinosis tissue is removed from the undersurface of the flexor pronator tendons. **F,** A rongeur is used to roughen the medial epicondyle to create a healing response. **G,** The ulnar nerve is identified and either simply decompressed or transposed, based on the presence and severity of preoperative ulnar nerve symptoms. **H,** The flexor pronator mass is securely repaired back to the medial epicondyle with No. 1 absorbable sutures.

brace can be worn for therapy and for more vigorous activities of daily living. Once painless full motion and strength are achieved, the patient is allowed to resume full sports participation without restrictions—usually at 3 to 4 months after surgery.

Pearls
- When detaching the flexor pronator origin, the surgeon must leave a healthy cuff of tissue to the medial epicondyle to permit a secure repair that will allow for early rehabilitation.
- The scratch test as described by Nirschl et al is an effective method to separate and remove the pathologic tissue from the healthy tendon.[4,5]
- Appropriate postoperative rehabilitation greatly aids the return of painless full elbow motion and strength.

© 2013 American Academy of Orthopaedic Surgeons

References

1. Vangsness CT Jr, Jobe FW: Surgical treatment of medial epicondylitis: Results in 35 elbows. *J Bone Joint Surg Br* 1991;73(3):409-411.
2. Baker CL Jr, Baker CL III: Long-term follow-up of arthroscopic treatment of lateral epicondylitis. *Am J Sports Med* 2008;36(2):254-260.
3. Szabo SJ, Savoie FH III, Field LD, Ramsey JR, Hosemann CD: Tendinosis of the extensor carpi radialis brevis: An evaluation of three methods of operative treatment. *J Shoulder Elbow Surg* 2006;15(6):721-727.
4. Nirschl RP, Pettrone FA: Tennis elbow: The surgical treatment of lateral epicondylitis. *J Bone Joint Surg Am* 1979;61(6A):832-839.
5. Dunn JH, Kim JJ, Davis L, Nirschl RP: Ten- to 14-year follow-up of the Nirschl surgical technique for lateral epicondylitis. *Am J Sports Med* 2008;36(2):261-266.
6. Ollivierre CO, Nirschl RP, Pettrone FA: Resection and repair for medial tennis elbow: A prospective analysis. *Am J Sports Med* 1995;23(2):214-221.
7. Kurvers H, Verhaar J: The results of operative treatment of medial epicondylitis. *J Bone Joint Surg Am* 1995;77(9):1374-1379.
8. Gabel GT, Morrey BF: Operative treatment of medial epicondylitis: Influence of concomitant ulnar neuropathy at the elbow. *J Bone Joint Surg Am* 1995;77(7):1065-1069.
9. Calfee RP, Patel A, DaSilva MF, Akelman E: Management of lateral epicondylitis: Current concepts. *J Am Acad Orthop Surg* 2008;16(1):19-29.

Chapter 8
Distal Biceps Repair

Lauren E. Geaney, MD   Robert A. Arciero, MD   Anthony A. Romeo, MD
Augustus D. Mazzocca, MS, MD

Patient Selection

Patients with an acute distal biceps tendon rupture usually describe a specific event of a sudden extension force on a flexed elbow and may report hearing a "pop" at the time of rupture.[1] Initially, the pain is sharp and tearing in the anterior forearm; it evolves into an aching pain persisting for weeks to months. Many have ecchymosis in the antecubital fossa and swelling and tenderness.[2] Morrey[3] described three criteria for diagnosis: (1) a history of a single traumatic event, (2) grossly palpable and visible signs of proximal retraction of the distal end of the biceps, and (3) weakness of flexion of the elbow and supination of the forearm. The O'Driscoll hook test may be used to identify an absence of the distal insertion:[4] The patient's arm is flexed to 90°, and the patient supinates the arm. If the distal tendon is intact, the examiner can hook a finger underneath. If absent, there is no structure to hook.

Most patients with an acute complete rupture of the distal biceps tendon should be offered surgery.[3] These are most often middle-aged, active men. Patients with significant comorbidities may be poor candidates. A discussion is conducted with all patients involving the risks and benefits of the procedure, and more sedentary patients may opt for nonsurgical treatment. In our practice, these patients are given a trial of physical therapy for 3 to 4 weeks and are encouraged to continue daily activities. If symptoms are unbearable at this time, they may undergo surgery. We recommend initial nonsurgical treatment of partial ruptures. If pain continues despite physical therapy, and weakness is unacceptable to the patient, surgical treatment is undertaken. Patients with chronic symptomatic ruptures are also offered surgery.[3]

Preoperative Imaging

AP and lateral radiographs are obtained to rule out fracture or other pathology. Occasionally, hypertrophy or avulsion of the radial tuberosity can be seen.[1,4,5] Diagnosis is primarily clinical, but MRI may be helpful for confirmation or in the case of partial ruptures. MRI can also help to identify the amount of tendon retraction for preoperative planning[2] (**Figures 1** and **2**).

Video 8.1 Cadaveric Demonstration: Distal Biceps Tendon Fixation. Anthony A. Romeo, MD; Augustus D. Mazzocca, MS, MD (32 min)

Procedure

Special Instruments/Equipment/Implants

Surgical techniques for distal biceps repairs are numerous, and a wide variety of fixation methods may be used. Our preferred method is a combination of a cortical button with interference screw fixation. We usually use an 8- × 12-mm interference screw. Other options include bone tunnels, suture anchors, and either a cortical button or interference screw alone.

Surgical Technique

Repair of the distal biceps may be nonanatomic or anatomic. The nonanatomic technique sutures the biceps tendon to the brachialis, in a simple procedure with limited dissection but which sacrifices supination power.[6] This is also a possible solution in cases of chronic ruptures where the tendon is retracted. Anatomic approaches reinsert the tendon to the radial tuberosity, restoring both supination and flexion strength. The initial approach was a single-incision anterior approach. However, a high incidence of nerve injuries were reported.[3]

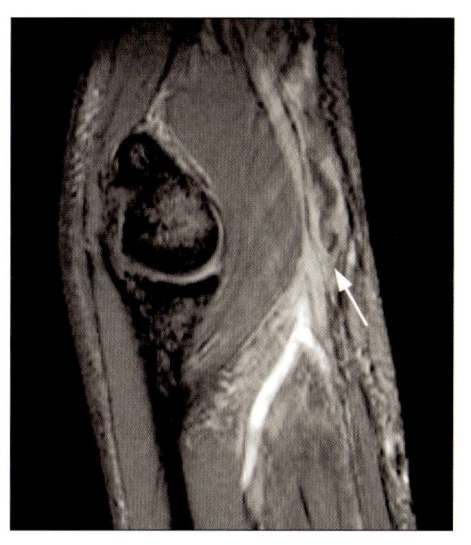

Figure 1 Sagittal MRI shows a torn biceps tendon (arrow) retracted 6 cm.

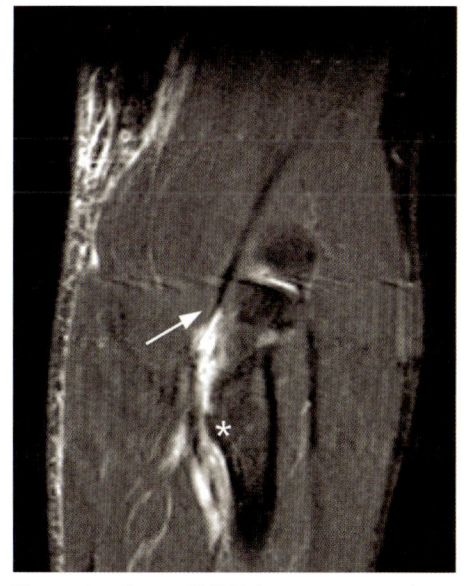

Figure 2 Coronal MRI shows a retracted biceps tendon (arrow) torn from the radial tuberosity (asterisk).

Dr. Geaney or an immediate family member serves as a board member, owner, officer, or committee member of the Connecticut Orthopaedic Society. Dr. Arciero or an immediate family member is a member of a speakers' bureau or has made paid presentations on behalf of Arthrex; has stock or stock options held in Soft Tissue Regeneration; and has received research or institutional support from Arthrex. Dr. Romeo or an immediate family member has received royalties from Arthrex; is a member of a speakers' bureau or has made paid presentations on behalf of Arthrex, DJ Orthopaedics, and the Joint Restoration Foundation; serves as a paid consultant to or is an employee of Arthrex; has received research or institutional support from Arthrex and DJ Orthopaedics; and serves as a board member, owner, officer, or committee member of the American Orthopaedic Society for Sports Medicine, the American Shoulder and Elbow Surgeons, and the Arthroscopy Association of North America. Dr. Mazzocca or an immediate family member serves as a paid consultant to or is an employee of Arthrex and has received research or institutional support from Arthrex and Arthrosurface.

Section 1: Sports Medicine

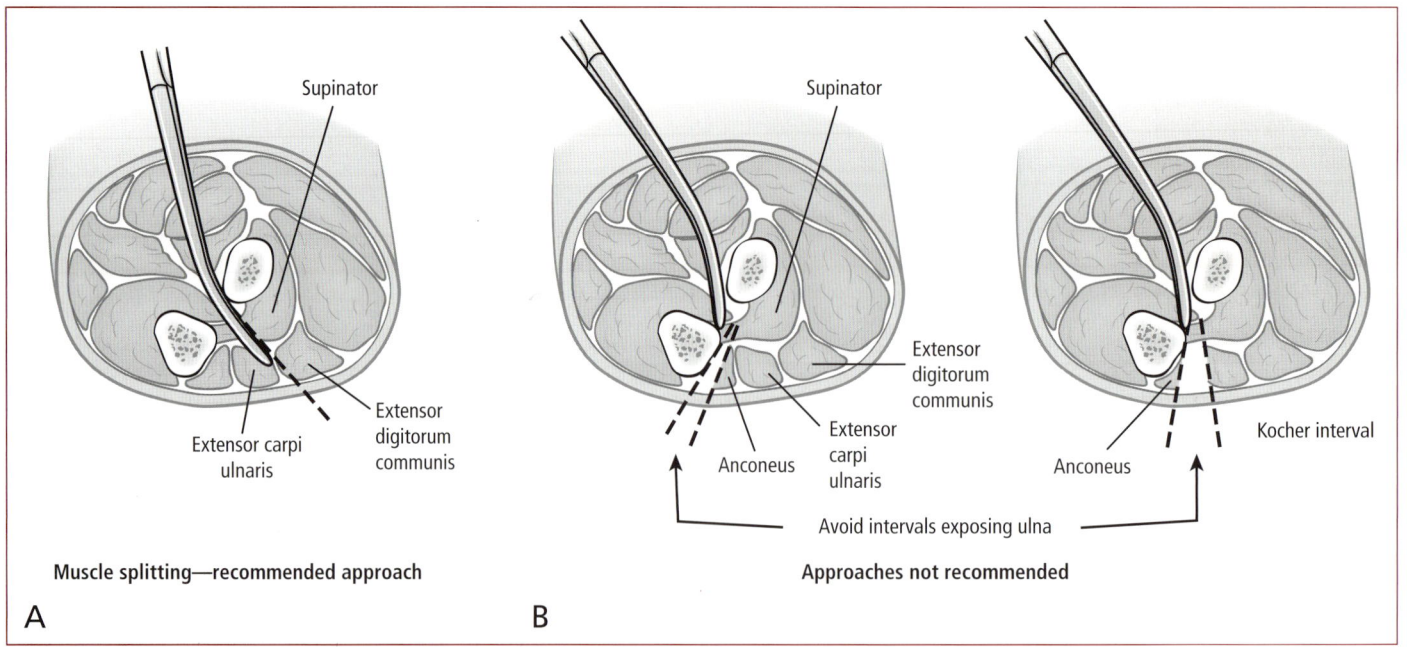

Figure 3 Illustrations demonstrate the two-incision approach for distal biceps repair. **A,** With the arm supinated, a clamp is advanced along the medial border of the radial tuberosity to the dorsolateral aspect of the proximal forearm. **B,** Exposure of the ulna should be avoided to reduce the risk of heterotopic ossification.

In 1961, trying to avoid these complications, Boyd and Anderson[7] introduced a method for reinserting the distal biceps tendon using a two-incision approach. Although their method reduced nerve injury, a higher rate of heterotopic ossification and radioulnar synostosis was reported.

In response, Morrey et al[8] modified the procedure to avoid subperiosteal elevation and advocated a muscle-splitting approach with copious irrigation to reduce the rates of heterotopic ossification and synostosis. However, complications continued to occur,[9] prompting the development of new one-incision anterior approaches, avoiding the extensive dissection necessary with two incisions.

Boyd and Anderson Two-Incision Approach

Boyd and Anderson[7] originally described an anterior S-shaped incision through which the tendon is identified and a posterolateral incision through which the lateral epicondylar extensor muscle group is detached and the radial tuberosity is exposed. Incisions now include the S incision, horizontal incisions, and vertical incisions, depending on surgeon preference.

A transverse incision about 2 to 4 cm long is made over the anterior elbow. Deep fascia is incised, and the biceps tendon is located and tagged with a heavy suture. The tendon is often retracted up to 7 cm. Care must be taken to protect the lateral antebrachial cutaneous nerve.[10] The nerve is identified in the antecubital fossa where it exits between the biceps and the brachioradialis.[5] Hemostasis is imperative at this point in the procedure. Dissection is then carried down to the radial tuberosity.

With the forearm fully supinated, a Kelly clamp is advanced along the medial border of the radial tuberosity to the dorsolateral aspect of the proximal forearm[2] (**Figure 3**). The elbow is flexed, and the second posterolateral incision is made over the palpated clamp. The fascia is again incised over the muscle mass. An interval is developed between the anconeus and the extensor carpi ulnaris.[10] Care is taken to avoid going too posteriorly and disrupting the periosteum. The supinator is sharply incised to expose the radial tuberosity, with the arm in maximal pronation to protect the posterior interosseous nerve (PIN) and expose the tuberosity.[2] This exposure may be used regardless of fixation beyond this point. If a bone bridge will be used, the tuberosity is burred down with holes drilled to pass tendon sutures from anterior to posterior and tied.

Single-Incision Approach

A transverse incision about 2 to 4 cm long is made over the anterior elbow, three fingerbreadths distal to the elbow crease. The subcutaneous tissue is dissected carefully to identify the lateral antebrachial cutaneous nerve.[10] The biceps

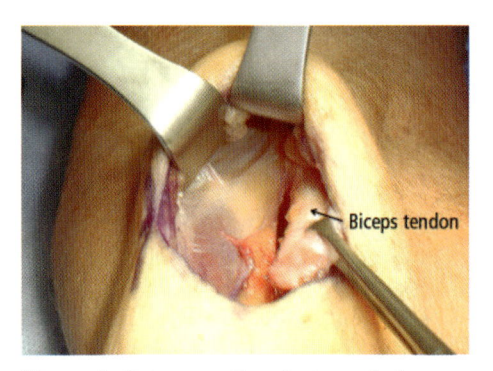

Figure 4 Intraoperative photograph shows single-incision approach for distal biceps repair. A transverse incision is made distal to the elbow crease and the biceps tendon is identified.

tendon can usually be located by tunneling under the skin (**Figure 4**). The tendon is often retracted up to 7 cm and can usually be found in the interval between the flexor and extensor muscle groups. If the tendon cannot be localized secondary to its chronicity and retraction, a second incision may be made proximally over the palpated stump. The nerve is identified in the antecubital fossa, where it exits between the biceps and the brachioradialis.[5] Hemostasis is imperative at this point in the procedure.

Dissection is then carried down to the radial tuberosity. The leash of Henry, an arcade of veins, is usually encountered in this dissection (**Figure 5**). The surgeon must be careful to avoid excessive radial retraction at this time to protect the PIN.

© 2013 American Academy of Orthopaedic Surgeons

Chapter 8: Distal Biceps Repair

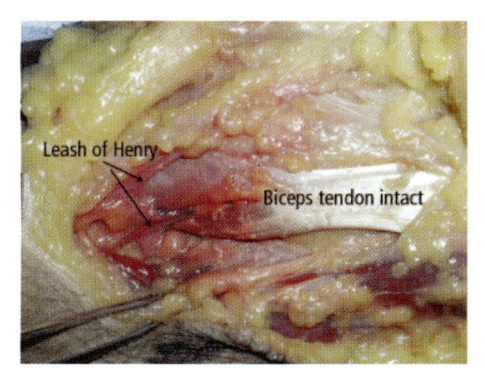

Figure 5 The leash of Henry, an arcade of veins, is identified during the dissection.

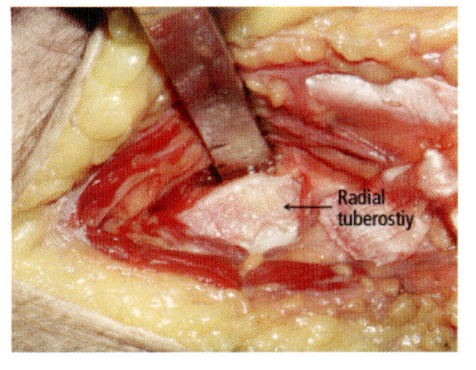

Figure 6 Dissection is carried down to the radial tuberosity, carefully avoiding the PIN.

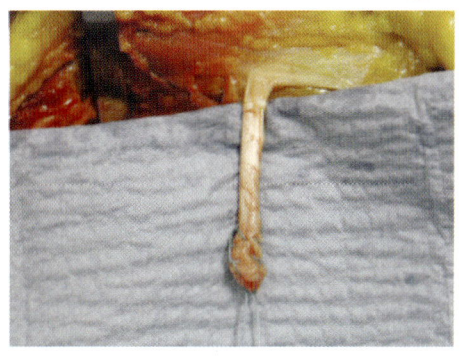

Figure 7 The biceps tendon is exposed and tagged.

Hypersupination allows for maximal exposure of the radial tuberosity (**Figure 6**). A blunt, small Hohmann retractor can be placed on the ulnar side, and any hard retraction on the radial side should be avoided.

Tendon Preparation
The tendon is identified, and any frayed edges should be resected and cleaned up (**Figure 7**). A standard Krackow locking stitch using high-strength nonabsorbable suture is placed in the distal tendon beginning 12 mm proximal to the end of the stump, traveling distally, and passed through the inner two holes of the cortical button 2 to 3 mm from the end. The second suture begins at the distal tendon, goes through the cortical button, and then travels proximally to the level of the first suture and again distally to meet the starting point (**Figure 8**). The longer end of the suture will be placed through the interference screw. Two nonabsorbable sutures are then placed in the outer two holes of the cortical button to pass it.

Alternatively, a FiberLoop, a Keith needle attached to a loop of No. 2 FiberWire (Arthrex), may be used, starting 3 cm from the end of the tendon. This is threaded distally in a Krackow-type fashion. The distal end can then be débrided into a bullet-shaped end. This is then supplemented with a No. 2 FiberWire traveling proximally and then distally—two or three stitches if an interference screw is to be used. The FiberLoop is cut and loaded through the center holes of the cortical button. This will allow the sutures to pass through the holes in the button and reduce the tendon into the hole.

Bone Preparation
The tuberosity is identified, and the proximal cortex is reamed (**Figure 9**). A guide pin for the cannulated reamers is placed into the central area of the tuberosity, making sure good bone (at least 2 mm)

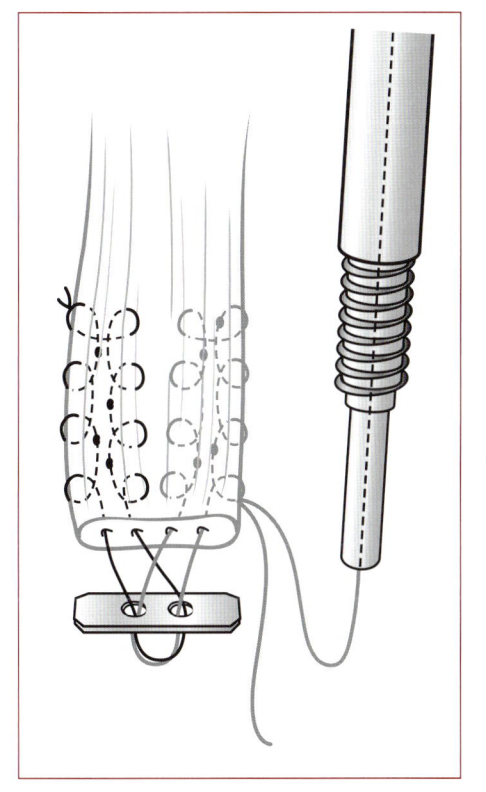

Figure 8 Illustration shows a locking stitch placed starting in the distal tendon, incorporating the cortical button and the interference screw.

is on either side. To ensure drilling is perpendicular to the tuberosity, the arm is placed in hypersupination, and a tunnel is prepared by reaming the near cortex in an ulnar direction. The 7- or 8-mm cannulated reamer is placed down the pin to make sure there will be no cortical blowout. The size of the reamer/screw (7 or 8 mm) is based on surgeon preference. Once the anterior cortex is drilled, the posterior cortex is prepared with a 3-mm spade-tip drill if using the Arthrex BicepsButton or a 4.5-mm tunnel if using an EndoButton (Smith & Nephew Endoscopy). The advantage of the BicepsButton is that passing sutures through the skin is not necessary. The disadvantage is in chronic cases where the tendon is re-

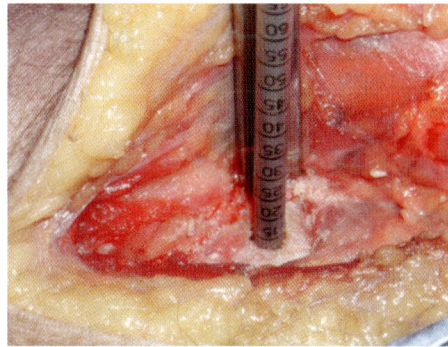

Figure 9 The proximal cortex is reamed perpendicular to the tuberosity with the arm in hypersupination.

tracted; the suture can break when trying to pull the tendon into the tunnel. In this case, the button is difficult to retrieve on the unexposed side of the radius. The EndoButton has the advantage in this situation, but the suture must be passed through the dorsal forearm. The ulnar direction is critical to avoid damaging the PIN. Copious irrigation is required after reaming to minimize the risk of heterotopic ossification. The bone tunnel is tapped.

Fixation
To pass the button if using the standard suture technique, the two outside holes are loaded with two sutures and delivered as described previously. These two outer sutures are passed through the eye of a Beath pin, which is passed through the tunnel. The arm is flexed, and the pin is passed through the dorsal skin. The cortical button is pulled through the dorsal cortex and then secured and confirmed by toggling.

If using the FiberLoop or Biceps Button, the button is passed through the anterior cortex with either a snap or an inserter device. The cortical button will then be deployed as it is passed. A mini C-arm can be used to confirm that the cortical button has appropriately

© 2013 American Academy of Orthopaedic Surgeons

Section 1: Sports Medicine

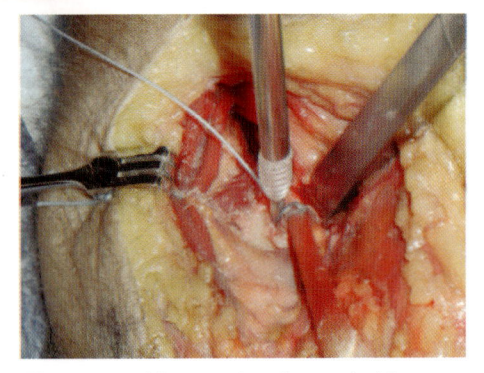

Figure 10 After passing the cortical button, the tendon is held in the bone tunnel while the screw is advanced.

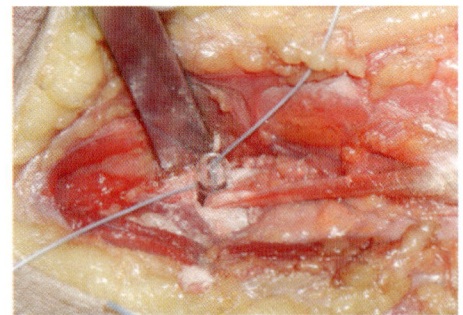

Figure 11 The interference screw is advanced.

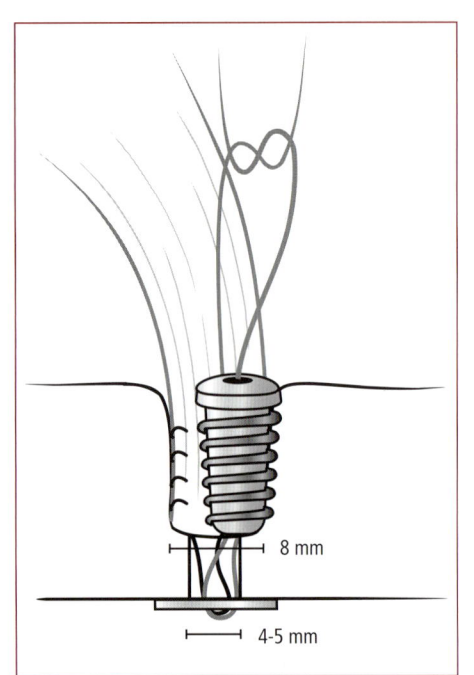

Figure 12 The final fixation of the biceps tendon.

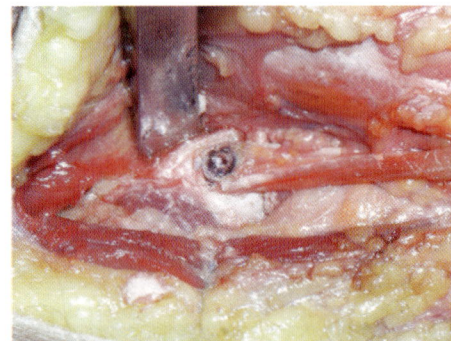

Figure 13 The suture is tied outside the screw after fixation.

caught the posterior cortex and has no soft-tissue interposition. The sutures are then pulled, delivering the tendon into the tunnel. Using an arthroscopic knot pusher, the sutures are tied deep in the tunnel.

The suture ends are then passed through the interference screw. The tendon is then held in the ulnar side of the bone tunnel by the tenodesis driver, and the screw is advanced over it (**Figures 10** and **11**). The suture through the cannulated screw is tied to that outside the screw[9,11] (**Figures 12** and **13**). The tendon should be anatomically fixed to the ulnar side with the screw radially.

Closure

Copious irrigation is essential before closure. The deep tissue of the extensor and flexor compartments is closed with an undyed absorbable suture. This will prevent hematoma and dehiscence. The skin is closed with subcuticular and running subcuticular absorbable suture. Adhesive strips and a soft dressing are then applied. The patient is allowed active assisted flexion and passive extension with gravity. The patient should have full range of motion by the first office visit at 7 days.

Complications

In most series, the most common complication is a nerve palsy of the lateral antebrachial cutaneous nerve, the PIN, or the superficial radial nerve. Lateral antebrachial cutaneous nerve palsy secondary to retraction or injury is reported in up to 5% to 7% of cases.[9]

Historically, nerve injuries were noted to be particularly frequent with the single-incision approach, driving the development of the two-incision approach. Although it addressed one concern, the Boyd and Anderson approach caused significant heterotopic ossification and synostosis. Hypothetically, copious irrigation minimizes the possibility of heterotopic ossification. In a recent retrospective review of 45 patients, 7 patients had nerve palsies, 3 had radioulnar synostosis, 5 had loss of motion, and 5 required reoperation.[12]

Postoperative Care and Rehabilitation

Following the procedure, the arm is placed in a soft dressing with immediate active-assisted flexion and active extension with gravity. Sutures are removed at 7 to 10 days. Full active range of motion commences at 3 to 4 weeks, with strength training at 10 weeks. We aim for a full range of motion at 2 to 3 weeks postoperatively. Most patients are allowed to return to work and full activities between 3 and 6 months.

Pearls

- The lateral antebrachial nerve usually travels with superficial veins, which will help with identification.
- The position of the bicipital tuberosity coincides with the position of the thenar eminence.
- Hypersupination allows maximal exposure of the tuberosity.
- Permanent retraction on the radial side should be avoided to minimize PIN injuries.
- The tunnel should be angled ulnarly to avoid damaging the PIN.
- The insertion of the distal biceps tendon is 2 mm × 14 mm. It twists 90° from the musculotendinous junction to the insertion on the ulnar side of the tuberosity.
- Every attempt should be made to re-create the anatomy after rupture with the tendon on the ulnar side.
- Polyetheretherketone (PEEK) screws are recommended because they are stronger and will not strip as easily as bioabsorbable screws.
- A tap should be used on the tuberosity.

References

1. Bernstein AD, Breslow MJ, Jazrawi LM: Distal biceps tendon ruptures: A historical perspective and current concepts. *Am J Orthop (Belle Mead NJ)* 2001;30(3): 193-200.
2. Mazzocca AD, Spang JT, Arciero RA: Distal biceps rupture. *Orthop Clin North Am* 2008;39(2):237-249, vii.
3. Morrey BF: Injury of the flexors of the elbow: Biceps tendon injury, in: Morrey BF, ed: *The Shoulder and Its Disorders*, ed 3. Philadelphia, PA, WB Saunders, 2000, pp 468-477.
4. O'Driscoll SW, Goncalves LB, Dietz P: The hook test for distal biceps tendon avulsion. *Am J Sports Med* 2007;35(11): 1865-1869.
5. Sutton KM, Dodds SD, Ahmad CS, Sethi PM: Surgical treatment of distal

biceps rupture. *J Am Acad Orthop Surg* 2010;18(3):139-148.

6. Vidal AF, Drakos MC, Allen AA: Biceps tendon and triceps tendon injuries. *Clin Sports Med* 2004;23(4):707-722, xi.

7. Boyd HB, Anderson LD: A method for reinsertion of the distal biceps brachii tendon. *J Bone Joint Surg Am* 1961;43(7):1041-1043.

8. Morrey BF, Askew LJ, An KN, Dobyns JH: Rupture of the distal tendon of the biceps brachii: A biomechanical study. *J Bone Joint Surg Am* 1985;67(3):418-421.

9. Kelly EW, Morrey BF, O'Driscoll SW: Complications of repair of the distal biceps tendon with the modified two-incision technique. *J Bone Joint Surg Am* 2000;82(11):1575-1581.

10. Rios CG, Mazzocca AD: Interference screw with cortical button for distal biceps repair. *Sports Med Arthrosc* 2008;16(3):136-142.

11. Mazzocca AD, Bicos J, Arciero RA, et al: Repair of distal biceps tendon ruptures using a combined anatomic interference screw and cortical button techniques in shoulder and elbow surgery. *Tech Shoulder Elbow Surg* 2005;6:108-115.

12. Bisson L, Moyer M, Lanighan K, Marzo J: Complications associated with repair of a distal biceps rupture using the modified two-incision technique. *J Shoulder Elbow Surg* 2008;17(1, suppl):67S-71S.

Chapter 9
Ulnar Collateral Ligament Reconstruction

Joshua S. Dines, MD   David W. Altchek, MD

Introduction

Injury to the elbow ulnar collateral ligament (UCL) in overhead athletes can be career ending. This ligament, which is composed of an anterior, posterior, and transverse bundle, originates at the inferior surface of the medial epicondyle of the humerus and inserts onto the sublime tubercle of the ulna. It is the anterior bundle that serves as the primary restraint to valgus forces of up to 290 N and angular velocities exceeding 3,100°/s that occur during the throwing of a baseball. Each pitch actually approaches the ultimate tensile strength of the ligament, so it is not surprising that repetitive throwing can cause microtrauma and, eventually, complete failure of the ligament.

Prior to Jobe et al[1] describing a technique for ligament reconstruction that successfully returned athletes to the previous level of play, there were no surgical options for UCL injuries. The technique of Jobe et al[1] involved submuscular transposition of the ulnar nerve, elevation of the flexor-pronator mass to expose the tunnel sites, and a figure-of-8 graft configuration through a tunnel on the ulnar side and three large holes in the medial epicondyle (**Figure 1, A**). Since this initial report, alternative reconstruction methods have been described, including the docking technique (**Figure 1, B**), interference screw fixation techniques, and the hybrid DANE TJ technique[2-4] (**Figure 1, C**).

The docking technique is performed through a muscle-splitting approach; instead of three large holes on the humeral side, a single bony tunnel with two small converging holes is used. We believe that this simplifies graft tensioning and decreases the risk of medial epicondyle fracture.[2,5] Additionally, arthroscopic evaluation of the elbow joint is used frequently in conjunction with the reconstruction, and the ulnar nerve is not routinely transposed.

At this point, most techniques for surgical reconstruction of the UCL reliably return athletes to their previous level of competition between 80% and 90% of the time.[4-7]

Patient Selection
Indications

Reconstruction is indicated in patients with medial-side elbow pain consistent with UCL insufficiency that prevents them from competing at their normal level. Although a complete discussion of the evaluation of medial elbow pain in an athlete is beyond the scope of this chapter, it is important to start with a thorough history. Athletes may report chronic medial-side pain or, less frequently, an acute event. The surgeon must ask about the location of the pain as well as the presence or absence of ulnar nerve symptoms.

During the physical examination, to diagnose UCL pathology, we routinely

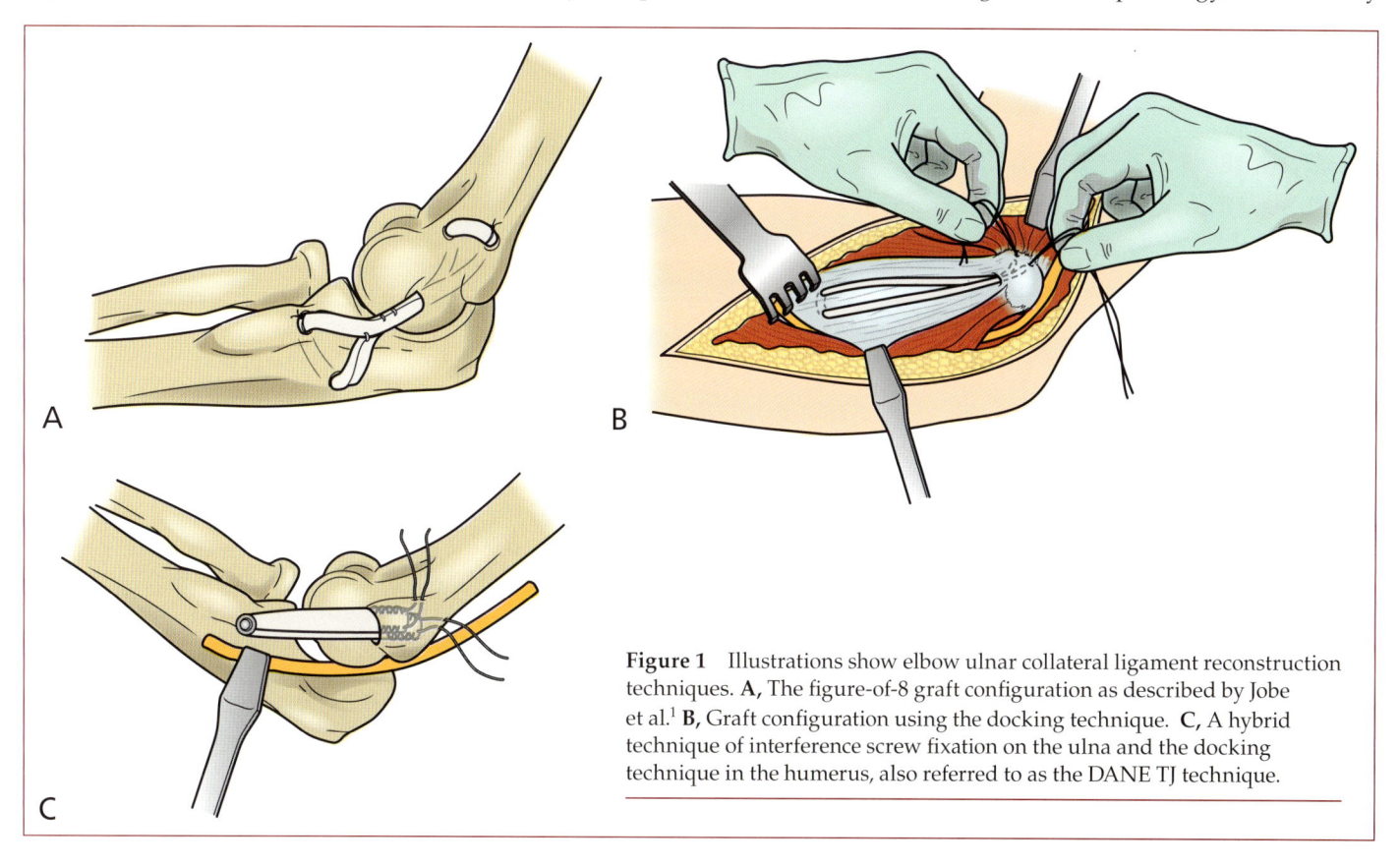

Figure 1 Illustrations show elbow ulnar collateral ligament reconstruction techniques. **A,** The figure-of-8 graft configuration as described by Jobe et al.[1] **B,** Graft configuration using the docking technique. **C,** A hybrid technique of interference screw fixation on the ulna and the docking technique in the humerus, also referred to as the DANE TJ technique.

Dr. Dines or an immediate family member has received royalties from Biomet, serves as a paid consultant to or is an employee of Biomimetic and Tornier, and has received research or institutional support from Biomimetic. Neither Dr. Altchek nor any immediate family member has received anything of value from or owns stock in a commercial company or institution related directly or indirectly to the subject of this chapter.

Section 1: Sports Medicine

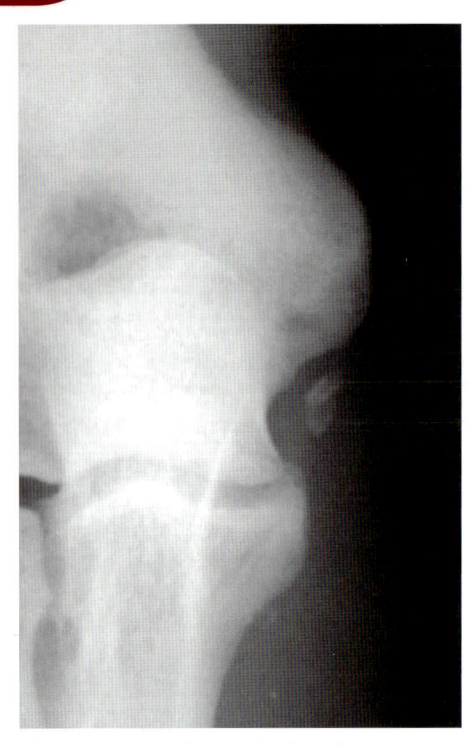

Figure 2 AP radiograph of an elbow shows ossification in the ulnar collateral ligament.

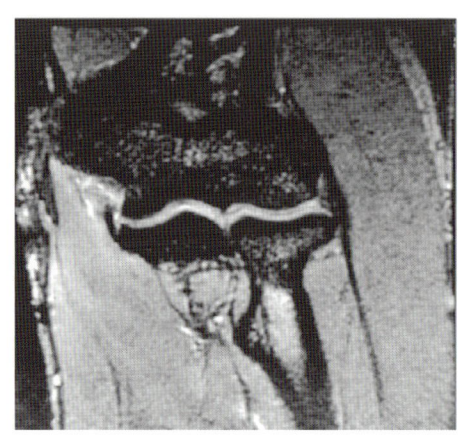

Figure 3 MRI shows a full-thickness tear of the ulnar collateral ligament in the coronal plane.

perform a valgus stress test (noting the presence of both pain and/or instability), the moving valgus stress test, and the milking maneuver. The surgeon should check for the presence of a palmaris longus tendon as a potential graft source. Imaging studies complement the history and physical examination. Radiographs may show calcification in the ligament, bone spurs, or avulsion fractures (**Figure 2**). MRI often confirms the diagnosis of UCL insufficiency and can identify associated injuries, such as flexor-pronator tears, loose bodies, and cartilage injury (**Figure 3**).

When indicated, our preference is to use the docking technique, given its excellent clinical track record and the technical benefits mentioned previously.[5,7]

Contraindications
In the one published study on nonsurgical treatment of UCL injuries, only 42% of the athletes returned to their previous level of play.[8] Therefore, in patients with physical examination and imaging findings consistent with UCL insufficiency affecting their ability to compete at their normal level, surgical reconstruction provides the most predictable outcome. However, if the athlete has no plans or options to continue playing the sport that bothers the elbow, surgery is usually not indicated. An example of this is the high-school senior pitcher who is not good enough to play in college. In situations like this, a change of position to one less stressful on the elbow (eg, from pitcher to first base or designated hitter) often allows the athlete to finish the season without surgery. Additionally, a successful outcome after surgery requires a lengthy course of rehabilitation. If patients are unwilling or unable to complete this year of therapy, surgery is contraindicated.

Video 9.1 Ulnar Collateral Ligament Reconstruction Using the Docking Technique. Joshua S. Dines, MD; David W. Altcheck, MD (5 min)

Procedure
Preoperative Planning
Prior to surgery, the type of graft to be used should be determined. The gracilis tendon and the palmaris longus tendon are the two most commonly used graft choices. Other grafts that have been used include a split segment of flexor carpi radialis, a toe extensor, or a plantaris tendon.

As originally described, the docking technique required arthroscopy at the time of reconstruction to address associated pathology.[2] Over the last few years, likely due to an increasing public awareness of UCL injuries, these injuries are being treated earlier in the disease spectrum; accordingly, concomitant injuries are less prevalent. We now reserve arthroscopy for patients with preoperative physical examination and imaging findings consistent with valgus extension overload.

Routine ulnar nerve transposition is not indicated. However, patients with persistent paresthesias, motor symptoms, or subluxation of the nerve preoperatively are indicated for an anterior subcutaneous ulnar nerve transposition.

Patient Positioning/Special Equipment
The procedure is performed with the patient supine and the affected arm prepped in sterile fashion and draped free on an arm board. For primary reconstructions, No. 1 nonabsorbable suture, a suture shuttling instrument (we prefer looped surgical steel on a curved needle), and several burrs (1.5 mm, 3.5 mm, 4 mm, and 4.5 mm) are the only special equipment necessary. In revision cases or cases of sublime tubercle fracture/insufficiency, one may need to use a Bio-Tenodesis screw (Arthrex) or an EndoButton (Smith & Nephew) for graft fixation.[9]

Surgical Technique
After successful administration of regional or general anesthesia, a nonsterile tourniquet is applied to the patient's upper arm. We begin by harvesting the previously determined graft. If the palmaris longus tendon is used, a transverse incision just proximal to the wrist flexor crease is made, and a No. 1 braided, nonabsorbable suture on an OS-2 needle is placed in Krackow fashion in the tendon (**Figure 4**). A tendon stripper is then used to harvest the tendon. A multiple-incision harvesting technique has also been described. In this situation, after the initial incision is made, two additional transverse incisions are made about 7 and 15 cm proximal to the wrist to expose the entire length of the tendon. The graft is amputated proximally at the musculotendinous junction. Once harvested, the graft is then placed in a moist sponge and protected on the back table. We then exsanguinate the arm and inflate the tourniquet.

A medial approach to the elbow beginning just proximal to the medial epicondyle extending distally over the UCL to a point about 2 cm past the sublime tubercle is used. Care must be taken to protect the medial antebrachial cutaneous nerve (**Figure 5**). A muscle-splitting approach through the posterior third of the common flexor mass within the anterior fibers of the flexor carpi ulnaris is used (**Figure 6, A**). A periosteal elevator is used to bluntly expose the anterior bundle of the ligament. The native ligament is then incised in line with its fibers, which exposes the joint (**Figure 6, B**). A 2-0 Vicryl suture (Ethicon) is placed on each side of the ligament to be used for repair later in the case. Care must be taken when

50 © 2013 American Academy of Orthopaedic Surgeons

Chapter 9: Ulnar Collateral Ligament Reconstruction

placing the suture in the posterior half of the ligament, because the ulnar nerve can be as close as a few millimeters from the ligament.

Next, attention should turn toward the creation of the ulnar tunnel. Again, care must be taken to protect the ulnar nerve posteriorly when exposing the sublime tubercle. Using a 3.5-mm burr, holes are made anterior and posterior to the tubercle, taking care to maintain at least a 1-cm bone bridge between the holes (**Figure 6, C**). The holes are connected with a curved curet. We use looped surgical steel on a curved needle to place a looped suture through the tunnel that will be used for passing the graft later in the case.

On the humeral side, a 4- or 4.5-mm burr (depending on graft size) is used to create the humeral socket in the origin of the UCL on the anterior-distal aspect of the medial epicondyle. It is important to not be too shallow in the epicondyle, as this would leave only a thin roof of bone over the graft and increase the risk for fracture. The socket is drilled longitudinally along the axis of the medial epicondyle to a depth of 15 mm. Two connecting puncture holes are made with a 1.5-mm burr anterior to the intermuscular septum. To ensure that the puncture holes connect, the authors leave a straight curet in the socket. This helps the surgeon's aim and allows the surgeon to hear when the burr contacts the curet. The exit punctures should be located about 10 mm apart on the anterior surface of the epicondyle. Separate shuttling sutures are brought through the humeral tunnel out each exit puncture and clamped for later use. Again, we prefer to use looped surgical steel to pass the shuttling sutures.

First, the graft is passed through the ulnar tunnel using the previously placed shuttling suture (**Figure 7, A**). We then repair the native ligament with the previously placed sutures while the arm is held in about 30° of elbow flexion and forearm supination and while applying a varus stress. Using the shuttling suture from the posterior humeral puncture hole, the posterior limb of graft is shuttled, "docking" it into the medial epicondylar socket (**Figure 7, B**). Application of tension through the grasping suture maintains "docking," or reduction of this limb of graft in the socket. Once again, by applying a varus force with the elbow flexed and the forearm supinated, the elbow is reduced while the graft is cycled

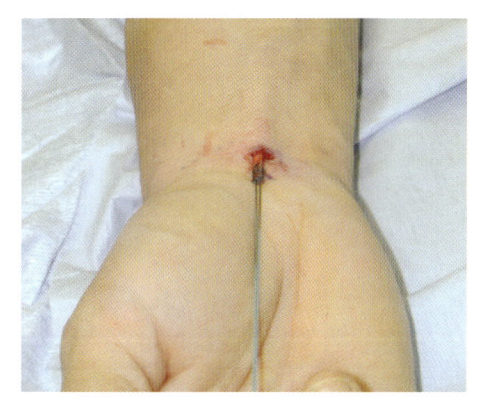

Figure 4 Photograph shows a palmaris longus graft harvested through a transverse incision. A Krackow stitch is placed in the end of the tendon before using a tendon stripper.

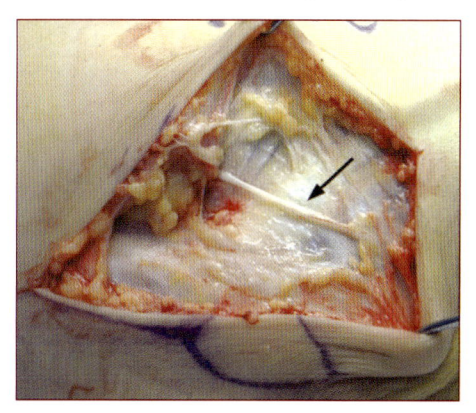

Figure 5 Intraoperative photograph shows the medial antebrachial cutaneous nerve (arrow), which frequently crosses the incision site. It should be protected throughout the case.

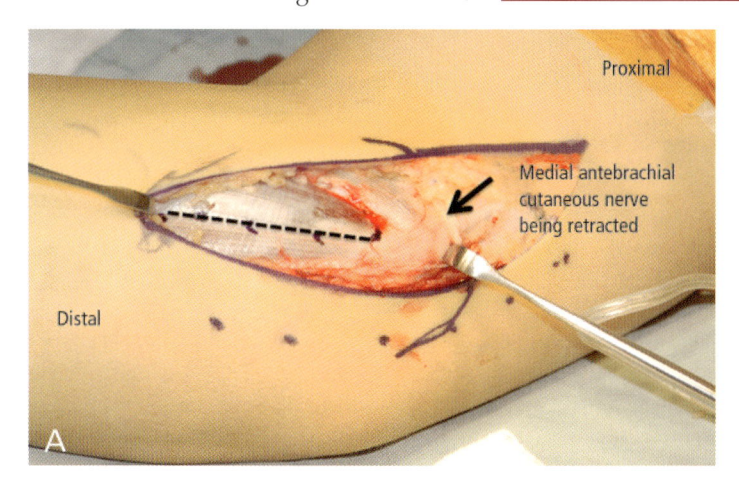

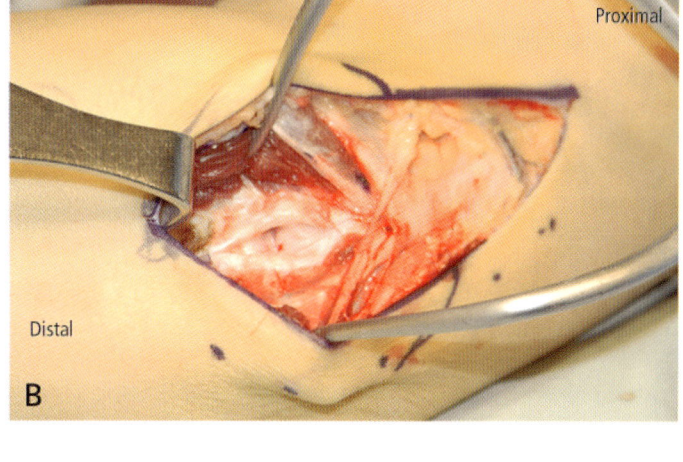

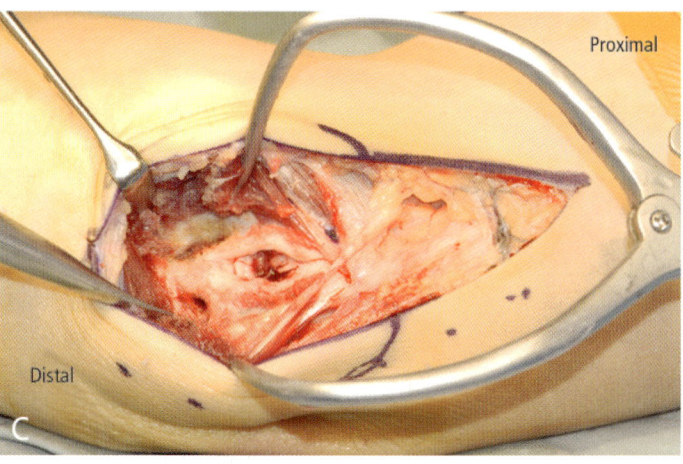

Figure 6 Intraoperative photographs show initial steps in the docking technique for elbow ulnar collateral ligament reconstruction. **A,** The dashed line shows the planned muscle-splitting approach through the posterior third of the common flexor mass within the anterior fibers of the flexor carpi ulnaris. **B,** The native ligament is exposed and then incised in line with its fibers. **C,** The ulnar tunnel has been created, taking care to preserve at least a 1-cm bone bridge between the holes.

© 2013 American Academy of Orthopaedic Surgeons

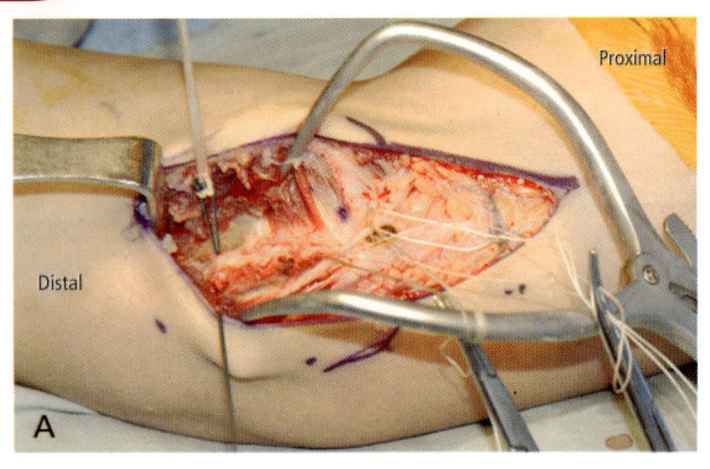

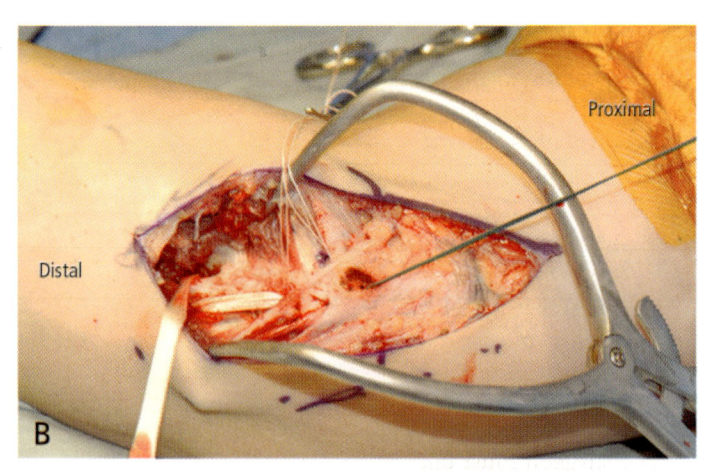

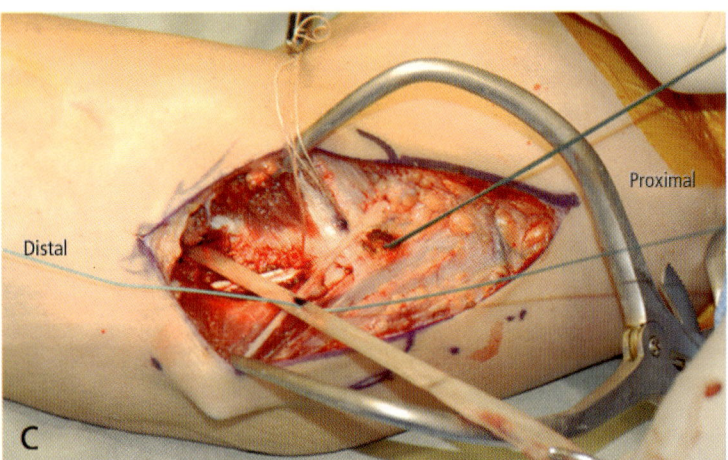

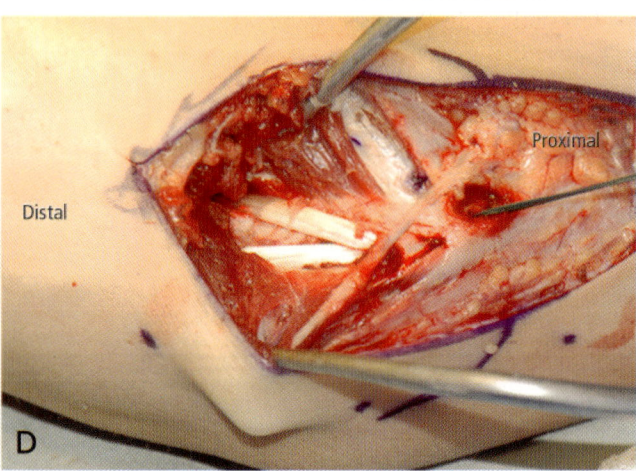

Figure 7 Intraoperative photographs show graft placement for the docking technique for elbow ulnar collateral ligament reconstruction. **A**, The graft is brought into the ulnar tunnel using the previously placed shuttling suture. **B**, The posterior limb of the graft is docked into the humeral socket, after which the anterior limb is marked where it will enter the socket. **C**, A running Krackow stitch is placed from the mark to a point 1 cm proximal. **D**, Final graft configuration.

and tensioned. After an appropriate amount of cycling of the graft to remove creep, the second (anterior) graft limb is then positioned next to the humeral tunnel to approximate the length of graft that will fit in the humeral socket. A No. 1 braided nonabsorbable suture is passed in Krackow fashion for the estimated length to be positioned in the tunnel, typically between 10 and 15 mm (**Figure 7, C**). With tension maintained on the posterior limb and the elbow reduced with varus stress and supination, the Krackow suture is brought through the humeral socket using the previously placed shuttling suture and out the anterior exit hole. Tension on the Krackow suture then "docks" the anterior limb adjacent to the posterior limb within the humeral socket. Final graft tensioning is confirmed, and the grasping sutures are then tied down over a bone bridge (**Figure 7, D**).

The tourniquet is deflated, and hemostasis is achieved. The fascia of the muscle-splitting approach is reapproximated with 0 Vicryl suture. The wound is then closed in layers, and the patient is placed in a posterior splint with the elbow flexed 45° and the forearm supinated.

Complications

The most common complications that can occur during UCL reconstruction are ulnar nerve injury, fracture of the ulnar bone bridge, and medial antebrachial cutaneous nerve injury. The ulnar nerve is particularly susceptible to injury during the drilling of the posterior ulnar tunnel and the posterior connection hole on the medial epicondyle. It is important to be cognizant of the nerve's proximity to the surgical field during these steps.

Fracture of the ulnar tunnel may happen intraoperatively but can also occur late during the postoperative period. The key to minimizing the risk of fracture involves preserving at least 1 cm of bone bridge between the anterior and posterior drill holes on the ulna. One should use a small curved curet to connect the two drill holes. If the fracture occurs intraoperatively, potential salvages, depending on the size of the hole in the ulna, include using a Bio-Tenodesis screw or an Endo-Button.

Medial antebrachial cutaneous nerve injury can lead to painful neuroma formation postoperatively. To minimize this risk, meticulous subcutaneous dissection should be performed, as the nerve almost always crosses the surgical field. Once identified, the nerve should be isolated and protected throughout the case.

Postoperative Care/Rehabilitation

At 1 week to 10 days postoperatively, patients are switched from the plaster splint to a hinged elbow brace with restrictions on range of motion. Initial motion allowed is from 40° to 90°. Motion is advanced to 15° to 105° by week 4. The goal is near-full motion, with discontinuation of the brace by 6 weeks postoperatively. During the first 3 to 4 months of recovery, physical therapy focuses on rotator cuff, forearm, core, and lower extremity strengthening. Any residual loss of elbow or shoulder motion is addressed. Most athletes begin an interval throwing program at approximately 4 months after surgery and progress to throwing off a mound at approximately 8 months. Many throwers find it helpful to work with a pitching coach early in the throwing program to optimize throwing mechanics. Competitive pitching is discouraged until 9 to 12 months after surgery.

Pearls

- Meticulous dissection during the surgical approach will help prevent medial antebrachial cutaneous nerve injury.
- Maintaining at least 1 cm of bone between the holes of the ulnar tunnel is important to prevent fracture.
- The surgeon must take care to not be too shallow in the medial epicondyle when drilling the humeral socket.
- After both limbs of the graft have been docked into the humerus, the arm is held in about 30° of flexion with the forearm supinated and a varus stress applied when tying the sutures.
- A structured postoperative protocol focusing on strengthening and motion of the elbow and shoulder, as well as throwing mechanics, is critical to achieving a successful outcome.

References

1. Jobe FW, Stark H, Lombardo SJ: Reconstruction of the ulnar collateral ligament in athletes. *J Bone Joint Surg Am* 1986;68(8):1158-1163.
2. Altchek DW, Hyman J, Williams R, et al: Management of MCL injuries of the elbow in throwers. *Tech Shoulder Elbow Surg* 2000;1:73-81.
3. Conway JE: The DANE TJ procedure for elbow medial ulnar collateral ligament insufficiency. *Tech Shoulder Elbow Surg* 2006;7:36-43.
4. Dines JS, ElAttrache NS, Conway J, Smith W, Ahmad CS: Clinical outcomes of the DANE TJ technique to treat ulnar collateral ligament insufficiency of the elbow. *Am J Sports Med* 2007;35:2039-2044.
5. Dodson CC, Thomas A, Dines JS, Nho SJ, Williams RJ III, Altchek DW: Medial ulnar collateral ligament reconstruction of the elbow in throwing athletes. *Am J Sports Med* 2006;34(12):1926-1932.
6. Thompson WH, Jobe FW, Yocum LA, Pink MM: Ulnar collateral ligament reconstruction in athletes: Muscle-splitting approach without transposition of the ulnar nerve. *J Shoulder Elbow Surg* 2001;10(2):152-157.
7. Bowers AL, Dines JS, Dines DM, Altchek DW: Elbow medial ulnar collateral ligament reconstruction: Clinical relevance and the docking technique. *J Shoulder Elbow Surg* 2010;19(2, suppl):110-117.
8. Rettig AC, Sherrill C, Snead DS, Mendler JC, Mieling P: Nonoperative treatment of ulnar collateral ligament injuries in throwing athletes. *Am J Sports Med* 2001;29(1):15-17.
9. Dines JS, Yocum LA, Frank JB, ElAttrache NS, Gambardella RA, Jobe FW: Revision surgery for failed elbow medial collateral ligament reconstruction. *Am J Sports Med* 2008;36(6):1061-1065.

Chapter 10
Arthroscopic Management of Femoroacetabular Impingement

Alexis Chiang Colvin, MD

Patient Selection

Femoroacetabular impingement (FAI) is a condition in which there is incongruity in the hip joint. This incongruity can originate from the femoral side (a cam lesion), the acetabular side (a pincer lesion), or both. Labral or cartilage tears or both can result, leading to pain. Patients typically report groin pain, but pain lateral and posterior to the hip can also occur. Pain occurs primarily with activity, such as walking, running, or sports. Patients may also have difficulty sitting for long periods of time and putting on socks and shoes. Some patients may experience a clicking or catching sensation in the hip joint.

When evaluating a patient for possible FAI, a complete history and physical examination should be performed. The history should include asking about any childhood hip abnormalities. The physical examination should evaluate both the range of motion of the hip and the strength of the hip muscle groups. Particular emphasis should be placed on the results of tests for intra-articular pathology, including the Stinchfield test, the anterior impingement test, the posterior impingement test, and the FABER (flexion, abduction, and external rotation) test. Ruling out other orthopaedic and nonorthopaedic sources of pain in the hip area, such as hernias, is also imperative. Responsiveness to an intra-articular anesthetic injection is highly correlated with an intra-articular abnormality.[1]

Indications

Arthroscopic treatment is indicated for FAI when nonsurgical treatment, including NSAIDs and physical therapy, does not relieve the patient's pain. Typically, nonsurgical treatments are tried for at least 6 weeks.

Contraindications

Absolute contraindications to hip arthroscopy include conditions that prevent access to the hip joint, such as advanced arthrofibrosis or ankylosis of the hip joint and severe obesity.[2] Hip arthroscopy is also contraindicated in patients with arthritis and advanced osteonecrosis.

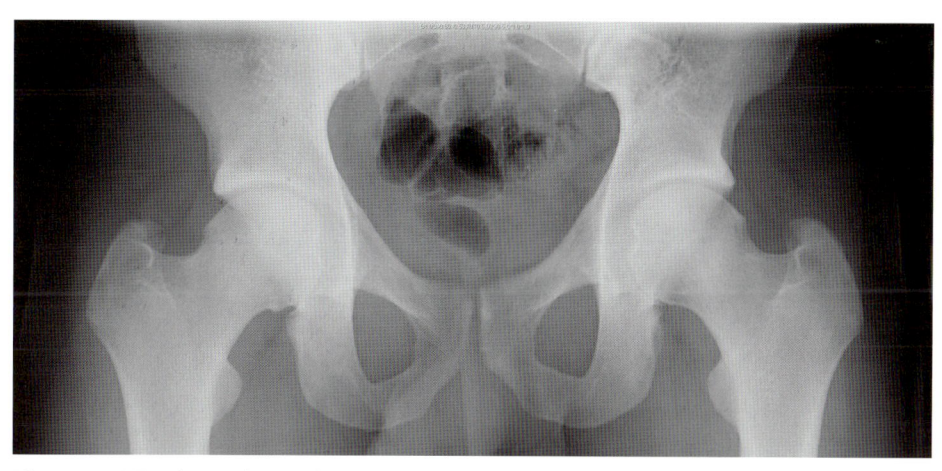

Figure 1 AP pelvis radiograph demonstrates bilateral cam lesions.

Preoperative Imaging

Standard AP pelvis and AP and frog-lateral or cross-table lateral hip radiographs should be obtained, with care taken to position the pelvis such that acetabular version can be assessed correctly. In males, the distance between the pubic symphysis and the tip of the sacrococcygeal junction should be 32 mm; in females, it should be 47 mm.[3] Measurement of the center-edge angle will quantify the amount of lateral coverage. A center-edge angle between 20° and 24° is considered borderline normal, and an angle less than 20° is considered dysplastic. Overcoverage of the femoral head by the acetabulum, known as pincer impingement, can be defined as a center-edge angle greater than 39°.[4] A false-profile view is useful for measuring the anterior center-edge angle. Images should be assessed for acetabular version as well as the presence or absence of a cam lesion (**Figure 1**), herniation pits in the femoral neck, joint space narrowing, and os acetabuli. CT with three-dimensional reconstructions also can be helpful in determining bony abnormalities.

Magnetic resonance arthrography has been found to have a better correlation (100%) with the identification of labral tears at arthroscopy than does conventional MRI (85%).[5] The two techniques are similar for the detection of cartilage abnormalities.[5] Other MRI findings of FAI include paralabral cysts (**Figure 2**), herniation pits at the head-neck junction, and os acetabuli.

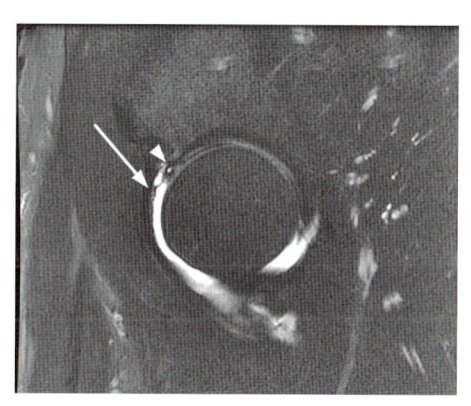

Figure 2 Sagittal T2-weighted magnetic resonance arthrogram demonstrates a paralabral cyst (arrow) and a perforation in the anterosuperior labrum (arrowhead).

Video 10.1 Arthroscopic Management of Pincer- and Cam-Type Femoroacetabular Impingement. Christopher M. Larson, MD; Rebecca M. Stone, ATC (8 min)

Procedure

Room Setup/Patient Positioning

The patient is positioned supine on a fracture table or a flat table using a hip distractor (**Figure 3**). After induction of anesthesia, an examination of the hip should be performed, assessing for any

Dr. Colvin or an immediate family member serves as a board member, owner, officer, or committee member of the American Academy of Orthopaedic Surgeons.

© 2013 American Academy of Orthopaedic Surgeons

Section 1: Sports Medicine

side-to-side differences in range of motion. The patient is then positioned as follows: The feet should be well padded. An oversized, well-padded peroneal post distances the post from the area of the pudendal nerve and helps to add a slight transverse component to the direction of the traction vector. The pelvis should be positioned at the level of the peroneal post and slid toward the nonsurgical side. The hip is positioned in approximately 20° of flexion, 30° of abduction, and neutral rotation. The ipsilateral arm is padded and positioned over the chest away from the surgical field. Slight traction should be placed on the nonsurgical leg before distracting the surgical side to stabilize the torso. Fluoroscopy is used to confirm that adequate distraction can be obtained on the hip. Traction is then released while preparation and draping are performed.

Special Instruments/Equipment/Implants

The instruments and equipment used to perform this procedure include large C-arm fluoroscopy, a fracture table or hip distractor, 30° and 70° arthroscopes, a slotted cannula, a concave extended-length 4.2-mm shaver, an arthroscopic 5.5-mm burr, a flexible electrothermal probe, a suture-passing device, and small biocomposite bone anchors.

Surgical Technique

Several portals have been described for hip arthroscopy (**Figure 4**). The anterolateral portal is marked at the anterior border of the superior aspect of the greater trochanter. The posterolateral portal is marked at the posterior border of the superior aspect of the greater trochanter. The posterolateral portal is marked but not necessarily used unless posterior pathology is present and needs to be addressed. Two anterior portals, the anterior and midanterior portals, are commonly used. The anterior portal is made at the intersection of a vertical line drawn distally from the anterior superior iliac spine and a horizontal line drawn medially from the top of the greater trochanter. Alternatively, a midanterior portal can be placed. This portal is marked at a location approximately 4 to 6 cm distal to the anterolateral portal at a 60° angle. Care should be taken to cut only the skin when placing the portals, especially the anterior portal, to avoid injuring the lateral femoral cutaneous nerve.

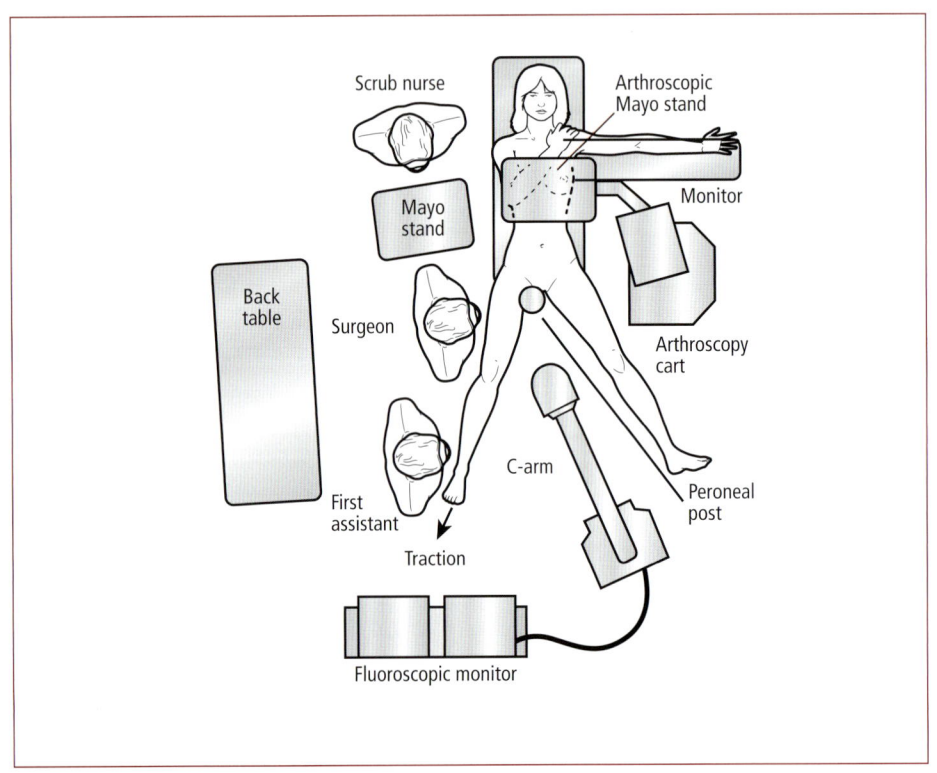

Figure 3 Illustration depicts the room setup for hip arthroscopy.

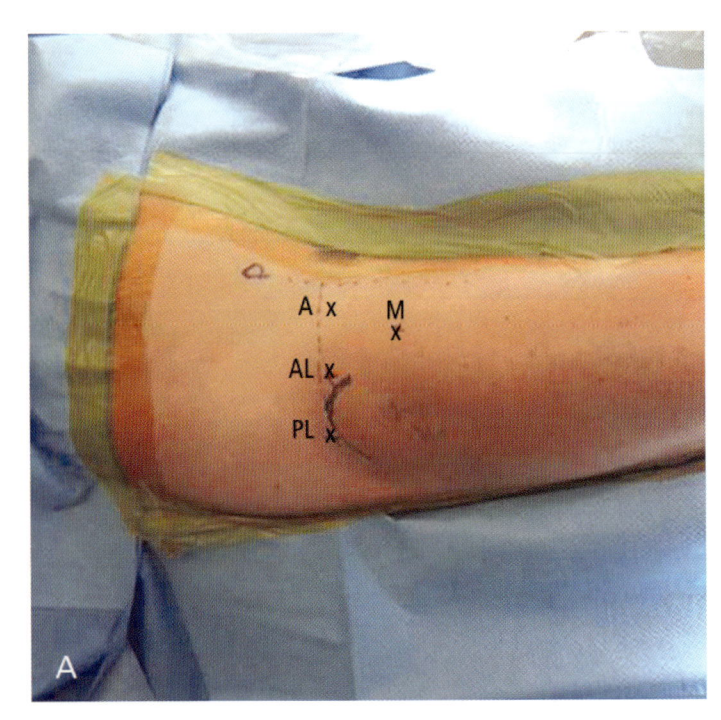

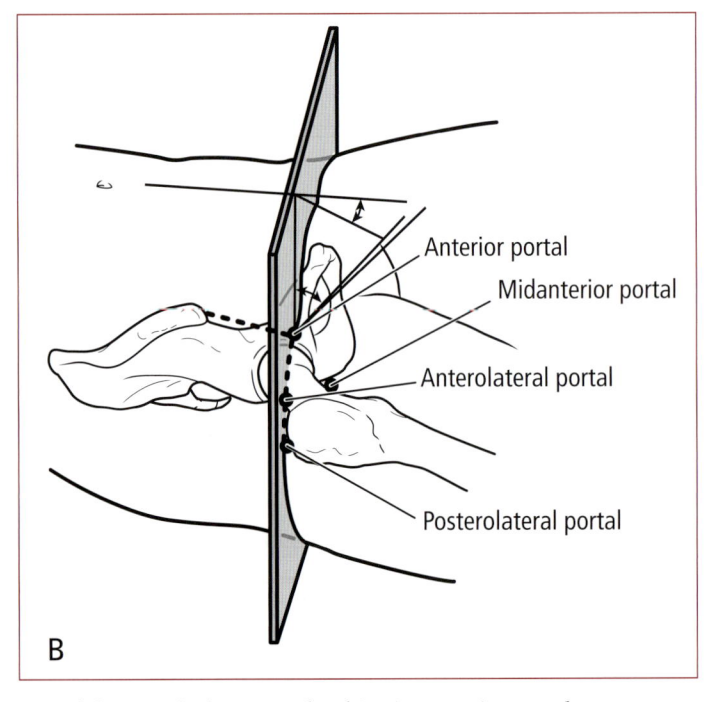

Figure 4 Portals used in hip arthroscopy. **A,** Photograph shows the locations of the portals drawn on the skin. A = anterior portal, AL = anterolateral portal, M = midanterior portal, PL = posterolateral portal. **B,** Illustration depicts the locations of commonly used portals.

The anterolateral portal is made first. Under fluoroscopy, a 17-gauge spinal needle is used to localize this portal. Once the stylet is removed, an air arthrogram can be visualized on fluoroscopy if the hip capsule has been entered successfully (Figure 5). The hip joint is insufflated with approximately 40 mL of normal saline mixed with 1% lidocaine with epinephrine. Care should be taken to avoid penetration into the labrum with the spinal needle. This can be ensured by checking that the needle does not stay superior when the joint distends. If this occurs, the needle should be repositioned. The bevel of the needle should be turned to avoid damaging the articular cartilage. A nitinol guidewire is passed through the spinal needle. Fluoroscopy is used to confirm that the guidewire does not go past the medial wall of the acetabulum. The portal should be dilated to an appropriate size, typically 5 or 6 mm, to allow for the insertion of the arthroscopy sheath.

The 70° arthroscope is used to directly visualize the placement of the midanterior portal. The triangle defined by the labrum, femoral head, and joint capsule should be visualized. The position of the anterolateral portal then should be visualized from the midanterior portal to ensure that the labrum has not been violated. A capsulotomy should be performed to allow better maneuverability of the instruments. With the arthroscope in the anterolateral portal, a beaver blade can be used in the midanterior portal to cut the capsule anteriorly. The arthroscope then is switched to the midanterior portal, the banana blade is inserted through the anterolateral portal to cut the capsule, and the cuts are connected. The capsule is débrided with a shaver to allow more space for maneuvering. A 90° arthroscopic ablator also can be useful when the capsule is particularly thickened.

Diagnostic arthroscopy is performed first through the anterolateral portal and then through the midanterior portal. The 70° arthroscope is best for visualizing the periphery of the hip joint, labrum, and inferior acetabular fossa. The 30° arthroscope is best for visualizing the central acetabulum, femoral head, and superior acetabular fossa.

First, the quality of the cartilage is assessed. At the chondrolabral junction, a wave sign, or bubbling of the cartilage, indicates unstable cartilage (Figure 6). Microfracture should be performed on focal Outerbridge grade IV chondral lesions, similar to those in the knee.

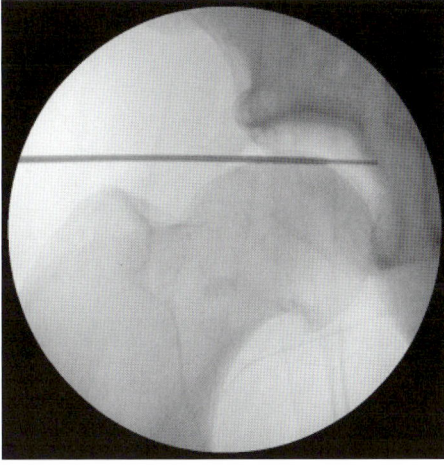

Figure 5 Air arthrogram visualized on fluoroscopy confirms intracapsular placement of the spinal needle.

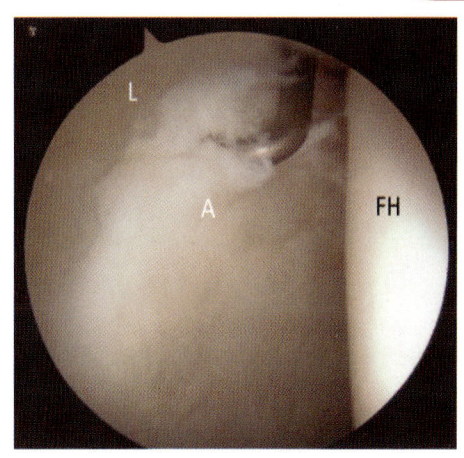

Figure 6 Arthroscopic view shows chondrolabral delamination in a right hip. A = acetabulum, L = labrum, FH = femoral head.

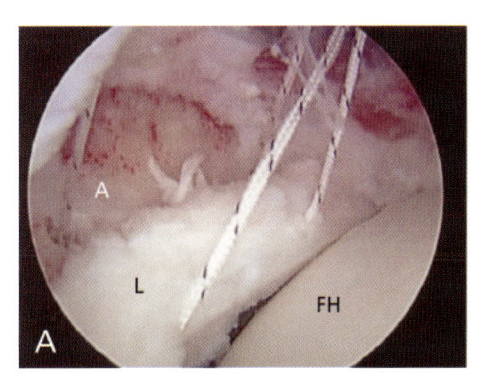

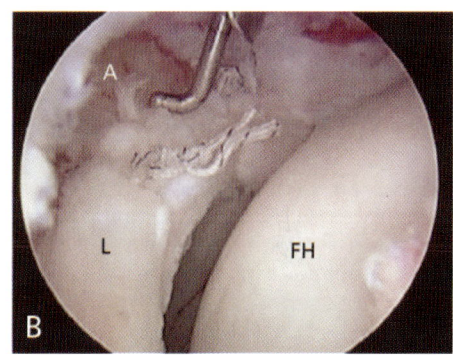

Figure 7 Arthroscopic views show labral repair in a right hip. **A,** The suture is placed in the labrum in a horizontal mattress configuration. **B,** The completed labral repair. A = acetabulum, L = labrum, FH = femoral head. (Courtesy of J.W. Byrd, MD, Nashville, TN.)

Next, the quality of the labrum is assessed. With the arthroscope in the anterolateral portal and the banana knife in the anterior portal, the labrum can be separated from the edge of the acetabulum. A shaver or burr can be used to prepare the edge of the acetabulum. If a pincer lesion is present, it can be addressed at this time. Under fluoroscopy, a burr is used to resect the prominent anterior wall until the anterior wall is medial to the posterior wall.[6] A punch or biter also can be used through the anterior portal to trim any unstable cartilage from the acetabular rim. An 8.5-mm cannula can be placed in the working portal to aid in the passage of instrumentation for repair.

Starting with the arthroscope in the midanterior portal, small anchors (3 mm or smaller) can be placed through the anterolateral portal, beginning superiorly on the acetabular rim. A suture anchor or knotless repair can be performed, using suture-passing devices of the surgeon's choice. The arthroscope then is placed into the anterolateral portal, and the remaining anchors are placed through the midanterior portal along the anterior rim of the acetabulum as needed (Figure 7). If the labral tissue is extremely degenerative and the repair cannot be performed, the labral tear should be débrided selectively to a stable transition zone.

Once the intra-articular work has been completed, the femoral head-neck junction is examined for a cam lesion. Traction is released and the hip is flexed to approximately 45° to allow inspection. Intraoperative fluoroscopy also is helpful for localizing a cam lesion, and if a cam lesion is present, ensuring that an appropriate amount of bone in the correct location has been resected. Often, the lesion can be identified by a change in the appearance of the cartilage (Figure 8, A). Internal rotation will allow visualization of the lateral aspect of the cam lesion, and external rotation will allow visualization of the medial aspect of the cam lesion. The lateral retinacular vessels should be identified (Figure 8, B), as well as the medial synovial fold. The resection should not proceed farther than these two land-

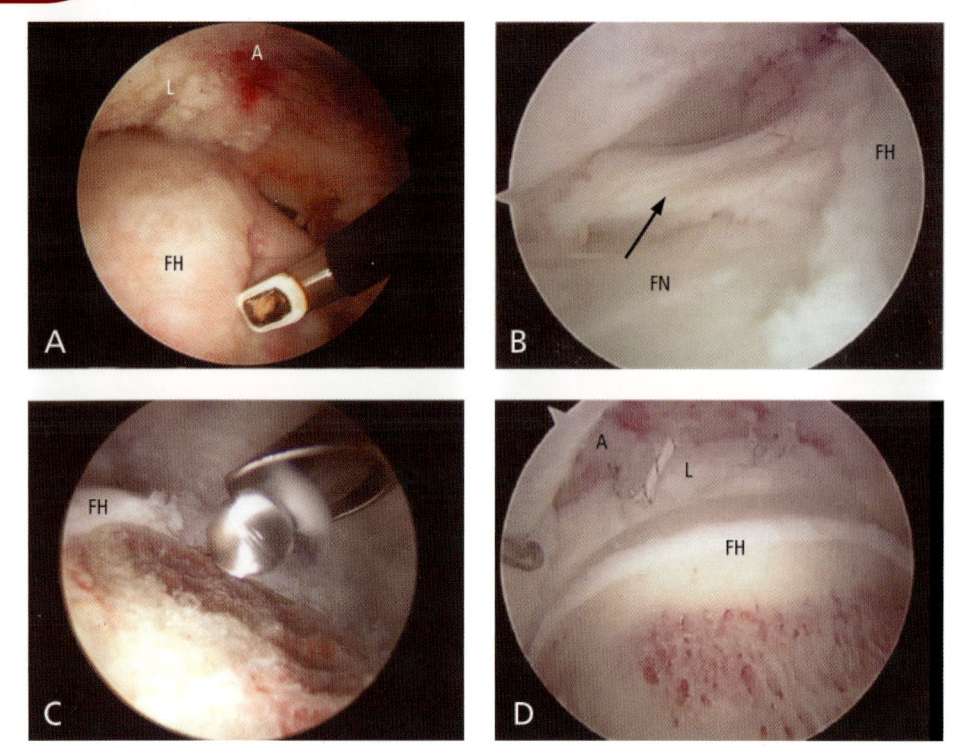

Figure 8 Arthroscopic views demonstrate repair of cam lesions in the right hips of two patients. **A**, Characteristic appearance of a cam lesion. **B**, The lateral retinacular vessels (arrow) are visualized. **C**, Resection of a cam lesion using a burr. **D**, Completed cam resection and labral repair. A = acetabulum, L = labrum, FH = femoral head, FN = femoral neck. (Panels B and D reproduced courtesy of J.W. Byrd, MD, Nashville, TN.)

marks. Care should be taken to avoid injury to the lateral retinacular vessels. A curet can be used to demarcate the line of resection; a 5.5-mm arthroscopic burr is then used for resection (**Figure 8, C**). The hip is extended gradually to reach more superior areas of the cam lesion. After completion of the cam resection (**Figure 8, D**), the hip should be taken through a full range of motion to ensure that no further impinging areas exist.

Complications

One of the most common reasons for the failure of surgery and the need for revision arthroscopy is incomplete resection of a cam lesion, a pincer lesion, or both.[7] Neurapraxia, which can affect the sciatic, pudendal, femoral, and/or lateral femoral cutaneous nerves, often results from poor positioning; typically, it resolves spontaneously.[7] Instrument breakage and iatrogenic cartilage injury also are possible.[7] Other less common complications that have been reported include fracture of the femoral neck after cam resection, postoperative dislocation, and fluid extravasation that leads to abdominal compartment syndrome.[7]

Postoperative Care and Rehabilitation

Patients are placed on a continuous passive motion machine as soon as possible after surgery. Physical therapy, beginning with passive range of motion, typically is begun by the second postoperative day. The patient also is permitted to use a stationary bike with no resistance.

Weight-bearing status depends on the procedure performed. For procedures with no osteoplasty/labral repair, such as loose body removal or labral débridement, the patient is limited to 20-lb foot-flat weight bearing for 2 weeks. When osteoplasty has been performed, weight bearing is restricted for 4 weeks. If microfracture has been performed, weight bearing is restricted for 6 to 8 weeks.

Progressive strengthening begins approximately 6 weeks after full weight bearing is allowed. Between 3 and 6 months, running and sport-specific training are begun.

Pearls

- Confirmation that adequate distraction can be obtained on the hip should be obtained under fluoroscopy before preparation and draping.
- A midanterior portal, rather than the anterior portal, often is helpful when both intra-articular pathology and a cam lesion need to be addressed.
- An adequate capsulotomy facilitates the use of instruments.
- If the hip has been under traction for 2 consecutive hours, the traction should be released. It can be reapplied later if the intra-articular work has not been completed.

References

1. Byrd JW, Jones KS: Diagnostic accuracy of clinical assessment, magnetic resonance imaging, magnetic resonance arthrography, and intra-articular injection in hip arthroscopy patients. *Am J Sports Med* 2004;32(7):1668-1674.
2. Byrd JW: Hip arthroscopy. *J Am Acad Orthop Surg* 2006;14(7):433-444.
3. Siebenrock KA, Kalbermatten DF, Ganz R: Effect of pelvic tilt on acetabular retroversion: A study of pelves from cadavers. *Clin Orthop Relat Res* 2003;407:241-248.
4. Tannast M, Siebenrock KA, Anderson SE: Femoroacetabular impingement: Radiographic diagnosis: What the radiologist should know. *AJR Am J Roentgenol* 2007;188(6):1540-1552.
5. Zlatkin MB, Pevsner D, Sanders TG, Hancock CR, Ceballos CE, Herrera MF: Acetabular labral tears and cartilage lesions of the hip: indirect MR arthrographic correlation with arthroscopy: A preliminary study. *AJR Am J Roentgenol* 2010;194(3):709-714.
6. Larson CM, Wulf CA: Intraoperative fluoroscopy for evaluation of bony resection during arthroscopic management of femoroacetabular impingement in the supine position. *Arthroscopy* 2009;25(10):1183-1192.
7. Ilizaliturri VM Jr: Complications of arthroscopic femoroacetabular impingement treatment: A review. *Clin Orthop Relat Res* 2009;467(3):760-768.

Video Reference

10.1 Larson CM, Stone RM: Video: *Arthroscopic Management of Pincer- and Cam-Type Femoroacetabular Impingement.* Edina, MN, 2011.

Chapter 11
Meniscectomy

Semon Bader, MD   Paul M. Saluan, MD   Richard D. Parker, MD

Introduction

Despite recent advances in meniscal repair and a greater understanding of the functional role of the meniscus, the majority of symptomatic meniscal tears observed at arthroscopy remain irreparable. Meniscal tears may be simple radial, vertical/longitudinal, or horizontal in orientation. More complex patterns include displaced bucket-handle, parrot-beak, multiplanar, degenerative, and meniscal root tears (**Figure 1**). Tears most often involve the posterior horn of the meniscus. The work done to identify the vascularity of the meniscus has been helpful in classifying tears, with peripheral tears, or red-red tears, occurring in an area of good vascular supply. Red-white tears and the most central white-white tears have less vascular penetration (**Figure 2**).

The menisci occupy 60% of the contact area between the tibia and the femur and transmit 50% of the compression forces across the joint.[1] The lateral meniscus plays a much greater role in force transmission than the medial meniscus; the medial meniscus provides secondary stability to anterior translation when the anterior cruciate ligament is torn. When possible, preservation of the menisci should be attempted because their importance in load transmission and as secondary stabilizers has been widely demonstrated. At our institution, meniscal repair is the treatment of choice for red-red and red-white tears in young patients. Radial tears extending into the red-red and even the red-white zone are treated with an attempt at repair as well, with meniscectomy of the central white-white component. Total lateral meniscectomy has been shown by Paletta et al[2] to result in a 235% to 335% increase in peak local contact pressure. Ahmed and Burke[3] found a linear correlation between the increase in peak stress on the tibial joint surface and the amount of medial meniscus excised.

The medial and lateral compartments of the knee appear to be affected to different degrees after meniscectomy. Because of the convexity of the lateral tibial plateau, point loading in the absence of the congruity imparted by the lateral meniscus leads to increases in peak contact pressures in the lateral compartment. This effect is not as profound in the medial compartment because of the relative maintenance of congruity, even in the absence of a medial meniscus.

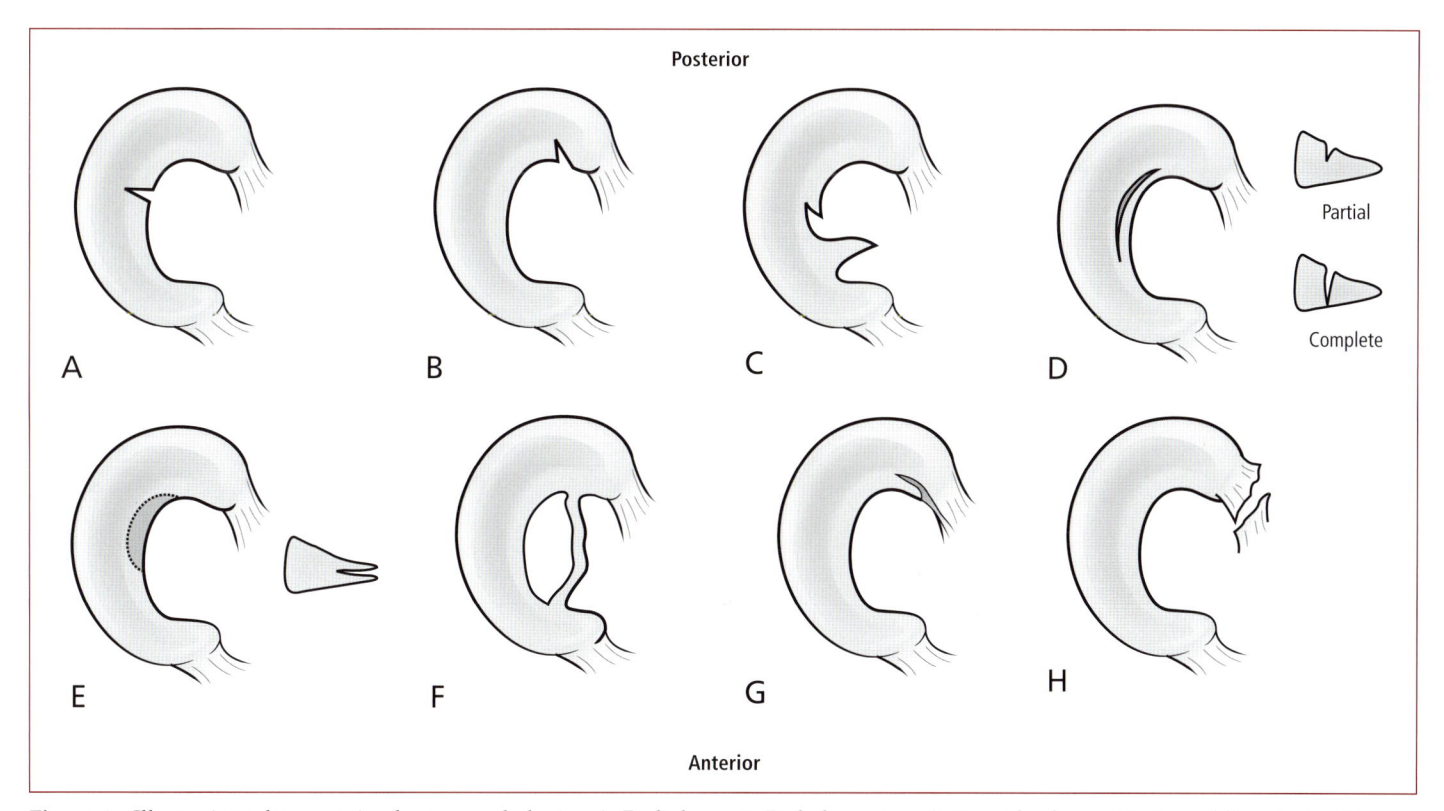

Figure 1 Illustrations show meniscal tear morphologies. **A**, Radial tear. **B**, Radial root tear. **C**, Parrot-beak tear. **D**, Vertical/longitudinal tears. **E**, Horizontal tear. **F**, Bucket-handle tear. **G**, Root tear. **H**, Root avulsion.

Dr. Saluan or an immediate family member is a member of a speakers' bureau or has made paid presentations on behalf of Arthrex; serves as an unpaid consultant to Triatrix; and has received research or institutional support from Zimmer. Dr. Parker or an immediate family member is a member of a speakers' bureau or has made paid presentations on behalf of Smith & Nephew Endoscopy and Zimmer; serves as a paid consultant to or is an employee of Zimmer and Smith & Nephew; and has received research or institutional support from Zimmer. Neither Dr. Bader nor any immediate family member has received anything of value from or has stock or stock options held in a commercial company or institution related directly or indirectly to the subject of this chapter.

Long-term clinical studies have shown radiographic degenerative changes and clinical deterioration of the knee after meniscectomy.[4] The effect is multifactorial; however, the role of the meniscus in pressure distribution via hoop stress is important. Disruption of the circumferential collagen fibers within the meniscal tissue, typically radial in orientation or from meniscal débridement, can prevent the formation of the hoop stresses that develop in the meniscus as it is loaded and may effectively represent a subtotal meniscectomy even after limited débridement. However, an in vitro study by Muriuki et al[5] demonstrated that the disruption to the posterior horn and root may have more impact on loads than disruption of the circumferential fibers caused by radial tears limited to the central two thirds of the meniscus (**Figure 3**). The load-bearing mechanics do not appear to be as significantly affected with longitudinal or horizontal tears.

Patient Selection

Débridement of meniscal tissue should be undertaken in irreparable tears due to significant degeneration, fragmentation, or tearing in avascular tissue. Complex or frayed white-white tears have the least healing potential and are best served with appropriate partial meniscectomy. Stable, partial-thickness vertical tears less than 10 mm in length in the peripheral third may be treated with abrasion or trephination or left alone if showing healing. Patient compliance and family dynamics in younger patients play a critical role in postoperative management and should be taken into account because the indications to repair a meniscus are not absolute. Higuchi et al[4] asserted that the goal is to resect irreparable and/or unstable meniscal tissue, leaving a contoured and smooth remnant of tissue, ideally preserving over 50% of the meniscal rim.

Diagnosis

Clinical evaluation should include a comprehensive history and physical examination. Symptoms of a meniscal tear include knee pain; mechanical symptoms; and pain or swelling with activities of daily living, work, and/or sports. A knee effusion is frequently present and an important indicator and can be associated with reduction in quadriceps strength. Joint-line tenderness and positive McMurray, Apley grind, and Thessaly tests, are also indicative of meniscal pathology. The Thessaly test, first described in 2005, has been shown by Karachalios et al[6] to have an accuracy greater than 94% in anterior cruciate ligament–intact knees. Loss of motion (particularly extension) may represent a displaced segment of meniscus. Discoid meniscal tears typically present in a child younger than 10 years, often with symptoms of intermittent painful episodes of dramatic popping or snapping within the knee. Frequently, the child is unable to achieve full extension, and a "clunk" can be elicited on examination with flexion, extension, and circumduction.

Preoperative Imaging

Standard radiographs should include 30° flexion lateral, Merchant, AP weight-bearing in extension, and 45° PA flexion weight-bearing views. Full-length weight-bearing radiographs can be used if malalignment is suspected and osteotomy is being considered. MRI, particularly 3-T MRI, gives excellent visualization of meniscal pathology and is excellent for ruling out other intra-articular pathology (**Figure 4**). Preoperative MRI is useful for delineating tear morphology and location and helps in predicting the likelihood of repair versus débridement. Matava et al[7] found a 74% accuracy in predicting tear repair based on MRI. Proton density-weighted, high-resolution, fast-spin-echo sequences are best for assessing both menisci and cartilage surfaces. Meniscal root tears require a higher index of suspicion, with meniscal extrusion being highly correlated.

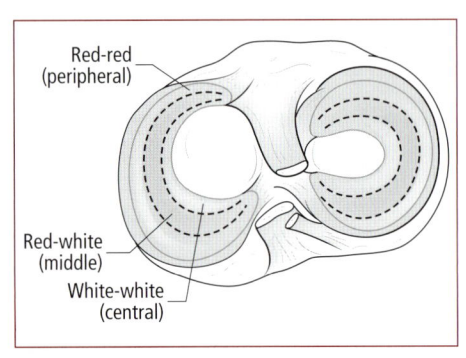

Figure 2 Illustration of the vascular zones of the meniscus. The medial meniscus is on the left, and the lateral meniscus is on the right.

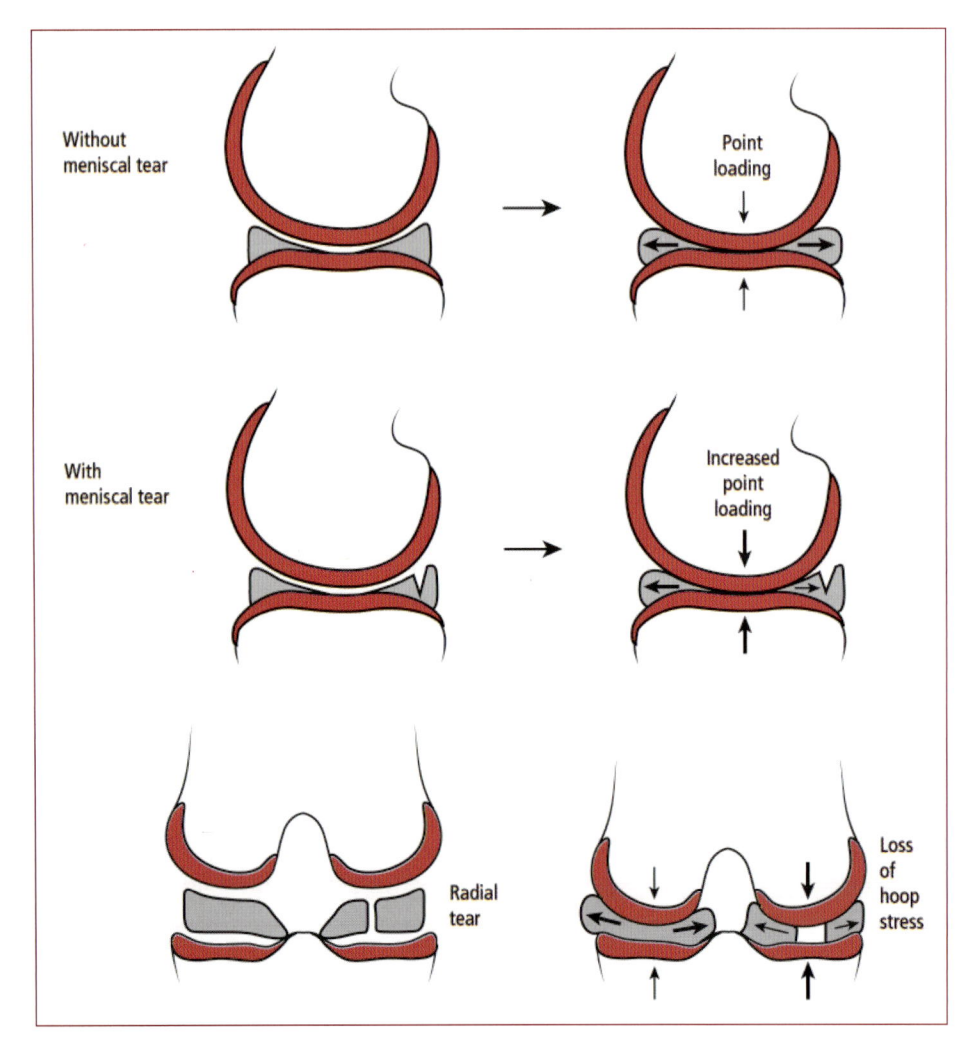

Figure 3 Illustrations demonstrate the maintenance of hoop stress on the uninjured side and loss of hoop stress on the injured side due to a radial meniscal tear.

Radiographic indicators of discoid meniscus may include tibial spine hypoplasia, widening of the lateral joint line, or flattening of the lateral femoral condyle on PA view. On MRI, an abnormally thickened "bow tie" on the coronal view or greater than three cuts with continuity of the anterior and posterior horn on a 5-mm–thick sagittal cut view are diagnostic for discoid meniscus.

Procedure
Setup/Equipment
In our institution, meniscal surgery is routinely performed on an outpatient basis. Patients are placed in the supine position under spinal, regional, or general anesthesia. Prophylactic antibiotic administration is variable among the orthopaedic surgeons at our institution. We typically do not use a tourniquet for routine arthroscopy. Preoperative examination under anesthesia is performed, focusing on ligamentous stability.

Preoperative intra-articular injection varies among the authors of this chapter but incorporates 10 to 50 mL of 1% lidocaine or 0.25% bupivacaine, both with at least 1:400,000 epinephrine. We prefer preoperative injection to allow for clearance of the analgesic during arthroscopy because of concerns over chondrotoxicity from prolonged exposure. One of the authors incorporates 4 mg of intra-articular morphine in the preoperative injection; others add an injection of 4 mg of morphine at the completion of the case.

We prefer a leg holder placed 5 to 8 cm proximal to the superior pole of the patella to maximize control of the limb; however, a post can suffice. The contralateral leg is placed in a well leg holder, and the foot of the operating table is dropped. Additionally, a sequential compression device is used on the contralateral limb as a nonpharmacologic and relatively safe prophylactic measure for deep venous thrombosis (DVT).

We use the standard arthroscopy pump, a motorized (4.5-mm or 5.0-mm) meniscal shaver, meniscal punches, and a toothed grasper. Straight, up-curved, and right- and left-curved punches are typically sufficient to complete meniscal débridement. A curved shaver may also be used to access the posterior rim and roots, minimizing articular injury when access to the posterior knee is limited. A backbiter and a 90° punch are useful for anterior work. We do not use radiofrequency devices for meniscal surgery because of a risk of injury to adjacent cartilage.

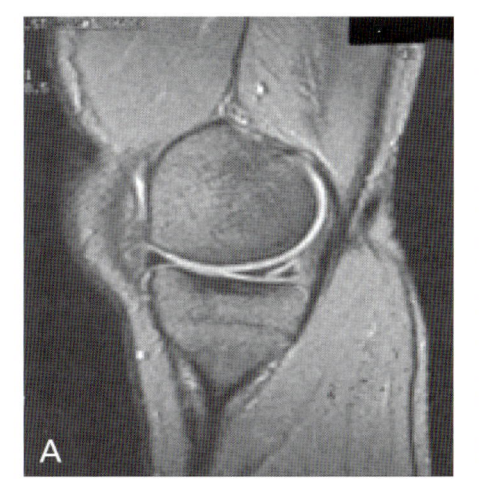

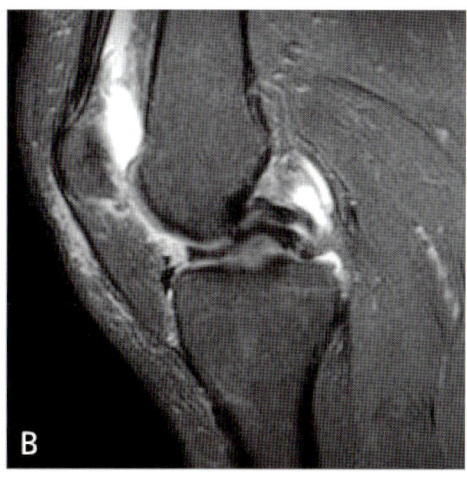

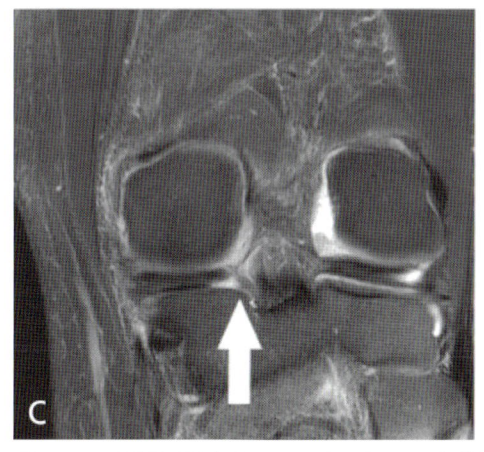

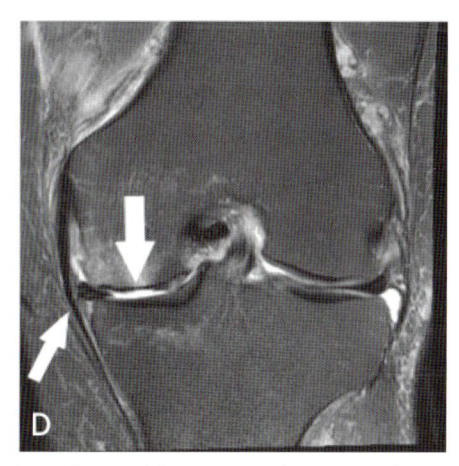

Figure 4 MRIs (3-T) show meniscal tears. **A,** Horizontal tear of the posterior horn extending to the inferior surface. **B,** Double posterior cruciate ligament sign, indicative of a displaced bucket-handle tear. **C,** Meniscal root tear on coronal view. **D,** A tear at the root (large arrow) and extrusion of the meniscus (small arrow).

Surgical Technique
Arthroscopy
Typical portal placement uses the inferior pole of the patella and the edges of the patellar tendon as landmarks. The vertical lateral portal is placed 0.5 to 1 cm off the lateral edge of the patellar tendon at the level of the inferior pole of the patella. This position allows for clearance of the tibial spine when visualizing the medial meniscus. The medial portal is placed in the soft spot approximately 1 to 2 cm off the medial edge of the patellar tendon. A variety of other portals have utility in specific circumstances. A posteromedial portal is useful for loose bodies in the back of the knee and can be created under direct visualization using a spinal needle inserted with a transillumination technique to avoid injury to the neurovascular structures. Rarely, a transpatellar portal is used to do work in the center of the knee.

The joint is insufflated through the anterolateral portal, and a standard superolateral or superomedial portal is placed to optimize flow. Routine diagnostic arthroscopy is performed, visualizing all compartments through the full range of motion. The anteromedial portal is created under direct visualization. Valgus stress is applied with the foot externally rotated; 10° to 20° of flexion improve visualization of the posterior horn. Stress relaxation of the collateral structures of the knee can be expected with gradual and steady force. The avoidance of abrupt changes in stress applied to the limb minimizes the risk of iatrogenic injury. Lateral meniscal inspection is facilitated with varus stress in a figure-of-4 position placed through the distal fibula rather than through the foot to avoid injury to the ankle. This technique can be facilitated by resting the lower leg on a well-padded Mayo stand with the knee at 45° to 90° of flexion.

Evaluation and Tear Morphology
We typically evaluate the menisci both visually and with tactile probing. A flounce sign is reassuring for an intact medial meniscus, as shown by Wright and Boyer.[8] Tactile probing of the meniscus is critical and allows for assessment of the stability of identified tears. Meniscal mobility

Section 1: Sports Medicine

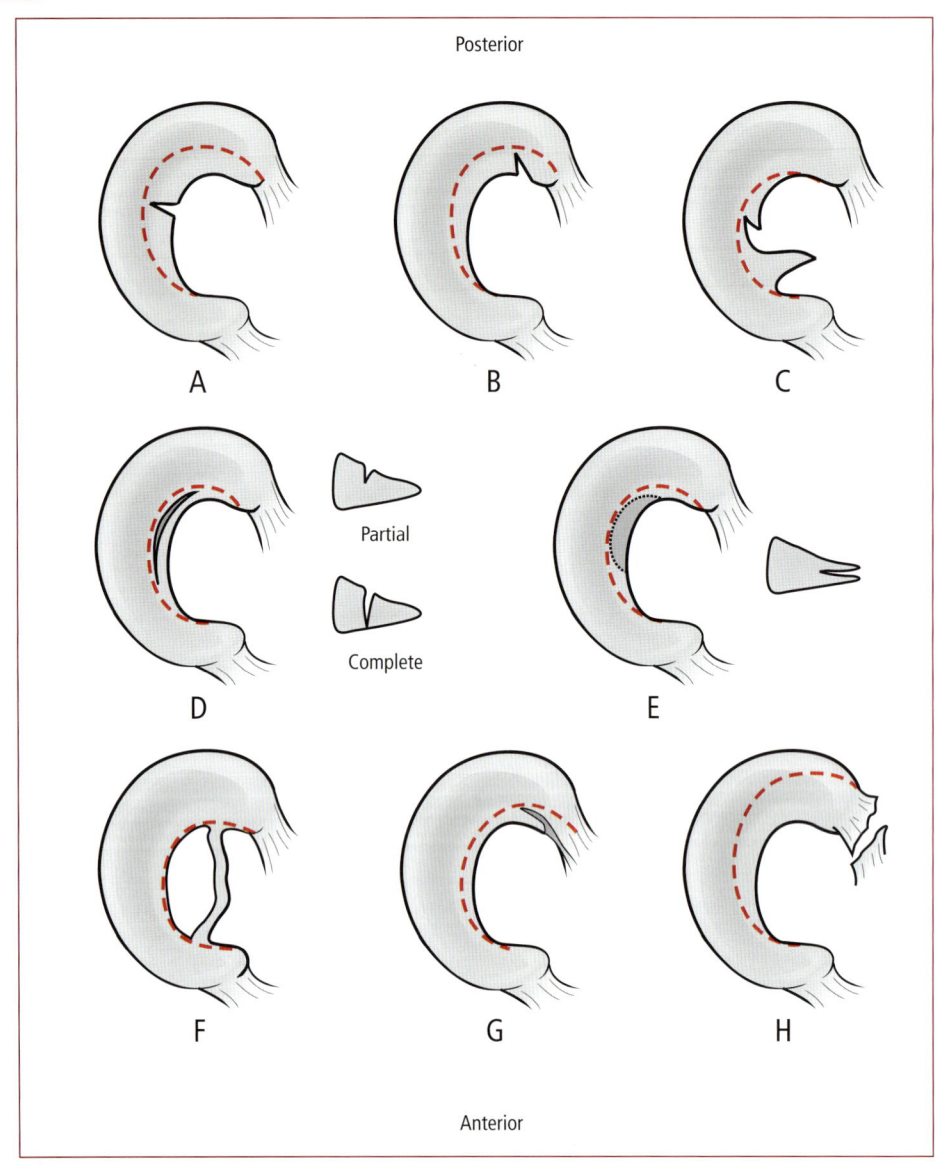

Figure 5 Illustrations show meniscal resections. **A** and **B**, Radial tears (**B** is radial root tear). **C**, Parrot-beak tear. **D**, Vertical/longitudinal tears. **E**, Horizontal tear. **F**, Bucket-handle tear. **G**, Root tear. **H**, Root avulsion. The resection line is shown by red dashes.

We use curved biters to optimize access to the meniscus, often removing much of the meniscus en bloc to minimize free body generation and improve the efficiency of resection. Care must be taken when pulling segments from the knee portals. The portal must be large enough to accommodate segment removal, and a firm hold of the segment with meniscal graspers avoids slippage of the tissue from the jaws. Alternatively, biters can be used, followed by a shaver to remove meniscal debris. Large 5.0-mm shavers are less apt to clog, and they add to the efficiency of clearance of the knee. The gutters should be carefully inspected at the conclusion of the case to confirm the removal of all meniscal debris.

For a lateral meniscal tear in a right knee, we begin with a right-curved or straight biter introduced from the medial portal. Resection begins anterior to the tear, creating a gentle contour to the remaining meniscus, with the peripheral extent of the tear as the target for the outermost resection. The segment posterior to the tear is removed with the biter in segments. The remnant tissue is sometimes débrided and smoothed with a high-speed shaver. A gradual transition from the residual segment of the meniscus minimizes unstable or acute edges that may cause symptoms or propagate new tears. If hybrid repair/débridement is being considered, resection should be more conservative, maintaining a stable segment for repair. Alternatively, repair of the peripheral segment of the tear can be performed, followed by resection of the more central irreparable tissue (**Figure 6**).

as noted by Vedi et al[9] can be expected to be approximately 4 mm for the posterior horns of the medial meniscus and 1 cm for the lateral meniscus. If a tear is found, the location, configuration, and vascularity are considered in the decision to repair or resect. Evaluation of the stability, size, and extent (partial or complete) of the tear is important in determining if any intervention is necessary. Pujol and Beaufils[10] noted that partial or stable tears along the periphery have shown good healing potential without treatment, particularly in conjunction with anterior cruciate ligament reconstruction. Typically, these tears are in the red-red or red-white zone of the meniscus, whereas tears in the inner margin or white-white zone have poor healing potential. **Figure 5** shows the areas of meniscal resection for various types of meniscal tears.

Radial Tears
There is evidence that some radial tears are amenable to repair, with clinical studies showing good rates of healing in more vascular zones.[11] For the most part, however, radial tears necessitate at least partial débridement, particularly of the central avascular zones of the menisci. Bedi et al[12] have shown that even with the disruption of hoop stress imparted by radial tears, the residual meniscus is functionally more capable of load transmission than after meniscectomy. Therefore, even in a case with avascular or degenerative tissue, judicial excision is prudent, and preservation of functional meniscal tissue is paramount. Hybrid repair/débridement techniques should be considered if radial tears extend into the red-red zone or the red-white zone, particularly in younger patients.

Horizontal Cleavage Tears
Débridement of horizontal cleavage tears is optimized when the larger leaf, either superior or inferior, is preserved and the unstable leaf of the horizontally torn meniscus is removed to the level of the peripheral margin of the tear (**Figure 5, E**). Haemer et al[13] demonstrated improved contact pressure if one leaf of a horizontal tear is preserved. Typically, we use biters to optimize access to the meniscus and the efficiency of the resection, later smoothing the residual meniscus and removing debris with a high-speed shaver. Alternatively, a high-speed shaver can be used for the entirety of the resection because horizontal tears tend to be of the degenerative type and are more readily resected with a shaver than other tear types. Smooth resectors tend to leave less

frayed remmant tissue. Tactile probing is performed to ensure that there is no unstable meniscal tissue flipped under or above the remaining tissue.

Vertical Tears

Assessment of vertical tears begins with the determination of the length and completeness of the tear. Tears less than 10 mm in length can be treated with trephination or abrasion, and smaller partial-thickness tears can be left alone. Tactile probing to confirm the stability of tears is important. Tears that are displaceable into the joint necessitate intervention. Vertical tears not amenable to repair due to fragmentation, degeneration, or patient factors are most easily excised by contoured resection of the most anterior and posterior attachment of the torn segment to stable tissue (**Figure 5, D**). Then a grasper and "gator" technique is used to remove large segments (locking the meniscal segment in a grasper and rolling the grasper in one direction as one exits the joint). Portal size may need to be enlarged to accommodate large segments of excised meniscus. Alternatively, resection of irreparable tissue can be undertaken from front-to-back or vice versa as long as a stable zone of transition is achieved. White-white tears are typically not repaired. Younger patients with healthy tissue are typically treated with an attempt at repair of red-white tears.

Displaced Bucket-Handle Tears

Attempts at reduction and repair of repairable bucket-handle tears at the periphery should be exhausted before resection. Prognostic indicators against repair include tears older than 6 months, patients older than 30 years, more central tear locations (white-white in young patients or red-white in older patients), and poor tear reducibility. More aggressive attempts at repair are typically made in patients younger than 30 years.

Displaced tears are most easily excised after reduction of the bucket-handle portion. Reduction can be achieved with a blunt trocar. Typically, for a medial bucket-handle tear, posterior pressure is applied to the displaced segment while simultaneously extending the knee to 20° with a valgus load. This maneuver offloads the posterior horn somewhat and relieves the tendency for the segment to displace anteriorly. Stable reduction of a displaced bucket-handle tear can sometimes be challenging, and variations of knee flexion angle can help facilitate the optimal position of the meniscal tissue for resection. Visibility can often be obstructed by displaced meniscal tissue.

If reduction is not possible, amputation of the most easily accessible attachment site can be undertaken to mobilize the tissue and expose the remaining attachment site. Removal en bloc can be accomplished after amputation of the most anterior and posterior attachment sites of the torn segment (**Figure 5, F**). This can be done with a biter or meniscal scissors. Then, using a grasper and the gator technique described earlier, the segment is removed. Portal size may need to be enlarged to accommodate larger segments of excised meniscus.

When access to the posterior horn is difficult, a posteromedial portal may be used. In this technique, the anterior attachment is released first. The remaining segment is grasped and controlled through the anteromedial portal. The posterior attachment is then released via a posteromedial portal. Alternatively, the anterior attachment may be released first, and a shaver can then be used to débride down segments attached to the posterior horn until the posterior attachment is visualized. The remnant meniscus can then be removed using a grasper with a firm twist and pull to avoid losing a fragment in the posterior compartment. The remaining free edges can be smoothed with a shaver.

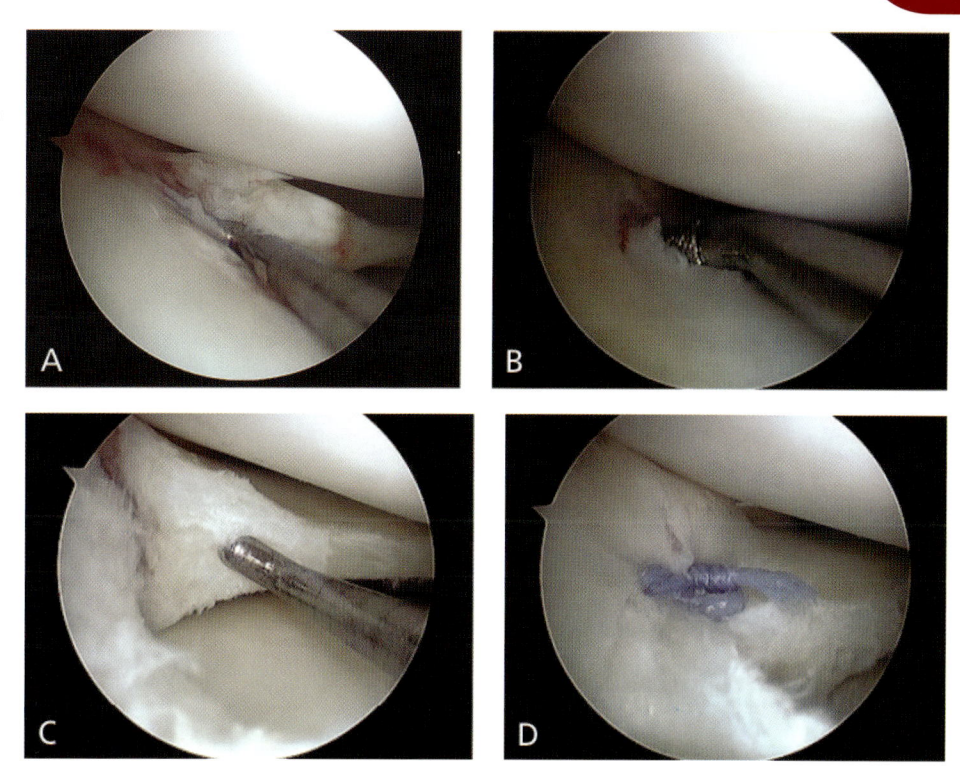

Figure 6 Arthroscopic views demonstrate repair of a radial meniscal tear. **A,** Radial tear of the lateral meniscus. **B,** Peripheral rasping. **C,** Central partial meniscectomy. **D,** All-inside repair of the remaining peripheral extent of the radial tear. (Courtesy of Paul M. Saluan, MD, Cleveland Clinic, Cleveland, OH.)

Meniscal Root Tears

Jones et al[14] showed that treatment should be undertaken cautiously in the setting of meniscal root tears, with preservation of as much stable root and posterior horn tissue as possible because rapidly progressive arthritic changes have been noted in this population after extensive resection. Patients should be counseled regarding the poorer prognosis after meniscal resection for root tears. Meniscal root tears have been shown to significantly increase peak contact pressures compared to the intact and repaired meniscus. Interestingly, Allaire et al[15] demonstrated little difference in the peak contact pressure between medial meniscal root tears and meniscectomized knees, underscoring the importance of meniscal repair when indicated in these tear patterns. Débridement should be undertaken with the goal of minimizing tissue removal while establishing a stable transition zone to normal tissue (**Figure 5, G** and **H**). Unfortunately, some tears with extensive involvement of the root and poor healing potential as a result of their degenerative nature often preclude repair as an option and may necessitate subtotal meniscectomy to achieve a stable remnant (**Figure 7**).

Discoid Meniscus

The most commonly used classification system of discoid meniscus is that of Watanabe.[16] He based the system on arthroscopic observations of the shape and tibial attachment of the meniscus. Type 1 and 2 discoid menisci have normal tibial attachment and differ only in the amount of tibial coverage, with type 1 completely covering the plateau, and type 2 being semilunar. Type 3, the Wrisberg ligament variant, does not have a discoid shape and has only a femoral attachment by the meniscofemoral ligament of Wrisberg. Type 3 variants are therefore much more mobile than are normal menisci. Intrasubstance degeneration that is not evident during arthroscopy can be detected on MRI, as demonstrated by Hamada et al.[17]

Treatment options are based on the frequency and severity of symptoms and the presence of a meniscal tear. Occasional and minor symptoms may not necessitate surgical intervention, whereas incidental asymptomatic discoid menisci found during arthroscopy need not be treated. Klingele et al[18] noted a high incidence of anterior horn instability; therefore, critical assessment of the anterior meniscus should always be completed. Symptomatic discoid menisci with central tearing and an intact peripheral rim are best treated with central partial débridement, or "saucerization." Care should be taken to preserve as much of the peripheral rim as possible to maintain some of the "shock absorption" capability of the meniscus (**Figure 8**). Saucerization is started at the free edge of the tear, resecting from back to front using standard biters and shavers until a smooth transition and stable edges are achieved to minimize the risk of retear. The remainder of the meniscus should be assessed for stability at completion. Repair or hybrid repair/débridement should be considered for tears extending into the red-red zone or the white-red zone. We are more aggressive with attempts at repair for the youngest patients, taking tear pattern, health of the tissue, complexity of the tear, and family dynamics into account.

Complications

Complications after knee arthroscopy are relatively rare. Measures to minimize the risk of DVT and pulmonary embolism (PE) include using a sequential compression device on the contralateral limb intraoperatively. Preoperative screening of patients helps to identify higher-risk patients in whom chemical prophylaxis may be indicated. They include those with a family or personal history of DVT or PE, a hypercoagulable state such as Factor V deficiency, or oral contraceptive use. Although the vast majority of patients do not need chemical prophylaxis after routine knee arthroscopy, it seems the most prudent and cost-effective approach is likely one incorporating thorough preoperative screening for risk factors for DVT and chemical prophylaxis in preoperatively identified high-risk patients.

Infections after knee arthroscopy typically present at about 7 to 10 days and are best treated with immediate aspiration for organism identification and urgent arthroscopic lavage. Patients should be placed on intravenous antibiotics for a period of 2 to 4 weeks. Early surgical intervention and maintenance of knee range of motion are paramount to achieving good outcome after this potentially devastating complication.[19]

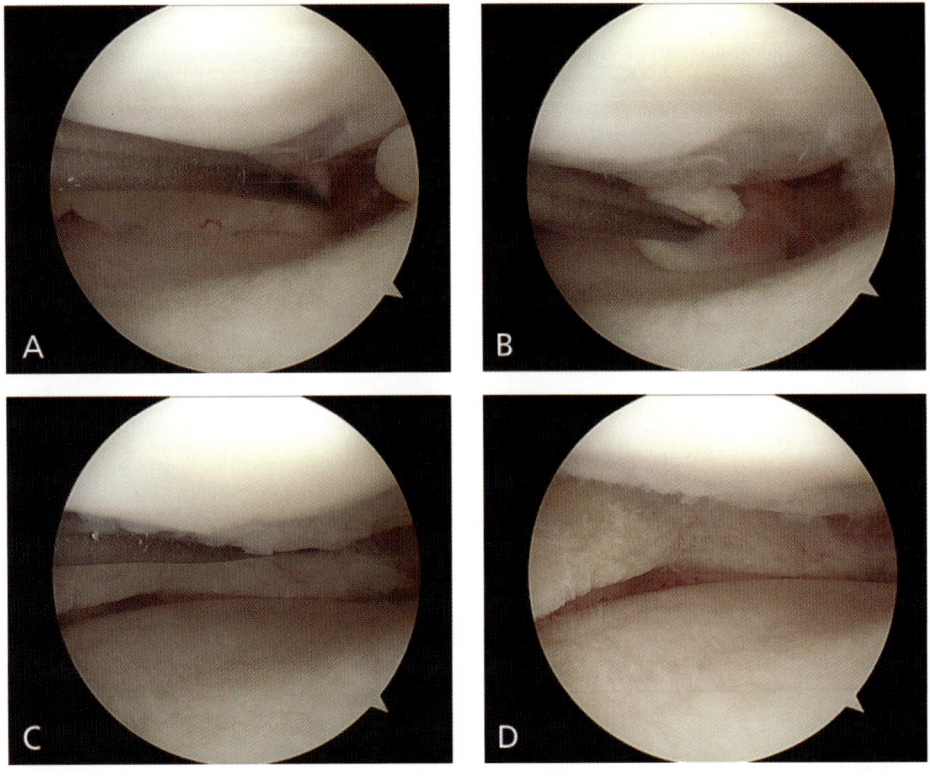

Figure 7 Arthroscopic views show meniscal root tears. **A**, Root avulsion. **B**, Demonstration of root instability. **C** and **D**, Subtotal meniscectomy for root tear.

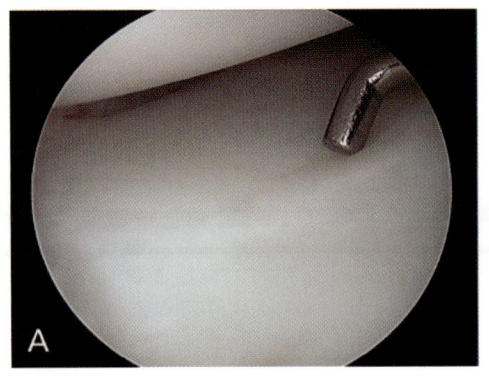

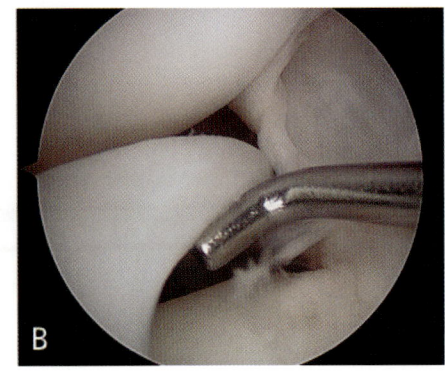

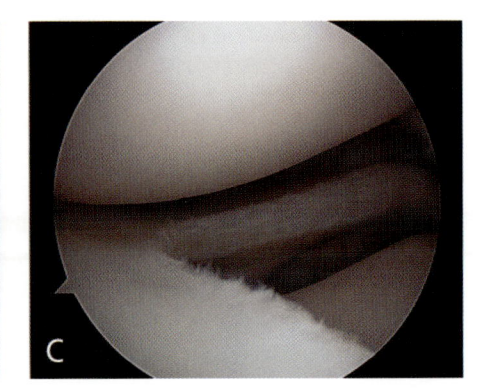

Figure 8 Arthroscopic views show discoid meniscus. **A**, Discoid lateral meniscus covering the entire tibial plateau. **B**, Redundant medial edge. **C**, Discoid meniscus after saucerization.

Postoperative Care and Considerations

After meniscal débridement, all patients are encouraged to mobilize immediately and are allowed weight bearing as tolerated with crutches. A thigh-high compression stocking on the surgical limb postoperatively helps reduce venous stasis, and chemical prophylaxis is initiated as dictated by the patient risk profile. Physical therapy may be initiated to regain mobility, range of motion, quadriceps function, and strength.

Patients with malalignment should be counseled regarding their increased risk of degenerative changes, particularly after subtotal meniscectomy in the more loaded compartment. Considerations for the use of unloading braces or future realignment procedures should be discussed during counseling. Ligamentous instability if symptomatic should also be discussed as a possible predisposing factor for future meniscal tears or even accelerated degenerative changes.

Pearls

- Placing the leg holder just proximal to the superior pole of the patella maximizes control of the limb.
- A well-padded Mayo stand placed under the lateral malleolus helps facilitate control of the limb for exposure of the lateral compartment.
- Tear morphology with respect to the zones of the meniscus must be considered, particularly with radial tears, because hybrid resection/repair techniques may help preserve the peripheral third if the tear extends to the capsule.
- The surgeon should attempt to preserve as much stable posterior horn and root attachment as possible when treating nonrepairable posterior horn and root tears.
- Patient status and tissue health should be taken into account when deciding when and how much meniscal resection is necessary.

References

1. Seedhom BB, Dowson D, Wright V: Proceedings: Functions of the menisci. A preliminary study. *Ann Rheum Dis* 1974;33(1):111.
2. Paletta GA Jr, Manning T, Snell E, Parker R, Bergfeld J: The effect of allograft meniscal replacement on intraarticular contact area and pressures in the human knee: A biomechanical study. *Am J Sports Med* 1997;25(5):692-698.
3. Ahmed AM, Burke DL: In-vitro measurement of static pressure distribution in synovial joints—Part I: Tibial surface of the knee. *J Biomech Eng* 1983;105(3):216-225.
4. Higuchi H, Kimura M, Shirakura K, Terauchi M, Takagishi K: Factors affecting long-term results after arthroscopic partial meniscectomy. *Clin Orthop Relat Res* 2000;377:161-168.
5. Muriuki MG, Tuason DA, Tucker BG, Harner CD: Changes in tibiofemoral contact mechanics following radial split and vertical tears of the medial meniscus an in vitro investigation of the efficacy of arthroscopic repair. *J Bone Joint Surg Am* 2011;93(12):1089-1095.
6. Karachalios T, Hantes M, Zibis AH, Zachos V, Karantanas AH, Malizos KN: Diagnostic accuracy of a new clinical test (the Thessaly test) for early detection of meniscal tears. *J Bone Joint Surg Am* 2005;87(5):955-962.
7. Matava MJ, Eck K, Totty W, Wright RW, Shively RA: Magnetic resonance imaging as a tool to predict meniscal reparability. *Am J Sports Med* 1999;27(4):436-443.
8. Wright RW, Boyer DS: Significance of the arthroscopic meniscal flounce sign: A prospective study. *Am J Sports Med* 2007;35(2):242-244.
9. Vedi V, Williams A, Tennant SJ, Spouse E, Hunt DM, Gedroyc WM: Meniscal movement: An in-vivo study using dynamic MRI. *J Bone Joint Surg Br* 1999;81(1):37-41.
10. Pujol N, Beaufils P: Healing results of meniscal tears left in situ during anterior cruciate ligament reconstruction: A review of clinical studies. *Knee Surg Sports Traumatol Arthrosc* 2009;17(4):396-401.
11. Choi NH, Kim TH, Son KM, Victoroff BN: Meniscal repair for radial tears of the midbody of the lateral meniscus. *Am J Sports Med* 2010;38(12):2472-2476.
12. Bedi A, Kelly NH, Baad M, et al: Dynamic contact mechanics of the medial meniscus as a function of radial tear, repair, and partial meniscectomy. *J Bone Joint Surg Am* 2010;92(6):1398-1408.
13. Haemer JM, Wang MJ, Carter DR, Giori NJ: Benefit of single-leaf resection for horizontal meniscus tear. *Clin Orthop Relat Res* 2007;457:194-202.
14. Jones AO, Houang MT, Low RS, Wood DG: Medial meniscus posterior root attachment injury and degeneration: MRI findings. *Australas Radiol* 2006;50(4):306-313.
15. Allaire R, Muriuki M, Gilbertson L, Harner CD: Biomechanical consequences of a tear of the posterior root of the medial meniscus: Similar to total meniscectomy. *J Bone Joint Surg Am* 2008;90(9):1922-1931.
16. Watanabe M: Arthroscopy of the knee joint, in: Helfet AJ, ed: *Disorders of the Knee*. Philadelphia, PA, JB Lippincott Co, 1974, pp 145-159.
17. Hamada M, Shino K, Kawano K, Araki Y, Matsui Y, Doi T: Usefulness of magnetic resonance imaging for detecting intrasubstance tear and/or degeneration of lateral discoid meniscus. *Arthroscopy* 1994;10(6):645-653.
18. Klingele KE, Kocher MS, Hresko MT, Gerbino P, Micheli LJ: Discoid lateral meniscus: Prevalence of peripheral rim instability. *J Pediatr Orthop* 2004;24(1):79-82.
19. Balabaud L, Gaudias J, Boeri C, Jenny JY, Kehr P: Results of treatment of septic knee arthritis: A retrospective series of 40 cases. *Knee Surg Sports Traumatol Arthrosc* 2007;15(4):387-392.

Chapter 12
Meniscal Repair

Karl F. Bowman, Jr, MD   Christopher D. Harner, MD

Patient Selection

Advances in the understanding of the role of the human meniscus in the transmission of forces across the knee joint and as a secondary stabilizer to pathologic motion have led to increased efforts to repair meniscal injuries. The meniscus provides a significant role in load bearing and shock absorption across the tibiofemoral joint by increasing the surface area for load transmission. Tears of the meniscus have been associated with progression of articular cartilage disease visible on imaging and arthroscopy, and a strong correlation exists between meniscectomy and the increased risk of developing radiographic signs of knee osteoarthritis.[1-4] The primary goal in meniscal preservation surgery is to protect the articular cartilage from the changes in joint contact pressures seen with meniscal deficiency.[5] Much of our philosophy in meniscal repairs is driven by more than 20 years of experience with meniscal transplantation and the rapid symptomatic deterioration of the meniscus-deficient athlete. We approach all meniscal tears as being potentially repairable and are increasingly aggressive about preserving the maximum amount of meniscal tissue with decreasing patient age.

Indications

The indications for meniscal repair are based on patient age, tear pattern, chronicity, and the presence of concomitant injuries. We initially approach every meniscal tear as repairable. The pattern and location of meniscal injury plays a significant role in selecting appropriate cases that are suitable for repair. Histologic studies have demonstrated that the vascular supply to the meniscus is provided by perforating vessels originating from the medial and lateral geniculate arteries. The peripheral capsular attachment of the meniscus has a robust blood supply, but the meniscus becomes increasingly avascular in the central portion. Three distinct zones have been described to classify tears according to their vascular supply, including the richly vascular red-red zone, the transitional red-white zone, and the avascular white-white zone.[6,7]

Classification of tear pattern helps to characterize the type of injury sustained to the meniscus and correlates with both the collagen fibers that are disrupted and the anticipated success of meniscal repair. The meniscus consists of longitudinal fibers running parallel to the long axis of the meniscus, radial tie fibers that bind the longitudinal fibers, and interstitial fibers that provide additional strength to the tissue.[8,9] Acute tears may be classified as longitudinal, or bucket-handle, tears; radial split tears; horizontal flap tears; or a combination of longitudinal and radial tears in a parrot beak pattern (**Figure 1**). Tears may be additionally classified as complex or degenerative in appearance. The ideal candidate for meniscal repair is a young patient with a longitudinal tear involving the vascular red-red zone without concomitant articular damage. Radial tears and parrot beak tears are also amenable to repair, especially in a young patient or if the tear involves the vascular portion of the meniscus. The expected success of meniscal healing is improved if a concomitant cruciate ligament is reconstructed at the time of surgery,[10] although isolated repairs can be augmented through the use of a fibrin clot, capsular rasping, or microfracture of the intercondylar notch.[11-13]

In the setting of a longitudinal meniscal tear that is displaced into the tibiofemoral compartment and blocks full range of motion, an attempt to reduce the displaced fragment should be performed. Displaced medial tears can be reduced by applying a valgus force on the knee at 20° to 30° of flexion while gradually bringing the knee into full extension. Lateral tears are reduced with a varus force applied at 40° to 60° of initial knee flexion followed by gradual extension. If the displaced fragment is able to be successfully reduced, the knee is immobilized in extension until surgery to prevent redisplacement or further meniscal damage. If the displaced fragment cannot be reduced, then a surgical reduction and repair is performed as soon as possible to minimize the risk of arthrofibrosis and chondral damage. Although controversial, in the setting of a displaced meniscal tear causing a block in range of motion, we will frequently delay cruciate ligament reconstruction for a period of 6 to 8 weeks following repair to allow for resolution of the acute inflammatory phase of injury, restoration of motion, and return of quadriceps strength/control.

Contraindications

Although we believe that no true contraindication to meniscal repair exists, tears involving significant intrasubstance degeneration, isolated tearing in the avascular white-white zone, the presence of tricompartmental arthritis, or unstable displaced meniscal fragments are less amenable to repair. Despite these relative contraindications, every attempt should be made to preserve the maximal amount of meniscal tissue to minimize the detrimental effects of meniscectomy on the articular cartilage.

Preoperative Imaging

Standard radiographs of both knees are obtained in all patients with suspected meniscal pathology to evaluate for fracture, associated arthritis, and joint congruency. The knee is also assessed for subtle findings including avulsion fracture, joint subluxation, and patellar height. MRI assists in the identification and classification of meniscal injury and associated pathology of the cruciate and collateral ligaments, chondral surfaces, and related structures[14] (**Figure 2**). Oblique coronal images in the plane of the anterior cruciate ligament are routinely obtained, and these sequences can be particularly useful to identify pathology

---

Dr. Harner or an immediate family member has received research or institutional support from DePuy and Smith & Nephew and serves as a board member, owner, officer, or committee member of the American Board of Orthopaedic Surgery, the American Orthopaedic Association, the American Academy of Orthopaedic Surgeons, and the American Orthopaedic Society for Sports Medicine. Neither Dr. Bowman nor any immediate family member has received anything of value from or owns stock in a commercial company or institution related directly or indirectly to the subject of this chapter.

© 2013 American Academy of Orthopaedic Surgeons

Section 1: Sports Medicine

1. Longitudinal tear (bucket-handle tear) —or— Displaced bucket-handle tear

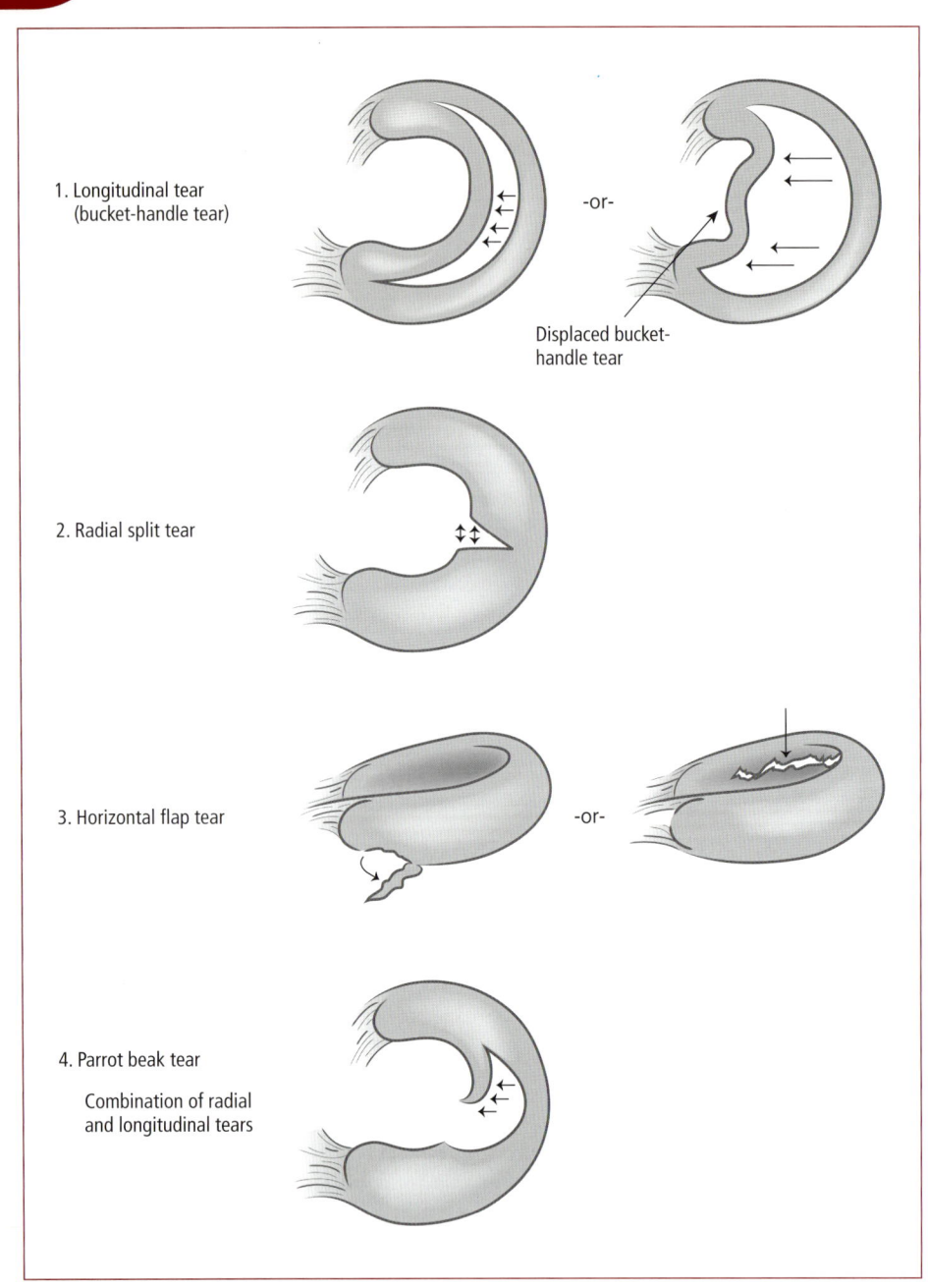

2. Radial split tear

3. Horizontal flap tear —or—

4. Parrot beak tear
   Combination of radial and longitudinal tears

Figure 1 Illustrations show acute meniscal tear patterns.

of the meniscal roots.[15] MRI findings are reviewed with the direct input of musculoskeletal radiologists before establishing an individualized treatment plan.

Procedure

Room Setup/Patient Positioning

The patient is identified in the preoperative holding area and the informed consent is reviewed. The surgical extremity is marked with the word "yes" and the surgeon's initials within the surgical field. A small bump is placed under the ipsilateral sacroiliac joint, and a lateral post is placed at the level of the greater trochanter. A 10-lb sandbag is secured to the operating table with tape to allow the limb to rest at 90° of knee flexion without manual assistance. We do not use a tourniquet. The contralateral extremity is padded to the level of the sacroiliac joint with surgical foam. Intravenous antibiotics are administered for routine prophylaxis within 60 minutes of the skin incision.

Special Instruments/Equipment/Implants

Our preference is to perform an inside-out repair technique with nonabsorbable sutures placed arthroscopically. Several instruments specifically designed for arthroscopic meniscal repair are commercially available (**Figure 3**). A standard meniscal repair surgical set consists of various rasps to freshen the tear edges and rasp the adjacent synovium. A Henning retractor is used to protect the soft-tissue structures and the surgeon's hands during suture needle passage. The retractor is also used to capture the needle tip as it exits the joint capsule and direct it

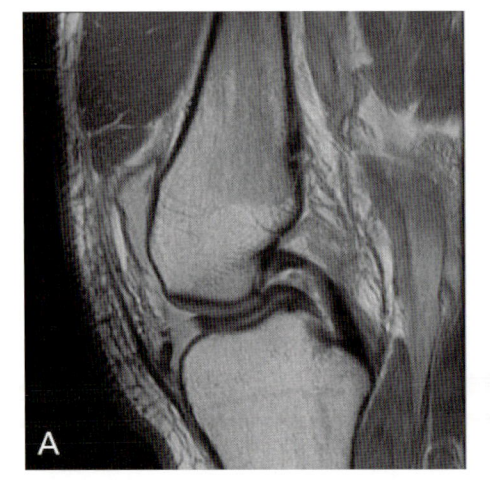

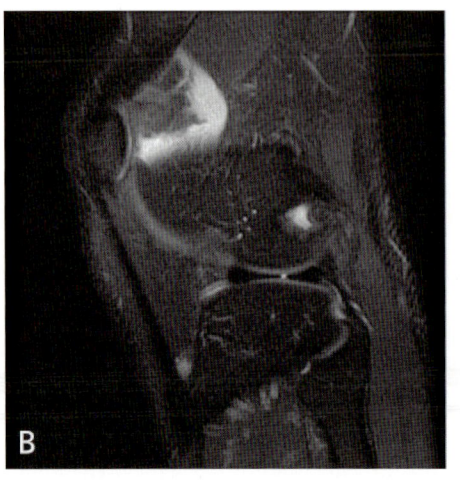

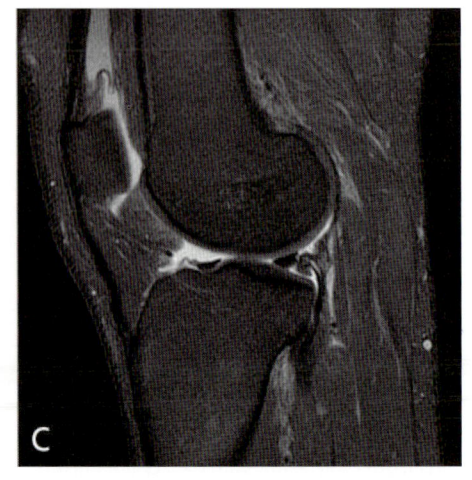

Figure 2 Sagittal MRIs demonstrate various meniscal tear patterns. **A,** T1-weighted MRI shows a displaced longitudinal (bucket-handle) tear of the medial meniscus. The displacement into the notch creates the classic "double posterior cruciate ligament" sign. **B,** A radial split tear of the lateral meniscus presents as a gap on the T2-weighted MRI. **C,** T2-weighted MRI shows a nondisplaced longitudinal tear of the lateral meniscus in the red-red zone.

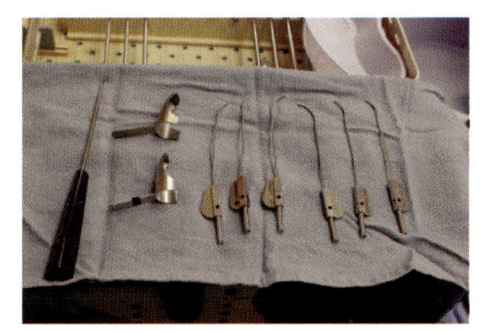

Figure 3 A standard meniscal repair instrument set.

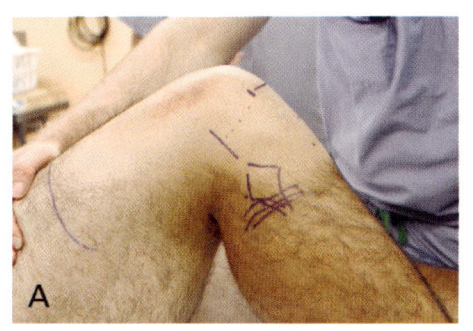

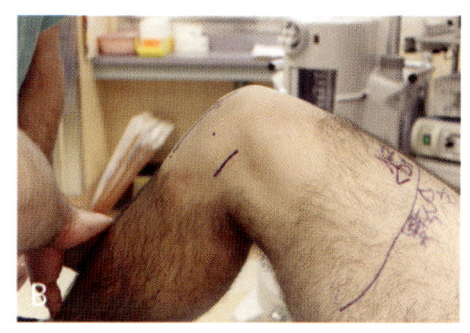

Figure 4 Photographs show skin markings for incisions for meniscal repair. **A,** Lateral meniscal procedures are performed through a 3- to 4-cm longitudinal incision placed posterior to the lateral collateral ligament at the junction of the middle and posterior thirds of the lateral femoral condyle. The incision is placed 1 cm proximal to the joint line and extended 2 to 3 cm distal to the joint line. **B,** Medial meniscal injuries are addressed through a 3- to 4-cm incision that is centered over the junction of the middle and posterior third of the medial femoral condyle.

toward the surgical incision for retrieval. Arthroscopic suture placement and passage is facilitated by the use of commercially available metallic cannulas that are pre-bent for zone-specific targeting of meniscal pathology. Multiple suture options exist for meniscal repair, with long nitinol wire needles fixed to a nonabsorbable suture material. We prefer to use a 2-0 nonabsorbable suture with a non-Kevlar core to prevent cutting of the delicate meniscal tissue during suture passage and knot tying.

Surgical Technique

The surface anatomy is identified and the planned surgical incisions are marked. Important landmarks include the inferior patellar pole, the tibial tubercle, the Gerdy tubercle, the fibular head, and the medial and lateral joint lines. The soft spot at the fibular neck is palpated and marked to correspond with the expected location of the peroneal nerve. The anterolateral portal is placed 2 to 3 mm lateral to the edge of the patellar tendon at the level of the inferior pole of the patella, and the anteromedial portal is placed 1 cm medial to the patellar tendon at the same level. A careful assessment of the presence of patella alta or baja is performed to allow consistent placement of the arthroscopic portals with respect to the joint line. A superolateral outflow portal is placed 1 cm proximal to the superior pole of the patella between the vastus lateralis and the iliotibial band. If a posteromedial portal is required, the site is determined during arthroscopy using a spinal needle. Lateral meniscal procedures are performed through a 3- to 4-cm longitudinal incision placed immediately posterior to the lateral collateral ligament (**Figure 4, A**). Palpation of the lateral collateral ligament is facilitated by placing the knee in the figure-of-4 position. Medial meniscal injuries are addressed through a 3- to 4-cm incision that is centered over the junction

of the middle and posterior third of the medial femoral condyle (**Figure 4, B**). The surgical incisions are injected with 0.25% bupivacaine and 1:100,000 epinephrine for hemostasis.

A routine diagnostic arthroscopy is performed through anteromedial and anterolateral portals. The arthroscope is placed into the intra-articular notch and advanced only under direct visualization into the suprapatellar pouch to avoid iatrogenic chondral injury to the trochlea. Inspection and careful probing of the chondral surfaces, cruciate ligaments, and medial and lateral menisci are performed. We carefully evaluate the presence and pattern of meniscal injury by probing both the superior and inferior meniscal surfaces and assessing any cleft for evidence of partial-thickness tearing. The medial meniscus is evaluated with the knee placed in 20° of flexion and a valgus load is applied through the lateral post. The foot is kept in an externally rotated position to maintain the valgus opening while minimizing further knee flexion. The 30° arthroscope is placed on the anteromedial tibial plateau with the lens angle directed into the posterior aspect of the compartment. This allows excellent visualization of the body and posterior horn of the medial meniscus. The meniscal root can be visualized via the Gillquist view by placing the arthroscope in the intercondylar notch through the interval between the medial condyle and the posterior cruciate ligament. Evaluation of the lateral meniscus is facilitated by placing the knee in the figure-of-4 position with the knee at 60° to 70° of flexion and the hip externally rotated. The foot is supported with a bolster, and a gentle varus force is applied to open up the lateral compartment.

The method of meniscal repair chosen depends on whether other procedures are performed in the same surgical setting. If the meniscal tear is identified and repaired during a cruciate reconstruction surgery, then the hemarthrosis produced from the bone tunnels is sufficient to provide exogenous factors to assist with clot formation and initiation of the healing cascade. If an isolated meniscal repair is being performed, we routinely augment the local tissue biology with a fibrin clot prepared on the surgical field and placed into the meniscal tear after suture placement. Preparation of the fibrin clot begins with the sterile collection of 60 mL of whole blood obtained from a fresh venipuncture. We do not use blood collected from a previously placed intravenous line because of the risk of contamination. The blood is then placed in a beaker and gently stirred with a frosted glass stir rod that is slowly rotated and moved from side to side. The fibrin products are then precipitated in the beaker. If the blood is stirred too quickly or vigorously, the clot will become very large and friable. Once the clot develops in the beaker, it is transferred onto a gauze sponge and gently compressed to produce a dense fibrous clot that is easily manipulated (**Figure 5**).

The surgical approach for lateral meniscus repair occurs through a 3- to 4-cm longitudinal incision placed posterior to the lateral collateral ligament. Two thirds of the incision should be inferior to the joint line and one third superior to the joint line. The skin is sharply incised, and fascial dissection is carried to the level of the biceps femoris musculature. The plane between the long and short heads of the biceps femoris is opened, and the underlying tendon of the lateral head of the gastrocnemius muscle is identified.

Section 1: Sports Medicine

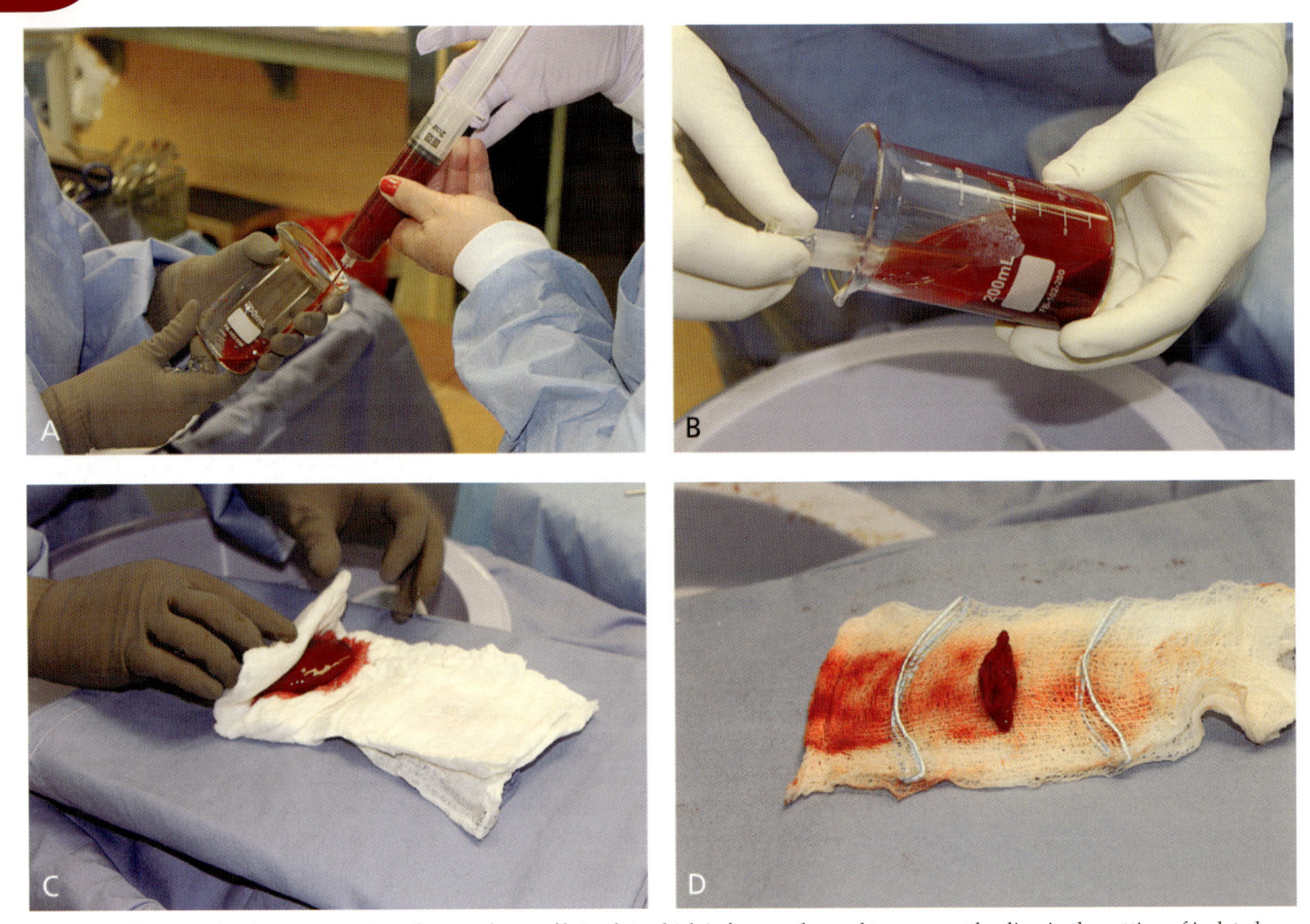

Figure 5 Photographs show preparation of an autologous fibrin clot, which is frequently used to augment healing in the setting of isolated meniscal repair. **A,** After harvesting from the patient, 60 mL of sterile venous blood is transferred to a beaker. **B,** The blood is gently rolled/stirred with a frosted glass stir rod to create the clot. The clot is gently compressed with gauze (**C**) into a fibrinous matrix (**D**).

A layer of adherent fascial tissue is frequently encountered and must be opened to facilitate gaining access to the space between the lateral joint capsule and the lateral head of the gastrocnemius muscle. The joint line is easily palpated through this interval, and a Henning retractor is placed for suture retrieval.

Medial meniscal repairs are performed through a 3- to 4-cm longitudinal incision centered over the junction of the middle and posterior thirds of the medial femoral condyle, with two thirds of the incision placed distal to the joint line. The skin is sharply incised, with dissection carried down to the first medial retinacular layer. The saphenous nerve and its branches are preserved and protected at all times during the exposure. The first retinacular layer is opened in line with the skin incision, and gentle blunt dissection is performed to identify the joint line and medial joint capsule. The space formed by the posteromedial capsule, medial head of the gastrocnemius, and the semimembranosus tendon is exploited, and a Henning retractor is placed within the interval.

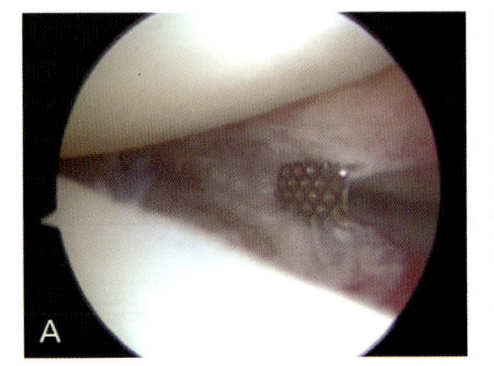

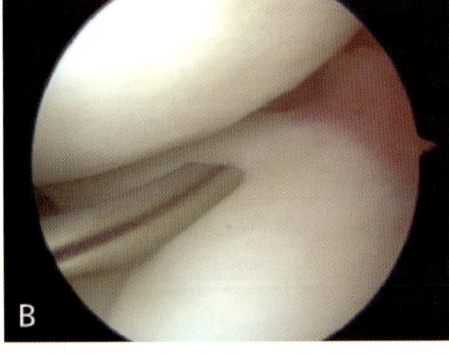

Figure 6 Arthroscopic views show meniscal repair. **A,** The meniscal edges and adjacent synovium are rasped before placement of sutures to freshen the tear edges and stimulate a vascular healing response. **B,** The arthroscope is placed into the portal adjacent to the meniscal tear, and the zone-specific cannula is placed through the contralateral portal. This allows the meniscal repair sutures to be advanced as perpendicular to the tissue as possible and the needle to be aimed away from the posterior neurovasculature.

Following the surgical approach, the edges of the meniscal tear are thoroughly rasped to freshen the tissue edges and facilitate healing. The adjacent synovium is also rasped to incite a local inflammatory response and stimulate synovial ingrowth to provide vascularity to the injury site (**Figure 6, A**). The arthroscope is placed in the portal adjacent to the site of repair; that is, medial repairs are visualized through the anteromedial portal, and lateral tears are visualized through the anterolateral portal (**Figure 6, B**). Arthroscopic cannulas are introduced into the knee from the contralateral portal to improve the suture angle and aim the needles toward the Henning retractor and away from the posterior

70 © 2013 American Academy of Orthopaedic Surgeons

Chapter 12: Meniscal Repair

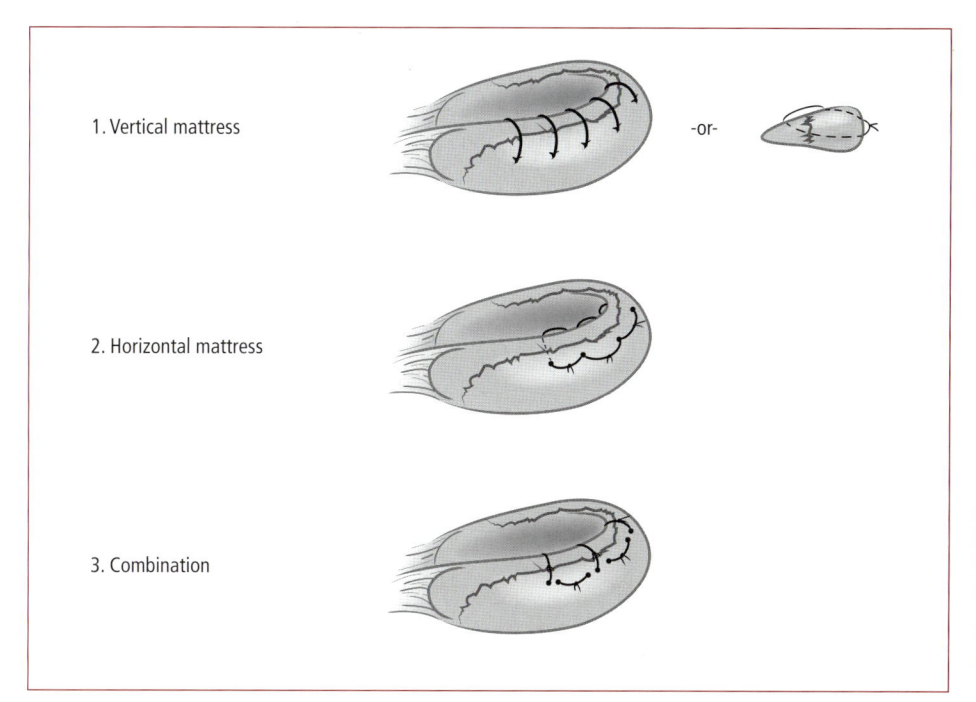

Figure 7 Illustration shows suture configurations for meniscal repair. Meniscal sutures are ideally placed in a vertical mattress fashion to maximize the biomechanical strength of the repair. Horizontal mattress sutures can also be used if the tibiofemoral compartment is tight or to augment the vertical mattress sutures for complete reapproximation of the tear edges.

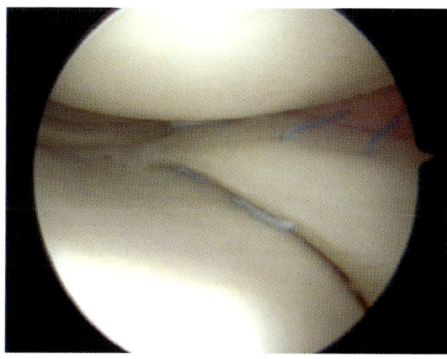

Figure 8 Arthroscopic image demonstrates a meniscal repair using a combination of vertical and horizontal mattress sutures to allow for complete reapproximation of the peripheral meniscal tissue.

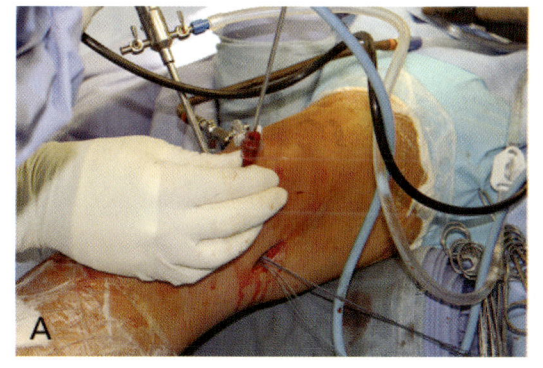

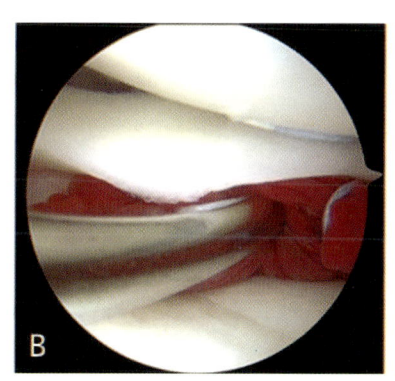

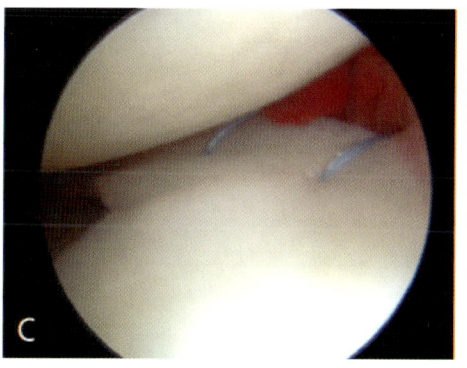

Figure 9 Placement of the fibrin clot during meniscal repair. **A,** Photograph shows introduction of the clot into the knee through a 5-mm cannula. The arthroscopic inflow is turned off to facilitate clot placement. **B,** Arthroscopic view shows the clot being manipulated into the meniscal repair. **C,** Arthroscopic view shows the clot secured with additional sutures.

neurovascular structures. The meniscal repair is performed from anterior to posterior, ideally using a vertical mattress suture configuration to reapproximate the meniscal edges. Horizontal mattress sutures are also acceptable for additional reinforcement if the compartment is tight and visualization is difficult or if the injury is a partial-thickness tear (**Figures 7** and **8**). The sutures are passed through the meniscus and capsular tissue and retrieved through the surgical incision, with care taken that no additional tissue intervenes between the suture knot and the joint capsule. If a fibrin clot is to be used, a 5-mm clear plastic cannula is placed through the working portal, and the arthroscopic fluid inflow is turned off. The knee is evacuated of fluid and a "dry scope" technique is used. The clot is pushed through the cannula with a blunt probe or switching stick into the compartment of the meniscal repair (**Figure 9, A**). The meniscal repair sutures are then pulled back and the meniscal tear is opened. The clot is manipulated into the tear and secured into the tear by applying tension through the sutures (**Figure 9, B**). The clot is then tucked into the defect and secured with one or two additional sutures (**Figure 9, C**). After placement of the meniscal repair sutures, any associated ligament reconstruction procedures are performed and tensioned. The knee is then brought to 20° of extension with a bolster under the popliteal fossa, and the sutures are tied onto the joint capsule. If necessary, the suture ends are retrieved before tying to avoid trapping additional tissue in the knots.

The wounds are copiously irrigated with an antibiotic solution, and a layered closure is performed. We prefer to use a 3-0 chromic gut suture in the deep dermal layers and a running subcuticular 4-0 absorbable monofilament suture. Skin glue is applied to seal the epidermal layer, followed by placement of a sterile dressing and a bias-cut wrap that incorporates a commercially available cooling device into the dressing. A hinged knee brace is placed. The brace is locked in 20° of flexion if an isolated meniscal repair was performed; it is locked in extension if an anterior cruciate ligament reconstruction was performed in conjunction with the meniscal repair.

Complications

Complications following arthroscopic meniscal repair are rare, but they may have significant consequences if not identified and treated promptly.

© 2013 American Academy of Orthopaedic Surgeons

Immediate postoperative complications include surgical-site infection, deep venous thrombosis (DVT), and stiffness. Patients are routinely seen within 5 to 7 days following surgery for a wound check and dressing change. Wound drainage or superficial dehiscence is monitored closely, with frequent dressing changes, clinical follow-up, and surgical débridement if necessary. Antibiotics are not routinely prescribed postoperatively. DVT prophylaxis with low-molecular-weight heparin is provided for individuals with an elevated risk because of previous DVT or pulmonary embolism history, active tobacco use, oral contraceptive use, or history of genetic clotting disorder. Symptoms of calf pain or swelling are evaluated urgently with a clinical examination and venous duplex ultrasonography. Postoperative knee range of motion is assessed at each clinical visit, and a protocol describing the expected progression of knee flexion is provided to the patient and physical therapist. If flexion or extension deficits are identified, the frequency of supervised physical therapy and postoperative clinical checks is increased. If a persistent extension or flexion deficit is not improved by 3 to 4 months following surgery, a manipulation under anesthesia, arthroscopic lysis of adhesions, and application of an extension drop-out cast is performed.

Postoperative Care and Rehabilitation

We use a standard postoperative protocol for all meniscal repairs. The knee is placed in a hinged knee brace as described previously. The patient is made non–weight bearing with crutches for a total of 6 weeks, with progressive transition to full weight bearing under the guidance of a physical therapist over the following 7 to 10 days. Knee flexion is restricted to 0° to 90° for 6 weeks, followed by progressive unrestricted knee flexion. The patient is instructed to begin home exercises consisting of isometric quadriceps sets, straight-leg raises, and ankle/calf pumps twice daily for the first week. A continuous passive motion machine is initiated 1 week following surgery, beginning at 0° to 45° and increasing by 5° per day to a maximum of 90° of flexion. After 6 weeks, the brace is discontinued and weight bearing and range of motion are advanced. A progressive strengthening program is initiated, and light jogging is allowed at 12 weeks. Return to sports is determined by a functional testing program performed by our physical therapists to evaluate core strength, quadriceps strength, and muscular endurance.

Pearls

- We approach all meniscal tears as being potentially repairable and are increasingly aggressive about preserving the maximum amount of meniscal tissue with younger patient age.
- The success of meniscal repair in the absence of a cruciate ligament reconstruction can be enhanced through the use of an autologous fibrin clot, meniscal rasping, or microfracture of the intercondylar notch.[13]
- As understanding of the importance of the meniscus increases, the indications for meniscus preservation surgery in the symptomatic athlete will continue to expand.

References

1. Magnussen RA, Mansour AA, Carey JL, Spindler KP: Meniscus status at anterior cruciate ligament reconstruction associated with radiographic signs of osteoarthritis at 5- to 10-year follow-up: A systematic review. *J Knee Surg* 2009;22(4):347-357.
2. Stein T, Mehling AP, Welsch F, von Eisenhart-Rothe R, Jäger A: Long-term outcome after arthroscopic meniscal repair versus arthroscopic partial meniscectomy for traumatic meniscal tears. *Am J Sports Med* 2010;38(8):1542-1548.
3. Brophy RH, Wright RW, David TS, et al; Multicenter ACL Revision Study (MARS) Group: Association between previous meniscal surgery and the incidence of chondral lesions at revision anterior cruciate ligament reconstruction. *Am J Sports Med* 2012;40(4):808-814.
4. Fairbank TJ: Knee joint changes after meniscectomy. *J Bone Joint Surg Br* 1948;30(4):664-670.
5. Logan M, Watts M, Owen J, Myers P: Meniscal repair in the elite athlete: Results of 45 repairs with a minimum 5-year follow-up. *Am J Sports Med* 2009;37(6):1131-1134.
6. Arnoczky SP, Warren RF: Microvasculature of the human meniscus. *Am J Sports Med* 1982;10(2):90-95.
7. DeHaven KE, Arnoczky SP: Meniscus repair: Basic science, indications for repair, and open repair. *Instr Course Lect* 1994;43:65-76.
8. Aspden RM, Yarker YE, Hukins DW: Collagen orientations in the meniscus of the knee joint. *J Anat* 1985;140(pt 3):371-380.
9. Wagner HJ: Architecture of collagen fibers in the meniscus of the human knee joint, with special reference to the medial meniscus and its connection to the articular ligaments [German]. *Z Mikrosk Anat Forsch* 1976;90(2):302-324.
10. Cannon WD Jr, Vittori JM: The incidence of healing in arthroscopic meniscal repairs in anterior cruciate ligament-reconstructed knees versus stable knees. *Am J Sports Med* 1992;20(2):176-181.
11. van Trommel MF, Simonian PT, Potter HG, Wickiewicz TL: Arthroscopic meniscal repair with fibrin clot of complete radial tears of the lateral meniscus in the avascular zone. *Arthroscopy* 1998;14(4):360-365.
12. Arnoczky SP, Warren RF: The microvasculature of the meniscus and its response to injury: An experimental study in the dog. *Am J Sports Med* 1983;11(3):131-141.
13. Arnoczky SP, Warren RF, Spivak JM: Meniscal repair using an exogenous fibrin clot: An experimental study in dogs. *J Bone Joint Surg Am* 1988;70(8):1209-1217.
14. Kuikka PI, Sillanpää P, Mattila VM, Niva MH, Pihlajamäki HK: Magnetic resonance imaging in acute traumatic and chronic meniscal tears of the knee: A diagnostic accuracy study in young adults. *Am J Sports Med* 2009;37(5):1003-1008.
15. Steckel H, Vadala G, Davis D, Fu FH: 2D and 3D 3-tesla magnetic resonance imaging of the double bundle structure in anterior cruciate ligament anatomy. *Knee Surg Sports Traumatol Arthrosc* 2006;14(11):1151-1158.

Chapter 13
Medial Meniscal Root Repair

Dharmesh Vyas, MD   Christopher D. Harner, MD

Introduction

The role of the meniscus is to disperse load, guide tibiofemoral contact, and act as a secondary stabilizer of the knee. A specific subset of meniscal injuries that have become increasingly recognized are tears of the posterior root of the medial meniscus, or medial meniscal root tears (MMRTs).[1-3] Meniscal root tears result in a loss of hoop stresses and expose cartilage to abnormal contact forces comparable to those after total meniscectomy.[4,5] The mechanisms of altered knee kinematics after an MMRT have been postulated to result from a predictable posteromedial displacement of femoral contact on the medial tibial plateau. Left untreated, they have been shown to result in meniscal extrusion, joint space narrowing, and rapidly progressive knee arthritis.[1,4,6,7]

Patient Selection

Indications for surgical management of meniscal root tears include (1) isolated symptomatic MMRTs with minimal arthritis, (2) failure of nonsurgical management with continued activity-limiting pain, and (3) lateral meniscal root tears concomitant with an anterior cruciate ligament (ACL) tear. (This chapter discusses MMRTs only.)

Contraindications to meniscal root repair are (1) medial joint space narrowing with Fairbank changes (on flexion weight-bearing PA radiographs), (2) asymmetric varus alignment (>3°) and medial joint space narrowing on long-cassette radiographs, and (3) diffuse International Cartilage Repair Society grade 3 or 4 chondral changes in the femoral condyle or tibial plateau articular cartilage identified at the time of surgery.

Preoperative Imaging
Radiographs

Diagnostic imaging begins with plain radiographs. These include 45° flexion weight-bearing PA views of both knees, a lateral view, and Merchant patella views (Figure 1). These radiographs are used to gauge the amount of joint space narrowing in the three compartments, patella height (lateral), and patellar tilt and subluxation (Merchant). A long-cassette AP view of the bilateral lower extremities is also obtained, and the overall limb alignment is determined by calculating the mechanical axis from the radiograph.

Magnetic Resonance Imaging

Based on the patient's history and physical examination, if a meniscal tear is suspected, then a noncontrast MRI of the knee is obtained. The meniscal root can be easily identified on contiguous coronal images as a band of low-signal-intensity tissue anchoring the meniscus to the underlying tibia (Figure 2). Although the root is also visible on sagittal images, its identification is more variable in these sequences.[2] Injury to the root varies from intrasubstance degeneration with mild fraying to full-thickness tears. A tear is identified by increased signal intensity within the meniscal root that extends to the articular surface on T2-weighted images. Additionally, root tears are often associated with extrusion of the meniscus more than 3 mm beyond the margin of the tibial plateau.[8] In the presence of a complete radial tear, the two fragments

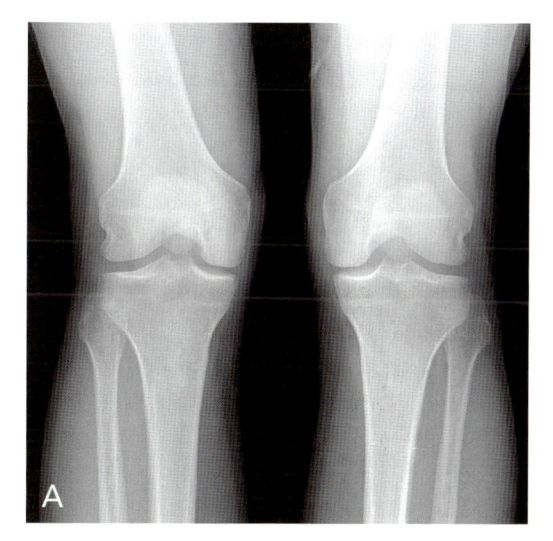

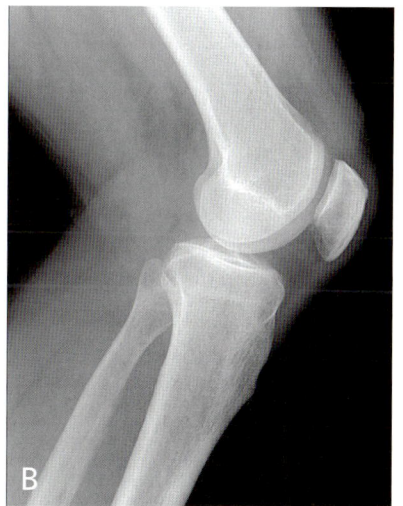

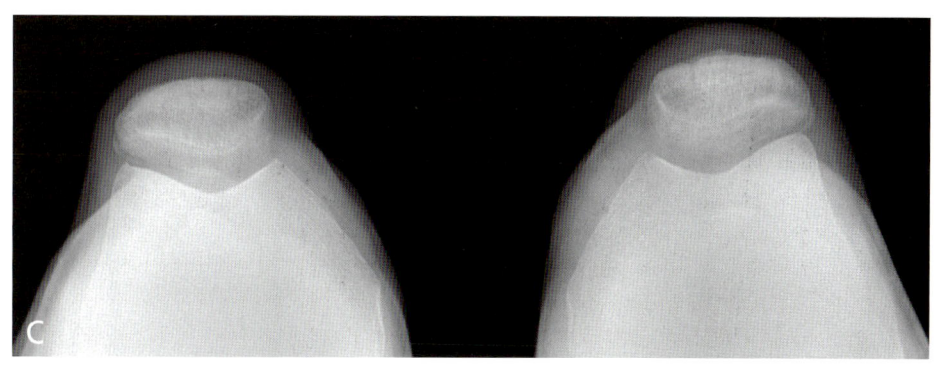

Figure 1 A 45° flexion weight-bearing PA view of both knees (**A**), a lateral view (**B**), and a Merchant patella view (**C**) demonstrate well-maintained joint spaces with mild early arthritic changes seen in the form of marginal osteophytes in all three compartments. Slight patella baja is also seen.

Dr. Harner or an immediate family member has received research or institutional support from DePuy and Smith & Nephew and serves as a board member, owner, officer, or committee member of the American Board of Orthopaedic Surgery, the American Orthopaedic Association, the American Academy of Orthopaedic Surgeons, and the American Orthopaedic Society for Sports Medicine. Neither Dr. Vyas nor any immediate family member has received anything of value from or owns stock in a commercial company or institution related directly or indirectly to the subject of this chapter.

Section 1: Sports Medicine

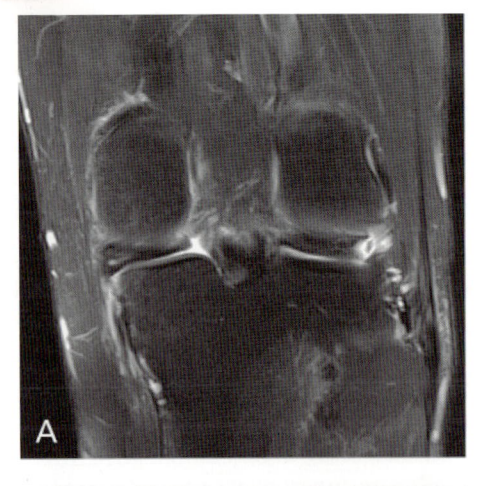

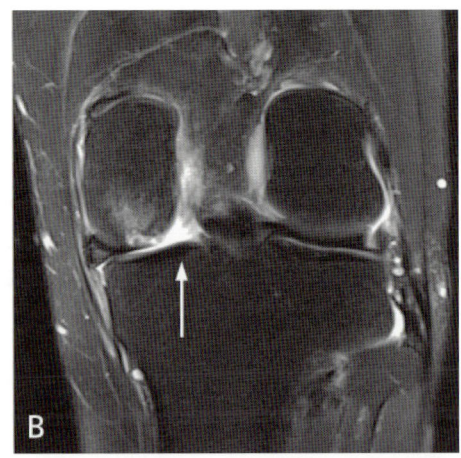

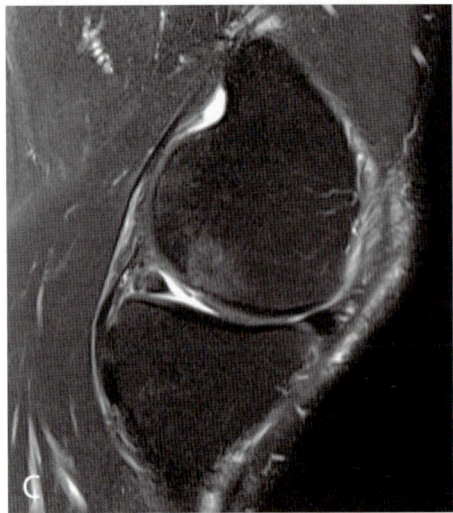

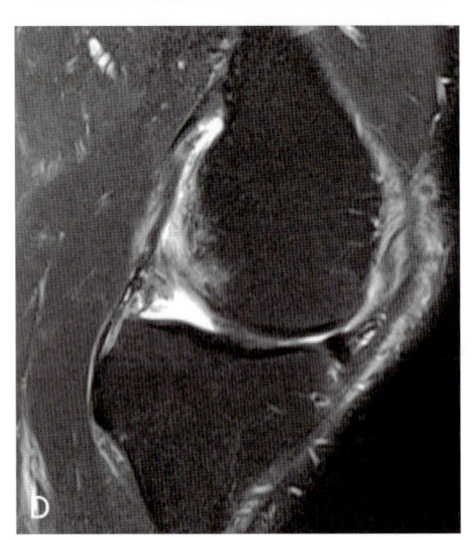

Figure 2 Coronal (**A** and **B**) and sagittal (**C** and **D**) T2-weighted MRIs demonstrate a medial meniscal root tear (MMRT) (arrow). This is identified by increased signal intensity within the meniscal root that extends to the articular surface. Also, extrusion of the medial meniscus is noted. As a result of a complete radial tear, the two fragments are separated and take on the appearance of an empty meniscal space (**C** and **D**). An associated medial femoral condyle articular cartilage lesion can also be seen.

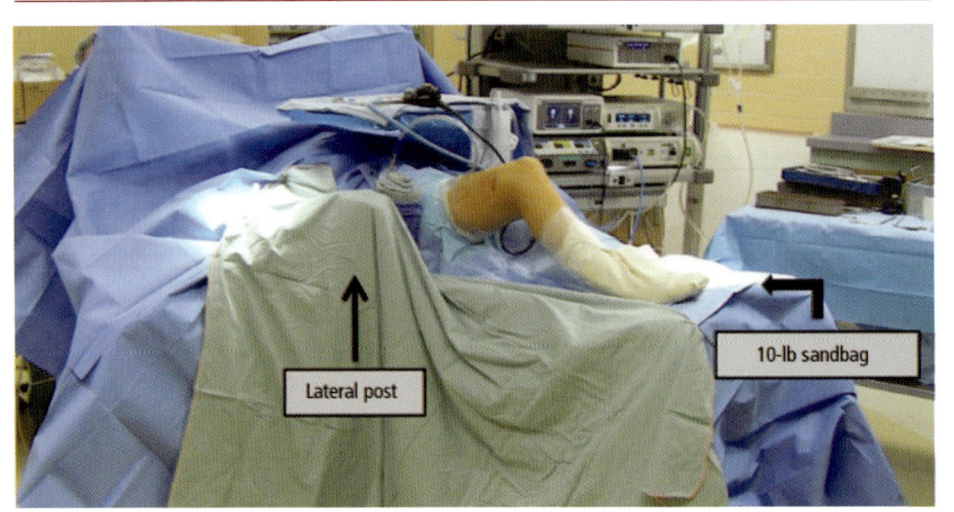

Figure 3 Photograph shows the surgical setup for MMRT repair. The patient is positioned supine with a bump under the ipsilateral hip. A sandbag and a lateral post are used to keep the leg at 90° of flexion.

may be separated and take on the appearance of an empty meniscal space or an empty meniscus sign.[9,10] Associated bone bruises and/or ligamentous injuries can also be identified on MRI.

Procedure

Room Setup/Patient Positioning
The patient is placed supine on the operating room table, and prophylactic antibiotics are administered. A soft gel bump is placed under the ipsilateral hip, and a 10-lb sandbag is taped to the table to support the knee at 90° of flexion (**Figure 3**). A lateral post is placed at the level of the midthigh to support the lower extremity. We do not use a tourniquet or a leg holder.

Special Instruments/Equipment/Implants
The procedure calls for the following equipment:
- 30° and 70° arthroscopes
- 4.5-mm full-radius resectors (straight and curved)
- ACL drill guide with guide pin
- Meniscal rasp
- 70° suture shuttle
- Hewson suture passer
- 8-mm clear cannula
- No. 2 nonabsorbable braided suture
- 6.5-mm cancellous screw with washer

Surgical Technique
Examination Under Anesthesia
An examination of both knees is performed after anesthesia is induced. Knee range of motion, the presence of an effusion, and ligamentous laxity are assessed and documented. Prior to preparation and draping of the limb, surface landmarks and incisions are drawn with a skin marker. To aid in hemostasis, the incisions are prepped with Betadine (povidone-iodine), and the skin is injected with 1% lidocaine with epinephrine (1:100,000). The extremity is then prepped in its entirety with Betadine and draped.

Landmarks
Key landmarks are the patella (inferior pole), the patellar tendon, the medial joint line, the Gerdy tubercle, and the tibial tubercle.

Portals and Incisions
The landmarks, arthroscopic portal sites, and skin incisions are marked on the skin (**Figure 4**). For the procedure, we use four portals: anterolateral, anteromedial, superolateral outflow, and posteromedial. A 5- to 7-cm skin incision is made medial to the tibial tubercle, starting 1 cm proximal to the patellar tendon attachment and extending distally. A 3-cm oblique incision is made on the anterolateral proximal tibia, distal to the Gerdy tubercle and proximal to the origin of the tibialis anterior muscle.

Diagnostic Arthroscopy
The diagnostic arthroscopy is performed with the arthroscope in the anterolat-

Chapter 13: Medial Meniscal Root Repair

eral portal and a probe placed through the anteromedial portal. After all three compartments have been evaluated and associated injuries ruled out, attention is turned to the posterior root of the medial meniscus. In some cases, the root of the medial meniscus is difficult to inspect arthroscopically. To assist in visualization of the posteromedial joint space, the arthroscope is positioned along the lateral aspect of the medial femoral condyle and under the posteromedial bundle of the posterior cruciate ligament (Gillquist view). From this position, both the posterior horn of the medial meniscus and the medial meniscal root insertion are inspected. Under direct visualization and tactile probing, the root is confirmed to be repairable (adequate quality remaining tissue with minimal retraction of the meniscus). At this point, a posteromedial portal is created if necessary to improve visualization of the root.

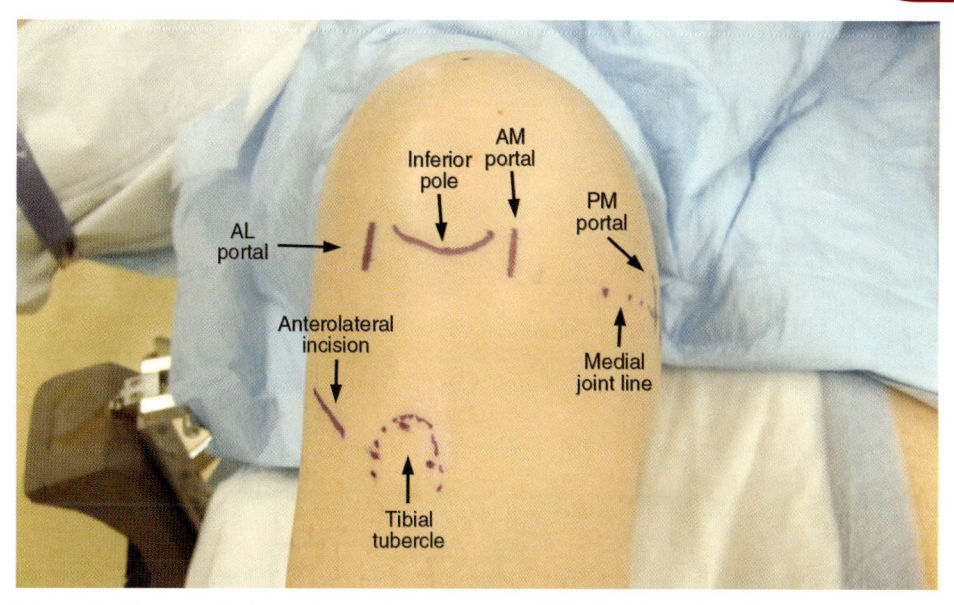

Figure 4 Photograph shows the surface anatomy and skin incisions for arthroscopic MMRT repair. Surface landmarks are marked and include the inferior pole of the patella, the medial joint line, and the tibial tubercle. Three of the four portals are shown: anterolateral (AL), anteromedial (AM), and posteromedial (PM—provisionally marked; the final position is determined by direct arthroscopic visualization). Not shown is the superolateral outflow portal. The anterolateral tibial incision is also marked.

Posteromedial Portal

The knee is maintained flexed at 90°, and the entry point is approximated at 10 mm proximal to the medial joint line and 5 mm behind the posterior edge of the femoral condyle. Under direct visualization from the Gillquist view, a spinal needle is inserted percutaneously to verify the entry point. When the entry point has been confirmed, the needle is withdrawn, and a vertical portal is made using a No. 11 blade (the incision is made through all soft-tissue layers, including the capsule). Using a switching stick, the arthroscope is then introduced into the posteromedial joint space through this portal.

Video 13.1 Posterior Horn Medial Meniscal Root Repair. Dharmesh Vyas, MD, PhD; Christopher D. Harner, MD (13 min)

Procedure

Figure 5 illustrates steps in arthroscopic meniscal root repair.

Exposure of the Root Tear and Insertion Site

After establishing all the necessary portals, the first step in the root repair is to provide adequate exposure to visualize the meniscal root and its insertion on the posterior tibial plateau. This is done using a 4.5-mm full-radius resector (shaver) to perform a reverse notchplasty of synovium and 3 to 5 mm of articular cartilage from the posteroinferior aspect of the medial femoral condyle. The utility of the reverse notchplasty is for visualization of the root and insertion, tunnel positioning, repair bed preparation, and root fixation.

Critical to the repair is preparation of a broad tibial insertion site down to bleeding bone. This is done with the arthroscope in the posteromedial portal and the curved shaver or meniscal rasp in the anterolateral portal. The surface is shaved until pinpoint bleeding sites or marrow fat globules are seen emanating from the prepared bed.

Suture Passage and Tunnel Preparation

After the tibial bed has been adequately prepared, suture capture of the meniscal root is performed. To facilitate the passage and control of the suture, an 8-mm clear cannula is used in the anterolateral portal. Visualized with the arthroscope in the anteromedial portal, the suture shuttle device is introduced via the cannula, and the meniscal root is pierced in a tibial-to-femoral surface direction. The monofilament loop is passed through the meniscal root, and the shuttle device is removed from the joint. The loop is then pulled out of the anterolateral portal, and the free ends of the monofilament are held to prevent them from advancing into the joint. Next, one end of the braided No. 2 suture is fed into the monofilament loop, and a braided loop is created by making the two ends equal. The monofilament is used to shuttle the braided loop through the meniscus and out the anterolateral portal. Outside the joint, the free ends of the braided suture are then fed through its loop and advanced down onto the meniscus, creating a tight loop stitch. This step is repeated to capture the root with a second loop stitch for added security and force distribution to prevent suture pull-out.

Tunnel preparation for the passage of the sutures begins with the arthroscope in the posteromedial portal. An ACL transtibial tip guide is inserted through the anterolateral portal, over the ACL, and positioned at the native root insertion site. The entry point of the guidewire is estimated using the drilling sleeve, and an oblique incision is made over the anterolateral tibial skin. The dissection is carried down to the anterior compartment fascia and the periosteum. Two to 3 cm of anterior compartment soft tissue is elevated off the tibia at a level just distal to the Gerdy tubercle. This is done to protect the soft tissue during drilling of the tunnel as well as placement of the screw/washer-post construct.

Next, the ACL tip guide is repositioned on the root insertion, and the drill sleeve is placed onto the anterolateral aspect of the tibia. A 3/32-in (2.4-mm) guide pin is drilled to (but not through) the posterior cortex of the tibia by power. Perforation of the far cortex is completed manually by tapping the guide pin with gentle mallet blows, thereby assuring steady control

© 2013 American Academy of Orthopaedic Surgeons

Section 1: Sports Medicine

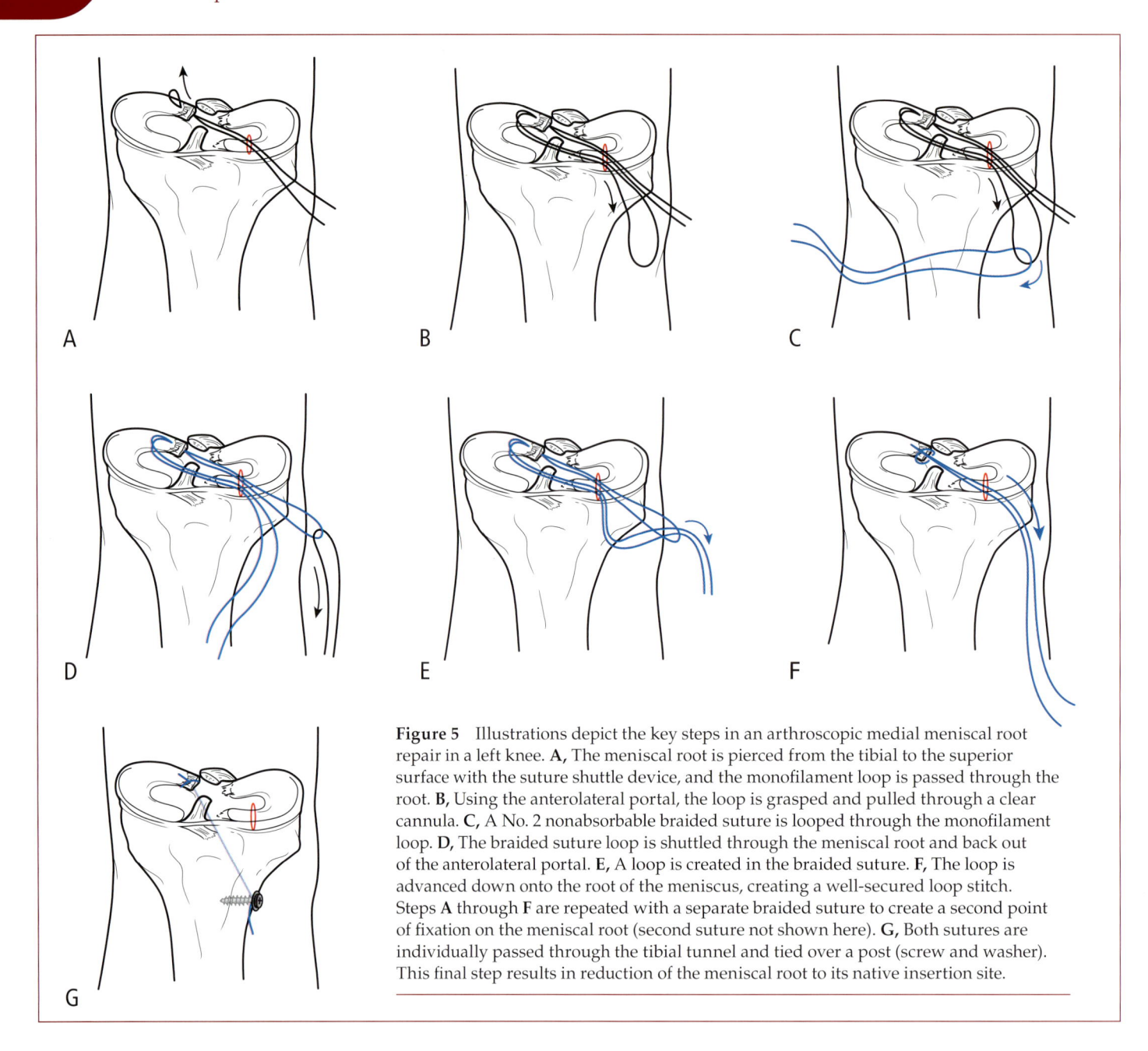

Figure 5 Illustrations depict the key steps in an arthroscopic medial meniscal root repair in a left knee. **A**, The meniscal root is pierced from the tibial to the superior surface with the suture shuttle device, and the monofilament loop is passed through the root. **B**, Using the anterolateral portal, the loop is grasped and pulled through a clear cannula. **C**, A No. 2 nonabsorbable braided suture is looped through the monofilament loop. **D**, The braided suture loop is shuttled through the meniscal root and back out of the anterolateral portal. **E**, A loop is created in the braided suture. **F**, The loop is advanced down onto the root of the meniscus, creating a well-secured loop stitch. Steps **A** through **F** are repeated with a separate braided suture to create a second point of fixation on the meniscal root (second suture not shown here). **G**, Both sutures are individually passed through the tibial tunnel and tied over a post (screw and washer). This final step results in reduction of the meniscal root to its native insertion site.

of the pin when in close proximity to the popliteal neurovascular bundle.

Tear Fixation
Having completed the tunnel, the guide pin is withdrawn and a Hewson suture passer is introduced in its place. Through the anterolateral portal, arthroscopic suture retrievers (ice tongs) are passed through the Hewson loop, and the braided suture is grasped and pulled out through the tunnel. To facilitate ease of passage, the ice tongs can be used as a pulley to improve the angle of suture retrieval through the tunnel entrance. Depending on the size of the posterior horn as well as the extent of the tear, a second suture may provide added fixation to the root tear. In that case, both sets of sutures can be retrieved through the same tunnel. Reduction of the root to its insertion should be arthroscopically verified by pulling tension on the sutures after they have been retrieved out the anterior tibia.

As the final step in the fixation, the sutures are tied over a post on the anterolateral aspect of the tibia using a 4.5-mm cancellous screw with a washer (**Figure 6**). This is accomplished with the knee in 30° of flexion to aid in proper reduction of the meniscus. The anterior compartment soft tissue is reapproximated using No. 0 Vicryl (Ethicon), and the skin is closed in the usual fashion.

Complications
Complications specific to meniscal root repair surgery can occur mostly from inadequate exposure of the repair bed (insufficient reverse notchplasty). This could result in an insufficient amount of root tissue captured with the repair stitch, iatrogenic damage to the ACL with frequent and vigorous passage of the tip guide, or even damage to the neurovascular bundle in the posterior knee with a poorly visualized pin passage. Other complications generally associated with knee surgery include postoperative infection, arthrofibrosis, deep venous thrombosis, and failure of meniscal root healing despite an otherwise properly executed repair.

Postoperative Care and Rehabilitation
Postoperatively, the patient is allowed partial weight bearing for the first 6 weeks. Progressive weight bearing is then begun, with a goal of full weight bearing by 8 weeks after surgery. In the immediate postoperative period, a continuous passive motion machine is used

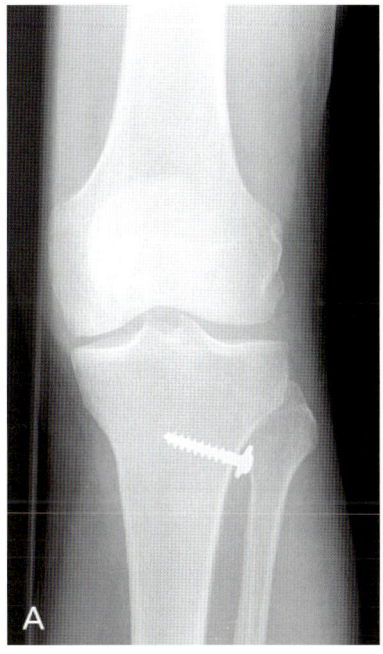

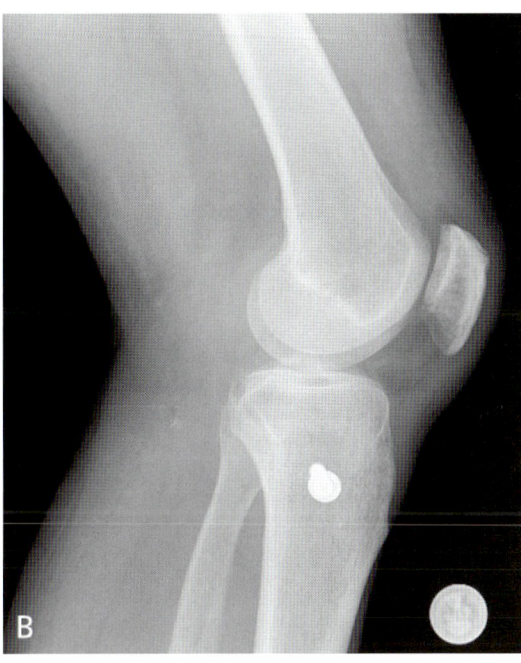

Figure 6 Postoperative AP (**A**) and lateral (**B**) radiographs demonste the position of the screw-and-washer construct used as a post to tie the meniscal root fixation sutures. Note that this is not a 45° flexion weight-bearing view, so it projects slightly differently from the preoperative views in Figure 1.

for the first 4 weeks (set at 0° to 90°). In the first month, physical therapy consists of straight-leg raises, quadriceps sets, heel slides, and calf pumps. Formal, supervised physical therapy can be prescribed during the second and third months after surgery. In most patients, return to full activity can be achieved by 4 months. Bracing is optional; it may be useful for the first week in the event of a regional block or weak quadriceps strength.

Pearls
- The majority of the procedure can be done with the knee at 90° of flexion and without the use of a tourniquet or leg holder.
- A posteromedial portal is often necessary for added visualization of the root and its insertion.
- A reverse notchplasty should be performed. Compromised arthroscopic visualization of the insertion site will make bed preparation, suture passage, and fixation very difficult.
- Multiple passes of the suture shuttle device through the meniscal root should be avoided because this will result in irreparable fraying of already injured tissue.
- If two sets of sutures are passed around the meniscus, the surgeon should not try to pass all four strands through the tunnel at the same time.

References
1. Harner CD, Mauro CS, Lesniak BP, Romanowski JR: Biomechanical consequences of a tear of the posterior root of the medial meniscus: Surgical technique. *J Bone Joint Surg Am* 2009;91(suppl 2): 257-270.
2. Koenig JH, Ranawat AS, Umans HR, Difelice GS: Meniscal root tears: Diagnosis and treatment. *Arthroscopy* 2009;25(9):1025-1032.
3. Rubinstein RA Jr, DeHaan A, Baldwin JL: Posterior medial meniscus detachment: A unique type of medial meniscal tear. *J Knee Surg* 2009;22(4):339-345.
4. Allaire R, Muriuki M, Gilbertson L, Harner CD: Biomechanical consequences of a tear of the posterior root of the medial meniscus: Similar to total meniscectomy. *J Bone Joint Surg Am* 2008;90(9):1922-1931.
5. Ding C, Martel-Pelletier J, Pelletier JP, et al: Knee meniscal extrusion in a largely non-osteoarthritic cohort: Association with greater loss of cartilage volume. *Arthritis Res Ther* 2007;9(2):R21.
6. Stärke C, Kopf S, Gröbel KH, Becker R: The effect of a nonanatomic repair of the meniscal horn attachment on meniscal tension: A biomechanical study. *Arthroscopy* 2010;26(3):358-365.
7. Lerer DB, Umans HR, Hu MX, Jones MH: The role of meniscal root pathology and radial meniscal tear in medial meniscal extrusion. *Skeletal Radiol* 2004;33(10): 569-574.
8. Brody JM, Lin HM, Hulstyn MJ, Tung GA: Lateral meniscus root tear and meniscus extrusion with anterior cruciate ligament tear. *Radiology* 2006;239(3): 805-810.
9. Choi CJ, Choi YJ, Lee JJ, Choi CH: Magnetic resonance imaging evidence of meniscal extrusion in medial meniscus posterior root tear. *Arthroscopy* 2010;26(12):1602-1606.
10. Lee SY, Jee WH, Kim JM: Radial tear of the medial meniscal root: Reliability and accuracy of MRI for diagnosis. *AJR Am J Roentgenol* 2008;191(1):81-85.

Chapter 14
Microfracture

Armando F. Vidal, MD   Jennifer FitzPatrick, MD

Introduction
Chondral lesions of the knee are frequently encountered during arthroscopic procedures and can commonly be a source of pain and recurrent effusions. In the young patient, the presence of chondral pathology can be complicated by instability, malalignment, and meniscal insufficiency. It has been known for decades that articular cartilage has limited intrinsic healing capacity, therefore, various different cartilage repair strategies have been developed. Broadly, these strategies have included marrow-stimulating techniques such as microfracture, autologous and allograft osteochondral transplants, and autologous chondrocyte implantation. Marrow-stimulating techniques rely on perforation of the subchondral plate, which allows pluripotential mesenchymal cells to fill the defect and create a hybrid fibrocartilage repair.

Patient Selection
For many patients, the microfracture technique is the first-line treatment of full-thickness cartilage lesions (Outerbridge grade IV) because of its success, relative ease, and cost effectiveness. In addition, when unsuccessful, it generally does not preclude the use of other cartilage restoration techniques as subsequent treatment options. The selection criteria for a successful outcome are very specific, however.

Indications
Clinically important parameters when considering the suitability of a patient for microfracture include size, location, and containment of the articular cartilage lesion; status of the meniscus; age of the patient; and body mass index. Although there is some controversy as to the maximum size of the lesion, many describe the "ideal" lesion as less than 2 cm^2 and not exceeding an area of 4 cm^2.[1-4] Additionally, the lesion should be unipolar and well contained. Microfracture is not indicated for degenerative, bipolar lesions. Femoral condylar lesions are ideal; however, microfracture can be performed on any articular surface. Generally, the results are less favorable for lesions in the patellofemoral compartment.[5] Additionally, the ability of these pluripotential cells to differentiate into cartilage is influenced by age. Several authors have shown better results in younger patients.[2,3,5-7] The age cutoff has generally been accepted as younger than 40 years. It is also essential to determine by history and physical examination which lesions are symptomatic, as focal grade IV cartilage defects have been found in asymptomatic elite athletes.[8]

Contraindications
Contraindications to microfracture include bipolar lesions, diffuse degenerative joint disease, uncorrected malalignment, significant loss of meniscal tissue, and patients who will not be able to fulfill or comply with the required postoperative protocol. Bipolar lesions preclude the appropriate healing environment because there are two incongruent surfaces in contact with one another.[9] Lesions with subchondral bone loss and uncontained lesions are not amenable to microfracture for similar reasons. Uncorrected malalignment will cause abnormal mechanics, which will place increased loads on the microfractured surface.[10] Longer duration of preoperative symptoms and a body mass index greater than 30 kg/m^2 may also have an association with poorer outcomes.[4,7]

Preoperative Imaging
The diagnostic imaging begins with plain radiographs. A standard series includes four views: weight-bearing AP, weight-bearing 45° PA, lateral, and Merchant. In patients with chronic or degenerative conditions, these views can help determine if the degree of arthrosis is too severe or diffuse to consider microfracture as a viable option. In an acute injury, these four views may reveal a donor site and a loose body consistent with an osteochondral fragment. When any cartilage repair technique is being considered, including microfracture, long-leg alignment radiographs must also be obtained to evaluate for any angular deformity that may require concomitant treatment. Focal cartilage lesions that satisfy these criteria in the setting of varus malalignment can be treated successfully with combined microfracture and high tibial osteotomy.[10]

MRI also has become a standard diagnostic imaging technique. Cartilage-specific MRI sequences can accurately diagnose cartilage injury[11] (**Figure 1**). Sequences recommended by the International Cartilage Repair Society are proton density–weighted fast spin-echo imaging with or without fat saturation, T2-weighted fast spin-echo imaging with or without fat saturation, and T1-weighted gradient-echo imaging with fat suppression.[11] In addition to the chondral injury, MRI will reveal any concomitant meniscal or ligamentous pathology that may need to be addressed.

Video 14.1 Microfracture: Technique and Pearls. Armando F. Vidal, MD (10 min)

Procedure
Setup/Patient Positioning
Microfracture can be performed under general, spinal, or regional block anesthesia. After anesthesia is administered, the patient is placed in the supine position, and the affected lower extremity is prepared for a standard knee arthroscopy based on the surgeon's preference. An examination under anesthesia is important, as with any cartilage or ligamentous procedure. A valgus stress post or leg holder can be used to provide access to the intended compartment as long as full range of motion of the knee is allowed. A tourniquet is not typically necessary but can be used per surgeon preference. The pressure created by the arthroscopic fluid is usually sufficient to tamponade bleed-

---

Dr. Vidal or an immediate family member is a member of a speakers' bureau or has made paid presentations on behalf of the Musculoskeletal Transplant Foundation. Neither Dr. FitzPatrick nor any immediate family member has received anything of value from or owns stock in a commercial company or institution related directly or indirectly to the subject of this chapter.

ing during the procedure. A standard diagnostic knee arthroscopy is then performed through anterolateral and anteromedial portals. Meniscal, chondral, and ligamentous pathologies are identified. Often, loose bodies are encountered with full-thickness cartilage lesions; these should be addressed.

Surgical Technique

In general, other pathology (meniscal tears, plica, loose bodies, etc) is addressed first, and the microfracture procedure is reserved for the end. This sequence is recommended because the bleeding caused by the microfracture may obscure visualization for the other parts of the procedure. However, it is recommended that ligamentous pathology be addressed after the microfracture procedure. Generally, the chondral lesion is easier to access before the ligament reconstruction; additionally, undue stress on the graft is avoided while accessing the chondral lesion.

Once the chondral lesion is identified, unstable cartilage flaps are débrided, and the factors mentioned earlier are assessed to determine if the lesion is amenable to microfracture treatment. If there is significant subchondral bone loss or an uncontained lesion without clear borders, then microfracture may not be indicated because the results will be suboptimal. The arc of motion in which the lesion is weight bearing is noted because this may have implications for the postoperative rehabilitation course. The débridement and preparation of the lesion is performed with a combination of an arthroscopic shaver and a curet. The shaver is used both on oscillate and on forward and reverse to help define the lesion and rid the joint of debris, which may later lead to loose bodies. It is important to create perpendicular edges at the transition between the lesion and stable, healthy cartilage. This step enhances the lesion's ability to contain the "super clot." Our preference is to use a ring curet that produces a vertical and stable shoulder to the lesion. After débridement, the calcified cartilage layer that remains must be débrided (**Figure 2**). Animal studies have shown this to be a critical step that enhances volume fill of the lesion and the ability of the repair tissue to bond to the underlying subchondral plate.[12] If a stable rim of healthy cartilage does not shoulder the lesion, achieving a stable clot may be more difficult.[4,13]

After débridement and preparation of the lesion, commercially available microfracture awls are used to create holes within the base of the lesion. The awls have conical-shaped tips and come in multiple angles to facilitate the creation of holes perpendicular to the subchondral plate (**Figure 3**). Accessory portals may also be necessary to achieve this, particularly for very posterior femoral condyle or patellar lesions. Typically, the 45° awl is used first. The holes are created in a systematic fashion, starting at the periphery and working in toward the center of the lesion. It is imperative that the awl is perpendicular to the surface to prevent skiving so that the holes do not become confluent with one another. It is also important to maintain adequate spacing (approximately 3 to 4 mm) when creating the holes to preserve the integrity of the subchondral bone between the holes. This will help to prevent the "macrofracture" complication, rather than the microfracture that is intended. The awls allow for controlled depth of penetration, approximately 2 to 4 mm. Adequate access to marrow elements is then assessed with the visualization of fat droplets or blood by clamping off the inflow or the negative pressure from the arthroscopic pump. An egress of blood and fat droplets from all holes confirms successful penetration with the awls. (The steps of the microfracture technique are shown in **Figure 4**.) It is important to perform this procedure without tourniquet control to assess the stimulation of blood from the subchondral plate. Bony debris created during the microfracture process is removed with a shaver.

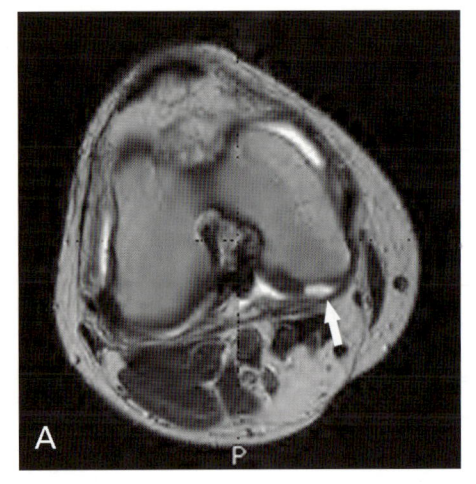

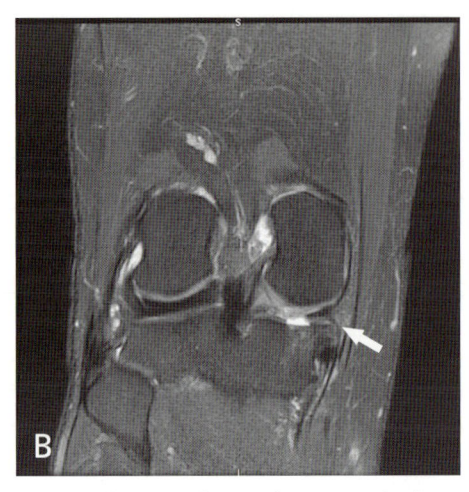

Figure 1 Cartilage-specific MRI sequences. **A,** Transaxial proton-density fast spin-echo fat-saturation MRI demonstrates a posterior femoral condyle lesion. **B,** Coronal proton density–weighted fat-saturation MRI demonstrates a medial tibial plateau lesion.

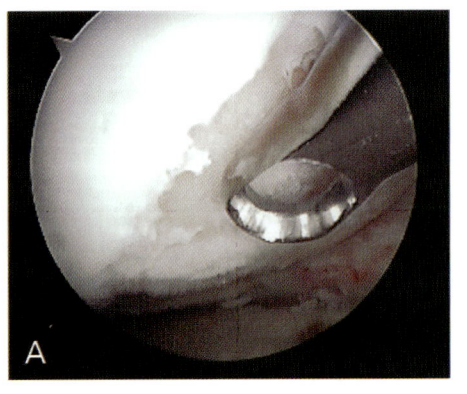

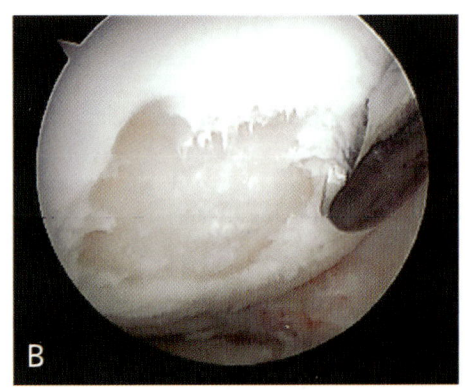

Figure 2 Arthroscopic views demonstrate débridement and preparation of a chondral lesion before microfracture. **A,** Ring curet removes the calcified cartilage layer. **B,** Ring curet creates shoulders.

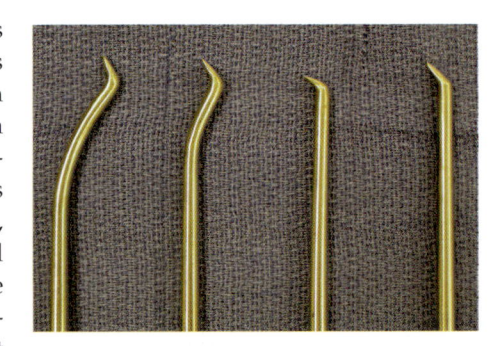

Figure 3 Photograph depicts microfracture awls of various angles.

Chapter 14: Microfracture

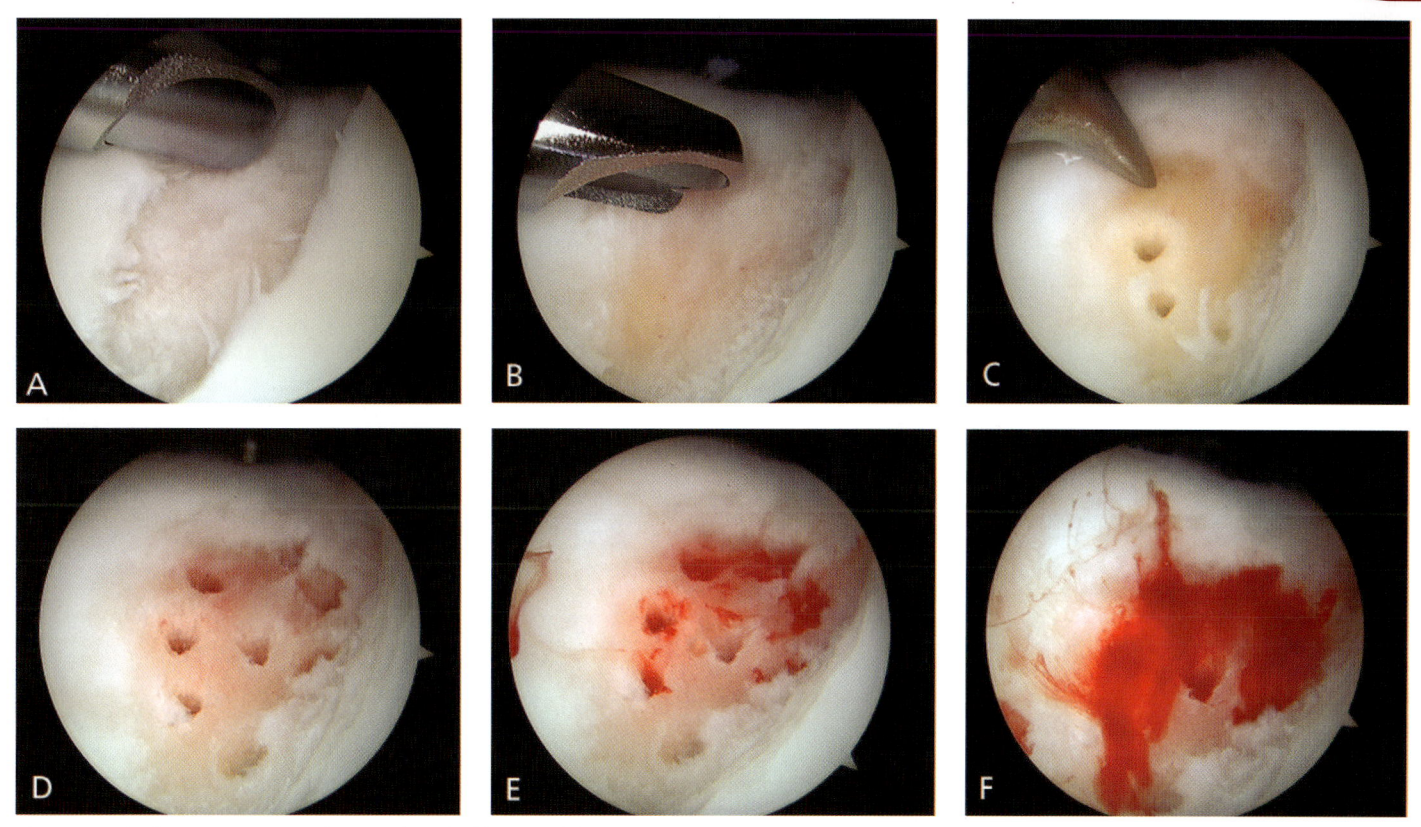

Figure 4 Arthroscopic views show a chondral lesion of the trochlea treated with the microfracture technique. **A,** Initial débridement of the lesion. **B,** A shaver is used to remove the calcified cartilage layer. **C,** Beginning at the periphery of the lesion, a microfracture awl is used to create holes perpendicular to the subchondral bone. **D,** The completed holes. **E** and **F,** Inflow has been clamped off, allowing visualization of blood emanating from the holes.

All arthroscopic instruments are then removed from the knee. Postoperative drains should not be used because they may dislodge or remove the mesenchymal cells that are intended for the super clot. A compressive wrap and cryotherapy cuff are applied to the knee to help with postoperative swelling and pain. A brace is typically not used for femoral condyle lesions. Knees treated for patellofemoral lesions are immobilized in a hinged knee brace locked in full extension.

Complications

One of the advantages of the microfracture procedure is that the associated complications are relatively few.

A joint effusion is typical for the first several weeks after surgery. A return of this effusion may occur at 6 to 8 weeks, when the patient begins full weight bearing and is becoming more active on the extremity. This effusion is generally painless and should not be alarming to the surgeon or patient because it usually resolves in a few weeks without any intervention.

Osseous overgrowth after microfracture has been noted on subsequent MRI studies in 25% to 49% of patients.[4] The repair cartilage overlying these areas is thinner, but it is unclear whether this plays a role in prognosis or patient outcome. Although the exact mechanism for osseous overgrowth has not been elucidated, excessive débridement of subchondral bone may be a contributing factor.[14] Although regenerative tissue following microfracture may be limited in terms of durability, intralesional bone formation and elevation of the subchondral bone plate seem to be characteristic problems of this technique. Additionally, although microfracture does not preclude other cartilage repair techniques in the future, the success of techniques such as autologous chondrocyte implantation may be compromised if performed as a revision procedure following microfracture rather than as a primary procedure.[14]

Because of the rehabilitation restrictions required, patients will develop some quadriceps weakness and atrophy. This frequently leads to anterior knee pain as the postoperative course progresses and patients begin to bear full weight and become more active. This pain resolves as quadriceps strength returns. After the treatment of patellofemoral lesions, patients may report mechanical symptoms during a range of motion. This also resolves as rehabilitation progresses.

Postoperative Care and Rehabilitation

The rehabilitation program is considered a critical component of the success of a microfracture procedure. Protocols are tailored somewhat, depending on the location of the chondral lesion, but the same basic principles apply to all microfracture patients: protected weight bearing and the use of a continuous passive motion (CPM) machine. However, rehabilitation protocols are mostly empirical because the effect of CPM and weight-bearing status has not been evaluated systematically.[7] The initial 7 to 10 days are focused on controlling edema and pain. A compressive bandage and a cryotherapy device are used. CPM use is started on the day of surgery. Patients are encouraged to avoid rigorous activity to allow the super clot to form and adhere. The goal is to provide the optimal environment for the mesenchymal cells of the super clot to differentiate into cartilage repair cells (**Figure 5**).

For lesions involving a femoral condyle or the tibial plateau, patients are started on a CPM machine immediately in the recovery room. The initial range-of-motion setting varies slightly based on surgeon preference, but frequently used protocols

© 2013 American Academy of Orthopaedic Surgeons 81

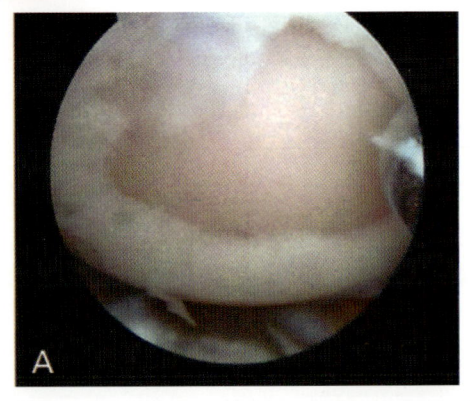

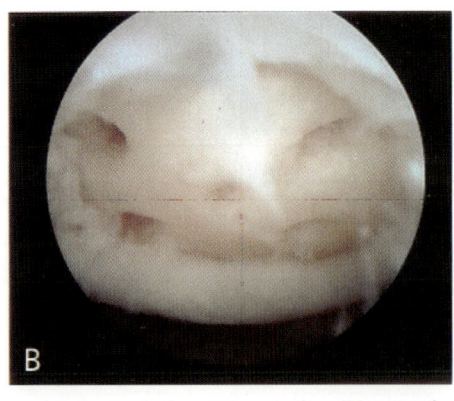

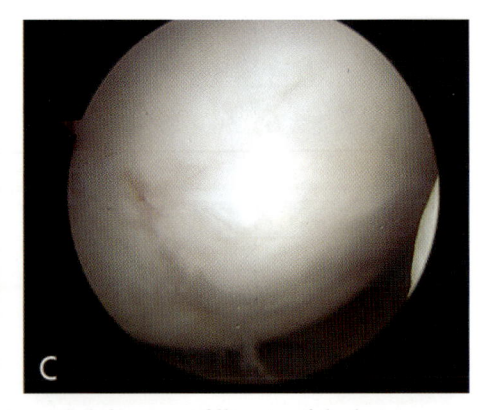

Figure 5 Arthroscopic images show a femoral condyle lesion before (**A**) and after (**B**) microfracture. **C**, Subsequent filling in of the lesion observed during a second-look arthroscopy.

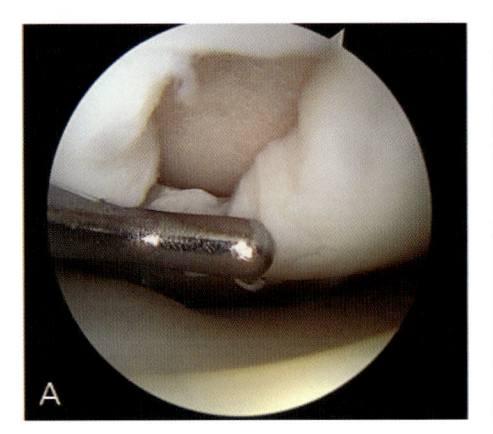

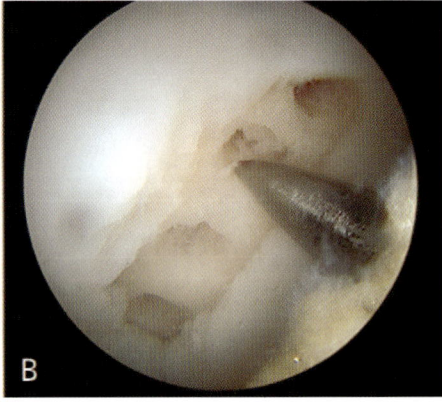

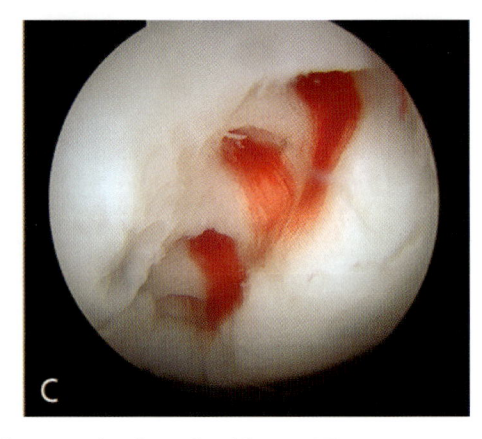

Figure 6 Arthroscopic views show microfracture. **A**, A small, well-contained femoral condyle lesion with robust shoulders. **B**, The same lesion after débridement and microfracture. **C**, Confirmation of penetration of the subchondral plate and bleeding from the microfracture holes. With small, well-shouldered lesions such as this, earlier weight bearing can be considered.

start at 0° to 60° or 30° to 70° at a rate of 1 cycle/min. The CPM machine is used for 6 to 8 hours per day for 6 to 8 weeks. Range of motion is advanced in 10° increments as tolerated by the patient until full passive range of motion is achieved. For those patients who cannot tolerate the CPM machine, a program of passive flexion and extension, with 500 repetitions three times a day, has been employed.[15]

Protected weight bearing is maintained for 6 to 8 weeks depending on the size of the lesion (**Figure 6**). Some authors prefer non–weight bearing with crutch assistance; others employ a touchdown weight-bearing protocol. With either protocol, the patient must understand the importance of protected weight bearing to avoid compressive forces that could jeopardize and dislodge the super clot. After the protected weight-bearing phase, patients are progressed to full weight bearing.

Strength training in the form of isometric quadriceps and hamstring strengthening can begin immediately. At 2 weeks, the patient can begin riding a stationary bike without resistance and commence exercises within the arc of motion that safely avoids compressive forces on the lesion. Progressive active strengthening begins at 8 weeks. Running is allowed at 3 to 4 months, but activities that involve any cutting or pivoting are restricted until 4 to 6 months after surgery.[9]

The rehabilitation guidelines for patellofemoral lesions differ slightly, but the same principles apply. To protect against compressive and shear forces on the super clot, a hinged knee brace is employed. Patients may weight-bear fully on the extremity with the knee brace locked in full extension for all weight-bearing activities.[9] The brace settings prevent the patella from engaging the trochlea while weight bearing. The CPM machine is begun immediately, and passive range of motion is allowed without the knee brace on. As with femoral condyle or tibial plateau lesions, early isometric strengthening is allowed. However, progressive strength training is limited to the arc of motion (noted at the time of surgery) in which the lesion is not subjected to compressive forces in the patellofemoral compartment.

Pearls
- The lesion should be defined with well-shouldered borders.
- The calcified cartilage layer that remains must be débrided.
- The lesion should be measured after débridement.
- Microfracture awls are used in systematic fashion, starting at the periphery and working centrally.
- Sharp microfracture awls should be used to avoid coalescence of the holes.
- The subchondral bone is perforated 2 to 4 mm apart and 2 to 4 mm deep.
- All holes should be checked for bleeding at the conclusion of the case. It is common for some of the microfracture holes to become impacted with bone, and preventing the marrow elements from emanating. All holes that do not actively bleed should be revised.

References
1. Asik M, Ciftci F, Sen C, Erdil M, Atalar A: The microfracture technique for the treatment of full-thickness articular cartilage lesions of the knee: Midterm results. *Arthroscopy* 2008;24(11):1214-1220.

2. Gobbi A, Nunag P, Malinowski K: Treatment of full thickness chondral lesions of the knee with microfracture in a group of athletes. *Knee Surg Sports Traumatol Arthrosc* 2005;13(3):213-221.

3. Knutsen G, Drogset JO, Engebretsen L, et al: A randomized trial comparing autologous chondrocyte implantation with microfracture: Findings at five years. *J Bone Joint Surg Am* 2007;89(10):2105-2112.

4. Mithoefer K, Williams RJ III, Warren RF, et al: The microfracture technique for the treatment of articular cartilage lesions in the knee: A prospective cohort study. *J Bone Joint Surg Am* 2005;87(9):1911-1920.

5. Kreuz PC, Steinwachs MR, Erggelet C, et al: Results after microfracture of full-thickness chondral defects in different compartments in the knee. *Osteoarthritis Cartilage* 2006;14(11):1119-1125.

6. Kreuz PC, Erggelet C, Steinwachs MR, et al: Is microfracture of chondral defects in the knee associated with different results in patients aged 40 years or younger? *Arthroscopy* 2006;22(11):1180-1186.

7. Mithoefer K, McAdams T, Williams RJ, Kreuz PC, Mandelbaum BR: Clinical efficacy of the microfracture technique for articular cartilage repair in the knee: An evidence-based systematic analysis. *Am J Sports Med* 2009;37(10):2053-2063.

8. Kaplan LD, Schurhoff MR, Selesnick H, Thorpe M, Uribe JW: Magnetic resonance imaging of the knee in asymptomatic professional basketball players. *Arthroscopy* 2005;21(5):557-561.

9. Steadman JR, Rodkey WG, Rodrigo JJ: Microfracture: Surgical technique and rehabilitation to treat chondral defects. *Clin Orthop Relat Res* 2001;391(suppl): S362-S369.

10. Sterett WI, Steadman JR, Huang MJ, Matheny LM, Briggs KK: Chondral resurfacing and high tibial osteotomy in the varus knee: Survivorship analysis. *Am J Sports Med* 2010;38(7):1420-1424.

11. Shindle MK, Foo LF, Kelly BT, et al: Magnetic resonance imaging of cartilage in the athlete: Current techniques and spectrum of disease. *J Bone Joint Surg Am* 2006;88(suppl 4):27-46.

12. Frisbie DD, Morisset S, Ho CP, Rodkey WG, Steadman JR, McIlwraith CW: Effects of calcified cartilage on healing of chondral defects treated with microfracture in horses. *Am J Sports Med* 2006;34(11):1824-1831.

13. Mithoefer K, Williams RJ III, Warren RF, et al: Chondral resurfacing of articular cartilage defects in the knee with the microfracture technique: Surgical technique. *J Bone Joint Surg Am* 2006; 88(suppl 1, pt 2):294-304.

14. Minas T, Gomoll AH, Rosenberger R, Royce RO, Bryant T: Increased failure rate of autologous chondrocyte implantation after previous treatment with marrow stimulation techniques. *Am J Sports Med* 2009;37(5):902-908.

15. Hurst JM, Steadman JR, O'Brien L, Rodkey WG, Briggs KK: Rehabilitation following microfracture for chondral injury in the knee. *Clin Sports Med* 2010;29(2):257-265, viii.

Chapter 15
Surgical Treatment of Osteochondritis Dissecans Lesions

Sarvottam Bajaj, BE   Michael J. Salata, MD   Brian J. Cole, MD, MBA

Introduction

Osteochondritis dissecans (OCD) is a pathologic joint disorder that affects the subchondral bone and the overlying articular cartilage.[1] The disease results in subchondral bone loss and destabilization of the overlying articular cartilage, leading to separation and increased susceptibility to stress and shear of the resultant fragment.[2] The true etiology is unknown, but this condition may be related to repetitive microtrauma, a single acute traumatic incident, ischemia, or endocrine and genetic predisposition.[3] Regardless of the etiology, the end result is fragmentation of both cartilage and bone that can progress to early degenerative changes and loss of function in the affected compartment. In its final stages, bipolar osteoarthritis can develop, leading to the need for arthroplasty in some instances.

The prevalence of OCD is estimated at 15 to 30 per 100,000, with most lesions occurring in the knee. Nearly 80% of the cases involve the medial femoral condyle (MFC), 15% involve the lateral femoral condyle, and 5% involve the patellofemoral region. More than 70% of all OCD lesions are found in the "classic" area of the lateral aspect of the MFC intersecting the intercondylar notch near the femoral footprint of the posterior cruciate ligament (PCL).[4]

In the case of a stable lesion and a short duration of symptoms, nonsurgical management can be successful. In the past, these lesions have been treated with immobilization and weight-bearing limitations. However, published studies have shown that prolonged immobilization can be detrimental to the health of the knee joint; thus, currently employed nonsurgical management should focus on a hiatus from sporting and high-impact activities for 6 to 8 weeks with allowance for normal weight bearing in a compliant patient.

Asking a patient to participate in "relative rest," much like the treatment recommendations for stress fractures, can maintain the health of the joint without compromising the healing potential of a symptomatic OCD lesion. The length of time required to render a patient asymptomatic and safe to return to high-level activities is highly variable and is a consideration when deciding to intervene with surgery.

In the case of failed nonsurgical management or in the setting of an unstable fragment, surgical intervention includes fragment removal, drilling (antegrade or retrograde), internal fixation,[2] marrow stimulation, autologous chondrocyte implantation (ACI), or osteochondral autograft/allograft transplantation to repair the lesion or supplement the area of cartilage loss. As a last resort, joint arthroplasty may be the only feasible solution in advanced cases.

Subtleties in Decision Making

Unique to OCD is the fact that patients with this pathology can have very little in the way of symptoms until the fragment becomes destabilized based on the endogenous natural history of that lesion or through acute or repetitive trauma. It is appropriate to consider symptomatic OCD with fragment instability as an intra-articular atrophic fracture nonunion. This concept is important to recognize because it relates to treatment decisions and the technical steps requisite to successful defect healing. Because the natural history of the isolated OCD lesion is not clarified in the body of existing literature nor in our contemporary experience, successful clinical treatment is often achieved through fragment removal, at least in the short and intermediate term. Although intuitively it is reasonable always to try to retain a viable fragment and provide rigid fixation to promote biologic union of any osteochondral fragment, the fact that many patients can clinically tolerate a concave, well-defined osteochondral defect is provocative to the extent that benign neglect following fragment removal remains a treatment option in some instances.

The resultant paucity of symptoms following fragment removal is explicable by the typical geometry and the relatively load-sparing location of these lesions, which allow the defect bed to become clinically silent simply because the surrounding osteoarticular environment can "shield" the lesion, rendering it less clinically relevant. The debate that remains is when to treat these lesions early with cartilage restoration procedures when initial fragment excision renders a patient clinically normal. Because no cartilage restoration procedure has been demonstrated to last "forever" nor been demonstrated to definitively prevent progression of osteoarthritis over time, decision making remains challenging for the patient presenting with the asymptomatic defect following fragment removal. This is especially true for the high-level competitive athlete who places a premium on the short- and intermediate-term maintenance of functional activity.

Patient Selection

A thorough history is mandatory and should elicit any inciting events, any underlying metabolic or systemic conditions that may have contributed to the OCD, the duration of symptoms, and previous attempts at treatment (both nonsurgical and surgical). The typical presentation of OCD in the knee includes pain and swelling related to activity.[1,3] Instability is usually not reported, although mechanical symptoms such as catching or locking can occur if the fragment has become completely detached and is acting as a loose body. On physical examination, patients typically have tenderness localized over the compartment where the OCD lesion is located.[1] The patient may walk

---

Dr. Salata or an immediate family member serves as a paid consultant to or is an employee of Linvatec, Mitek, and Smith & Nephew. Dr. Cole or an immediate family member has received royalties from Arthrex, DJ Orthopaedics, Lippincott, and Elsevier; is a member of a speakers' bureau or has made paid presentations on behalf of Genzyme; serves as a paid consultant to or is an employee of Zimmer, Arthrex, Carticept, Biomimetic, Allosource, and DePuy; and has received research or institutional support from Regentis, Arthrex, Smith & Nephew, DJ Orthopaedics, Zimmer, and DePuy. Neither Mr. Bajaj nor any immediate family member has received anything of value from or has stock or stock options held in a commercial company or institution related directly or indirectly to the subject of this chapter.

with an antalgic gait or with the leg externally rotated (Wilson sign) to decrease pressure over the lesion. With external rotation, a lesion located on the MFC will not impinge with the medial tibial eminence, which decreases the pain associated with motion at the lesion interface. Joint effusion, decreased range of motion, loose-body symptoms, and quadriceps atrophy are variably present, depending on the extent of the lesion and the duration of symptoms.

When contemplating surgical intervention, it is important to consider the site of the lesion. Certain sites, such as the classic location on the MFC, have a spontaneous resolution rate of less than 30%, whereas nonclassic locations are much more likely to heal in the adolescent population, with 88% to 100% healing rates reported with nonsurgical management.[4]

The ideal candidate for primary repair is an unstable lesion in an active, symptomatic patient. The ideal patient is willing to comply with the postoperative weight-bearing limitations and activity restrictions and understands the potential need for a second procedure for implant removal. Patients with open physes on radiographs and in whom nonsurgical therapy for a stable fragment fails to achieve symptomatic and radiographic improvement should be considered for retrograde or antegrade drilling. Arthroscopically stable, symptomatic lesions might benefit from bioabsorbable screw fixation, with the screw heads buried just below the level of the subchondral plate as an adjunct to drilling through an extra-articular or periarticular location. Primary surgical fixation is not recommended if the lesion is free-floating as a loose body and the underlying subchondral bone is compromised. An initial strategy in this patient population should include loose body removal and possible chondrocyte biopsy for subsequent ACI if the patient demonstrates persistent symptoms attributable to the resultant chondral defect. In such cases, primary marrow stimulation can also be considered on a case-by-case basis. Should these initial treatments fail to resolve symptoms, definitive cartilage restoration (osteochondral autografting, osteochondral allograft transplantation, or ACI) can be considered.

Preoperative Imaging

Because the physical findings of OCD are often vague and nonspecific, a physical examination cannot be used in isolation to diagnose this type of pathology. Imaging is crucial in the evaluation of patients

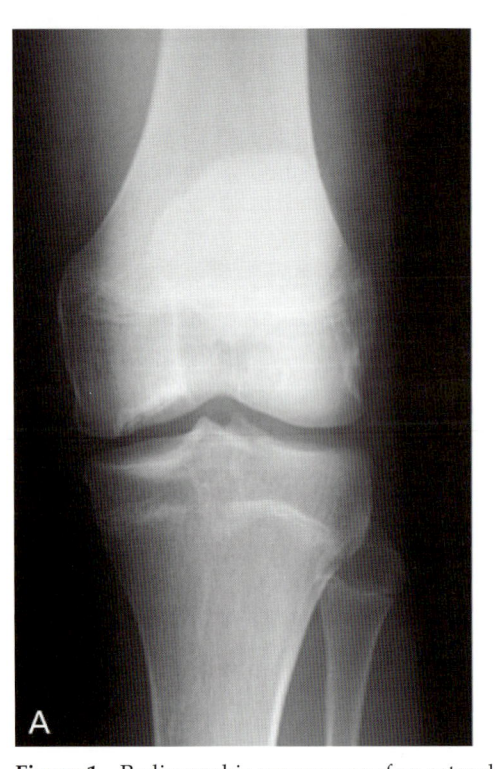

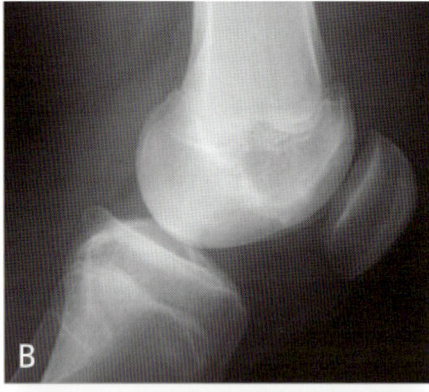

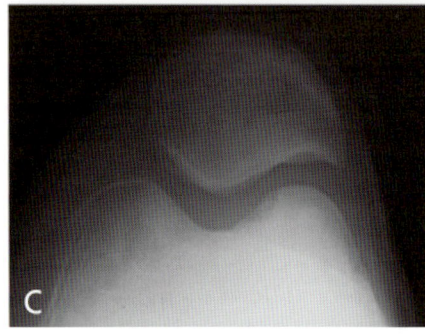

Figure 1 Radiographic appearance of an osteochondritis dissecans (OCD) lesion. **A,** Weight-bearing AP radiograph of a left knee depicts an OCD lesion on the medial femoral condyle (MFC). **B,** Lateral view at 45° flexion. **C,** Merchant view. The area of lucency on the MFC can be best appreciated on the AP and lateral views.

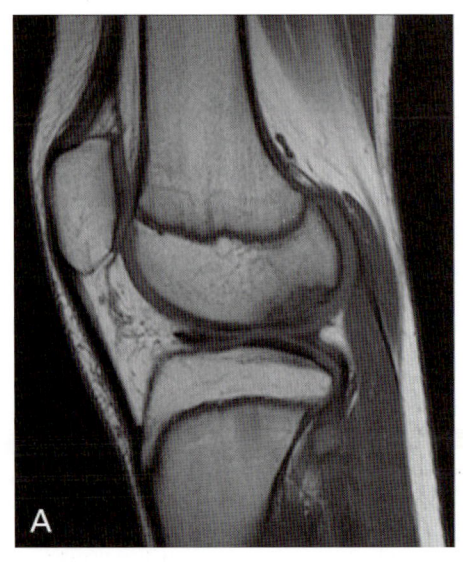

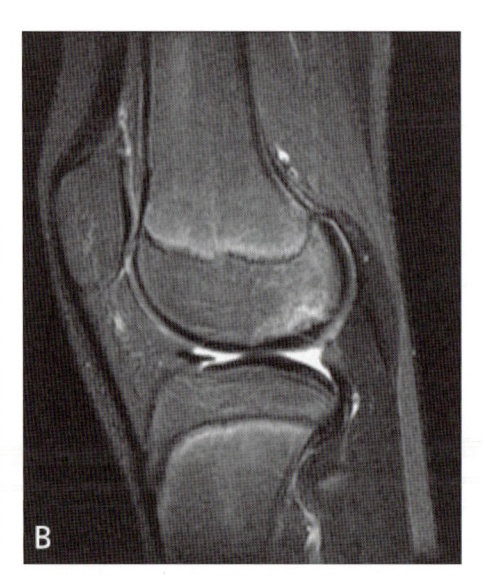

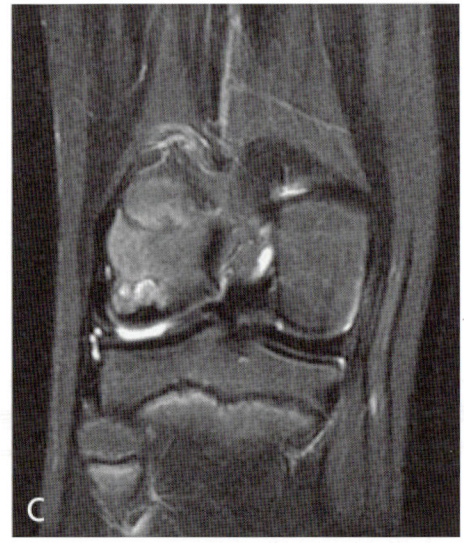

Figure 2 MRI appearance of an osteochondritis dissecans (OCD) lesion. **A,** T1-weighted sagittal view. **B,** T2-weighted sagittal view. **C,** T2-weighted coronal view of an OCD lesion presenting concomitantly with compromised subchondral bone. An area of high signal intensity between the OCD lesion and the subchondral bone suggests instability.

Chapter 15: Surgical Treatment for Osteochondritis Dissecans Lesions

presenting with these symptoms and should include a plain radiographic series and often a subsequent MRI.

Preliminary radiographs should be standard and include AP weight-bearing knee, weight-bearing 45° flexion PA, lateral, and Merchant views[3] (**Figure 1**). The flexion weight-bearing PA view should be obtained in addition to standard AP because it allows for better visualization of lesions along the posterolateral aspect of the MFC. Open physes are a positive predictor for healing of an OCD lesion and should be noted on the plain radiographs.

MRI is often required in the diagnosis of OCD lesions because it is the most informative imaging modality. Specifically, an evaluation for the presence of bone edema, subchondral separation, cartilage breakdown, lesion size, and location can be assessed using MRI before treatment.[5] The MRI scans are assessed based on the criteria presented below, in which meeting one of the four criteria offers up to 97% sensitivity and 100% specificity in predicting lesion stability[2] (**Figure 2**):

1. A thin, ill-defined, or well-demarcated line of high signal intensity, measuring 5 mm or more in length at the interface between the lesion and the underlying subchondral bone

2. A discrete, rounded area of homogeneous high signal intensity

3. A focal defect with a width of 5 mm or more in the articular surface of the lesion

4. A high signal intensity line traversing the articular cartilage and subchondral bone plate into the lesion

Procedure

Most adult OCD cases arise from established but untreated or asymptomatic juvenile OCD. Spontaneous healing has been reported in such cases with nonsurgical treatment options. However, for lesions presenting in the classic location of the lateral aspect of the MFC or lesions that persist after adequate nonsurgical treatment, an array of surgical options is available.

The overall goal of surgical intervention is to enhance the healing potential of the subchondral bone, fix the unstable fragment, or replace the abnormal cartilage and bone with implantable tissue.[2]

The type and extent of surgery necessary for OCD depends on myriad factors, including patient age, lesion characteristics (the quality of the articular cartilage; the size of the associated subchondral bone; and the shape, thickness, and location of the lesion), lesion stability, and surgeon preference (**Figure 3**).

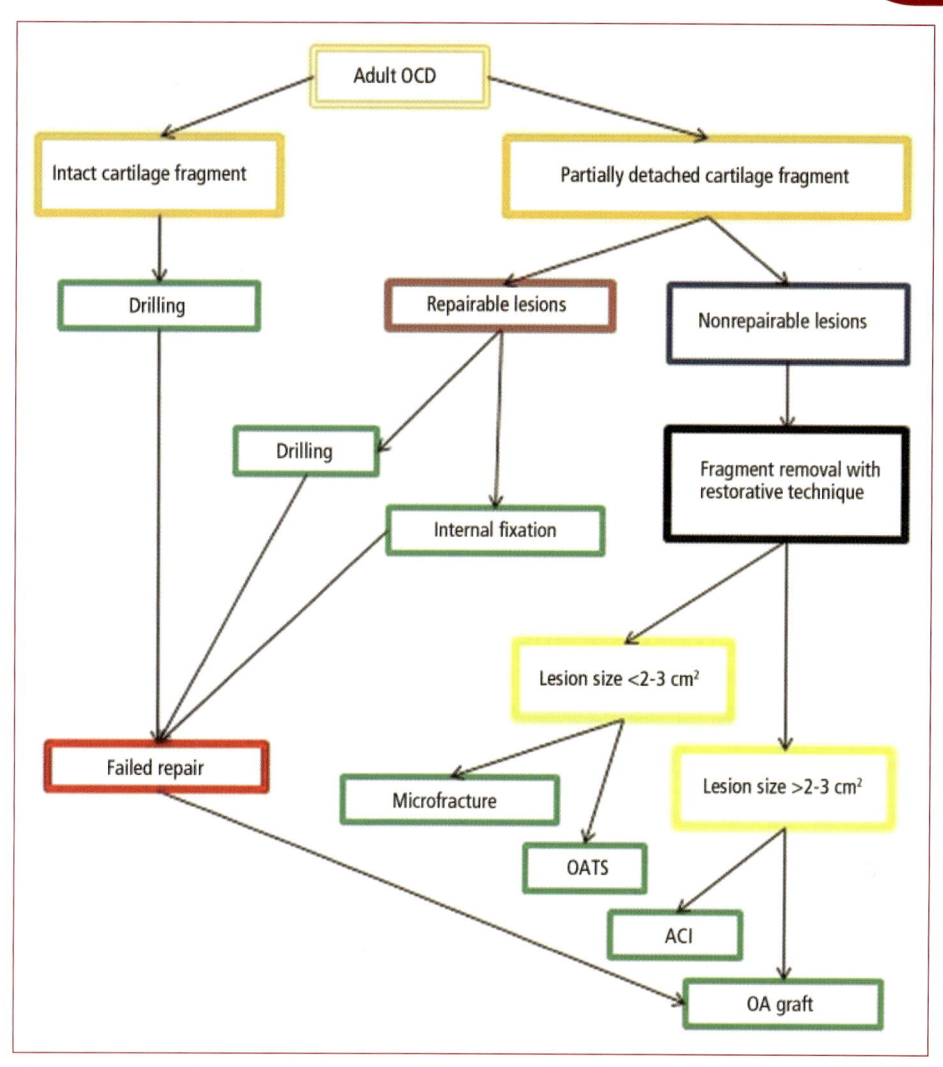

Figure 3 Surgical treatment algorithm for osteochondritis dissecans. The surgical goals should always incorporate an attempt to reestablish the joint surface using the least invasive procedure first. OA graft = osteochondral allograft, OATS = osteochondral autograft transfer system, ACI = autologous chondrocyte implantation.

Room Setup/Patient Positioning

A supine position, with the affected leg placed within a leg holder allowing full flexion, allows complete access to femoral condyle lesions that might require hyperflexion or a figure-of-4 position to optimize arthroscopic lesion preparation and fixation. The contralateral extremity is positioned in an obstetric-type well leg holder with adequate padding around the common peroneal nerve. The affected joint is draped to the proximal thigh, and a well-padded nonsterile pneumatic tourniquet is applied before draping. An examination under anesthesia is performed to assess range of motion and ligamentous stability. Depending on the lesion site and size, an arthroscopic or a mini-open technique is used. Lesions on the condyles are often easily accessed with the use of arthroscopic techniques and through satellite portal placement wherever needed. Patellofemoral and tibial lesions can be more difficult to access arthroscopically and may require an arthrotomy or mini-arthrotomy for adequate visualization and treatment.

Surgical Technique

A complete arthroscopic evaluation of each compartment and its structure is performed to determine all intra-articular sources of pain. A standard arthroscopic probe is used to assess the boundaries and the stability of the lesion (**Figure 4**). In the case of a lesion with intact articular cartilage, the lesion will be ballottable, and a "trampoline" effect will be appreciated when the lesion is probed. This clinical scenario is more common in very young patients who present with

© 2013 American Academy of Orthopaedic Surgeons

Section 1: Sports Medicine

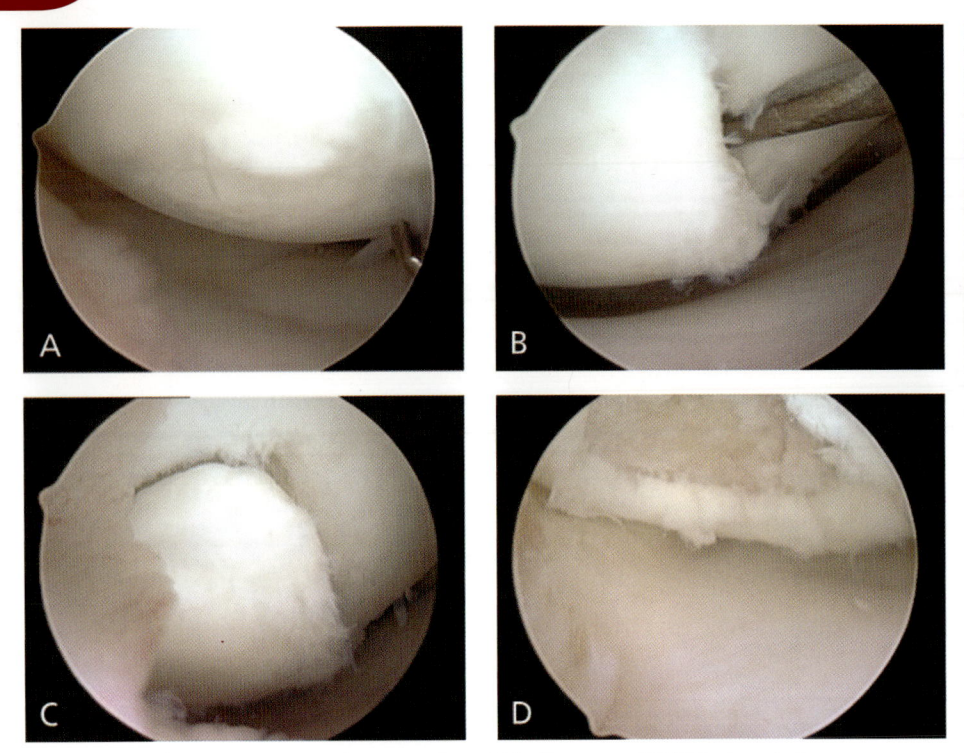

Figure 4 Arthroscopic views of an osteochondritis dissecans (OCD) lesion. **A**, Large OCD lesion with fibrillation and fissuring demarcating the lesion border. **B**, Arthroscopic assessment of lesion stability performed using a standard probe. **C**, Detached OCD lesion with demarcated border. **D**, Subchondral base of the detached OCD lesion, which will be débrided using a shaver or burr.

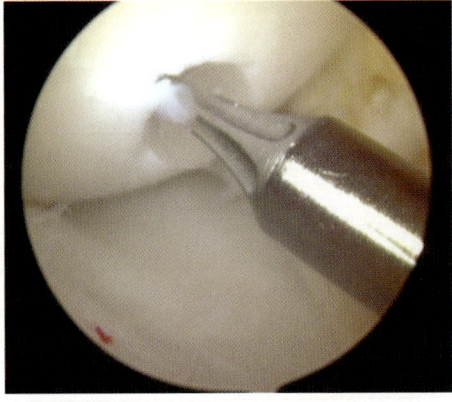

Figure 5 Arthroscopic view shows osteochondritis dissecans (OCD) lesion fixation using a bioabsorbable screw. This is used for intact OCD lesions that are neither ballottable nor displaceable at the time of surgical intervention.

activity-related pain without effusions and with fluid behind the lesion on MRI. However, in many cases, there are fissures or fibrillations that mark a distinct transition from a firm to a soft segment of cartilage that can be appreciated as one moves the elbow of a probe from normal cartilage to the overlying cartilage of an OCD lesion. Often, for classic OCD of the MFC, access can occur at the leading edge of the femoral origin of the PCL using an electrocautery device and elevator to expose a fissure that enters the intercondylar notch in this area.

With the lesion identified and classified, the following surgical techniques can be used to alleviate a patient's symptoms.

Reparative Procedures

The goal of a reparative procedure is to restore the integrity of the subchondral bone and preserve the overlying articular cartilage. This generally is a primary reduction and fixation of the fragment. It is often accompanied by a removal of fibrocartilaginous scar at the interface between the lesion and underlying subchondral bone, coupled with restoration of blood flow to the lesion by microfracture or drilling of the host tissue bed. In the presence of cystic changes or attritional bone loss, local bone graft procedures that harvest cancellous bone from the Gerdy tubercle or the distal femur using a small-diameter osteochondral autograft harvesting tube are effective.

Drilling

In the setting of a stable lesion with intact articular cartilage that remains symptomatic despite appropriate nonsurgical management, retrograde or antegrade drilling can restore blood supply to the fragment. This technique serves to create vascular channels that can provide adequate blood flow to the affected region, allowing for healing.[5] This technique is less likely to be successful with true fragment instability. Understanding that these lesions often hurt because of micromotion due to "fracture nonunion" principles can help surgeons avoid implementation of subtherapeutic treatment that might inevitably lead to repeated surgical intervention if the lesions become macroscopically unstable.

Antegrade drilling has been described as being performed from within the joint through the articular cartilage and into the subchondral bone. Lesions of the MFC can be drilled through an anterolateral or anteromedial portal, whereas lesions of the lateral femoral condyle are usually accessible through the anterolateral portal. If the lesion is not accessible via standard portals, accessory portals are created to obtain an orthogonal drilling angle. Holes are drilled uniformly using a Kirschner wire (K-wire), and blood and fat droplets from the drilled region are used to confirm the depth of the penetration.[6] Anterograde drilling violates the articular cartilage surface, with the resultant gap filled in with fibrocartilage, tissue similar to the cartilage created with a microfracture. We prefer to avoid direct penetration of intact healthy articular cartilage overlying the fragment and drill just behind the lesion through the intercondylar notch or through the juxta-articular osseous surfaces, which is more analogous to retrograde drilling. In addition, consideration should be given to the use of third-generation small-diameter bioabsorbable, variably pitched screws (Bio-Compression Screw, Arthrex) placed directly through the lesion, which will essentially provide a combined approach of antegrade drilling with fracture fixation, even if the fragment is only "microscopically" unstable (**Figure 5**). Surgeons must consider that, despite being bioabsorbable, these devices will remain intact for up to several years; therefore, their heads must be advanced to or beyond the subchondral plate to avoid inadvertent damage to opposing articular surfaces either primarily or following potential fragment subsidence over time.

The argument supporting extra-articular or retrograde drilling is to avoid fibrocartilage formation at the fragment site and damage to intact, healthy cartilage in general. In this procedure, the drill enters proximal to the lesion and penetrates the sclerotic proximal border of the lesion without violating the overlying articular cartilage. Fluoroscopic guidance is extremely helpful when performing ret-

Chapter 15: Surgical Treatment for Osteochondritis Dissecans Lesions

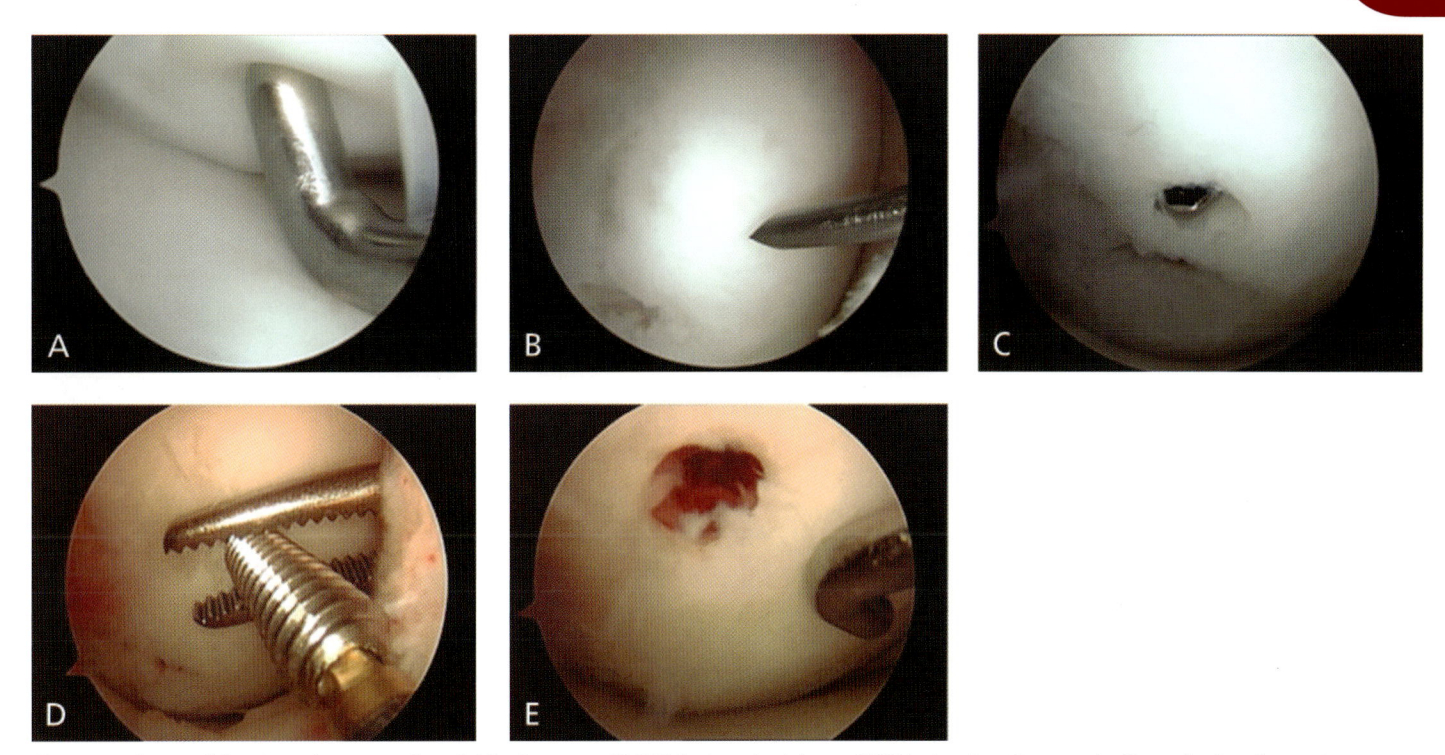

Figure 6 Internal fixation of an osteochondritis dissecans (OCD) lesion. **A**, A large OCD lesion is arthroscopically probed to determine stability. **B**, Guidewires are placed to control rotation during fixation. **C**, OCD lesion affixed using a nonabsorbable, cannulated, headless variable-pitch compression screw. **D**, Removal of the cannulated, headless compression screw. A hemostat is used to prevent loss of the screw in the joint, fat pad, or extra-articular soft tissue. **E**, Assessing lesion stability after removal of fixation.

rograde drilling. A definitive "plunge" is felt when passing the K-wire through the sclerotic border, which can be used to confirm that this border has been appropriately perforated.

Overall outcomes of OCD drilling are generally favorable in the younger population. Donaldson and Wojtys[7] compared outcomes of juvenile OCD to adult OCD, reporting a higher level of radiographic healing and favorable relief of symptoms in the younger population.

As noted previously, drilling should be used only when the defect is categorically stable to palpation. When possible, drilling should be performed through the intercondylar notch (ie, adjacent to the PCL femoral origin for OCD of the MFC) or along the lateral nonarticulating border of the distal femur using a 4.5-mm K-wire.[6] Occasionally, in the setting of larger lesions, we augment the treatment of these lesions by using one or two bioabsorbable compression screws that are buried deep to the level of the subchondral plate in an effort to stimulate biologic healing and stabilize the osteochondral fragment.

Internal Fixation

OCD lesions that have detached from the subchondral bone may present with articular cartilage flaps or loose bodies. If the lesion has sufficient subchondral bone to provide biologic and mechanical support for fixation, every attempt to perform a reduction (arthroscopic or open) and fixation should be made.[2] With all types of fixation, the bed of the defect should be prepared to optimize healing.[8] In the setting of a flap, the fragment can be hinged open, and the bed can be cleared of fibrocartilaginous scar using a curet and microfractured to restore vascular channels.

Internal fixation can be achieved using a variety of fixative devices, such as cannulated screws, metal pins/K-wires, and bioabsorbable pins and screws.[6] The method of fixation is largely based on surgeon preference. Some surgeons bury the head of these screws to prevent subsequent damage to the opposing tibial surfaces; however, when repairing grossly unstable osteochondral fragments that are mobile and hinged open during defect preparation, we prefer to use a cannulated variable-pitched metal screw placed deep to the level of the subchondral cortical bone. A second surgical procedure is planned 8 weeks after the first operation to assess for healing and for hardware removal (**Figure 6**).

Bioabsorbable screws have been recommended by some to avoid removal, but the degree of compression provided by these devices is probably inferior to traditional metal screws, and the long-term effects of this implant material require consideration by the surgeon before use.[2] In addition, these devices must be considered prolonged absorbable and will remain intact for at least 12 months; thus, they can still become noxious mechanical devices and lead to opposing surface damage if implanted incorrectly or following fragment subsidence.

Once the sclerotic bed is prepared appropriately (using a curet, a shaver, and a microfracture awl), a guidewire is drilled through the fragment into the femoral condyle to provide provisional fixation. It is often necessary to trim the edges of the fragment because the borders often become rounded and may hypertrophy, making an anatomic reduction difficult.[8] As mentioned previously, cystic changes or cumulative bone loss within the bed can be grafted first by arthroscopically harvesting and morcellizing small-diameter osteochondral autograft plugs from the intercondylar notch, the trochlear ridge, or the Gerdy tubercle before stabilization. Once the guidewires are placed, they are exchanged for a compression screw.

In general, at least two fixation points are used to ensure compression and rotational stability. Screws are tightened until the fragment is compressed, but overtightening should be avoided to prevent fragment fracture or implant failure.[2] All devices with a prominent head should be recessed beneath the articular cartilage to avoid further injury to the articulating surface of the tibia. As mentioned

© 2013 American Academy of Orthopaedic Surgeons

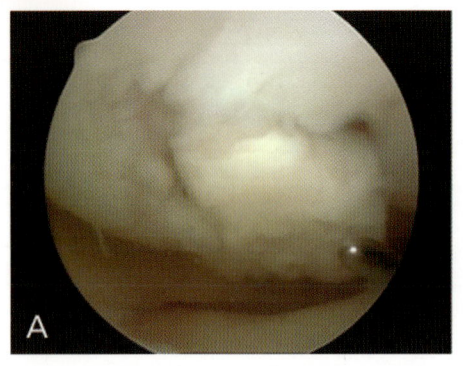

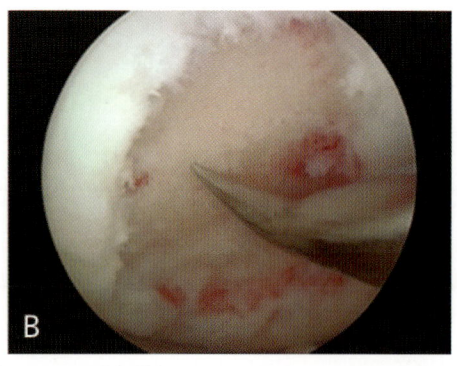

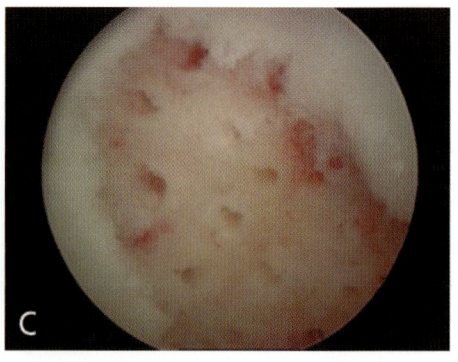

Figure 7 Microfracture of an osteochondritis dissecans (OCD) lesion. **A,** Arthroscopic view of an unstable OCD lesion. **B,** Defect site is prepared with vertical wall formation. A surgical awl is used to penetrate the subchondral bone. **C,** Completed microfracture; the holes are about 3 to 4 mm apart. Microfracture holes are started at the periphery, adjacent to the stable cartilage rim.

previously, nonabsorbable screws often require a second procedure for hardware removal; however, an advantage of this is that it allows a second look at the lesion site to verify healing. Although screw removal obviously requires a subsequent procedure, it offers the opportunity to remove any fragments that fail to unite and can help the surgeon determine the source of persistent symptoms following fragment fixation once patients are allowed to return to higher level activities.

Following any OCD procedure treated with internal fixation, the knee should be ranged to ensure that the screw head does not abrade the opposing articular surface.[2] Patients are made heel-touch weight bearing and use continuous passive motion (CPM) for 6 hours per day for up to 6 weeks.

Despite the screws being "headless," we prefer to remove them to prevent them from becoming proud with settling of the fragment and to determine which part of the fragments may not have healed entirely. Following screw removal, patients are asked to avoid high-impact activities for at least an additional 8 weeks.

Bioabsorbable screws are also an option, especially when only one screw is needed for adequate stabilization. In this case, a second-look arthroscopy is generally not performed, but the screw must be recessed completely within bone.

With strict postoperative rehabilitation, favorable outcomes have been reported after internal fixation of OCD fragments using absorbable and nonabsorbable screws.[9]

Restorative Procedures

Restorative procedures attempt to replace the damaged articular cartilage with hyaline or hyaline-like tissue.[6] These techniques should be considered if the reparative options have failed and the patient presents with recurrent joint effusion, pain, and reduced range of motion or if the fragment at the time of the index procedure is determined to be unsuitable for primary reduction and fixation.[2] Multiple restorative techniques can be employed for the treatment of OCD; however, the treatment algorithm should start with the least invasive and progress to the most invasive options. Practically speaking, although not necessarily appropriate, the decision to repair an OCD lesion or perform microfracture is rarely associated with a decision to simultaneously address concomitant pathology, such as meniscal deficiency or malalignment. In contrast, higher-level procedures, such as ACI or osteochondral grafting for OCD lesions, are often undertaken simultaneously with meniscal allograft transplantation and osteotomy when appropriate. This distinction must be kept in mind when using the literature to make decisions for patients being treated surgically because there is considerable treatment bias inherent in the specific options being offered.

Marrow Stimulation (Microfracture)

Microfracture involves perforation of the subchondral bone, allowing for an egress of pluripotent stem cells from the marrow (**Figure 7**). This influx results in the formation of a super clot and allows for subsequent cell differentiation and the formation of fibrocartilage.[1] The decision of when to perform microfracture in a patient with OCD is complex and takes into consideration multiple variables. Despite the fact that most microfracture procedures performed for OCD are conducted at the time the fragment is removed or as a primary revision treatment of the empty defect without consideration for relevant comorbidities (meniscal deficiency and malalignment), good results following microfracture of OCD lesions have been reported. The real challenge in decision making for treatment of the patient in whom a fragment must be removed is whether the literature and our experience is sufficient to help us decide if a concave defect with associated bone loss will behave any differently clinically with or without microfracture after the fragment is removed, which is often all that is required to render a patient initially less symptomatic or asymptomatic. Postoperative rehabilitation requires 6 weeks of protected weight bearing with the use of CPM for 6 hours a day. In a randomized clinical trial, Knutsen et al[10] randomized femoral condyle (28% with OCD lesions) cartilage defects to treatment with microfracture or ACI. Both groups demonstrated satisfactory results in 77% of the patients at 5 years, with younger patients reporting better outcomes.[10] Overall, microfracture should be considered as a first-line treatment, especially in the setting of fragment removal in small, shallow defects.

Because microfracture is often entertained as a first-line treatment of the defect bed at the time of fragment removal or considered as an option if the empty defect becomes symptomatic later, several concepts must be considered during the decision-making process before recommending a microfracture procedure. Implicit in this decision making is a desire to reduce symptoms in the "here and now" versus a desire to change the natural history of what might otherwise remain an asymptomatic lesion. If the patient's symptoms are acute on a chronic, previously asymptomatic, never-treated OCD lesion, then fragment removal might lead to complete and prolonged symptom resolution. There is no formal guidance on the long-term benefits of performing microfracture in these patients because only low levels of research evidence exists in this regard. Thus, a decision to perform microfracture in the patient undergoing fragment removal is highly individualized, with considerations of defect location, defect containment, the condition of the bone, and the size and depth of the lesion. Given the rehabilitation required following microfracture, the decision is not taken lightly. Even beyond the initial period of protected weight bearing and CPM, if the surgeon truly follows the existing recommendations about return to sport for these patients, they would not be allowed to return to high-level activities for at least 6 to 8 months. Thus, it can be challenging to hold active patients back when all that might have been required was fragment removal to render them symptom free.

A weight-bearing, shallow, small, contained defect with a healthy subchondral (ie, nonsclerotic) bed represents the ideal defect for microfracture. Alternatively, a deep, sclerotic, uncontained defect presents a challenging mechanical and biologic environment where microfracture may have little to no benefit. Thus, we microfracture the bed (of a recently removed fragment) only if it includes the ideal defect characteristics, assuming the patient understands and consents to the postoperative program. Although this decision making is somewhat intuitive, it is not supported by any literature that demonstrates that with this exact clinical scenario the symptoms will be reduced further than fragment removal alone, that symptom onset will be prevented or delayed, or that the natural history of the defect will be altered in any way.

In conclusion, it must be remembered that the decision to perform microfracture may have no bearing on the future progression of the defect—either structurally or clinically—because neither the literature nor our experience offers us guidance in this regard.

Osteochondral Autograft Transfer System

Scenarios in which the underlying subchondral bone integrity has been significantly compromised do not perform well with a marrow stimulation technique and require restorative procedures to address both the underlying structural support of the subchondral plate and the articular surface to be successful. The osteochondral autograft transfer system (OATS) involves transplantation of osteochondral autograft tissue from a non–weight-bearing region of the joint to the defect site[8] (**Figure 8**). A single autograft plug is preferred for defects smaller than 1 cm[2]; however, some clinicians perform a mo-

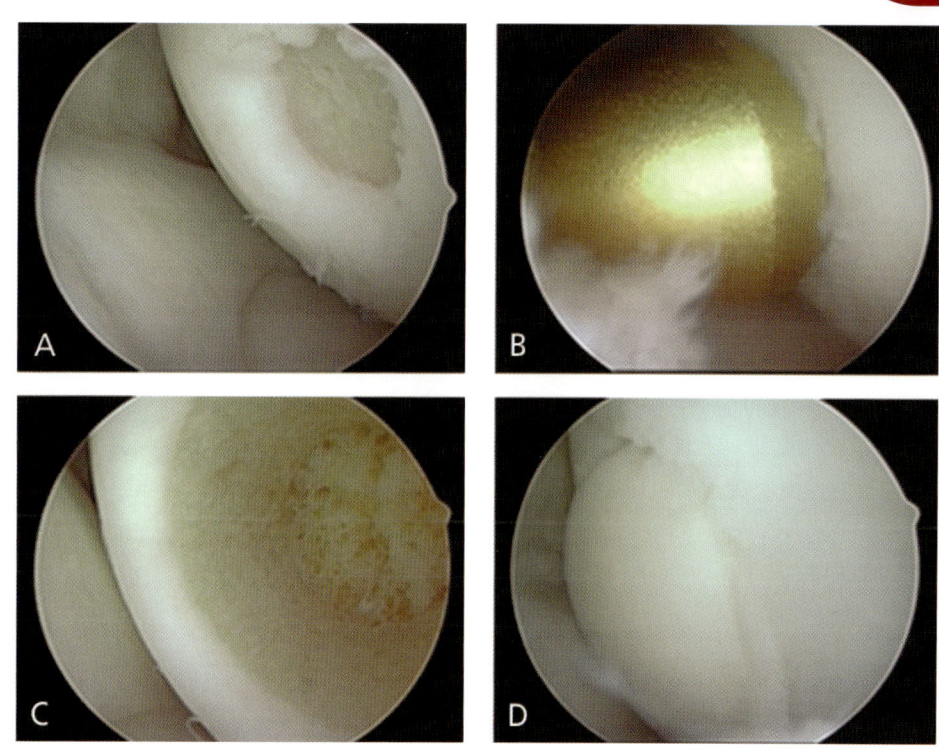

Figure 8 Osteochondral autograft for an osteochondritis dissecans (OCD) lesion. **A,** Arthroscopic view of an unstable OCD lesion. **B,** Using the osteochondral autograft transfer system (OATS) transfer tool, the defect site is prepared to an appropriate depth. **C,** Arthroscopic view of the recipient site. **D,** Implantation of a donor osteochondral plug into the recipient site.

saicplasty with multiple smaller plugs for larger defects. In general, OATS is limited to small lesions because of a limited supply of donor tissue and donor-site morbidity. Typically, restorative treatment of OCD using OATS has limited utility because of the size and the geometry of most lesions. A novel technique of using an osteochondral autograft plug as a biologic splint has been reported by Miniaci and Tytherleigh-Strong[11] and remains a consideration for a defect that has an intact, relatively stable fragment within the defect bed.

Postoperative rehabilitation consists of immediate CPM with protected weight bearing for 4 to 6 weeks. Return to normal activities of daily living and sport activity is considered at 8 to 12 months. Good clinical outcomes have been reported for OATS techniques, with Miniaci and Tytherleigh-Strong[11] reporting normal postoperative knee scores at 18 months for all 20 OCD patients. Osteochondral plugs taken from the ipsilateral lateral patella to treat patients with large osteochondral defects allowed 81% of the cohort to return to a high level of function.[11] However, as stated earlier, OATS is limited to small lesions because of limited donor tissue supply and donor-site morbidity.

In general, most OCD lesions that require further treatment beyond initial repair, débridement, or microfracture are relatively large, deep, and uncontained. Thus, the use of OATS is relatively limited for the treatment of this pathology, other than the approach described using an osteochondral plug as a biologic splint.[11]

Autologous Chondrocyte Implantation

For large, isolated osteochondral defects measuring up to 10 cm[2], we employ the ACI technique. This two-step procedure involves an initial healthy chondrocyte biopsy, performed arthroscopically with tissue extracted from the non–weight-bearing intercondylar notch region;[6] or, in the setting of an irreparable OCD, the biopsy can be taken from the excised loose body as long as the fragment is grossly healthy. Extracted cells are dedifferentiated in vitro over 4 to 6 weeks and reimplanted at the lesion site. At the time of implantation, defect preparation involves preservation of the calcified cartilage layer and creation of a vertically walled defect to act as a reservoir for the implanted cells and better distribute force at the edges of the lesion.[12] Either periosteum or a synthetic collagen patch (off-label usage) is attached to the perimeter of the healthy articular cartilage using 6-0 Vicryl sutures (Ethicon).[6] The edges are sealed using fibrin glue, and the cultured cells are injected beneath the patch[12]

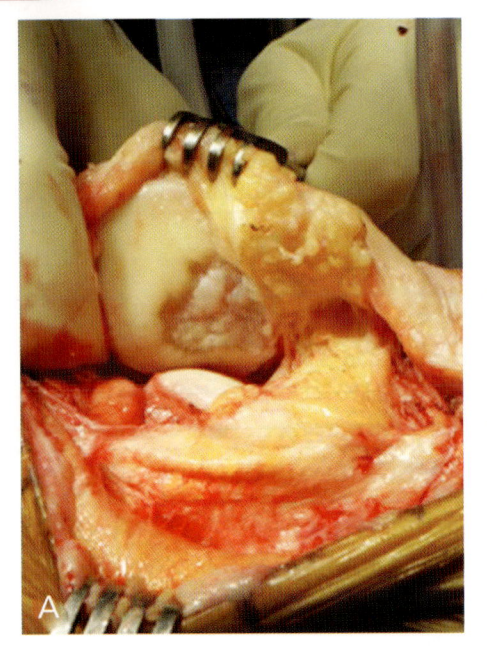

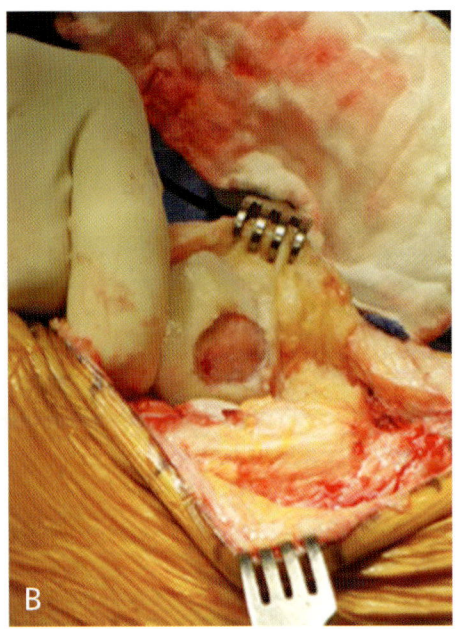

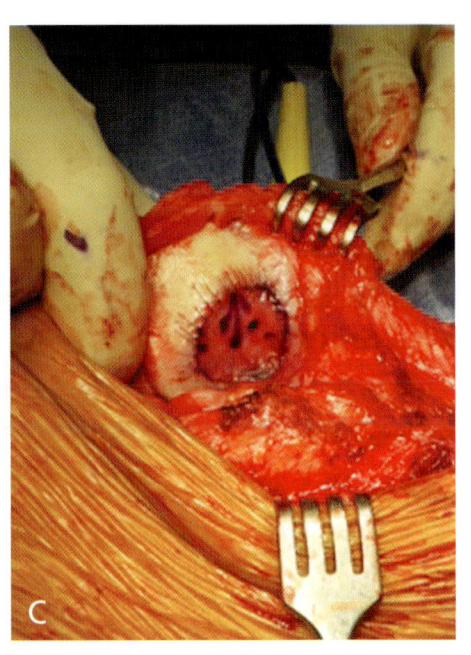

Figure 9 Autologous chondrocyte implantation (ACI) for an osteochondritis dissecans lesion. **A**, Patellar defect. **B**, The defect site after vertical wall formation, ready for suturing of the type I/III collagen patch. The patch is sutured with 6-0 Vicryl. **C**, The lesion following injection of the dedifferentiated cultured chondrocytes and suturing and gluing of the collagen patch. The patch is sutured and then glued over the defect using a fibrin glue.

(**Figure 9**). Similar to a microfracture, 6 weeks of postoperative non–weight bearing and CPM are indicated for both OATS and ACI.

Defects deeper than 8 to 10 mm can still be treated with ACI; however, a concomitant or staged bone grafting is recommended. Prior to bone grafting, drilling through the subchondral bed following débridement allows appropriate blood flow into the defect site, optimizing the incorporation of the bone graft into the defect site. When bone grafting is performed as a primary procedure in an effort to stage for definitive treatment with ACI, it is customary to wait a minimum of 6 months to allow bone graft incorporation before implantation of the cultured chondrocytes.

Because this is a long interval for patients to endure, an alternative method of ACI can be implemented in a deep lesion that requires bone grafting. A bilayer collagen membrane (periosteal "sandwich" technique) can be employed without the need to stage the ACI. A layer of collagen membrane is used to seal the bone graft and is fixed using a 6-0 Vicryl suture. A second layer is placed on top of the first and is similarly sewn, followed by injection of the cultured cell in between the two layers. However, limited experience exists with this technique.[13] Results following ACI for OCD lesions have been well described in the literature, with Bentley et al[14] reporting good to excellent outcomes in 88% of the cohort from a large patient population undergoing ACI for OCD lesions. Similarly, Knutsen et al[10] reported 77% satisfactory results in patients with femoral condyle lesions treated with ACI.

Postoperatively, patients who undergo ACI for femoral condyle lesions require protected weight bearing with CPM for up to 6 weeks. Following ACI for a patellofemoral lesion, patients are permitted to fully weight-bear with the knee in extension as long as a tibial tuberosity osteotomy was not performed, which would require some degree of weight-bearing protection to prevent a postoperative tibia fracture.

Patients whose initial treatment fails, who remain symptomatic or become symptomatic over time, and who are young with relatively shallow contained OCD lesions, especially of the patellofemoral joint, represent some of the best candidates for ACI. The challenges in decision making include defects that are cavitating, are cystic, and/or have a sclerotic base that presents a difficult biologic environment for ACI to successfully integrate. These patients may be better candidates for osteochondral allograft transplantation because the bone represents a greater clinical and biomechanical challenge than the cartilage surface.

Osteochondral Allograft

Large OCD lesions may be treated with osteochondral allograft transplantation. This is a salvage procedure that should rarely be used as the first-line treatment[2] because this technique requires further violation of the subchondral architecture, limiting future treatment options should the procedure prove unsuccessful. An advantage of the osteochondral allograft is that this technique has the ability to resurface larger and deeper defects with mature hyaline cartilage while concomitantly addressing the underlying subchondral bone deficiency. Commercially available systems convert the host defect to a cylindrical socket. A prolonged fresh allograft is then shaped into a plug that matches the diameter and depth of the resultant socket. Ideally, the allograft tissue should be implanted before 28 days of donor asystole to maximize the viability of the donor articular cartilage.[15] At the time of implantation, minimal force should be used to place the donor plug because the donor chondrocytes can be adversely affected by increased levels of force.[16] To ensure proper fixation, a bioabsorbable compression screw is implanted in the center of the graft with the head advanced to the level of the subchondral bone[6] (**Figure 10**). This osteochondral allograft technique can be seen on the video supplement.

Video 15.1 Fresh Osteochondral Allografting to the Knee for Osteochondritis Dissecans. Joseph Yu, MD; William Bugbee, MD (8 min)

Fresh osteochondral allograft transplantation has demonstrated good to excellent clinical outcomes with long-term follow-up. For a group of OCD lesions presenting on the femoral condyle, Garrett[17] reported successful outcomes at a mean follow-up of 3 years in 94% of the patients. In a larger study of 66 OCD lesions in 64 patients, treatment with fresh osteochondral allograft yielded good to excellent results in 72% of patients.[18] Postoperative rehabilitation is similar to that used with the OATS or ACI procedures. After rehabilitation, significant improvements are observed in the majority of patients, with approximately 88% of them showing excellent graft incorporation on radiographic examination.[19]

Patients whose initial treatment has failed and who have deeper, cavitating lesions with poor quality subchondral bone represent ideal candidates for osteochondral allograft treatment. While engaging in a treatment strategy that "burns no bridges," our experience suggests that osteochondral allografts rarely fail; when they do, it is typically a clinical failure (ie, symptoms persist) despite graft incorporation and maintenance of the articular surface. Revising a failed osteochondral allograft with another osteochondral allograft should it fail to integrate represents a reasonable treatment option as well, but typically failure results from the extent of subchondral bone involvement, which can initially be addressed with restoration using autograft bone grafting, allowing a minimum of 6 to 8 months to incorporate before definitive treatment with an osteochondral allograft. Because of the complex and variable geometry of the patellofemoral joint, in addition to the fact that most OCD lesions at this location tend to be relatively shallow, we reserve large osteochondral allografting for revisions of failed ACI procedures. Notably, this decision making is not universal among surgeons who perform cartilage restoration procedures.

Comorbidities

Combined pathologies such as meniscal injury or deficiency, malalignment, and ligamentous instability are frequently encountered when treating articular cartilage defects. These pathologies are notoriously known to contribute to the development of articular lesions, and a correcting surgical intervention is crucial for an effective and durable cartilage repair. Studies have reported that surgically addressing these combined pathologies ensures the integrity of the primary cartilage repair without affecting the patient's ability to return to day-to-day activities. It is also advantageous to address these combined pathologies at the time of primary cartilage repair to avoid prolonged rehabilitation.

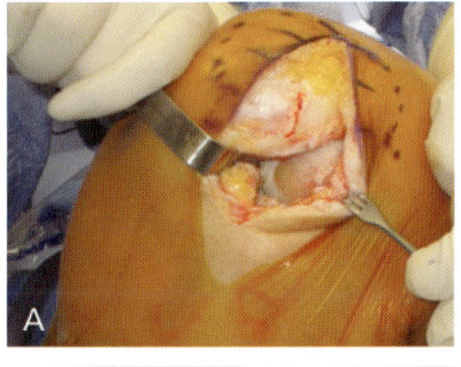

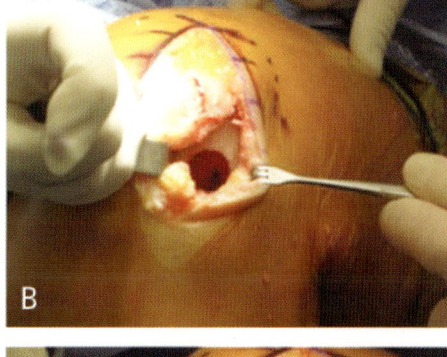

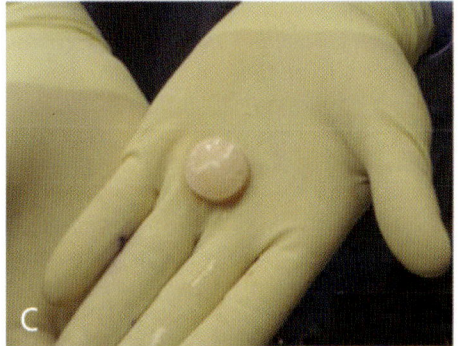

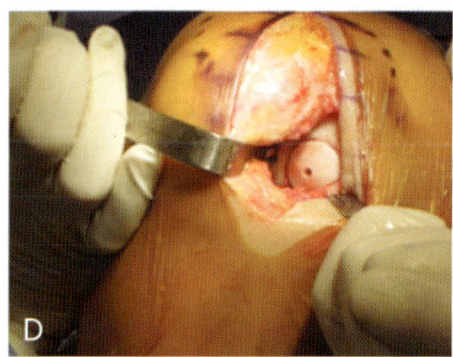

Figure 10 Osteochondral allografting for an osteochondritis dissecans (OCD) lesion. **A**, Arthrotomy reveals the chondral defect. **B**, The defect site is prepared to receive a donor cartilage plug. A counterbore is used to drill to a depth of 6 to 8 mm or until a bleeding bone is established. **C**, A donor cartilage plug is procured from a donor condyle that has been sized and contour matched to the recipient site. **D**, The donor plug is press-fit into place, and a bioabsorbable compression screw is used to ensure fixation.

Pearls

- Early recognition is important, and treatment should be initiated once the diagnosis of a symptomatic OCD lesion is rendered.
- Advanced imaging, including MRI, is helpful in making the diagnosis and determining the relative stability of the lesion.
- In skeletally immature patients, initial nonsurgical therapy can be employed with some success, but persistently painful lesions may still require surgical fixation despite skeletal immaturity.
- In the case of an unstable lesion that is favorable for repair, every effort should be made to preserve the fragment; the treatment concepts are somewhat analogous to treating an atrophic fracture nonunion.
- If the fragment is irreparable, the initial step should be removal of the fragment with or without a concomitant microfracture procedure and ultimately considering a trial of return to activities to allow the patient to determine a persistent or recurrent problem. An ACI biopsy can be performed at the time of the fragment removal.
- The condition of the subchondral bone and the size of the lesion should be used to select the appropriate cartilage augmentation or restoration procedure.
- Comorbidities such as malalignment, meniscal deficiency, or ligament deficiency should be addressed with the same decision making as any cartilage repair procedure.

References

1. Bedi A, Feeley BT, Williams RJ III: Management of articular cartilage defects of the knee. *J Bone Joint Surg Am* 2010;92(4):994-1009.
2. McCarty LP III: Primary repair of osteochondritis dissecans in the knee, in Cole BJ, Sekiya JK, eds: *Surgical Techniques of the Shoulder, Elbow, and Knee in Sports Medicine*. Philadelphia, PA, Saunders Elsevier, 2008, pp 517-526.
3. Aichroth P: Osteochondritis dissecans of the knee: A clinical survey. *J Bone Joint Surg Br* 1971;53(3):440-447.

4. Steinhagen J, Bruns J, Deuretzbacher G, Ruether W, Fuerst M, Niggemeyer O: Treatment of osteochondritis dissecans of the femoral condyle with autologous bone grafts and matrix-supported autologous chondrocytes. *Int Orthop* 2010;34(6): 819-825.

5. Adachi N, Deie M, Nakamae A, Ishikawa M, Motoyama M, Ochi M: Functional and radiographic outcome of stable juvenile osteochondritis dissecans of the knee treated with retroarticular drilling without bone grafting. *Arthroscopy* 2009;25(2):145-152.

6. Cole BJ, Pascual-Garrido C, Grumet RC: Surgical management of articular cartilage defects in the knee. *J Bone Joint Surg Am* 2009;91(7):1778-1790.

7. Donaldson LD, Wojtys EM: Extraarticular drilling for stable osteochondritis dissecans in the skeletally immature knee. *J Pediatr Orthop* 2008;28(8):831-835.

8. Magnussen RA, Carey JL, Spindler KP: Does operative fixation of an osteochondritis dissecans loose body result in healing and long-term maintenance of knee function? *Am J Sports Med* 2009;37(4): 754-759.

9. Pascual-Garrido C, Friel NA, Kirk SS, et al: Midterm results of surgical treatment for adult osteochondritis dissecans of the knee. *Am J Sports Med* 2009; 37(suppl 1):125S-130S.

10. Knutsen G, Drogset JO, Engebretsen L, et al: A randomized trial comparing autologous chondrocyte implantation with microfracture: Findings at five years. *J Bone Joint Surg Am* 2007;89(10): 2105-2112.

11. Miniaci A, Tytherleigh-Strong G: Fixation of unstable osteochondritis dissecans lesions of the knee using arthroscopic autogenous osteochondral grafting (mosaicplasty). *Arthroscopy* 2007;23(8): 845-851.

12. Day JB, Gillogly SD: Autologous chondrocyte implantation in the knee, in Cole BJ, Sekiya JK, eds: *Surgical Techniques of the Shoulder, Elbow, and Knee in Sports Medicine*. Philadelphia, PA, Saunders Elsevier, 2008, pp 559-566.

13. Bartlett W, Gooding CR, Carrington RW, Skinner JA, Briggs TW, Bentley G: Autologous chondrocyte implantation at the knee using a bilayer collagen membrane with bone graft: A preliminary report. *J Bone Joint Surg Br* 2005;87(3):330-332.

14. Bentley G, Biant LC, Carrington RW, et al: A prospective, randomised comparison of autologous chondrocyte implantation versus mosaicplasty for osteochondral defects in the knee. *J Bone Joint Surg Br* 2003;85(2):223-230.

15. Williams JM, Virdi AS, Pylawka TK, Edwards RB III, Markel MD, Cole BJ: Prolonged-fresh preservation of intact whole canine femoral condyles for the potential use as osteochondral allografts. *J Orthop Res* 2005;23(4):831-837.

16. Kang RW, Friel NA, Williams JM, Cole BJ, Wimmer MA: Effect of impaction sequence on osteochondral graft damage: The role of repeated and varying loads. *Am J Sports Med* 2010;38(1):105-113.

17. Garrett JC: Fresh osteochondral allografts for treatment of articular defects in osteochondritis dissecans of the lateral femoral condyle in adults. *Clin Orthop Relat Res* 1994;303:33-37.

18. Kang RW, Gomoll AH, Cole BJ: Osteochondral allografting in the knee, in Cole BJ, Sekiya JK, eds: *Surgical Techniques of the Shoulder, Elbow, and Knee in Sports Medicine*. Philadelphia, PA, Saunders Elsiever, 2008, pp 549-557.

19. McCulloch PC, Kang RW, Sobhy MH, Hayden JK, Cole BJ: Prospective evaluation of prolonged fresh osteochondral allograft transplantation of the femoral condyle: Minimum 2-year follow-up. *Am J Sports Med* 2007;35(3):411-420.

Video Reference

15.1 Yu J, Bugbee W: DVD-Video: *Fresh Osteochondral Allografting to the Knee for Osteochondritis Dissecans*. Rosemont, IL, American Academy of Orthopaedic Surgeons, 2005.

Chapter 16
Anterior Cruciate Ligament Reconstruction: Single-Bundle Transtibial Technique

Eric J. Strauss, MD   Adam B. Yanke, MD   Bernard R. Bach, Jr, MD

Introduction

Injuries to the anterior cruciate ligament (ACL) are common, typically occurring in association with participation in athletic activities. For active patients, surgical reconstruction of the ACL following injury is recommended in an effort to restore stability and normal knee kinematics that will lead to an improvement in function and a return to an active lifestyle. Various reconstruction techniques and graft options are available for ACL reconstruction, including autograft (bone-patellar tendon-bone [BPTB], quadriceps tendon, and hamstring) and allograft (BPTB, hamstring, anterior and posterior tibialis tendons, and Achilles tendon) tissue.[1,2] For the past 25 years, patellar tendon autograft reconstruction has been the most commonly used technique secondary to its biomechanical strength, accessibility and ease of graft harvest, bone-to-bone healing, rigid initial interference screw fixation, and its track record of clinical success.[1-7] This chapter describes the surgical technique for endoscopic ACL reconstruction with BPTB autograft using a single-bundle transtibial approach. This endoscopic technique can be used with patellar tendon autograft tissue, enabling the creation of a femoral tunnel that replicates a portion of both the posterolateral and anteromedial bundles, thereby eliminating both the abnormal Lachman test results and, more importantly, the pivot-shift phenomenon.

Patient Selection

Indications

The ideal patient for ACL reconstruction using a BPTB autograft is young (<40 years) with an active, athletic lifestyle. Other considerations include the specific type of sports involvement, the hours of sports involvement weekly, KT-1000 arthrometer (MEDmetric) instrumented side-to-side differences, concomitant meniscal pathology, the failure of nonsurgical care, and the ability to participate in a structured postoperative physical therapy program. In our practice, approximately 15% of patients are over 40 years of age, and for these patients, different graft sources are generally recommended, preferably patellar tendon allograft. Surgical intervention is delayed until the patient's postinjury effusion has fully resolved, full knee range of motion has been regained, quadriceps control is achieved, and personal and professional issues are "under control" so that the patient is physically and psychologically prepared for surgery. In our practice, if patients have normal or nearly normal motion recovery before surgery, the incidence of reoperation for symptomatic scar tissue/arthrofibrosis has averaged 1% to 2% since 1986. Ideally, the patient should have no evidence of patellar tendon disease, should have no patellar malalignment or antecedent patellofemoral symptoms, and should not be employed in a profession that requires repetitive or prolonged kneeling secondary to the potential incidence of postoperative anterior knee pain or kneeling pain following graft harvest.

Contraindications

BPTB autograft reconstruction is contraindicated in patients with open physes and those with symptomatic preoperative patellar tendon disease. In adolescents, we use a variety of factors—onset of menses in females, skeletal bone age as determined by a PA radiograph of the hand, parent height, and Tanner characteristics—to guide the recommendation for ACL surgery and graft choice. Relative contraindications include radiographic evidence of degenerative joint disease, a sedentary or inactive lifestyle, and an unwillingness or inability to comply with the required rigorous postoperative rehabilitation protocol.

Preoperative Imaging

During the initial evaluation of patients with ACL injuries, radiographs are obtained to assess the quality of the joint space, the bony alignment, and the notch architecture. The four-view series includes a weight-bearing AP view in full extension, a weight-bearing PA 45° flexion view, a non–weight-bearing 45° flexion lateral view, and a Merchant view of the patellofemoral joint. Plain radiographs may identify a Segond fracture consistent with a lateral capsular avulsion, a tibial spine fracture, a "lateral notch" sign, or loose bodies present within the joint.

Although the KT-1000 arthrometer does not measure rotational translations and for this reason some authors question its value, we have used the KT-1000 arthrometer in our practice since 1986. It gives valuable information both preoperatively and postoperatively. Anterior translations greater than 10 mm or side-to-side differences exceeding 3 mm are highly suggestive of an ACL injury.

MRI is used as an adjunct to the patient's history and physical examination to support the diagnosis of an ACL tear. However, our experience suggests that it is extremely unusual to require MRI to establish the diagnosis of an ACL injury. It is critical to emphasize that the physical history and physical examination, along with a KT-1000 arthrometer measurement, establishes the diagnosis of ACL injury in over 98% of our patients. Nevertheless, MRI has been demonstrated to be both sensitive and specific for ACL injuries in addition to providing information about the status of other intra-articular structures, such as the menisci, posterior cruciate ligament, medial collateral ligament, lateral collateral ligament, and chondral surfaces. Bone bruises associated with ACL injury are often readily identifiable on MRI, typically presenting in the midportion of the lateral femoral condyle and in the posterior aspect of the lateral tibial plateau. A careful review of the preoperative MRI can alert the treating orthopaedic surgeon to concomitant

---

Dr. Bach or an immediate family member has received nonincome support (such as equipment or services), commercially derived honoraria, or other non–research-related funding (such as paid travel) from Arthrex, Smith & Nephew, Conmed Linvatec, and Össur. Neither of the following authors nor any immediate family member has received anything of value from or has stock or stock options held in a commercial company or institution related directly or indirectly to the subject of this chapter: Dr. Strauss and Dr. Yanke.

Section 1: Sports Medicine

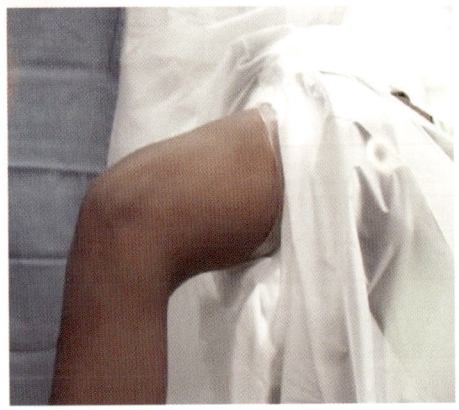

Figure 1 Photograph shows positioning of a left lower extremity for anterior cruciate ligament reconstruction. With the foot of the operating room table flexed completely, the surgical knee is capable of at least 110° of flexion.

Video 16.1 Anterior Cruciate Ligament Reconstruction: Single-Bundle Transtibial Technique. Eric J. Strauss, MD; Adam Yanke, MD; Bernard R. Bach, Jr, MD (19 min)

injuries that may need to be addressed during the ACL reconstruction.

Procedure
Room Setup/Patient Positioning
Following the induction of anesthesia, the patient is positioned supine on the operating room table. The waist of the operating table is flexed to reduce the amount of lumbar extension and, subsequent to the examination under anesthesia, the opposite leg is placed in a gynecological leg holder to protect the femoral and peroneal nerves. The surgical knee is carefully examined under anesthesia, evaluating the amount of translation present with the anterior and posterior drawer tests and the Lachman test, knee stability with applied varus and valgus stress, and whether a pivot-shift phenomenon is present. The status of the posterolateral corner is assessed for asymmetric external rotation at both 30° and 90° of knee flexion, with comparison made to the contralateral side. If a pivot-shift is noted during the examination under anesthesia, the BPTB graft harvest can proceed before diagnostic arthroscopy.

A tourniquet is then placed on the thigh, and the surgical lower extremity is placed in an arthroscopic leg holder. Although some surgeons routinely use a tourniquet, we rarely inflate it during the procedure. The foot of the operating room table

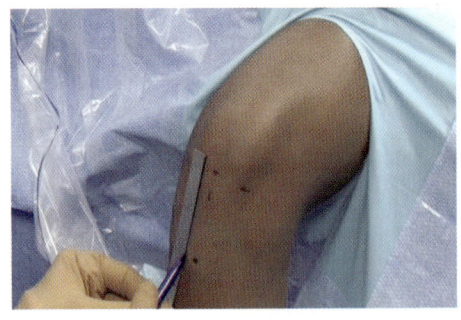

Figure 2 Photograph shows the incision for autologous bone–patellar tendon–bone anterior cruciate ligament reconstruction. The incision extends from the distal aspect of the patella to 2 cm distal to the tibial tubercle just medial to the midline.

is flexed completely, allowing the surgical knee to flex to at least 110° (**Figure 1**). The leg is then prepped and draped, and a preoperative dose of a first-generation cephalosporin is administered.

Special Instruments/Equipment/Implants
The single-bundle transtibial BPTB autograft ACL reconstruction is performed using a standard arthroscopy setup and instruments, including arthroscopic scissors and a basket. For the graft harvest, a No. 10 scalpel, forceps with teeth, two Senn retractors, an Army-Navy retractor, a metal ruler, 3/8- and 1/4-in curved osteotomes, a mallet, and Metzenbaum scissors are required. The bone plugs are created using an oscillating saw with a 10-mm–wide blade (No. 238 blade). For graft preparation, a rongeur, 10- and 11-mm sizing tubes, a Kirschner-wire (K-wire) driver with 0.062-in smooth K-wires, and two No. 5 sutures are needed. A tibial aiming device (we prefer the elbow aimer to the tip aimer) for the tibial tunnel and a 7-mm offset aimer are required for drilling the femoral tunnel, using 11-mm and 10-mm acorn reamers, respectively. A chamfer reamer and a hand rasp are used to aid in tibial tunnel preparation. A large shaver, a 1/4-in (7-mm) curved osteotome, and a large spherical burr are needed for clearing and preparing the intercondylar notch. A satellite pusher is used to aid in graft passage, and for graft fixation, a 14-in hyperflex nitinol wire and 7 × 25-mm metal interference screw are used for the femoral tunnel, and a 9 × 20-mm screw is used for the tibial tunnel.

Surgical Technique
Graft Harvest
Prior to making the surgical incision, anatomic landmarks, including the distal

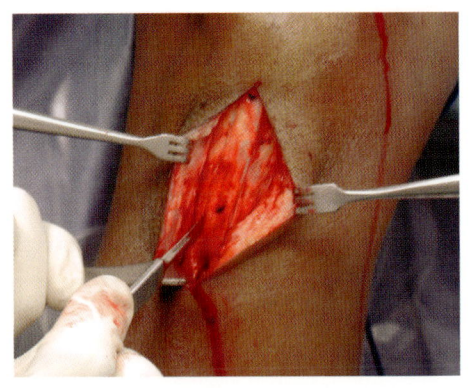

Figure 3 Photograph shows a central-third bone–patellar tendon–bone autograft harvest using a No. 10 scalpel blade starting on the patella and continuing into the patellar tendon.

aspect of the patella, the tibial tubercle, and the borders of the patellar tendon, are marked using a surgical marking pen. The BPTB autograft is harvested through an 8-cm incision extending from the distal patellar pole to the tibial tubercle region, paralleling the medial edge of the patellar tendon (**Figure 2**). This incision allows for both graft harvest and tibial tunnel drilling through the same approach. The incision is taken down to the transverse fibers of the patellar tendon paratenon. At this level, medial and lateral skin flaps are created. A No. 15 scalpel is then used to make a midline, longitudinal incision in the paratenon, which is extended both proximally and distally with Metzenbaum scissors. The Metzenbaum scissors are then used to elevate the paratenon off the patellar tendon both medially and laterally, fully exposing the patellar tendon. The tendon width is measured and recorded in the surgical report.

The ideal BPTB autograft is 10 mm wide with 10 × 25-mm bone plugs. The center of the inferior pole of the patella and the center of the distal patellar tendon at the tibial tubercle are marked with a surgical marking pen, and a curved 3/8-in osteotome (which is roughly 10 mm in width) is used as a cutting guide for the central third of the patellar tendon. With the Army-Navy retractor placed proximally, parallel longitudinal incisions are made using a No. 10 scalpel, starting on the patella and continuing into the patellar tendon. Once the midpoint of the patellar tendon is reached, the Army-Navy retractor is switched to the inferior aspect of the wound to protect the skin as the incision is extended distally 2.5 cm past the tendo-osseous junction on the tibial tubercle (**Figure 3**).

Chapter 16: Anterior Cruciate Ligament Reconstruction: Single-Bundle Transtibial Technique

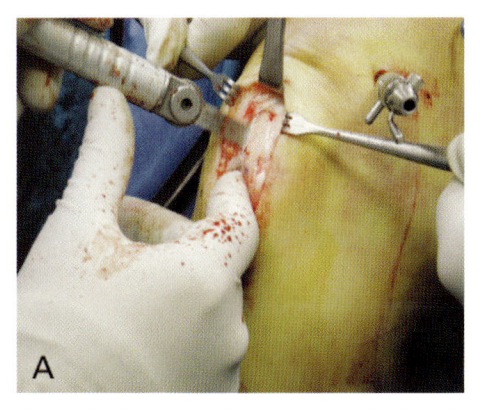

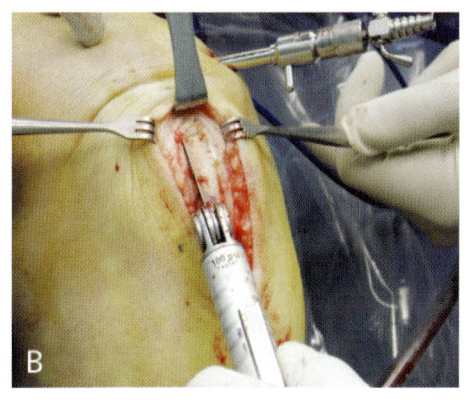

Figure 4 Intraoperative photographs show bone cuts made using an oscillating saw with a 10-mm (No. 238) blade. Cuts on the right side are made with the saw in the surgeon's right hand (**A**) and those on the left are made with the saw in the surgeon's left hand (**B**).

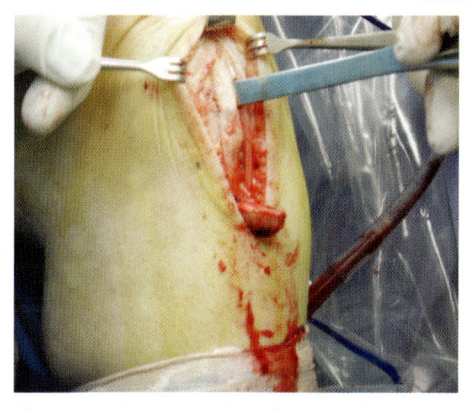

Figure 5 Intraoperative photograph shows the patellar bone plug being freed from its osseous bed with an osteotome.

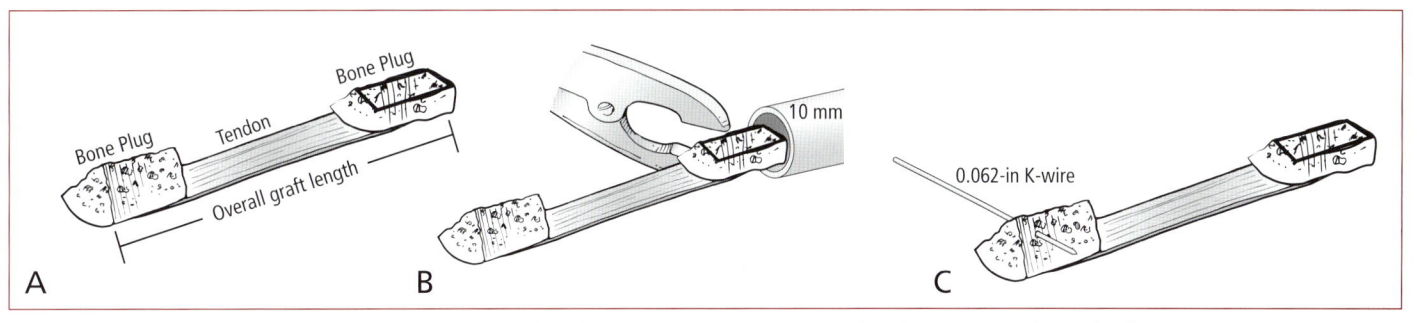

Figure 6 Illustrations demonstrate the preparation of the harvested bone–patellar tendon–bone autograft. **A**, The first step is measurement of the overall graft length, the length of its tendinous portion, and then the length of each bone plug. **B**, Fine tuning of the bone plugs is performed using a rongeur, ensuring that each bone plug fits in the 10-mm sizing tube. **C**, Two drill holes are made in the tibial bone plug using a smooth 0.062-in K-wire with a No. 5 suture passed through each hole.

This process is repeated on the other side, creating a 10-mm–wide graft.

Bone cuts are then made using an oscillating saw with a 10-mm (No. 238) blade, starting on the tibial side. Cuts on the right side of the graft are made with the saw in the surgeon's right hand and those on the left with the saw in the surgeon's left hand (**Figure 4**). With the saw supported by the surgeon's thumb and the graft protected with the index finger, the oscillating saw is used to first score the cortex, starting at the tendo-osseous junction, followed by angling of the saw to create a plug with an equilateral triangle profile. The transverse bony cut is then made with the saw angled 45°, using the corner of the blade on each side of the graft to avoid the creation of stress risers. The patellar bone plug is then cut in similar fashion, angling the saw during the longitudinal cuts to create a plug that is trapezoidal in shape. The saw blade should not penetrate deeper than 6 to 7 mm, to avoid injury to the patellar articular surface. The transverse bony cut is similarly made with the saw angled 45°. The tibial bone plug is then carefully freed from its osseous bed using 3/8- and 1/4-in osteotomes, without levering. A lap sponge is then placed around the freed tibial plug to apply traction on the graft as Metzenbaum scissors are used to remove any remaining connections to the underlying fat pad. The patellar bone plug is then similarly freed from its osseous bed (**Figure 5**), and the harvested graft is wrapped in a moist sponge and walked to the back table by the operating surgeon.

Graft Preparation

The first assistant prepares the BPTB autograft, fashioning the graft's bone plugs to 10 × 25-mm dimensions. The first step is the measurement and documentation of the overall graft length, the length of its tendinous portion, and the length of each bone plug (**Figure 6, A**). Fine tuning of the bone plugs is performed using a rongeur to allow for passage through the 10-mm sizing tube (**Figure 6, B**). Excess bone removed during the preparation process should be saved for later bone grafting of the harvest sites. Once appropriately sized, two drill holes are made in the tibial bone plug using a smooth 0.062-in K-wire, parallel to its cortex (**Figure 6, C**). A No. 5 suture is then placed through each hole. Because we prefer to use a push-in technique for graft passage, no drill holes are created in the femoral bone plug. A surgical marking pen is then used to mark the tendo-osseous junction on the femoral side of the graft to aid in assessing the full seating of the graft in the femoral tunnel, and the distal cortical edge of the tibial plug is marked to assist in graft orientation. The prepared BPTB graft is then wrapped in a moist sponge and safely set aside in a kidney basin. It is critical that all operating room staff know where the graft has been placed so it is not inadvertently passed off the field.

Diagnostic Arthroscopy and Notch Preparation

A superomedial outflow portal is created proximally, and the standard inferolateral and inferomedial portals are created within the graft harvest site. A diagnostic arthroscopy is performed to assess the patellofemoral joint, the lateral and medial gutters, and the medial and lateral compartments, assessing for associated meniscal injury, loose bodies, and articular cartilage injury. In the absence of associated pathology that requires surgical management, attention is turned to the intercondylar notch. Once in the notch, the status of the posterior cruciate ligament can be evaluated and the nature of the ACL injury can be documented.

© 2013 American Academy of Orthopaedic Surgeons

Section 1: Sports Medicine

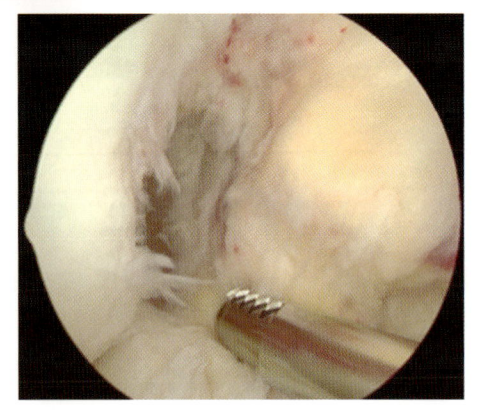

Figure 7 Arthroscopic view demonstrates débridement of the remnant of the torn anterior cruciate ligament.

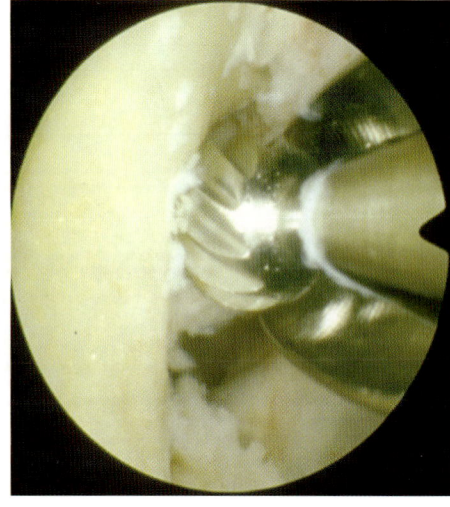

Figure 8 Arthroscopic view demonstrates notchplasty. A 5.5-mm spherical burr is used to widen the notch in an anterior-to-posterior direction, working toward the over-the-top position.

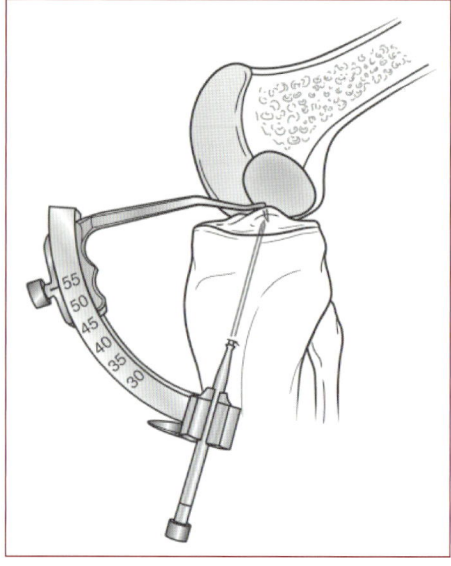

Figure 9 Illustration shows a variable-angle tibial aimer used for the creation of the tibial tunnel.

The interval between the remnant ACL and the posterior cruciate ligament is developed and any remaining ACL tissue is removed using a combination of arthroscopic scissors, an arthroscopic basket, and a large motorized shaver (**Figure 7**). The lateral wall of the notch is cleared of soft tissue using the shaver or a curet. Any fat pad or ligamentum mucosum that is impeding visualization can also be removed from the intercondylar notch.

Notchplasty is performed if necessary to improve visualization of the "over-the-top" position posteriorly and limit the possibility of graft impingement, especially with the knee in the extended position. A 1/4-in curved osteotome is inserted through the medial portal and used to begin the notchplasty at the level of the articular surface of the lateral wall, with the fragments removed with an arthroscopic grasper. These fragments are saved for later use as graft for the distal patellar and tibial tubercle defects. Next, a 5.5-mm spherical burr is used to widen the notch in an anterior-to-posterior direction, working toward the over-the-top position (**Figure 8**). The adequacy of the notchplasty is checked with an arthroscopic probe, ensuring that the probe can be hooked around the sharp edge of the posterior wall of the notch.

Tibial Tunnel Placement

To create the tibial tunnel, a variable-angle tibial aimer is used, with the angle selected dependent on the length of the soft-tissue component of the BPTB graft (**Figure 9**). Generally, we use an "N + 10" rule for setting the angle of the tibial aimer (45 mm of tendon length equates to a 55° setting on the aimer). However, we do not use less than 55° for shorter tendon lengths. The major criticism of the transtibial technique is that surgeons do not create enough obliquity with the tibial tunnel, leading to a femoral tunnel that is drilled with an orientation that is too vertical. A vertically oriented femoral tunnel is the most common technical error we have encountered in failed endoscopic reconstructions. Some authors have advocated drilling through an accessory portal to create a femoral tunnel along the lateral intercondylar wall.[8-10] Other authors have maintained that a two-incision technique with independent tunnel creation will obviate the potential for a vertically oriented femoral tunnel.[11-13] Still other authors have advocated the use of a double-bundle technique to more anatomically replicate the anteromedial and posterolateral ACL femoral bundles.[14,15] We have developed an alternative approach, whereby an accessory incision is placed through the patellar tendon rent, 1 cm distal and 1 cm lateral to the standard inferomedial portal. This portal allows easier rotation of the tibial aimer and a more distal starting point on the tibia, which reduces the likelihood of graft tunnel mismatch and allows for the creation of a tibial tunnel that is obliquely oriented such that the subsequent femoral tunnel can be created to replicate portions of both the posterolateral and anteromedial bundles of the ACL. The tip of the tibial aimer is inserted through this accessory midpatellar portal, created following spinal needle localization. An ideal guide-pin placement is just lateral to the medial tibial spine at the level of the posterior aspect of the anterior horn of the lateral meniscus and/or 7 mm anterior to the posterior cruciate ligament. We use the posterior edge of the anterior horn of the lateral meniscus as a coronal plane landmark for placement of the pin within the midregion of the former ACL insertion. Once the tip of the tibial aimer is appropriately localized intra-articularly, the cannulated portion of the aimer is rotated into position using the upper border of the pes anserine and the anterior edge of the superficial edge of the medial collateral ligament as anatomic landmarks. Provisional guide-pin placement is performed using a 3/32-in smooth Steinmann pin (**Figure 10**). Once the pin is advanced into the joint, its position is checked arthroscopically, ensuring that no impingement on the superior notch occurs with knee extension; the pin should be posterior to the apex of the intercondylar notch with the knee in complete extension. With the knee returned to the flexed position, the guide pin is advanced with a mallet until it reaches the lateral wall of the intercondylar notch, to stabilize it during the reaming process.

Next, the appropriately sized cannulated acorn reamer is used over the guide pin. We typically ream the tibial tunnel with an 11-mm reamer for a 10-mm bone plug to ease the process of graft passage and reduce the likelihood of graft delamination. During the reaming process, the arthroscopic pump is turned off, and a cannulated bone chip collector is placed over the tibial reamer, allowing bone chips from reaming to be collected for later grafting of the harvest sites. After the reamer is advanced into the joint, the pump is turned back on, and additional

Chapter 16: Anterior Cruciate Ligament Reconstruction: Single-Bundle Transtibial Technique

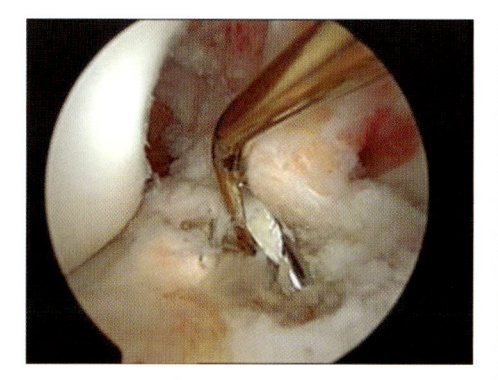

Figure 10 Arthroscopic view shows provisional guide pin placement performed using a 3/32-in smooth Steinmann pin.

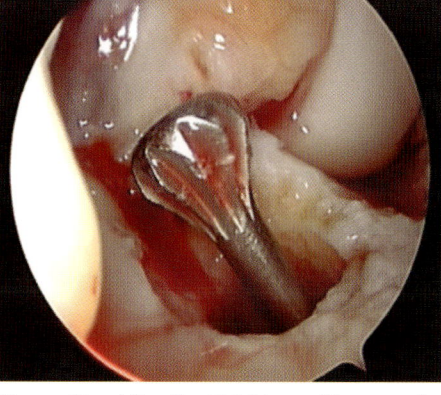

Figure 11 After the tibial tunnel is reamed using an 11-mm acorn reamer, a chamfer reamer is used to smooth the posterolateral edge of the tunnel.

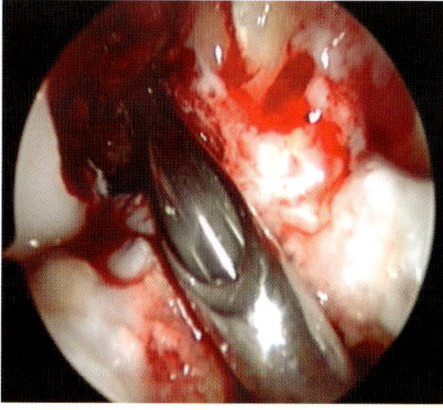

Figure 12 Arthroscopic view shows a 7-mm offset aimer inserted through the tibial tunnel into the intercondylar notch, with its tip hooked around the back wall and rotated laterally, to allow for guide-pin placement low on the lateral wall at the anatomic femoral footprint of the anterior cruciate ligament.

bone from the reaming process is collected using fine-mesh burn gauze. Once the tibial tunnel has been created, its posterior edge is smoothed with a chamfer reamer and finished with an arthroscopic hand rasp (**Figure 11**). Any overhanging soft tissue can be removed with a large shaver.

Femoral Tunnel Placement
For the femoral tunnel, a 7-mm offset aimer is inserted through the tibial tunnel into the intercondylar notch, with the knee flexed to approximately 80° to 90°. The tip of the aimer is hooked around the posterior wall of the over-the-top position and rotated laterally to allow for guide-pin placement lower on the lateral wall of the notch (**Figure 12**). A smooth 3/32-in Steinmann pin is drilled into the lateral wall to a depth of 3 cm. With the arthroscopic pump turned off, the guide pin is then overreamed using a 10-mm reamer, initially advanced 1 cm and then backed off to allow for visual confirmation of maintained posterior wall integrity (**Figure 13**). Ideally, 1 to 2 mm of posterior cortex should remain. Reaming of the femoral tunnel is then completed to a depth of 30 to 35 mm. The arthroscopic pump is then turned back on, so that reamings can once again be collected using fine-mesh burn gauze. The overall integrity of the femoral tunnel can be visually inspected by inserting the arthroscope retrograde through the tibial tunnel into the femoral tunnel. This is important to make certain that an intratunnel perforation has not occurred.

Graft Passage and Interference Screw Fixation
Following intercondylar notch preparation, notchplasty, and tibial and femoral tunnel creation, attention is directed to graft passage and fixation. The BPTB autograft is advanced into the joint using a push-in technique. With this technique, the graft is inserted into the tibial tunnel with a two-pronged pusher placed at the base of the femoral bone plug. A hemostat is inserted through the medial portal, grasping the femoral bone plug at the junction of the proximal and middle thirds, guiding the plug into the femoral tunnel with the cortical surface of the plug facing posteriorly (**Figure 14**). The femoral bone plug is seated into the tunnel approximately 75%, leaving room for placement of the 14-inch hyperflex nitinol wire. A small pilot hole for wire placement can be created using a hemostat or a tunnel-notching device. The nitinol wire is then inserted at the 1-o'clock (left knee) or 11-o'clock (right knee) position of the graft, the knee is further flexed, and the wire is advanced into the depth of the tunnel. With the nitinol wire in position, the femoral bone plug can then be advanced and fully seated using a satellite pusher. Prior to interference screw placement, the tibial bone plug should be evaluated for any graft-tunnel mismatch that may be present. If mismatch is present, the femoral bone plug can be further recessed with the satellite pusher. With the femoral bone plug in its final position, the knee is hyperflexed to 100° to 115°, and the 7 × 25-mm metal interference screw is advanced over the nitinol wire. Care should be taken to remove the wire once the screw has been inserted halfway (**Figure 15**).

With the femoral bone plug secured, tension is held on the tibial bone plug sutures and the "rock test" is performed. Enough tension is placed on the graft to rock the patient on the operating table, confirming stable fixation of the femoral bone plug. Gross isometry is then checked by the surgeon by placing a thumb at the tibial tunnel aperture, with tension held on the tibial bone-plug sutures. As the knee is extended from 90° to full extension, 1 to 2 mm of graft shortening is typically noted during the terminal 20° of extension. The graft is then cycled, and attention is turned to tibial bone-plug fixation. With the knee in full extension and an axial load applied, a hemostat is used to externally rotate the tibial bone plug 180°, such that the cortical surface of the plug is facing anteriorly. The nitinol wire is inserted anterior to the tibial bone plug, and a 9 × 20-mm metal interference screw is inserted while tension is held on the tibial bone-plug sutures. The screw is advanced until it is seated just below the cortical surface of the tibia. Following tibial-side fixation, the arthroscope is placed back into the lateral portal to visually inspect and probe the graft to ensure proper graft tension (**Figure 16**). A Lachman test and pivot-shift test are performed to confirm knee stability.

Closure
The wound is copiously irrigated, and the patellar tendon is reapproximated using three or four interrupted No. 1 Vicryl sutures (Ethicon) with the knee in flexion to avoid excessive shortening. Bone graft that was collected from the reaming process and graft preparation are placed into the patellar and tibial bony defects. The patellar tendon paratenon is closed with a running 2-0 Vicryl suture. Skin closure is then performed with subcutaneous 2-0 Vicryl sutures followed by a running 3-0 Prolene pullout stitch (Ethicon). The superomedial outflow arthroscopic portal

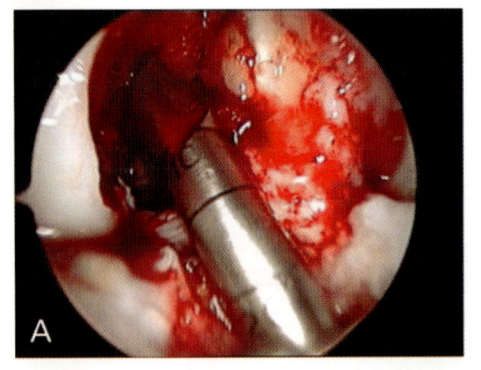

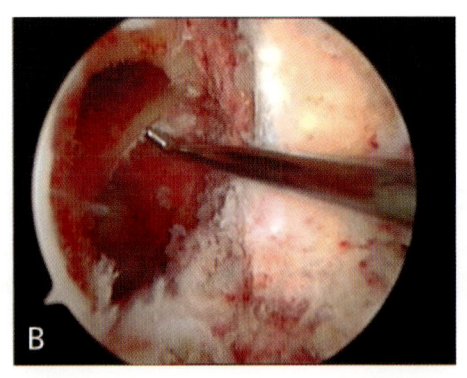

Figure 13 Arthroscopic views show overreaming of the guide pin. A 10-mm reamer is initially advanced 1 cm (**A**) and then backed off to allow for visual confirmation of maintained posterior wall integrity (**B**).

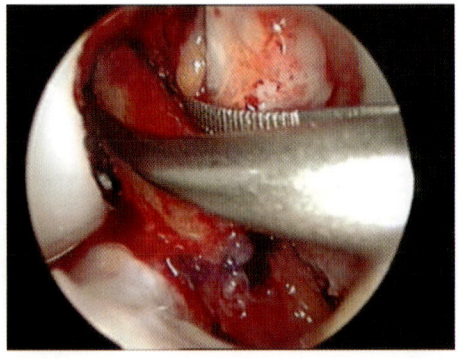

Figure 14 Arthoscopic view demonstrates the push-in technique for femoral bone plug insertion. A hemostat inserted through the medial portal guides the plug into the femoral tunnel, with the cortical surface of the plug facing posteriorly.

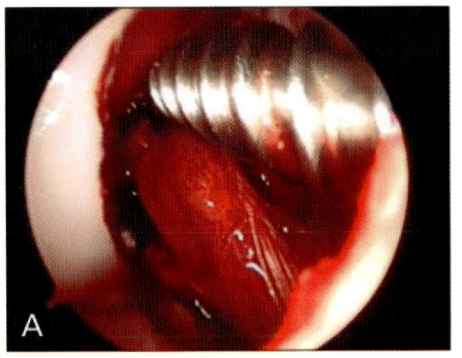

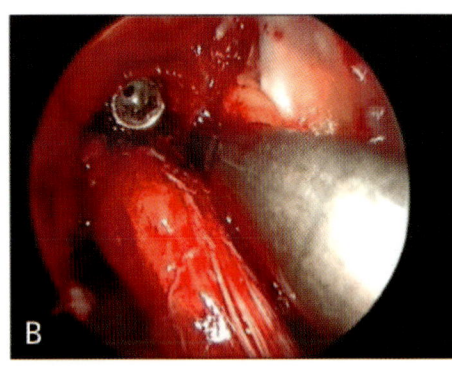

Figure 15 **A,** The 7 × 25-mm metal screw is advanced over a nitinol wire for interference screw fixation. Once the screw is advanced halfway, the wire is removed because removal is more difficult once the screw is fully seated. Care should be taken to avoid fraying of the soft-tissue component. **B,** With the driver and wire removed, the screw is slightly recessed, and there is no evidence of graft damage during insertion.

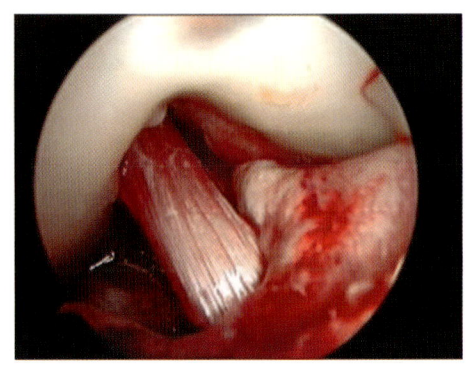

Figure 16 Arthroscopic view shows the final anterior cruciate ligament reconstruction.

is closed with a simple 3-0 Prolene suture. The surgical incision is injected with 0.5% bupivacaine and covered with adhesive skin closure strips and sterile dressings. A cryotherapy device is placed over a gauze bandage and overwrapped with a compressive elastic wrap. Finally, the leg is placed in a hinged knee brace locked in extension but allowing full range of motion as tolerated.

Complications

Potential postoperative complications following ACL reconstruction using BPTB autograft include arthrofibrosis, infection, patellar fracture, anterior knee pain, deep venous thrombosis, complex regional pain syndrome, and compartment syndrome. In a literature review of ACL reconstructions using BPTB autografts, Nedeff and Bach[16] reported an overall reoperation rate of 13% following the procedure, with reported mean incidences of arthrofibrosis and infection of 7% and 0.4%, respectively. Specifically, the incidence of intraoperative or postoperative patellar fracture is approximately 1 in 300; patellar tendon rupture, 1 in 1,000; and infection, 1 in 300. Our reoperation rate for symptomatic knee flexion contractures or arthrofibrosis has averaged 1% to 2% since 1986. The senior author's (B.R.B's) overall personal revision rate has been 1.7% based on 1,809 primary ACL reconstructions performed between July 1986 and March 2012. Two thirds of these were autografts, and one third were allograft BPTB reconstructions. No differences were noted in the personal revision rates of autograft versus allograft BPTB (1.6% vs. 2.0%), and no differences were noted between nonirradiated allograft versus low-dose (1.5-mRad) BPTB allograft. However, the mean age for primary autograft ACL reconstruction was 26 years, whereas the mean age for primary allograft was 36 years. Our personal revision rate between 2002 and 2009 was as follows: four fellowship-trained surgeons performed 1,944 ACL reconstructions and personally revised 28 patients (1.4%). In previous studies, we reported patellofemoral pain symptoms ranging from 12% to 18%, with the majority of patients reporting minimal to mild pain. In previously reported studies, approximately 95% of patients were either completely or mostly satisfied.[3,5,17,18]

Postoperative Care and Rehabilitation

Following ACL reconstruction using a BPTB autograft, we employ an accelerated protocol, including closed-chain exercises, with the goal of regaining full active knee range of motion while maintaining stability and avoiding symptoms related to the patellofemoral joint. In the immediate postoperative period, patients are allowed to fully weight-bear with the hinged knee brace locked in extension. The brace is used specifically to protect the donor site should the patient slip or fall. It is removed for motion activities. Supervised physical therapy is started at 1 week postoperatively, at which point quadriceps sets, straight-leg raises, and patellar mobilizations are performed with the knee in extension. We emphasize regaining complete extension or hyperextension within the first 10 days postoperatively; a secondary goal is to have 80° to 90° of knee flexion. From weeks 2 through 4, closed-chain extension exercises are initiated along with hamstring curls and the use of a stationary bicycle. From weeks 4 through 6, the goal of knee flexion to 120° is usually obtained, and patients are advanced to using a stair climber for continued quadriceps strengthening. At 8 to 10 weeks postoperatively, patients are advanced to light jogging and outdoor biking while continuing to perform closed-chain strengthening exercises. Sport-specific exercises and a gradual return to play are allowed at 4 to 6 months postoperatively. Open-chain exercises and isokinetic strengthening are not used in our postoperative rehabilitation program.

Patients are seen at 10 days postoperatively for suture removal and evaluation of range of motion. If they have achieved full extension and flexion to 90° at this visit, patients are seen again at 6 weeks postoperatively. If their range of motion is short of this goal, patients are seen weekly until motion recovery is acceptable. Starting at the 6-week time point, patients are seen at 6-week intervals until the 6-month postoperative visit, with KT-1000 arthrometer testing performed at each visit. Patients are then seen at 9 months and 1 year postoperatively, at which point they are discharged from care.

Pearls

- The patient should be positioned so that once the foot of the operating room table is dropped, the knee is able to flex to 110°; this will avoid difficulty with drilling of the femoral tunnel and placement of the femoral interference screw.
- The surgical incision should be 8 cm long, extending from the distal aspect of the patella to 2 cm distal to the tibial tubercle, just medial to the midline, so that both graft harvest and tibial tunnel drilling can be performed through the same approach.
- During the graft harvest, a curved 3/8-in osteotome (which is effectively 10 mm wide) can be used as a template for the central third of the patellar tendon.
- The surgeon should use both hands when making the bone cuts during the graft harvest (cuts on the right side of the graft are made with the saw in the surgeon's right hand and those on the left with the saw in the surgeon's left hand); this improves visualization during the harvest process.
- For placement of the tibial aiming guide, an accessory midpatellar portal can improve the surgeon's effort to improve the obliquity of the tibial tunnel.
- Reaming the tibial tunnel with an 11-mm reamer for a 10-mm bone plug can make graft passage easier.
- Placing the arthroscope through the tibial tunnel and into the femoral tunnel allows visual confirmation of the integrity of the posterior wall throughout its length.
- With the femoral plug seated in the femoral tunnel, the tibial bone plug should be checked for evidence of graft-tunnel mismatch; if present, recession of the femoral bone plug can be performed to improve tibial plug position.
- The tibial bone plug should be externally rotated such that the cortical surface is facing anteriorly; this allows for anterior placement of the tibial interference screw, which keeps the graft posterior, avoiding potential impingement in extension.
- The patellar tendon is reapproximated with the knee in flexion to avoid excessive shortening.

References

1. Miller SL, Gladstone JN: Graft selection in anterior cruciate ligament reconstruction. *Orthop Clin North Am* 2002;33(4):675-683.
2. West RV, Harner CD: Graft selection in anterior cruciate ligament reconstruction. *J Am Acad Orthop Surg* 2005;13(3):197-207.
3. Bach BR Jr, Levy ME, Bojchuk J, Tradonsky S, Bush-Joseph CA, Khan NH: Single-incision endoscopic anterior cruciate ligament reconstruction using patellar tendon autograft: Minimum two-year follow-up evaluation. *Am J Sports Med* 1998;26(1):30-40.
4. Deehan DJ, Salmon LJ, Webb VJ, Davies A, Pinczewski LA: Endoscopic reconstruction of the anterior cruciate ligament with an ipsilateral patellar tendon autograft: A prospective longitudinal five-year study. *J Bone Joint Surg Br* 2000;82(7):984-991.
5. Bach BR Jr, Tradonsky S, Bojchuk J, Levy ME, Bush-Joseph CA, Khan NH: Arthroscopically assisted anterior cruciate ligament reconstruction using patellar tendon autograft: Five- to nine-year follow-up evaluation. *Am J Sports Med* 1998;26(1):20-29.
6. Fox JA, Nedeff DD, Bach BR Jr, Spindler KP: Anterior cruciate ligament reconstruction with patellar autograft tendon. *Clin Orthop Relat Res* 2002;402:53-63.
7. Novak PJ, Bach BR Jr, Hager CA: Clinical and functional outcome of anterior cruciate ligament reconstruction in the recreational athlete over the age of 35. *Am J Knee Surg* 1996;9(3):111-116.
8. Bedi A, Musahl V, Steuber V, et al: Transtibial versus anteromedial portal reaming in anterior cruciate ligament reconstruction: An anatomic and biomechanical evaluation of surgical technique. *Arthroscopy* 2011;27(3):380-390.
9. Silva A, Sampaio R, Pinto E: ACL reconstruction: Comparison between transtibial and anteromedial portal techniques. *Knee Surg Sports Traumatol Arthrosc* 2012;20(5):896-903.
10. Harner CD, Honkamp NJ, Ranawat AS: Anteromedial portal technique for creating the anterior cruciate ligament femoral tunnel. *Arthroscopy* 2008;24(1):113-115.
11. Garofalo R, Moretti B, Kombot C, Moretti L, Mouhsine E: Femoral tunnel placement in anterior cruciate ligament reconstruction: Rationale of the two incision technique. *J Orthop Surg Res* 2007;2:10.
12. Gill TJ, Steadman JR: Anterior cruciate ligament reconstruction the two-incision technique. *Orthop Clin North Am* 2002;33(4):727-735, vii.
13. Harner CD, Marks PH, Fu FH, Irrgang JJ, Silby MB, Mengato R: Anterior cruciate ligament reconstruction: Endoscopic versus two-incision technique. *Arthroscopy* 1994;10(5):502-512.
14. Steckel H, Starman JS, Baums MH, Klinger HM, Schultz W, Fu FH: The double-bundle technique for anterior cruciate ligament reconstruction: A systematic overview. *Scand J Med Sci Sports* 2007;17(2):99-108.
15. Cha PS, Brucker PU, West RV, et al: Arthroscopic double-bundle anterior cruciate ligament reconstruction: An anatomic approach. *Arthroscopy* 2005;21(10):1275.
16. Nedeff DD, Bach BR Jr: Arthroscopic anterior cruciate ligament reconstruction using patellar tendon autografts: A comprehensive review of contemporary literature. *Am J Knee Surg* 2001;14(4):243-258.
17. Bach BR Jr, Jones GT, Sweet FA, Hager CA: Arthroscopy-assisted anterior cruciate ligament reconstruction using patellar tendon substitution: Two- to four-year follow-up results. *Am J Sports Med* 1994;22(6):758-767.
18. Bach BR Jr, Aadalen KJ, Dennis M, et al: Primary anterior cruciate ligament reconstruction using fresh-frozen nonirradiated patellar tendon allograft: Minimum 2-year follow-up. *Am J Sports Med* 2005;32(2):284-292.

Video Reference

16.1 Strauss EJ, Yanke A, Bach BR Jr: Anterior Cruciate Ligament Reconstruction: Single-Bundle Transtibial Technique, in Fu FH, Howell SM, eds: Video: *Arthroscopic Surgical Techniques: Anterior Cruciate Ligament Reconstruction*. Rosemont, IL, American Academy of Orthopaedic Surgeons, 2010.

Chapter 17
Anterior Cruciate Ligament Reconstruction: Two-Tunnel Technique

Dharmesh Vyas, MD   Christopher D. Harner, MD

Introduction

The anterior cruciate ligament (ACL) has been shown to play a critical role in the maintenance of knee stability. Leaving an ACL-deficient knee untreated can result in recurrent instability, meniscal pathology, and articular cartilage damage.[1] Despite the fact that ACL injury has become one of the most popular topics of study in orthopaedic sports medicine, significant disagreement exists on the appropriate management of this injury.[2,3] Despite adherence to strict surgical principles, the inability to predict long-term articular cartilage degeneration after ACL reconstruction (ACLR) has raised questions about the choice of surgical technique, graft choices, fixation, and rehabilitation. In this chapter, we present our preference for ACLR, which is based on a single-bundle reconstruction primarily using a bone–patellar tendon–bone (BTB) autograft. The procedure takes advantage of the medial portal technique (versus transtibial) for femoral tunnel placement.[4,5] Unique to this technique is its versatility, being appropriate for all autograft and allograft types as well as fixation methods.[4]

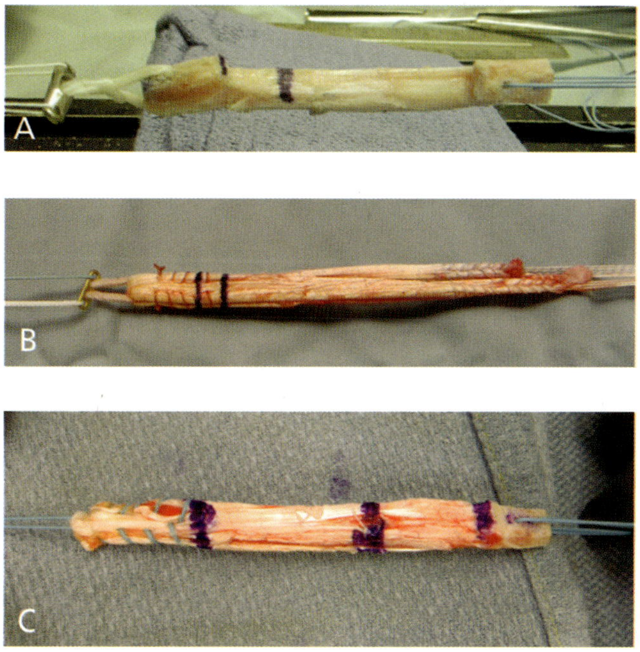

Patient Selection

The decision to proceed with an ACLR begins with a comprehensive history and physical examination. This includes a demonstration of ACL insufficiency and an assessment of the patient's expectations, activity level, and comorbidities. Surgical indications are founded on three major criteria: the degree of perceived instability, associated knee injuries (meniscus or multiligament), and chronicity of the ligament insufficiency.

Prior to surgical intervention, the patient is enrolled in physical therapy, emphasizing the achievement of full range of motion, symmetric quadriceps strength, and decreased effusion. Generally, most patients meet these criteria within 3 to 4 weeks. In the context of an associated medial collateral ligament (MCL) injury amenable to nonsurgical management, we delay surgery for up to 6 weeks to allow time for the MCL to heal. Contraindications to ACLR include (1) partial tears with minimal reported instability and no joint laxity on examination; (2) elderly, low-demand patients with minimal instability; and (3) comorbidities that make surgical intervention unsafe for the patient.

Graft Choice

Graft options are individualized for each patient and are contingent on age, activity level, the grade of injury (partial versus complete), associated injuries, and the return-to-play timeline. In most cases, autografts are recommended for patients younger than 35 years, and allografts are reserved for older patients.[6] This is based on the notion that younger patients generally have more active lifestyles.

Figure 1 Photographs depict autograft options. **A,** Bone–patellar tendon–bone: femoral side with EndoButton CL BTB (Smith & Nephew Endoscopy) and tibial side with Ethibond (Ethicon) lead sutures. The first blue mark is at the bone-tendon junction, and the second marks the amount of graft needed in the femoral tunnel for the EndoButton to engage the lateral femoral cortex. **B,** Quadrupled hamstring: semitendinosus and gracilis. **C,** Quadriceps with patellar bone block.

We prefer to use BTB in younger, active athletes, especially if they are involved in cutting sports (eg, football, soccer, basketball), and in larger patients[7] (Figure 1). Hamstring grafts are used in patients who require single-bundle augmentation, those with contraindications to BTB, and females with donor-site incisional cosmesis concerns (unless the activity level dictates otherwise). In select revision cases, we use quadriceps tendon graft.

Preoperative Imaging
Radiography

Diagnostic imaging begins with plain radiographs. These include 45° flexion weight-bearing PA views of both knees, a lateral view, and Merchant patella views. These radiographs are used to identify associated fractures (avulsion, plateau, or subchondral impaction), gauge the amount of joint-space narrowing in the three compartments, and assess patellar height (lateral view), tilt, and subluxation (Merchant view). Determination of patella alta versus patella baja is critical for medial portal ACLR because it influences the correct position of the portals. Furthermore, radiographs are a prerequisite in pediatric patients to assess the status of the growth plate. In these patients, hand and wrist radiographs are often

---

Dr. Harner or an immediate family member has received research or institutional support from DePuy and Smith & Nephew and serves as a board member, owner, officer, or committee member of the American Board of Orthopaedic Surgery, the American Orthopaedic Association, the American Academy of Orthopaedic Surgeons, and the American Orthopaedic Society for Sports Medicine. Neither Dr. Vyas nor any immediate family member has received anything of value from or owns stock in a commercial company or institution related directly or indirectly to the subject of this chapter.

Section 1: **Sports Medicine**

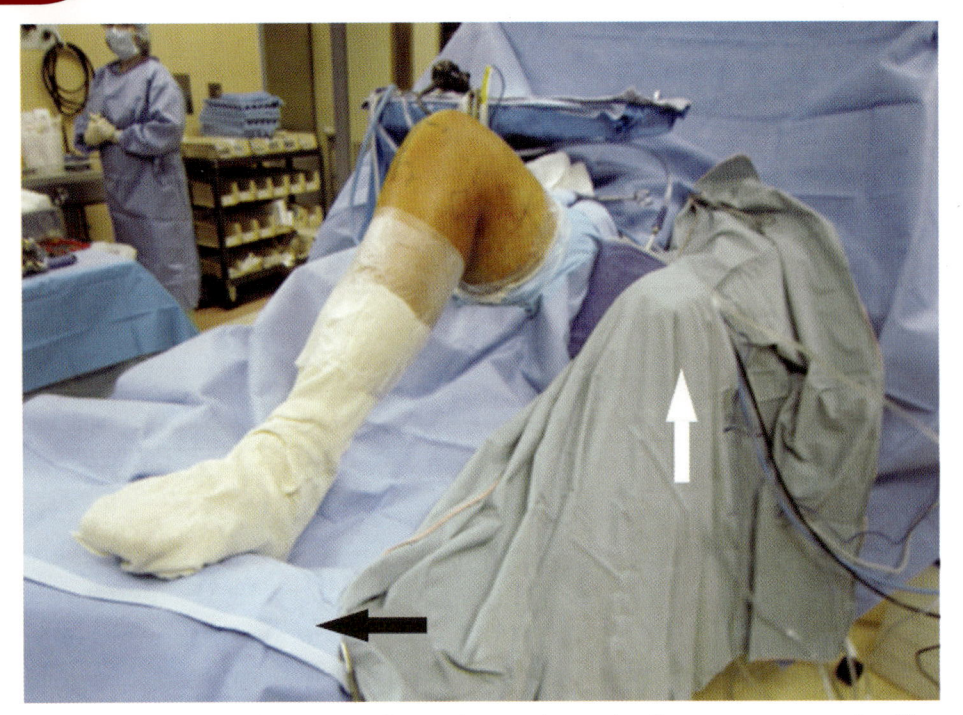

Figure 2 Photograph shows surgical setup for anterior cruciate ligament reconstruction. The patient is positioned supine with a bump under the ipsilateral hip. A sandbag (black arrow) and a lateral post (white arrow) are used to keep the leg at 90° of flexion for most of the case.

obtained to assist in the determination of skeletal age.[8]

Magnetic Resonance Imaging
Based on the patient's history and physical examination, if an ACL tear is suspected, then a noncontrast MRI scan of the knee is obtained in most cases. Discontinuity of the ACL in the coronal and sagittal planes on either the T1 or T2 image sequences is a reliable indication of an ACL tear. Importantly, MRI helps the clinician identify associated injuries of the knee, such as meniscal tears, chondral damage including bone bruises, and associated ligament injuries. This is especially important in the patient with an acute knee injury when the physical examination for associated injuries can be limited by pain and swelling.

Procedure
Room Setup/Patient Positioning
On the day of surgery, laterality is marked and consent is reviewed with the patient in the preoperative holding area. A combined femoral and sciatic nerve block is administered for postoperative pain control. The sciatic block is maintained for 3 days postoperatively with an indwelling catheter. The procedure is performed under either monitored or general anesthesia as determined by the anesthesiologist. The patient is placed supine on the operating room table, and prophylactic antibiotics are administered. The lower extremity is positioned in neutral rotation with the use of a soft gel bump under the ipsilateral hip. A 10-lb sandbag is taped to the table to support the knee at 90° of flexion (**Figure 2**). A lateral post is placed at the level of the midthigh to support the lower extremity. We do not use a tourniquet or a leg holder. The nonoperative side is well padded to prevent pressure points and nerve palsies.

Special Instruments/Equipment/Implants
The procedure calls for the following equipment:
- 30° arthroscope
- 30° Steadman awl
- ACL drill guide with 3/32-in Kirschner wire (K-wire) guide pin
- EndoButton CL BTB (Smith & Nephew)
- 3.2-mm EndoButton cannulated drill
- Cannulated compaction reamer
- Tunnel dilators (round, 0.5-mm increments)
- Beath pin
- 4.5-mm cortical screw with washer
- 0.25% bupivacaine hydrochloride with 1:200,000 epinephrine (subcutaneous injection for local anesthesia and hemostasis)

Surgical Technique
Examination Under Anesthesia
An examination of both knees is performed after anesthesia is induced. Knee range of motion, presence of an effusion, and ligamentous laxity are assessed and documented. The Lachman, anterior drawer, and pivot shift tests are documented, as is any ligamentous laxity in the coronal plane. Prior to preparation and draping of the limb, surface landmarks and incisions are drawn with a skin marker. To aid in hemostasis, the skin is injected with 0.25% bupivacaine hydrochloride with epinephrine (1:100,000). The extremity is then prepped in its entirety with povidone-iodine and draped.

Landmarks
Key landmarks are the patella (inferior pole), the medial and lateral joint lines (assess for patella alta or baja), the tibial tubercle, the medial parapatellar skin incision for BTB autograft harvest, and the anteromedial tibial skin incision (approximately 3 cm below the joint line for hamstring tendon harvest).

The meniscal repair landmarks are: medial, medial joint line, and posterior border of superficial MCL; and lateral, lateral joint line, and fibular head.

Portals and Incisions
The landmarks and arthroscopic portal sites and skin incisions are marked on the skin (**Figure 3**).

For the procedure, we use three portals: anterolateral (AL; viewing), (AM; working), and superolateral (outflow). An accessory medial portal is not required with this technique. The AL and AM portals are made with the knee in 90° of flexion and in line with their respective joint lines and approximately 1 cm from the patellar tendon edges. The medial portal is made under direct arthroscopic visualization, using a spinal needle to identify the appropriate location. This is done not only to avoid damaging the medial meniscus, but also to allow adequate clearance from the medial femoral condyle (important to avoid articular cartilage damage during passage of the reamer for femoral tunnel drilling). Furthermore, correct positioning of the medial portal will allow a proper trajectory for the reamer into the anatomic location on the wall of the lateral femoral condyle. The superolateral portal is made with the knee in extension and 2 cm proximal to the superior pole of the patella and lateral to the quadriceps tendon.

Incisions for the BTB or hamstring autograft harvest sites are marked and shown in **Figure 1**. The tibial tunnel is drilled using these incisions. If using allograft, a

Chapter 17: Anterior Cruciate Ligament Reconstruction: Two-Tunnel Technique

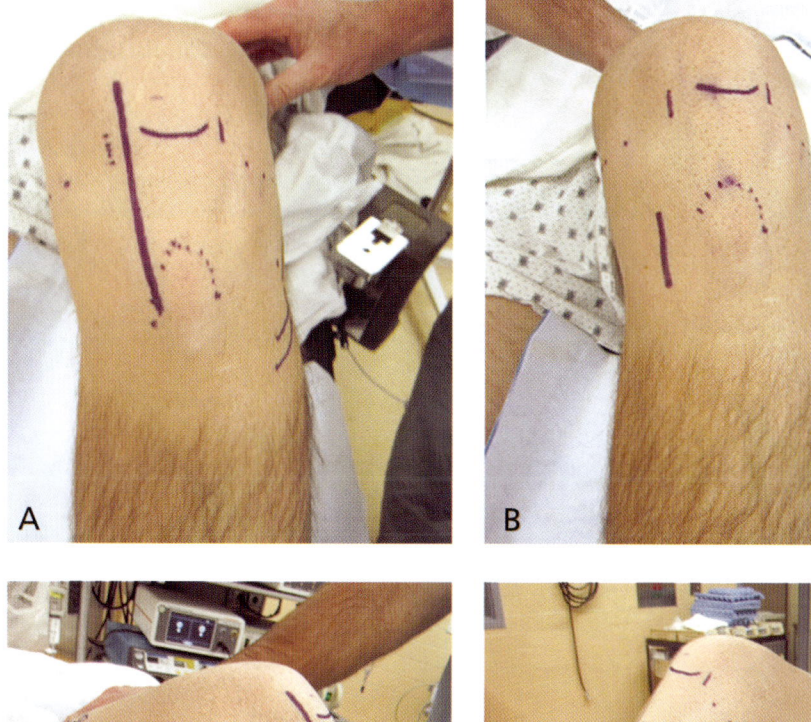

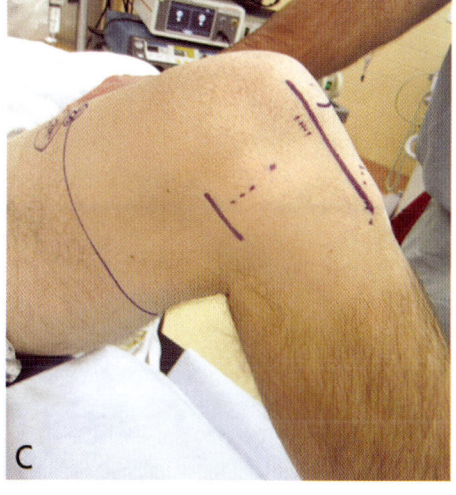

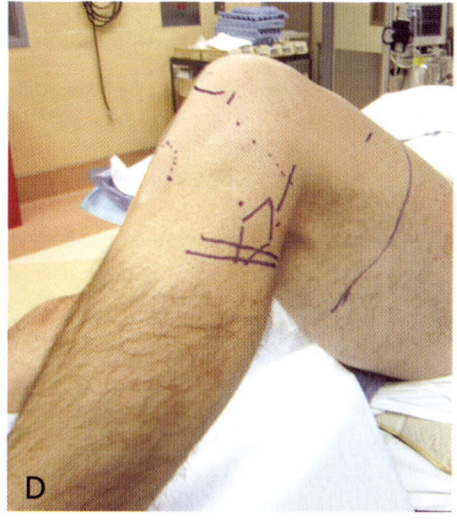

Figure 3 Photographs show surface anatomy and skin incisions marked on skin for anterior cruciate ligament reconstruction procedures. **A,** BTB autograft. Marked are the inferior pole of the patella, the tibial tubercle, the graft harvest incision, the medial and lateral joint lines, the lateral portal, and the provisional position of the medial portal. This portal is made through the BTB incision and only after identification of the appropriate location with a spinal needle. **B,** Hamstring autograft. **C,** Medial meniscus inside-out repair (as needed). **D,** Lateral meniscus inside-out repair (as needed). Markings include the lateral joint line, the fibular head and neck, and the position of the peroneal nerve.

3-cm vertical incision is made later in the procedure, with its position estimated by provisional placement of the tibial tunnel ACL guide.

Diagnostic Arthroscopy

Prior to graft harvest, a diagnostic arthroscopy is performed with the arthroscope in the AL portal. All three compartments are inspected for articular cartilage damage, medial and/or lateral meniscal tears, and verification of the ACL injury. Only after the ACL tear has been confirmed do we proceed with the graft harvest. If a repairable meniscus tear is encountered, an inside-out technique is most frequently used. The sutures are passed but not tied until after the ACLR is completed, thereby preventing repair failure during hyperflexion of the knee for the femoral tunnel drilling. Focal articular cartilage injuries are treated with microfracture if indicated.

Video 17.1 Anterior Cruciate Ligament Reconstruction: Medial Portal Technique. Dharmesh Vyas, MD, PhD; Christopher D. Harner, MD (16 min)

Graft Harvest and Preparation

Autograft harvest is performed after an ACL tear is confirmed during the diagnostic arthroscopy. Our preference is a BTB graft;[9] however, in select cases, we use hamstring or quadriceps tendon autografts. All three grafts are harvested in the standard fashion, but only the BTB will be described here.

For the BTB harvest, a 5- to 6-cm skin incision is made just medial to the midline. Full-thickness flaps are developed and limited by the medial and lateral borders of the patellar tendon. Next, a midline vertical incision is made in the paratenon, and it is meticulously lifted off the tendon. This layer is preserved and closed after the tendon is harvested. A 10-mm–wide middle-third tendon segment is harvested with 20-mm bone plugs. The plugs are designed to be trapezoidal in shape (not triangular), and the leading plug is tapered to facilitate graft passage. Two 1.5-mm holes are drilled in the tibial bone plug and a No. 5 braided nonabsorbable suture is threaded through the holes. These will be used to secure final plug fixation over a post. On the femoral bone plug, an EndoButton CL BTB is attached via a 1.5-mm drill hole in the plug. The EndoButton loop size necessary to allow the entirety of the plug to reside in the femoral tunnel is not determined until after the tunnel has been drilled and measured. After the bone plugs have been sized, any extra trimmed bone is replaced into the patella bone harvest site, and the paratenon is closed in its entire length with a No. 0 Vicryl suture (Ethicon) in a running fashion.

Femoral and Tibial Insertion Site Preparation

With the arthroscope in the AL portal and working instruments in the AM portal, the ACL tear pattern is evaluated. The fat pad is left intact to prevent postoperative scarring, patellar entrapment, and pain. In the context of a partial tear with a preserved AM or posterolateral bundle, we may choose to augment the deficient bundle if indicated. On the femoral side, and using the location of the torn ACL remnant as a guide, we mark the center of the anatomic ACL insertion site with a 30° Steadman awl. Next, the ACL remnant is removed and the wall of the lateral femoral condyle is exposed using a combination of a shaver and an arthroscopic burner. In contrast, on the tibial side, a significant portion of the ACL stump is preserved to enhance proprioceptive and vascular properties.[10] We do not routinely perform a notchplasty unless needed for better visualization (1 to 2 mm) or to alleviate graft impingement.

© 2013 American Academy of Orthopaedic Surgeons

Section 1: Sports Medicine

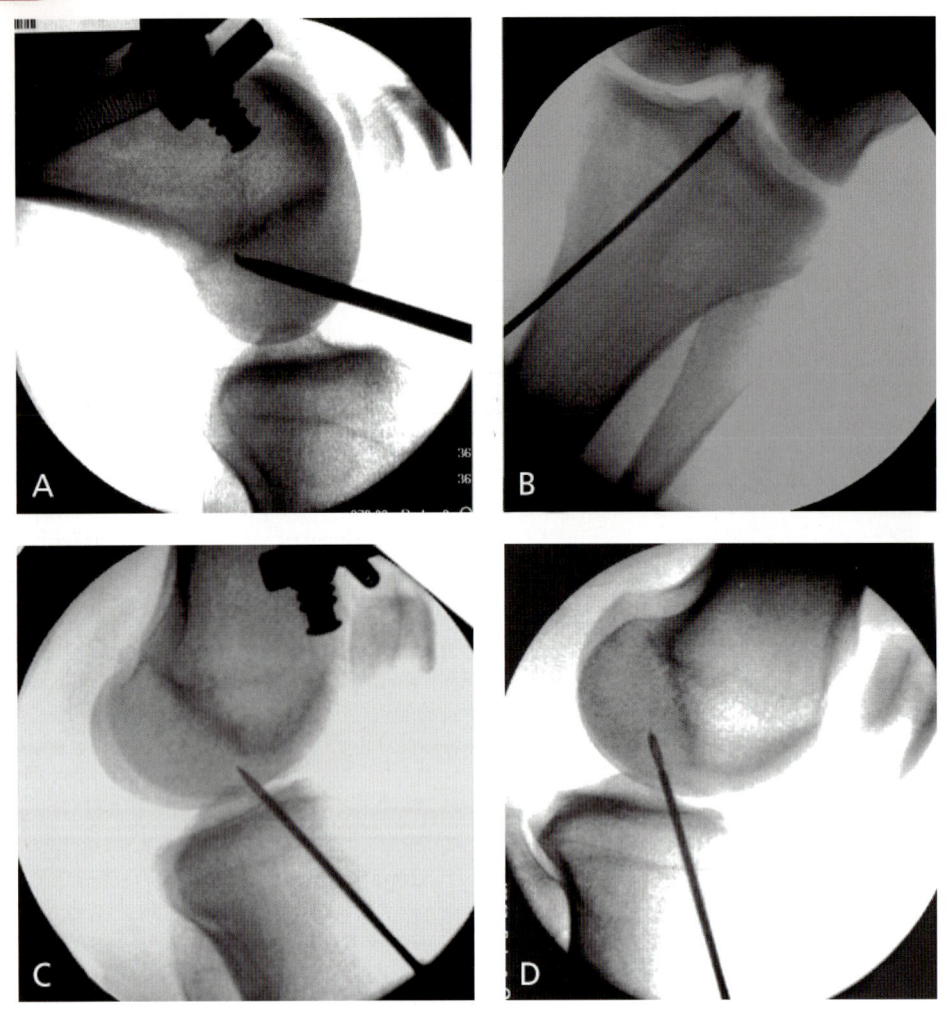

Figure 4 Intraoperative fluoroscopy used to verify tunnel positions before drilling. **A,** Position of the femoral tunnel as marked using the Steadman awl through the medial portal. The awl is used to mark the center of the anterior cruciate ligament footprint, with the goal being anatomic positioning of the tunnel. **B,** AP view of the knee shows correct guidewire placement in the coronal plane. This corresponds to the midpoint between the tibial spines. **C,** Lateral image of the knee shows correct position of the tibial guidewire for bone–patellar tendon–bone grafts. The proper placement is parallel and in line with the Blumensaat line. **D,** Lateral view of the knee shows the correct position of the tibial guidewire for soft-tissue grafts. Proper placement is parallel and 2 to 4 mm posterior to the Blumensaat line.

Femoral and Tibial Tunnel Placement

We strongly recommend that all tunnel positions be confirmed by intraoperative fluoroscopy before drilling[11] (**Figure 4**).

Femoral Tunnel

We aim for anatomic placement of the femoral and tibial tunnels. The femoral tunnel placement is done via the medial portal, allowing placement of its position independent of the tibial tunnel (transtibial technique). This technique may be used in all cases of primary ACLR (single- or double-bundle, or augmentation) or revision ACLR and is not dependent on the choice of graft, instrumentation, or final fixation. Importantly, placement of the femoral tunnel through the medial portal has been shown to decrease tunnel widening and minimize divergence when using interference screw fixation.[12]

As described previously, the femoral insertion of the ACL is marked using an awl before débridement of the lateral notch. The native ACL footprint, although variable in each individual, is generally 4 to 6 mm anterior to the posterior femoral cortex with the knee at 90° of flexion. Thorough débridement of the wall of overlying periosteum allows adequate visualization of the posterior cortex ("back wall") and confirms, proper placement of the femoral tunnel. If necessary, and for additional perspective, the provisional tunnel mark can be visualized with the arthroscope temporarily placed in the medial portal. Appropriate tunnel position is further confirmed via intraoperative fluoroscopy by taking a lateral image of the knee (90° flexion and overlapping condyles) with the awl left in position (**Figure 4, A**). The knee is flexed maximally (>120°), and through the medial portal a guide pin is malleted into the position marked by the awl. A 0.5- to 1-cm undersized cannulated acorn reamer is drilled over the guidewire, and special care is taken not to damage the cartilage of the medial femoral condyle during insertion into the joint. By hand, a shallow provisional footprint of the reamer is made on the medial wall and evaluated to ensure accurate position and safe distance away from the posterior wall (to prevent posterior femoral wall compromise). If acceptable, the reamer is connected to power and drilled to a predetermined depth for the fixation technique of choice. In 0.5-mm increments and using the round dilators, the tunnel is then sequentially dilated to a size 1 mm larger than the bone block diameter. Finally, a 3.2-mm EndoButton drill is used to breach the lateral femoral cortex.

Tibial Tunnel

Anatomic tibial tunnel positioning is also accomplished using a combination of visual arthroscopic landmarks and fluoroscopic imaging (**Figure 4, B** through **D**). An ACL tip-guide is set at 50° to 55° and positioned at the intersection between the free edge of the anterior horn of the lateral meniscus and the midline between the tibial spines. The usual tunnel length is 30 to 45 mm; however, in cases of patella alta (longer BTB tendinous portion), a longer tunnel is required. The guidewire is inserted at a point approximately 3 cm below the medial joint line and 1.5 to 2 cm medial to the tibial tubercle. A 3/32-in K-wire is advanced until the tip is visible in the joint under direct arthroscopic visualization. The wire (and subsequent tunnel) placement can be accomplished through the previous BTB or hamstring harvest incisions. If allograft is used, a 4- to 5-cm incision is made in the corresponding area.

Anatomic placement of the K-wire is verified both arthroscopically and with fluoroscopy. The knee is then brought into full extension to check for guide pin impingement on the notch. Next, AP and lateral images of the knee are taken. In the AP view, the wire should be placed directly between the two tibial spines. On the lateral view, the authors aim for placement of the pin within the anterior 20% to 40% of the tibial plateau and parallel to the Blumensaat line (in line for BTB grafts, 2 to 4 mm posterior for hamstring or quadriceps soft-tissue grafts) (**Figure 4, C** and **D**). If minor adjustments

Chapter 17: Anterior Cruciate Ligament Reconstruction: Two-Tunnel Technique

are needed in any plane, a 3- or 5-mm offset K-wire guide is used for corrections.

Following satisfactory placement of the tibial guide pin, a cannulated compaction reamer (0.5 to 1 cm smaller than the final graft size) is used to drill the tunnel. In 0.5-mm increments, the tunnel is dilated to a final size 0.5 mm larger than the bone block. At this point, a Beath pin with attached suture loop is passed from the medial portal into the femoral tunnel and out the skin on the lateral thigh. The suture loop is pulled through the tibial tunnel using an arthroscopic grasper.

Graft Passage and Fixation

Using the looped Beath pin, the passing sutures from the femoral side of the graft are pulled out through the lateral side of the thigh. The graft is advanced up the tibial tunnel, and the tendinous portion of the BTB graft is maintained in the posterior aspect of both tunnels. After clearing the lateral femoral cortex with the EndoButton, the device is engaged and seated on the cortex, preventing antegrade passage back into the tunnel. Tension is applied to the tibial sutures, and the knee is cycled to minimize graft creep. Graft impingement and isometry are checked as the final step before tibial fixation.

The tibial fixation for graft choices is tying over a post (4.5-mm AO fully threaded cortical screw over a washer, bicortical purchase). The screw is placed 1 to 2 cm below the tunnel, and the sutures are individually tied around the post with the knee in full extension. Range-of-motion, Lachman, and pivot-shift testing are performed to confirm restoration of normal knee laxity. If a meniscal repair is performed, it is at this point in the surgery that the inside-out sutures are tied over the capsule. Closure of the incisions is performed in the standard fashion.

Complications

Complications specific to the medial portal technique for ACLR can occur secondary to incorrect placement of the medial portal and resultant damage to the medial femoral condyle. This is usually the result of inadequate clearance from the medial femoral condyle for safe passage of the guide pins and drill bits. The use of half acorn reamers (introduced into the joint with the nonfluted side facing the condyle) has significantly helped avoid this complication. Other complications generally associated with arthroscopic ACLR include iatrogenic injury to the menisci, articular cartilage, and tibial spines

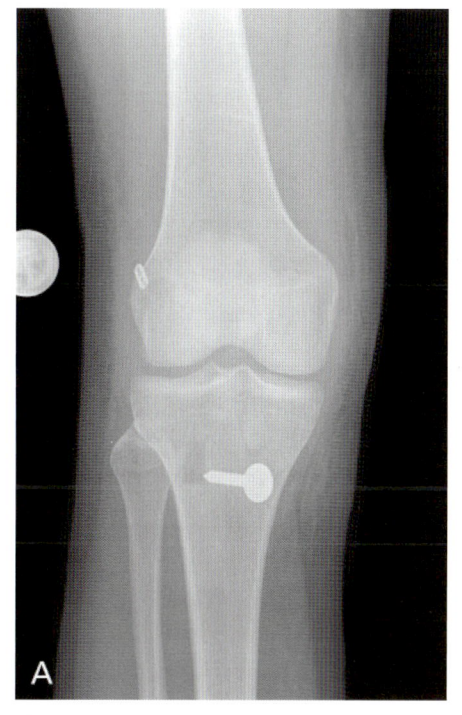

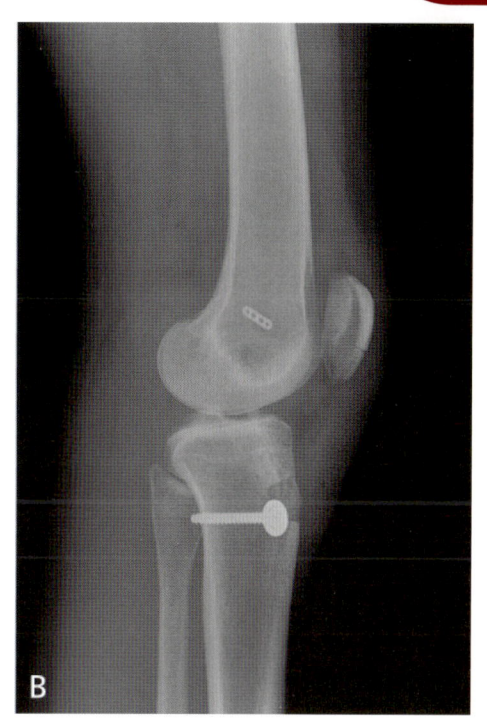

Figure 5 Postoperative AP (**A**) and lateral (**B**) radiographs demonstrate femoral and tibial fixation and tunnel positions.

(especially the medial tibial spine). Also included are postoperative infection, arthrofibrosis, deep venous thrombosis, or failure of graft healing despite an otherwise properly executed reconstruction. It is our philosophy to use enoxaparin as prophylaxis against deep venous thrombosis in patients who smoke or have a personal or family history of blood clots, or in females patients.

Postoperative Care and Rehabilitation

Postoperatively for the first week, the patients are asked to bear weight with crutches and with their brace locked in full extension.[13] Basic home exercises include quadriceps sets, straight-leg raises, calf pumps, and heel slides. The goal is protection of the graft while regaining quadriceps strength and knee extension. At the first postoperative visit (1 week), the incisions are checked, radiographs are obtained (**Figure 5**), and formal physical therapy is started with the brace unlocked. The patient is allowed to wean off crutches at 1 month and begin running at 6 months. The expected return to full activity is projected at 9 to 12 months postoperatively. This time is extended in the context of allograft use.

Pearls

- The medial portal technique is universal to all autograft and allograft choices. An accessory medial portal is not necessary.
- The majority of the procedure can be done with the knee at 90° of flexion; final fixation on the tibia is accomplished with the knee in full extension.
- We do not use a tourniquet or leg holder.
- Positioning of the BTB vertical incision just medial to the midline minimizes scar-induced anterior knee pain during kneeling.
- Closure of the paratenon over the patellar tendon helps restore normal anatomic fascial planes.
- The medial portal is made under direct arthroscopic visualization with a spinal needle. This provides three benefits: avoidance of iatrogenic damage to the medial meniscus; adequate clearance of the medial femoral condyle articular cartilage, prevention of damage during the passage of reamers; and facilitation of the proper angle for direct access to the anatomic positioning of the graft on the lateral femoral condyle.
- Use of half acorn reamers also helps to minimize the chances of iatrogenic damage to the medial femoral condyle during passage of the drill bits.
- Use of intraoperative fluoroscopy ensures precise and reproducible positioning of the femoral and tibial tunnels.
- Minor adjustments to the tibial guidewire positioning can be made quickly and easily using a 3- or 5-mm offset drill guide.

© 2013 American Academy of Orthopaedic Surgeons

- Intraoperative fluoroscopy is critical to verify that the EndoButton has seated and engaged the lateral femoral cortex.
- The tibial and femoral tunnels are dilated 0.5 mm larger than the BTB bone block size to facilitate easy passage of the graft.
- Meniscal repair sutures are passed before the ACLR is undertaken but are not tied until after the graft is passed and secured. This avoids tearing of the repair sutures during hyperflexion of the knee for the femoral tunnel drilling.

References

1. Maletius W, Messner K: Eighteen- to twenty-four-year follow-up after complete rupture of the anterior cruciate ligament. *Am J Sports Med* 1999;27(6):711-717.
2. McCulloch PC, Lattermann C, Boland AL, Bach BR Jr: An illustrated history of anterior cruciate ligament surgery. *J Knee Surg* 2007;20(2):95-104.
3. Marx RG, Jones EC, Angel M, Wickiewicz TL, Warren RF: Beliefs and attitudes of members of the American Academy of Orthopaedic Surgeons regarding the treatment of anterior cruciate ligament injury. *Arthroscopy* 2003;19(7):762-770.
4. Harner CD, Honkamp NJ, Ranawat AS: Anteromedial portal technique for creating the anterior cruciate ligament femoral tunnel. *Arthroscopy* 2008;24(1):113-115.
5. Bedi A, Musahl V, Steuber V, et al: Transtibial versus anteromedial portal reaming in anterior cruciate ligament reconstruction: An anatomic and biomechanical evaluation of surgical technique. *Arthroscopy* 2011;27(3):380-390.
6. Harner CD, Lo MY: Future of allografts in sports medicine. *Clin Sports Med* 2009;28(2):327-340, ix.
7. Greis PE, Burks RT, Bachus K, Luker MG: The influence of tendon length and fit on the strength of a tendon-bone tunnel complex: A biomechanical and histologic study in the dog. *Am J Sports Med* 2001;29(4):493-497.
8. Greulich WW, Pyle SI: *Radiographic Atlas of Skeletal Development of the Hand and Wrist*. Stanford, CA, Stanford University Press, 1959.
9. Nedeff DD, Bach BR Jr: Arthroscopic anterior cruciate ligament reconstruction using patellar tendon autografts. *Orthopedics* 2002;25(3):343-359.
10. Lee BI, Min KD, Choi HS, Kim JB, Kim ST: Arthroscopic anterior cruciate ligament reconstruction with the tibial-remnant preserving technique using a hamstring graft. *Arthroscopy* 2006;22(3):e1-e7.
11. Singh AP, Singh BK: The use of intraoperative image intensifier control for the ACL surgeon. *Knee* 2011;18(6):379-381.
12. Chhabra A, Kline AJ, Nilles KM, Harner CD: Tunnel expansion after anterior cruciate ligament reconstruction with autogenous hamstrings: A comparison of the medial portal and transtibial techniques. *Arthroscopy* 2006;22(10):1107-1112.
13. Harner CD, Sandoval CM: Anterior cruciate ligament injuries: Evaluation and management. *Oper Tech Sports Med* 2009;17:32-38.

Chapter 18
Anatomic Anterior Cruciate Ligament Double-Bundle Reconstruction

Jeffrey Macalena, MD   Carola van Eck, MD, PhD   Freddie H. Fu, MD

Introduction

Injury to the anterior cruciate ligament (ACL) is common. Each year, more than 100,000 ACL reconstructions are done in the United States alone.[1] Traditionally, only one of the two native bundles of the ACL is reconstructed. These traditional "single-bundle" reconstructions place the ACL outside the native insertion site area, in a nonanatomic position.[2,3] They have been shown to return the knee to normal International Knee Documentation Committee (IKDC) scores in only 61% to 67% of patients.[4] Anatomic double-bundle reconstruction better re-creates the native knee kinematics and function.[5,6] Further, we believe that performing anatomic reconstruction and respecting the native anatomy will improve the long-term health of the knee and decrease the risk of degenerative arthritis.

Patient Selection

Ruptures to the ACL are diagnosed based on the patient's history and physical examination. A detailed history is of utmost importance to the diagnosis of ACL injuries. Most ACL ruptures are secondary to noncontact trauma to the knee sustained during cutting or pivoting sports. Athletes frequently report hearing a pop and noticing an immediate effusion.

The physical examination is also important to the workup of athletes with an injured knee. Attention to Lachman and pivot-shift testing is very important. Isolated injuries to the posterolateral (PL) bundle are suggested by the presence of a positive pivot-shift test with an intact end point on Lachman testing. Isolated injuries to the anteromedial (AM) bundle are indicated by increased anterior translation without a firm end point on Lachman testing and a negative pivot-shift examination. KT-1000 and KT-2000 arthrometer testing (MEDmetric) can be used to further objectify the physical examination.

Indications

The indications for anatomic ACL double-bundle reconstruction are an ACL-deficient knee with symptomatic instability or in a patient who desires to return to cutting and pivoting sports. For decision making on the course of treatment of individual patients, the anatomic single- and double-bundle ACL reconstruction algorithm can be followed (**Figure 1**).[7-15]

Contraindications

Relative contraindications to anatomic ACL double-bundle reconstruction include the following:

- A small femoral or tibial insertion site. Tibial insertion sites smaller than 14 mm will not support the bone tunnels necessary for anatomic double-bundle reconstruction. This can be determined on MRI preoperatively, but the ultimate decision is made at the time of surgery by arthroscopic measurement of the ACL insertion site. When the insertion site is smaller than 14 mm, an anatomic single-bundle reconstruction is performed.
- Notch size of less than 12 mm in the medial-to-lateral dimension.[16,17] Small notch widths do not allow for the placement of both tunnels, and an anatomic single-bundle reconstruction is preferred.

As with all surgical procedures, absolute contraindications to ACL reconstruction exist. Active infection is an absolute contraindication to ACL reconstruction, as is malalignment in the setting of a chronic ACL-deficient knee. In knees with a chronic ACL deficiency, any malalignment needs to be corrected before proceeding with ACL reconstruction. Malalignment is best judged on standing pelvis-to-ankle radiographs on a 32-in cassette. Instability to varus or valgus stress also needs to be evaluated and corrected if present. ACL reconstructions performed in the setting of incompetency of the posterior cruciate ligament, the posterolateral corner, or the medial collateral ligament complex will increase the rate of failure. Meniscal tears should be treated with either repair or partial meniscectomy as clinically indicated. Osteochondritis dissecans lesions should be evaluated and treated accordingly.

Preoperative Imaging

Plain radiographs are evaluated for fractures and dislocations, as well as the presence of a Segond fracture. A Segond fracture is an avulsion injury to the lateral meniscotibial ligament and is pathognomonic for an ACL injury. MRI is used to evaluate for concomitant ligament injury as well as associated meniscal or chondral pathology. MRI can be used for preoperative planning. Using special planes, such as the oblique sagittal and oblique coronal planes,[18] both the AM and the PL bundles of the ACL can be adequately evaluated. In addition, measurements of the ACL femoral and tibial insertion sites can be performed. If MRI of the contralateral knee is available, the native ACL inclination angle can be measured (**Figure 2**). MRI can also be used to determine autograft length and the diameter of the quadriceps and bone–patellar tendon–bone graft.

Dr. Fu or an immediate family member has received royalties from Arthrocare; serves as a paid consultant to or is an employee of Stryker; has stock or stock options held in Stryker; and serves as a board member, owner, officer, or committee member of the American Academy of Orthopaedic Surgeons; the American Orthopaedic Society for Sports Medicine; the International Society of Arthroscopy, Knee Surgery, and Orthopaedic Sports Medicine; and the Orthopaedic Research and Education Foundation. Neither of the following authors nor any immediate family member has received anything of value from or owns stock in a commercial company or institution related directly or indirectly to the subject of this chapter: Dr. Macalena and Dr. van Eck.

Video 18.1 Anatomic Single- and Double-Bundle Anterior Cruciate Ligament Reconstruction. Jeffrey Macalena, MD; Carola van Eck, MD, PhD; Freddie H. Fu, MD (11 min)

Section 1: Sports Medicine

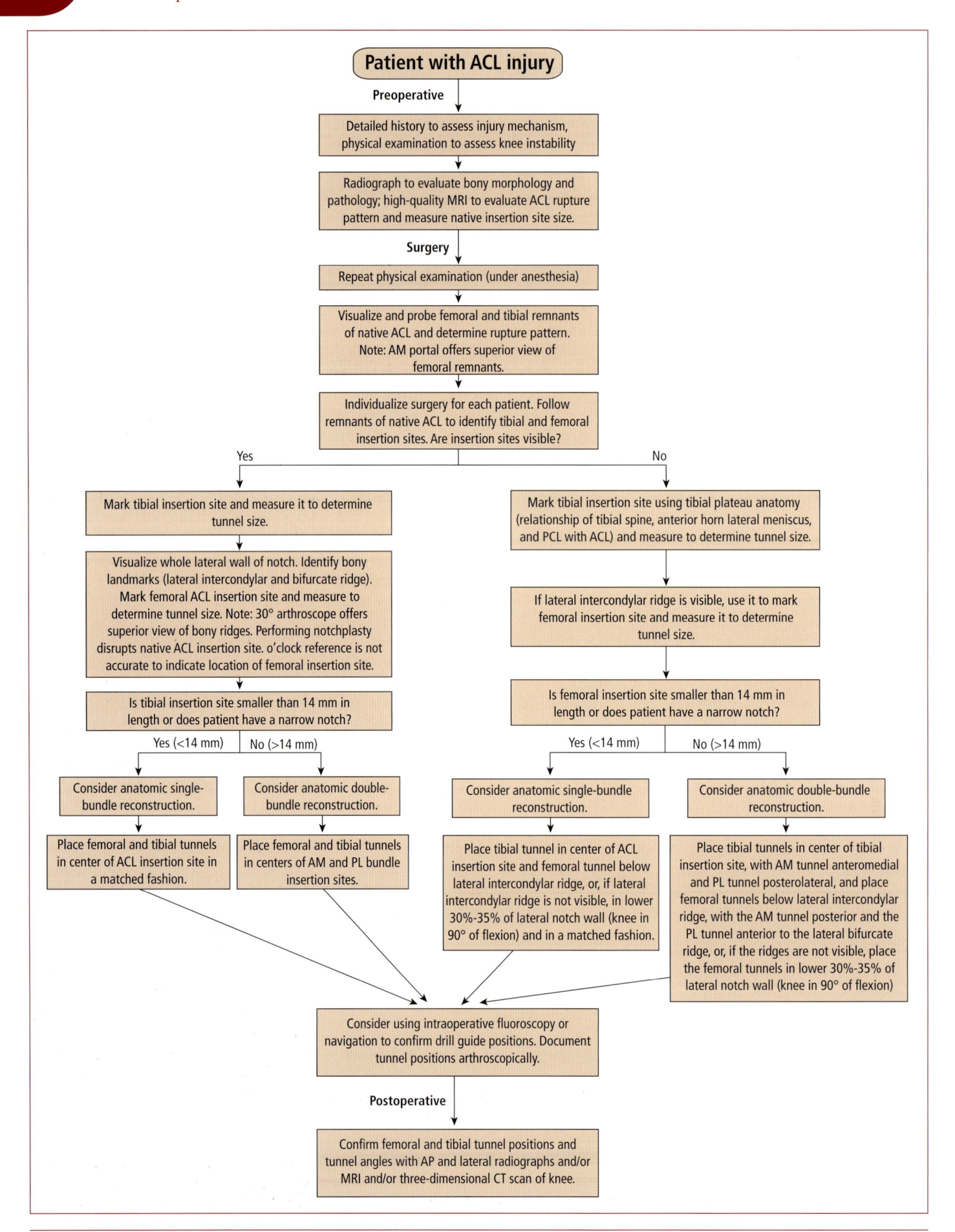

```
                    ┌─────────────────────┐
                    │ Patient with ACL injury │
                    └─────────────────────┘
                          Preoperative
                               ↓
        Detailed history to assess injury mechanism,
        physical examination to assess knee instability
                               ↓
        Radiograph to evaluate bony morphology and
        pathology; high-quality MRI to evaluate ACL rupture
        pattern and measure native insertion site size.
                            Surgery
                               ↓
        Repeat physical examination (under anesthesia)
                               ↓
        Visualize and probe femoral and tibial remnants
        of native ACL and determine rupture pattern.
        Note: AM portal offers superior view of
        femoral remnants.
                               ↓
        Individualize surgery for each patient. Follow
        remnants of native ACL to identify tibial and femoral
        insertion sites. Are insertion sites visible?
              Yes ↙                           ↘ No
```

Yes branch:
- Mark tibial insertion site and measure it to determine tunnel size.
- Visualize whole lateral wall of notch. Identify bony landmarks (lateral intercondylar and bifurcate ridge). Mark femoral ACL insertion site and measure to determine tunnel size. Note: 30° arthroscope offers superior view of bony ridges. Performing notchplasty disrupts native ACL insertion site. o'clock reference is not accurate to indicate location of femoral insertion site.
- Is tibial insertion site smaller than 14 mm in length or does patient have a narrow notch?
  - Yes (<14 mm): Consider anatomic single-bundle reconstruction. → Place femoral and tibial tunnels in center of ACL insertion site in a matched fashion.
  - No (>14 mm): Consider anatomic double-bundle reconstruction. → Place femoral and tibial tunnels in centers of AM and PL bundle insertion sites.

No branch:
- Mark tibial insertion site using tibial plateau anatomy (relationship of tibial spine, anterior horn lateral meniscus, and PCL with ACL) and measure to determine tunnel size.
- If lateral intercondylar ridge is visible, use it to mark femoral insertion site and measure it to determine tunnel size.
- Is femoral insertion site smaller than 14 mm in length or does patient have a narrow notch?
  - Yes (<14 mm): Consider anatomic single-bundle reconstruction. → Place tibial tunnel in center of ACL insertion site and femoral tunnel below lateral intercondylar ridge, or, if lateral intercondylar ridge is not visible, in lower 30%-35% of lateral notch wall (knee in 90° of flexion) and in a matched fashion.
  - No (>14 mm): Consider anatomic double-bundle reconstruction. → Place tibial tunnels in center of tibial insertion site, with AM tunnel anteromedial and PL tunnel posterolateral, and place femoral tunnels below lateral intercondylar ridge, with the AM tunnel posterior and the PL tunnel anterior to the lateral bifurcate ridge, or, if the ridges are not visible, place the femoral tunnels in lower 30%-35% of lateral notch wall (knee in 90° of flexion)

Consider using intraoperative fluoroscopy or navigation to confirm drill guide positions. Document tunnel positions arthroscopically.

Postoperative

Confirm femoral and tibial tunnel positions and tunnel angles with AP and lateral radiographs and/or MRI and/or three-dimensional CT scan of knee.

Figure 1 Algorithm for anatomic single- and double-bundle ACL reconstruction.[7-15] ACL = anterior cruciate ligament, AM = anteromedial, PCL = posterior cruciate ligament, PL = posterolateral. (Adapted with permission from van Eck C, Lesniak B, Schreiber V, Fu F: Anatomic single- and double-bundle anterior cruciate ligament flowchart. *Arthroscopy* 2010;26[2]:258-268.)

Chapter 18: Anatomic Anterior Cruciate Ligament Double-Bundle Reconstruction

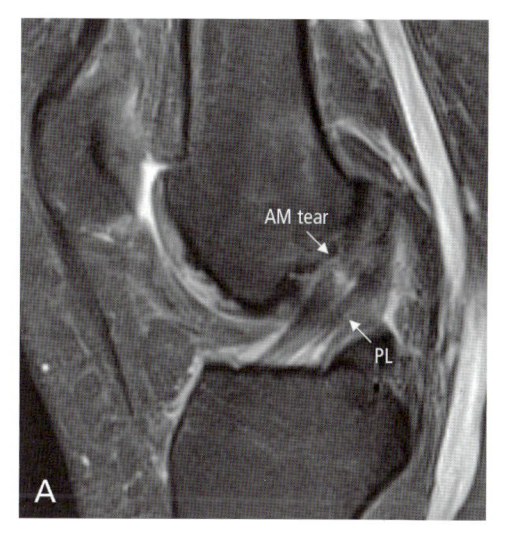

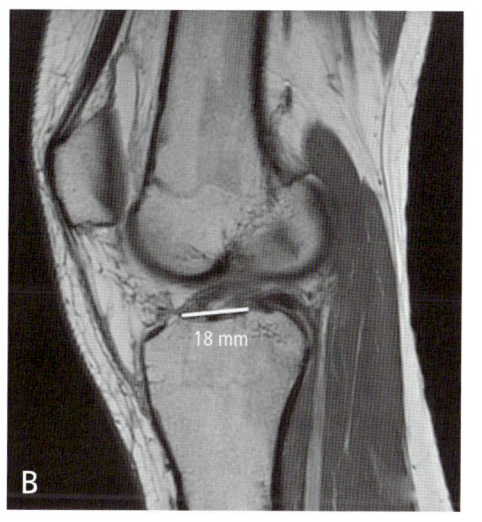

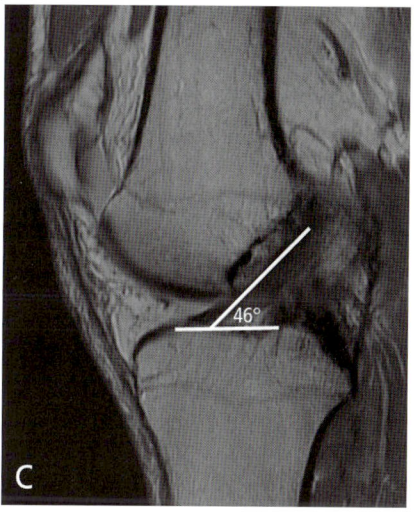

Figure 2 Sagittal MRIs of the knee, showing a cut through the anterior cruciate ligament (ACL). **A,** The two-bundle anatomy of the ACL can be observed, as well as the presence of an isolated anteromedial (AM) bundle tear; the posterolateral (PL) bundle remains intact. **B,** The ACL insertion site is measured on MRI; it measures 18 mm in this patient. **C,** The inclination angle of the ACL is measured on MRI; it measures 46° in this patient.

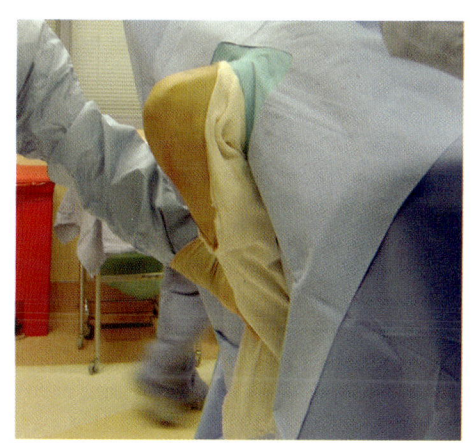

Figure 3 Photograph shows the surgical setup for anterior cruciate ligament reconstruction. The left (surgical) knee is in a leg holder. This allows maximum knee flexion (more than 125°) during femoral tunnel drilling.

Procedure

Anesthesia
Regional anesthesia is used whenever possible. Femoral and sciatic nerve blocks are frequently used, as well as spinal anesthesia. Laryngeal mask airway or general endotracheal anesthesia is used per the discretion of the anesthesiologist.

Examination Under Anesthesia
After adequate anesthesia and sedation are achieved, a detailed examination under anesthesia is performed. Passive range of motion is assessed, and Lachman (for both translation and end point) and pivot-shift examinations are performed. These results are always compared with the contralateral side. Varus, valgus, and posterior drawer testing are also performed to clinically evaluate for concurrent ligamentous injuries.

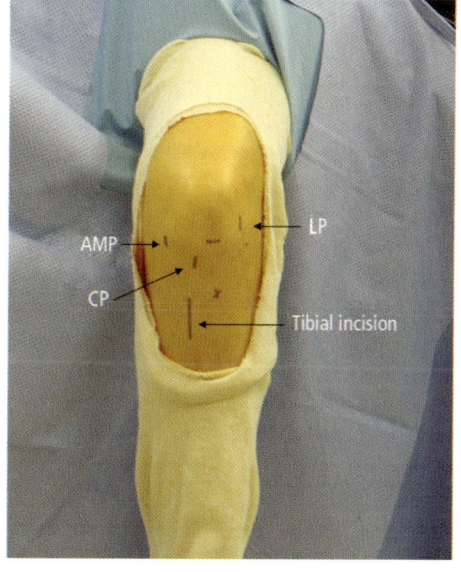

Figure 4 Photograph shows markings on the knee for the three-portal technique for anterior cruciate ligament reconstruction. The locations of the anterolateral portal (LP), the central portal (CP), and the accessory medial portal (AMP) are shown, as well as the location of the tibial incision for drilling the tibial tunnels and possible hamstring tendon harvest.

Room Setup/Patient Positioning
A standard operating room table is used for anatomic ACL reconstructions. A well-padded tourniquet is placed high on the surgical extremity. A leg holder is used, and the foot of the operating table is dropped to allow the surgical leg to be flexed to greater than 125° (**Figure 3**). The table height is raised, and monitors are positioned so that the surgeon can assume an ergonomic posture during the case.

Surgical Technique

Portals and Diagnostic Arthroscopy
Three portals are used during anatomic double-bundle reconstructions: anterolateral, central, and accessory medial (**Figure 4**). The anterolateral portal is made first. It is located high (above the tibiofemoral joint line and approximately 2 cm lateral to the patella), as this provides a panoramic view of the tibial insertion site (**Figure 5**). After placement of the anterolateral portal, a diagnostic arthroscopy is performed.

Under direct localization with a spinal needle, the central and accessory medial portals are placed. The central portal is placed just above the meniscus on either the medial border of the patellar tendon or through the medial half of the patellar tendon. The central portal provides improved visualization of the notch. The accessory medial portal is located at the level of the joint line and approximately 2 cm medial to the patellar tendon. This accessory medial portal allows drilling of the femoral tunnels while viewing through the central portal. A spinal needle should be able to pass into the notch with approximately 2 mm of clearance between the needle and the medial femoral condyle. A standard incision over the proximal medial tibia is used for drilling the tibial tunnel. Bone patellar tendon bone autograft or hamstring (semitendinosus/gracilis) autograft is harvested through this same incision. A separate midline incision centered over the quadriceps tendon is used when quadriceps autograft is harvested.

After completion of the diagnostic arthroscopy and confirmation of the dis-

© 2013 American Academy of Orthopaedic Surgeons

111

Section 1: Sports Medicine

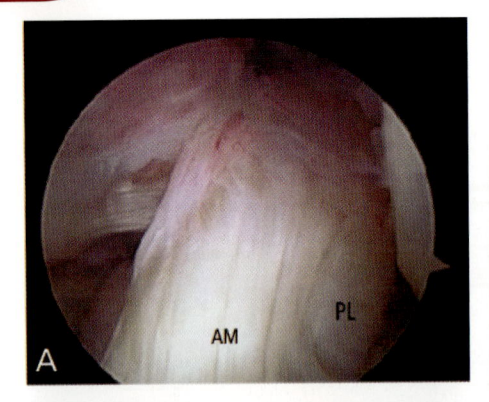

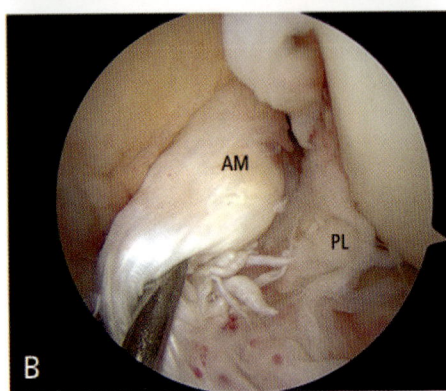

Figure 5 Anterolateral portal view of the left knee in 90° of flexion. **A,** Intact native anterior cruciate ligament (ACL), displaying the two-bundle anatomy. **B,** Torn ACL; the anteromedial (AM) and posterolateral (PL) bundles are both ruptured and separated from each other.

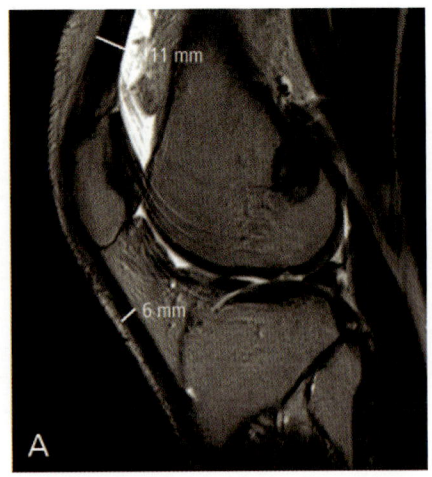

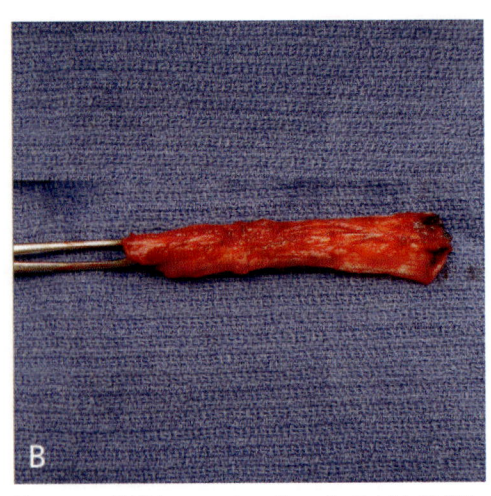

Figure 6 Graft selection for anterior cruciate ligament (ACL) reconstruction. **A,** Sagittal MRI shows the quadriceps tendon and the patellar tendon. The size of these tendons for use as autograft material for ACL reconstruction can be measured. In most patients, the quadriceps tendon (11 mm in this patient) is larger than the patellar tendon (6 mm in this patient). **B,** Photograph shows freshly harvested soft-tissue–only quadriceps tendon.

rupted ACL by probe palpation and an arthroscopically visualized Lachman, the autograft is harvested and prepared on the back table. At this time, any meniscal pathology present is addressed.

Graft Preparation

Both autograft and allograft tissue can be used for anatomic double-bundle ACL reconstruction. The risks and benefits of both allograft and autograft are discussed with all patients before surgery. Quadriceps autograft has the benefit that its size can be assessed preoperatively, and, because of its large width and length, it is often of sufficient size for double-bundle reconstruction (**Figure 6**). When quadriceps tendon is used, it is harvested through a standard midline incision beginning 1 cm proximal to the superior pole of the patellar tendon and extending 5 cm proximal. A 1-cm transverse incision through the tendon is made 8 cm proximal to the superior pole of the patella, and the lateral incision is made. At this time, a rectangle 20 mm in length by 10 mm in width is marked on the anterior surface of the patella, soft tissue is removed with a knife and electrocautery, and the bone block is harvested.

This is sized to the appropriate tunnel size, and a drill hole for passing sutures is placed. The graft is split longitudinally up to the bone block through the natural cleavage plane between the vastus intermedius and the rectus femoris. A modified Bunnell locking stitch is placed within both tails of the graft, which will become the AM and PL grafts. The PL bundle is marked. The femoral side is routinely fixed with an EndoButton (Smith & Nephew Endoscopy) or by tying it over a post. An interference screw is not routinely used on the femoral side because distortion of the reconstructed femoral footprint has been observed. Quadriceps autograft can also be harvested without bone block. In this situation, the graft is harvested just to the level of the superior pole of the patella. This soft-tissue graft is usually fixed with an EndoButton. When a quadriceps autograft is used for anatomic double-bundle reconstruction, a single femoral tunnel is drilled at the center of the AM and PL femoral tunnels. Two tibial tunnels are drilled to receive each tail (AM and PL) of the autograft.

Autograft or allograft hamstring or allograft tibialis anterior can also be used. Soft-tissue grafts are doubled over for both the AM and PL reconstruction. Standard fixation techniques on the femoral side include tying over a post or using an EndoButton. Interference screws, reinforced with either staples or a post and washer, are used on the tibial side.

For anatomic double-bundle reconstruction, any graft can be used. Most importantly, the graft choice must be tailored to the individual patient. Age, sports in which the patient participates, lifestyle, career aspirations, and patient preference all must be considered. The pros and cons of each graft choice should be discussed with each individual patient, and a combined decision-making approach should be used.

Soft-Tissue Débridement

After completion of the diagnostic arthroscopy and preparation of the grafts, the native ACL is evaluated and the tear pattern is recorded. The individual bundles are evaluated for isolated tear patterns, and the arthroscopic examination is coupled with the physical examination and imaging studies. If the AM bundle is found to be intact and the PL bundle is found to be ruptured, an isolated PL bundle reconstruction is performed. This is also true for isolated tears to the AM bundle. Once the tear pattern has been identified, the remnants of the native ACL are used to determine the location for the AM and PL tibial and femoral tunnels (**Figure 7**). Subsequently, measurements of the native ACL are performed, as well as of the width, height, and depth of the notch. In our experience, a notch width and depth larger than 12 mm is necessary to allow for an anatomic ACL double-bundle reconstruction. The steps of the double-bundle procedure are illustrated in **Figure 8**.

Alternating between the motorized oscillating shaver and the electrocautery (set to a low level), the residual ACL is removed, and the anatomy of the lateral femoral condyle is identified. Care is taken to preserve the local bony anatomy. The lateral bifurcate ridge separating the AM and PL bundles and the lateral

Chapter 18: Anatomic Anterior Cruciate Ligament Double-Bundle Reconstruction

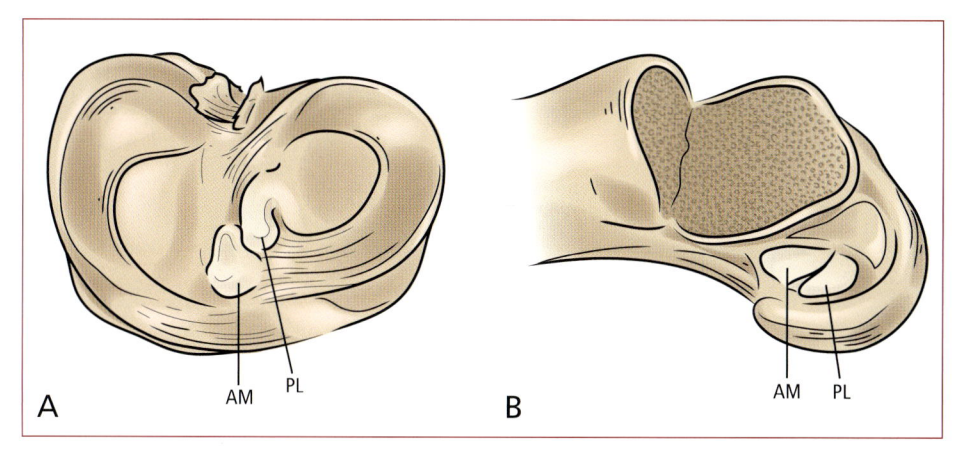

Figure 7 Illustrations show the two-bundle anatomy of the anterior cruciate ligament. **A,** Tibial anteromedial (AM) and posterolateral (PL) bundle insertion site locations. **B,** Femoral AM and PL bundle insertion site locations.

intercondylar ridge (resident's ridge) are identified.[16,19] During this portion of the procedure, the anteromedial portal and accessory medial portal are both used as viewing and working portals to ensure complete visualization of the femoral ACL footprint.

Femoral Tunnel: Posterolateral

After the femoral footprints are identified, the center of the footprint is marked with a Steadman awl, and a guidewire is placed within the awl punch site from the accessory medial portal. During femoral tunnel preparation, the arthroscope is placed through the central portal. With the knee in hyperflexion (>125°), a mallet is used to impact the guidewire. The position is checked with the camera in both the central and accessory medial portals. When satisfactory position of the guide pin has been confirmed, the knee is hyperflexed and the femoral PL tunnel is drilled with a size 6 reamer. The tunnels are drilled to a depth of 20 to 25 mm. An EndoButton reamer is then used to break the lateral cortex. The tunnel is inspected arthroscopically, confirming that the lateral cortex is intact. Dilation of the tunnel to the desired size is performed by hand.

Tibial Tunnels

With the arthroscope in the anterolateral portal, the ACL guide is introduced through the accessory medial portal. The guide is set to 45° for the PL bundle and 55° for the AM bundle. A 3- to 4-cm incision is made over the anteromedial tibia midway between the tibial tubercle and the palpable posterior border of the tibia. Soft tissue is removed from the bone, and care is taken to not elevate the medial collateral ligament, which is located at the posterior aspect of the incision. The ACL guide is set, and two guide pins, one for the AM tunnel and one for the PL tunnel, are advanced. The position is checked with the arthroscope to ensure that the guide pins enter the knee joint at the center of the previously marked tibial AM and PL insertion sites. The guide pins are drilled with a size 6 reamer. Dilation by hand with round dilators is performed until the final diameter is reached. A rasp is used to smooth the posterior aspect of each tunnel, and a motorized shaver is used to remove any soft tissue that will prevent graft passage.

Femoral Tunnel: Anteromedial

Attention is returned to the AM femoral tunnel. The surgeon can check if the femoral AM tunnel can be drilled through either the PL tibial tunnel (possible in 60%

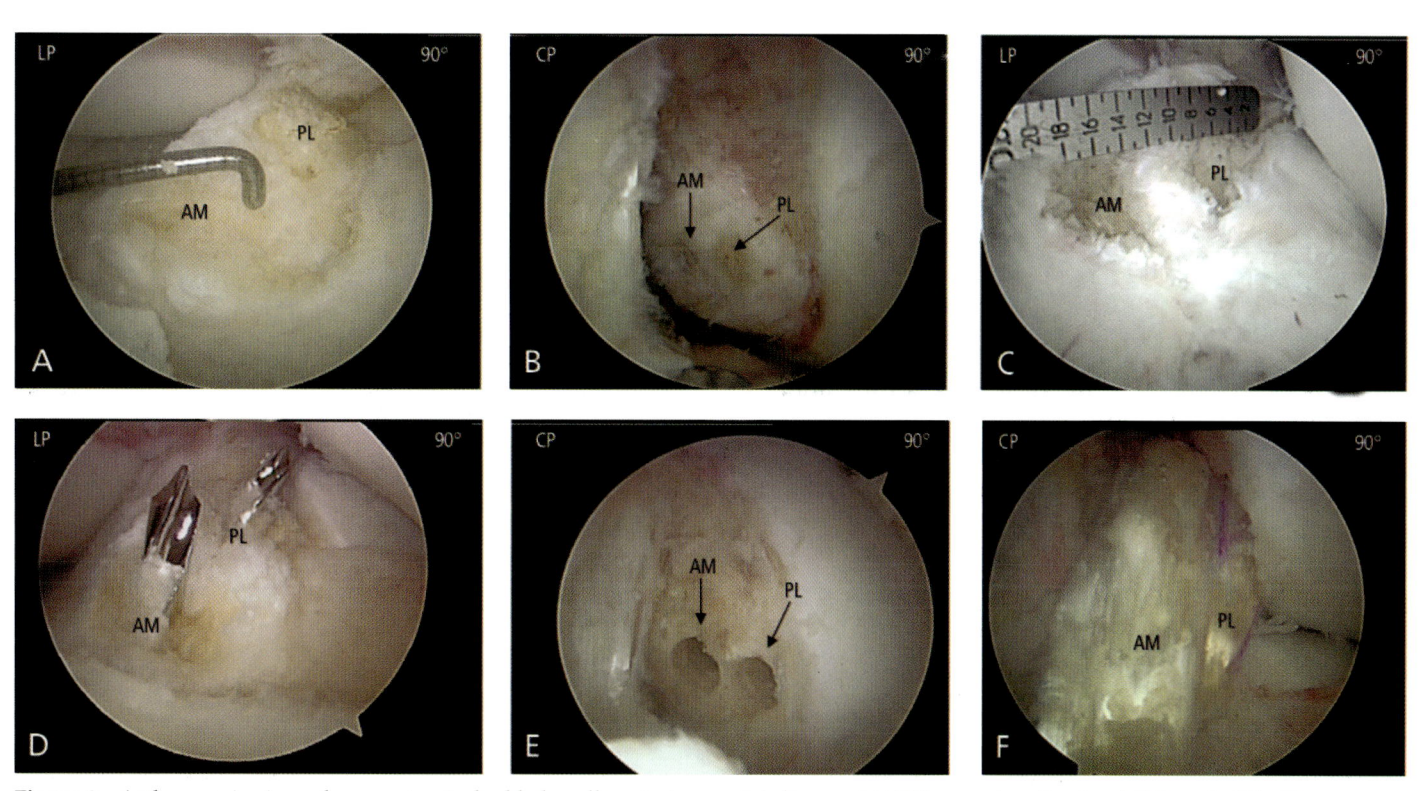

Figure 8 Arthroscopic views show anatomic double-bundle anterior cruciate ligament (ACL) reconstruction in a left knee in 90° of knee flexion. The tibial (**A**) and femoral (**B**) ACL insertion sites are marked. **C,** The tibial insertion site is measured; in this patient, it is 20 mm. Two tibial (**D**) and two femoral (**E**) tunnels are created. **F,** The AM and PL grafts are passed, and the two-bundle anatomy is restored. AM = anteromedial, CP = central portal view, LP = anterolateral portal view, PL = posterolateral.

© 2013 American Academy of Orthopaedic Surgeons

Section 1: Sports Medicine

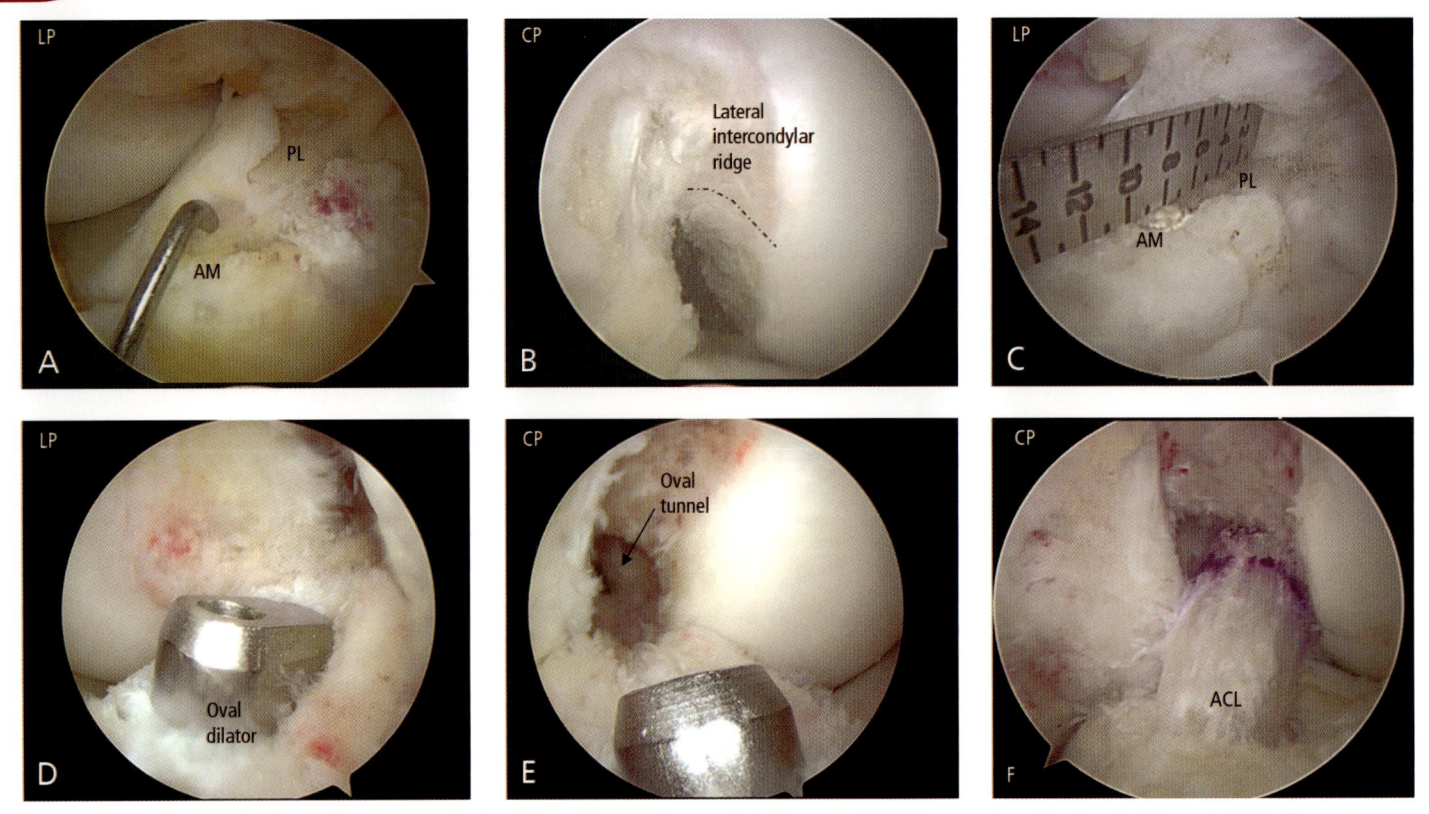

Figure 9 Arthroscopic views show anatomic single-bundle anterior cruciate ligament (ACL) reconstruction in a left knee in 90° of knee flexion. The tibial (**A**) and femoral (**B**) ACL insertion sites are marked; on the femoral side, the lateral intercondylar ridge can be observed as the superior border of the ACL insertion site. **C**, The tibial insertion site is measured; in this patient, it is only 12 mm. Oval-shaped single tibial (**D**) and femoral (**E**) tunnels are created. **F**, The ACL graft is passed. AM = anteromedial, CP = central portal view, LP = anterolateral portal view, PL = posterolateral.

of cases) or the AM tibial tunnel (possible in about 5% of cases). A guide pin is used to check the position. If a transtibial approach does not result in an anatomic position, the femoral AM tunnel can be drilled through the accessory medial portal (possible in 99% of cases). The tunnel is then drilled to a size 6 and dilated by hand to the final diameter.

Routing the Grafts
The PL graft is routed first. Beath pins with No. 5 Ethibond sutures (Ethicon) are passed from the accessory medial portal and out the PL and AM tunnels. The suture is retrieved from the respective tibial tunnel, and the graft is passed. It should be confirmed that the graft passes smoothly through the sizing guide before passing the graft in situ.

Femoral Fixation
An EndoButton is routinely used for femoral fixation. After it is delivered over the lateral cortex, the EndoButton is toggled. An intraoperative radiograph is always obtained to confirm that the EndoButton is "flipped" and in good position. If there is concern for the integrity of the lateral cortex, a post-and-washer technique can be used.

Cycling the Graft
The grafts are then cycled 25 times, with tension held on the grafts as they exit the tibial tunnel. The grafts are viewed arthroscopically through both the lateral and central portals to ensure that there is no impingement along the roof in full extension or along the posterior cruciate ligament.

Tibial Fixation
Tibial fixation is performed with the knee in 45° of flexion for the AM bundle and 0° to 10° of flexion for the PL bundle. The PL bundle is tensioned first. A bioabsorbable interference screw is used, of equal diameter to the final dilated tunnel diameter. Palpation of the lateral cortex is performed to ensure that the screw is not prominent; the grafts are viewed arthroscopically to ensure that the tip of the screw is not prominent in the notch. Finally, an arthroscopic anterior drawer and palpation of the graft with a probe are performed to ensure appropriate tension of the grafts.

Single-Bundle Anatomic Reconstruction
An anatomic single-bundle ACL reconstruction is performed when indicated by the patient's anatomy. A tibial insertion site of less than 14 mm for both the AM and PL bundles or a notch width of less than 12 mm is an indication for anatomic single-bundle ACL reconstruction. The tunnels are prepared in a manner similar to that for double-bundle reconstruction. Oval dilators are then used to better approximate the local anatomy of the femoral ACL footprint. The steps of the single-bundle procedure are illustrated in **Figure 9**.

Closure
The wounds are closed in a layered manner. The periosteum and deep fascia over the tibial incision are closed with 0 Vicryl (Ethicon). The subcutaneous tissue is closed with 2-0 Vicryl, and the skin is closed with absorbable monofilament. The portals are closed with 3-0 nylon suture. Sterile dressings are applied, as well as an elastic bandage starting at the foot. An ice pack over the knee and a hinged knee brace locked in full extension are also placed before transfer to the recovery room.

Complications
One of the most feared complications of ACL reconstruction is graft failure. Rates of functional graft failure are reported

to be between 0% and 27.3%.[20] The main cause of graft failure is related to malposition of the tunnel (eg, placing the tibial tunnel too anteriorly or placing the graft too vertically). Poor biologic incorporation of the graft, recurrent trauma, or early return to sport may also lead to graft failure. Other complications are rare; they include infection, deep venous thrombosis, and pulmonary embolism. To prevent the latter two, early mobilization is encouraged.

Postoperative Care and Rehabilitation

Patients are allowed to be discharged home when they meet the same-day discharge criteria of our surgery center. The patient is restricted to toe-touch weight bearing for 1 week after the surgery. For this week, the hinged knee brace is kept locked in full extension. The patient is provided narcotic pain medication. The first postoperative visit is at approximately 1 week. At this time, sutures are removed and new dressings are placed. The hinged knee brace is refit and range of motion is allowed from 0° to full extension. Weight bearing is allowed, although crutches are continued until the patient can walk without a limp (approximately 3 to 4 weeks). The hinged knee brace is continued until 6 weeks postoperatively. Physical therapy for quadriceps activation and range of motion is initiated during this second week. A continuous passive motion machine is used starting 1 week postoperatively. A protocol is initiated in which motion is begun from 0° to 45° and advanced 10° per day to a goal of 0° to 100°. A goal of 2 hours twice per day on the machine is desirable. Chemical deep venous thrombosis prophylaxis is not routinely used unless specific risk factors are present; when specific risk factors are present, daily aspirin (325 mg) or daily low-molecular-weight heparin is used. Running is not permitted until 3 months postoperatively, and return to sport is not allowed until 9 to 12 months after surgery. A functional ACL brace for sports is recommended until 2 years after the ACL reconstruction.

Pearls

- The ability to hyperflex the surgical knee to greater than 125° should be ensured. This allows for adequate femoral tunnel length.
- When looking at the tibial insertion site, the arthroscope should be placed in the anterolateral portal, withdrawn as far as possible, and the optics aimed inferior to provide a panoramic view of the tibial insertion site.
- The femoral insertion site is best viewed through the central portal, with the optics aimed slightly superior and lateral to visualize the bony ridges.
- The femoral notch width should be 12 mm for an anatomic double-bundle reconstruction; if the notch is smaller, an anatomic single-bundle reconstruction should be considered.
- The tibial footprint should be 14 mm for an anatomic double-bundle reconstruction; if it is smaller, an anatomic single-bundle reconstruction should be considered.
- The width of the quadriceps tendon should be measured on preoperative MRI to ensure that it is wider than 8 mm before autograft harvest.
- The femoral tunnel position should be checked from both the central and medial portals before reaming of the femoral tunnel.
- Prior to drilling the AM tunnel from the medial portal, a guide pin should be used to check if an anatomic position can be obtained through the PL or AM tibial tunnel.
- The posterior lateral graft should be routed first.
- Intraoperative radiographs are imperative to confirm the correct position of EndoButton fixation.
- The PL graft should be tensioned in 0° of flexion and the AM graft in 45° of flexion.
- After fixation of both the femoral and tibial sides, the knee should be re-scoped to evaluate graft tension. If the ACL graft is loose, the graft should be retensioned.
- If there is concern for femoral or tibial fixation, a post-and-washer construct can be used as secondary fixation.
- After final fixation, the knee should be taken through a full range of motion while visualizing the graft with the arthroscope, to make sure the graft does not impinge.

References

1. Lyman S, Koulouvaris P, Sherman S, Do H, Mandl LA, Marx RG: Epidemiology of anterior cruciate ligament reconstruction: Trends, readmissions, and subsequent knee surgery. *J Bone Joint Surg Am* 2009;91(10):2321-2328.
2. Kopf S, Forsythe B, Wong AK, et al: Nonanatomic tunnel position in traditional transtibial single-bundle anterior cruciate ligament reconstruction evaluated by three-dimensional computed tomography. *J Bone Joint Surg Am* 2010;92(6):1427-1431.
3. Forsythe B, Kopf S, Wong AK, et al: The location of femoral and tibial tunnels in anatomic double-bundle anterior cruciate ligament reconstruction analyzed by three-dimensional computed tomography models. *J Bone Joint Surg Am* 2010;92(6):1418-1426.
4. Biau DJ, Tournoux C, Katsahian S, Schranz P, Nizard R: ACL reconstruction: A meta-analysis of functional scores. *Clin Orthop Relat Res* 2007;458:180-187.
5. Yagi M, Wong EK, Kanamori A, Debski RE, Fu FH, Woo SL: Biomechanical analysis of an anatomic anterior cruciate ligament reconstruction. *Am J Sports Med* 2002;30(5):660-666.
6. Yamamoto Y, Hsu WH, Woo SL, Van Scyoc AH, Takakura Y, Debski RE: Knee stability and graft function after anterior cruciate ligament reconstruction: A comparison of a lateral and an anatomical femoral tunnel placement. *Am J Sports Med* 2004;32(8):1825-1832.
7. Zantop T, Brucker PU, Vidal A, Zelle BA, Fu FH: Intraarticular rupture pattern of the ACL. *Clin Orthop Relat Res* 2007;454:48-53.
8. Wittstein J, Kaseta M, Sullivan R, Garrett WE: Incidence of the remnant femoral attachment of the ruptured ACL. *Clin Orthop Relat Res* 2009;467(10):2691-2694.
9. Cohen SB, Fu FH: Three-portal technique for anterior cruciate ligament reconstruction: Use of a central medial portal. *Arthroscopy* 2007;23(3):325.e1-5.
10. Edwards A, Bull AM, Amis AA: The attachments of the anteromedial and posterolateral fibre bundles of the anterior cruciate ligament: Part 1. Tibial attachment. *Knee Surg Sports Traumatol Arthrosc* 2007;15(12):1414-1421.
11. Ferretti M, Ekdahl M, Shen W, Fu FH: Osseous landmarks of the femoral attachment of the anterior cruciate ligament: An anatomic study. *Arthroscopy* 2007;23(11):1218-1225.
12. Fu FH: The clock-face reference: Simple but nonanatomic. *Arthroscopy* 2008;24(12):1433, author reply 1434.
13. Shen W, Forsythe B, Ingham SM, Honkamp NJ, Fu FH: Application of the anatomic double-bundle reconstruction concept to revision and augmentation anterior cruciate ligament surgeries. *J Bone Joint Surg Am* 2008;90(suppl 4):20-34.
14. Pombo MW, Shen W, Fu FH: Anatomic double-bundle anterior cruciate ligament

reconstruction: Where are we today? *Arthroscopy* 2008;24(10):1168-1177.

15. Martins CA, Kropf EJ, Shen W, van Eck CF, Fu FH: The concept of anatomic anterior cruciate ligament reconstruction. *Oper Tech Sports Med* 2008;16:104-115.

16. van Eck CF, Martins CA, Vyas SM, Celentano U, van Dijk CN, Fu FH: Femoral intercondylar notch shape and dimensions in ACL-injured patients. *Knee Surg Sports Traumatol Arthrosc* 2010;18(9):1257-1262.

17. van Eck CF, Martins CA, Lorenz SG, Fu FH, Smolinski P: Assessment of correlation between knee notch width index and the three-dimensional notch volume. *Knee Surg Sports Traumatol Arthrosc* 2010;18(9):1239-1244.

18. Casagranda BU, Maxwell NJ, Kavanagh EC, Towers JD, Shen W, Fu FH: Normal appearance and complications of double-bundle and selective-bundle anterior cruciate ligament reconstructions using optimal MRI techniques. *AJR Am J Roentgenol* 2009;192(5):1407-1415.

19. Fu FH, Jordan SS: The lateral intercondylar ridge: A key to anatomic anterior cruciate ligament reconstruction. *J Bone Joint Surg Am* 2007;89(10):2103-2104.

20. Reinhardt KR, Hetsroni I, Marx RG: Graft selection for anterior cruciate ligament reconstruction: A level I systematic review comparing failure rates and functional outcomes. *Orthop Clin North Am* 2010;41(2):249-262.

Chapter 19
Pediatric Anterior Cruciate Ligament Reconstruction

*Davide Edoardo Bonasia, MD   Roberto Rossi, MD   Brian R. Wolf, MD, MS
Annunziato Amendola, MD*

Introduction

Although the exact incidence of anterior cruciate ligament (ACL) tears in skeletally immature patients is still unknown, the higher participation rate of children and adolescents in competitive sports has led to an increase of ACL injuries in the past decade.[1] The treatment of ACL tears in patients with open physes remains controversial, and the debated issues mainly involve surgical timing (early versus delayed reconstruction) and the most reliable surgical technique.

Early ACL reconstruction may improve knee function, avoid strict activity modification in competitive athletes, and reduce progressive chondral and meniscal injuries due to recurrent instability.[2] However, a wide range of growth disturbances have been reported in animal and clinical studies.[3] Many techniques have been described for pediatric ACL reconstruction in an attempt to reduce the risk of growth plate injury. These can be grouped into (1) physeal-sparing techniques (intra-articular, extra-articular, and combined intra-/extra-articular), (2) partial transphyseal techniques, and (3) complete transphyseal techniques (Figure 1).

Extra-articular and combined intra-/extra-articular procedures are nonanatomic types of ACL reconstruction.[4,5] Poor outcomes were reported for extra-articular tenodesis, which for this reason did not rise in popularity.[4,5]

Intra-articular physeal-sparing procedures have been developed to help provide ligamentous restraint similar to adult-type reconstruction, with all-epiphyseal femoral/tibial tunnels and without damage to the physes.[3]

The partial transphyseal techniques are a hybrid of the physeal-sparing and adult-type reconstructive procedures. Either the tibial or, most commonly, the femoral physis is left intact in an attempt to decrease the risk of growth disturbance. The graft is passed through a 6- to 8-mm drill hole that involves the physis for less than 5% of its cross-sectional area. The tunnel is placed more vertically than normal to further decrease growth plate damage.[3]

The femoral physis is left intact through epiphyseal tunnel drilling, as described for the physeal-sparing procedures. Alternatively, the femoral growth plate is left intact with an over-the-top positioning of the graft. A partial transphyseal technique with proximal over-the-top positioning of the graft will be described in this chapter and shown step by step in the video. Complete transphyseal reconstruction is comparable to conventional adult-type reconstruction.[3]

Direct repair also has been described for the treatment of ACL lesions, with inferior outcomes reported compared with

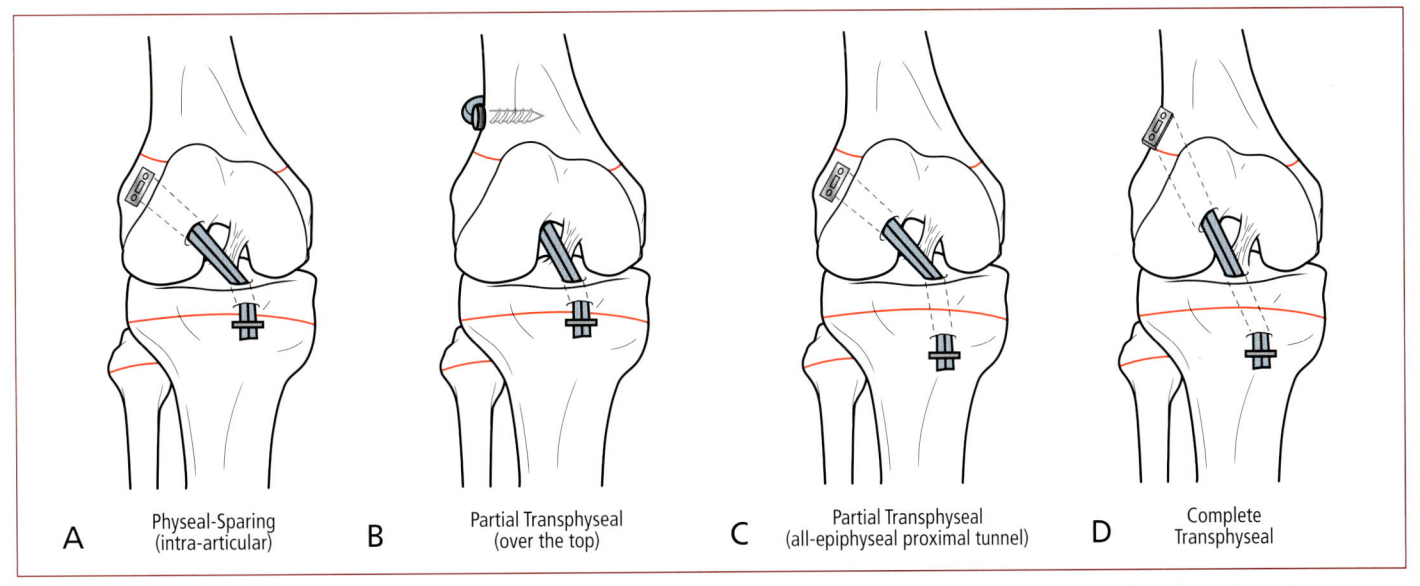

Figure 1 Illustrations show the most commonly used techniques for pediatric ACL reconstruction. **A,** Intra-articular physeal-sparing technique. **B,** Partial transphyseal technique, with proximal over-the-top positioning of the graft. **C,** Partial transphyseal technique, with all-epiphyseal proximal tunnel drilling. **D,** Complete transphyseal technique.

Dr. Wolf or an immediate family member serves as a board member, owner, officer, or committee member of the American Orthopaedic Society for Sports Medicine and the Arthroscopy Association of North America. Dr. Amendola or an immediate family member has received royalties from Arthrex and Arthrosurface; serves as a paid consultant to or is an employee of Arthrex; serves as an unpaid consultant to MTP Solutions; owns stock or stock options held in Arthrosurface and MTP Solutions; and serves as a board member, owner, officer, or committee member of the American Academy of Orthopaedic Surgeons, the American Board of Orthopaedic Surgery, the American Society for Sports Medicine, and the International Society of Arthroscopy, Knee Surgery, and Orthopaedic Sports Medicine. Neither of the following authors or any immediate family member has received anything of value or owns stock in a commercial company or institution related directly or indirectly to the subject of this chapter: Dr. Bonasia and Dr. Rossi.

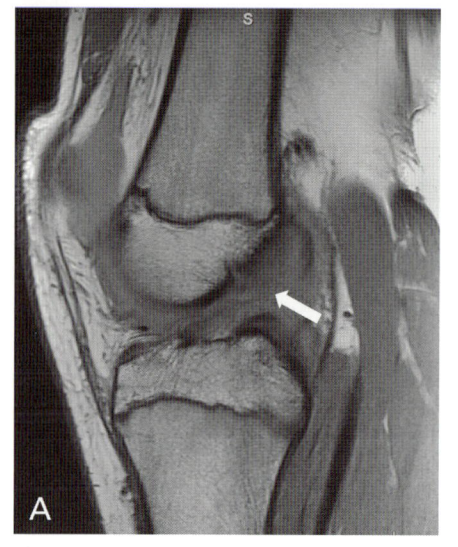

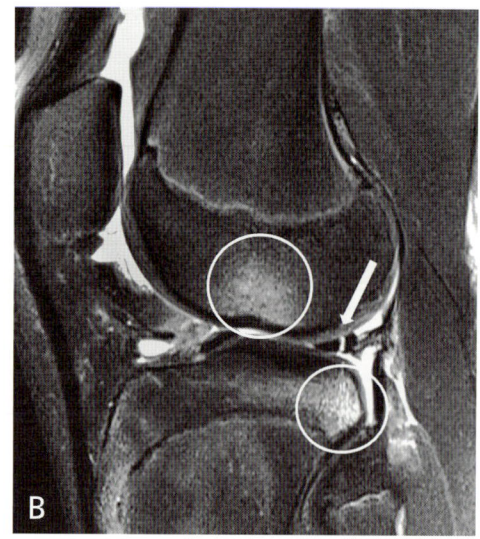

Figure 2 Preoperative sagittal MRIs of an ACL tear in a patient with open physes. **A,** T1-weighted image shows ACL tear (arrow). **B,** Short tau inversion recovery image shows impaction edema (circles) and lateral meniscus posterior horn tear (arrow) associated with the ACL tear.

reconstruction, most of all for midsubstance tears.[3]

Patient Selection

Clinical examination begins with a thorough history investigation. Patients commonly report an audible pop at the time of injury and the rapid onset of hemarthrosis. The mechanism of injury should be evaluated as well, with flexion-valgus–external rotation being the most common. The examination of an injured knee in children is more difficult than in adults. The patients are often in acute pain, frightened, and unable to relax. Joint effusion should be noted. Bony and soft-tissue palpation should pinpoint the areas of tenderness and rule out possible bony and growth plate injuries. Meniscal signs should be noted, if present. Range of motion and instability in all planes should be evaluated. Lachman, drawer, pivot-shift, and varus/valgus stress tests should be performed.

Nonsurgical treatment entails range-of-motion exercises, muscle strengthening, proprioception, functional braces, and activity modification. Considering the lack of evidence regarding pediatric ACL reconstruction and the postoperative risks of growth disturbance,[1] nonsurgical management with ACL reconstruction at skeletal maturity should always be mentioned as a possible treatment, especially for inactive patients.

Surgery is usually recommended when (1) the nonsurgical treatment fails (characterized by persistent effusion, pain, and recurrent episodes of instability), (2) the patient is unwilling or unable to modify activity levels, and (3) meniscal tears are associated with the ACL tear. In older adolescents with closing physes (Tanner stage 5, males >16 years of age, females >14 years of age), a complete transphyseal technique with either hamstring or patellar tendon can be used, although the surgeon must approach this cautiously because many of these patients may still have significant growth remaining. In younger adolescents with open physes (Tanner stage <3, males ≤16 years of age, females ≤14 years of age), the technique remains a matter of preference of the surgeon. Either physeal-sparing or partial transphyseal techniques with hamstring autograft can be used. In these techniques, the surgeon is making a compromise between the best reconstructive option and the technique with the least chance of physeal injury.

Our preferred procedure in patients with open physes is a partial transphyseal technique with proximal over-the-top positioning of semitendinosus tendon autograft.

In cases of acute proximal or distal avulsion of the ACL, a pull-out technique can be used for repair, with or without autologous graft augmentation.

ACL reconstruction is contraindicated in tibial spine avulsions. When completely displaced or inadequately reduced, these need to be reduced and fixed back to their bony bed with rigid fixation (screws) or pull-out techniques.

Preoperative Imaging

Imaging evaluation of the knee begins with a routine four-view radiographic series (AP, lateral, Merchant, and tunnel views) of both knees. Plain radiographs are used to rule out (1) tibial and/or femoral epiphyseal fractures, (2) tibial spine avulsions, and (3) malformation in the tibial spine and/or femoral notch, which is a common finding in patients with congenital absence of the ACL. The amount of tibial and femoral physeal closure can also be evaluated on routine radiographs.

MRI is very useful in (1) demonstrating the ACL tear, when the diagnosis at physical examination is in question; (2) assessing combined soft-tissue injuries and meniscal injury when suspected; (3) evaluating the status of maturity of the femoral and tibial epiphyses when needed; and (4) evaluating the location of injury (eg, proximal femoral avulsion) for a possible direct repair (**Figure 2**).

Video 19.1 Pediatric Anterior Cruciate Ligament Reconstruction. Davide Edoardo Bonasia, MD; Roberto Rossi, MD; Brian R. Wolf, MD; Annunziato Amendola, MD (18 min)

Procedure

Room Setup/Patient Positioning

The patient is administered spinal or general anesthesia and positioned supine on the operating table. A tourniquet is positioned on the proximal thigh. Intravenous antibiotic prophylaxis is administered. The surgical leg is stabilized with an arthroscopic leg holder, and the distal extremity of the bed is dropped down. The table is slightly reflexed to achieve 10° of hip flexion and reduce the tension on the neurovascular structures of the anterior thigh.

Alternatively, a lateral post can be used with the bed intact, to obtain leg abduction away from the table and knee flexion up to 120°.

Surgical Technique

Considering the previously mentioned inferior accuracy of clinical examination and MRI in children compared to adults, a thorough examination under anesthesia is essential.

The indication to proceed with graft harvesting is if the surgeon is satisfied that there is complete ACL disruption (ie, an anterior tibial translation >5 mm on the injured side without an end point, compared to the uninjured side, and a positive pivot-shift test). Otherwise, a di-

Chapter 19: Pediatric Anterior Cruciate Ligament Reconstruction

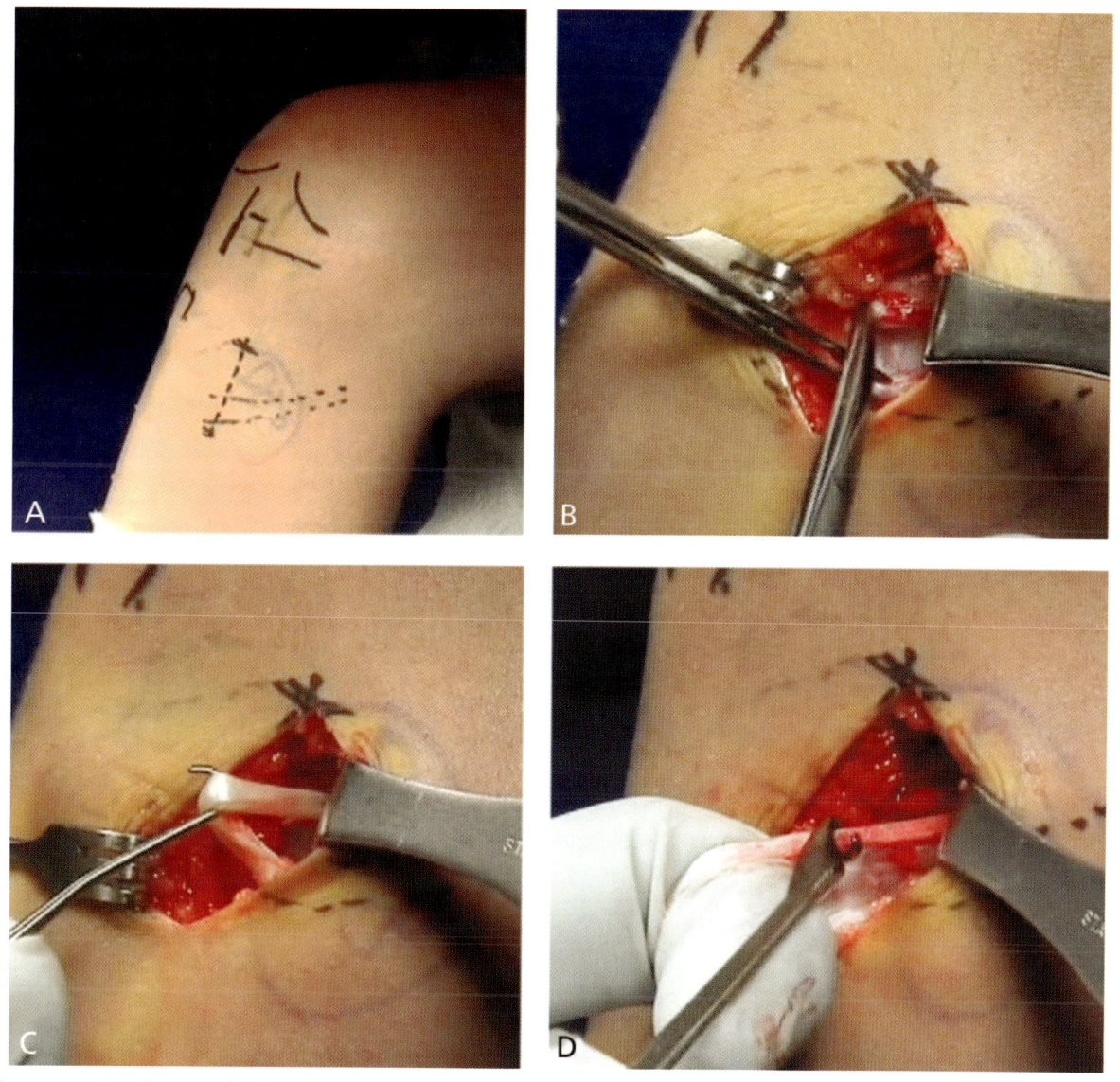

Figure 3 Intraoperative photographs demonstrate semitendinosus graft harvesting. **A,** The incision is placed 2 cm medial to the tibial tubercle, started 3 cm below the joint line, and prolonged 3 to 4 cm distally. **B,** The sartorial fascia is incised proximally and parallel to the tendons with a No. 15 blade first and then with Metzenbaum scissors. **C,** The semitendinosus tendon is then pulled out with a blunt hook, and all the vincula are released proximally, distally, medially, and laterally. **D,** An open tendon stripper is used to harvest the semitendinosus.

agnostic arthroscopy is performed first to confirm the diagnosis.

Harvesting

The tourniquet is inflated after leg elevation. A 3- to 4-cm longitudinal skin incision is made on the anteromedial aspect of the tibia (**Figure 3, A**). The incision is placed 2 cm medial to the tibial tubercle, started 3 cm below the joint line, and prolonged distally. In thinner patients, the pes anserinus can be palpated with a thumb and the incision centered on the tendons.

Once on the sartorial fascia, the hamstrings (mainly the semitendinosus tendon) can be palpated with a thumb or forceps. The sartorial fascia is incised proximally and parallel to the tendons with a No. 15 blade first and then with Metzenbaum scissors (**Figure 3, B**). Deep to the retracted sartorial fascia, the gracilis tendon proximally and the semitendinosus tendon distally are visualized. The semitendinosus is then pulled out with a blunt hook (**Figure 3, C**). The vinculum to the medial head of the gastrocnemius and all the other minor vincula of the tendon should be released proximally, distally, medially, and laterally. If the tendon has been completely released, when pulling it with one hand, movement of the hamstrings can be appreciated with the other hand in the medial popliteal fossa. When the distal insertion of the tendon is left intact, as in this technique, an open tendon stripper is used to harvest the semitendinosus (**Figure 3, D**). Alternatively, the tendon can be distally detached, armed with a leading suture, and harvested with a closed tendon stripper. Then the periosteum at the base of the graft is vertically incised with a scalpel and traction is applied to the tendon to harvest the whole distal insertion.

Graft Preparation

The graft is taken to the back table to be prepared. The residual vincula and muscle are removed. The graft is doubled after passing it through a closed loop device. The distal ends are armed together with No. 2 nonabsorbable braided suture. The graft is then sized and pretensioned at approximately 15 N. A 2-0 bioabsorbable suture is used to arm the remnant of the graft and maintain part of the tension, once the graft is removed from the workstation (**Figure 4**). The tendon is kept in a moist sponge.

Knee Balance

A complete diagnostic arthroscopy is performed through standard anterome-

© 2013 American Academy of Orthopaedic Surgeons

Section 1: Sports Medicine

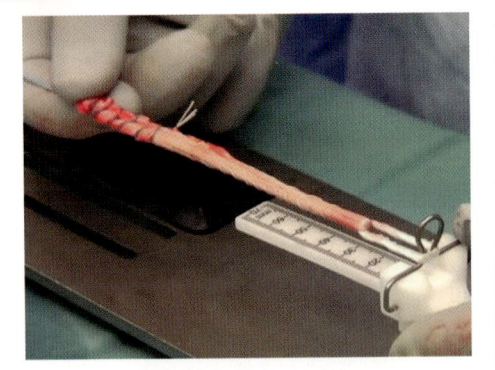

Figure 4 Photograph demonstrates the preparation of a semitendinosus graft for reconstruction of the ACL.

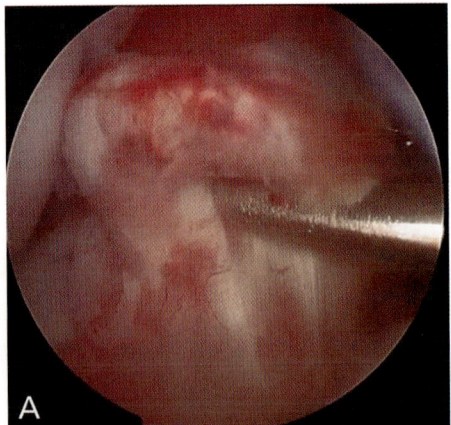

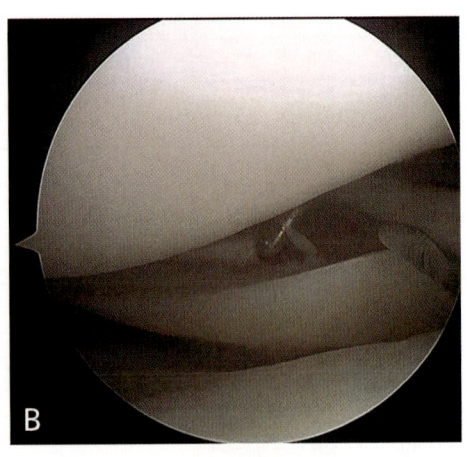

Figure 5 Arthroscopic evaluation of knee balance. **A,** The length of the ACL stump is assessed. **B,** Associated lesions are evaluated. Note the lateral meniscus posterior horn tear.

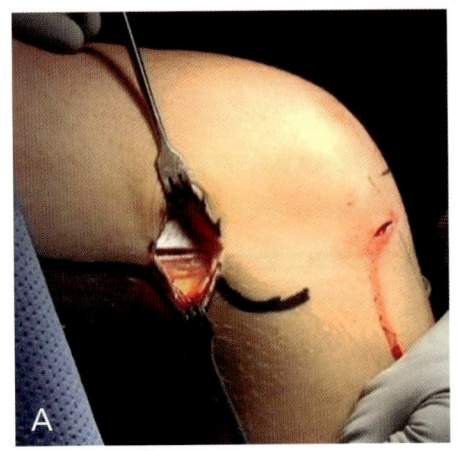

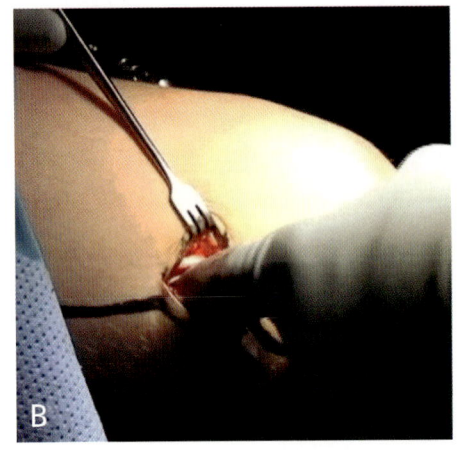

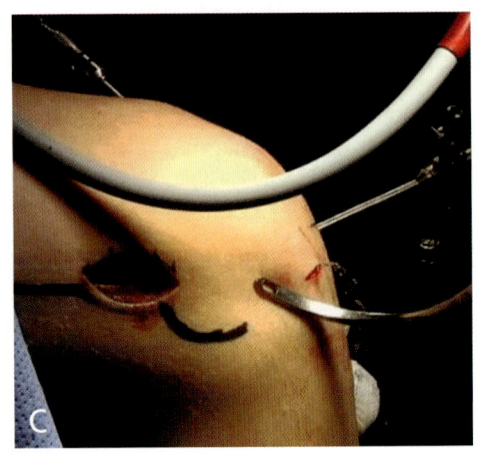

Figure 6 Intraoperative photographs demonstrate the lateral femoral approach for ACL reconstruction. **A,** A 3- to 4-cm skin incision is performed at the level of the posterior femoral cortex, proximal to the lateral femoral condyle, and the iliotibial band is incised longitudinally. **B,** Metzenbaum scissors and a finger are used to create an opening in the intermuscular septum, posterior to the vastus lateralis. **C,** A gaff hook (or a curved Kelly clamp) is passed from the anterolateral portal into the notch.

dial and anterolateral portals. The length of the ACL stump is evaluated (**Figure 5**). When possible, an ACL repair with semitendinosus autograft augmentation is performed. Any associated pathology (eg, meniscal tears or chondral injuries) is identified and treated at this point (**Figure 5**). The remaining ACL stump is left in place if there is no notch impingement in extension; otherwise, it is removed with a mechanical shaver until it is no longer impinging. Our preference is to leave the stump and incorporate it into the reconstruction. Notch preparation or notchplasty is not performed.

Lateral Approach
A 3- to 4-cm skin incision to the lateral femur is performed at the level of the posterior femoral cortex proximal to the lateral femoral condyle (**Figure 6, A**). The iliotibial band is incised longitudinally. The vastus lateralis is bluntly separated from the intermuscular septum and retracted anteriorly. Metzenbaum scissors are used to bluntly create a hole in the septum. The scissors must be kept in contact with the posterior femoral cortex, aiming toward the intercondylar notch, to avoid damage to the neurovascular bundle. A finger is used to enlarge the septum opening until the posterior aspect of the condyles and the posterior capsule can be palpated (**Figure 6, B**).

Proximal Over-the-Top Preparation
A gaff hook or a curved Kelly clamp is passed from the anterolateral portal into the notch (**Figure 6, C**). The tip of the hook is placed in contact with the posterior femoral cortex and against the posterior capsule. The tip of the hook can be palpated from the lateral approach with a finger (**Figure 7, A and B**). It is very important to palpate the passage of the metal hook along the posterior cortex as it comes out laterally to prevent popliteal vessel injury. The hook is then pushed through the posterior capsule and guided with the finger outside the lateral incision. A suture loop is placed into the tip of the hook and retrieved anteriorly through the anterolateral portal (**Figure 7, C through F**).

Tibial Tunnel Preparation
An ACL guide is inserted into the joint through the anteromedial portal and positioned on the native ACL footprint. A guide pin is then drilled into the proximal tibia in a more vertical position compared to conventional adult ACL reconstruction (**Figure 8, A**). A tibial tunnel of the same size as the graft (usually approximately 6 mm) is drilled over the guide pin. If the guide pin is seen advancing into the joint, a curet is used to keep it distal until the tibial tunnel drilling is completed. An arthroscopic grasper is inserted into the joint through the tibial tunnel, and the loop of the shuttle suture, previously positioned over the top, is retrieved out of the anteromedial tibia (**Figure 8, B**). The shuttle suture is used to pull the proximal graft leading suture out of the lateral

120 © 2013 American Academy of Orthopaedic Surgeons

Chapter 19: Pediatric Anterior Cruciate Ligament Reconstruction

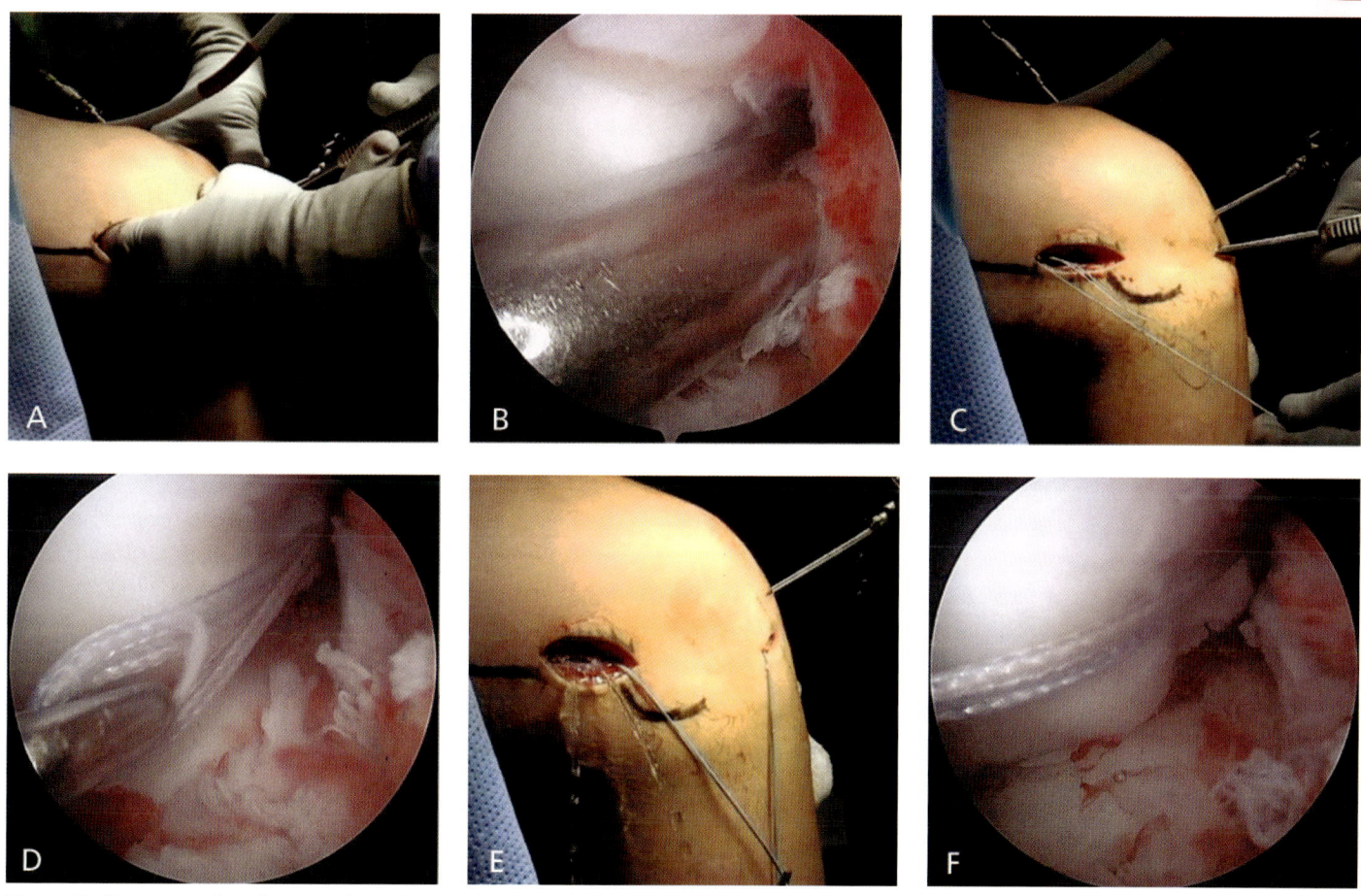

Figure 7 Intraoperative photographs and corresponding arthroscopic views demonstrate proximal over-the-top preparation. **A** and **B,** Once the tip of the hook is placed in contact with the posterior femoral cortex and against the posterior capsule, it can be palpated from the lateral approach with a finger. **C** and **D,** The hook is then pushed through the posterior capsule and guided with the finger outside the lateral incision. **E** and **F,** A suture loop is placed into the tip of the hook and retrieved anteriorly through the anterolateral portal.

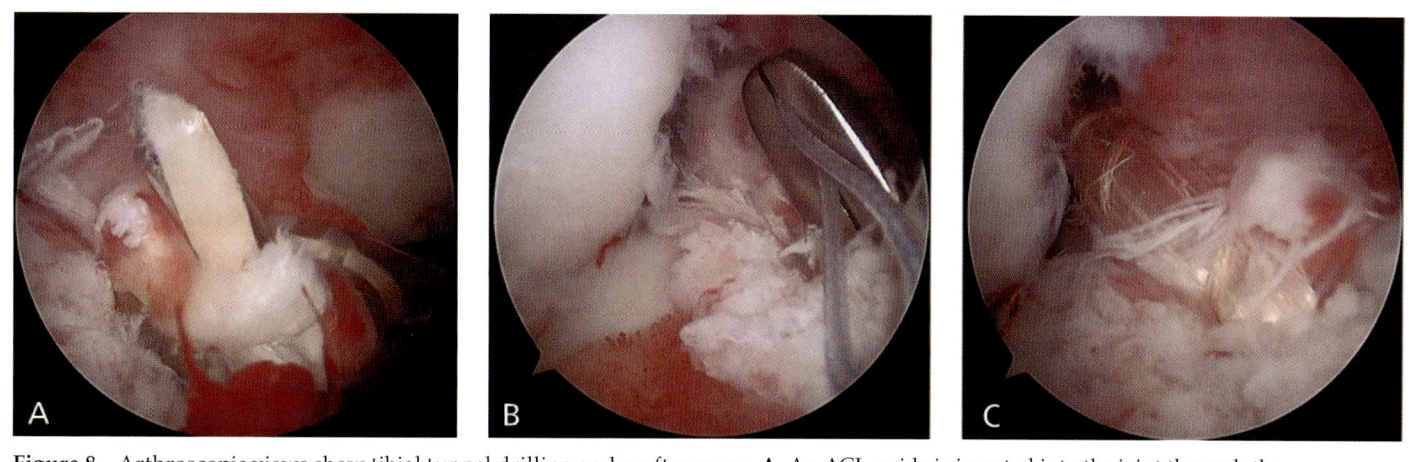

Figure 8 Arthroscopic views show tibial tunnel drilling and graft passage. **A,** An ACL guide is inserted into the joint through the anteromedial portal and positioned on the native ACL footprint. A guide pin is then drilled into the proximal tibia in an almost vertical position. A tibial tunnel of the same size as the graft (approximately 6 mm) is drilled over the guide pin. **B,** An arthroscopic grasper is inserted into the joint through the tibial tunnel, and the loop of the shuttle suture, previously positioned over the top, is retrieved out of the anteromedial tibia. **C,** The graft is then pulled into the joint.

incision. The graft is then pulled into the joint (**Figure 8, C**).

Proximal Fixation
The loop device for the proximal fixation of the graft is visualized from the proximal incision. The lateral femoral cortex is then exposed. A drill tip is used to palpate the anterior and posterior femoral cortices and drill a hole at the center of the shaft. A screw with a soft-tissue washer is then inserted into the femur but is not tightened at this point (**Figure 9, A**). The loop is then placed around the screw. Some tension is applied to the graft to allow the loop to sit in a correct position around the screw (**Figure 9, B**). The screw is then tightened.

Distal Fixation
The graft is tensioned distally with traction and knee flexion/extension maneuvers. A soft-tissue staple is positioned distal to the growth plate to fix the graft (**Figure 9, C**). The remnant of the graft is then trimmed, the stability and range of motion of the knee are evaluated, and the wounds are closed.

© 2013 American Academy of Orthopaedic Surgeons

Section 1: Sports Medicine

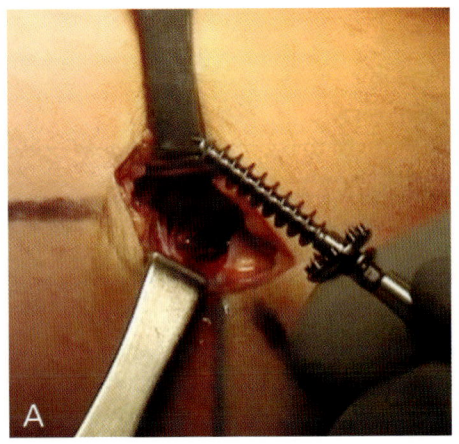

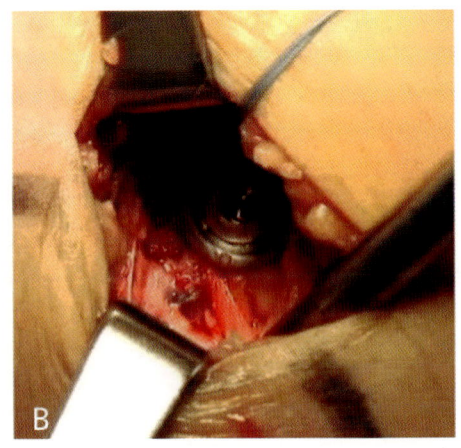

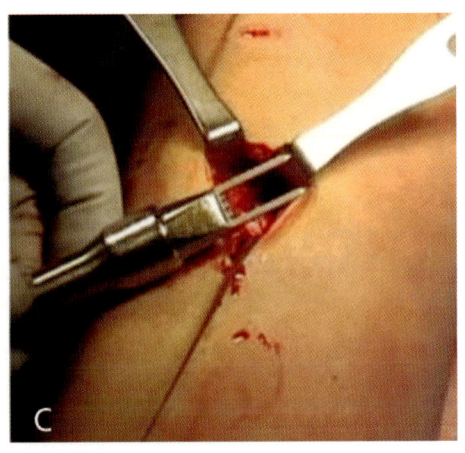

Figure 9 Intraoperative photographs demonstrate proximal and distal fixation of the graft. **A**, A 6.5-mm cancellous screw with a soft-tissue washer is used to fix the loop device, previously placed in the proximal part of the graft. **B**, The screw is shown in position. **C**, Distally, the graft is fixed with a soft-tissue staple.

Complications

The exact incidence of complications after pediatric ACL reconstruction is unknown because of the small case series available in the literature. In addition to the complications commonly related to any ACL reconstruction (eg, infection, residual instability, incorrect tunnel placement, stiffness), growth disturbance (limb-length discrepancy and axial deformity) is an actual risk specific to pediatric patients.

Kocher et al[6] investigated the management and complications of pediatric ACL injuries by surveying members of the Herodicus Society and the ACL Study Group; they found large practice variation in initial management and ACL reconstruction technique. The complications included 15 reported cases of growth disturbance: 8 cases of distal femoral valgus deformity with arrest of the lateral distal femoral physis, 3 cases of tibial recurvatum with arrest of the tibial tubercle apophysis, 2 cases of genu valgum without arrest, and 2 cases of limb-length discrepancy. In 11 of 15 cases, the growth disturbance was associated with technical errors, including fixation hardware across the lateral distal femoral physis (3 cases), bone plugs of a patellar tendon graft across the distal femoral physis (3 cases), large (12-mm) tunnels (2 cases), and fixation hardware across the tibial tubercle apophysis (3 cases). Proximal over-the-top positioning of the graft and extra-articular tenodesis procedures were reported to have complications as well. There was one case of distal femoral valgus deformity with a bony bar associated with over-the-top graft placement. There were two cases of genu valgum without a bony bar associated with lateral extra-articular tenodesis procedures.[6]

Postoperative Care and Rehabilitation

Postoperatively, immediate weight bearing and full range of motion are allowed. A knee brace is usually not necessary. During the first 6 weeks, full range of motion should be achieved, and strengthening exercises are commenced. Noncutting and nontwisting sports such as swimming, biking, and running in a straight line are allowed at 12 weeks after surgery. Return to full activity is usually allowed at 6 months postoperatively. Exceptions to this protocol may be dictated by combined chondral or meniscal repair procedures, age, and compliance of the patient.

Pearls

Considering the complications related to technical errors, a careful and thorough surgical technique is essential to reduce the risk of growth disturbance.

- When harvesting hamstring autograft, care should be taken to completely release the major and minor vincula of the tendons medially, laterally, proximally, and distally. Inadequate release of the tendons may result in insufficient harvesting and short grafts.
- During the preparation for the proximal over-the-top positioning of the graft, care should be taken to not place the lateral femoral incision too proximal. This can result in a difficult approach to the posterior femoral condyles and too-proximal fixation, with inadequate graft length for the tibial fixation. In addition, the hook or the Kelly clamp, passed inside out through the anterolateral portal, must be kept against the posterior femoral cortex and guided through the posterior capsule with a finger placed into the lateral incision to avoid posterior neurovascular damage.
- During tibial drilling, a small vertical tunnel (6- to 8-mm) should be made to minimize the damage to the growth plate and reduce the risk of growth disturbance.
- During the fixation of the graft, it is essential to avoid hardware placement at the level of the physes (**Figure 10**). Hardware positioning can be verified fluoroscopically. Excessive tensioning of the graft should be avoided as well, to minimize the risk of axial deformities.

Conclusions/Results

As previously mentioned, limited strong evidence is available regarding ACL reconstruction in pediatric patients. For all patients, the possible treatment options, complications, and outcomes need to be clearly communicated. Although the risk of growth disturbance is possible, in most cases this seems to be related to technical errors. Therefore, an accurate surgical technique is essential to avoid pitfalls.

Although the natural history of ACL deficiency in children seems to entail recurrent instability with progressive chondral and meniscal injuries, absolute indications for reconstruction are unclear. Children are very active, and controlling their activity level is very difficult; accordingly, they can actually be treated like high-level athletes at risk of reinjury with an unstable knee. Based on the literature and our experience, we recommend surgical stabilization in highly active children with open growth plates. Symptomatic meniscal injury is a definite indication for surgical intervention.

Mainly case series and level IV studies are available regarding this topic. In a

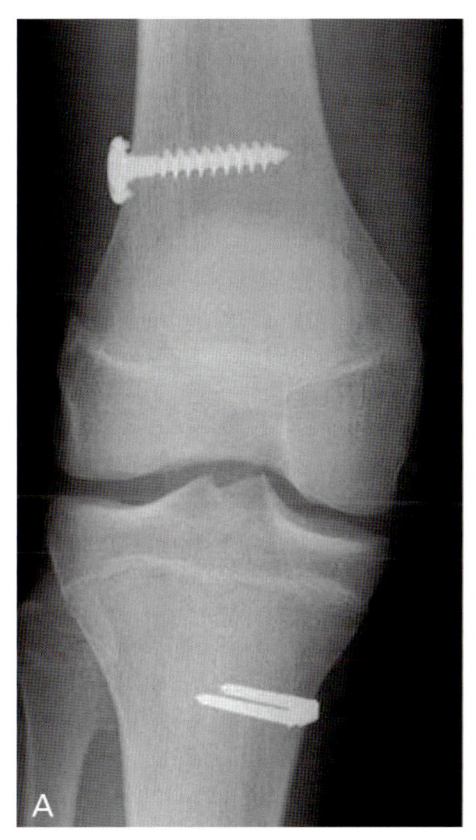

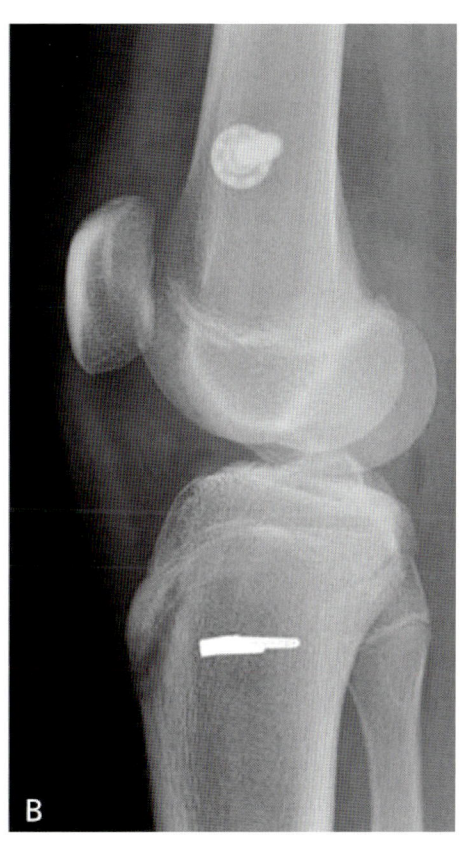

Figure 10 Postoperative AP (**A**) and lateral (**B**) radiographs following ACL reconstruction in a pediatric patient show hardware placement that avoids the level of the physes.

prognostic study, Aichroth et al[7] reported the results of 23 patients, who sustained an ACL tear and underwent nonsurgical treatment. At a mean 72-month follow-up, seven patients required medial or lateral meniscectomy and 10 patients showed radiographic arthritic changes at final review.

Andrews et al[8] reported the results of allograft ACL reconstruction in eight patients at a mean 58-month follow-up. A partial transphyseal technique with proximal over-the-top positioning of the graft was used. They reported six excellent, one good, and one fair result. No growth disturbances were reported.

Lo et al[9] reported the results of ACL reconstruction in eight pediatric patients at a mean 7.4-year follow-up. A partial transphyseal technique with proximal over-the-top positioning of the graft was used. Hamstring or quadriceps tendon autograft was used in all the cases. They reported excellent results. Poor outcome was described for only one patient, who sustained a subsequent patellofemoral injury. No limb-length discrepancy was reported. Similar results have been reported for the other techniques.[10]

References

1. Mohtadi N, Grant J: Managing anterior cruciate ligament deficiency in the skeletally immature individual: A systematic review of the literature. *Clin J Sport Med* 2006;16(6):457-464.
2. Henry J, Chotel F, Chouteau J, Fessy MH, Bérard J, Moyen B: Rupture of the anterior cruciate ligament in children: Early reconstruction with open physes or delayed reconstruction to skeletal maturity? *Knee Surg Sports Traumatol Arthrosc* 2009;17(7):748-755.
3. Larsen MW, Garrett WE Jr, Delee JC, Moorman CT III: Surgical management of anterior cruciate ligament injuries in patients with open physes. *J Am Acad Orthop Surg* 2006;14(13):736-744.
4. Kocher MS, Garg S, Micheli LJ: Physeal sparing reconstruction of the anterior cruciate ligament in skeletally immature prepubescent children and adolescents: Surgical technique. *J Bone Joint Surg Am* 2006;88(suppl 1, pt 2):283-293.
5. Kocher MS, Garg S, Micheli LJ: Physeal sparing reconstruction of the anterior cruciate ligament in skeletally immature prepubescent children and adolescents. *J Bone Joint Surg Am* 2005;87(11):2371-2379.
6. Kocher MS, Saxon HS, Hovis WD, Hawkins RJ: Management and complications of anterior cruciate ligament injuries in skeletally immature patients: Survey of the Herodicus Society and the ACL Study Group. *J Pediatr Orthop* 2002;22(4):452-457.
7. Aichroth PM, Patel DV, Zorrilla P: The natural history and treatment of rupture of the anterior cruciate ligament in children and adolescents: A prospective review. *J Bone Joint Surg Br* 2002;84(1):38-41.
8. Andrews M, Noyes FR, Barber-Westin SD: Anterior cruciate ligament allograft reconstruction in the skeletally immature athlete. *Am J Sports Med* 1994;22(1):48-54.
9. Lo IK, Kirkley A, Fowler PJ, Miniaci A: The outcome of operatively treated anterior cruciate ligament disruptions in the skeletally immature child. *Arthroscopy* 1997;13(5):627-634.
10. Kaeding CC, Flanigan D, Donaldson C: Surgical techniques and outcomes after anterior cruciate ligament reconstruction in preadolescent patients. *Arthroscopy* 2010;26(11):1530-1538.

Video Reference

19.1 Adapted from Bonasia DE, Rossi R, Wolf B, Amendola A: Video: *ACL: Pediatric Anterior Cruciate Ligament Reconstruction*. Rosemont, IL, American Academy of Orthopaedic Surgeons, 2011.

Chapter 20
Medial Patellofemoral Ligament Reconstruction for Recurrent Patellar Instability

Andrew J. Cosgarea, MD   Miho J. Tanaka, MD   John J. Elias, PhD

Introduction

The medial patellofemoral ligament (MPFL) is the most important passive soft-tissue restraint to lateral patellar instability.[1] It has been shown both clinically and radiographically that the MPFL tears when the patella dislocates.[2] The other crucial stabilizing components of the knee extensor mechanism are the bony restraints (especially the lateral trochlear ridge) and the dynamic soft-tissue restraints (especially the vastus medialis obliquus). MPFL reconstruction is one of a large number of different surgical procedures that have been described to restore patellar stability. Studies reporting short-term and midterm results of MPFL reconstruction confirm excellent patient satisfaction and low recurrent instability rates.[3-5] Sometimes other procedures are better suited to addressing the pathoanatomy. For example, patients with excessive tibial tuberosity lateralization may need a medializing tibial tuberosity osteotomy, and patients with extreme patella alta may need a distalizing osteotomy.

Patient Selection
Indications

MPFL reconstruction is indicated for patients with symptomatic recurrent patellar instability when the primary etiologic factor is medial soft-tissue insufficiency. MPFL reconstruction may also be indicated as a concomitant procedure when tibial tuberosity osteotomy alone is not sufficient to restore functional stability.

A thorough assessment of the patient's history, description of symptoms, and physical examination are crucial in determining when to perform surgical stabilization. Patients who report recurrent painful episodes of lateral subluxation or dislocation associated with the classic twisting mechanism and exhibit apprehension with lateral translation on physical examination are the best candidates. A course of physical therapy designed to strengthen core, hip, and quadriceps musculature may negate the need for surgery, especially for patients with demonstrable weakness and only one or two previous instability episodes. Patients with substantial patellofemoral pain independent of instability episodes are likely to have continued anterior knee pain even after successful stabilization.

Contraindications

The primary contraindication to MPFL reconstruction is medial patellar instability; this instability is usually an iatrogenic problem found after overaggressive lateral retinacular release, but it may also be seen as a primary problem, especially in patients with hyperlaxity syndromes. Active infection is another contraindication to MPFL reconstruction. Patients who are skeletally immature require a modification of this procedure to minimize the risk of growth plate injury at the femoral attachment site adjacent to the distal femoral physis.[6]

Preoperative Imaging

It is crucial that the appropriate radiographic studies be obtained before recommending a specific surgical procedure. In addition to standard AP and notch views, the sunrise view is obtained at 45° and the lateral view is obtained at 30° of knee flexion. For patients in whom tibiofemoral osteoarthritis is suspected, the notch view is replaced by a PA view in 45° of flexion. The lateral radiograph is used to quantify the relative patellar height (**Figure 1**). Patients with extreme patella alta (Insall-Salvati ratio >1.50) may benefit from a distalizing tibial tuberosity osteotomy. Trochlear dysplasia can also be seen on the lateral radiograph as the "crossing sign" (**Figure 2**). Patellofemoral degenerative changes and joint space narrowing seen on the sunrise view may suggest the need for an anteromedializing osteotomy to decrease joint reactive forces.

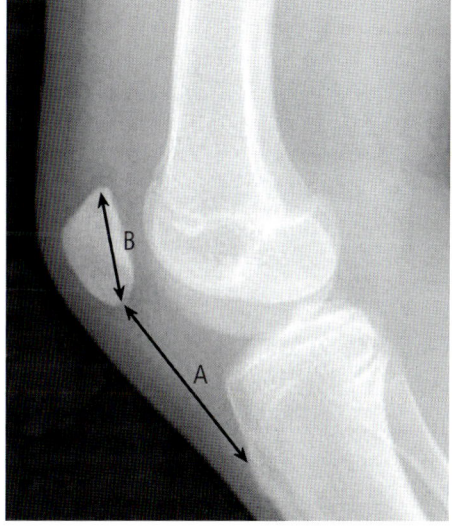

Figure 1 The lateral radiograph is used to determine relative patellar height. This patient has patella alta: Insall-Salvati ratio (A/B) >1.20. Line A is the length of the patellar tendon, and line B is the length of the patella.

MRI is most useful for assessing the integrity of the articular surfaces. If localized high-grade chondral lesions are identified, then the surgeon can plan for concomitant cartilage débridement, marrow stimulation, or osteochondral replacement procedures. When high-grade lateral patellofemoral chondral abnormalities are noted, an osteotomy that unloads the lateral patellofemoral joint (eg, an Elmslie-Trillat medialization osteotomy) may be indicated as an isolated or concomitant procedure. When a high-grade inferior pole lesion is noted, an osteotomy that unloads the inferior pole (eg, Fulkerson anteromedialization osteotomy) may be considered.

CT scans are particularly useful for determining trochlear morphology and measuring malalignment, as determined by tibial tuberosity lateralization. The tibial tuberosity–trochlear groove (TT-TG) distance is measured on superimposed axial CT cuts through the distal femur at

---

Dr. Cosgarea or an immediate family member has received research or institutional support from Toshiba and serves as a board member, owner, officer, or committee member of the American Orthopaedic Society for Sports Medicine and the American Academy of Orthopaedic Surgeons. Dr. Elias has received research or institutional support from the National Institutes of Health (NIAMS & NICHD), Toshiba, and Intuitive Surgical Systems. Neither Dr. Tanaka nor any immediate family member has received anything of value from or owns stock in a commercial company or institution related directly or indirectly to the subject of this chapter.

Section 1: Sports Medicine

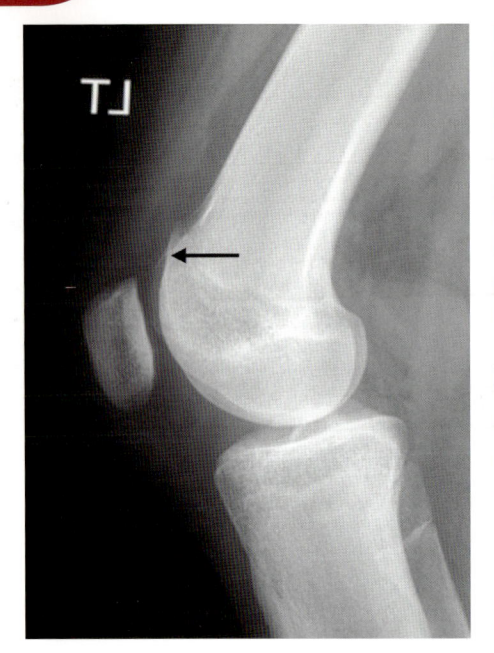

Figure 2 Lateral radiograph of a knee shows the "crossing sign" (arrow), indicative of trochlear dysplasia.

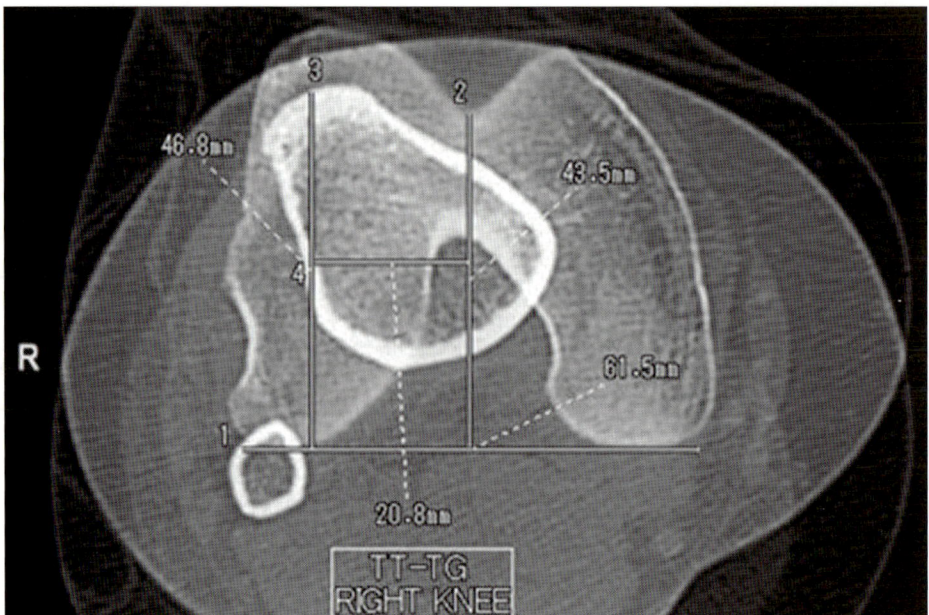

Figure 3 CT scan of a knee with superimposed axial cuts through the level of the trochlear groove and tibial tuberosity. The tibial tuberosity–trochlear groove (TT-TG) distance is the distance between vertical lines drawn through these landmarks.

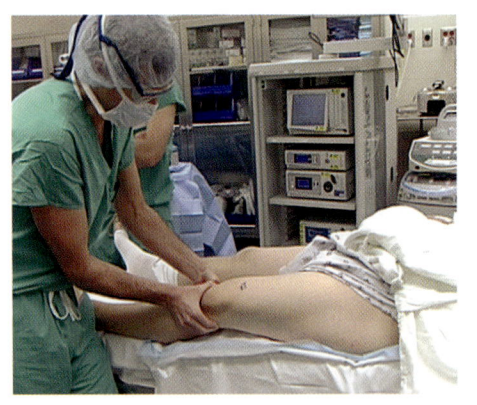

Figure 4 Photograph shows the glide test, which is performed during the examination under anesthesia to determine passive lateral patellar translation.

the level of the Roman arch and the proximal tibia at the level where the tuberosity is most prominent (**Figure 3**). The distance between vertical lines drawn through the base of the trochlear groove and the anterior prominence of the tuberosity is measured. Normal values are up to 15 mm. More recently, dynamic CT scanning has been used to assess maltracking. In contrast to traditional CT scans, where static images are obtained at specific flexion angles, dynamic CT scans are imaged while the patient actively flexes and extends the knee, which allows the surgeon to not only quantify the amount of maltracking but also determine the flexion angle where the lateral translation of the patella is greatest.

Video 20.1 Medial Patellofemoral Ligament Reconstruction Using Single Strand Hamstring Graft and Interference Screw Fixation. Andrew J. Cosgarea, MD; Miho J. Tanaka, MD (8 min)

Procedure

Patient Positioning/Examination Under Anesthesia

The patient is placed supine on the operating table. The procedure always begins with an examination under anesthesia, including assessment of limb alignment, hip rotation measurement, and a formal knee ligament evaluation. A crucial part of the examination under anesthesia is the glide test, which is used to manually assess the amount of lateral translation of the patella (**Figure 4**). Lateral translation is quantified in quadrants (100% lateral translation equals four quadrants). It is very important to compare this translation to that of the contralateral knee. Assuming that the contralateral knee has normal lateral translation (no previous episodes of instability), the goal will be to set the tension of the MPFL graft on the surgical side to allow an amount of translation equal to that of the normal side. The tilt test is used to determine the tightness of the lateral retinaculum. The examiner should be able to evert the patella to a horizontal position by pushing up manually on the lateral facet of the patella. Although usually not necessary, a lateral retinacular release may be performed using an open or arthroscopic technique if the lateral retinaculum is determined to be excessively tight.

Surgical Technique

After prophylactic intravenous antibiotics are administered and a tourniquet is placed around the thigh, a diagnostic arthroscopy is performed. Arthroscopic evaluation is necessary to assess patellar tracking and, in particular, to determine the location and degree of any chondral abnormalities. If high-grade (Outerbridge grade 3 or 4) chondral lesions are noted on the lateral facet or the inferior pole of the patella, consideration should be given to performing a concomitant medializing (eg, Elmslie-Trillat) or anteromedializing (eg, Fulkerson) tibial tuberosity osteotomy. If an osteotomy is indicated, it should be performed before the MPFL reconstruction.

After the examination under anesthesia and diagnostic arthroscopy are completed, bony landmarks are marked on the surface of the skin (**Figure 5, A**). The leg is exsanguinated with an elastic bandage, and the tourniquet is inflated. Hamstring graft harvest begins with an incision directly over the pes anserine bursa. Blunt dissection is performed, small vessels are electrocauterized, and the superior edge of the sartorial fascia is exposed. The tips of the scissors are placed under the sartorial fascia, which is then sharply released off its insertion on the proximal medial tibia. The sartorial fascia is everted, exposing the underlying gracilis tendon.

Chapter 20: Medial Patellofemoral Ligament Reconstruction for Recurrent Patellar Instability

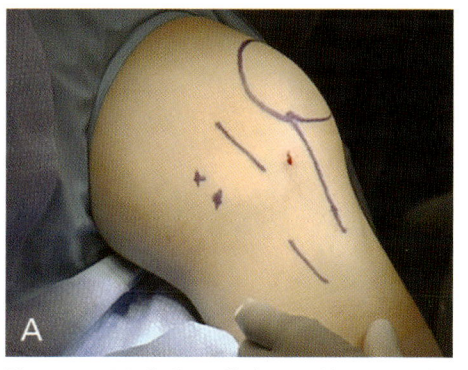

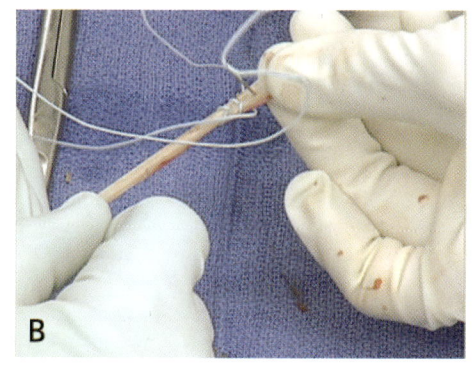

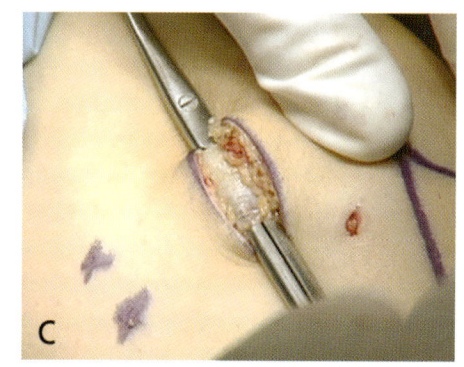

Figure 5 Medial patellofemoral ligament (MPFL) reconstruction. **A,** Bony landmarks are marked on the surface of the skin. The proximal X is over the adductor tubercle, and the distal X is over the medial femoral epicondyle. **B,** A locking stitch is woven through the patellar end of the graft. **C,** The residual attenuated MPFL tissue is exposed through a longitudinal incision midway between the patella and the medial epicondyle.

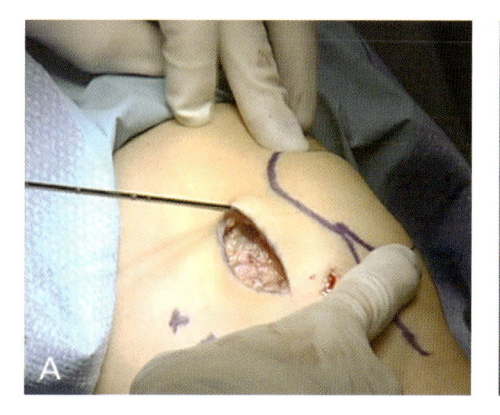

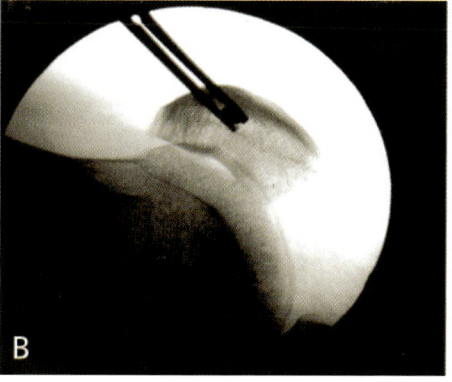

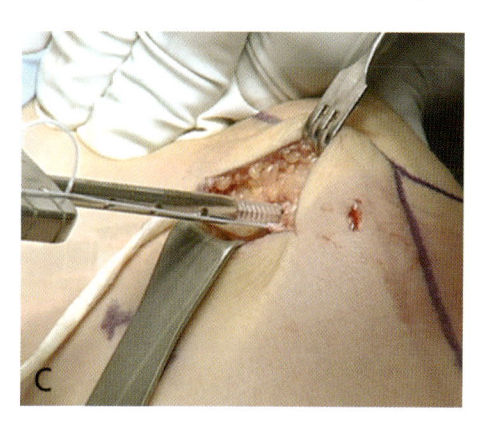

Figure 6 Intraoperative photographs and a fluoroscopic view demonstrate the placement of the patellar tunnel. **A,** The superior and inferior poles of the patella are palpated to confirm the position of the drill bit. **B,** Appropriate positioning of the Kirschner wire in the patella is confirmed with lateral fluoroscopy (mini C-arm). **C,** Patellar fixation is achieved with a tenodesis screw.

The gracilis tendon is dissected free from the sartorial fascia and semitendinosus tendon. If the gracilis is too small, the semitendinosus is harvested. The end of the tendon is tagged with a locking stitch. An open-ended tendon stripper is then used to harvest the tendon. The surgeon must be careful during harvest to release any accessory bands that can promote premature transection of the hamstring tendon. Hamstring allograft may be preferable in patients undergoing revision surgery or in those with connective tissue disorders.

The graft is brought to the rear table for preparation. Muscle is scraped off the hamstring tendon at the musculotendinous junction using curved scissors. Additional tissue is then débrided sharply to create a smooth graft of the appropriate size. The graft is then passed through a sizer to measure its diameter. A 4- to 5-mm diameter is more than adequate. A No. 2 nonabsorbable suture is woven through the distal end of the graft using a locking technique (**Figure 5, B**).

After the graft harvest is completed, an incision is made directly over the MPFL, midway between its femoral and patellar attachments. The attenuated native MPFL is identified and exposed just distal and deep to the vastus medialis obliquus muscle (**Figure 5, C**). Alternatively, two smaller incisions can be used: one along the medial border of the patella and one just anterior to the medial femoral epicondyle and adductor tubercle. The medial border of the patella is exposed, and a rongeur is used to clear soft tissue from an area just proximal to its equator. A 2.5-mm drill bit is passed from medial to lateral, ensuring that the anterior cortex and articular surface of the patella are not violated. Safe placement can be confirmed by palpating the articular surface through a small medial capsular window. The superior and inferior poles are palpated to confirm the position of the drill bit just proximal to the equator of the patella (**Figure 6, A**). A mini C-arm fluoroscopy unit can also be used to confirm the appropriate position of the patellar tunnel (**Figure 6, B**). The drill bit is exchanged for an eyelet Kirschner wire (K-wire), which is then overdrilled with a cannulated drill bit, 0.5 mm larger than the diameter of the graft. Patellar fixation is achieved with interference or tenodesis screw techniques (**Figure 6, C**). The screw is inserted deep enough into the tunnel so that it is flush with the medial edge of the patella. Adequate fixation is confirmed by tugging aggressively on the free end of the graft.

Alternatively, patellar fixation may be achieved via the docking technique. A blind tunnel is drilled approximately 15 mm deep into the patella. Two diverging eyelet K-wires are then drilled laterally through the end of the tunnel, exiting the lateral cortex of the patella. One end of the suture is passed through each K-wire, and the knot is tied over a bony bridge. The advantage of the docking technique is that the femoral tunnel tends to be smaller, and no implants are necessary.[7]

The locations of the adductor tubercle and the medial epicondyle are identified by palpation. Sharp and blunt dissection are used to expose both anatomic landmarks. Small vessels are electrocauterized, and care is taken to protect the saphenous nerve. A 2.5-mm drill bit is placed just anterior to the medial epicondyle (**Figure 7, A**), and the mini C-arm can be used again to confirm

© 2013 American Academy of Orthopaedic Surgeons

Section 1: Sports Medicine

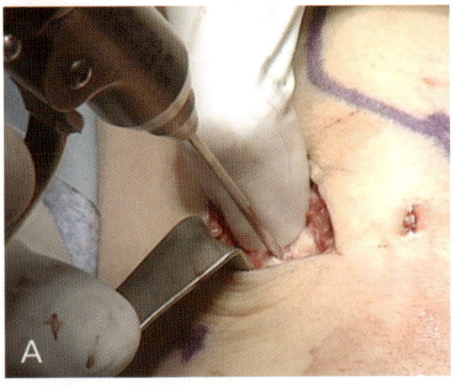

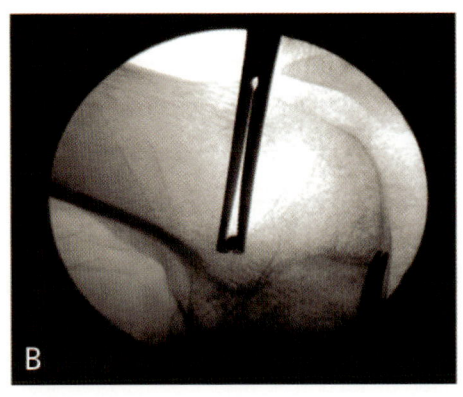

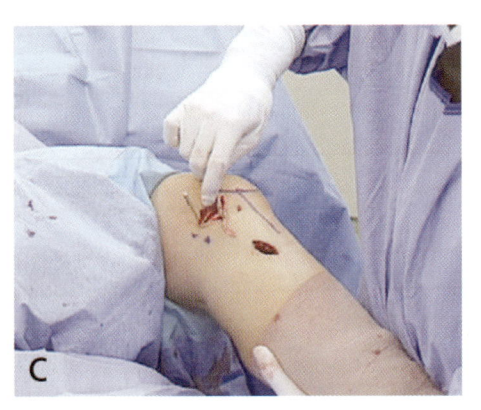

Figure 7 Intraoperative photographs and a fluoroscopic view demonstrate femoral tunnel position. **A,** Preliminary femoral tunnel position is determined by placing a Kirschner wire just anterior to the palpable medial femoral epicondyle. **B,** The position of the drill bit is confirmed with fluoroscopy. **C,** The graft is wrapped around the drill bit, and knee range of motion is assessed to confirm appropriate isometry.

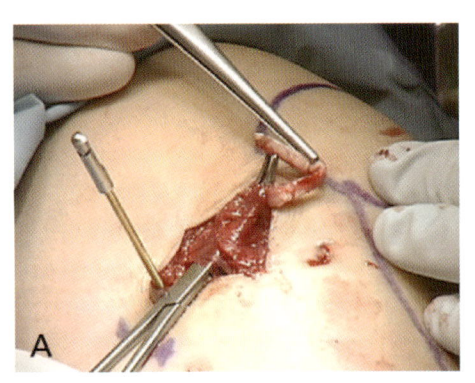

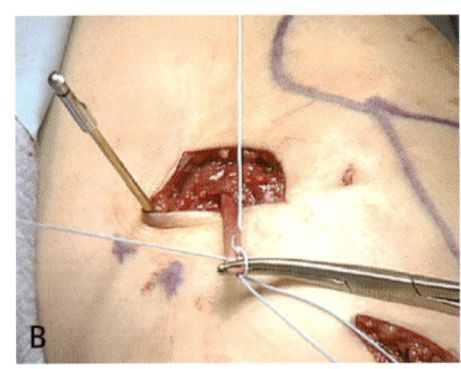

Figure 8 Intraoperative photographs demonstrate graft placement. **A,** The graft is passed through a soft-tissue tunnel deep to the residual medial patellofemoral ligament and medial retinaculum and superficial to the capsule. **B,** The pull-out suture is passed through a loop (at the tip of the hemostat) created in the locking stitch on the femoral end of the graft.

positioning of the drill bit (**Figure 7, B**). Appropriate positioning of the femoral tunnel is crucial because malpositioning has been shown to result in excessive patellofemoral joint surface loads.[8] The femoral end of the graft is wrapped around the 2.5-mm drill bit.

Graft tension is monitored as the knee is taken through a range of motion to confirm that the position is isometrically appropriate for the femoral tunnel (**Figure 7, C**). The tunnel position can be modified if necessary by altering the position of the drill bit. One common mistake is to place the femoral tunnel too proximal. This error has been shown to be surprisingly common, even with experienced surgeons.[9] A graft placed too proximal will develop excessive tension as the knee is flexed, which can result in motion loss, graft failure, or excessive joint forces.[8]

Once the optimal femoral tunnel position has been confirmed, the graft is cut so as to leave an additional 2 cm in length to be buried in the blind tunnel. The graft is then passed in the soft-tissue plane deep to the residual MPFL and superficial to the joint capsule (**Figure 8, A**). A nonabsorbable No. 2 suture is passed through the femoral end of the graft with a locking technique. A loop is created at the end of the grafts, allowing for passage of a pull-out suture (**Figure 8, B**). This loop allows the pull-out suture to be removed after fixation of the graft in the blind femoral tunnel. The drill bit is exchanged for an eyelet K-wire, which is drilled in a direction that is proximal and anterior to the lateral epicondyle so as to protect the common peroneal nerve. The blind femoral tunnel is drilled 25 mm deep using a cannulated drill bit with a diameter 0.5 mm larger than the diameter of the graft. The graft pull-out suture is threaded through the eyelet of the K-wire, which is advanced out the lateral side of the distal thigh. By pulling on the pull-out suture, the graft is docked into the blind femoral tunnel (**Figure 9**).

The most crucial part of MPFL reconstruction surgery is to determine the appropriate tension of the graft. An interference screw 1 to 2 mm larger than the diameter of the femoral tunnel is placed over a guidewire and advanced to the opening of the femoral tunnel. The appropriate amount of lateral patellar translation is confirmed before the screw is inserted in the femoral tunnel. It is particularly important not to fix the graft too tightly because doing so can overconstrain the patella and lead to excessively elevated patellofemoral joint forces.[8,10]

With tension placed on the free lateral pull-out sutures, the surgeon takes the knee through a range-of-motion cycle. The knee should have full, unrestricted range of motion. Tension in the graft can be determined directly by visualization and palpation of the graft and indirectly by feeling the tension in the lateral pull-out sutures. The native MPFL becomes looser with flexion beyond 70°, and so should the MPFL graft. At this point, it is important to repeat the glide test and confirm that the amount of lateral translation is similar to that of the normal contralateral knee. For patients with instability or excessive laxity of the contralateral knee, the goal should be to reestablish two to three quadrants of lateral translation. Once these parameters are achieved, the femoral screw is advanced (**Figure 10**) and the pull-out suture is removed.

The wounds are closed in layers. Judicious use of local anesthetic and cryotherapy devices facilitates surgery on an outpatient basis. A drain may be used if desired. Adhesive skin closure strips are applied, followed by a cryotherapy unit and a loosely applied compression dressing and thromboembolic stocking. A hinged brace is then applied to facilitate progression to full weight bearing as soon as possible (**Figure 11**). Formal physical therapy is recommended to promote quadriceps strengthening and knee range-of-motion exercises.

Complications

The most common complication after MPFL reconstruction is loss of motion. The risk of developing arthrofibrosis is

Chapter 20: Medial Patellofemoral Ligament Reconstruction for Recurrent Patellar Instability

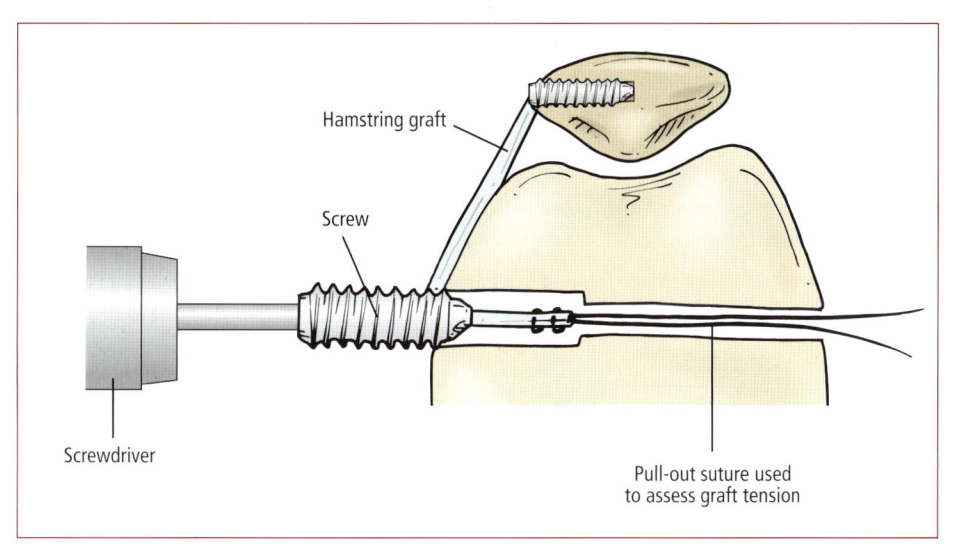

Figure 9 Illustration shows fixation in the femoral tunnel. The graft is first fixed to the patella, then into the blind femoral tunnel. With manual traction placed on the pull-out suture, the surgeon assesses knee range of motion to confirm appropriate graft tension and isometry before fixation with the femoral screw.

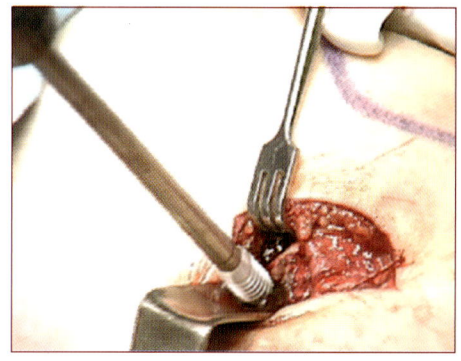

Figure 10 Intraoperative photograph demonstrates femoral screw advancement into the femur after appropriate graft tension is confirmed.

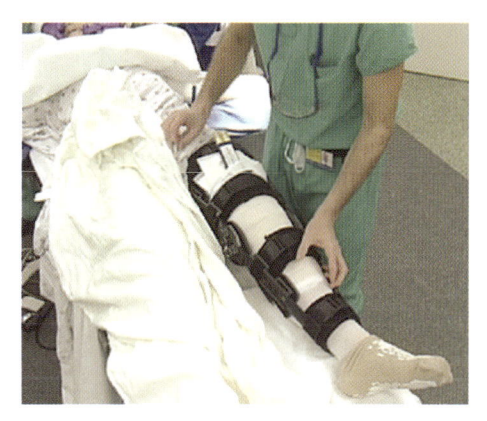

Figure 11 After medial patellofemoral ligament reconstruction, a cryotherapy unit is placed over a sterile dressing, followed by a hinged brace locked in full extension.

minimized by providing adequate pain medication, controlling swelling, and initiating range-of-motion exercises in the first few days after surgery. Technical errors, such as femoral tunnel malpositioning or overtensioning of the graft, can also result in restricted motion.[11] Because of the cam shape of the medial femoral condyle, graft tension relationships are more sensitive to femoral tunnel position than to patellar tunnel position.[12] MPFL isometry is normally maintained during the first 50° to 70° of flexion and then loosens slightly with greater flexion angles. Proximal malpositioning of the femoral tunnel can cause excessive graft tension with greater flexion angles.[8] If the femoral tunnel is positioned too far proximally, the graft will tighten with increasing flexion, which will eventually result in loss of flexion, articular cartilage overload, or graft failure.

Fixing the graft in place with excessive tension will result in decreased lateral patellar excursion, increased pressure on the patellofemoral cartilage, and possibly iatrogenic medial subluxation. Beck et al[10] showed that 2 N of graft tension restored normal patellar translation; higher loads (10 and 40 N) significantly restricted motion and increased medial patellofemoral contact pressure. Iatrogenic medial patellar subluxation is one potential cause of residual postoperative symptoms. Patients report pain and a feeling of lateral patellar translation when the knee begins to flex from an extended position. This diagnosis can be confirmed using the medial subluxation test. The test is performed by flexing the knee while a medial translation force is manually applied to the patella, which usually dramatically reproduces the symptoms. Both potential technical errors (malpositioning of the femoral tunnel and overtightening of the graft) could overload the medial patellofemoral joint surface and result in arthrosis.[8]

Fixation of the femoral end of the graft is of particular concern in the pediatric patient because drilling the femoral tunnel places an open physis at risk for injury. Adequate alternative fixation can be achieved by suturing a loop of the femoral end of the graft around the proximal superficial medial collateral ligament. Other complications after MPFL reconstruction include recurrent instability, implant pain,[5,13] and patellar fracture.[14,15]

Postoperative Care and Rehabilitation

In the recovery room, just hours after MPFL reconstruction surgery, patients are taught quadriceps contraction exercises, straight-leg raises, and partial weight bearing by a physical therapist. For each patient, a hinged range-of-motion brace is applied and locked in full extension for safe ambulation. One week after surgery, the brace is unlocked for physical therapy and home exercises. We prefer a formal structured physical therapy program three times a week. Patients quickly progress to full weight bearing, and the brace is unlocked for ambulation as soon as quadriceps function allows, with a goal for patients to have full extension immediately postoperatively, 120° of flexion by 4 weeks, and full knee flexion by 8 weeks. The brace can usually be discontinued after 6 weeks, and jogging can usually be resumed by 12 weeks. Sport-specific drills are then initiated, and athletes are generally cleared to return to sports by 4 to 5 months.

For patients undergoing concomitant tibial tuberosity osteotomy, the rehabilitation must be modified. To minimize the risk of tibial fracture, patients remain on crutches for 6 weeks, until the tuberosity osteotomy begins to heal. Jogging is usually resumed by 4 months, and full return to sports usually occurs by 6 to 8 months.

Pearls

- The indication for MPFL reconstruction is symptomatic recurrent lateral patellar instability unresponsive to nonsurgical treatment in patients who have medial soft-tissue insufficiency as the primary cause.
- Tibial tuberosity osteotomy may be a preferred surgical approach in patients with excessive tuberosity lateralization, patella alta, or high-grade inferior or lateral chondral lesions. After completing the osteotomy, a concomitant MPFL reconstruction can be performed if the patella is still unstable.

- Surgical stabilization can reliably prevent recurrent instability in most cases but is less reliable in treating concomitant anterior knee pain unrelated to instability episodes.
- If the patient's symptoms, preoperative radiographs, and physical examination are consistent with excessive lateral pressure, then a concomitant arthroscopic lateral retinacular release should be considered.
- A common technical error is to place the femoral tunnel too proximal. Malpositioning the femoral tunnel by as little as 5 mm can result in substantially increased graft force and pressure applied to the medial patellofemoral cartilage.
- After fixing the patellar end of the graft in place, the femoral end is wrapped around a drill bit placed just anterior to the medial femoral epicondyle. If graft isometry is not optimal (tension should decrease with flexion beyond 70°), the position of the drill bit should be modified before drilling the femoral tunnel.
- The glide test is used to determine the normal amount of lateral patellar translation in the asymptomatic contralateral knee. This amount of excursion is reproduced in the graft on the symptomatic knee before final graft fixation.
- Femoral fixation may be achieved in skeletally immature patients by suturing a loop at the femoral end of the graft to the proximal medial collateral ligament so that the distal femoral growth plate is not placed at risk.
- The most common postoperative complication is loss of motion. Motion deficits may be the result of inadequate postoperative rehabilitation or intraoperative technical errors such as malpositioning the femoral tunnel or overtensioning the graft.

References

1. Conlan T, Garth WP Jr, Lemons JE: Evaluation of the medial soft-tissue restraints of the extensor mechanism of the knee. *J Bone Joint Surg Am* 1993;75(5):682-693.
2. Sallay PI, Poggi J, Speer KP, Garrett WE: Acute dislocation of the patella: A correlative pathoanatomic study. *Am J Sports Med* 1996;24(1):52-60.
3. Ahmad CS, Brown GD, Stein BS: The docking technique for medial patellofemoral ligament reconstruction: Surgical technique and clinical outcome. *Am J Sports Med* 2009;37(10):2021-2027.
4. Ronga M, Oliva F, Longo UG, Testa V, Capasso G, Maffulli N: Isolated medial patellofemoral ligament reconstruction for recurrent patellar dislocation. *Am J Sports Med* 2009;37(9):1735-1742.
5. Steiner TM, Torga-Spak R, Teitge RA: Medial patellofemoral ligament reconstruction in patients with lateral patellar instability and trochlear dysplasia. *Am J Sports Med* 2006;34(8):1254-1261.
6. Deie M, Ochi M, Sumen Y, Yasumoto M, Kobayashi K, Kimura H: Reconstruction of the medial patellofemoral ligament for the treatment of habitual or recurrent dislocation of the patella in children. *J Bone Joint Surg Br* 2003;85(6):887-890.
7. Brown GD, Ahmad CS: The docking technique for medial patellofemoral ligament reconstruction. *Oper Tech Orthop* 2007;17:216-222.
8. Elias JJ, Cosgarea AJ: Technical errors during medial patellofemoral ligament reconstruction could overload medial patellofemoral cartilage: A computational analysis. *Am J Sports Med* 2006;34(9):1478-1485.
9. Servien E, Verdonk PC, Neyret P: Tibial tuberosity transfer for episodic patellar dislocation. *Sports Med Arthrosc* 2007;15(2):61-67.
10. Beck P, Brown NA, Greis PE, Burks RT: Patellofemoral contact pressures and lateral patellar translation after medial patellofemoral ligament reconstruction. *Am J Sports Med* 2007;35(9):1557-1563.
11. Thaunat M, Erasmus PJ: Management of overtight medial patellofemoral ligament reconstruction. *Knee Surg Sports Traumatol Arthrosc* 2009;17(5):480-483.
12. Farr J, Schepsis AA: Reconstruction of the medial patellofemoral ligament for recurrent patellar instability. *J Knee Surg* 2006;19(4):307-316.
13. Christiansen SE, Jacobsen BW, Lund B, Lind M: Reconstruction of the medial patellofemoral ligament with gracilis tendon autograft in transverse patellar drill holes. *Arthroscopy* 2008;24(1):82-87.
14. Mikashima Y, Kimura M, Kobayashi Y, Miyawaki M, Tomatsu T: Clinical results of isolated reconstruction of the medial patellofemoral ligament for recurrent dislocation and subluxation of the patella. *Acta Orthop Belg* 2006;72(1):65-71.
15. Thaunat M, Erasmus PJ: Recurrent patellar dislocation after medial patellofemoral ligament reconstruction. *Knee Surg Sports Traumatol Arthrosc* 2008;16(1):40-43.

Chapter 21
Realignment for Patellofemoral Arthritis

Albert Lin, MD   Robin West, MD

Patient Selection

Patellofemoral arthritis is a common and often debilitating cause of anterior knee pain. Causes of patellofemoral arthritis may be related to limb alignment, the bony architecture of the trochlea and the patella, and the integrity of the surrounding soft tissues.[1-3] Because of these multifactorial causes, treatment options may be particularly challenging. Surgical treatment may be indicated for patients in whom nonsurgical management—consisting of activity modification, bracing, physical therapy, medications, and injections—fails. The surgical treatment is variable, depending on the patient's age and activity level, the degree and location of chondral damage, and the association with tibiofemoral arthritis.[4-6] Current procedures include lateral release, cartilage restoration, patellofemoral arthroplasty, total knee arthroplasty, and patellar realignment. Patellar realignment consisting of anteromedialization of the tibial tubercle with osteotomy, as first described by Fulkerson for patellar instability, is an excellent option for patients with isolated lateral facet arthritis.[1,5]

The indications for anteromedialization of the tibial tubercle for patellofemoral arthritis and pain include isolated distal/lateral patella facet or lateral trochlear chondrosis with no chondrosis of the proximal/medial patellofemoral joint.[5] Other indications may include more central patellar wear in patients with patellar subluxation seen on radiographs, where the central patella is articulating with the lateral trochlear ridge throughout the early flexion zones. These patients may or may not have associated symptoms of patellar instability or an increased tibial tuberosity–to–trochlear groove (TT-TG) distance.[2]

Contraindications to tibial tubercle anteromedialization include severe medial and/or proximal patellar chondrosis that would be subject to increased loading after transfer. Standard contraindications to osteotomy around the knee include osteoporosis, nicotine use, nonspecific pain, complex regional pain syndrome, infection, inflammatory arthropathies, patella baja, or arthrofibrosis. A relative contraindication is the presence of a varus knee, medial compartment arthritis, or the post–medial meniscectomy knee, because the peak pressure will increase in the medial tibiofemoral joint space after medialization of the tibial tubercle.[7] Another relative contraindication is the presence of severe medial and/or lateral compartment arthritis of the knee, which would require a more global procedure, such as a total knee arthroplasty, to address all pathologies.[1]

Preoperative Imaging
Radiographs

We take standard 45° flexion weight-bearing PA, lateral, and Merchant views of both knees (**Figure 1**). The weight-bearing flexion radiographs show the degree of tibiofemoral joint space narrowing. The Merchant view is used to assess patellar tilt, subluxation, and trochlear dysplasia. The lateral view is used to evaluate the patellar height and trochlear dysplasia.

Magnetic Resonance Imaging

MRI is useful in evaluating injury to the medial patellofemoral ligament and the degree and location of articular cartilage loss. Bone bruise patterns and other associated ligamentous or meniscal injuries can also be identified. MRI can also be used to assess the lateral offset of the tibial tuberosity from the deepest point in the trochlear groove (TT-TG distance). A distance greater than 20 mm is nearly always associated with patellar instability and can be addressed with a tibial tubercle realignment as well.[2]

Computed Tomography

Cross-sectional imaging with CT slices at different positions along the lower limb can provide a three-dimensional view of the patellofemoral joint. These CT cuts can be used to assess the TT-TG distance, femoral anteversion, and patellar tracking at different flexion angles. We rarely order a CT scan in the treatment of patellofemoral arthritis and occasionally order a CT scan in the treatment of patellofemoral instability in patients with correlating femoral anteversion, increased tibial torsion, and patellar maltracking. MRI is equally as reliable as CT in assessing the TT-TG distance.[8]

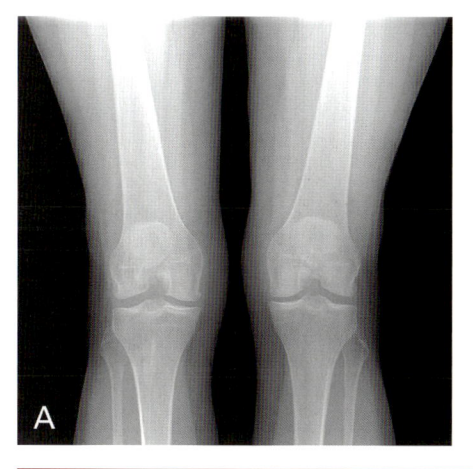

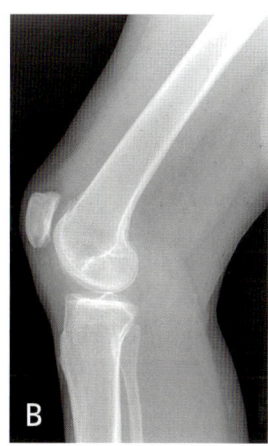

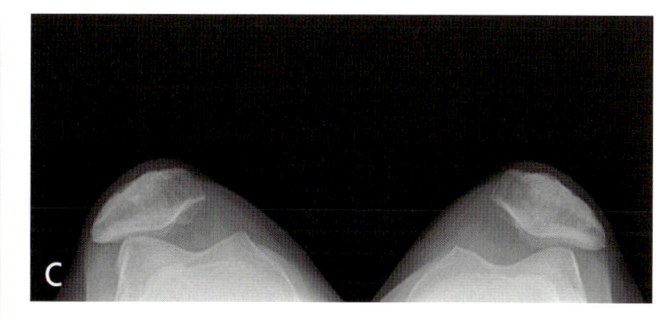

Figure 1 Preoperative radiographs obtained before realignment for patellofemoral arthritis include 45° flexion weight-bearing PA (**A**), 30° lateral (**B**), and Merchant (**C**) views.

Dr. West or an immediate family member serves as a board member, owner, officer, or committee member of the American Academy of Orthopaedic Surgeons and the American Orthopaedic Society for Sports Medicine. Neither Dr. Lin nor any immediate family member has received anything of value from or owns stock in a commercial company or institution related directly or indirectly to the subject of this chapter.

Section 1: Sports Medicine

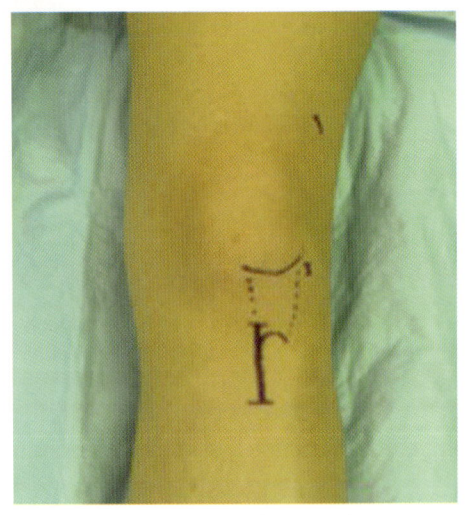

Figure 2 Preoperative photograph shows the standard incisions used for patellofemoral realignment, including a superolateral and an inferolateral portal site marked on the skin.

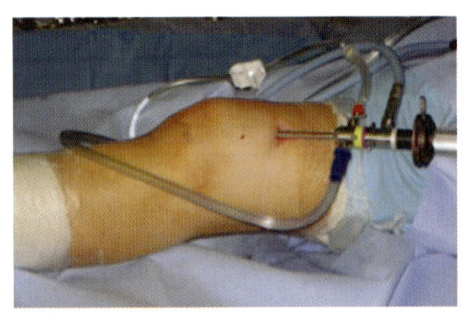

Figure 3 The 70° arthroscope is shown in the superolateral portal.

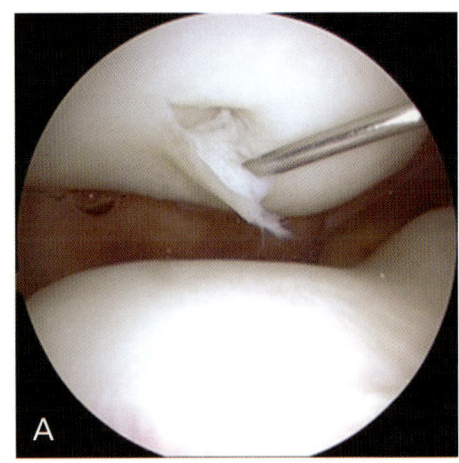

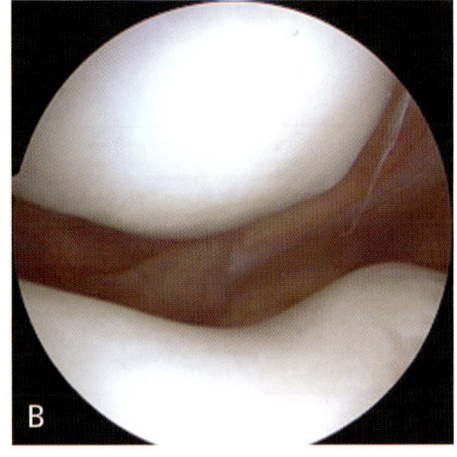

Figure 4 Arthroscopic views from the superolateral portal with the 70° arthroscope of a patellar articular cartilage defect (**A**) and the proximal patella and trochlea (**B**).

Procedure
Room Setup/Patient Positioning
The affected extremity is identified and signed in the preoperative holding area. The patient is placed supine on the operating room table. All bony prominences are well padded. A tourniquet is applied, and the leg is prepped and draped. A surgical time-out is called at this time prior to the skin incision.

Video 21.1 Anterior Medialization via Tibial Tubercle Osteotomy. Albert Lin, MD; Robin West, MD (21 min)

Special Instrumentation/Equipment/Implants
The following instruments and equipment should be available for this procedure: 30° and 70° arthroscopes; a microsagittal saw; standard Steinmann pins and Kirschner wires (K-wires); 4.5- and 3.2-mm drill bits; and 4.5-mm fully threaded, standard AO cortical screws.

Surgical Technique
Examination Under Anesthesia
Under anesthesia, both knees are examined and compared. The range of motion, presence of effusion, generalized ligamentous examination, and patellar tracking/tilt/crepitus/glide are all documented. The patellar examination should be performed with the knee in full extension and then again at 20° to 30° of flexion (when the patella is engaged in the trochlea).

Landmarks, Portals, and Incisions
The landmarks for this procedure are the patella, the patellar tendon attachment on the tibial tubercle, the Gerdy tubercle, and the tibial crest. The landmarks, arthroscopic portal sites, and skin incisions are marked on the skin (**Figure 2**).

The best viewing portal for the patellofemoral joint is the superolateral portal. A 70° arthroscope is used to assess the articular cartilage in the patellofemoral joint and evaluate patellofemoral tracking/glide/tilt.

Diagnostic Arthroscopy
The diagnostic arthroscopy typically involves two portals. The superolateral portal is used with the 70° arthroscope to evaluate the patellofemoral joint (**Figure 3**). This portal gives excellent visualization of the articular cartilage throughout the patellofemoral joint (**Figure 4**). Patellar tracking and glide can be examined from this portal. An approximation of correction in vivo can be estimated as well because patellar tracking can be visualized while the knee is taken through a range of motion and the patella is manually displaced medially. Confirmation that there is no contraindication to realignment of the tubercle can be determined at this time. Contraindications would include the presence of significant chondrosis of the proximal/medial patellar facet or trochlea that would result in significant overload following the tubercle osteotomy. The standard anterolateral portal is then used with the 30° arthroscope for completion of the full diagnostic examination of the knee.

Realignment
Initially, the diagnostic arthroscopy is performed to assess the articular cartilage status and confirm that there is no contraindication to the realignment. An open lateral release is performed only if the retinaculum is exceptionally taut (negative patellar tilt) and tilt cannot be passively restored to neutral (**Figure 5**). This release is performed through a 2 to 3-cm longitudinal incision from the midportion of the patella to just proximal to the superior pole. The release confirms that the retinaculum will not tether the patella after the tibial tubercle transfer. The release should not be too extensive and should be done only from the inferior pole to the superior pole, taking care not to injure the insertion of the vastus lateralis obliquus. A tourniquet set at 250 mm Hg is used only for the osteotomy portion of the case and released before wound closure.

The incision is made just medial to the tibial tubercle and is 5 to 7 cm in length, extending from 1 cm proximal to the patellar tendon insertion and extending distally. The fascia is exposed and then elevated off the lateral tibia to expose the anterolateral tibial crest and the Gerdy tubercle. The edges of the patellar tendon are identified. An Army-Navy retractor is placed under the patellar tendon. The osteotomy site is marked with a Bovie on the anteromedial tibial crest, starting at the medial edge of the patellar tendon

Chapter 21: Realignment for Patellofemoral Arthriis

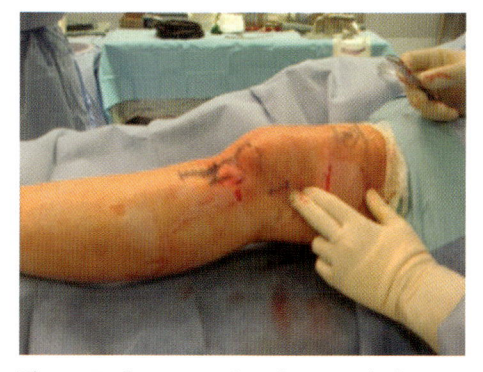

Figure 5 Intraoperative photograph shows the incision for the open lateral release.

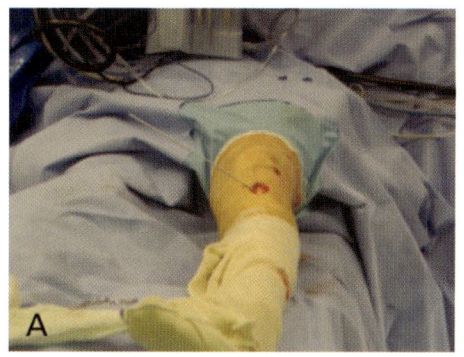

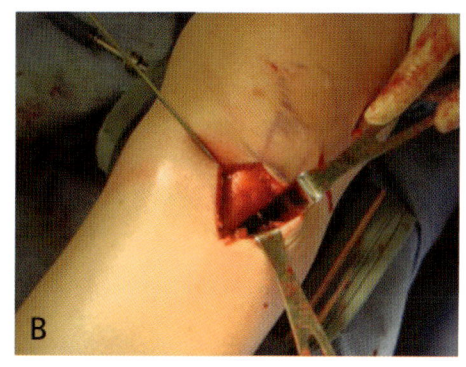

Figure 6 Intraoperative photographs show use of a Steinmann pin to mark the osteotomy angle for patellofemoral realignment. **A,** View from the end of the table with the Steinmann pin in place. **B,** Close-up view with the Steinmann pin exiting the lateral tibial cortex.

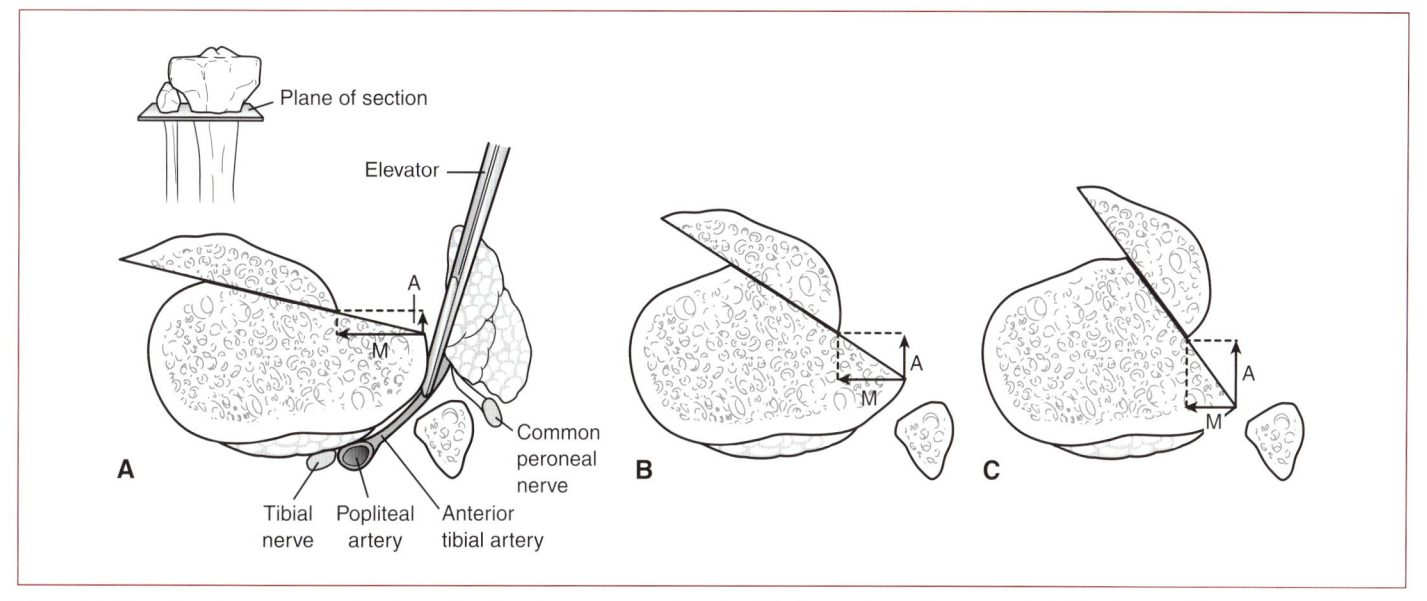

Figure 7 Drawing demonstrates the determination of osteotomy slope for tibial tubercle realignment. **A,** A flat (no-angle) osteotomy allows medialization of the tibial tubercle. The elevator protects the neurovascular bundle. **B,** A steeper cut provides equal anteriorization and medialization of the tibial tubercle. **C,** A very steep cut provides maximum anteriorization of the tibial tubercle with less medialization. A = distance of anteriorization, M = distance of medialization.

insertion and extending distally about 5 cm.

The osteotomy is performed freehand. With the tibial tubercle pointing directly at the ceiling (the foot is usually internally rotated), a Steinmann pin is placed from the medial tibial crest at the proximal portion of the osteotomy. The slope of the pin indicates the slope of the osteotomy (**Figure 6**). The slope is determined based on the amount of patellofemoral chondrosis and can be adjusted for more medialization or anteriorization (**Figure 7**). Once the slope of the osteotomy is determined, a microsagittal saw is used to perform the osteotomy (**Figure 8, A** and **B**).

The osteotomy is completed with a 1/4-inch curved osteotome proximally at the patellar tendon insertion in a transverse fashion (**Figure 8, C**). This maneuver helps to prevent fracture extension into the lateral plateau. The osteotomy is hinged distally and is completed only if patella alta is identified on the preoperative radiographs, using the modified Insall-Salvati and Caton-Deschamps ratios.

The tibial tubercle is then shifted anteromedially up to about 1 cm. Care is taken to make sure the tubercle has at least 50% contact with the underlying tibia to ensure good healing potential. The tuberosity is temporarily fixed with a K-wire and then permanently fixed with two 4.5-mm fully threaded screws, using the AO compression technique (**Figure 9**). It is helpful to countersink these screws to prevent painful, prominent hardware. A mini C-arm is used to confirm good position and length of the two screws before wound closure (**Figure 10**).

The fascial layer is closed in an interrupted fashion, followed by a subcutaneous closure and then a subcuticular closure. Care is taken to provide hemostasis after releasing the tourniquet and before wound closure. A drain is not routinely used.

Complications

Complications specific to the procedure include detachment of the vastus lateralis obliquus and resultant quadriceps weakness, dysfunction, and/or medial patellar instability from overzealous lateral release, injury to the patella tendon, and iatrogenic tibial metaphyseal fracture. Other remaining complications are similar to those of any bony work around the knee, including infection, nonunion, malunion, compartment syndrome, arthrofibrosis, patella baja, and worsening or no improvement in symptoms.[1,4]

Postoperative Care and Rehabilitation

Our patients are immediately fully weight bearing with crutches and a brace locked in full extension. Formal radiographs are

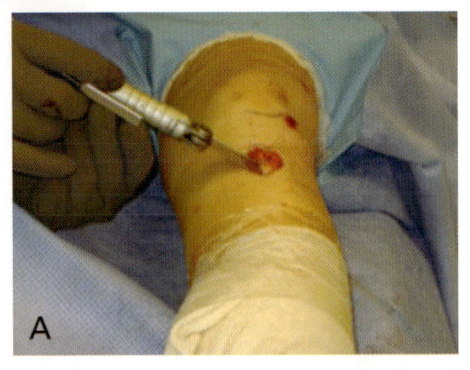

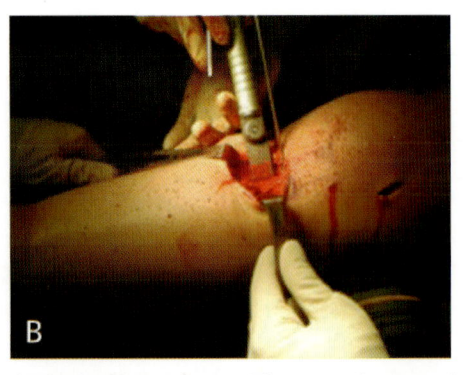

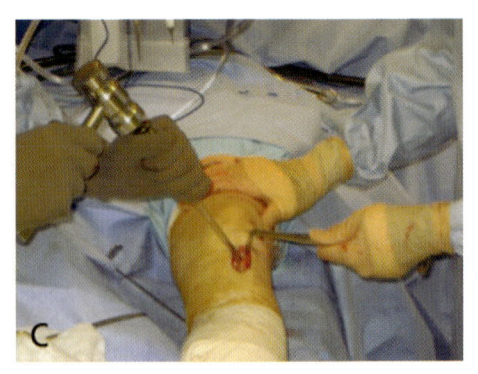

Figure 8 Intraoperative photographs show the tibial tubercle osteotomy. The sagittal saw angle from the end of the table (**A**) and from the side (**B**). **C**, The proximal transverse cut is completed under the patella with the 1/4-inch curved osteotome.

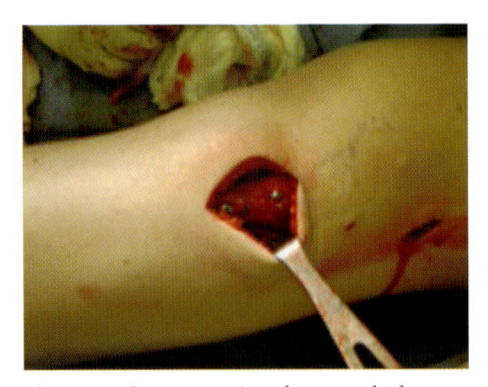

Figure 9 Intraoperative photograph shows the two bicortical screws in place.

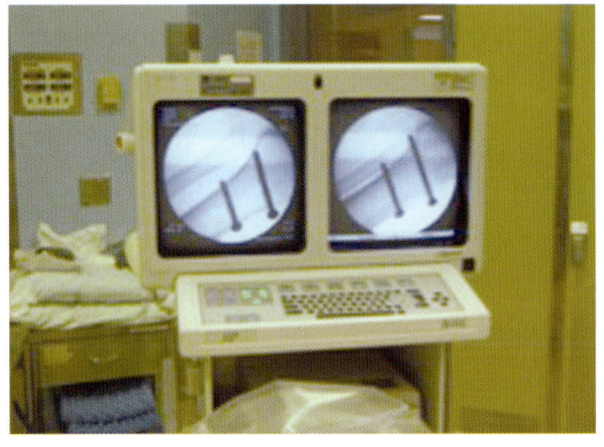

Figure 10 The C-arm is used to check the lengths of the screws and confirm that the osteotomy has not extended distally.

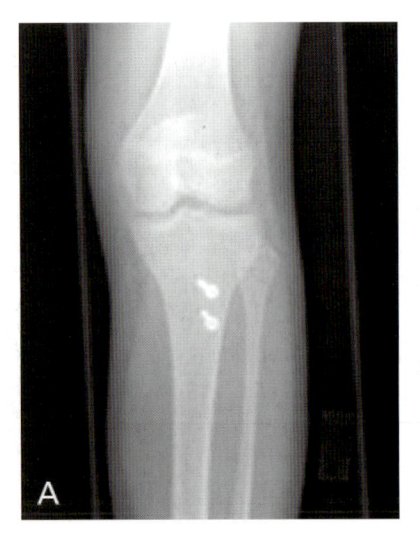

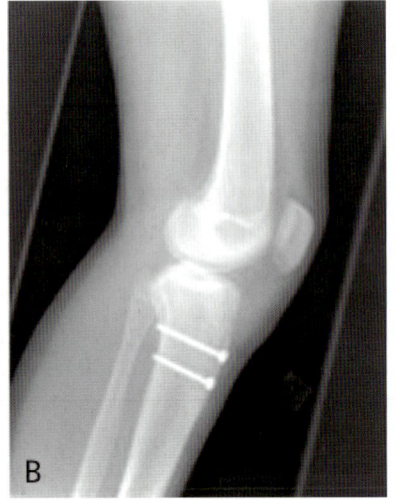

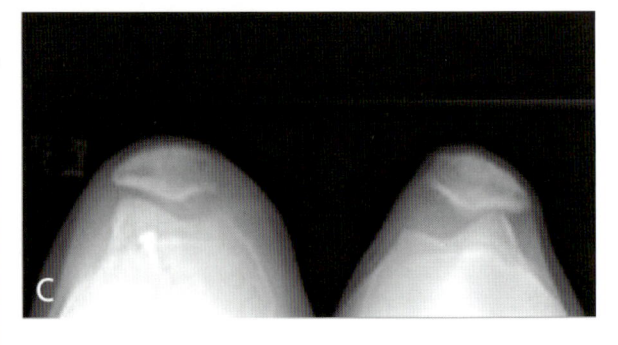

Figure 11 Postoperative non–weight-bearing AP (**A**), lateral (**B**), and Merchant (**C**) radiographs of the same patient shown in Figure 1.

obtained at the first postoperative visit to confirm screw lengths and the position of the osteotomy as well as patellar tilt and subluxation (**Figure 11**). The brace is unlocked at 6 weeks or when the osteotomy is radiographically healed and is discontinued when the patient has excellent quadriceps control. A continuous passive motion machine is started within a few days after surgery, and heel slides are allowed to 90° of knee flexion until the osteotomy is healed. Physical therapy is started immediately to help regain quadriceps control and patellar mobility, control swelling, and begin a comprehensive core stabilization program.

Once the osteotomy is healed, activity is progressed from strengthening to functional training and jogging and finally return to sports without restrictions at 4 to 5 months postoperatively.

Pearls
- The lateral release is done in conjunction with the tibial tubercle transfer to help "balance" the soft tissues. Overzealous lateral release can lead to poor quadriceps function, medial patellar instability, and increased lateral laxity. The surgeon must be sure to preserve the vastus lateralis obliquus insertion.
- Fracture at the osteotomy site can occur in patients who have osteoporosis or use nicotine.
- The osteotomy is completed proximally with a 1/4-inch curved osteotome to avoid fracture extension into the lateral plateau.
- The screws are countersunk to avoid prominent, painful hardware.
- To aid in healing, 50% contact between the tubercle and the tibia is maintained after the tubercle transfer.
- Full weight bearing is allowed postoperatively only with the brace locked in full extension to avoid excessive force across the osteotomy site.

References

1. Carofino BC, Fulkerson JP: Anteromedialization of the tibial tubercle for patellofemoral arthritis in patients > 50 years. *J Knee Surg* 2008;21(2):101-105.
2. Dejour H, Walch G, Nove-Josserand L, Guier C: Factors of patellar instability: An anatomic radiographic study. *Knee Surg Sports Traumatol Arthrosc* 1994;2(1):19-26.
3. Fithian DC, Paxton EW, Stone ML, et al: Epidemiology and natural history of acute patellar dislocation. *Am J Sports Med* 2004;32(5):1114-1121.
4. Buuck DA, Fulkerson JP: Anteromedialization of the tibial tubercle: A 4 to 12 year follow-up. *Oper Tech Sports Med* 2000;8:131-137.
5. Fulkerson JP, Becker GJ, Meaney JA, Miranda M, Folcik MA: Anteromedial tibial tubercle transfer without bone graft. *Am J Sports Med* 1990;18(5):490-496, discussion 496-497.
6. Ramappa AJ, Apreleva M, Harrold FR, Fitzgibbons PG, Wilson DR, Gill TJ: The effects of medialization and anteromedialization of the tibial tubercle on patellofemoral mechanics and kinematics. *Am J Sports Med* 2006;34(5):749-756.
7. Kuroda R, Kambic H, Valdevit A, Andrish JT: Articular cartilage contact pressure after tibial tuberosity transfer: A cadaveric study. *Am J Sports Med* 2001;29(4):403-409.
8. Schoettle PB, Zanetti M, Seifert B, Pfirrmann CW, Fucentese SF, Romero J: The tibial tuberosity-trochlear groove distance: A comparative study between CT and MRI scanning. *Knee* 2006;13(1):26-31.

Chapter 22

Surgical Treatment of Traumatic Quadriceps and Patellar Tendon Injuries of the Knee

Patrick Schottel, MD   Keith R. Reinhardt, MD   Gregory S. DiFelice, MD   Anil S. Ranawat, MD

Introduction

Ruptures of the extensor mechanism of the knee are debilitating injuries that typically require surgery and prolonged physical therapy. The severity of this injury is due in part to the central role that knee extension plays in the activities of daily living. Anatomically, the knee extensor mechanism is composed of four principal components: the quadriceps femoris muscles (rectus femoris, vastus lateralis, vastus medialis, vastus intermedius), the quadriceps tendon, the patella, and the patellar tendon (**Figure 1**). The tendinous portions of the quadriceps muscles typically coalesce into the quadriceps tendon 3 cm proximal to the superior pole of the patella.[1] From the patellar insertion, the anteriormost rectus femoris component of the quadriceps tendon continues over the anterior surface of the patella, joining the patellar tendon at the inferior patellar pole. The patellar tendon subsequently inserts into the tibial tubercle.

Patellar fractures are the most common cause of extensor mechanism failure.[2] Quadriceps and patellar tendon injuries occur less frequently. The infrequency of tendinous rupture is due in part to the relative strength of the tendons. Biomechanical studies have estimated that the force required to disrupt the knee extensor mechanism is approximately 17.5 times body weight.[3] Therefore, when nondirect traumatic tendinous rupture does occur, it is likely to occur through an area of pathologic change. Conditions known to predispose patients to tendon rupture include end-stage renal disease, diabetes mellitus, rheumatoid arthritis, gout, obesity, hyperparathyroidism, systemic lupus erythematosus, systemic steroid use, infection, and repetitive microtrauma. Reports vary, but the incidence of such systemic conditions has been reported to be as high as 70% in cases of bilateral quadriceps tendon ruptures and 20% in unilateral ruptures.[4]

In addition to predisposing systemic diseases, the vascular density of the tendon may be another component explaining the location and reason for tendon failure. Using cadaver models, Yepes et al[5] showed that the poorest area of tendinous blood supply was a zone 1 to 2 cm from the patellar insertion site of the quadriceps tendon. This finding corroborates the observation that most quadriceps tendon ruptures occur within 2 cm of the superior patellar pole. The same study also reported that the most vascular zone was the area of tendon within 1 cm of the superior patellar pole.

Finally, it is important to recognize that quadriceps and patellar tendon ruptures have a characteristic demographic presentation. Siwek and Rao[6] first reported this relationship after studying nearly a

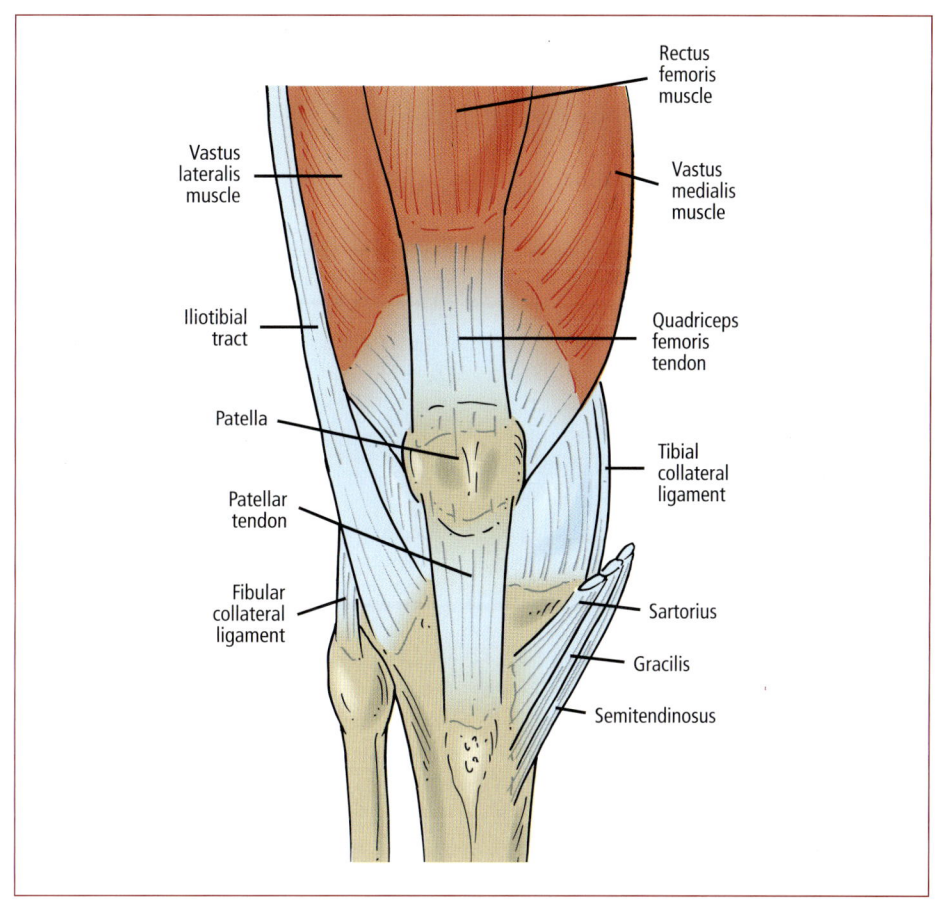

Figure 1 Illustration shows the musculoskeletal anatomy of the knee, including the four normal components of the knee extensor mechanism: the quadriceps femoris muscles, the quadriceps tendon, the patella, and the patellar tendon.

Dr. DiFelice or an immediate family member is a member of a speakers' bureau or has made paid presentations on behalf of Arthrex and serves as a paid consultant to or is an employee of Arthrex. Dr. Ranawat or an immediate family member has received royalties from DePuy and Stryker; is a member of a speakers' bureau or has made paid presentations on behalf of Mako, Conformis, NOVA Surgical, DePuy, and Stryker; serves as a paid consultant to or is an employee of Mako, DePuy, and Stryker; serves as an unpaid consultant to Conformis; has stock or stock options held in Conformis and NOVA Surgical; has received research or institutional support from Mako, DePuy, and Stryker; has received nonincome support (such as equipment or services), commercially derived honoraria, or other non–research-related funding (such as paid travel) from DePuy and Stryker; and serves as a board member, owner, officer, or committee member of the Eastern Orthopaedic Association. Neither of the following authors nor any immediate family member has received anything of value from or has stock or stock options held in a commercial company or institution related directly or indirectly to the subject of this chapter: Dr. Schottel and Dr. Reinhardt.

century's worth of literature. They noted that most quadriceps tendon ruptures occurred in patients who were older than 40 years, whereas most patellar tendon ruptures occurred in patients younger than 40 years.

Patient Selection
Complete quadriceps and patellar tendon ruptures usually exhibit the classic clinical triad of pain, inability to perform a straight-leg raise due to a lack of active knee extension, and a palpable suprapatellar or infrapatellar defect. Additionally, patients typically present with a large knee effusion and ecchymosis.

Complete tendon tears require surgical repair for optimal functional results. Although randomized trials comparing surgical and nonsurgical treatment have not been performed, little debate exists regarding the superiority of surgical repair versus nonsurgical management for complete tears.

The timing of surgical repair also has been shown to be important. Siwek and Rao[6] observed that extensor mechanism rupture repairs performed more than 2 weeks after injury were associated with increased surgical complexity and led to more unsatisfactory results, as determined by knee range of motion (ROM) and quadriceps strength. Based on these observations, they advocated early surgical repair. Although other studies have attempted to define the optimal timing of surgery or whether early repair does, in fact, lead to better clinical outcomes, no clear consensus has yet been reached.[4,6-8] Nonetheless, our recommendation and practice are to repair all extensor mechanism ruptures in an acute fashion—within 3 weeks, when possible.

Numerous relative contraindications exist for the tendinous repair of the extensor mechanism. Although each particular clinical scenario needs to be assessed carefully by the surgeon, we believe that nonsurgical management should be strongly considered for nonambulatory patients and for patients with significant medical comorbidities; compromised soft tissues around the knee as a result of infection, trauma, or radiation; a known history of noncompliance with rehabilitation; chronic irreparable tears; and insignificant partial tears. Surgical repair is almost always advocated for complete tears, but one of the few instances in which nonsurgical treatment is acceptable is in cases of incomplete extensor mechanism tendon tears. Incomplete tears are diagnosed when patients retain active knee extension against gravity while supine but demonstrate compromised extension against resistance while in a seated position. Although these patients typically present with an effusion, they lack the large palpable tendinous defect and the common radiographic findings of patella baja or patella alta that are seen in patients with complete tears. A common treatment regimen for a partial tear includes elevation, ice, compression, anti-inflammatory medications, and brace immobilization with the knee locked in extension, along with progressive ROM and strengthening exercises.

Preoperative Imaging
In addition to the clinical examination and patient history, imaging studies are important not only in confirming the diagnosis of an extensor mechanism tendon rupture but also in evaluating for concomitant injuries. Common imaging modalities include plain radiography, ultrasonography, and MRI.

Radiographs should be the initial imaging modality for a patient presenting with knee pain. At a minimum, an AP and lateral view should be obtained, with additional imaging such as Merchant and oblique views, depending on the clinical scenario. Characteristic findings on plain radiographs in patients with quadriceps tendon tears include patella baja,

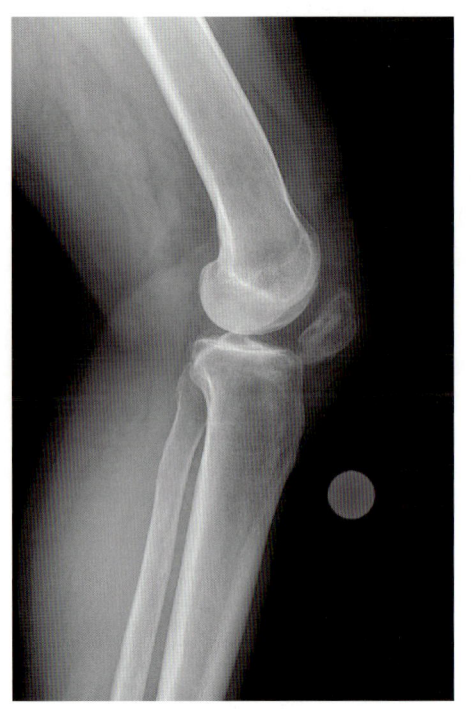

Figure 2 Lateral radiograph of the right knee of a patient with a rupture of the quadriceps tendon. The patella is below the Blumensaat line, indicating patella baja.

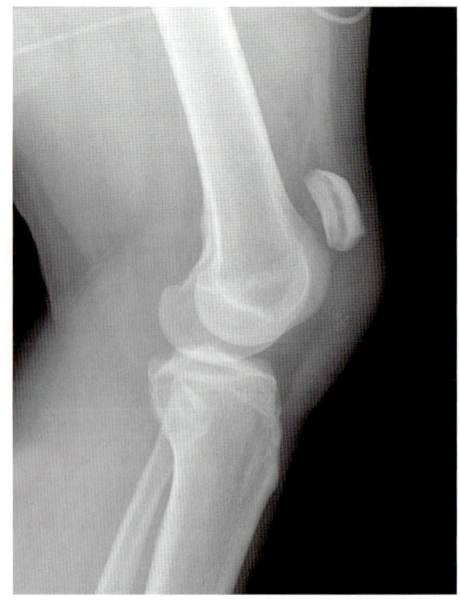

Figure 3 Lateral radiograph of the left knee of a patient with an acute rupture of the patellar tendon. The image clearly demonstrates patella alta, with the entire patella above the Blumensaat line.

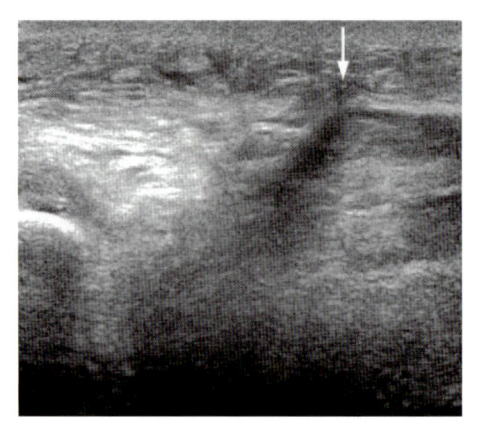

Figure 4 Sagittal ultrasonographic image of a ruptured quadriceps tendon. The anechoic shadow within the substance of the tendon (arrow) represents the rupture.

interruption of the quadriceps tendon soft-tissue shadow, and a suprapatellar soft-tissue mass (**Figure 2**). In cases of patellar tendon rupture, patella alta is the most characteristic radiographic finding. Patella alta can be identified by the patella being located superior to the Blumensaat line on the lateral image or as defined by the Insall-Salvati ratio (**Figure 3**).

Ultrasonography is another means of diagnosing a quadriceps or patellar tendon tear. Although this modality is operator dependent, it is an expeditious and relatively inexpensive way to determine the location and completeness of the tear, as judged by the presence and extent of an anechoic shadow (**Figure 4**).

MRI is used not only to accurately diagnose difficult to evaluate cases, but also

Chapter 22: Surgical Treatment of Traumatic Quadriceps and Patellar Tendon Injuries of the Knee

to identify concomitant injuries. A recent study examining extensor mechanism ruptures and concomitant knee injuries using MRI found that patients with a patellar tendon rupture had a 30% incidence of an associated injury and those with a quadriceps tendon rupture had a 10% incidence of a concomitant knee injury, with anterior cruciate ligament and medial meniscus tears being the most common findings.[9] Although MRI is expensive and may potentially delay treatment, its ability to confirm a clinical diagnosis and provide additional anatomic information, facilitating the formulation of a more accurate surgical plan and the identification of concomitant injury, can be invaluable (**Figure 5**).

Video 22.1 Repair of Injuries to the Extensor Mechanism: Quadriceps and Patellar Tendons. Spero G. Karas, MD; Richard J. Hawkins, MD, FRCSC; J. Richard Steadman, MD (10 min)

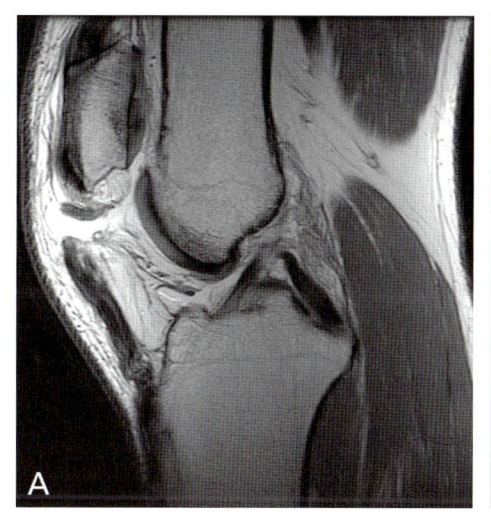

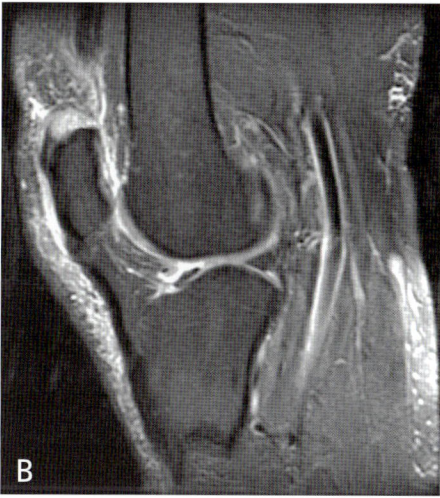

Figure 5 Extensor mechanism injuries of the knee. **A**, Sagittal T1-weighted MRI demonstrates an acute patellar tendon rupture. **B**, Sagittal fluid-sensitive, fat-suppressed MRI demonstrates an acute quadriceps tendon tear.

Procedure
Surgical Technique
Under regional anesthesia, the patient is positioned supine with a bump under the hip of the surgical extremity. A tourniquet is placed as proximal on the surgical extremity as possible, and the patient is prepared and draped in the usual sterile fashion. An examination under anesthesia is conducted to evaluate for soft-tissue injuries or confirm the presence and extent of such injuries identified in preoperative imaging. Antibiotic administration is confirmed, and the tourniquet is inflated after exsanguination of the extremity.

Quadriceps Tendon Repair
Numerous methods have been described for the repair of quadriceps tendon tears. Although the location, extent, and chronicity of the tear may dictate the use of one method over another, the most commonly used technique is a transosseous tunnel technique. It involves placing interlocking sutures through the proximal tendon and then passing them through longitudinal transosseous patellar drill holes and subsequently tying them over a patellar bone bridge (**Figure 6**). This method is best used for tears that occur at or near the osteotendinous junction. An end-to-end primary repair with interrupted nonabsorbable sutures may be used for midsubstance tears with sufficient proximal and distal tendon remaining. Variations of these two techniques, including the use of suture anchors or reinforcement of the repair with a partial-thickness turndown of the quadriceps tendon, known as the Scuderi technique, have been described in the literature.[8,10] This section describes our preferred surgical technique for repair using transosseous tunnels.

A midline longitudinal skin incision is made starting 5 cm proximal to the superior border of the patella and extending to the inferior pole of the patella distally. The incision is subsequently carried down through the subcutaneous tissue until the extensor mechanism is identified, with close attention paid to creating full-thickness skin flaps during the approach. Depending on the length of time between the injury and surgery, either a hematoma or loosely organized scar tissue will be encountered. This is removed, followed by copious wound irrigation (**Figure 7, A**). The tourniquet is deflated to allow full mobilization of the quadriceps, and hemostasis is subsequently achieved with the use of electrocautery.

Attention is then turned to the proximal tendon segment, where any degenerative

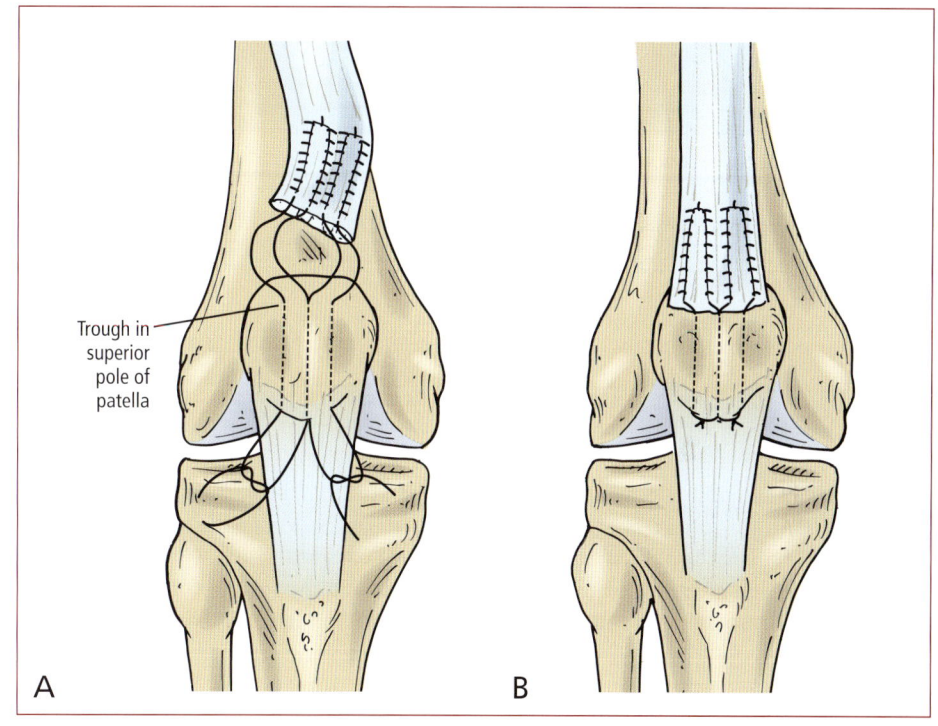

Figure 6 Illustrations show acute quadriceps tendon repair. **A**, The four suture limbs of the Krackow stitch are passed through the three transosseous drill holes. **B**, The suture limbs are tied together over the patellar bone bridge.

© 2013 American Academy of Orthopaedic Surgeons

Section 1: Sports Medicine

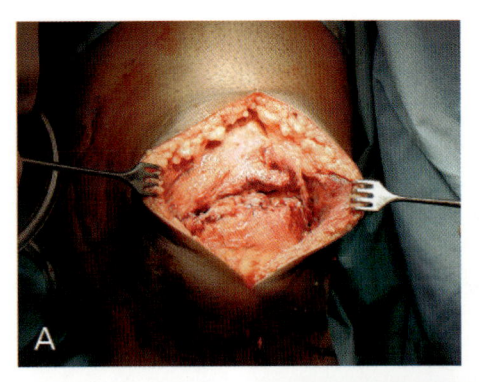

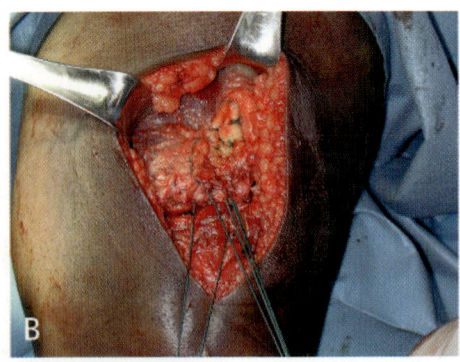

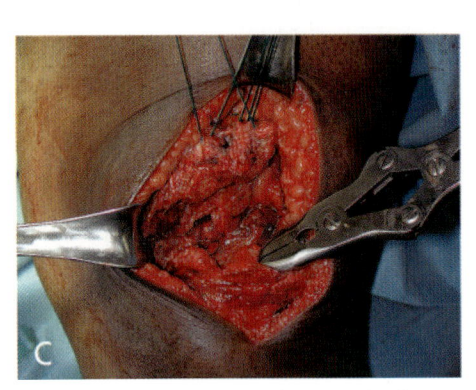

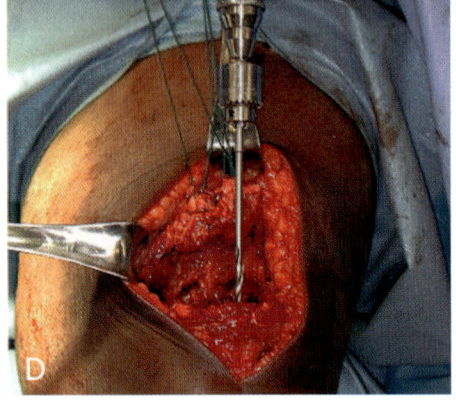

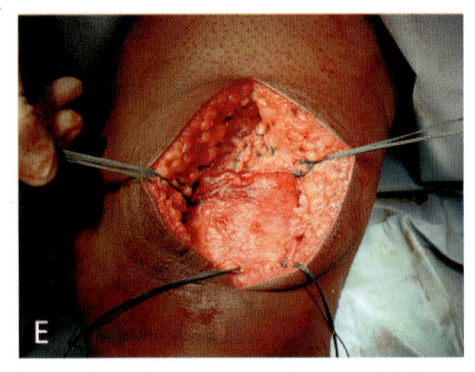

Figure 7 Intraoperative photographs demonstrate the surgical repair of an acute quadriceps tendon rupture. **A,** Exposure of the tear. **B,** The quadriceps tendon is mobilized after two sutures are placed in the tendon using a Krackow stitch. **C,** Débridement of the superior patellar pole. **D,** Creation of the transosseous patellar tunnels using a 2.5-mm drill. Careful attention is paid to drill orientation to avoid iatrogenically violating the articular cartilage. **E,** Medial and lateral retinaculum repair.

tendon is débrided, and all adhesions to the surrounding soft tissues are disrupted. Two No. 5 nonabsorbable sutures are then placed using a Krackow stitch through the full-thickness medial and lateral aspects of the tendon. With the placement of these two sutures, the quadriceps tendon is captured and mobilized (**Figure 7, B**). It is critical to maximize the number of sutures across the tendon. In certain cases, three sutures can be used, but this should not be done if it compromises the vascular integrity of the tendon. At this point, the superior pole of the patella is débrided of any remaining tendon, and a bleeding cancellous bone bed is created with a burr, curet, or rongeur (**Figure 7, C**). A 2.5-mm drill is used to create medial, middle, and lateral longitudinal holes through the patella (**Figure 7, D**). It is best to err in drilling in an anterior and midline trajectory to avoid iatrogenic patellar cartilage damage. Next, a suture passer is used to pull the four suture limbs through the bone tunnels. At this point, with the knee in full extension and the patella maximally elevated superiorly with a bone clamp, the sutures are tied over the patellar bone bridges (**Figure 7, E**).

Following the tendon repair, attention is turned to the medial and lateral retinaculum. Tears are identified and closed using No. 2 nonabsorbable sutures, using a figure-of-8 stitch technique. The knee is taken through a gentle ROM from 0° to 90° to assess the tension on the repair. A surgical drain is placed subfascially and attention then is turned toward the superficial closure. After irrigation of the wound, interrupted 0 and 2-0 absorbable sutures are used for the closure of the deep fascia and superficial subcutaneous tissue. Finally, the skin is closed with interrupted 3-0 nylon sutures and covered with a sterile dressing. A hinged knee brace, locked in extension, is then fitted to the surgical extremity.

Acute Patellar Tendon Repair

As with a quadriceps tendon tear, the location and chronicity of a patellar tendon rupture dictates the appropriate surgical procedure. The most commonly encountered clinical scenario is an acute disruption within the vicinity of the patella–patellar tendon junction. These injuries typically are repaired with a locking stitch through the tendinous component that is then passed through longitudinal transosseous patellar drill holes and tied over a patellar bone bridge proximally (**Figure 8**).

Other infrequently encountered acute injuries include midsubstance and distal patellar tendon tears. Distal disruptions in proximity to the tibial tubercle attachment are repaired with locking sutures inserted through the proximal portion of the tendon and then passed through tibial drill holes and tied. Midsubstance tears typically are repaired by direct reopposition of the torn edges. For acute midsubstance tears that cannot be reliably repaired primarily, however, augmentation using semitendinosis autograft or a tendinous allograft can be performed. This technique involves passing the tendon graft through horizontal tibial and patellar drill holes and suturing the graft to itself as well as to the remnants of the native patellar tendon. In cases of deficient remaining native tendon and a likely tenuous soft-tissue graft repair, reconstruction is accomplished using a chronic tear repair technique, described in the next section. Another uncommon injury that deserves mention is an avulsion fracture of the nonarticulating inferior pole of the patella. When comminuted, these frac-

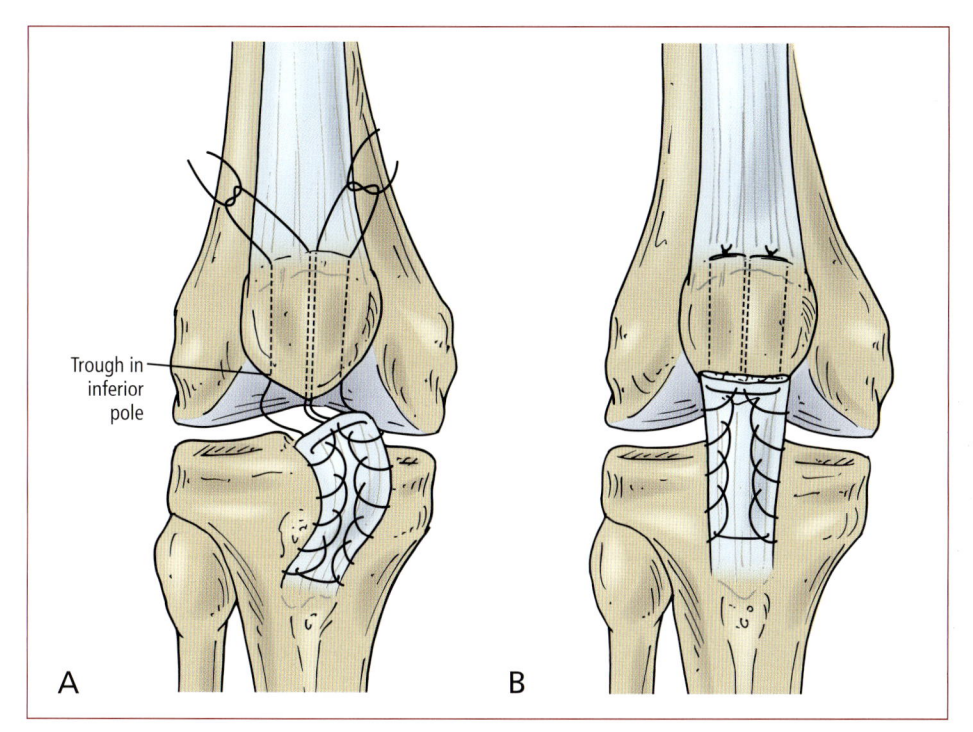

Figure 8 Illustrations demonstrate acute patellar tendon repair. **A,** The four suture limbs are passed through the three transosseous drill holes. **B,** The sutures are tied over the patellar bone bridge, reapproximating the torn superior portion of the patellar tendon with the patella.

tures are typically treated by resection of the distal fragments. The patellar tendon is subsequently reattached in a manner similar to that used for acute disruptions, which is described later. In cases of minimal comminution and/or nonosteoporotic bone, Veselko and Kastelec[11] have shown promising outcomes with open reduction and internal fixation using a basket plate and screws.

At this time, we prefer to perform internal fixation if the quality and amount of bone are adequate for reliable fixation. If significant osteoporosis and comminution are present, however, then an osteotendinous repair can be performed, with close attention paid to the avoiding subsequent patella baja. The following paragraphs describe our preferred surgical technique for acute patellar tendon tears at the proximal osteotendinous junction.

Patients are identified, positioned, and prepared in a fashion similar to that used for the quadriceps rupture repair procedure discussed previously. Likewise, an examination under anesthesia is conducted, and perioperative antibiotics are administered. The tourniquet is inflated, and a midline longitudinal skin incision is made starting 2 cm proximal to the superior border of the patella and extending distally to the tibial tubercle. The incision is carried down sharply through the subcutaneous tissue until the patella and the patellar tendon rupture are identified. If the paratenon is identified, it is preserved for possible repair later. Once the exposure is complete, the tourniquet is deflated to allow full mobilization of the extensor mechanism, and hemostasis is obtained. It should be noted, however, that some surgeons keep the tourniquet on until the sutures have been passed through the patellar drill holes. This is acceptable as long as the tourniquet is deflated before tensioning of the repair.

At this point, the inferior pole of the patella is addressed. It is débrided of any remaining tendon until a bed of bleeding cancellous bone is obtained. This can be accomplished with either a burr drill or curet. Two No. 5 nonabsorbable sutures are sewn using a Krackow stitch through the full-thickness medial and lateral aspects of the patellar tendon. As stated previously, it is critical to maximize the number of sutures across the tendon. In certain cases, three sutures can be used, but not at the expense of compromising the tendon. A 2.5-mm drill then is used to create medial, middle, and lateral longitudinal tunnels through the patella (**Figure 9, A**). A suture passer is used to pull the suture ends through the bone tunnels proximally (**Figure 9, B**). The sutures are then tied to each other over bone bridges with the knee in full extension (**Figure 9, C**).

Following the tendon repair, attention is turned to any medial or lateral retinaculum tears as well as an augmentation suture. First, if any retinaculum tears are present, they are closed with No. 2 nonabsorbable sutures using a figure-of-8 technique. If a question exists as to the patient's compliance or the stability of the repair, an angiocatheter is used to pass a No. 5 nonabsorbable suture through the distal quadriceps muscle and tendon immediately proximal to the superior pole of the patella. This suture is tied in a figure-of-8 pattern through a tibial drill hole using a 2.5-mm drill bit with the knee in 45° of flexion (**Figure 9, D**). The purpose of this augmentation suture is to take tension off the repair by preventing patella alta until the tendon has healed.

Finally, the knee is taken through a gentle ROM to assess tension on the repair. A surgical drain is placed subfascially, and the wound is closed in a fashion similar to that used in a quadriceps tendon rupture repair, using deep interrupted 0 absorbable sutures for fascial closure, followed by interrupted 2-0 absorbable sutures for the superficial subcutaneous tissue and interrupted 3-0 nylon sutures for skin closure. A sterile dressing is applied and a hinged knee brace, locked in extension, is fitted to the surgical extremity.

Chronic Quadriceps and Patellar Tendon Repairs

Chronic quadriceps and patellar tendon ruptures or failed repairs are rare but disabling injuries that represent a technically difficult treatment dilemma for the orthopaedic surgeon. The difficulty of these repairs is due to a combination of factors, including retraction of the patella, adhesions of the extensor mechanism to the surrounding tissue, quadriceps atrophy, and, most importantly, a relative paucity of native tendon to use for the repair. Numerous surgical techniques have been described in the literature to overcome these potential obstacles, such as augmentation with wire or additional nonabsorbable sutures when the revision repair is tenuous, or a V-Y quadricepsplasty when muscular contraction prevents adequate tissue apposition. More advanced techniques use autograft or allograft for reconstruction of the deficient suprapatellar or infrapatellar tendon. Two of the more common autograft options for deficient patellar tendons are contralateral bone–patellar tendon–bone autograft with double-wire loop reinforcement or autologous ipsilateral semitendinosus and/or gracilis tendon transfers with or without wire augmentation.[12-15] Various reconstruc-

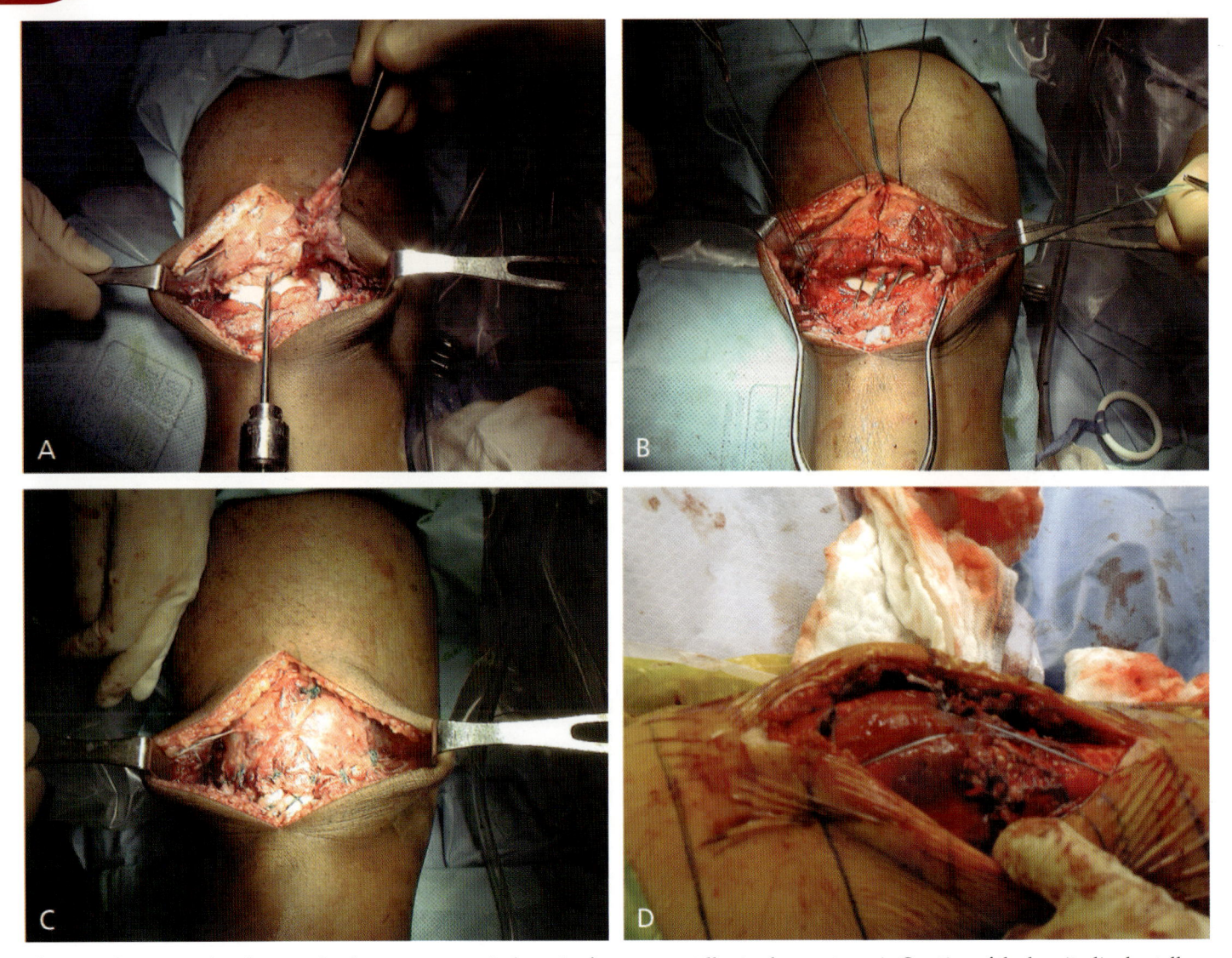

Figure 9 Intraoperative photographs demonstrate surgical repair of an acute patellar tendon rupture. **A,** Creation of the longitudinal patellar tunnels. **B,** Passage of the patellar tendon sutures. It is important to ensure that the tourniquet is deflated before tightening the repair, to facilitate adequate mobilization of the proximal portion of the knee extensor mechanism. **C,** Completed repair of the patellar tendon and retinaculum. **D,** Figure-of-8 augmentation suture. The suture is passed around the superior patellar pole and through a tibial drill hole before tightening to take tension off the patellar tendon repair.

tion techniques using allograft also have been described. Most commonly, Achilles tendon–bone allograft is used in various ways, with the bone plug secured into the patella or proximal tibia and the allograft tendon used to reconstruct the patellar or quadriceps tendons.[16-18] Unfortunately, no consensus currently exists among surgeons regarding the optimal method of reconstruction. Thus, the choice of an autograft, allograft, or synthetic material is one the surgeon needs to make based on the clinical scenario, graft availability, and surgical experience. The following paragraphs describe our preferred method for the repair of chronic patellar tendon ruptures.

Exposure of the patella and patellar tendon is completed in a fashion identical to that described previously for acute patellar tendon rupture repair. After hemostasis is achieved, the extensive scar and adhesions that typically are present are débrided and lysed. If adequate tendon remains, a repair similar to that described previously for acute patellar tendon rupture should be attempted. If the native tendon is in any way deficient, however, resulting in patella baja and/or a perceived tenuous repair, then Achilles allograft is used (**Figure 10**). To prepare the sites for allograft insertion, the inferior pole of the patella first is débrided until a bleeding cancellous bone bed is obtained. Next, an anterior cruciate ligament tibial tunnel guide system is used to drill a 10-mm hole centrally in the inferior patellar pole to a depth of approximately 30 mm. Distally, a similar 10 × 30 mm drill hole is made just inferior to the tibial tubercle in the anterior cortex of the tibia. With the bone beds prepared, attention is turned to the Achilles allograft.

On a back table, the Achilles tendon–bone allograft is fashioned with an oscillating saw into a calcaneal bone plug of approximately 10 × 25 mm. This bone plug is placed within the inferior drill hole of the patella and secured with a 7 × 25 mm metal interference screw. Next, using a docking technique, the Achilles allograft is measured and whipstitched distally with a No. 2 nonabsorbable suture. The tendon is docked into the tibial drill hole and secured in place with a 9 × 30 mm absorbable interference screw. Of importance, fluoroscopic imaging is used intraoperatively during this step to determine the correct patellar height, as judged by the Insall-Salvati ratio. The target ratio should be determined by measurements made on preoperative radiographs of the contralateral knee (**Figure 11**). If any difficulty is encountered in correcting patella alta and restoring the

Chapter 22: Surgical Treatment of Traumatic Quadriceps and Patellar Tendon Injuries of the Knee

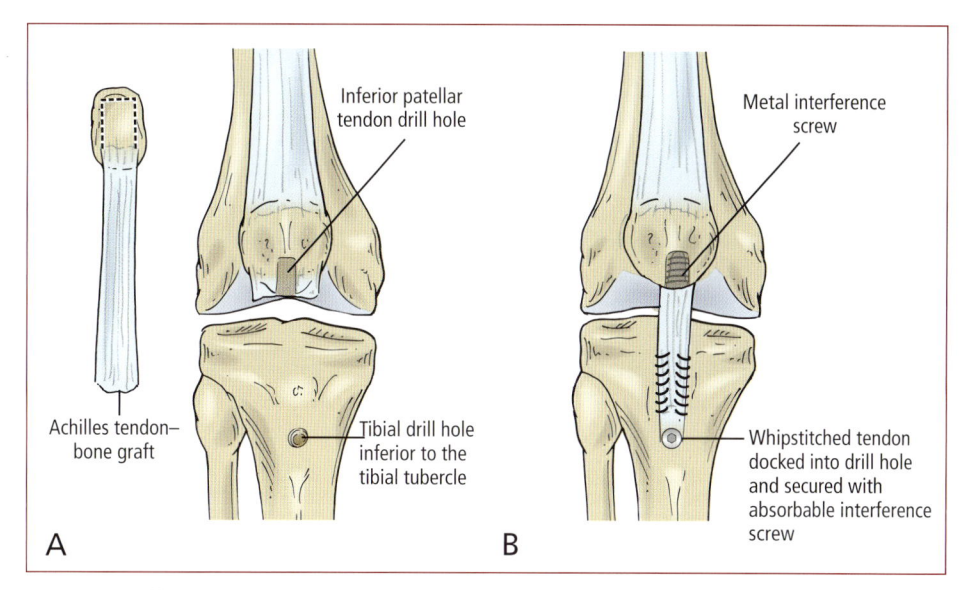

Figure 10 Illustrations demonstrate patellar tendon allograft reconstruction. **A,** The inferior patellar and tibial drill holes are made, and an Achilles tendon–bone allograft is prepared. **B,** The bone plug is fitted into the inferior patellar drill hole and secured with an interference screw. The distal tendinous portion of the graft is whipstitched and seated in the tibial drill hole using a docking technique.

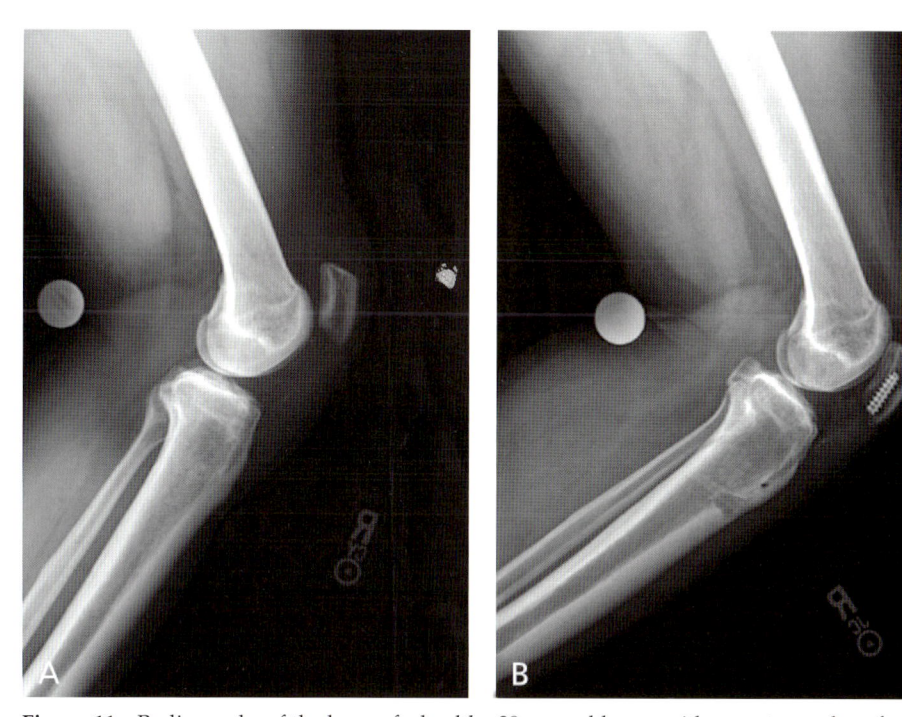

Figure 11 Radiographs of the knee of a healthy 39-year-old man with an extensor lag after a failed patellar tendon repair. **A,** Lateral view of the right knee demonstrates patella alta. **B,** Postoperative lateral radiograph of the right knee after a revision patellar tendon repair using an Achilles allograft. The patient regained all extension and a normal patellar height.

tibial drill hole with the knee in 45° of flexion. The wound is closed in a similar manner to that for an acute extensor mechanism rupture repair, covered in a sterile dressing, and placed in a hinged knee brace, which is locked in extension.

Extensor Mechanism Disruptions After Total Knee Arthroplasty

Rupture of the quadriceps or patellar tendon is an uncommon complication of total knee arthroplasty (TKA). The published incidence of such injuries in two large institutional case series is 0.1% for quadriceps tendon tears and 0.17% for patellar tendon ruptures.[19,20] Ruptures can occur intraoperatively as a result of a difficult exposure, immediately postoperatively if aggressive manipulation of a stiff extremity is undertaken, or as a delayed complication caused by component malalignment, leading to chronic degeneration of the tendon. Repairs of such ruptures occasionally can be accomplished with a technique similar to that described previously for direct repair with nonabsorbable sutures or via transosseous bone tunnels. For more complicated cases, however, autograft or allograft augmentation or complete allograft reconstruction has been described. One particular allograft reconstruction technique, first advocated by Emerson et al,[21] uses a quadriceps tendon–patella–patellar tendon–tibial tubercle graft. These repairs often are fraught with complications and should be attempted only by experienced adult reconstruction surgeons.

Complications

Complications are relatively uncommon in extensor mechanism surgery. The most frequently encountered complication is postoperative quadriceps atrophy and weakness. A relative paucity of data on this exists, but Siwek and Rao[6] noted that 75% of patients with an acutely repaired quadriceps tendon had 2 to 4 cm of persistent atrophy measured on follow-up examination. Rougraff et al[7] reported that 3 of 20 patients (15%) with unilateral quadriceps tendon repair had a more than 20% deficit in extensor peak torque function compared with the contralateral uninjured extremity in isokinetic testing. Additional common complications include quadriceps lag and anterior knee pain. Other more rare potential complications of extensor mechanism rupture repair include rerupture, wound infection or dehiscence, and patellar fracture. In a case series of 51 acutely repaired quadri-

native Insall-Salvati ratio secondary to quadriceps contracture, a Z-plasty or V-Y lengthening procedure can be performed (**Figure 12**). V-Y lengthening is achieved by making a full-thickness inverted V-shaped incision in the quadriceps with the distal portions of the incision ending approximately 1.3 cm proximal to the superior pole of the patella or, if used for quadriceps tendon rupture repair, 1 cm proximal to the site of tendon repair (**Figure 13, A and B**). Once adequate tendon length is gained, as determined by fluoroscopy, the incision is repaired with nonabsorbable sutures, resulting in the creation of the Y-shaped repair (**Figure 13, C**).

With proper patellar height confirmed, attention is turned to augmenting the repair. As in acute patellar tendon rupture repairs, an angiocatheter is used to pass a No. 5 nonabsorbable suture around the superior pole of the patella that then is tied in a figure-of-8 pattern through a

ceps tendon repairs, Konrath et al[4] reported one case of delayed wound healing and one case of rerupture. In addition, Rougraff et al[7] described 1 case of superficial wound infection and 2 reruptures in 53 cases of acutely repaired quadriceps tendon ruptures.

In our experience, patellar tendon repairs heal faster than quadriceps repairs but have a higher risk of developing patella baja. The patellar tendon rupture patients also typically report more knee stiffness, especially in cases of inferior patellar avulsion fracture repair. Quadriceps repair, on the other hand, typically involves tendon of a more degenerative nature, and repairs are at a higher risk of stretching out over time. Finally, although no case series are large enough from which to draw any meaningful conclusions, our experience is that chronic tendon reconstructions have a much higher rate of complications compared to acute repairs, including fixation failure and infection.

Postoperative Care and Rehabilitation

Postoperative care and rehabilitation should be tailored to each patient but typically include three phases of care: a period of immobilization, passive ROM, and active ROM with functional training. The immobilization phase begins immediately in the recovery room with adequate pain control, ice, therapy, and bracing. Subsequently, most patients are instructed for the first postoperative month to ambulate fully weight bearing with crutches and a hinged knee brace locked in extension at all times. Additionally, patients are encouraged to attempt quadriceps isometric exercises—with or without the help of electrical stimulation therapy—along with calf pumps and hamstring stretching. The length of the immobilization phase depends on numerous factors, including the nature of the injury and repair. For example, we typically start motion sooner in cases of inferior pole patellar fracture fixation, but we may be more conservative for noncompliant patients with quadriceps tendon rupture repairs.

The second phase of rehabilitation, the passive ROM phase, typically begins after the first postoperative month. In this phase, patients begin passive ROM and quadriceps strengthening exercises, including mini squats, wall slide mini squats, and hamstring curls out of the brace. All exercises are conducted with low weight and high repetitions. Although passive ROM is permitted in this stage, no isolated active knee extension is performed.

The third phase is the active ROM and functional training phase. Patients continue the previously described activities with the addition of active knee extension exercises, as well as unlocking of the knee brace and a focus on gait training and walking without a limp. After a month of these activities, the patient is weaned slowly from the crutches and brace. The patient is started with closed-chain quadriceps exercises, such as a stationary bike or elliptical trainer, and advanced to jogging, with the initiation of running, cutting, jumping, and pivoting maneuvers by the fifth postoperative month. From this point, therapy is advanced to weight strengthening, including exercises such as leg presses, squats, leg curls, and lunges, with a gradual return to previous activities under controlled conditions.

When considering whether it is safe for a patient to return to sports and full activities, five criteria must be met. They

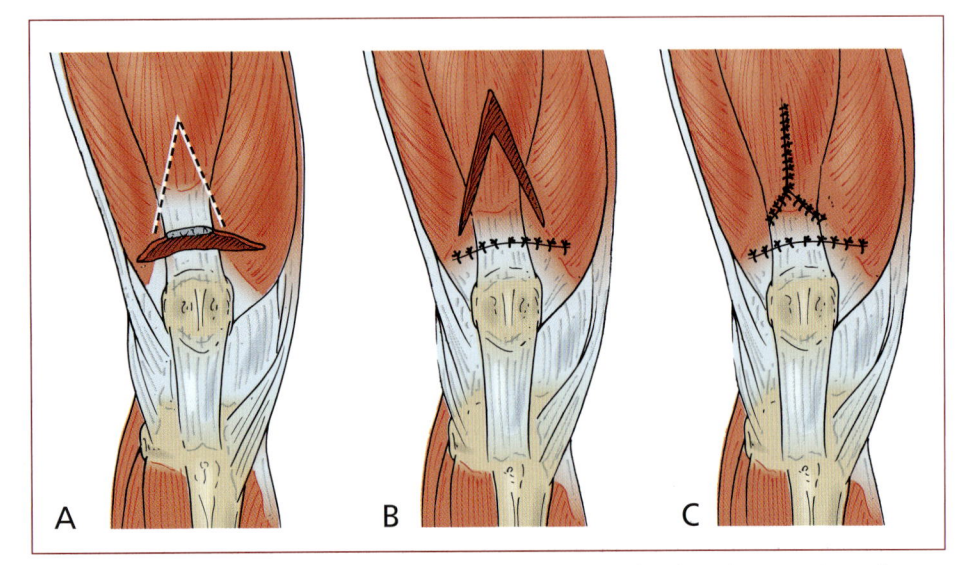

Figure 12 Illustrations show V-Y lengthening. **A,** An inverted V-shaped incision is made proximal to the traumatic rupture to allow mobilization of the quadriceps tendon. **B,** The quadriceps tear is repaired. **C,** The V-shaped incision is sutured closed, creating a Y-shaped repair.

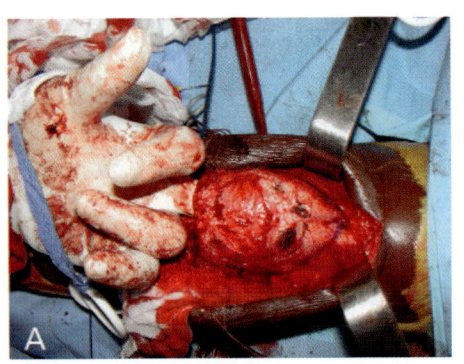

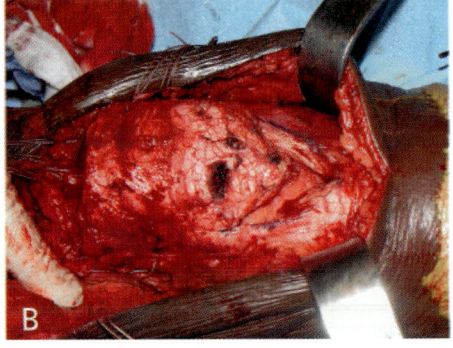

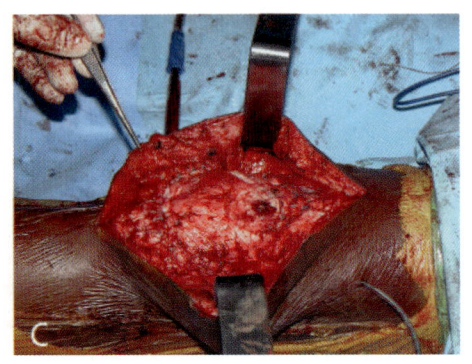

Figure 13 Intraoperative photographs demonstrate V-Y lengthening in a patellar tendon rupture with quadriceps contracture. **A,** The gap between the remaining patellar tendon and the patella is demonstrated. This gap is due to quadriceps contracture, resulting in the inability to adequately mobilize the proximal knee extensor mechanism component. **B,** A full-thickness inverted V-shaped incision is made in the quadriceps tendon approximately 1.3 cm cephalad to the superior patellar pole, allowing adequate mobilization of the proximal extensor mechanism. **C,** The completed patellar tendon repair.

include quadriceps strength greater than 90% of that of the contralateral leg; a one-leg hop test and vertical jump greater than 90% of that of the contralateral leg; demonstration of jogging, full-speed run, shuttle run, and figure-of-8 running without a limp; the ability to rise from a full squat; and no visible effusion or quadriceps atrophy.

Pearls

- An accurate diagnosis can be achieved with a thorough history and physical examination and radiographs.
- MRI is a useful adjunct only if the surgeon has a high index of suspicion for concomitant injury.
- Quadriceps tendon tears are more degenerative in nature than are patellar tendon ruptures and typically occur in patients who are older than 40 years.
- Inferior pole of the patella fractures with significant comminution are patellar tendon rupture variants and can be fixed in a similar manner; however, the surgeon must avoid creating patella baja.
- Although suture anchors are an option for repairs of quadriceps or patellar tendon ruptures, repairs using a transosseous technique are less technically demanding and have known long-term results compared with newer techniques.
- The strength of a repair depends on the number of sutures that cross the repair site. In some cases, three sutures can be used, but this should not be done if it compromises the vascular and structural integrity of the tendon.
- Chronic repairs or reruptures are best treated with allograft augmentation.
- Complications such as infection, loss of knee ROM, decreased quadriceps strength, or patellar fracture can occur in acute extensor mechanism rupture repairs but are more frequent in cases of chronic tendon rupture repair.

- Physical therapy should be individualized to the patient, but three phases should be emphasized: immobilization, passive ROM, and active ROM with functional training.

References

1. Ilan DI, Tejwani N, Keschner M, Leibman M: Quadriceps tendon rupture. *J Am Acad Orthop Surg* 2003;11(3):192-200.
2. Kerin C, Hopgood P, Banks AJ: Delayed repair of the quadriceps using the Mitek anchor system: A case report and review of the literature. *Knee* 2006;13(2):161-163.
3. Zernicke RF, Garhammer J, Jobe FW: Human patellar-tendon rupture. *J Bone Joint Surg Am* 1977;59(2):179-183.
4. Konrath GA, Chen D, Lock T, et al: Outcomes following repair of quadriceps tendon ruptures. *J Orthop Trauma* 1998;12(4):273-279.
5. Yepes H, Tang M, Morris SF, Stanish WD: Relationship between hypovascular zones and patterns of ruptures of the quadriceps tendon. *J Bone Joint Surg Am* 2008;90(10):2135-2141.
6. Siwek CW, Rao JP: Ruptures of the extensor mechanism of the knee joint. *J Bone Joint Surg Am* 1981;63(6):932-937.
7. Rougraff BT, Reeck CC, Essenmacher J: Complete quadriceps tendon ruptures. *Orthopedics* 1996;19(6):509-514.
8. Scuderi C: Ruptures of the quadriceps tendon: Study of twenty tendon ruptures. *Am J Surg* 1958;95(4):626-634.
9. McKinney B, Cherney S, Penna J: Intra-articular knee injuries in patients with knee extensor mechanism ruptures. *Knee Surg Sports Traumatol Arthrosc* 2008;16(7):633-638.
10. Richards DP, Barber FA: Repair of quadriceps tendon ruptures using suture anchors. *Arthroscopy* 2002;18(5):556-559.
11. Veselko M, Kastelec M: Inferior patellar pole avulsion fractures: Osteosynthesis compared with pole resection. Surgical technique. *J Bone Joint Surg Am* 2005;87 (pt 1, suppl 1):113-121.
12. Milankov MZ, Miljkovic N, Stankovic M: Reconstruction of chronic patellar tendon rupture with contralateral BTB autograft: A case report. *Knee Surg Sports Traumatol Arthrosc* 2007;15(12):1445-1448.
13. Ecker ML, Lotke PA, Glazer RM: Late reconstruction of the patellar tendon. *J Bone Joint Surg Am* 1979;61(6):884-886.
14. Casey MT Jr, Tietjens BR: Neglected ruptures of the patellar tendon: A case series of four patients. *Am J Sports Med* 2001;29(4):457-460.
15. Nsouli AZ, Nsouli TA, Haidar R: Late reconstruction of the patellar tendon: Case report with a new method of repair. *J Trauma* 1991;31(9):1319-1321.
16. Falconiero RP, Pallis MP: Chronic rupture of a patellar tendon: A technique for reconstruction with Achilles allograft. *Arthroscopy* 1996;12(5):623-626.
17. McNally PD, Marcelli EA: Achilles allograft reconstruction of a chronic patellar tendon rupture. *Arthroscopy* 1998;14(3):340-344.
18. Lewis PB, Rue JP, Bach BR Jr: Chronic patellar tendon rupture: Surgical reconstruction technique using 2 Achilles tendon allografts. *J Knee Surg* 2008;21(2):130-135.
19. Rand JA, Morrey BF, Bryan RS: Patellar tendon rupture after total knee arthroplasty. *Clin Orthop Relat Res* 1989;244:233-238.
20. Dobbs RE, Hanssen AD, Lewallen DG, Pagnano MW: Quadriceps tendon rupture after total knee arthroplasty: Prevalence, complications, and outcomes. *J Bone Joint Surg Am* 2005;87(1):37-45.
21. Emerson RH Jr, Head WC, Malinin TI: Extensor mechanism reconstruction with an allograft after total knee arthroplasty. *Clin Orthop Relat Res* 1994;303:79-85.

Video Reference

22.1 Karas SG, Hawkins RJ, Steadman JR: Video: *Repair of Injuries to the Extensor Mechanism: Quadriceps & Patellar Tendons*. Rosemont, IL, American Academy of Orthopaedic Surgeons, 2000.

Shoulder and Elbow

Section Editor
John W. Sperling, MD, MBA

23 Arthroscopic Subacromial Decompression and
Distal Clavicle Resection 149
Albert Lin, MD; Mark William Rodosky, MD

24 Arthroscopic Management of Frozen Shoulder 153
*Peter N. Chalmers, MD; Seth L. Sherman, MD;
Neil Ghodadra, MD; Gregory P. Nicholson, MD*

25 Arthroscopic Rotator Cuff Repair 159
Thomas R. Duquin, MD; Donald W. Hohman, Jr, MD

26 Percutaneous Pinning of Proximal Humerus Fractures 169
Bradford O. Parsons, MD

27 Fixation of Proximal Humerus Fractures 175
Michael E. Torchia, MD; Thomas S. Obermeyer, MD

28 Hemiarthroplasty for Proximal Humerus Fractures 183
Arnaldo I. Rodriguez-Santiago, MD; T. Bradley Edwards, MD

29 Total Shoulder Arthroplasty for Osteoarthritis 191
Stephanie H. Hsu, MD; Louis U. Bigliani, MD

30 Reverse Total Shoulder Arthroplasty for
Rotator Cuff Arthropathy 197
Peter Silvero, MD; Michael A. Wirth, MD

31 Arthroscopy of the Elbow 203
*Thomas V. Giel III, MD; Larry D. Field, MD;
Felix H. Savoie III, MD*

32   **Open Treatment of Radial Head Fractures and Olecranon Fractures** 211
Julie E. Adams, MD, MS; Scott P. Steinmann, MD

33   **Open Reduction and Internal Fixation of Distal Humerus Fractures** 219
Michael David McKee, MD, FRCSC

34   **Total Elbow Arthroplasty** 225
Peter Johnston, MD; Matthew L. Ramsey, MD

Chapter 23
Arthroscopic Subacromial Decompression and Distal Clavicle Resection

Albert Lin, MD   Mark William Rodosky, MD

Patient Selection
Subacromial impingement and degenerative changes of the acromioclavicular joint are common causes of shoulder pain. Repetitive overhead use can lead to a painful inflammatory process, termed impingement, of the subacromial bursa and the supraspinatus as they traverse a bony outlet under the acromion.[1,2] These patients often report pain with overhead activities, lateral shoulder pain, night pain, and pain with abduction and internal rotation.[2] Likewise, hypertrophic changes from a degenerative acromioclavicular joint can lead to localized pain as well as impingement of the underlying rotator cuff. In these patients, anterosuperior pain that worsens with cross-body adduction or reaching behind the back may be more typical.[3,4]

Surgical intervention, either open or arthroscopic, may be indicated in patients in whom nonsurgical management fails. The advantages of all-arthroscopic techniques include decreased surgical pain and, often, faster postoperative recovery, improved cosmesis, less trauma to the deltoid, and decreased blood loss.[2] Arthroscopic subacromial decompression and distal clavicle resection are excellent options for impingement and acromioclavicular degenerative joint disease and can be performed at the same time for concomitant pathology.[4]

Indications for surgery include failure of a 3- to 6-month course of nonsurgical management that includes anti-inflammatory medications such as steroid injections and NSAIDs, physical therapy that includes a rotator cuff strengthening protocol, and activity modification. In patients with a massive and irreparable rotator cuff tear or with rotator cuff arthropathy, disruption of the coracoacromial ligament is contraindicated.[1,2] Distal clavicle resection without a stabilizing procedure is also contraindicated in patients with grade III or higher acromioclavicular joint instability.[3]

Preoperative Imaging
Radiography
A radiographic series for impingement should include a true AP view of the glenohumeral joint (to assess for glenohumeral arthritis), an outlet view to evaluate the acromion (**Figure 1, A**), and an axillary lateral view to rule out an os acromiale. A Zanca view is best for evaluating the acromioclavicular joint for degenerative changes and osteolysis (**Figure 1, B**). Radiographs of the asymptomatic shoulder can allow side-to-side comparison.

Magnetic Resonance Imaging
MRI may be helpful in assessing the condition of the rotator cuff, including tendinopathy, partial tearing, or full-thickness tearing as well as any associated pathologies. Increased signal intensity or inflammatory changes around the acromioclavicular joint seen on MRI may also aid in confirming a suspected diagnosis based on history and physical examination.

Video 23.1 Subacromial Decompression and Distal Clavicle Resection. Mark Rodosky, MD; Albert Lin, MD (6 min)

Procedure
Room Setup/Patient Positioning
The patient is placed in an upright beach-chair position with the acromion parallel to the floor (**Figure 2**). Bony prominences are well padded.

Special Instruments/Equipment/Implants
The following equipment should be on hand for this procedure: a 30° arthroscope, 4.5- and 5.5-mm arthroscopic shavers, a 5.5-mm arthroscopic burr, a standard arthroscopic electrocautery device, and a hooked arthroscopic electrocautery device.

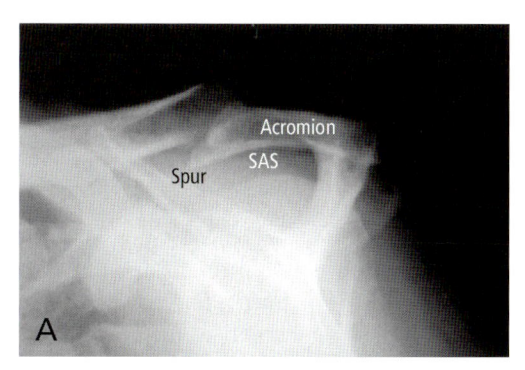

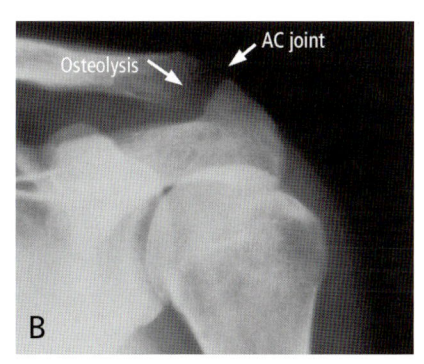

Figure 1 Radiographs of a shoulder obtained before arthroscopic subacromial decompression and distal clavicle resection. **A**, Outlet view shows an undersurface acromial spur encroaching on the subacromial space (SAS). **B**, Zanca view shows osteolysis of the acromioclavicular (AC) joint.

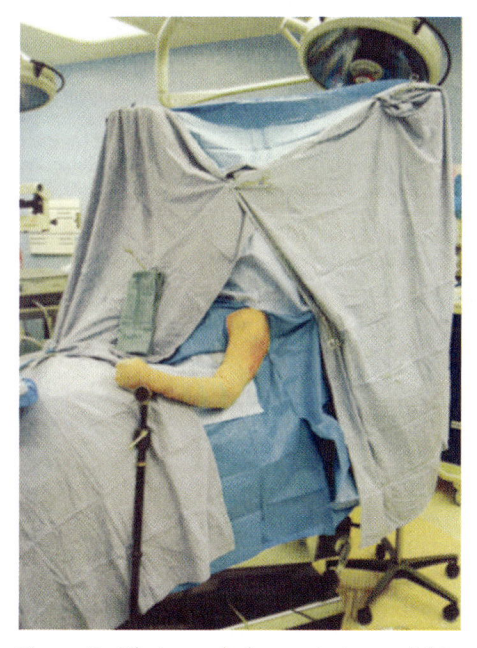

Figure 2 Photograph demonstrates upright beach-chair positioning of a patient for arthroscopic subacromial decompression and distal clavicle resection.

Neither of the following authors nor any immediate family member has received anything of value from or owns stock in a commercial company or institution related directly or indirectly to the subject of this chapter: Dr. Lin and Dr. Rodosky.

Section 2: Shoulder and Elbow

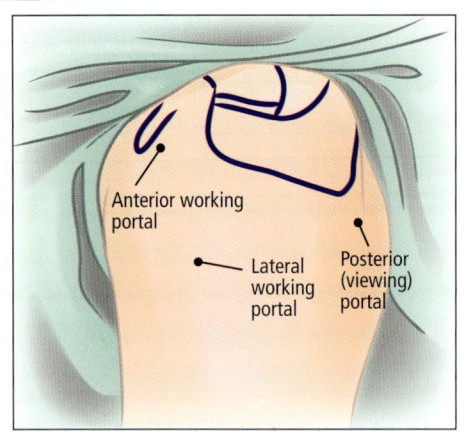

Figure 3 Illustration shows the location of the anterior working portal, lateral working portal, and posterior (viewing) portal in relationship to the coracoid, clavicle, acromion, and scapular spine, which are marked on the skin.

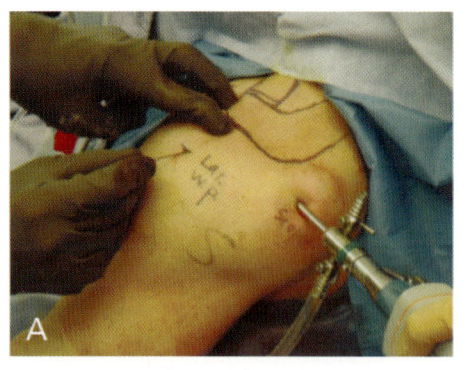

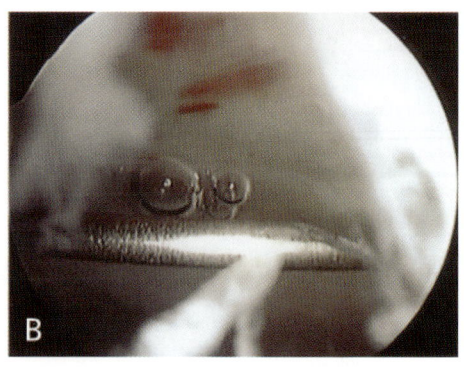

Figure 4 Portals used for arthroscopic subacromial decompression and distal clavicle resection. **A**, Photograph shows an 18-gauge spinal needle used to localize the lateral working portal and the arthroscope in the posterior portal, beneath the acromion. **B**, Arthroscopic view shows the spinal needle inside the subacromial space, coming laterally underneath the acromion.

Surgical Technique
Examination Under Anesthesia
A thorough examination under anesthesia (EUA) should be performed to evaluate range of motion and ligamentous laxity. One advantage of performing an EUA before preparing and draping the patient is that a side-to-side comparison with the nonsurgical limb can be performed.

Landmarks/Portals
The arthroscopic portal sites as well as landmarks (clavicle, acromion, scapular spine, and coracoids) are marked on the skin (**Figure 3**). Three portals are used: an anterior working portal, a posterior (viewing) portal, and a lateral working portal. Arthroscopic subacromial decompression is best accomplished by placing the arthroscope through the posterior viewing portal and instrumentation through the lateral working portal. Arthroscopic distal clavicle resection is best accomplished by placing the arthroscope through the lateral working portal and instrumentation through the anterior working portal.

Diagnostic Arthroscopy
Diagnostic arthroscopy through the posterior viewing portal is important in evaluating associated intra-articular and subacromial pathologies such as loose bodies, labral tears, and rotator cuff tears. The skin incision for the posterior viewing portal is made 2 to 3 cm inferior, in line with the posterolateral corner of the acromion. This area corresponds to the "soft spot" of the posterior shoulder. Before introducing the arthroscope, it is often advantageous to mark the anterior portal just lateral to the tip of the coracoid (**Figure 3**). This site will be collinear with the glenohumeral joint and can also serve as an aiming point when the arthroscope is introduced into the joint from the posterior portal. The anterior portal, however, is always made under direct visualization with the arthroscope, usually using a spinal needle first to confirm position. The final portal position can vary depending on the associated pathologies that need to be addressed. When an arthroscopic distal clavicle resection is being performed, the anterior portal should be parallel to the acromioclavicular joint; this is almost always achieved when the portal is made just lateral to the coracoid tip. Once within the joint, a systematic evaluation should be performed to assess the cartilage, labrum, capsuloligamentous structures, biceps, and rotator cuff.

When the glenohumeral arthroscopy is completed, the joint fluid is evacuated, and the arthroscope is placed in the subacromial space. The arthroscope should hug the undersurface of the acromion because this serves to keep the bursa below the entry site. It is also helpful to use the trocar for the arthroscope to bluntly break up subacromial adhesions with a sweeping motion under the acromion before placing the arthroscope in the subacromial space. The anterolateral corner of the acromion should be visualized before making the lateral working portal. A spinal needle should be used before making the portal to verify that the portal is parallel and slightly inferior to the undersurface of the anterior third of the acromion and in line with the front edge of the acromion (**Figure 4**). An anterior position is preferred for the lateral working portal because it is closer to the area of work for subacromial decompression (the anterior third of the acromion) and adjacent to the most common area for rotator cuff tears, the leading edge of the supraspinatus tendon. It is also better to err on being low than high. A low portal can be corrected with arm abduction, but a high portal makes it difficult—if not impossible—to access the medial acromion and also limits visualization of the acromioclavicular joint. The lateral portal should be no more than 3 to 4 cm inferior to the lateral edge of the acromion to avoid injury to the axillary nerve.

After the diagnostic glenohumeral arthroscopy has been performed as described previously to identify and address concomitant pathologies, the arthroscope is introduced into the subacromial space. Anterior and lateral working portals are established as described previously.

Acromioplasty and Subacromial Decompression
A 5.5-mm arthroscopic shaver is used to perform a bursectomy and expose the undersurface of the acromion (**Figure 5**). Exposing the area under the anterolateral aspect of the acromion first helps identify the position of the shaver within the subacromial space and avoid injury to the undersurface of the deltoid. Once visualization and a working area have been established, the débridement proceeds in a posterior and medial direction until the scapular spine is visualized. This will expose the anterior two thirds of the acromion and help to avoid leaving ridges behind at the margins of the subacromial decompression.

If a deficient rotator cuff or an irreparable cuff tear is present, the coracoacromial ligament should be preserved. In all other cases, the ligament is released from the front edge of the acromion with an arthroscopic electrocautery device. Incising the ligament first at the anterolateral

Chapter 23: Arthroscopic Subacromial Decompression and Distal Clavicle Resection

corner of the acromion in a line parallel with the deltoid muscle fibers establishes the depth of the fibers without risking injury to the deltoid fibers perpendicular to their length. Once the depth of the deltoid is known, it can be released safely around the front and lateral edges of the acromion. Once the acromion is well exposed, a subacromial decompression can be performed.

A 5.5-mm arthroscopic burr is placed through the lateral working portal to perform the acromioplasty for the subacromial decompression. The acromioplasty should start at the front edge of the anterolateral aspect of the acromion (**Figure 6, A** and **B**). The arthroscopic burr is used to flatten the lateral half of the anterior third of the acromion until it is collinear with the middle third of the acromion (**Figure 6, C**). In most patients, the depth of the acromioplasty will be equal to the entire width of the burr. The lateral half is then used as a template for the medial half. The medial half is resected in the same fashion until the entire front third of the acromion is flattened to the level of the middle third of the acromion (**Figure 6, D**). This effectively converts the acromion into a type I acromion. Bone particles are then removed with the arthroscopic shaver. This completes the subacromial decompression and acromioplasty.

Distal Clavicle Resection

If a distal clavicle resection is also being performed, the acromioclavicular joint is exposed after the subacromial decompression is completed. With the arthroscope still in the posterior portal, an anterior working portal is established in the subacromial space. In most patients, the routine anterior glenohumeral working portal will line up directly with the acromioclavicular joint. This portal is established using a blunt trocar, which also serves to verify its position immediately under the acromioclavicular joint. With the trocar in position, the arthroscope is then switched to the lateral working portal, which gives an end-on view of the acromioclavicular joint and distal clavicle.

With the arthroscope in the lateral portal, a 5.5-mm arthroscopic shaver is then placed through the anterior portal (**Figure 7, A**). The inferior and anterior capsule and intra-articular fibrocartilaginous disk are resected. The arthritic distal clavicle cartilage is exposed and removed with the shaver. A hooked electrocautery device is then used to elevate the capsule from the edge of the clavicle. Particular care is taken to preserve the posterior and superior capsule as it is being elevated because it is critical for maintaining the stability of the acromioclavicular joint. Exposure of the superior distal clavicle is also important to ensure that the entire width of the distal clavicle is resected because inadequate resection, particularly superiorly, may lead to residual pain in the acromioclavicular joint.

After exposure of the distal clavicle, a 5.5-mm arthroscopic burr is placed in the anterior portal and used to resect 1 cm of the distal clavicle to a smooth, flat surface. The front half is resected first, which allows measurement of the depth of resection against the intact posterior half and can also serve as a template for resection (**Figure 7, B**). No more than 1 cm of distal clavicle should be removed to maintain the integrity of the posterior and superior capsule (which is important for anterior-posterior stability of the acromioclavicular joint) and the coracoclavicular ligaments (which are important for superior-inferior stability).[3] A rasp with known dimensions can be used to verify level, orientation, and depth of resection (**Figure 7, C**).

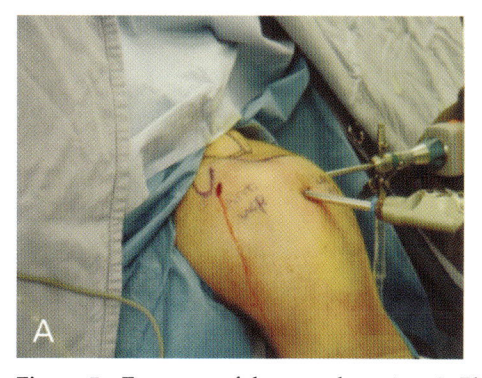

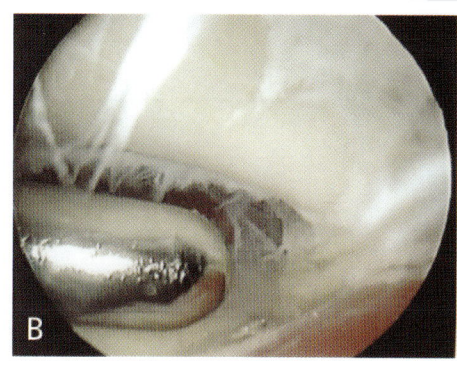

Figure 5 Exposure of the scapular spine. **A,** Photograph shows a 5.5-mm arthroscopic shaver in the lateral working portal in the subacromial space and the arthroscope in the posterior portal under the acromion. **B,** Arthroscopic view shows the motorized shaver exposing the scapular spine.

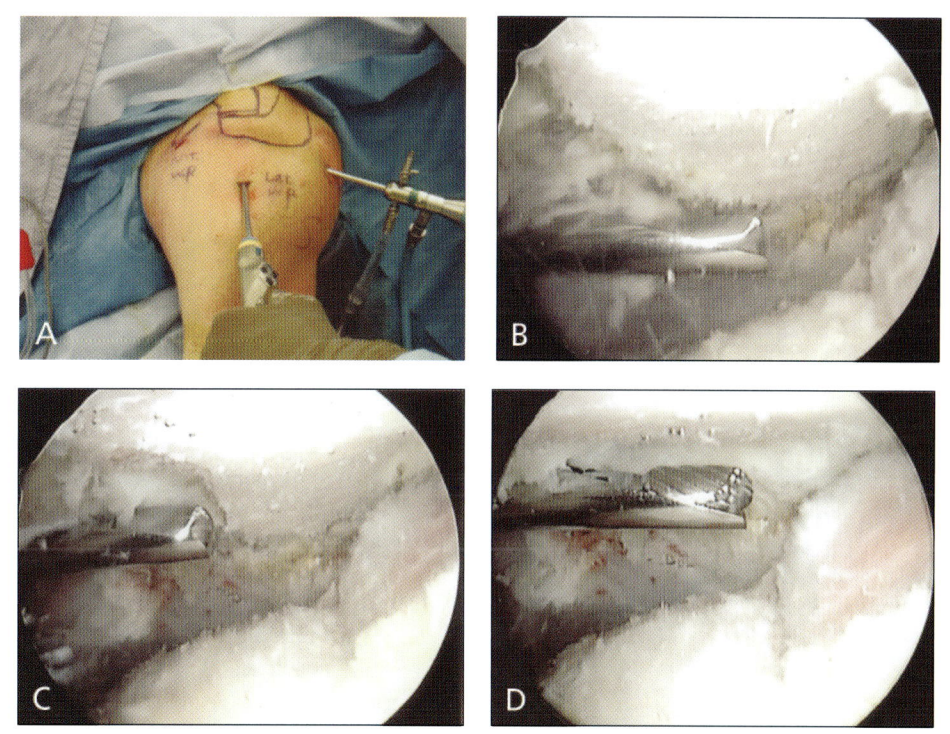

Figure 6 Acromioplasty for subacromial decompression. **A,** Photograph shows the arthroscope in the posterior portal and the 5.5-mm arthroscopic burr entering the subacromial space through the lateral working portal. **B,** Arthroscopic view demonstrates that the burr is parallel to the undersurface of the anterior third of the acromion and is immediately posterior to the anterior edge. **C,** The lateral half of the anterior third of the acromion is flattened with a 5.5-mm arthroscopic burr to the level of the middle third and can be used as a template for the medial portion of the acromioplasty. **D,** A completed acromioplasty is shown, demonstrating an entirely flat surface with no hidden ridges.

© 2013 American Academy of Orthopaedic Surgeons

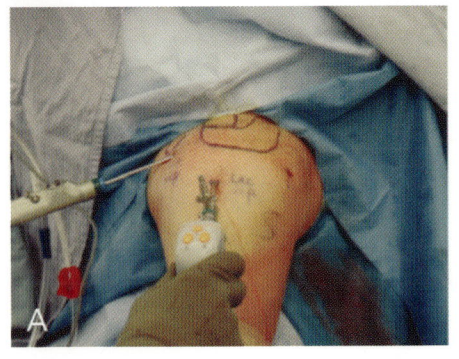

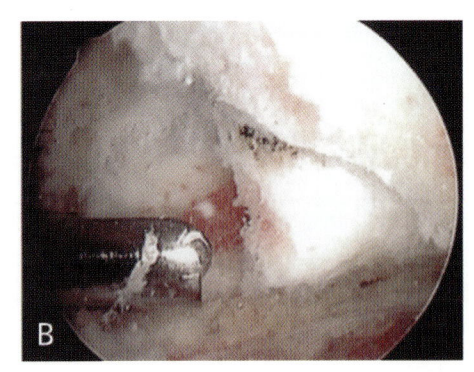

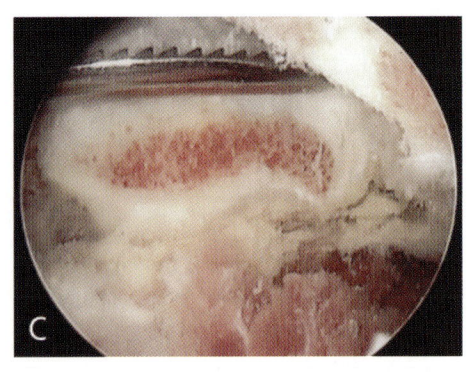

Figure 7 Distal clavicle resection. **A,** Photograph shows the arthroscope in the lateral working portal and the 5.5-mm arthroscopic burr in the anterior working portal. **B,** Arthroscopic view demonstrates the position of the burr at the distal clavicle. The anterior half has been resected from superior to inferior. **C,** At the completion of the distal clavicle resection, a rasp of known dimension is used to verify the width and angle of resection.

Conclusion of Procedure

Fluid is suctioned from the subacromial space, and the portal sites are closed with buried monofilament absorbable sutures. Standard dressings and a sling are applied, as well as a compressive cooling device.

Complications

Complications specific to the procedure include incomplete resection of the acromion or distal clavicle, regrowth of the acromion or distal clavicle, and continued pain. Overzealous distal clavicle resection of more than 1 cm can result in acromioclavicular joint instability.[3] Other complications are similar to those associated with all shoulder arthroscopies, including infection, adhesive capsulitis, and neurovascular injury, particularly of the axillary nerve and the acromial branch of the thoracoacromial artery. Brachial plexus or axillary artery injuries are exceedingly rare.

Postoperative Care and Rehabilitation

A sling and a compressive cold device are used for the first 48 hours for comfort. Pendulum exercises are started immediately, and formal physical therapy is initiated within the first 24 to 48 hours. Progressive passive and active range-of-motion exercises in all planes of motion are initiated immediately, with strengthening starting within a few weeks once full range of motion is achieved and the patient can tolerate strengthening exercises. Return to most activities is expected within 6 weeks. Full return to strenuous activities, including intensive labor and sports, is expected by 3 to 6 months.

Pearls

- In establishing a lateral working portal for a subacromial decompression, a common mistake is to make the portal too high. This is particularly relevant in heavier or obese patients. Improper portal placement can be avoided by using a spinal needle under direct visualization to localize the lateral working portal and paying strict attention to the bony landmarks.
- The use of an arthroscopic pump is helpful in allowing the surgeon to change the pressure for visualization and adjusting for variability in the patient's blood pressure.
- Complete exposure of the anterior two thirds of the scapula and the scapular spine before acromioplasty will help avoid leaving behind ridges (and inadequate decompression) at the margins of decompression.
- When subacromial decompression is performed in patients with a deficient rotator cuff or an irreparable rotator cuff tear, the coracoacromial ligament should be preserved.
- For arthroscopic distal clavicle resections, placing the anterior working portal parallel to the acromioclavicular joint makes resection easier.
- The capsule should be fully released before performing a distal clavicle resection, and resection should proceed from superior to inferior. This prevents inadequate resection, particularly superiorly. It also helps avoid leaving small parcels of bone behind in the joint capsule, which may grow larger and become a source of residual or recurrent pain.
- Particular care should be taken to avoid resecting more than 1 cm of the distal clavicle because this will destabilize the acromioclavicular joint.

References

1. Bigliani LU, Levine WN: Subacromial impingement syndrome. *J Bone Joint Surg Am* 1997;79(12):1854-1868.
2. McFarland EG, Selhi HS, Keyurapan E: Clinical evaluation of impingement: What to do and what works. *J Bone Joint Surg Am* 2006;88(2):432-441.
3. Blazar PE, Iannotti JP, Williams GR: Anteroposterior instability of the distal clavicle after distal clavicle resection. *Clin Orthop Relat Res* 1998;348:114-120.
4. Kay SP, Dragoo JL, Lee R: Long-term results of arthroscopic resection of the distal clavicle with concomitant subacromial decompression. *Arthroscopy* 2003;19(8):805-809.

Chapter 24
Arthroscopic Management of Frozen Shoulder

Peter N. Chalmers, MD   Seth L. Sherman, MD   Neil Ghodadra, MD
Gregory P. Nicholson, MD

Patient Selection

Frozen shoulder is defined by loss of range of motion of the shoulder, impairing the patient's ability to sleep, work, perform activities of daily living, or perform desired recreational activities. Etiology, pathology, natural history, diagnosis, and treatment have been debated.[1-4] Cytokines, myofibroblasts, growth factors, and matrix metalloproteinases have all been implicated, and similarities to both Dupuytren contracture and Peyronie disease have been described.[3,4] Frozen shoulder may be the end-stage manifestation of several primary conditions, including trauma, surgery, prolonged immobilization, endocrine disorders such as hypothyroidism or diabetes mellitus, and idiopathic causes.[5] This condition generally affects patients 40 to 60 years of age and occurs in roughly 2% of the population but up to 18% of diabetic patients.[1,2] The natural history of idiopathic frozen shoulder is variable but generally progresses in three stages, each 6 to 9 months in length: (1) inflammation (freezing), (2) fibrosis with disorganization and contracture (frozen), and (3) resolution (thawing).[1,2] Although resolution generally occurs within 2 to 3 years in idiopathic frozen shoulder, some limitation of range of motion of questionable functional significance may be permanent.[1] Because of the combination of inflammation and fibrosis seen on pathology, the terms *frozen shoulder* and *adhesive capsulitis* have been used interchangeably.

Frozen shoulder is a clinical diagnosis. The primary maneuver used to diagnose frozen shoulder is the assessment of range of motion before and after the injection of local anesthetic into the glenohumeral joint. If limitation in range of motion resolves after the injection of local anesthetic, other conditions must be considered, but if range of motion limitation persists, then a diagnosis of frozen shoulder is more likely. Evaluation of range of motion after subacromial injection can also be useful to exclude impingement as the primary pathology limiting shoulder mobility. Other conditions, such as rotator cuff tears, acromioclavicular joint pathology, subacromial impingement, and cervical spine pathology, should all be excluded before diagnosing a patient with frozen shoulder.

A variety of treatments have been described for frozen shoulder, including benign neglect, nonsteroidal anti-inflammatory drugs (NSAIDs), oral steroids, steroid injections, home stretching regimens, supervised physical therapy, brisement, manipulation under anesthesia (MUA), arthroscopic synovectomy, arthroscopic subacromial decompression, arthroscopic capsular release, open capsular release, and combinations thereof.[2,5-10] Nonsurgical measures, including NSAIDs, oral steroids, steroid injections, home stretching, and physical therapy by a therapist with an understanding of frozen shoulder should be pursued for at least 6 weeks to 3 months before surgical intervention. Almost 90% of patients respond to nonsurgical treatment.[7,8] If patients have had symptoms for 3 to 6 months, had nonsurgical treatment for a known diagnosis of shoulder stiffness for at least 6 to 8 weeks, and still continue to experience pain and decreased range of motion interfering with their ability to sleep, work, complete activities of daily living, or participate in sporting activities as they desire, surgical intervention should be considered.

Arthroscopic capsular release has been demonstrated to decrease pain, improve range of motion, improve function, and possibly shorten the natural history of the disorder.[2,3,5,10,11] Contraindications to arthroscopic capsular release include an indwelling prosthesis or a history of instability. A controversial relative contraindication to arthroscopic capsular release is a history of open surgical intervention. In this circumstance, range of motion limitation may be secondary to scarring between tissue layers, which can be a more technically demanding arthroscopic procedure.

Historically, MUA was performed for these indications and has been shown to be effective in a recent meta-analysis.[6] Advantages of arthroscopic capsular release over MUA include (1) additional diagnostic information gained by arthroscopy with respect to the subacromial space, the state of the articular cartilage, and other intra-articular pathology; (2) a more controlled and precise capsular release of the structures selected, instead of the ripping avulsion of the weakest structures produced by MUA; (3) the ability to perform a simultaneous brisement of the joint via insufflation; (4) the ability to perform concomitant synovial débridement, which has been discussed as the possible mediator of the pathologic process, and which was performed in 80% of shoulders in the series reported by one of the authors (G.P.N.);[5] and (5) the ability to perform subacromial decompression, which was performed in 33% of shoulders in that series.[5] Additionally, MUA has been associated with proximal humeral fracture, axillary nerve neurapraxias, labral injuries, subscapularis tears, superior labral anterior-to-posterior (SLAP) tears, and articular cartilage injuries.[9,12] Arthroscopic release also has several advantages over open release, including decreased surgical morbidity, decreased length of stay, decreased postoperative pain, and improved ability to address the posterior capsule. Because of these advantages, arthroscopic capsular release has become the standard surgical approach to frozen shoulder.

Preoperative Imaging

Although frozen shoulder is a clinical diagnosis, it is also one of exclusion; thus imaging can be helpful to exclude other pathology. AP, lateral, outlet, and Zanca

---

Dr. Nicholson or an immediate family member has received royalties from Innomed and Zimmer; serves as a paid consultant to or is an employee of Zimmer and Tornier; owns stock or stock options held in Zimmer; and has received research or institutional support from EBI, Tornier, and Zimmer. None of the following authors or any immediate family member has received anything of value from or owns stock in a commercial company or institution related directly or indirectly to the subject of this chapter: Dr. Chalmers, Dr. Sherman, and Dr. Ghodadra.

Section 2: Shoulder and Elbow

views of the shoulder can be used to evaluate for glenohumeral arthritis, fracture, locked dislocation, chondrolysis, calcific tendinitis, acromioclavicular arthrosis, abnormal acromial morphology, and other disorders. Shoulder MRI can be useful to evaluate the rotator cuff, biceps tendon, and glenohumeral and coracohumeral ligaments. Shoulder arthrography was traditionally used to document decreased joint volume, but this method is currently only of historical interest.

Video 24.1 Arthroscopic Management of the Frozen Shoulder. Peter N. Chalmers, MD; Seth L. Sherman, MD; Neil Ghodadra, MD; Gregory P. Nicholson, MD (4 min)

Procedure
Patient/Positioning/Equipment
Capsular release for frozen shoulder is among the more difficult arthroscopic procedures in the shoulder. Contracted capsule can limit both visualization and the mobility of instruments within the joint. The surgeon must be patient and recognize the limited visualization for this procedure without becoming frustrated. In addition to general arthroscopy equipment, an insufflation pump that allows control of flow and pressure, an articulated arm holder, and 90° bipolar electrocautery can greatly assist the surgeon.

In addition to a scalene block with a long-acting local anesthetic or a scalene catheter to allow postoperative pain control, patients also receive general anesthesia to assist in muscular relaxation. Hypotensive anesthesia decreases intraoperative bleeding. Both the beach-chair position and the lateral decubitus position with axial traction have been described. The beach-chair position allows subtle rotational positioning changes and eases conversion to an open procedure (**Figure 1**). A rolled towel is placed beneath the medial border of the scapula. An articulated arm holder is attached to the operating table and covered with a sterile drape to facilitate finding and maintaining the subtle positioning changes that allow visualization of the joint and the excursion of instruments within it.

An experienced assistant aids greatly with arm positioning. The acromion, distal clavicle, and coracoid are marked (**Figure 2**). After anesthesia has been

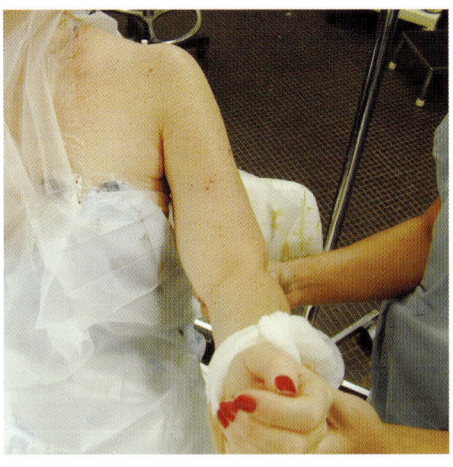

Figure 1 Preoperative photograph shows the patient placed in the beach-chair position. Range of motion under anesthesia should be documented, including elevation, external rotation in adduction, external rotation in abduction, and internal rotation. This patient demonstrated marked limitation to external rotation in adduction.

administered, range of motion is documented, including elevation, external rotation in adduction, external rotation in abduction, and internal rotation. Internal rotation may be sufficiently limited to make measurement in adduction difficult. Internal rotation also should be measured in 40° of abduction in the scapular plane. Manipulation of the joint before arthroscopy causes hemorrhage, making subsequent joint visualization difficult.[12] We do not routinely manipulate before arthroscopy.

Surgical Technique
The joint is entered posteriorly with an 18-gauge spinal needle 2 cm medial and inferior to the posterolateral corner of the acromion, aiming toward the coracoid. The joint is insufflated to 20 mm Hg using a flow rate of 200 mL/hour. Insufflation fluid with dilute (1:300,000) epinephrine improves visualization intraoperatively. A stab wound is made, and a blunt obturator is introduced into the joint, aiming toward the labral attachment of the long head of the biceps. This trajectory allows more of the sheath to enter and avoids articular cartilage damage. Resistance may be encountered because the capsule is often thickened and contracted. Intra-articular positioning is confirmed with fluid flow through the sheath. The arthroscope is then introduced. Although previous authors have described use of a 3.5-mm arthroscope to ease mobility of the arthroscope within a contracted joint, we have not encountered difficulty with the standard arthroscope. Alternate ir-

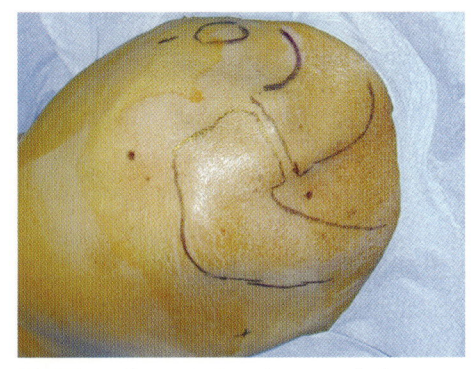

Figure 2 Preoperative photograph shows marking of the acromion, distal clavicle, and coracoid to assist with portal placement.

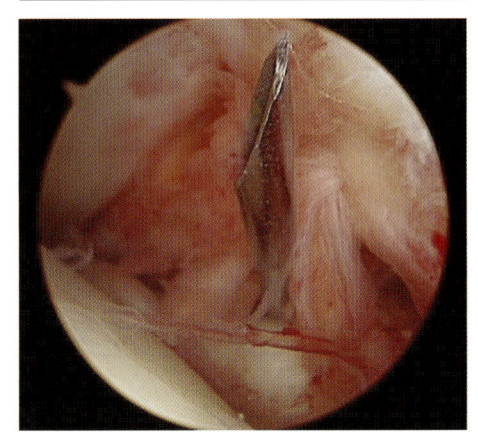

Figure 3 Arthroscopic view shows proliferative hypertrophic synovial tissue in the rotator interval. A spinal needle is seen entering the joint for the placement of the anterior portal.

rigation and suctioning is commonly required to improve visualization initially.

The arthroscopic triangle between the long head of the biceps, the superior edge of the subscapularis, and the glenoid is first examined. Red, filmy, gelatinous proliferative hypertrophic synovial tissue with neovascularization is often seen within the rotator interval and within the axillary pouch. An anterior portal is then introduced using the "outside-in" technique, inserting a spinal needle lateral to the tip of the coracoid (**Figure 3**). Once the needle is visualized, a stab wound in made in the skin and a 7-mm smooth cannula is introduced into the joint. Once fluid flow is confirmed, a 4.0-mm or 4.5-mm shaver is introduced into the joint. The synovial hyperplasia is resected. The shaver and smooth cannula are then extracted, and the electrocautery device is inserted through the anterior tract.

The electrocautery we prefer is a 3.5-mm 90° bipolar device that does not have suction capability. It has the best shape and stiffness for effective and efficient tissue release (**Figure 4, A**). Other devices, such as monopolar electrocautery, baskets,

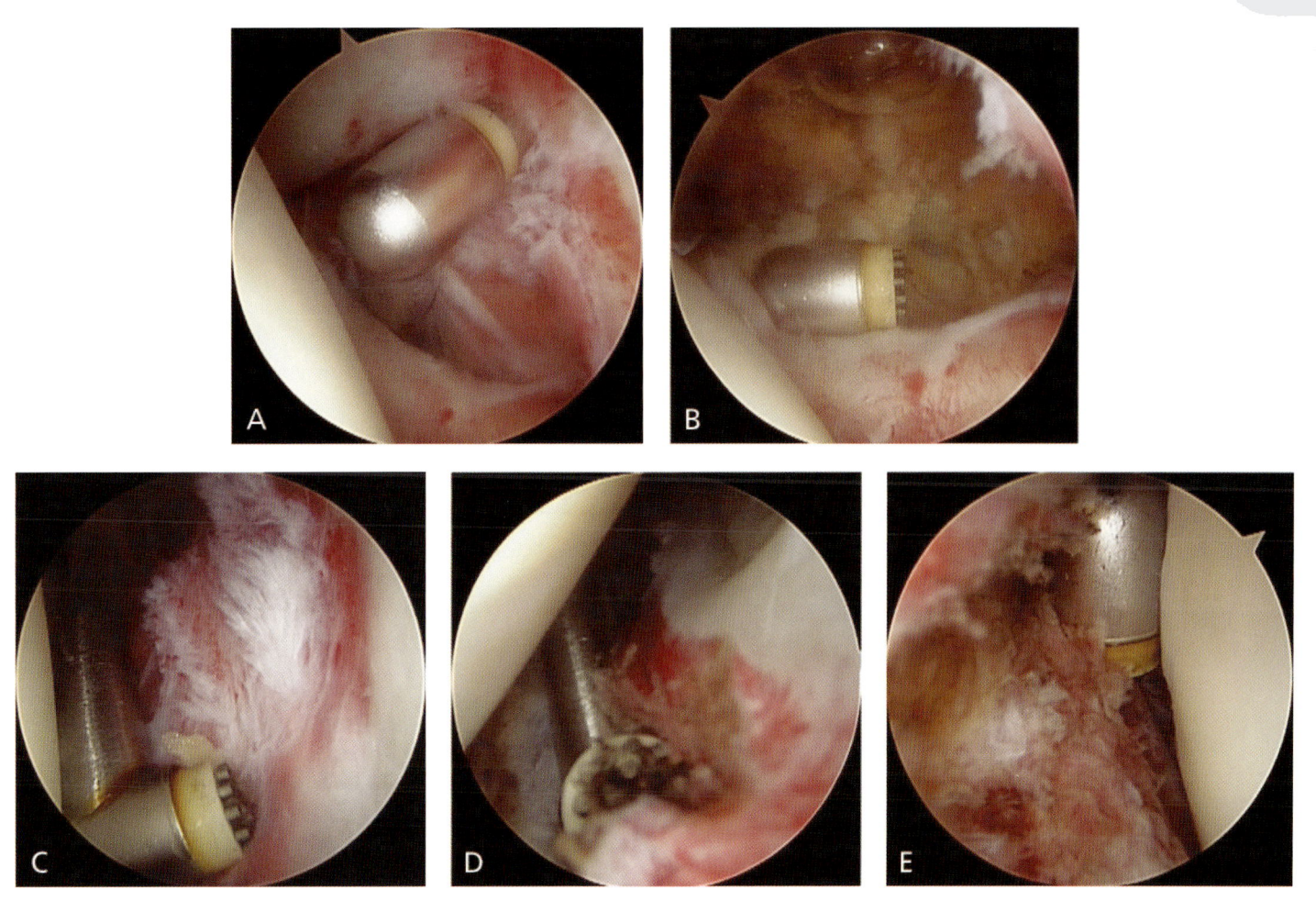

Figure 4 Arthroscopic views show capsular release for frozen shoulder. **A,** The electrocautery is inserted through the anterior portal. The ArthroWand allows the surgeon to cut into the capsule directly adjacent to where the electrocautery device enters the joint. **B,** The release begins just below the long head of the biceps and proceeds inferiorly to the superior edge of the subscapularis, including the coracohumeral ligament and the superior glenohumeral ligament. **C,** Inferior to the subscapularis tendon, the lower region of the middle glenohumeral ligament and the anterior band of the inferior glenohumeral ligaments are released as part of the capsular release. **D,** Once the 5-o'clock position is reached, the orientation of the electrocautery is changed such that the head points superiorly and the angle points inferiorly, to prevent axillary nerve damage. **E,** Similar to the anterior release, the posterior release proceeds from superiorly at the posterior border of the long head of the biceps tendon to inferiorly meet the anterior release.

shavers, radiofrequency ablation, or a combination of these methods, have also been used with success.

Release is performed anteriorly from superior to inferior and then posterior in the same fashion. The release is performed in an extralabral fashion, as close to the glenoid rim as possible without injuring the labrum. The release begins just below the long head of the biceps and proceeds inferiorly to the superior edge of the subscapularis, including the coracohumeral ligament and superior glenohumeral ligament (**Figure 4, B**). The release proceeds inferiorly, thus "unzipping" the anterior capsule. This allows access and visualization to proceed inferiorly. The release can also be carried across the top of the subscapularis tendon horizontally, releasing the upper region of the middle glenohumeral ligament if needed. During rotator interval release, visualization is often improved by placing the joint in 30° to 40° of abduction and alternating between 30° of internal and external rotation. Release of the intra-articular portion of the subscapularis tendon is controversial.[5,10,11,13] Subscapularis release may not adversely affect postoperative shoulder function or internal rotation strength.[13] For refractory cases in which global capsular release does not allow acceptable external rotation, release of the intra-articular portion of the subscapularis tendon could be considered. We prefer not to perform subscapularis release routinely.

Inferior to the subscapularis tendon, the lower region of the middle glenohumeral ligament and the anterior band of the inferior glenohumeral ligaments are released as part of the capsular release (**Figure 4, C**). Humeral traction can improve visualization in this region. As release proceeds, visualization within the joint should improve. Once the 5-o'clock position is reached, the orientation of the electrocautery is changed such that the head points superiorly and the angle points inferiorly, to prevent axillary nerve damage (**Figure 4, D**). Previous studies have shown the distance between the glenoid rim and the axillary nerve to be 7 mm from the axillary nerve.[14]

Once release is complete to the 6-o'clock position, the arthroscope is switched to the anterior portal and the electrocautery device to the posterior portal. Similar to the anterior release, the posterior release proceeds from superiorly at the posterior border of the long head of the biceps tendon to inferiorly meet the anterior release (**Figure 4, E**). Release of the posterosuperior recess above the long head of the biceps tendon and the superior labrum edge can be particularly helpful in improving range of motion because the supraspinatus may be adherent to the capsule, particularly in postoperative stiffness such as after SLAP repairs or rotator cuff repairs. Posterior release may or may not be required, depending

Section 2: Shoulder and Elbow

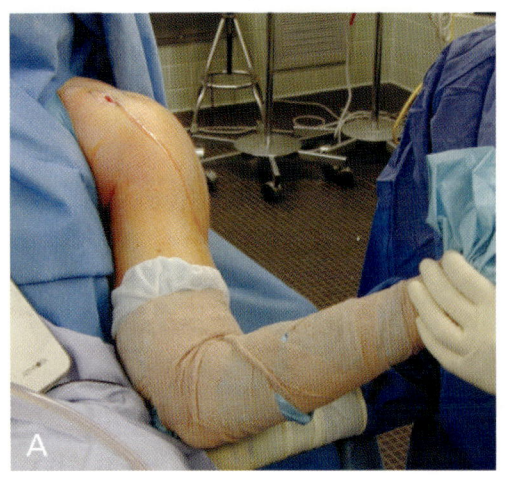

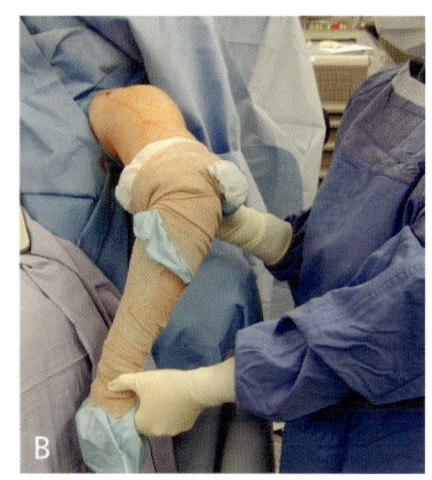

Figure 5 Intraoperative photographs demonstrate range of motion performed at the completion of capsular release. This examination demonstrates improvements in external rotation in adduction (**A**) and internal rotation in abduction (**B**).

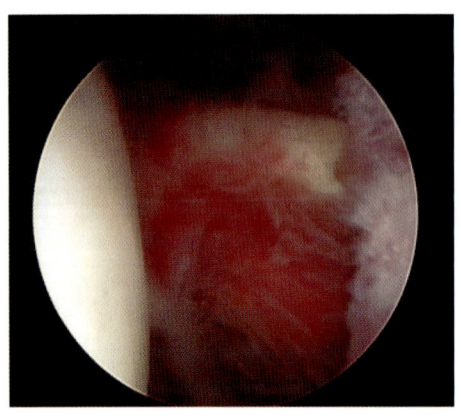

Figure 6 After capsular release and gentle range of motion, the subscapularis tendon should be visible.

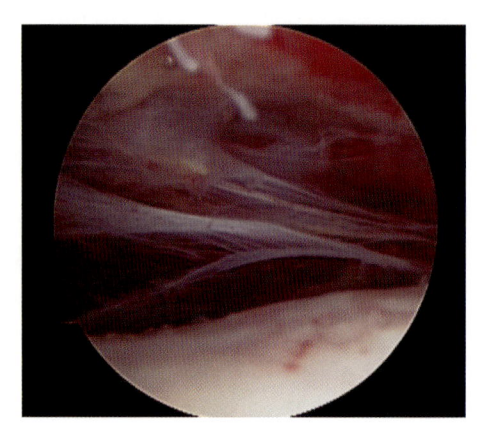

Figure 7 Evaluation of the subacromial space is critical. If subacromial involvement is present, then adhesiolysis, bursectomy, and acromioplasty are commonly required.

on the patient's range of motion.[10] Posterior release is indicated for limitation of internal rotation. In the series reported by Nicholson,[5] 66% of patients required posterior release. A shaver may be useful once the capsule has been divided to trim the capsular edges.

At the completion of the capsular release, the joint is gently ranged sequentially through abduction, elevation, external rotation in adduction, external rotation in abduction, and internal rotation (**Figure 5**). This maneuver completes the release. Another useful technique is to translate the humeral head parallel to the glenoid joint surface in the posterior, anterior, and inferior directions. This can release the remaining tethers to motion without significant force on the proximal humerus. We perform this maneuver before putting the shoulder through a range of motion and typically do not perform a true MUA. With each movement, some small giving way will be felt but not the definite snap traditionally felt.

The joint is re-entered with the arthroscope after ranging to evaluate the subacromial space as well as to survey the results of capsular release. The infraspinatus and the free subscapularis tendon should be visible (**Figure 6**). Persistent impingement pathology has been associated with frozen shoulder, thus evaluation of the subacromial space is critical[5] (**Figure 7**). Debate exists within the literature about whether subacromial impingement could cause frozen shoulder.[15] If subacromial involvement is present, then adhesiolysis, bursectomy, and acromioplasty are commonly required. If not addressed, postoperative subacromial impingement can cause continued pain and interfere with home exercises and physical therapy.

Various authors have described different extents of capsular release, from release of the rotator interval alone to 360° release. Tailoring the procedure to be performed to the specific range-of-motion deficits of the patient has also been described, as have repeat examinations during the procedure after each release, to decide whether further release is necessary.[2,3,10,11]

Complications

Complications after arthroscopic capsular release are rare. Several series have reported no major complications.[2,3,10,11] Even with good technique, we have found that approximately 20% of patients will develop transient decrease in motion 3 to 5 weeks after the procedure. The shoulder motion becomes less flexible and can actually become very "rubbery" and painful. This is an inflammatory flare-up that should be recognized; the patient should be reassured and treated with patience and anti-inflammatory medication in the form of a prescription for a methylprednisolone dose pack (if not contraindicated) or an intra-articular steroid injection. These symptoms usually resolve in 3 to 6 weeks.[5]

Although damage to the axillary nerve, posterior humeral circumflex artery, and brachial artery are all theoretical risks, these complications have not been commonly encountered.[2,3,10,11] These structures could be damaged directly intraoperatively or because of the increased excursion of the joint postoperatively. In addition, instability, although theoretically possible, has not been described.[2,3,10,11]

Outcomes following arthroscopic capsular release are generally excellent. In several studies, American Shoulder and Elbow Surgeons scores ranged preoperatively from 23.5 to 25.5 and improved to 57 to 93 postoperatively.[5,11,13] In the series reported by Nicholson,[5] Constant scores improved from 17.7 preoperatively to 82.8 postoperatively; simple shoulder test scores improved from 3 preoperatively to 10 postoperatively; and visual analog scale scores for pain improved from 6 preoperatively to 0 postoperatively. Elevation improved from 76° preoperatively to 165° postoperatively for a change of 26° to 79°.[5,11,13] Internal rotation in abduction improved from 23° preoperatively to 41° postoperatively.[5,11] Internal rotation in adduction improved 7 spinal segments.[5,11] External rotation in adduction improved from 12° preoperatively to 58° postoperatively for a change of 29° to 40°.[5,11,13] Abduction improved from 66° preoperatively to 142° postoperatively for a change of 76°.[13] Expected outcome may or not may not depend on etiology.[5,11] Diabetes may confer worse outcomes.[5] Whether arthroscopic capsular release influences the natural history of the disorder is unclear, but within the results reported by Nicholson,[5] the average time to pain-free range of motion was 6 to 10 weeks and the time for which therapy was deemed necessary was 10 weeks, whereas the average duration of stiffness in patients treated nonsurgically has been described as 4 years or longer.[1]

Postoperative Care and Rehabilitation

Postoperatively, patients are placed in a sling and swathe with a derotational wedge to ensure neutral rotation and avoid internal rotation. As the technique and results have become more consistent, most patients are now treated with outpatient surgery, with physical therapy beginning within 1 or 2 days of the surgery. However, it can also be advantageous for patients with profound stiffness who undergo arthroscopic capsular release to be admitted for 23-hour observation. Hospital admission allows the patient to undergo inpatient physical therapy while under scalene block. Arthroscopy for frozen shoulder is scheduled as the first case of the day or early in the morning, to allow the patient to undergo two sessions of physical therapy on the day of surgery. These hospital therapy sessions are critical to the success of the operation, because they demonstrate to the patient normal pain-free range of motion. The psychological relief this provides motivates the patient for therapy. In addition to repeat scalene block for the duration of hospitalization, patients are provided with intramuscular and oral narcotic pain medications and intramuscular ketorolac while in the hospital. We provide patients with oral ketorolac for 4 days after discharge as well as oral narcotics to be taken as needed. Home continuous passive motion machines are reserved for patients who have required repeat capsular release in whom previous MUA has failed, diabetic patients with severe limitations in range of motion preoperatively, and other patients for whom the risk of treatment failure is deemed high.

Patients are encouraged to use the shoulder out of the sling for dressing, eating, and other activities of daily living. Discharge with a pulley and a stick facilitates home exercises, which include pendulums, pulley exercises, elevation, and passive external and internal rotation with a stick. These exercises are prescribed for 15 to 20 minutes three or four times per day, with warm moist heat before and ice afterward. Supervised physical therapy is recommended three times per week for 3 weeks and then two times per week for 3 weeks. Return to modified work activities typically occurs within 3 weeks. All therapy consists of range-of-motion exercises initially; even light resistance is discouraged until 6 to 8 weeks or until the patient achieves pain-free, flexible, and consistent range of motion.

Pearls

- Arthroscopic capsular release for frozen shoulder is a challenging procedure requiring patience on the part of the surgeon.
- The beach-chair position, a pump system with independent control of flow and pressure with which the surgeon is well acquainted, and a 90° 3.5-mm bipolar electrocautery can all increase the likelihood of success.
- Selective capsular resection of the rotator interval or of the anterior capsule alone should be reserved for patients with solitary deficits of external rotation and with documented full range of motion intraoperatively after selective capsular resection. Most patients will require completion of inferior and posterior capsular release to regain range of motion comparable with the contralateral shoulder.
- Release of the intra-articular portion of the subscapularis tendon should be reserved for cases in which global capsular release does not provide sufficient external rotation.
- Aggressive shoulder manipulation before arthroscopic capsular release should be avoided because the ensuing hemorrhage can compromise intra-articular visibility.

References

1. Binder AI, Bulgen DY, Hazleman BL, Roberts S: Frozen shoulder: A long-term prospective study. *Ann Rheum Dis* 1984;43(3):361-364.
2. Hannafin JA, Chiaia TA: Adhesive capsulitis: A treatment approach. *Clin Orthop Relat Res* 2000;372:95-109.
3. Neviaser AS, Hannafin JA: Adhesive capsulitis: A review of current treatment. *Am J Sports Med* 2010;38(11):2346-2356.
4. Rodeo SA, Hannafin JA, Tom J, Warren RF, Wickiewicz TL: Immunolocalization of cytokines and their receptors in adhesive capsulitis of the shoulder. *J Orthop Res* 1997;15(3):427-436.
5. Nicholson GP: Arthroscopic capsular release for stiff shoulders: Effect of etiology on outcomes. *Arthroscopy* 2003;19(1):40-49.
6. Buchbinder R, Green S, Youd JM, Johnston RV, Cumpston M: Arthrographic distension for adhesive capsulitis (frozen shoulder). *Cochrane Database Syst Rev* 2008;1:CD007005.
7. Griggs SM, Ahn A, Green A: Idiopathic adhesive capsulitis: A prospective functional outcome study of nonoperative treatment. *J Bone Joint Surg Am* 2000;82(10):1398-1407.
8. Levine WN, Kashyap CP, Bak SF, Ahmad CS, Blaine TA, Bigliani LU: Nonoperative management of idiopathic adhesive capsulitis. *J Shoulder Elbow Surg* 2007;16(5):569-573.
9. Parker RD, Froimson AI, Winsberg DD, Arsham NZ: Frozen shoulder: Part II. Treatment by manipulation under anesthesia. *Orthopedics* 1989;12(7):989-990.
10. Warner JJ: Frozen shoulder: Diagnosis and management. *J Am Acad Orthop Surg* 1997;5(3):130-140.
11. Holloway GB, Schenk T, Williams GR, Ramsey ML, Iannotti JP: Arthroscopic capsular release for the treatment of refractory postoperative or post-fracture shoulder stiffness. *J Bone Joint Surg Am* 2001;83(11):1682-1687.
12. Loew M, Heichel TO, Lehner B: Intraarticular lesions in primary frozen shoulder after manipulation under general anesthesia. *J Shoulder Elbow Surg* 2005;14(1):16-21.
13. Liem D, Meier F, Thorwesten L, Marquardt B, Steinbeck J, Poetzl W: The influence of arthroscopic subscapularis tendon and capsule release on internal rotation strength in treatment of frozen shoulder. *Am J Sports Med* 2008;36(5):921-926.
14. Zanotti RM, Kuhn JE: Arthroscopic capsular release for the stiff shoulder: Description of technique and anatomic considerations. *Am J Sports Med* 1997;25(3):294-298.
15. Richards DP, Glogau AI, Schwartz M, Harn J: Relation between adhesive capsulitis and acromial morphology. *Arthroscopy* 2004;20(6):614-619.

Chapter 25
Arthroscopic Rotator Cuff Repair

Thomas R. Duquin, MD   Donald W. Hohman, Jr, MD

Introduction

Disorders of the rotator cuff represent one of the most common reasons for shoulder pain. Although many causative factors have been implicated, the true pathogenesis remains controversial. The most common and central factors include age-related degeneration of the tendons, mechanical impingement, and changes in the vascularity of the rotator cuff tendon.[1] The natural history of rotator cuff disease has been recognized as a continuum, progressing from simple tendinitis to partial- and full-thickness rotator cuff tears.[2]

This chapter provides an overview of the arthroscopic management of rotator cuff pathology. Special consideration is given to the evaluation of the patient with a suspected rotator cuff tear, as well as preoperative planning, surgical management, and postoperative rehabilitation.

Patient Selection

Patients with rotator cuff disorders often present with an insidious onset of pain that is located in the anterior and lateral aspect of the shoulder and upper arm. Pain is exacerbated by overhead and lifting activities, and nighttime symptoms that interfere with sleep are common. Each patient must undergo a thorough history and physical examination, with special attention paid to the acuity of symptoms, the nature of the pain, and the degree of functional limitations. The initial management of patients with suspected rotator cuff pathology includes a variety of nonsurgical modalities such

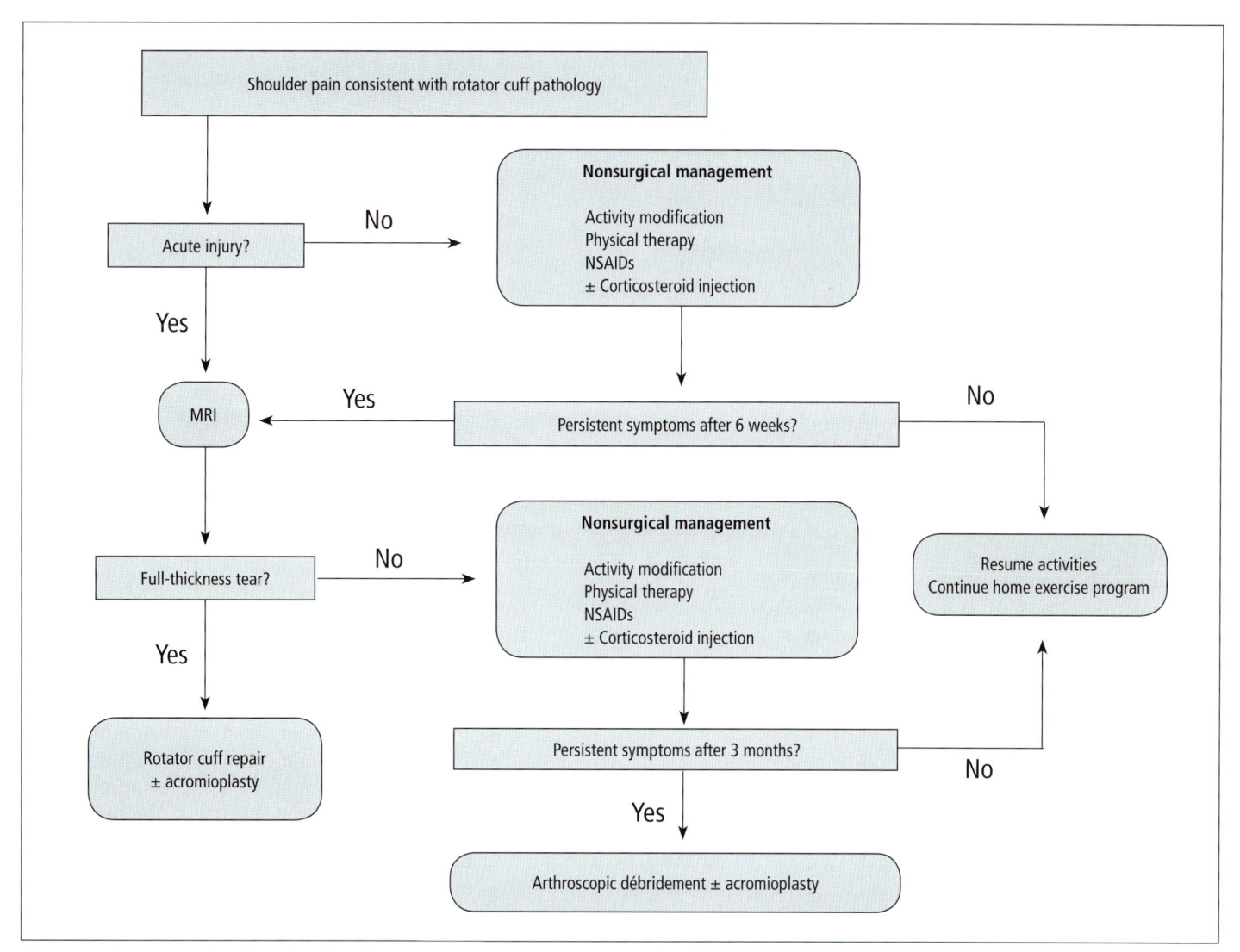

Figure 1 Treatment algorithm for shoulder pain consistent with rotator cuff pathology. (Adapted with permission from Duquin TR, Sperling JW: Rotator cuff disorders, in Margheritini F, Rossi R: *Orthopedic Sports Medicine: Principles and Practice.* Milan, Italy, Springer-Verlag, 2011, pp 211-225.)

Dr. Duquin or an immediate family member serves as a paid consultant to or is an employee of Biomet and Arthrex. Neither Dr. Hohman nor any immediate family member has received anything of value from or owns stock in a commercial company or institution related directly or indirectly to the subject of this chapter.

Section 2: Shoulder and Elbow

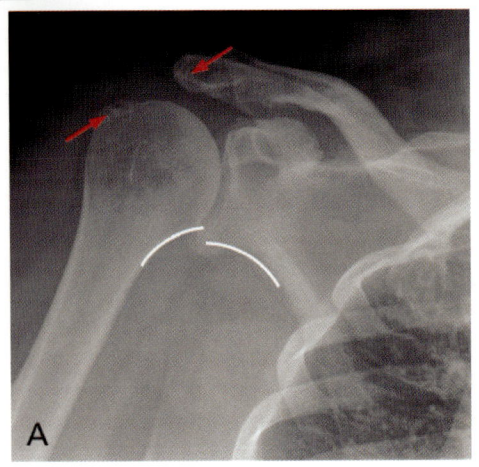

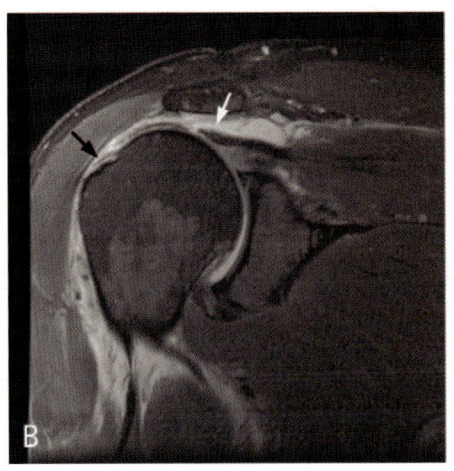

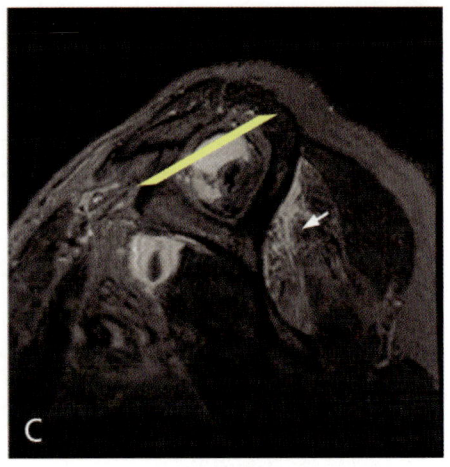

Figure 2 Signs of rotator cuff pathology on imaging. **A,** AP radiograph of the shoulder demonstrates the radiographic signs of a rotator cuff tear: sclerosis and cystic change of the greater tuberosity and acromion (red arrows) and subtle superior migration of the humeral head, indicated by a loss of the Gothic arch (white lines). **B,** The greater tuberosity rotator cuff footprint (black arrow) and the torn and retracted rotator cuff tear of the supraspinatus tendon (white arrow) are seen on a T2-weighted coronal oblique MRI of a right shoulder. **C,** Severe atrophy of the supraspinatus indicated by a positive tangent sign (yellow line) and fatty infiltration of the infraspinatus (white arrow) are seen on a T2-weighted sagittal MRI. (Panel A reproduced with permission from Duquin TR, Sperling JW: Rotator cuff disorders, in Margheritini F, Rossi R: *Orthopedic Sports Medicine: Principles and Practice.* Milan, Italy, Springer-Verlag, 2011, pp 211-225.)

as activity modification, nonsteroidal anti-inflammatory drugs, physical therapy, and corticosteroid injections (**Figure 1**). With these measures, symptoms will improve in most individuals who do not have full-thickness tears. Lack of improvement after 4 to 6 weeks of nonsurgical management is an indication for further investigation of the cause of the symptoms, with MRI to evaluate the rotator cuff.

As arthroscopic techniques have improved, so has the instrumentation, resulting in expanded indications for arthroscopic rotator cuff repair. The results of arthroscopic rotator cuff repair are comparable to those of open repair, without the disadvantage of deltoid detachment.[3] Anecdotal reports indicate that patients have less pain in the initial postoperative period after arthroscopic repair than after traditional open repairs. A relatively steep learning curve is associated with arthroscopic repairs of the rotator cuff, and the surgeon should have advanced skills in shoulder arthroscopy.

Indications

Patients with full-thickness or high-grade partial-thickness tears of the rotator cuff who have pain and limited function despite an appropriate interval of nonsurgical management are candidates for arthroscopic repair. The primary indication is for the relief of pain, with improved strength and mobility being a secondary goal. Although the presence of a full-thickness rotator cuff tear does not obligate the need for repair, the patient should be counseled about the risk of tear progression and muscle atrophy resulting in an irreparable rotator cuff. Patients with asymptomatic rotator cuff tears do not need surgery but should be monitored for signs or symptoms of tear progression.

Contraindications

Absolute contraindications include the presence of acute infection, end-stage arthritis, arthropathy with fixed superior migration of the humeral head, an inability to tolerate anesthesia because of medical comorbidities, or an inability to comply with postoperative rehabilitation. Relative contraindications to repair include massive retracted tears, poor tendon quality, fatty atrophy of the muscle belly, and advanced patient age.[4]

Preoperative Imaging
Radiography

Plain radiographs of the shoulder, including AP, scapular Y, and axillary views, should be obtained. The morphology of the acromion can be assessed on the scapular Y view; rotator cuff impingement should be suspected when a type III acromion is seen. In patients with rotator cuff impingement, subtle or nonspecific findings often are found, including sclerosis of the greater tuberosity and the undersurface of the acromion (**Figure 2, A**). Radiographic signs of large or massive tears include superior migration of the humeral head, which results in a loss of continuity of the Gothic arch formed by the medial neck of the proximal humerus and the inferior aspect of the glenoid neck, and a decrease in the acromiohumeral distance, which is normally greater than 6 mm).

Magnetic Resonance Imaging

MRI, including the evaluation of both T1-weighted and T2-weighted images in the coronal, sagittal, and oblique planes, is the gold standard for the assessment of rotator cuff disorders. The tear pattern, size, and retraction, as well as the quality of the tendon and muscle, are important factors in the determination of the ability to perform arthroscopic repair. It is important to include the entire scapula on the MRI so that assessment of the atrophy and fatty infiltration of the rotator cuff muscles can be performed (**Figure 2, B**). The tangent sign described by Zanetti et al[5] is used to quantify the degree of supraspinatus atrophy, with poor results documented in patients with a supraspinatus muscle that does not intersect the line drawn from the scapular spine to the coracoid process (**Figure 2, C**).

Ultrasonography

Ultrasonography is an accepted alternative to MRI for the assessment of rotator cuff pathology and is useful in patients with metal implants from prior surgeries. Multiple studies have shown that the sensitivity and specificity of ultrasonography approaches that of MRI, with the added benefit of dynamic examination. This modality is extremely operator-dependent, however, and requires considerable expertise in performing and interpreting musculoskeletal ultrasonography to ensure accurate results.

Chapter 25: Arthroscopic Rotator Cuff Repair

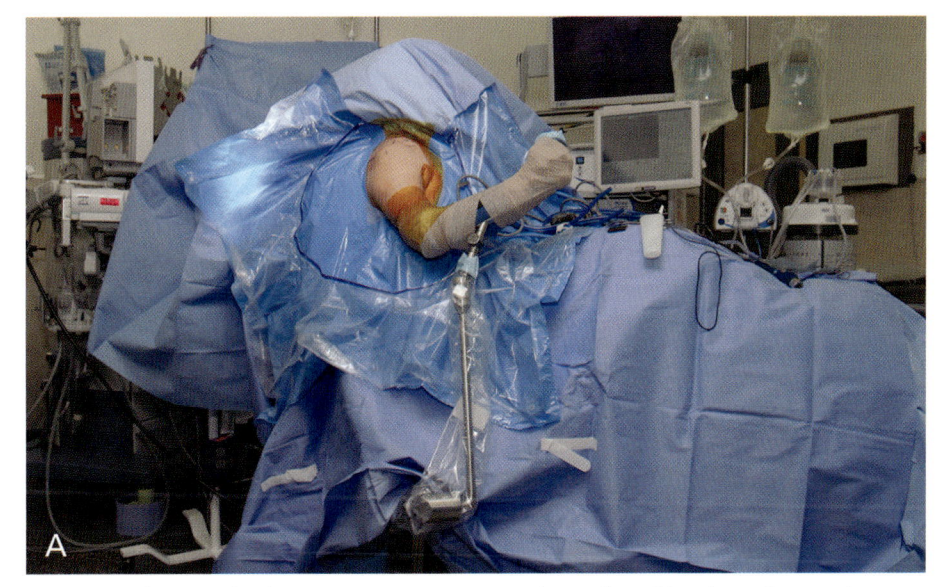

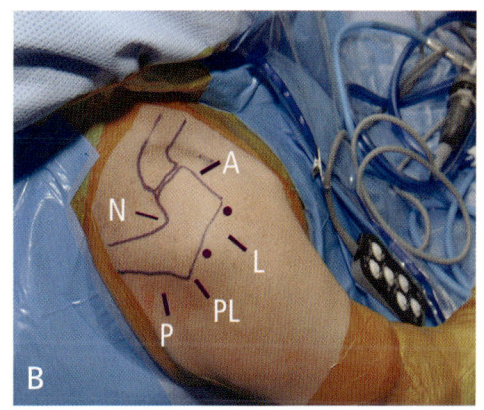

Figure 3 Photographs show patient positioning and portal marking for arthroscopic rotator cuff repair. **A,** The arthroscopic beach-chair position, with standard draping and room setup. **B,** Anatomic landmarks and the location of arthroscopic portals are marked on the skin. The circles represent stab incision locations for anchor introduction. A = anterior portal, L = lateral portal, N = Neviaser portal, P = posterior portal, PL = posterolateral portal.

Procedure

Special Instruments/Equipment/Implants Required

A description of all the available devices for arthroscopic rotator cuff repair is beyond the scope of this chapter. The essential tools include a 30° arthroscope, a fluid pump system, and standard arthroscopic instruments including suture passing, suture retrieving, and knot-tying devices, arthroscopic shavers and burrs, and a radiofrequency ablation wand. Arthroscopic cannulas and retractors can aid greatly in the successful performance of the operation.

Suture anchors used for rotator cuff repair come in a variety of materials, including metal, bioabsorbable plastic (polylactic acid), nonbioabsorbable plastic (polyetheretherketone), and biocomposite (70% polylactide coglycolide and 30% tricalcium phosphate). Each material has been used with varying degrees of success and attendant risks, but all have been shown to have similar strengths of fixation.[6] Anchors also come in a variety of sizes, mechanisms of fixation, and suture materials. Anchor designs that do not require an arthroscopically tied knot (knotless anchors) are available, but mode of failure and reliability of fixation remain concerns.[7]

Our current preference is a biocomposite anchor, which has the advantages of a biodegradable implant. This anchor is associated with a lower risk of the bone destruction that has been described with the use of the all–polylactic acid implants.

For single-row repairs and the medial row of a double-row repair, we use 5.5-mm anchors double-loaded with high-tensile-strength suture. Lateral-row fixation is accomplished with a knotless anchor to create a suture-bridge construct.

Video 25.1 Arthroscopic Rotator Cuff Repair. Thomas R. Duquin, MD; Donald W. Hohman, MD (30 min)

Surgical Technique

Performing a successful arthroscopic rotator cuff repair involves ten steps (**Table 1**). It is important to complete the steps in sequence.

1. Patient Positioning and Examination Under Anesthesia

Appropriate room setup and patient positioning are essential for successful arthroscopic rotator cuff repair. Many technologic advances have occurred in arthroscopic shoulder surgery, and the development of a simple and reproducible method using the resources available at the surgeon's institution is essential. Having surgical staff members who are experienced in arthroscopic surgery greatly improves the ability to perform all arthroscopic rotator cuff repairs.

Examination under anesthesia is performed on every shoulder before the initiation of surgery. The correlation of preoperative pain and physical examination findings may be corroborated with the examination under anesthesia, and the presence of a joint contracture or instability may alter the course of treatment.

Both the beach-chair position and the lateral decubitus position have been described for rotator cuff repair. Our preference is to place the patient in the beach-chair position with the head of the bed elevated to 80° (**Figure 3, A**). Care must be taken to pad all bony prominences of the extremities and position the head and neck in neutral alignment in both the

Table 1 Steps in Arthroscopic Rotator Cuff Repair

1. Patient positioning and examination under anesthesia
2. Intra-articular arthroscopy and débridement
3. Subacromial bursectomy and acromioplasty
4. Rotator cuff tear characterization and mobilization
5. Tuberosity and tendon preparation
6. Marginal convergence sutures (if required)
7. Anchor placement and suture passage
8. Knot tying
9. Lateral-row repair (if required)
10. Closure and perioperative care

© 2013 American Academy of Orthopaedic Surgeons

Table 2 Tips for Portal Placement for Arthroscopic Rotator Cuff Repair

Portal	Tip/Pearl	Location
Posterior portal	Provides best visualization of the shoulder joint; placement too far lateral should be avoided or joint visualization will be difficult	1-3 cm distal and 1-2 cm medial to the posterolateral tip of the acromion
Anterior portal	Working portal for instruments and suture management; placed using the outside-in technique under arthroscopic visualization and spinal needle localization into the triangle formed by the labrum (medial border), biceps tendon (superior border), and subscapularis (inferior border)	Halfway between the acromioclavicular joint and the lateral aspect of the coracoid; pierces the anterior fibers of the deltoid and enters the joint in the interval between the supraspinatus and subscapularis
Lateral portal	Working portal for the subacromial space; used to visualize the subacromial space; if placed too posteriorly in a large or muscular patient, it will be difficult for the instruments to "turn the corner" to reach the anterior acromion.	Placed laterally, in line with the midclavicle and 2-3 cm lateral to its lateral edge
Posterolateral portal	Visualization of the subacromial space during rotator cuff repair	1 cm distal to the posterolateral corner of the acromion
Neviaser	Working portal for the subacromial space; useful for suture passage in rotator cuff repair	Superomedial portal bordered by the clavicle, the acromioclavicular joint, and the spine of the scapula

coronal and sagittal planes. Access to the posterior aspect of the shoulder is essential, and the entire scapula should be free from the edge of the table. The surgical arm is placed in an articulated hydraulic arm holder that facilitates exposure. This is especially helpful when surgical assistants are limited or inexperienced.

2. Intra-articular Arthroscopy and Débridement

The acromion, distal clavicle, and coracoid process are outlined with a marking pen, and the locations of the standard posterior, anterior, and lateral portals are marked (**Figure 3, B**). Tips for the successful placement of all portals are provided in **Table 2**. The posterior viewing portal (2 cm medial and inferior to the posterolateral corner of the acromion) is established using a blunt trocar, with the arm placed in 15° of abduction and 30° of forward flexion and with the assistant providing a gentle lateral distraction to avoid damage to the articular surfaces. The 30° arthroscope is introduced, and diagnostic arthroscopic examination of the joint is performed.

Thorough evaluation includes visualization of the articular cartilage of the humeral head and glenoid; the labrum; the biceps tendon; the inferior recess; the articular surface; and the insertion of the subscapularis, supraspinatus, infraspinatus, and teres minor. In most instances, degenerative labral tears, synovitis, or cartilage lesions are present and need to be débrided. In these cases, an anterior working portal is established high in the rotator interval, and a 7-mm cannula is placed using an outside-in technique after localization with an 18-gauge spinal needle. A 4.5-mm full-radius shaver is used to perform intra-articular débridement as indicated. Biceps tendon pathology is treated as indicated with débridement, tenotomy, or tenodesis, depending on the degree of injury and surgeon preference. The initial débridement of the rotator cuff tear is performed with the arthroscope in the joint and a full-radius shaver in the anterior portal. The amount of débridement and preparation of the tuberosity that is possible will depend on the size and extent of the rotator cuff tear. Full-thickness tears allow access to the entire footprint of the tuberosity, which is débrided of all soft tissue using the full-radius resector and radiofrequency ablation wand before moving to the subacromial space.

3. Subacromial Bursectomy and Acromioplasty

After completion of the intra-articular débridement, the arthroscope is moved to the subacromial space. This is done using the same posterior portal but using the arthroscope trocar to slide just under the acromion, over the posterior rotator cuff. The trocar is then swept across the undersurface of the acromion and through the lateral gutter to break up adhesions in the bursa and create a space for arthroscopic evaluation. The arthroscope is introduced, and the subacromial space is inspected. In most symptomatic rotator cuff tendon tears, the bursa is inflamed and thickened, which can compromise visualization.

The first landmark to be identified is the coracoacromial ligament, which is in the anterior aspect of the subacromial space. After adequate visualization, a lateral working portal is created through the deltoid muscle in line with the posterior aspect of the distal clavicle and 2 to 3 cm lateral to the edge of the acromion. Localization is performed initially with a spinal needle, followed by insertion of an 8.25-mm threaded cannula. Then the full-radius shaver is used to perform a complete bursectomy. It is important to remove as much bursa as possible to provide adequate space to perform the rotator cuff repair.

The bursa and soft tissue are removed from the undersurface of the acromion using the radiofrequency ablation wand. The anterior aspects of the acromion and coracoacromial ligament are examined. If evidence of impingement is present or if the subacromial space is too small to allow arthroscopic rotator cuff repair, then an acromioplasty is performed. If an acromioplasty is required, partial resection of the coracoacromial ligament is performed with the ablation wand to expose the entire anterior aspect of the acromion.

Our preferred technique for acromioplasty is to use a 4.5-mm barrel-shaped burr through the lateral portal. The acromioplasty is started at the anterolateral corner, and 5 to 8 mm of bone is removed, taking care to preserve the fascial fibers of the deltoid muscle. The depth of bone removal is estimated based on the width of the burr, with a goal of removing 1.5 times the width of the burr.

After the depth of resection is established laterally, the resection is carried medially to the acromioclavicular joint. Avoiding overresection is important to prevent destabilization of the deltoid insertion. The resection is made level by sweeping the burr from anterior to posterior, creating a flat undersurface of the acromion. The arthroscope is then moved to the lateral portal, and the acromioplasty is made level by placing the burr in the posterior portal and sweeping in a medial-to-lateral direction.

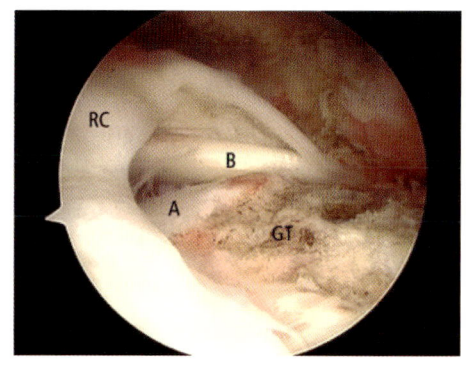

Figure 4 Arthroscopic view depicts a large crescentic rotator cuff tear viewed from the posterolateral portal. RC = rotator cuff tendon, A = articular surface, B = biceps tendon, GT = greater tuberosity.

4. Rotator Cuff Tear Characterization and Mobilization

Following complete bursectomy and acromioplasty, attention is directed to the rotator cuff tendon tear. The importance of visualizing the tear cannot be overemphasized; moving the arthroscope from the posterior portal to the posterolateral portal facilitates inspection. This portal is made 2 cm distal to the posterolateral corner of the acromion. A 7-mm cannula is placed in the posterior portal and will be used for suture passage and docking.

Débridement of any remaining devitalized or diseased tendon tissue is performed, followed by an assessment of the tear. Multiple tear patterns have been described, including crescent-, L-, reverse L-, and U-shaped patterns (**Figures 4** and **5**). The size of the tear, the degree of retraction, the quality of the tendon tissue, and the excursion of the tendon are important factors in the arthroscopic assessment of a rotator cuff tear. Using a tendon-grasping instrument or placing a traction suture through the lateral portal can be very helpful in assessing the tear pattern and tendon mobility. Within each tear pattern, the mobility of the tear must be assessed, and soft-tissue releases may be required to attain reduction of the tendon to the tuberosity before the initiation of repair. Tension-free repair may require the evaluation and dissection of both the bursal and articular side of the tendon. Specifically, the tear pattern, chronicity, degree of retraction, and mobility of the tendon may warrant the release of adhesions on both sides of the tendon. This also may include the release of the rotator interval, thereby increasing tendon excursion. These maneuvers may be performed effectively with either electrocautery or a tissue elevator. Coracohumeral ligament release (interval slide) from a retracted supraspinatus tendon is simple in principle and can significantly enhance the mobility of a retracted rotator cuff tear.

A complete description of these techniques has been published in the literature.[8-10] For the surgeon who is transitioning to arthroscopic rotator cuff repair and encounters a large retracted tear, we recommend converting to the surgeon's preferred method of open or mini-open repair.

5. Tuberosity and Tendon Preparation

After mobilization and characterization of the tear type, repair of the rotator cuff tear can be initiated. The first step is to prepare the tendon and tuberosity. Healing rates following rotator cuff repair range from 30% to 100% in the literature and have been associated with patient factors, tear size, amount of retraction, fatty atrophy, tendon quality, and repair technique.[4,11,12] Appropriate preparation of the tendon and tuberosity is essential for healing. A devascularized tendon cannot be expected to heal to a tuberosity covered with avascular scar tissue no matter how strong the fixation.

Débridement of the tendon to healthy tissue and creation of a bleeding bone surface on the tuberosity must be performed before anchor placement and repair of the tendon. The tendon and tuberosity are prepared with the arthroscope in the posterolateral portal and the instruments in the lateral portal. The tendon can be débrided with arthroscopic basket resectors or a full-radius shaver. The tuberos-

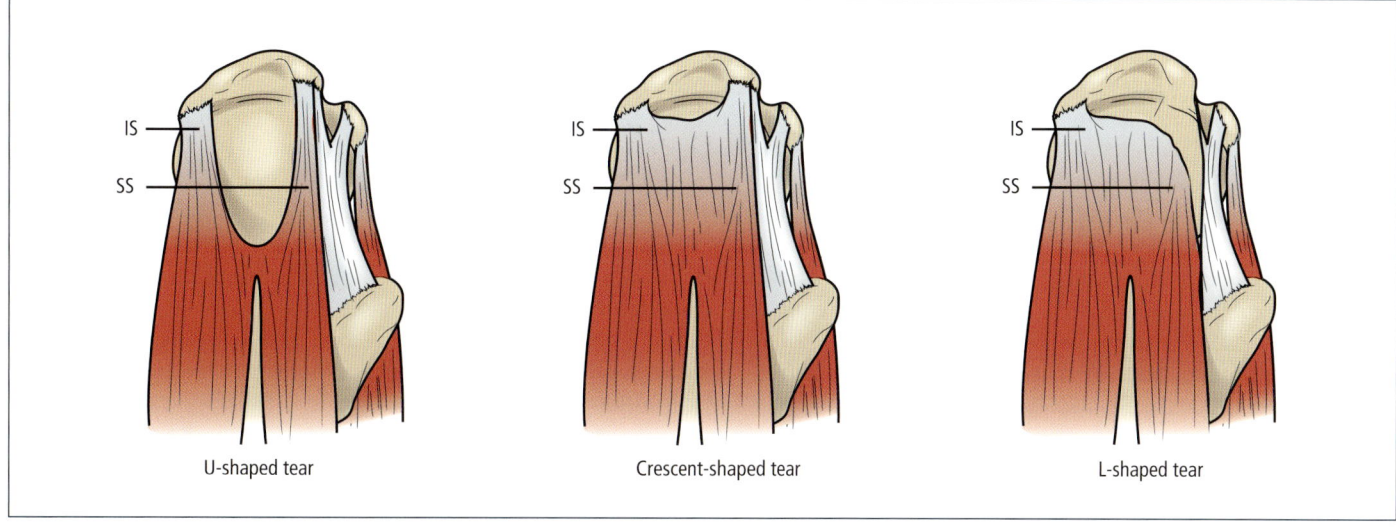

Figure 5 Illustration shows types of rotator cuff tears. IS = infraspinatus, SS = supraspinatus.

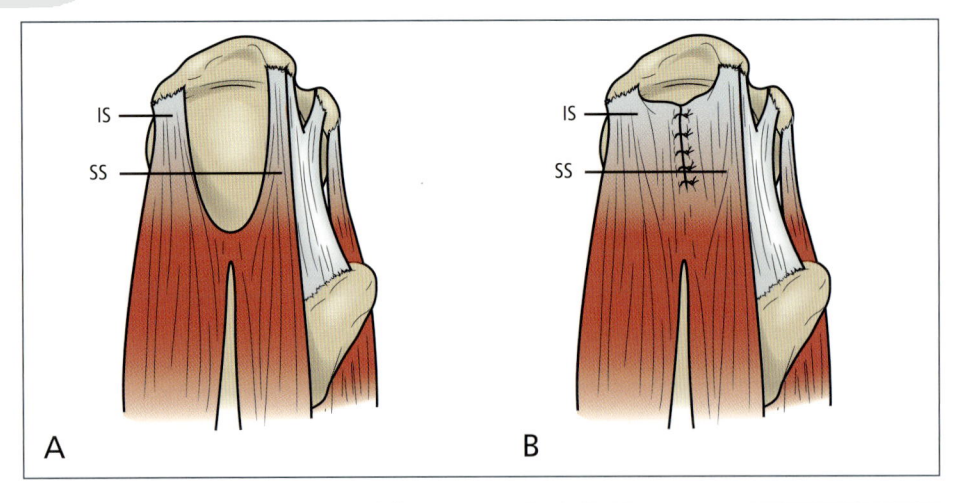

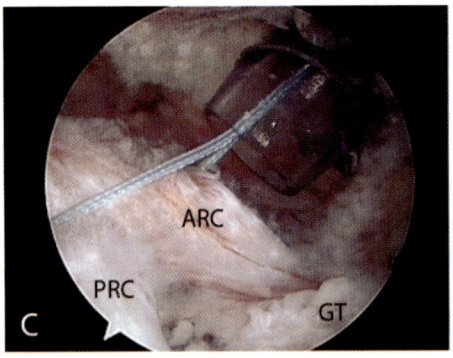

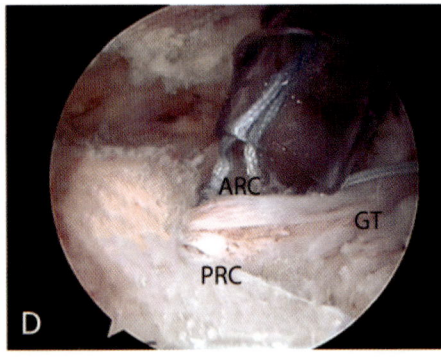

Figure 6 The use of marginal convergence sutures to repair a rotator cuff tear. Illustrations show a U-shaped rotator cuff tear pattern amenable to marginal convergence suture placement before (**A**) and after (**B**) placement of the sutures. **C,** Arthroscopic view depicts marginal convergence suture placement viewed from the posterolateral portal. A free suture is passed through the anterior and posterior margins of the longitudinal portion of the tear. **D,** Knot tying results in closure of the longitudinal split in the tendon, reducing the tendon defect. IS = infraspinatus, SS = supraspinatus, ARC = anterior rotator cuff leaflet, PRC = posterior rotator cuff leaflet, GT = greater tuberosity.

ity should be cleared of soft tissue with the ablation wand, and then a burr can be used to create a bleeding bone surface. It is important to not remove all the cortical bone from the tuberosity, because this will result in difficulty in obtaining adequate fixation of the suture anchors.

6. Marginal Convergence Sutures
Certain tear patterns require the placement of marginal convergence sutures (**Figure 6, A** and **B**). These are tendon-to-tendon sutures not included in an anchor that are meant to reduce longitudinal tears in the tendon fibers. The tear types that are most amenable to this type of repair are the L-, reverse L-, and U-shaped tears. Marginal convergence sutures greatly reduce the size of the tear and the amount of strain on the tendon at the tuberosity repair.

The passage of marginal convergence sutures can be performed using sharp suture-passing instruments, suture shuttle devices, or antegrade suture-passing devices. Our preferred method is to use a sharp suture-passing instrument loaded with a high-tensile-strength free suture through the anterior portal to penetrate the anterior leaf of the tear and a second suture-passing instrument from the posterior portal to penetrate the posterior leaf of the tear. Then, the free suture is passed from the anterior instrument to the posterior device and then pulled through the posterior portal (**Figure 6, C** and **D**). Both limbs of the suture can then be retrieved through the lateral portal and tied to complete the marginal convergence stitch.

Careful planning and placement of marginal convergence sutures is essential to prevent malreduction of the tendon tissue. Although marginal convergence is a powerful tool in many cases, it is important to note that its use is not indicated in all tear patterns. Using this technique when not indicated will result in significant bunching of the tendon and the creation of "dog ears," which can cause impingement of the tendon on the acromion and limit the surface area of the tendon for healing.

7. Anchor Placement and Suture Passage
Several methods of anchor placement and suture passage have been described. The first decision that must be made is the type of repair to be performed. Extensive research has been performed on various types of repair, including single-row suture anchor, single-row transosseous, and double-row suture anchor and suture-bridge repairs. Despite compelling biomechanical data indicating superior fixation and increased surface area contact/compression using double-row repairs compared with single-row repairs, no studies have shown superior clinical outcomes associated with double-row repairs.[13] A systematic review of the literature has demonstrated improved healing rates in tears greater than 1 cm with double-row techniques, however.[14] We prefer to perform double-row repairs for all tears greater than 1 cm in size.

No matter the type of repair chosen, anchor insertion is facilitated by using an accessory transdeltoid portal just off the lateral margin of the acromion. This allows for an optimal angle for anchor insertion. Each anchor should be placed with an approximately 45° orientation to facilitate fixation and prevent pullout (**Figure 7**). The localization and trajectory of anchor placement should be verified using a spinal needle, followed by a small stab incision and placement of the anchor without the use of a cannula. Multiple stab incisions can be used for anchor placement in various regions of the tuberosity.

In single-row repairs (**Figure 8, A**), suture anchors should be placed at the lateral aspect of the tuberosity. One limb of the double-loaded anchor is placed in a horizontal mattress configuration, and the other limb is passed as a simple suture medial to the horizontal mattress, resulting in a modified Mason-Allen stitch, with the horizontal limb preventing suture cutout.

In double-row repairs (**Figure 8, B**), the medial row of suture anchors is placed at the medial aspect of the tuberosity just off the articular margin. These sutures are passed in a horizontal mattress fashion and then tied to secure the tendon to the medial aspect of the tuberosity. Our preference is to perform a suture-bridge double-row repair (**Figure 8, C**). This involves taking the suture limbs from the medial row and incorporating them into a knotless anchor placed lateral to the greater tuberosity, resulting in secure

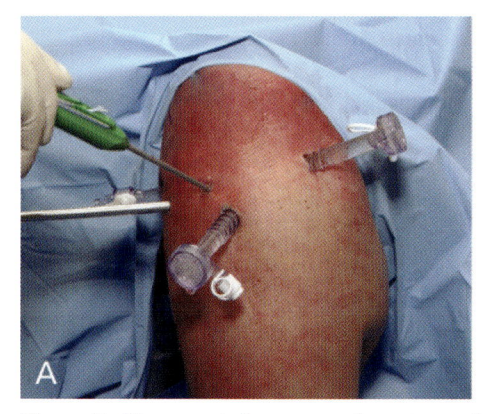

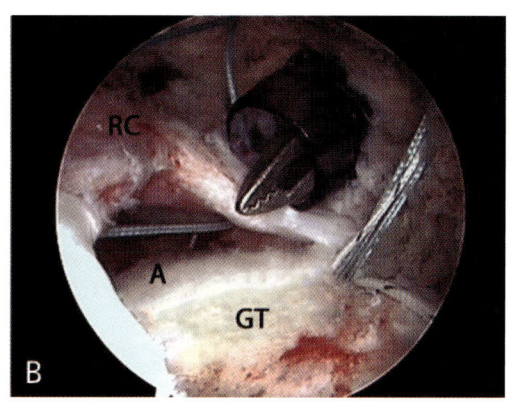

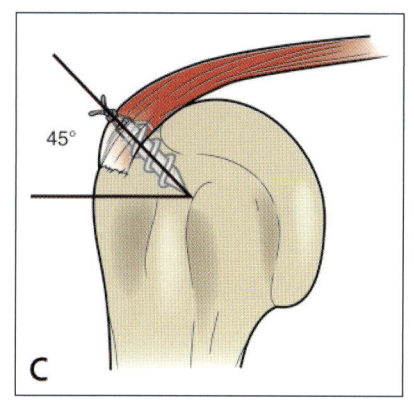

Figure 7 Placement of suture anchors to repair a rotator cuff tear. **A,** Intraoperative photograph shows the suture anchors placed using a stab incision at the margin of the acromion to achieve a 45° angle of insertion at the medial border of the greater tuberosity. **B,** Arthroscopic view from a posterolateral portal demonstrates the positioning of a medial-row suture anchor. Note the 45° angle of anchor insertion at the margin of the articular surface. **C,** Illustration shows the appropriate angle of anchor insertion (the deadman's angle). RC = rotator cuff tendon, A = articular surface, GT = greater tuberosity.

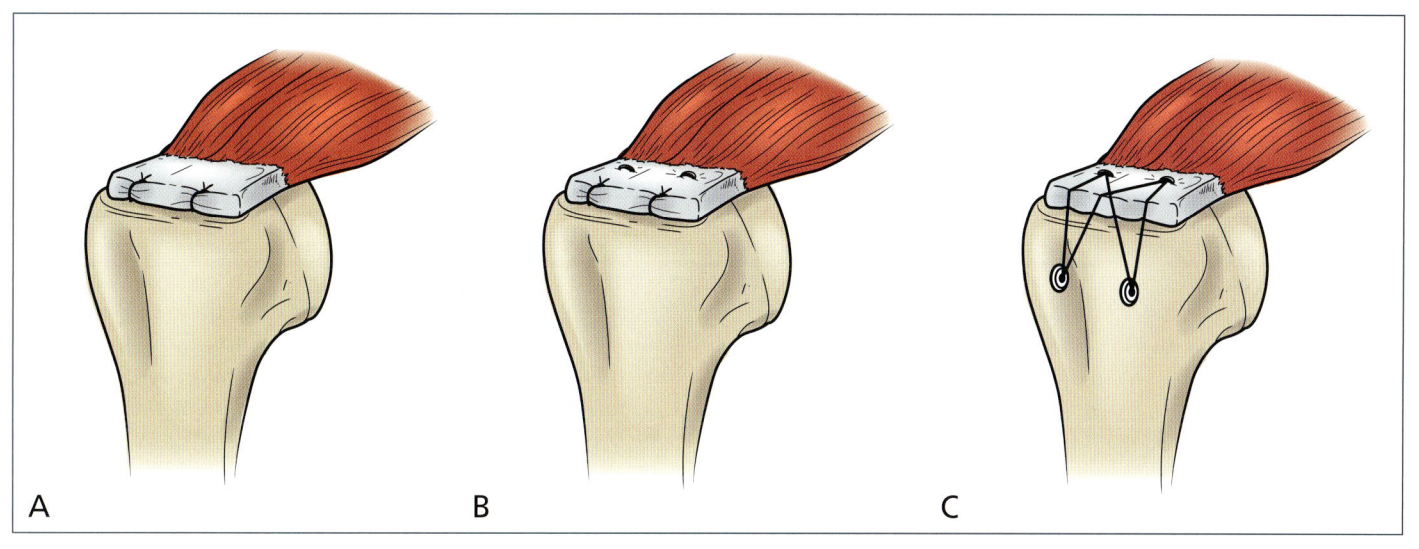

Figure 8 Illustrations depict types of arthroscopic rotator cuff repair. **A,** Single-row repair. **B,** Double-row repair. **C,** Suture-bridge repair.

fixation and compression of the tendon to the footprint of the tuberosity. The number of anchors and the configuration of the medial and lateral rows depend on the size of the tear. In general, a medium-sized tear (1 to 3 cm) will require one medial-row anchor and two lateral-row anchors; a large tear (3 to 5 cm) will use two medial-row anchors and two or three lateral-row anchors; and massive tears (> 5 cm) require three medial-row anchors and two or three lateral-row anchors.

Numerous devices are available for suture passage, including sharp suture-passing instruments, suture shuttles, and antegrade suture-passing instruments. We prefer to use an instrument that allows multiple antegrade sutures to be passed with a single loading. We have found this to be the most efficient and simple way to pass the horizontal mattress sutures that we use in both single-row and double-row repairs. In some instances, the use of suture shuttle devices through the anterior, posterior, or Neviaser portal can be helpful.

8. Knot Tying

The ability to tie a secure arthroscopic knot is a requirement for arthroscopic rotator cuff repair. Arthroscopic knots can be categorized as simple knots, sliding knots, or sliding-locking knots (**Figure 9**). At the minimum, a surgeon should be competent in tying a simple knot and a sliding or sliding-locking knot.

We prefer to use a sliding-locking knot (a Tennessee slider), followed by three alternating half hitches. If the suture will not slide easily through the suture anchor, we use a standard Revo knot (three half hitches with the same post followed by three half hitches with alternating posts).

9. Lateral-Row Repair

As mentioned previously, using a lateral row increases the biomechanical

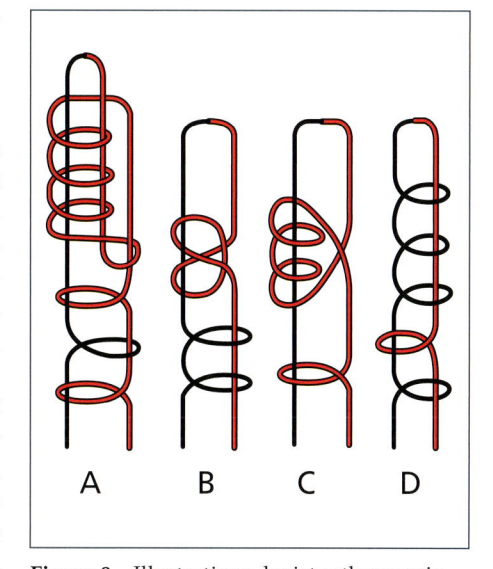

Figure 9 Illustrations depict arthroscopic knots. **A,** The Duncan loop, backed with alternating post half hitches (a nonlocking sliding knot). **B,** The Tennessee slider knot (a sliding-locking knot). **C,** The midshipman's hitch knot (a sliding-locking knot). **D,** The Revo knot (a nonsliding knot).

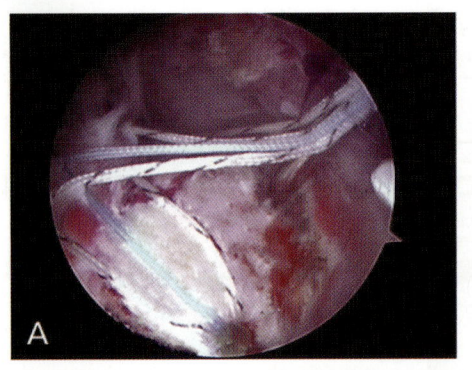

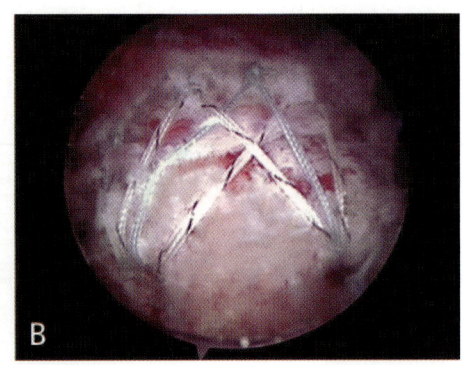

Figure 10 Arthroscopic views show a suture-bridge repair. **A,** View from the posterolateral portal shows the insertion of the lateral-row anchor 1 cm lateral to the greater tuberosity. **B,** Reduction of the rotator cuff tear and compression to the tuberosity is achieved with a double-row suture-bridge repair.

properties of a rotator cuff repair, but the clinical benefit has yet to be proven.[13] The options for lateral-row fixation include the placement of suture anchors or the creation of a suture-bridge construct using a knotless anchor.

If standard suture anchors are used, they should be placed at the lateral margin of the tuberosity, and sutures should be passed before tying the medial-row repair. Whether to tie the medial-row sutures or lateral-row sutures first has been debated; in our opinion, fixation of the lateral row first, followed by the medial row, appears to offer the most biomechanically sound method of fixation.

In a suture-bridge repair, the limbs of the tied medial-row mattress sutures are fixed to the lateral aspect of the proximal humerus using a knotless anchor. Multiple knotless devices are available, with techniques specific to each device. In general, the sutures from the medial row, usually one from each medial knot, are retrieved through the lateral portal and then passed into a knotless anchor. The anchor is placed 1 cm lateral to the tuberosity (**Figure 10, A**). Débridement of the bursa over the lateral aspect of the proximal humerus will facilitate anchor insertion, and careful planning must be performed to space the anchors at least 1 cm apart. Compression of the tendon tissue to the tuberosity is important (**Figure 10, B**), but overtightening of the suture bridge may result in compromise of the blood supply to the tendon tissue, negatively affecting the healing of the tendon.

10. Closure and Perioperative Care

After the rotator cuff is repaired, any ancillary procedures are performed and hemostasis is obtained. The arthroscopic portals are closed with an absorbable buried stitch, and adhesive skin closure strips and a topical skin adhesive are applied for skin closure. Dry sterile dressings are applied. While on the operating room table, the patient is placed in a sling with an abduction pillow and is awakened from anesthesia with deep extubation to prevent bucking or movement of the surgical extremity. The patient is discharged home after meeting postoperative care unit criteria. The dressings are left intact for 72 hours, at which time they are removed and showering is permitted. The patient is seen for initial follow-up and wound check 10 to 14 days following the repair.

Complications

Complications after arthroscopic rotator cuff repair are similar to those of open rotator cuff repair. The overall complication rate following rotator cuff repair is estimated to be approximately 10% (**Table 3**). This is based on a large review of 40 published series on rotator cuff repairs.[15] Complications include shoulder stiffness, failure of healing, infection, reflex sympathetic dystrophy, deep venous thrombosis, and death.

Persistent stiffness and arthrofibrosis are the most common sequelae following rotator cuff repair. Risk factors include preoperative joint contracture and a history of arthrofibrosis after prior operations. Stiffness and loss of motion following arthroscopic rotator cuff repair are expected and, in some series, have been associated with increased rates of tendon healing. Physical therapy usually resolves even moderate stiffness over the course of several months following surgery. Refractory postoperative stiffness may be managed with manipulation under anesthesia, arthroscopic lysis of adhesions, and capsular release.

Failures of tendon repair and rerupture are well recognized and have been associated with larger tear size, poor tendon quality, and fatty atrophy of the muscle. Failure of tendon healing after rotator cuff repair has been shown to result in reasonable pain relief but inferior functional results. Most individuals with failure of tendon healing are satisfied with the outcome and do not require additional surgical intervention. If revision surgery is proposed, specific goals need to be identified based on individual patient pathology and expectations. Persistent pain is the most common indication for reoperation; the preoperative identification of the etiology of the patient's symptoms is essential for successful revision surgery. The results following revision rotator cuff repair are compromised compared with primary repair.[16] Patient expectations need to be appropriate because strength deficits may persist, particularly in the setting of permanent atrophic tendon or in the presence of fatty atrophy within the cuff muscles, identified in the preoperative evaluation.

As with any surgical procedure, medical complications following arthroscopic or open rotator cuff surgery have been reported. They include, but are not limited to, pneumonia, myocardial infarction, cerebrovascular ischemia, deep venous thrombosis, pulmonary embolus, and postoperative depression. Superficial wound infection also has been reported, but the incidence is exceedingly low, and the rate of deep infection represents an even lower rate of occurrence.[15,17]

Hypotensive anesthesia, with systolic pressures of 100 to 110 mm Hg, has been associated with potential problems with cerebral perfusion, especially in patients with preoperative hypertension.[18]

Postoperative Care and Rehabilitation

Postoperative protocols often are very surgeon-specific, with some advocating early motion to prevent stiffness and faster recovery of function and others recommending very limited activity to allow tendon healing. Recent studies on rehabilitation programs following rotator cuff repair have shown no difference in range of motion or function with accelerated rehabilitation protocols but have shown increased rates of recurrent tearing on postoperative MRI at 1 year.[19] Our current protocol involves three phases of

Table 3 Reported Complications of Rotator Cuff Repair

Complication	No. of Shoulders (%)
Failed tendon repair	182 (6.2)
Nerve injury	33 (1.1)
Infection	31 (1.1)
Deltoid avulsion	16 (0.5)
Frozen shoulder	16 (0.5)
Suture granuloma	14 (0.5)
Wound hematoma	11 (0.4)
Dislocation	3 (0.1)
Reflex dystrophy	2 (0.1)
Greater tuberosity fracture	1 (0.1)
Acromion fracture	1 (0.1)
Total	310 (10.5)

Reproduced with permission from Mansat P, Cofield RH, Kersten TE, Rowland CM: Complications of rotator cuff repair. *Orthop Clin North Am* 1997;28(2):205-213.

rehabilitation. The exact duration of each phase is modified slightly, depending on the size of the tear, the quality of the tissues, and the strength of the repair.

Healing Phase (Weeks 0 to 5)

The patient is placed in a sling with an abduction pillow immediately following surgery. The patient is instructed to remove the sling to perform hand, wrist, and elbow range-of-motion and pendulum exercises 2 to 3 times daily. The sling may be removed for hygiene activities and dressing, being careful to not use the arm for any active motion. The patient is instructed in how to perform the exercises before leaving the hospital and, in most cases, formal physical therapy is not required during this phase. For patients who develop severe stiffness or have difficulty complying with the home exercise program, formal physical therapy is initiated after the first postoperative visit, at 2 weeks after the repair. Physical therapy at this time is focused on pendulum and gentle passive range-of-motion exercises.

Recovery of Motion Phase (Weeks 6 to 12)

The sling is discontinued 6 weeks after surgery, and the patient is allowed to use the arm for activities of daily living with strict instructions to not lift anything heavier than 2 lb. Physical therapy is begun at this time if it has not already been initiated, focusing on active and active-assisted range-of-motion exercises. At the conclusion of this phase, the patient should have full range of motion and the ability to use the arm for all activities of daily living. Soft-tissue discomfort and weakness of the shoulder girdle often remain, however.

Strengthening Phase (Weeks 12–)

At 12 weeks after surgery, the patient is started on a formal rotator cuff strengthening program. Recovery of full strength and function often takes several months, and ultimate recovery frequently is not obtained until 12 to 18 months following repair.

Pearls

The ultimate goal of repair is to create a tension-free anatomic restoration of the rotator cuff tendon insertion. This goal must not be compromised by the desire to perform an all-arthroscopic repair. Conversion to a mini-open repair is done easily by extending the lateral working portal by 2 to 3 cm and splitting the deltoid fibers. In our experience, this has not resulted in any increased morbidity or compromised outcome.

For successful arthroscopic repair, adequate visualization; accurate assessment of the tear pattern and a plan for the method of repair; and a simple and reproducible plan for anchor placement; suture passage, docking, and knot tying are essential. The following pearls will help achieve these goals.

To minimize swelling and fluid extravasation and facilitate visualization:
- The total arthroscopy time should be less than 2 hours.
- Cannulas should be used for all working portals.
- Low fluid pressure and flow (40 to 50 mm Hg) should be maintained.
- A radiofrequency probe should be used to cauterize bleeding tissues.
- Retractors can be used to help improve visualization in the presence of significant swelling or fluid extravasation.
- Hypotensive anesthesia (a systolic blood pressure of 100 to 110 mm Hg) can be used.

To facilitate accurate assessment of the tear pattern and a plan for the method of repair:
- The subacromial bursa should be resected completely, taking care to delineate the plane between the cuff and the bursal tissue to help prevent damage to the tendon.
- Acromioplasty should be performed before starting the repair to help increase the working space.
- Traction sutures can be placed in the tendon to facilitate mobilization and reduction.
- The release of adhesions on the bursal and articular sides of the tendon and the rotator interval may be required in retracted tears.
- Marginal convergence sutures can be placed to help close longitudinal tears and relieve tension from the tuberosity repair.

The following techniques will help facilitate the placement and management of sutures:
- When placing multiple anchors, start with the most anterior anchor and work in a posterior direction.
- The sutures from each anchor are passed and docked in the anterior portal before the next anchor is inserted.
- Knot tying is performed once all sutures have been passed, starting with the most posterior suture and proceeding anteriorly.
- For single-row repairs, each suture is cut following the knot tying; in suture-bridge repairs, the sutures are docked in the posterior portal.

References

1. Rudzki JR, Adler RS, Warren RF, et al: Contrast-enhanced ultrasound characterization of the vascularity of the rotator

cuff tendon: Age- and activity-related changes in the intact asymptomatic rotator cuff. *J Shoulder Elbow Surg* 2008;17(1, suppl):96S-100S.

2. Mall NA, Kim HM, Keener JD, et al: Symptomatic progression of asymptomatic rotator cuff tears: A prospective study of clinical and sonographic variables. *J Bone Joint Surg Am* 2010;92(16):2623-2633.

3. Buess E, Steuber KU, Waibl B: Open versus arthroscopic rotator cuff repair: A comparative view of 96 cases. *Arthroscopy* 2005;21(5):597-604.

4. Melis B, DeFranco MJ, Chuinard C, Walch G: Natural history of fatty infiltration and atrophy of the supraspinatus muscle in rotator cuff tears. *Clin Orthop Relat Res* 2010;468(6):1498-1505.

5. Zanetti M, Gerber C, Hodler J: Quantitative assessment of the muscles of the rotator cuff with magnetic resonance imaging. *Invest Radiol* 1998;33(3):163-170.

6. Barber FA, Hapa O, Bynum JA: Comparative testing by cyclic loading of rotator cuff suture anchors containing multiple high-strength sutures. *Arthroscopy* 2010;26(9, suppl):S134-S141.

7. Hayashida K, Yoneda M, Mizuno N, Fukushima S, Nakagawa S: Arthroscopic Bankart repair with knotless suture anchor for traumatic anterior shoulder instability: Results of short-term follow-up. *Arthroscopy* 2006;22(6):620-626.

8. Burkhart SS, Lo IK: Arthroscopic rotator cuff repair. *J Am Acad Orthop Surg* 2006;14(6):333-346.

9. Huijsmans PE, Pritchard MP, Berghs BM, van Rooyen KS, Wallace AL, de Beer JF: Arthroscopic rotator cuff repair with double-row fixation. *J Bone Joint Surg Am* 2007;89(6):1248-1257.

10. Nho SJ, Ghodadra N, Provencher MT, Reiff S, Romeo AA: Anatomic reduction and next-generation fixation constructs for arthroscopic repair of crescent, L-shaped, and U-shaped rotator cuff tears. *Arthroscopy* 2009;25(5):553-559.

11. Lafosse L, Brzoska R, Toussaint B, Gobezie R: The outcome and structural integrity of arthroscopic rotator cuff repair with use of the double-row suture anchor technique: Surgical technique. *J Bone Joint Surg Am* 2008;90(suppl 2 pt 2):275-286.

12. Zumstein MA, Jost B, Hempel J, Hodler J, Gerber C: The clinical and structural long-term results of open repair of massive tears of the rotator cuff. *J Bone Joint Surg Am* 2008;90(11):2423-2431.

13. Saridakis P, Jones G: Outcomes of single-row and double-row arthroscopic rotator cuff repair: A systematic review. *J Bone Joint Surg Am* 2010;92(3):732-742.

14. Duquin TR, Buyea C, Bisson LJ: Which method of rotator cuff repair leads to the highest rate of structural healing? A systematic review. *Am J Sports Med* 2010;38(4):835-841.

15. Mansat P, Cofield RH, Kersten TE, Rowland CM: Complications of rotator cuff repair. *Orthop Clin North Am* 1997;28(2):205-213.

16. Cofield RH, Parvizi J, Hoffmeyer PJ, Lanzer WL, Ilstrup DM, Rowland CM: Surgical repair of chronic rotator cuff tears: A prospective long-term study. *J Bone Joint Surg Am* 2001;83(1):71-77.

17. Brislin KJ, Field LD, Savoie FH III: Complications after arthroscopic rotator cuff repair. *Arthroscopy* 2007;23(2):124-128.

18. Rains DD, Rooke GA, Wahl CJ: Pathomechanisms and complications related to patient positioning and anesthesia during shoulder arthroscopy. *Arthroscopy* 2011;27(4):532-541.

19. Cuff DJ, Pupello DR: Prospective randomized study of arthroscopic rotator cuff repair using an early versus delayed postoperative physical therapy protocol. *J Shoulder Elbow Surg* 2012;21(11):1450-1455.

Chapter 26
Percutaneous Pinning of Proximal Humerus Fractures

Bradford O. Parsons, MD

Patient Selection
Indications

Percutaneous pinning is indicated for select displaced two-, three-, and four-part fractures and in select patients. Originally described by Jaberg et al,[1] it has gained popularity and has proven efficacious, enabling a minimally invasive approach to fracture reduction, fixation, and restoration of functional outcome.[2-8] Optimal fracture patterns include displaced surgical neck fractures without calcar or medial hinge comminution, select three-part fractures in which humeral head version and tuberosity height can be anatomically restored, and the valgus-impacted four-part fracture in which the medial hinge and calcar are intact[3-5] (**Figure 1**). The timing of surgical management has an impact on the success of this technique; late reduction (>1 week from injury) may be difficult because hematoma and scarring diminish fracture fragment mobility and reduction.

Contraindications

Although percutaneous pinning has been successfully performed in elderly patients, osteopenic bone may pose a relative contraindication, as deficient bone quality may preclude sufficient fixation strength of percutaneously placed pin or screw fixation.[2] Additionally, fractures with extensive comminution of the tuberosities, medial calcar, or head segment are often not amenable to percutaneous pin and screw fixation because sufficient fixation is not afforded with this technique (**Figure 2**). Varus-displaced fractures, with loss of medial bone integrity, also are contraindicated because pin fixation is often insufficient to prevent redisplacement of the varus fracture fragments. Further, true three- and four-part fracture-dislocations or head-split fractures are often not amenable to percutaneous treatment. These more complex fractures with diminished bone quality, comminution, and varus displacement are indicated for formal open reduction and internal fixation with locking-plate fixation or arthroplasty reconstruction.

Preoperative Imaging

Preoperative imaging requires three orthogonal plain radiographs: the true AP view with the shoulder in neutral rotation taken in the plane of the scapula (Grashey view) the scapular lateral view, and the axillary lateral view (**Figure 3**). Often, CT aids in the assessment of fracture fragment positioning, angulation, and comminution and can be very helpful (**Figure 4**). MRI is not usually necessary or indicated.

Video 26.1 Percutaneous Pinning: When and How to Do It. Jonathan P. Braman, MD; Evan L. Flatow, MD (7 min)

Procedure
Room Setup/Patient Positioning

Patients are positioned in the beach-chair position, with the injured arm freely mobile and lateral to the table. An articulating arm positioner is routinely used. The entire forequarter is draped free. Patients are routinely anesthetized with an interscalene regional block, and general anesthesia is not usually required. Critical to the success of percutaneous management of proximal humerus fractures is the ability to obtain precise, multiplanar fluoroscopic images.[9] A large C-arm is brought into the surgical field from the contralateral side such that a Grashey

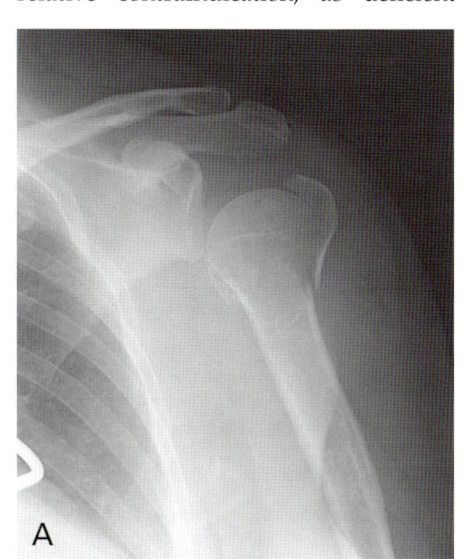

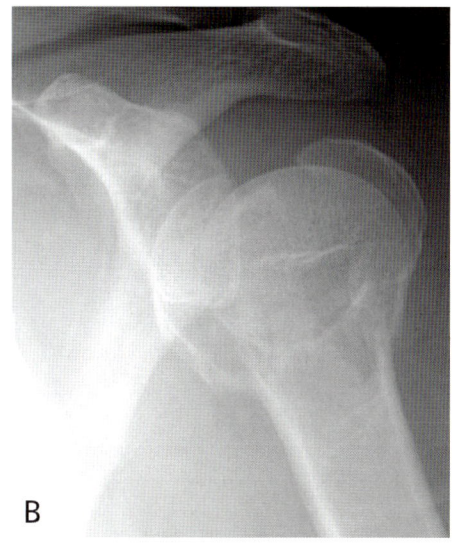

Figure 1 Grashey (**A**) and AP (**B**) views of the shoulder demonstrate a valgus-impacted four-part proximal humerus fracture.

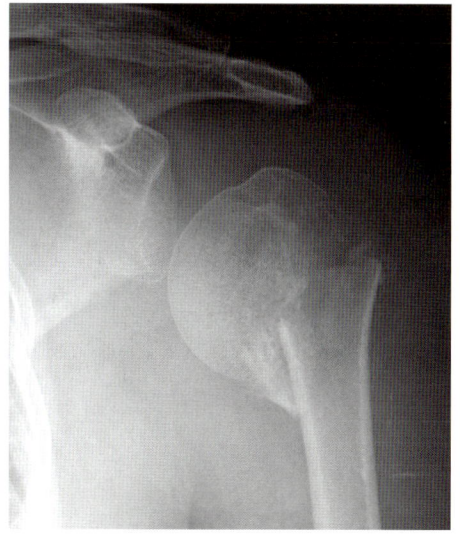

Figure 2 Grashey view demonstrates a varus-displaced surgical neck fracture with medial calcar comminution. This fracture pattern is at high risk for redisplacement and is most often not amenable to percutaneous fixation. Proximal humeral locking-plate fixation is most often advocated for such fractures.

Dr. Parsons or an immediate family member is a member of a speakers' bureau or has made paid presentations on behalf of Zimmer and Arthrex; serves as a paid consultant to or is an employee of Zimmer and Arthrex; and has received research or institutional support from Wyeth.

Section 2: Shoulder and Elbow

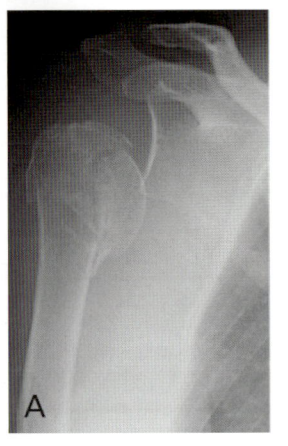

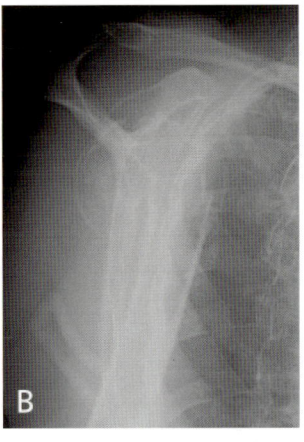

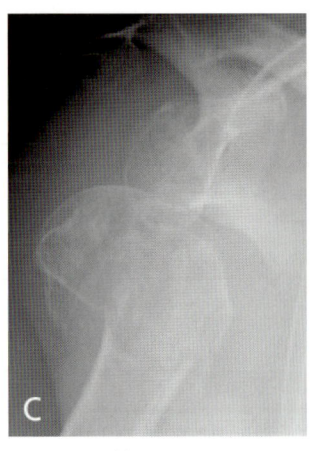

Figure 3 Typical trauma series of radiographs required to assess proximal humerus fractures, including a Grashey view (**A**), a scapular lateral view (**B**), and an axillary lateral view (**C**). The head-split component of this fracture is most evident on the axillary lateral view.

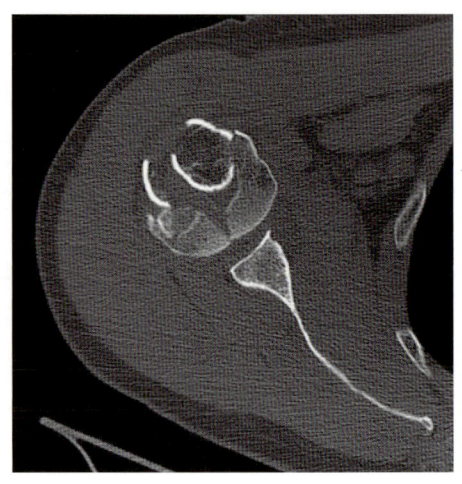

Figure 4 Axial CT scan of the shoulder shows a head-split fracture.

view, a scapular lateral view, and an axillary lateral view can be obtained (**Figure 5**). Positioning of the operating table, patient, drapes, and C-arm in a fashion that enables seamless fluoroscopic imaging of all three planes is critical; if this imaging cannot be obtained, percutaneous techniques may not be warranted. Although the steps in the video are nearly identical to those outlined here, one minor difference is the use of a mini C-arm imager, as opposed to a larger imager, which is currently routinely used.

Special Instruments/Equipment/Implants

Equipment necessary for this technique includes small elevators (eg, Cobb, Freer); bone tamps (small and large); small bone/skin hooks; and surgical clamps, which allow for portal dilation, fracture fragment mobilization, and reduction. Routinely, 3.5-/4.0-mm partially threaded cannulated screws are used to fix tuberosity fragments to the medial calcar bone, and often screw lengths of over 50 mm may be necessary in larger patients. Soft-tissue drill sleeves are critical to protect deep tissues. Rigid, terminally threaded 2.4- or 2.8-mm pins are used for shaft-to-head fixation. A large pin cutter is required to cut 2.4-/2.8-mm pins beneath the skin at the completion of fracture reduction and fixation. A commercial equipment set that contains the aforementioned instrumentation and screws/pins necessary for percutaneous fixation is presently available from Arthrex.

Surgical Technique

After the patient is appropriately positioned and the affected extremity is prepped and draped, the osseous landmarks are marked on the skin. Portals are marked for fracture reduction and proximal screw fixation, as well as the orientation of the axillary nerve relative to the lateral edge of the acromion. Typical portals are marked along the lateral edge of the acromion for proximal tuberosity fixation, and the reduction portal is positioned 2 to 3 cm distal to the anterolateral acromial corner (**Figure 6**).

With the fractured arm in neutral to slight external rotation, the reduction portal is developed and blunt dissection through the deltoid down to the proxi-

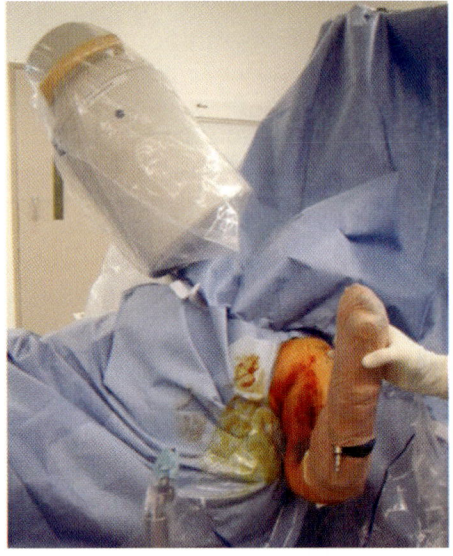

Figure 5 Intraoperative photograph shows the recommended room setup, which is critical to successful percutaneous fixation of proximal humerus fractures. A beach-chair position is routinely used, as well as an arm holder. To enable precise, multiplanar fluoroscopic views, including Grashey, outlet, and axillary views, a large C-arm imager that comes from the contralateral side can be used.

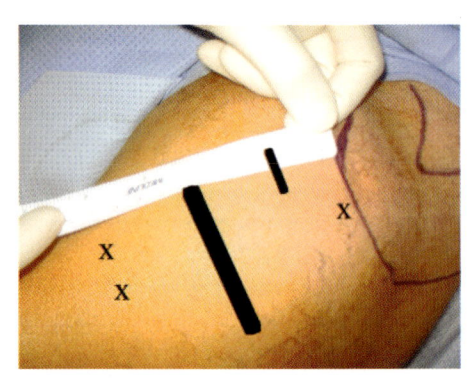

Figure 6 Photograph shows markings for placement of portals (X) for fracture reduction and pin placement, including the distal portals for placement of 2.8-mm pins into the shaft and head. The tuberosity Kirschner-wire portal, next to the lateral acromion, is denoted by the purple line. The short black line denotes placement of the reduction portal, usually 2 to 3 cm distal to the anterolateral acromial corner. The long black line denotes the typical course of the axillary nerve, approximately 5 cm distal to the lateral edge of the acromion.

mal humerus is performed. Typically, the fracture plane between the head, the tuberosities, and the shaft occurs just posterior to the bicipital groove in three- and four-part fractures. Under fluoroscopic guidance, a small elevator is placed into the fracture site to develop the fracture plane, followed by a small tamp that is used to elevate the humeral head segment from the valgus-impacted position (**Figure 7**). Isolated, displaced surgical neck fractures can similarly be reduced along the surgical neck fracture plane.

Once anatomic articular segment reduction is obtained, including restoration of neck-shaft angle and version, the head segment is pinned with a 2.8-mm terminally threaded wire placed in a retrograde fashion from the humeral shaft

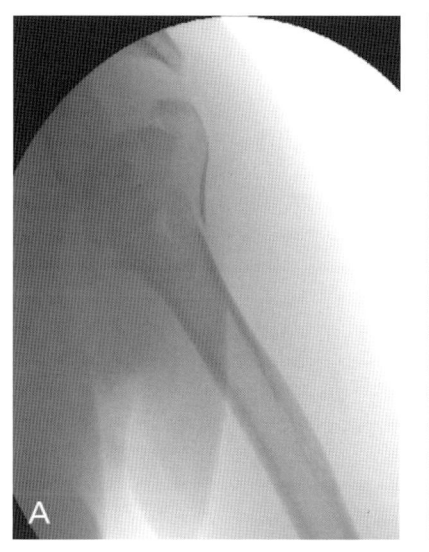

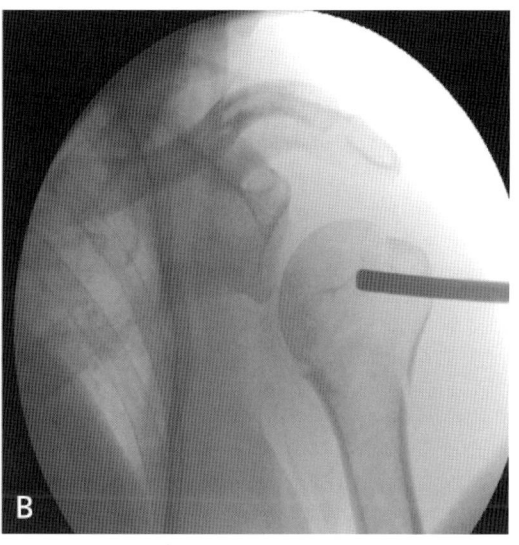

Figure 7 Fluoroscopic images of a valgus-impacted fracture. **A,** Preoperative image demonstrates tuberosity malposition. **B,** A small bone tamp is placed into the fracture plane beneath the humeral head, and impaction is used to anatomically reduce the humeral head into appropriate inclination and version.

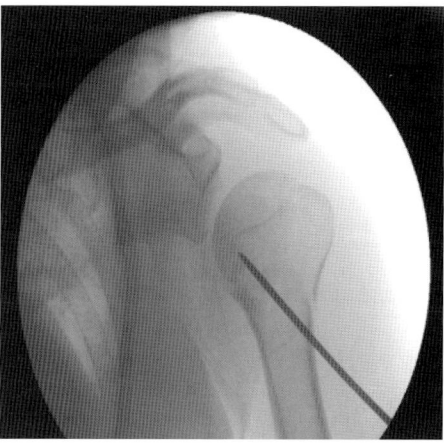

Figure 8 Fluoroscopic image shows placement of a 2.8-mm terminally threaded pin via the distal skin portals into the shaft and humeral head in a retrograde fashion. Once appropriate angulation into the head is confirmed by fluoroscopy, pins are advanced by hand with care to prevent penetration through the subchondral bone into the joint.

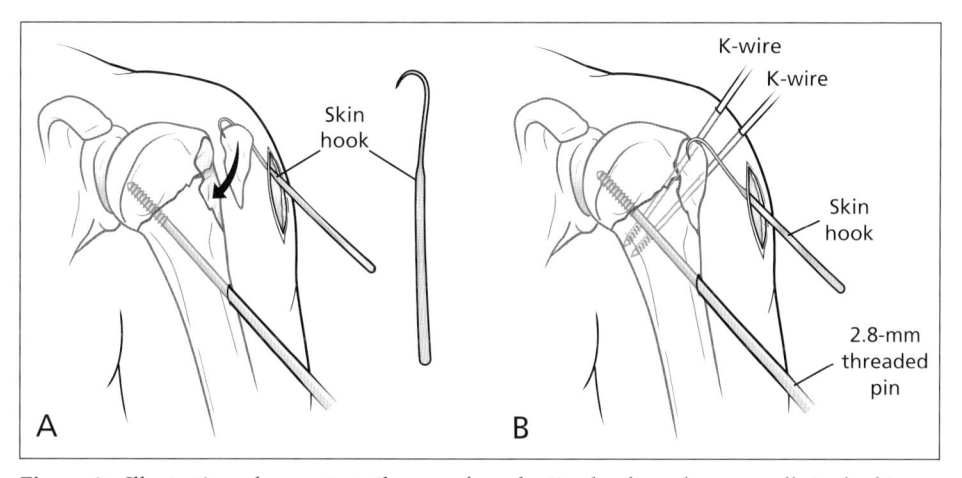

Figure 9 Illustrations demonstrate the use of a reduction hook, such as a small single skin hook, which is placed through the reduction portal into the subacromial space onto the greater tuberosity. Often the tuberosity is superiorly and posteriorly displaced, and by anteroinferior pull with the hook, the fracture can be reduced (**A**) and held until provisional Kirschner-wire (K-wire) fixation is obtained (**B**).

into the head (**Figure 8**). Distal pins are placed through small (<1 cm) portals in the anterolateral brachium, distal to the course of the axillary nerve. After pin penetration of the lateral humeral cortex, the pin is advanced by hand to prevent articular segment penetration. The use of a soft-tissue sleeve is paramount in preventing soft-tissue injury during pin passage.[9-11] After confirmation of appropriate reduction and pin placement, length is confirmed on multiplanar fluoroscopy. A second pin parallel to the first is placed in a similar fashion, usually 2 to 3 cm apart.[10] In some situations, a third pin may be placed in select fractures.

Once the humeral head is securely fixed to the shaft, attention is focused on reduction of the greater and/or lesser tuberosities. In two-part fractures involving the surgical neck, this step is not required, but it is necessary for three- and four-part fractures. Often, when anatomic reduction of the articular segment is obtained, the tuberosities will spontaneously reduce. If reduction is required, the greater tuberosity is reduced first. Using the fracture reduction portal, a small skin hook or clamp is placed deep to the deltoid into the subacromial space and is used to reduce the greater tuberosity anatomically relative to the humeral head (**Figure 9**). Provisional fixation is then made with two percutaneously placed 1.6-mm Kirschner wires (K-wires), which will later be overdrilled and replaced by cannulated screws. Pin/screw orientation should be from the top of the tuberosity, aimed distally into the medial humeral calcar and cortical bone[11] (**Figure 10**). Bicortical screw fixation is critical for these fragments. As calcar comminution may preclude such fixation, fractures with calcar comminution and varus displacement are often contraindicated for percutaneous management. Two K-wires are routinely placed in the greater tuberosity to prevent loss of reduction when the K-wire is overdrilled. Ultimately, two partially threaded cannulated screws are placed through small (<1 cm) portals over the K-wires with appropriate length and orientation confirmed on multiplanar fluoroscopic imaging.

If the lesser tuberosity remains displaced following reduction of the articular segment and the greater tuberosity, it is now reduced. In many four-part valgus-impacted fractures, the lesser tuberosity will spontaneously reduce following reduction of the humeral articular surface and the greater tuberosity, and in such situations, formal reduction or fixation is not necessary. Stability of the lesser tuberosity is often maintained by soft-tissue attachments of the rotator interval and rotator cuff tissues between the tuberosities and head. Using the reduction portal and reduction hooks, the lesser tuberosity is reduced (**Figure 11**). Most often, this requires visualization of the fragment on scapular lateral or axillary radiographs for full assessment of fracture position. Once reduction is confirmed, lesser tuberosity fixation is obtained in a similar fashion as for the greater tuberosity, with pin placement followed by cannulated screw fixation. However, in some cases,

Section 2: Shoulder and Elbow

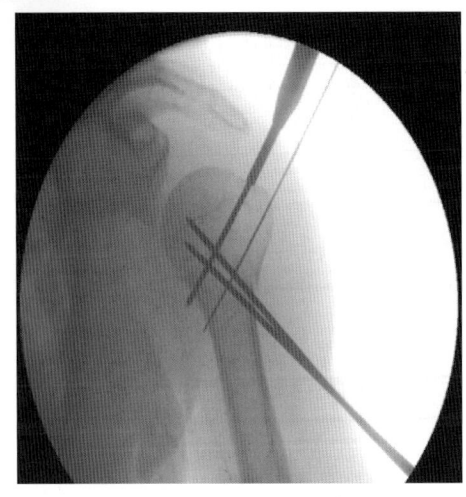

Figure 10 Fluoroscopic image shows placement of two Kirschner wires (K-wires) for provisional fixation after tuberosity reduction. K-wires are routinely placed distally into the humeral medial calcar for optimal fixation.

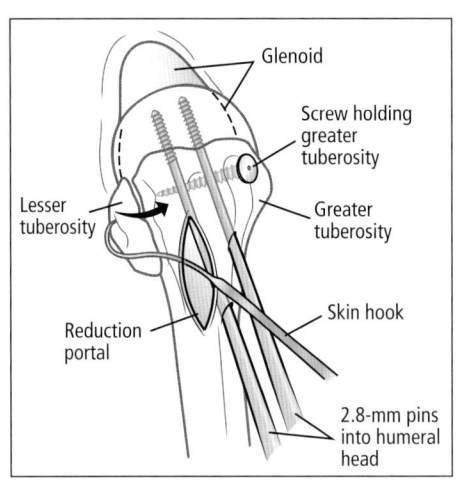

Figure 11 Illustration demonstrates the use of a small skin hook to reduce the lesser tuberosity following reduction and fixation of the humeral head and greater tuberosity in a valgus-impacted four-part fracture.

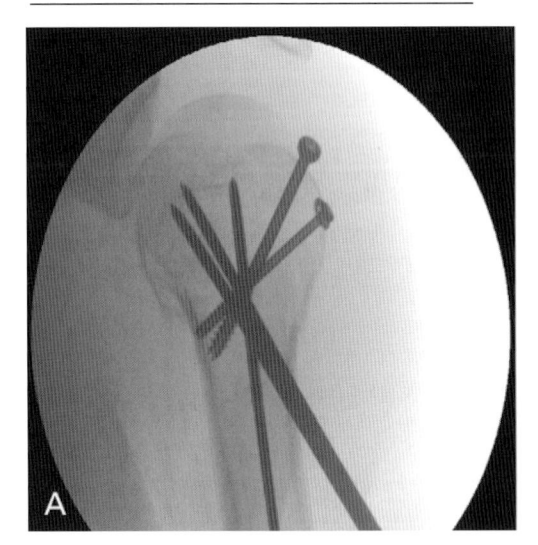

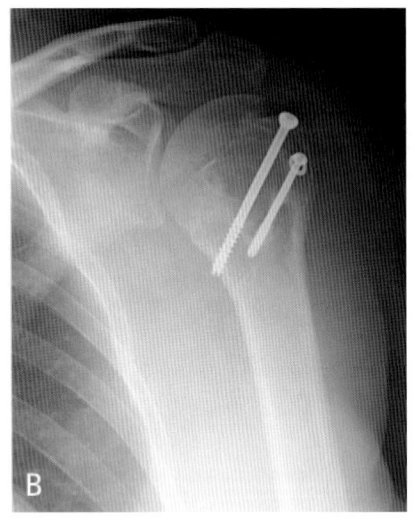

Figure 12 Final fluoroscopic image (**A**) demonstrates pin placement and screw fixation of a valgus-impacted four-part proximal humerus fracture. Postoperative AP radiograph (**B**) obtained at 6 months demonstrates the healed fracture and retained cannulated screws. Pins are routinely removed at 4 weeks under fluoroscopic image guidance in the operating room.

the lesser tuberosity fragment orientation relative to the other fracture planes enables only unicortical or cancellous fixation within the humeral head, in which case a partially threaded 4.0-mm cancellous screw is used.

After definitive screw fixation of the tuberosities is complete, the shoulder is brought through a range of motion under fluoroscopy to critically analyze anatomic fracture reduction and ensure that sufficient fracture fixation has been obtained. Careful fluoroscopic examination for hardware penetration of the joint should be performed. Observation of any crepitus should also be evaluated for prominent intra-articular hardware. Most often, hardware is likely to penetrate the posterosuperior quadrant of the humeral head, which may be observed only with extreme externally rotated AP imaging or axillary imaging.[9] When reduction and appropriate hardware placement/fixation are confirmed, the K-wires are removed from the cannulated screws, and the 2.8-mm pins are cut beneath the skin. Portals are closed with buried interrupted absorbable suture and dressed with adhesive skin closure strips and gauze. A final fluoroscopic examination is performed, and the arm is placed in a sling at the side (**Figure 12**).

Complications

Major complications are rare with this procedure. Reported series yield nearly a 100% union rate and low rates of complications, which include loss of reduction, malunion, hardware failure, and late osteonecrosis.[1-8] Loss of fracture reduction and hardware failure can occur, especially in older patients with osteoporotic bone or in patients who fail to comply with postoperative immobilization. Tuberosity failure is most often secondary to screw pullout if bicortical fixation into the calcar is not obtained (**Figure 13**). Some authors advocate greater tuberosity fixation into the humeral head, but in my experience, this may not be robust enough, leading to loss of fixation. I now routinely use the humeral calcar. Certain fractures may not be amenable to percutaneous fixation, especially varus, comminuted fractures, because these fractures are at high risk for hardware failure and redisplacement.

Pin penetration into the joint may occur and is most often missed when pins are placed in the posterosuperior quadrant of the humeral head. Careful fluoroscopic assessment of fracture reduction and hardware placement is critical to avoid intra-articular hardware. Secondarily, some pins that are cut beneath the skin may become prominent before 4 weeks postoperatively, possibly as arm swelling diminishes, or in cases of hardware failure or pin migration. Pins that become prominent may be removed if the fracture is stable.

Osteonecrosis can also occur, especially in four-part fractures, as late as a few years following treatment. In a series by Keener et al,[5] osteonecrosis was observed in 3 of 27 patients following percutaneous pinning of two-, three-, and four-part fractures. Recently, the intermediate outcome of this series of patients was reevaluated with longer term follow-up, and the results were presented at the 11th International Congress of Shoulder and Elbow Surgery.[12] Interestingly, osteonecrosis rates had increased to 26% (7 patients), representing 50% of the four-part fractures, with some developing symptomatic osteonecrosis more than 2 years postoperatively[12] (**Figure 14**).

Postoperative Care and Rehabilitation

The surgical arm is immobilized in a sling for 4 weeks. At 4 weeks, the 2.8-mm pins are removed under sedation and local anesthesia in the operating room, and a gentle examination under anesthesia is performed to assess fracture stability and guide therapy goals. Following pin removal, active-assisted and passive range-of-motion exercises typically are begun, with transition to active range of motion between 6 and 8 weeks after

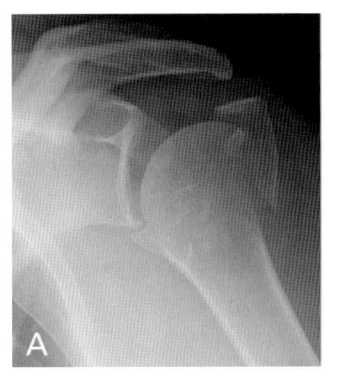

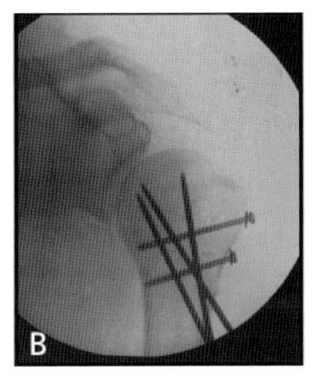

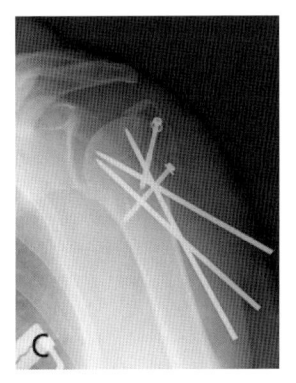

Figure 13 Images of the shoulder in a patient with a displaced three-part proximal humerus fracture. **A,** Preoperative AP radiograph. **B,** Intraoperative AP fluoroscopic image following percutaneous reduction and fixation. Note the questionable lack of bicortical fixation of the tuberosity screws into the humeral calcar distally. The patient fell postoperatively at 7 days and presented with loss of fixation and tuberosity redisplacement at 9 days postoperatively (**C**). Critical to success is stout fixation of the greater tuberosity with bicortical screw fixation into the humeral calcar.

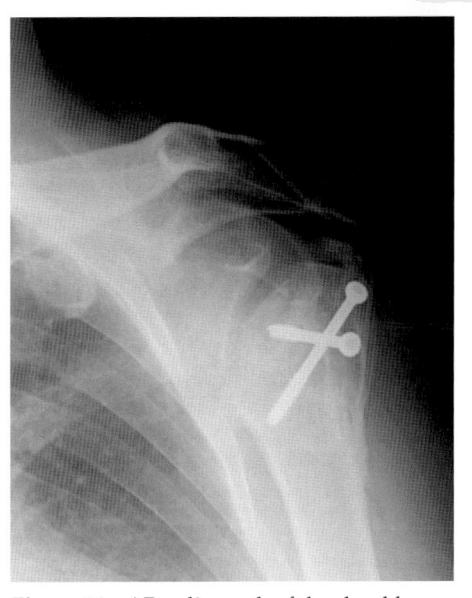

Figure 14 AP radiograph of the shoulder following percutaneous pinning of a four-part proximal humerus fracture. Patients such as this one, with posttraumatic changes and with persistent symptoms, may ultimately require arthroplasty reconstruction.

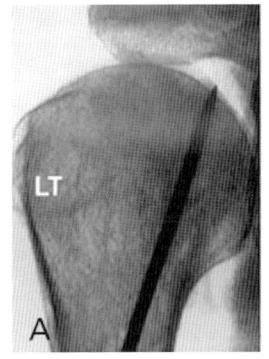

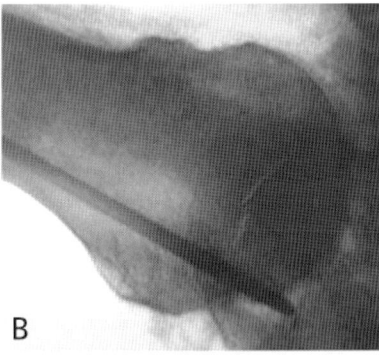

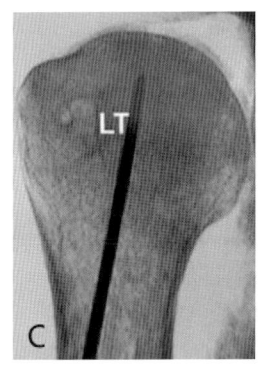

Figure 15 Fluoroscopic images demonstrate pin placement in the humeral head. Klepps et al[9] found that pin penetration most commonly occurred in the posterior quadrant of the humeral head and could be observed only in a 60° Grashey view (**A**) or cephalad tilt axillary view (**B**), as opposed to the standard neutral AP image (**C**). LT = lesser tuberosity. (Reproduced with permission from Klepps SJ, Miller SL, Lin J, Gladstone J, Flatow EL: Determination of radiographic guidelines for percutaneous fixation of proximal humerus fractures using a cadaveric model. *Orthopedics* 2007;30[8]:636-641.)

percutaneous pinning. Strengthening of the shoulder is begun at 12 weeks postoperatively.

Pearls

Critical to the success of percutaneous reduction and fixation of proximal humerus fractures is timing and being prepared. Optimally, patients are operated on with this technique within a few (up to 5 to 7) days following injury. Longer delay often results in early adhesions of fracture fragments, impeding reduction and often requiring open techniques. Second, bailout to an open plating or hemiarthroplasty may be necessary, and appropriate planning and equipment for this are required.

This technique has a learning curve, and certain fracture patterns are easier to treat percutaneously than others, notably surgical neck fractures without varus displacement or medial calcar comminution and true valgus-impacted four-part fractures. Surgeons who are gaining experience with this technique are more likely to have success managing these fracture patterns percutaneously before moving on to more complex patterns such as three-part fractures with altered version and comminuted fractures.

Technical pearls include portal placement, the identification of fracture planes, reduction techniques, and optimal hardware placement. The reduction portal is placed directly off the anterolateral corner of the acromion because this position is often directly over the biceps groove when the arm is in neutral or slight external rotation. Most commonly, the fracture plane between the greater and lesser tuberosity lies slightly posterior to the biceps groove, and the surgical neck fracture plane lies at the base of the biceps groove.

After an elevator is placed within the fracture plane and is beneath the humeral head, the next key step is to elevate the head out of valgus. This requires placement of an elevator or small tamp directly onto the cortical edge of the top of the humeral head. As the head is elevated, the tuberosities often will spontaneously reduce, indicating appropriate head reduction.

Finally, care must be taken to critically assess hardware placement, especially within the humeral head. Anatomic studies have shown that the posterior aspect of the head is the most common location of hardware prominence. An AP fluoroscopic view with the shoulder in greater than 60° of external rotation or an axillary view with cephalad tilt may aid in visualizing posteriorly penetrated pins[9] (**Figure 15**).

References

1. Jaberg H, Warner JJ, Jakob RP: Percutaneous stabilization of unstable fractures of the humerus. *J Bone Joint Surg Am* 1992;74(4):508-515.
2. Blonna D, Castoldi F, Scelsi M, Rossi R, Falcone G, Assom M: The hybrid technique: Potential reduction in complications related to pins mobilization in the treatment of proximal humeral fractures. *J Shoulder Elbow Surg* 2010;19(8):1218-1229.
3. Bogner R, Hübner C, Matis N, Auffarth A, Lederer S, Resch H: Minimally-invasive treatment of three- and four-part fractures of the proximal humerus in elderly patients. *J Bone Joint Surg Br* 2008;90(12):1602-1607.
4. Calvo E, de Miguel I, de la Cruz JJ, López-Martín N: Percutaneous fixation

of displaced proximal humeral fractures: Indications based on the correlation between clinical and radiographic results. *J Shoulder Elbow Surg* 2007;16(6):774-781.

5. Keener JD, Parsons BO, Flatow EL, Rogers K, Williams GR, Galatz LM: Outcomes after percutaneous reduction and fixation of proximal humeral fractures. *J Shoulder Elbow Surg* 2007;16(3):330-338.

6. Magovern B, Ramsey ML: Percutaneous fixation of proximal humerus fractures. *Orthop Clin North Am* 2008;39(4): 405-416, v.

7. Resch H, Povacz P, Fröhlich R, Wambacher M: Percutaneous fixation of three- and four-part fractures of the proximal humerus. *J Bone Joint Surg Br* 1997;79(2):295-300.

8. Soete PJ, Clayson PE, Costenoble VH: Transitory percutaneous pinning in fractures of the proximal humerus. *J Shoulder Elbow Surg* 1999;8(6):569-573.

9. Klepps SJ, Miller SL, Lin J, Gladstone J, Flatow EL: Determination of radiographic guidelines for percutaneous fixation of proximal humerus fractures using a cadaveric model. *Orthopedics* 2007;30(8): 636-641.

10. Jiang C, Zhu Y, Wang M, Rong G: Biomechanical comparison of different pin configurations during percutaneous pinning for the treatment of proximal humeral fractures. *J Shoulder Elbow Surg* 2007;16(2):235-239.

11. Rowles DJ, McGrory JE: Percutaneous pinning of the proximal part of the humerus. An anatomic study. *J Bone Joint Surg Am* 2001;83(11):1695-1699.

12. Harrison AK, Gruson KI, Zmistowski B, Keener J, Galatz L, Williams G, Parsons BO, Flatow EL: Intermediate outcomes following percutaneous fixation of proximal humerus fractures. *J Bone Joint Surg Am*, in press.

Video Reference

26.1 Braman JP, Flatow EL: Video. *Percutaneous Pinning of Proximal Humerus Fractures: When and How to Do It*. Rosemont, IL, American Academy of Orthopaedic Surgeons, 2006.

Chapter 27
Fixation of Proximal Humerus Fractures

Michael E. Torchia, MD   Thomas S. Obermeyer, MD

Introduction
Interest in the fixation of proximal humerus fractures has grown worldwide during the past several years. This change in practice has been driven by several factors, including (1) recognition that humeral head replacement after an acute fracture has an unpredictable outcome;[1] (2) understanding that posttraumatic osteonecrosis of the humeral head is not a clinical disaster;[2] (3) more accurate preoperative imaging using three-dimensional CT scans; (4) improvements in fluoroscopy; (5) refined reduction maneuvers;[3-5] and (6) improved implants, in the form of contoured locking plates. Despite these advances, clinical results are inconsistent, and the reported rates of surgical complications remain far too high.[6-10] Most reoperations are due to technical problems that can be avoided with good surgical technique. This chapter focuses on techniques that have proven successful for achieving fixation of these fractures.

Patient Selection
Indications
Neer's guidelines, published almost 40 years ago, remain useful.[11,12] Minimally displaced one-part fractures are treated nonsurgically. Most displaced fractures typically are treated with surgery. If the anticipated demands on the extremity are very low, however, it is reasonable to allow a displaced fracture to malunite and accept the motion loss caused by tuberosity impingement. Most two- and three-part fractures can be reliably fixed using modern methods, even in patients with poor bone quality. Some four-part fractures also can be treated with open reduction and internal fixation (ORIF).[10,13,14] It was recently suggested that the outcome of a properly done osteosynthesis may be better than that of humeral head replacement.[10]

Contraindications
There are very few absolute contraindications to fixation of proximal humerus fractures. In general, patients with minimally displaced one-part fractures do not benefit from surgical treatment. Additionally, very low demand patients and the infirm typically are more likely to be considered for nonsurgical treatment. Many of the more severe fracture patterns do not have reliable outcomes with ORIF; these include four-part fracture-dislocations and most head-splitting fractures. Three-dimensional CT has shown that some so-called head-splitting fractures involve only a few millimeters of the humeral head and are actually a variation of the three-part patterns. These three-part variants can be treated with ORIF if the articular fracture can be visualized by opening the rotator cuff interval and/or dividing the upper portion of the subscapularis tendon and anterior capsule, preserving the circumflex vessels. We have learned that excellent fixation of proximal humerus fractures requires not only modern hardware but also traditional tension band sutures. Thus, we generally do not attempt ORIF in patients who have associated rotator cuff tear arthropathy. Finally, the surgeon occasionally encounters elderly patients with proximal humerus fractures who have associated severe glenohumeral arthritis. Although fixation is technically feasible, arthroplasty might be a better option in this uncommon situation.

Preoperative Imaging
When fixing proximal humerus fractures, it should be recognized that osteoporotic bone is crushed. This crushing precludes the use of "cortical reads" to reduce the fracture. Rather, the surgeon must rely on intraoperative fluoroscopic imaging to assess the quality of reduction of the tuberosities and of the head fragment on the humeral shaft. Because the anatomy of the proximal humerus is variable, a comparison radiograph of the opposite shoulder is valuable for intraoperative assessment of the quality of the reduction (**Figure 1**). A well-centered AP view of the scapula with the arm in external rotation clearly demonstrates the position of the greater tuberosity relative to the head (**Figure 1, B**). Checking this relationship intraoperatively provides the surgeon with a method of avoiding varus reductions (one of the most common complications after ORIF).[4,7,10,15,16]

Two-dimensional CT will often reveal the magnitude of traumatic bone loss and guide decision making about the need for bone grafting. Three-dimensional CT scans can also be useful for understanding the geometry of more complex fractures and fracture-dislocations. Subtraction views show bony Bankart lesions and articular fractures of the humeral head that may be difficult to detect on some two-dimensional images. For three- or four-part fractures, three-dimensional CT also reveals what, if any, part of the greater or lesser tuberosity is attached to the head segment. Any area of continuity between the tuberosities and head segment may serve as a "handle" to indirectly reduce the head segment with traction sutures placed at the bone-tendon junction of the rotator cuff (the so-called string-puppet reduction technique). The use of three-dimensional CT has made it possible to plan all aspects of the case, including the exposure, reduction maneuvers, and placement of the hardware, including occasional supplemental minifragment antiglide plating (**Figure 2**).

Procedure
Room Setup for Fluoroscopic Imaging/Patient Positioning
The optimal operating room setup allows unrestricted access to the shoulder for fluoroscopic imaging. Most surgeons prefer using a standard operating table and some variation of the familiar beach-chair patient position. The table is turned 90° after induction of anesthesia, so that the injured shoulder is opposite the anesthesia team and the equipment. This

---

Neither of the following authors nor any immediate family member has received anything of value from or owns stock in a commercial company or institution related directly or indirectly to the subject of this chapter: Dr. Torchia and Dr. Obermeyer.

Adapted from Torchia ME: Technical tips for fixation of proximal humeral fractures in elderly patients. Instr Course Lect *2010;59:553-561.*

Section 2: Shoulder and Elbow

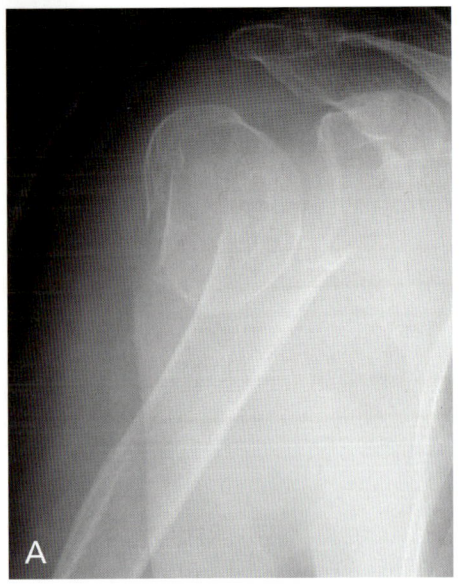

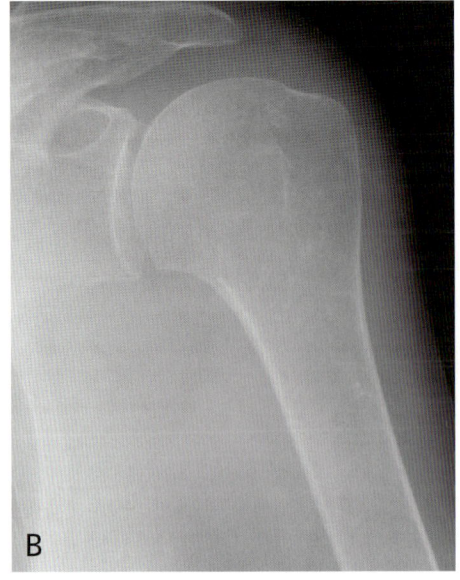

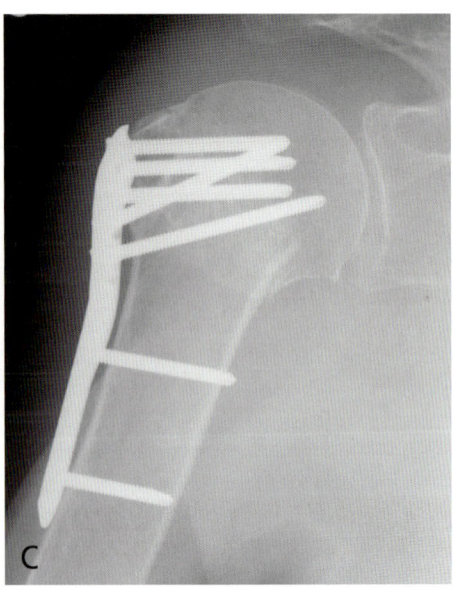

Figure 1 Two-part proximal humerus fracture in a 95-year-old woman. **A,** Preoperative AP radiograph. **B,** AP radiograph of the contralateral shoulder with the arm in external rotation. This comparison view serves as a template for reduction. **C,** AP external rotation radiograph taken at follow-up. Despite shortening to gain stability, the neck-shaft angle and the position of the greater tuberosity were restored. (Reproduced from Torchia ME: Technical tips for fixation of proximal humeral fractures in elderly patients. *Instr Course Lect* 2010;59:553-561.)

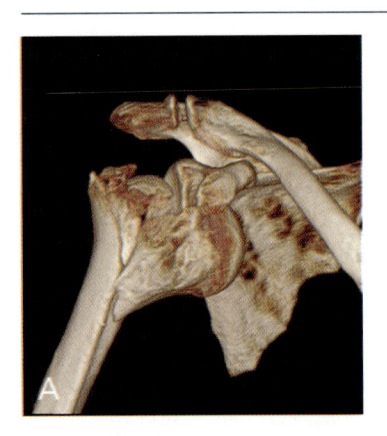

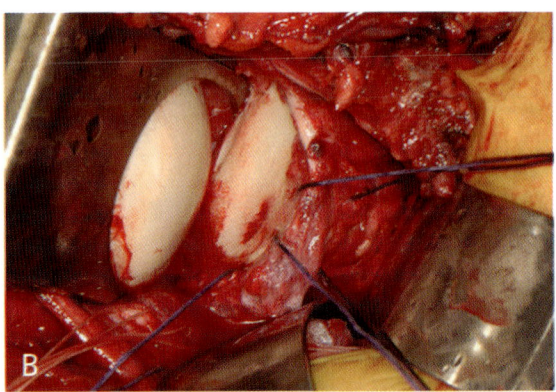

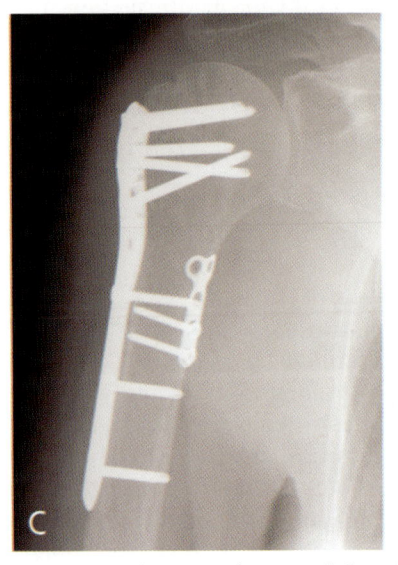

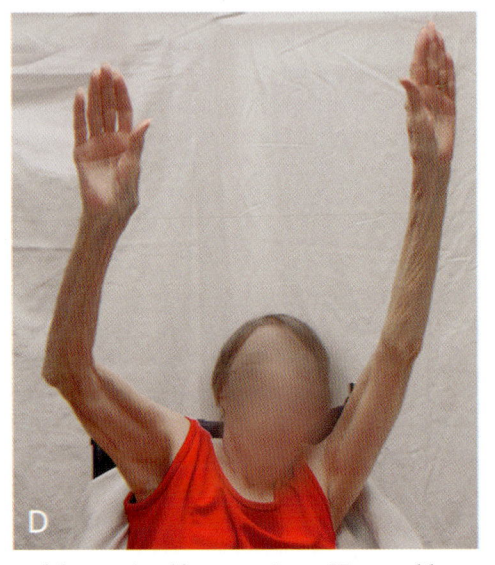

Figure 2 Three-part fracture-dislocation of the proximal humerus in an 87-year-old woman. **A,** Three-dimensional CT scan used in planning the surgical exposure and positioning the implants. **B,** Intraoperative photograph shows an anterior arthrotomy, used for access to the glenoid rim fracture and placement of transosseous sutures. **C,** Postoperative AP radiograph shows placement of a minifragment antiglide plate along the medial aspect of the humerus; the pectoralis major tendon was divided and later repaired after the medial plate application. Note that the medial plate is placed well below the humeral head to preserve blood supply. **D,** Clinical photograph of the patient (taken at 3-month follow-up) demonstrating overhead elevation of the arm. (Reproduced from Torchia ME: Technical tips for fixation of proximal humeral fractures in elderly patients. *Instr Course Lect* 2010;59:553-561.)

position allows the C-arm to enter and exit the field from the head of the operating table. Regardless of the setup and patient positioning, it is wise to verify before draping that a minimum of two high-quality fluoroscopic views can be obtained (**Figure 3**). This step is critical for the prevention of intraoperative screw penetration. When treating fracture-dislocations, it seems wise to also obtain a true axillary view to verify the position of the humeral head relative to the glenoid. The true axillary view is also preferred when reducing and stabilizing the lesser tuberosity.

Special Instruments/Equipment/Implants

- Intraoperative fluoroscopy is essential for the assessment of fracture reduction and evaluation of screw length with reference to the subchondral bone of the humeral head.
- A large Weber or "lobster claw" bone clamp is used to control the shaft segment. Heavy suture should be available to assist in tuberosity reduction and fixation.
- A precontoured low-profile locking plate is the implant of choice. Smooth holes at the periphery of the plate can be used as anchor points for tension-band sutures.
- Kirschner wires and Steinmann pins are useful for holding provisional reduction before definitive fixation. Larger Steinmann pins can also be used as "joysticks" to control the head segment.

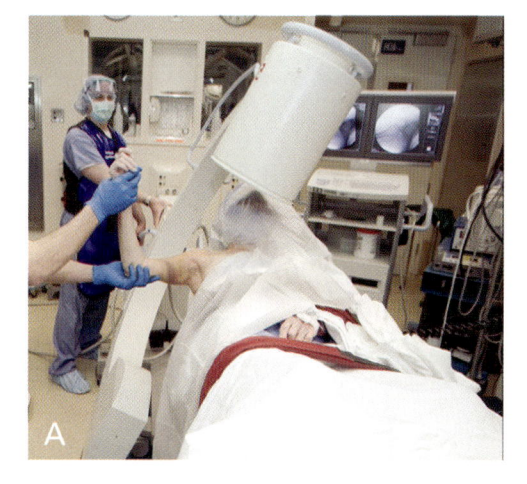

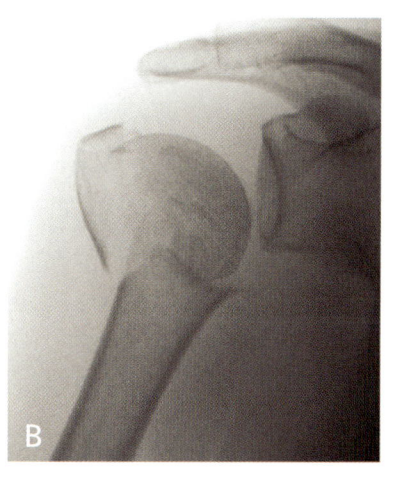

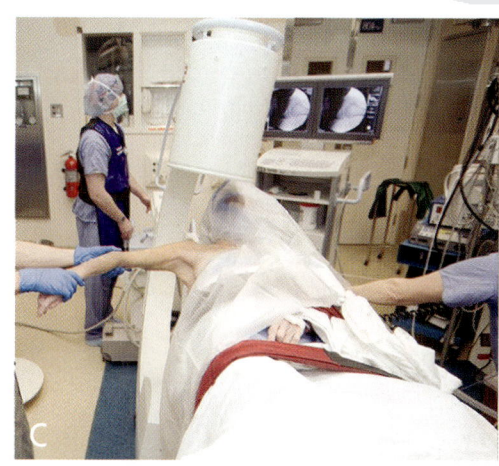

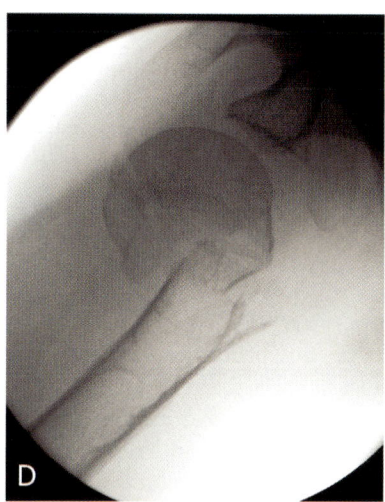

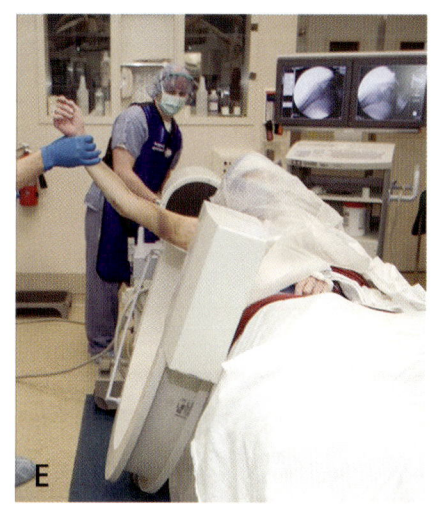

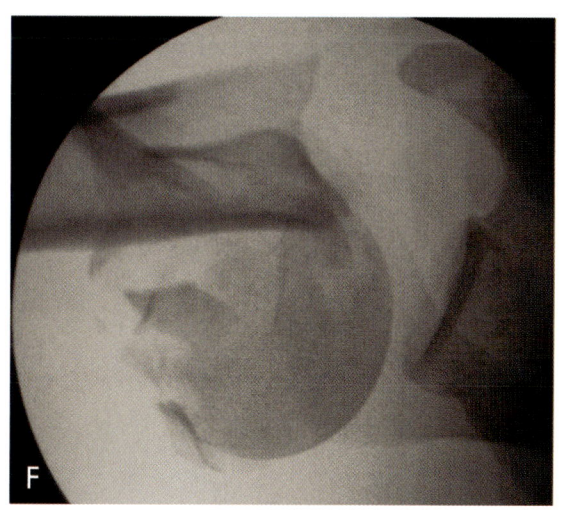

Figure 3 Operating room setup for fixation of a proximal humerus fracture. **A,** Photograph shows positioning of the fluoroscopic imaging device to direct the fluoroscopic beam perpendicular to the scapula, with the patient's arm held in external rotation. **B,** Preoperative AP external rotation fluoroscopic view. The relationship among the humeral shaft, the humeral head, and the greater tuberosity can be seen. **C,** Patient positioning for the Velpeau axillary view taken with the arm held in internal rotation and slight longitudinal traction. Gentle traction lateralizes the scapula away from the operating room table and the patient's head. This allows unobstructed imaging of the proximal humerus and glenoid. **D,** Preoperative Velpeau axillary internal rotation fluoroscopic view. Note the typical apex anterior angulation between the shaft and head segment. **E,** Patient positioning for the standard axillary view taken with the arm held in neutral rotation and longitudinal traction. **F,** Preoperative fluoroscopic axillary view. This view shows the position of the lesser tuberosity and the relationship of the humeral head to the glenoid. (Reproduced from Torchia ME: Technical tips for fixation of proximal humeral fractures in elderly patients. *Instr Course Lect* 2010;59:553-561.)

- A Cobb or periosteal elevator placed laterally may help to disimpact the head from the shaft and facilitate reduction of the humeral head.
- In varus fracture patterns, a miniature malleable retractor ("brain retractor") can be placed between the head and shaft segments. The small, thin malleable retractor can then be used like a shoehorn to assist in placement of the shaft under the head.
- Bone void filler may be helpful to support the osteoporotic head segment and thus minimize the risk of fracture settling and subsequent screw penetration.
- In selected fractures with no medial support, an allograft fibular strut may be beneficial. Proximal fibular allografts fit very well within the intramedullary canal of the proximal humerus and can be drilled and fixed with locking screws. We make an effort to medialize the allograft and use the convex curve of the allograft to reproduce the "calcar" of the proximal humerus. In many shoulders, the physiologic curve of the medial calcar (Shenton line) can be used to approximate the appropriate location of the humeral head in relation to the humeral shaft, with the intervening deficient segments reconstructed with allograft strut.
- For cases in which there is a question regarding the viability and condition of the humeral head, a fracture prosthesis for conversion to hemiarthroplasty or reverse arthroplasty should be available intraoperatively.

Surgical Technique
Exposure
The extended deltopectoral approach is preferred because of the options for extensile exposure to address almost any proximal humerus fracture pattern, including fracture-dislocations. The interval from the clavicle to the deltoid insertion is developed while preserving the muscle origin and releasing a portion of the insertion as needed. The subdeltoid space is mobilized with care to avoid the terminal branches of the axillary nerve. Efforts are made to correctly identify the position of the axillary nerve via the "tug test," because normal anatomic planes may be distorted from the injury. A Brown deltoid retractor is placed. Abduction of the arm relaxes the deltoid and allows access to the entire greater

tuberosity and rotator cuff.[17] The rotator interval is incised for several centimeters from the humeral head to the level of the glenoid, and the biceps is tenotomized intra-articularly and delivered distally so that it may be later tenodesed to the top of the pectoralis tendon. During the exposure and placement of hardware, every attempt is made to protect the primary blood supply to the humeral head.

Extensile Maneuvers
Fractures of the proximal humerus occasionally extend into the diaphysis. For this pattern, the exposure is carried distally (the Henry approach), and a long plate is applied to the lateral aspect of the humerus. In this situation, the anterior fibers of the deltoid insertion are released, but doing so does not appear to have any clinical sequelae, in the absence of a brachial plexopathy.[18] Conversely, dissection can be extended proximally and medially to enter the glenohumeral joint so that a humeral head articular fracture or glenoid rim fracture can be treated. In patients with neurovascular injury, the brachial plexus and axillary artery can be explored through the deltopectoral interval.

Reduction Maneuvers
Reduction maneuvers are determined by the fracture pattern. Impacted fractures are elevated using the method described by Jakob et al[5] (**Figure 4**). Unimpacted fractures are compressed using the "parachute technique" for valgus impaction osteotomy described by Banco et al[3] (**Figure 5**). A valgus impaction osteotomy allows balanced compression of the head segment on the shaft. This technique relies on tension-band sutures and is ideally suited for reducing two-part surgical neck fractures. The method also can be used to reduce three-part fractures if the anterior portion of the greater tuberosity is connected to the head segment.

Although the principles of the parachute technique can be applied to most proximal humerus fractures, contraindications do exist. The reduction method depends on an intact rotator cuff and cannot be

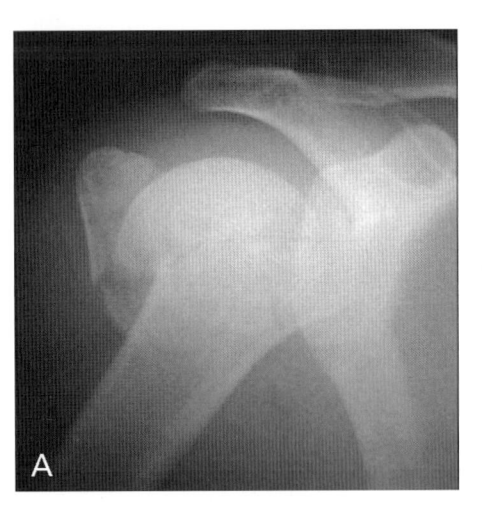

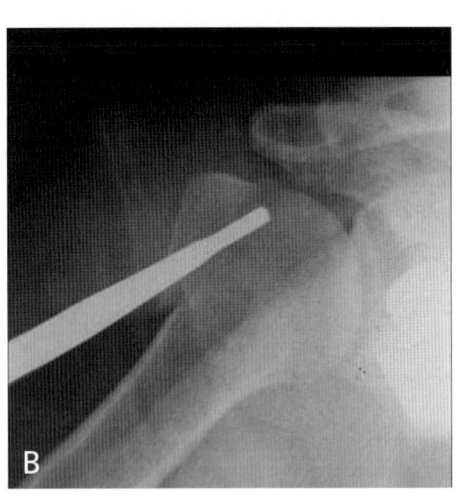

Figure 4 Valgus-impacted four-part fracture of the proximal humerus. **A,** Preoperative AP radiograph. **B,** Intraoperative fluoroscopic image shows elevation of the humeral head using a square-tipped impactor placed through a coronal split in the greater tuberosity. (Reproduced from Torchia ME: Technical tips for fixation of proximal humeral fractures in elderly patients. *Instr Course Lect* 2010;59:553-561.)

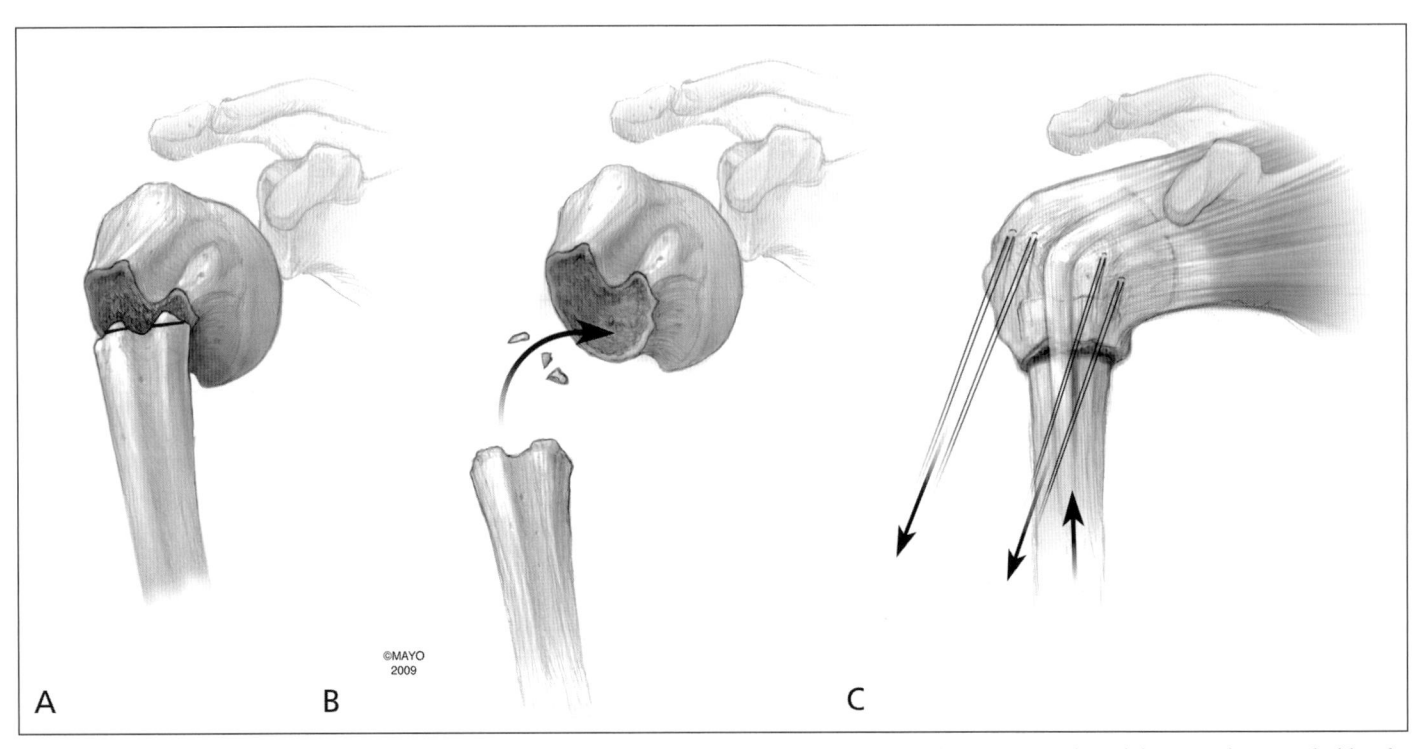

Figure 5 Illustrations show Banco's parachute technique for valgus impaction osteotomy. **A,** The transverse line delineates the intended level of the osteotomy. Prominent edges of the shaft anteriorly and laterally are trimmed with a rongeur to create a relatively flat surface that will allow balanced compression of the head segment. **B,** The "trimmings" are placed into the head segment and function as local bone graft. **C,** The head segment is supported by upward impaction of the shaft. The position of the head segment is adjusted with traction sutures placed at the bone-tendon junction of the subscapularis and supraspinatus tendons. (Reproduced with permission from the Mayo Foundation of Medical Education and Research, Rochester, MN.)

Chapter 27: Fixation of Proximal Humerus Fractures

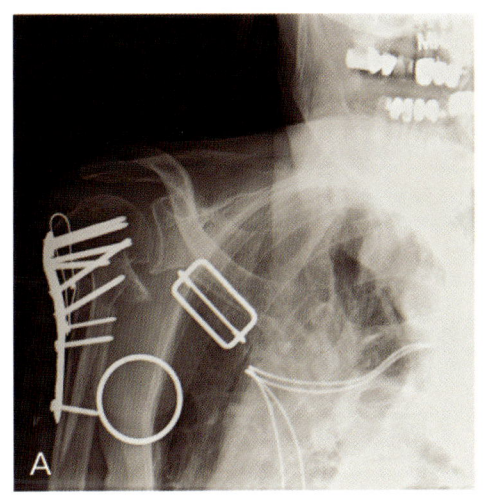

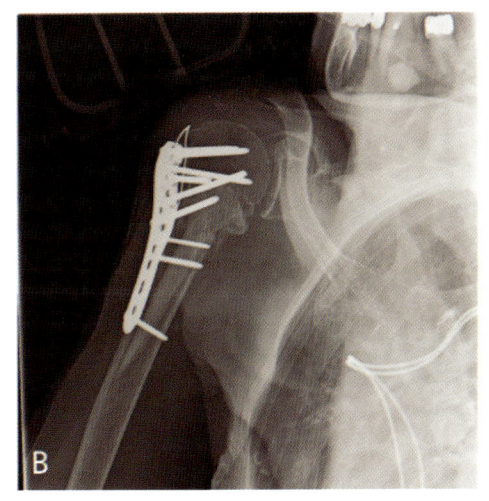

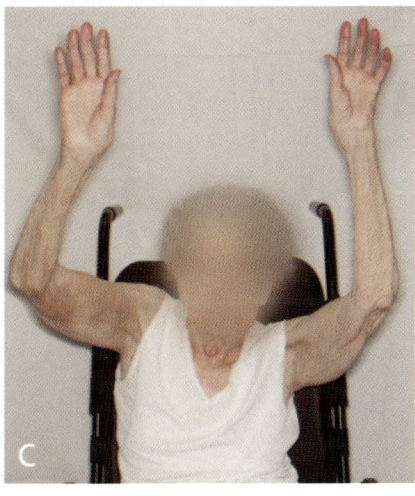

Figure 6 Use of a fibular allograft in a 90-year-old patient with a proximal humerus fracture with severe metaphyseal comminution. **A**, Postoperative AP radiograph shows the intramedullary allograft positioned along the medial cortex to provide medial support and recreate the calcar. In this case, the allograft was initially stabilized with a 2.7-mm screw. Given the poor bone quality and anticipated postoperative noncompliance, an 18-gauge tension-band wire was used (in addition to sutures) to neutralize the deforming force of the supraspinatus tendon and protect the locking plate fixation. **B**, Postoperative radiograph obtained at 6-month follow-up demonstrates consolidation of the calcar. **C**, Photograph shows the clinical result at 6 months.

used in fractures in which the tuberosities are detached from the head segment, impacted fracture patterns, and fractures with severe metaphyseal comminution. In fractures with metaphyseal comminution, the parachute technique can result in excessive humeral shortening and inferior instability. In this situation, humeral length can be restored with an intramedullary fibular allograft. This powerful method not only addresses the bone loss but also adds structural integrity to the fixation construct[4] (**Figure 6**). Restoration of humeral length is also important in treating complex anterior fracture-dislocations in which the proximal humerus and glenoid are fractured. If humeral length is not restored, it can be difficult to keep the humeral head concentrically reduced in the postoperative period. This situation is particularly problematic in patients with an associated axillary nerve injury.

Humeral Head Support

The concept of humeral head support has been emphasized by several authors.[3,6,19] When the soft humeral head is supported only by rigid hardware, it tends to settle onto the metal. The result is secondary screw or peg cutout, which is a frequently reported reason for revision surgery.[7-10] This problem can be avoided with appropriate head support. Most often, the degree of traumatic bone loss is only mild and the head segment can be supported by the shaft of the humerus. If there is moderate bone loss, then a small quantity of bone graft or bone graft substitute can be used, dissipating the stress concentration of the tips of the locking screws. In cases with severe bone loss, an intramedullary fibular allograft can be useful.[4]

Provisional Fixation

After the initial reduction, provisional fixation is achieved with a Steinmann pin or pins placed just posterior to the long head of the biceps tendon. Alternatively, pins are placed through stabs in the skin just distal to the inferior aspect of the surgical incision, which provides an appropriate vector between the humeral shaft and humeral head. Either method avoids interference with the plate that will later occupy the lateral surface of the proximal humerus. The traction sutures are tensioned and tied to the pin (**Figure 7**). This form of robust temporary tension-band fixation allows the arm to be rotated so that the reduction can be fluoroscopically assessed in multiple planes.

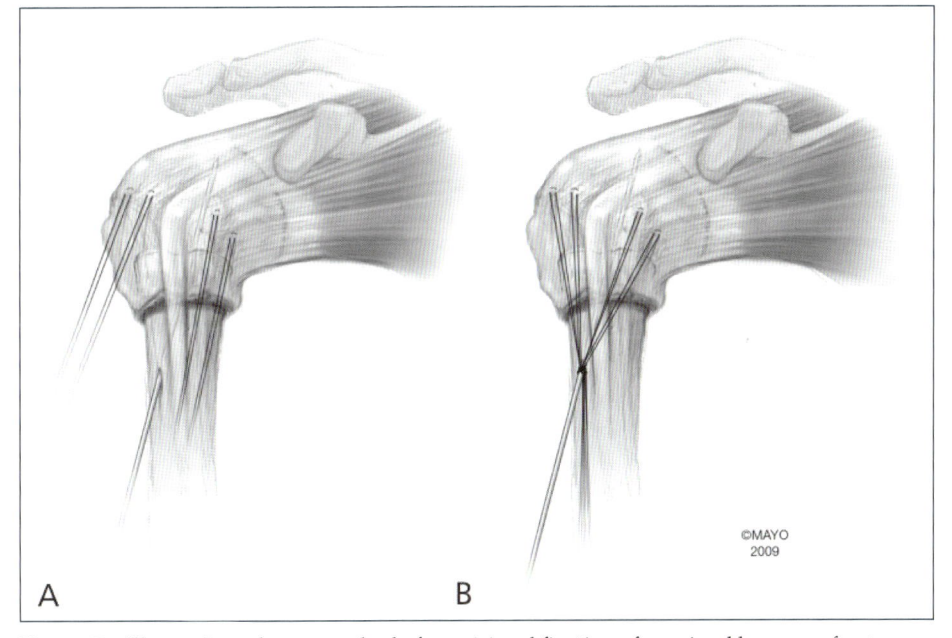

Figure 7 Illustrations show a method of provisional fixation of proximal humerus fractures using pin and tension-band suture fixation. This form of robust provisional fixation allows rotation of the arm for high-quality fluoroscopic imaging to assess the reduction in multiple planes. **A**, A long Steinmann pin is placed from the shaft into the head segment. **B**, Traction sutures are tensioned and tied to the pin. Tensioning the sutures pulls the head segment out of varus. (Reproduced with permission from the Mayo Foundation of Medical Education and Research, Rochester, MN.)

© 2013 American Academy of Orthopaedic Surgeons

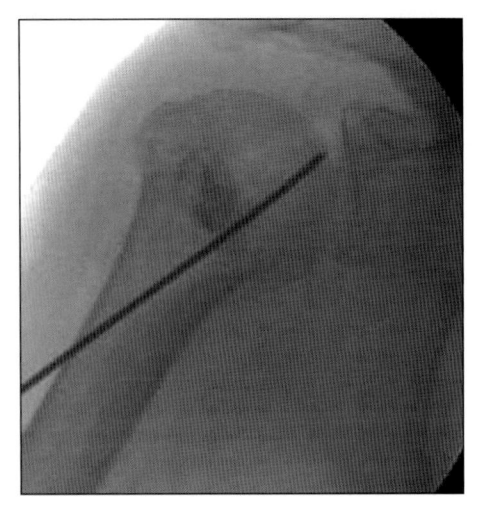

Figure 8 AP external rotation fluoroscopic image shows a provisional reduction of a three-part proximal humerus fracture with a Steinmann pin and tension-band sutures. A small amount of bone graft substitute was used to help support the humeral head. (Reproduced from Torchia ME: Technical tips for fixation of proximal humeral fractures in elderly patients. *Instr Course Lect* 2010;59: 553-561.)

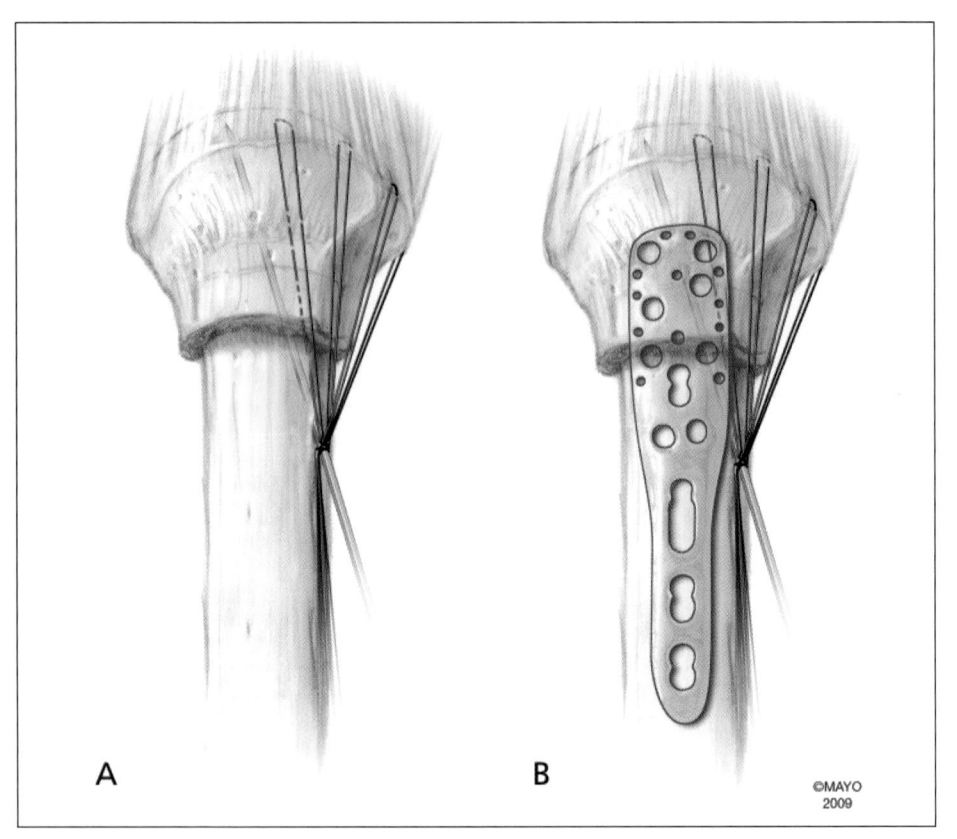

Figure 9 Definitive plate fixation of a proximal humerus fracture. The position of the pin and sutures used in the provisional fixation (**A**) allows unobstructed access for definitive fixation with a precontoured locking plate (**B**). It is important to recognize that with this technique the plate is applied to a fracture that has already been reduced, compressed, and provisionally fixed. (Reproduced with permission from the Mayo Foundation of Medical Education and Research, Rochester, MN.)

Assessment of Reduction

The position of the shaft, head, and tuberosities is assessed with high-quality fluoroscopic imaging. On the AP external rotation fluoroscopic view (**Figure 8**), the shaft of the humerus should be under the humeral head, the greater tuberosity should be approximately 5 to 10 mm below the top of the head, and the articular surface should point toward the upper portion of the glenoid (RH Cofield, MD, Rochester MN, personal communication, 1998). Additional precision can be gained by referencing the image of the opposite shoulder. A reasonable attempt should be made to match the tuberosity height and neck-shaft angle of the opposite shoulder. Additional fluoroscopic views are used as necessary to assess translation and angulation of the humeral shaft relative to the head, the position of the lesser tuberosity, and the position of the head segment relative to the glenoid. The course of the long head of the biceps tendon is checked to confirm the rotational accuracy of the reduction. The provisional reduction should be scrutinized, and final adjustments should be made before the hardware is placed. The most common pitfall is the persistent varus position of the head segment. In most instances, this problem is easily resolved by slightly backing out the provisional Steinmann pin and adding additional provisional tension band sutures extending from the bone-tendon junction of the supraspinatus to the provisional pin.

Definitive Fixation

A precontoured locking plate is applied laterally (**Figure 9**) and held with a push-pull reduction device (the so-called whirlybird). It is important to note that the plate is applied to the fracture after it is reduced and compressed. Hardware position is primarily assessed from the external rotation view (**Figure 10**). If the plate is positioned too high, it will cause impingement; if it is too low, the screw trajectory may be suboptimal. Gaps between the plate and the bone in the metadiaphysis are acceptable, and no attempt is made to contour the plate. This technique is quite different from the use of the plate as a reduction tool. Pulling the bone to the plate with screws or sutures tends to leave the head unsupported and at risk for varus drift or secondary screw penetration.[7,15] When the plate position is optimal, screws are placed into the osteoporotic humeral head. Because bone quality is often poor in this elderly patient population, only the outer cortex is drilled. The depth gauge is then inserted and gently advanced to the desired depth under fluoroscopic control (**Figure 11**). It is important to understand that if the head is supported and tension-band sutures are used, the subchondral bone of the head need not be engaged. Placing shorter screws lowers the risk of screw penetration[7] (**Figure 12**). Following plate application, the provisional pin and suture fixation is removed. Next, definitive tension band sutures are placed, using any open holes in the plate as anchor points (**Figure 13**). It is preferable to use smooth holes to minimize the risk of suture abrasion.

Complications

Most complications can be avoided with good surgical technique. Perhaps the most frequent problem is inadequate reduction. Many fractures are fixed with residual varus deformity. This can be avoided by referencing a comparison radiograph or fluoroscopic image of the opposite shoulder with the arm in external rotation. In almost all cases, the greater tuberosity will be below the top of the humeral head. Conversely, if the fluoroscopic image of the provisional reduc-

Chapter 27: Fixation of Proximal Humerus Fractures

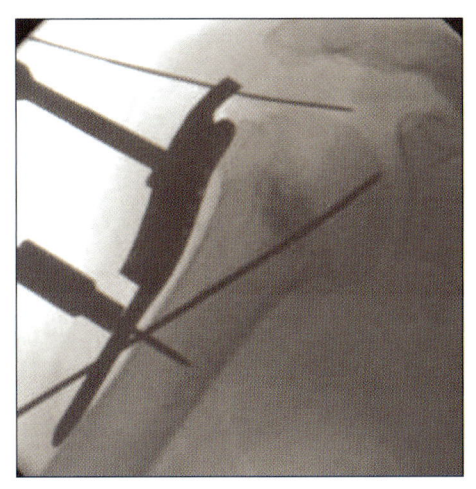

Figure 10 AP external rotation view fluoroscopic image shows plate positioning below the top of the humeral head. (Reproduced from Torchia ME: Technical tips for fixation of proximal humeral fractures in elderly patients. *Instr Course Lect* 2010;59: 553-561.)

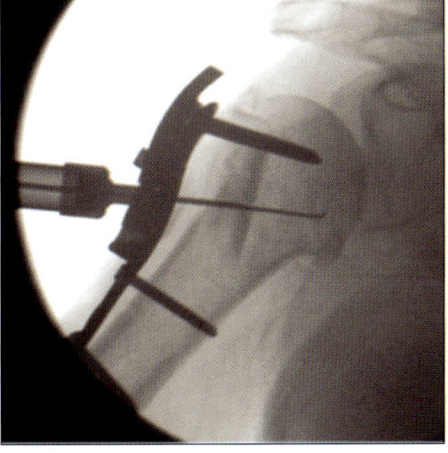

Figure 11 Intraoperative fluoroscopic image demonstrates a method of determining screw length in geriatric patients. Only the outer cortex is drilled. The depth gauge is then pushed into the osteoporotic humeral head until resistance is encountered and fluoroscopic imaging is done to verify appropriate length. No attempt is made to engage the subchondral bone. (Reproduced with permission from the Mayo Foundation of Medical Education and Research, Rochester, MN.)

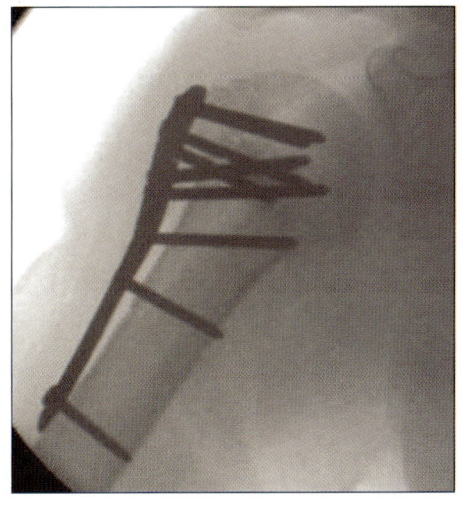

Figure 12 AP fluoroscopic image shows a method of screw placement that minimizes the risk of primary or secondary penetration. The arm is rotated under the fluoroscopy machine to check screw length in multiple planes. (Reproduced from Torchia ME: Technical tips for fixation of proximal humeral fractures in elderly patients. *Instr Course Lect* 2010;59:553-561.)

tion shows the greater tuberosity above the head, then the fracture is almost certainly in varus.

Another common problem is intraoperative screw penetration. Screw penetration through the humeral head most commonly occurs in the posterosuperior humeral head, where it may be difficult to accurately assess screw length on the AP view. This can be avoided by checking an intraoperative Velpeau axillary lateral view. The two static orthogonal views (AP and Velpeau axillary) allow much of the head to be seen. Rotating the arm on each of these views allows almost all surfaces of the humeral head to be imaged. Another method to evaluate for articular screw penetration is for the surgeon to place his/her finger through a rent in the rotator interval to palpate the articular surface of the humeral head directly. Screw penetration after fixation is typically due to inadequate head support or osteonecrosis. This problem may be treated with hardware removal or conversion to arthroplasty. Axillary nerve palsy or brachial plexopathy may occur with fracture-dislocations, and a good preoperative neurologic examination is critical to documenting baseline function. Infection is uncommon if prophylactic antibiotics are used. Osteonecrosis rarely occurs after ORIF of two- and three-part fractures. This problem is more common in four-part fractures with a small medial hinge.

The most underemphasized complication is inadequate protection of the hardware construct. The hardware can be protected in several ways, including supporting the head segment, liberal use of tension-band sutures, and immobilization in a sling in the postoperative period. Aggressive postoperative physical therapy after ORIF of proximal humerus fractures can contribute to fixation failure.

Postoperative Care and Rehabilitation

Experience with caring for elderly patients in whom these osteoporotic fractures are common suggests that cognitive impairment should be considered when planning the postoperative rehabilitative program. Many patients older than 75 years have limited understanding of their condition and are unable to participate in the gentle, passive range-of-motion program used in younger patients with good bone quality. Aggressive range-of-motion and strengthening exercises done before union of the fracture may increase the risk of fixation failure. With these concerns in mind, a variation of Neer's limited goals rehabilitation program seems appropriate for this patient population.[17,20] The primary focus of the program is protection of the fixation construct. Motion and strength are restored gradually over months.

During the first 6 weeks after surgery, patients are directed to wear a sling full time. After 6 weeks, supine active-assisted range-of-motion exercises are initiated. Radiographs taken 12 weeks after surgery usually show fracture con-

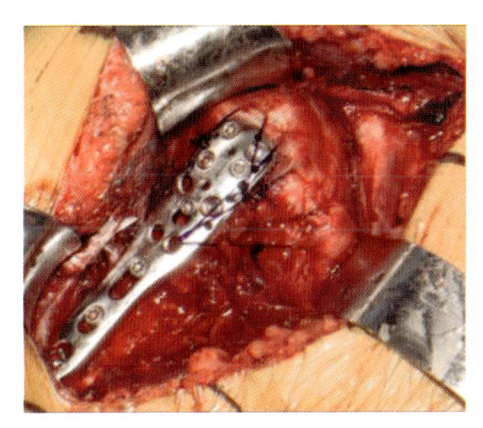

Figure 13 Intraoperative photograph shows the final construct. Heavy monofilament absorbable tension-band sutures are applied liberally using empty holes in the plate as anchor points. The sutures are placed in the anterior supraspinatus and superior subscapularis to neutralize the deforming forces of these tendons, which produce varus and apex anterior angulation of the fracture. (Reproduced from Torchia ME: Technical tips for fixation of proximal humeral fractures in elderly patients. *Instr Course Lect* 2010;59: 553-561.)

solidation (**Figure 14**). At this point, use of the sling is discontinued, and the patient is encouraged to use the arm for light daily activities, including driving and shopping. More forceful activities, such as yard work, tennis, and golf, are avoided for 6 months.

Pearls

- Good intraoperative radiographs/fluoroscopic images are essential, and

© 2013 *American Academy of Orthopaedic Surgeons*

Section 2: Shoulder and Elbow

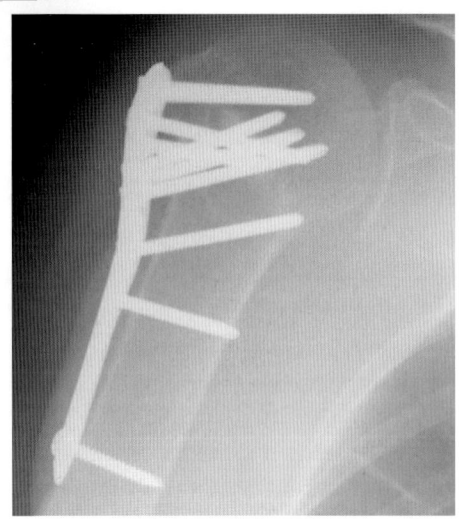

Figure 14 A typical 3-month follow-up AP external rotation radiograph of the proximal humerus shows consolidation of a two-part fracture following treatment with the method described in this chapter. (Reproduced from Torchia ME: Technical tips for fixation of proximal humeral fractures in elderly patients. *Instr Course Lect* 2010;59:553-561.)

time during setup should ensure that quality C-arm images are available.
- Temporary traction sutures placed at the bone-tendon junction of the rotator cuff facilitate mobilization and reduction of the tuberosities. In two-part fractures and many three-part fractures, strategically placed rotator cuff traction sutures can be used to indirectly reduce the humeral head. Traction on the anterosuperior portion of the rotator cuff corrects the varus, apex anterior angular deformity typical of most two- and three-part fractures.
- Support of the osteoporotic humeral head is essential and can be achieved with the proximal humeral shaft or with a structural bone graft in cases with metaphyseal comminution.
- Varus malreduction of the humeral head will lead to malunion and loss of motion postoperatively. This is avoided with careful scrutiny of intraoperative images and comparison with the contralateral shoulder radiographs.
- Placing the plate too proximally will lead to subacromial impingement and should be avoided. The anterior-posterior plate position should be carefully assessed. Placing the plate just posterior to the bicipital groove avoids disturbance of the circumflex vessels.
- The plate should be applied after the fracture has been reduced, compressed, and provisionally fixed with pins and tension-band sutures.
- Appropriate screw length is critical. Screws that are too short risk inadequate head fixation and secondary displacement, and screws that are too long may lead to articular penetration and damage to the glenoid surface.
- Improved screw purchase in the osteoporotic head segment can be achieved by drilling only the lateral cortex and pushing the depth gauge to the desired screw length with fluoroscopic control. This "underdrilling" results in improved compaction of the bone around the screw.
- Proper screw trajectory into the plate should be evaluated, as improper screw trajectory may lead to improper locking into the plate and later loosening or cold welding.
- Tension-band sutures neutralize the deforming forces of the rotator cuff and should be used liberally.
- In elderly patients, hardware can be protected with a 6-week period of immobilization, which in our experience has not led to disabling stiffness.

References

1. Antuña SA, Sperling JW, Cofield RH: Shoulder hemiarthroplasty for acute fractures of the proximal humerus: A minimum five-year follow-up. *J Shoulder Elbow Surg* 2008;17(2):202-209.
2. Gerber C, Hersche O, Berberat C: The clinical relevance of posttraumatic avascular necrosis of the humeral head. *J Shoulder Elbow Surg* 1998;7(6):586-590.
3. Banco SP, Andrisani D, Ramsey M, Frieman B, Fenlin JM Jr: The parachute technique: Valgus impaction osteotomy for two-part fractures of the surgical neck of the humerus. *J Bone Joint Surg Am* 2001;83(pt 1, suppl 2):38-42.
4. Gardner MJ, Boraiah S, Helfet DL, Lorich DG: Indirect medial reduction and strut support of proximal humerus fractures using an endosteal implant. *J Orthop Trauma* 2008;22(3):195-200.
5. Jakob RP, Miniaci A, Anson PS, Jaberg H, Osterwalder A, Ganz R: Four-part valgus impacted fractures of the proximal humerus. *J Bone Joint Surg Br* 1991;73(2):295-298.
6. Rose PS, Adams CR, Torchia ME, Jacofsky DJ, Haidukewych GG, Steinmann SP: Locking plate fixation for proximal humeral fractures: Initial results with a new implant. *J Shoulder Elbow Surg* 2007;16(2):202-207.
7. Brunner F, Sommer C, Bahrs C, et al: Open reduction and internal fixation of proximal humerus fractures using a proximal humeral locked plate: A prospective multicenter analysis. *J Orthop Trauma* 2009;23(3):163-172.
8. Egol KA, Ong CC, Walsh M, Jazrawi LM, Tejwani NC, Zuckerman JD: Early complications in proximal humerus fractures (OTA Types 11) treated with locked plates. *J Orthop Trauma* 2008;22(3):159-164.
9. Owsley KC, Gorczyca JT: Fracture displacement and screw cutout after open reduction and locked plate fixation of proximal humeral fractures [corrected]. *J Bone Joint Surg Am* 2008;90(2):233-240.
10. Solberg BD, Moon CN, Franco DP, Paiement GD: Locked plating of 3- and 4-part proximal humerus fractures in older patients: The effect of initial fracture pattern on outcome. *J Orthop Trauma* 2009;23(2):113-119.
11. Neer CS II: Displaced proximal humeral fractures: I. Classification and evaluation. *J Bone Joint Surg Am* 1970;52(6):1077-1089.
12. Neer CS II: Displaced proximal humeral fractures: II. Treatment of three-part and four-part displacement. *J Bone Joint Surg Am* 1970;52(6):1090-1103.
13. Esser RD: Treatment of three- and four-part fractures of the proximal humerus with a modified cloverleaf plate. *J Orthop Trauma* 1994;8(1):15-22.
14. Robinson CM, Page RS: Severely impacted valgus proximal humeral fractures. *J Bone Joint Surg Am* 2004;86(pt 2, suppl 1):143-155.
15. Agudelo J, Schürmann M, Stahel P, et al: Analysis of efficacy and failure in proximal humerus fractures treated with locking plates. *J Orthop Trauma* 2007;21(10):676-681.
16. Südkamp N, Bayer J, Hepp P, et al: Open reduction and internal fixation of proximal humeral fractures with use of the locking proximal humerus plate: Results of a prospective, multicenter, observational study. *J Bone Joint Surg Am* 2009;91(6):1320-1328.
17. Neer CS: Shoulder Reconstruction. Philadelphia, PA, WB Saunders, 1990, pp 170-173.
18. Gill DR, Torchia ME: The spiral compression plate for proximal humeral shaft nonunion: A case report and description of a new technique. *J Orthop Trauma* 1999;13(2):141-144.
19. Gardner MJ, Weil Y, Barker JU, Kelly BT, Helfet DL, Lorich DG: The importance of medial support in locked plating of proximal humerus fractures. *J Orthop Trauma* 2007;21(3):185-191.
20. Barlow JD, Sanchez-Sotelo J, Torchia M: Proximal humerus fractures in the elderly can be reliably fixed with a "hybrid" locked-plating technique. *Clin Orthop Relat Res* 2011;469(12):3281-3291.

Chapter 28
Hemiarthroplasty for Proximal Humerus Fractures

Arnaldo I. Rodriguez-Santiago, MD   T. Bradley Edwards, MD

Patient Selection
Hemiarthroplasty is a useful procedure for many acute displaced proximal humerus fractures. Certain fracture patterns preclude the ability to use internal fixation techniques to reconstruct the proximal humerus, particularly in patients with poor bone quality.

Indications
The indications for unconstrained humeral head replacement are severely displaced four-part fractures, fracture-dislocations (**Figure 1**), head-splitting fractures, impression articular fractures involving over 40% of the articular surface, dislocation present for more than 6 months, a humeral head fragment devoid of soft-tissue attachment, and selected three-part fractures not amenable to surgical fixation.[1]

Contraindications
Contraindications to this procedure are nondisplaced fractures, fractures amenable to open reduction and internal fixation, active soft-tissue infection, and chronic osteomyelitis. Relative contraindications include massive rotator cuff tear, uncontrolled shoulder spasticity, and poor general patient health precluding surgical treatment.

History and Physical Examination
A thorough history is taken from the antecedent trauma responsible for the fracture. Presence of any shoulder problems before the fracture should be noted in the history. Performance of physical examination in a patient with an acute proximal humerus fracture is limited so that the patient is not unnecessarily subjected to pain. A detailed neurovascular examination is performed with specific attention to the sensory and motor functions of the axillary nerve. The sensory function of the axillary nerve can be evaluated by testing sensibility to touch of the posterior aspect of the upper part of the arm (superior lateral brachial cutaneous branch). Motor function may be more difficult to evaluate because pain induced by the fracture may inhibit deltoid contraction. The condition of the soft tissues, particularly anterior at the planned surgical site, is meticulously evaluated.

Preoperative Imaging
Three radiographic views are obtained in all patients with a proximal humerus fracture: an AP view of the glenohumeral joint with the arm in neutral rotation, an axillary view, and a scapular outlet view. These radiographs are used to evaluate the fracture pattern (two-part, three-part, four-part), the amount of displacement of the fracture fragments, the presence of humeral head dislocation, and the presence of a split in the humeral head fragment. AP full-length radiographs of the humerus of both the affected and unaffected extremity, taken with the arm in neutral rotation, are obtained for use in preoperative determination of appropriate humeral head height. These radiographs must include the entire length of the humerus and must be controlled for magnification.

CT is performed in all patients with substantially displaced proximal humerus fractures. This study allows further elucidation of the fracture pattern and assessment of the amount of displacement of the fracture fragments. Additionally, the position of the tuberosities and the humeral head is visualized, thereby allowing easier identification at the time of surgery.

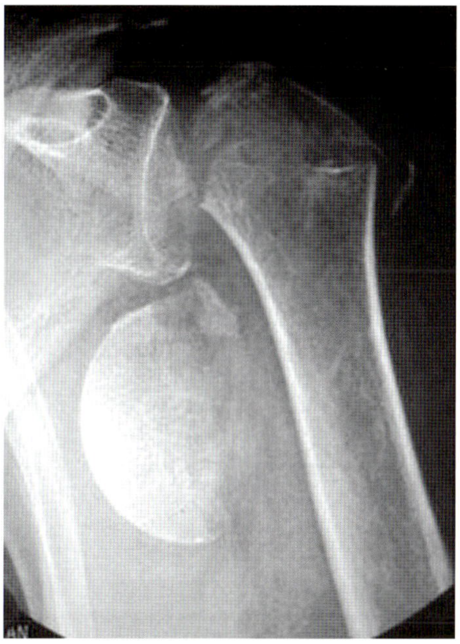

Figure 1 AP radiograph shows a four-part humeral fracture-dislocation, a typical indication for hemiarthroplasty.

Placement of the prosthesis at the correct height and version remains one of the most difficult challenges when performing hemiarthroplasty for a fracture. The authors prefer the Gothic arch technique popularized by Krishnan et al.[2] In preoperative planning for the Gothic arch technique, AP full-length humeral radiographs of the affected and unaffected arm are required. From the radiograph of the unaffected arm, the length of the humerus from the superior aspect of the humeral head to the transepicondylar axis is measured and normalized for magnification (**Figure 2, A**). This measurement is obtained by first establishing the prosthetic axis proximally within the humeral canal. This is done by measuring the center point of the proximal diaphysis at two locations and connecting these points with a line running the length of the humerus. Next, a line perpendicular to the prosthetic axis is drawn at the superior aspect of the humeral head. A third line is drawn at the transepicondylar axis of the distal humerus. The distance between the superior aspect of the humeral head and the transepicondylar axis is measured in centimeters along the prosthetic axis.

Dr. Edwards or an immediate family member has received royalties from Tornier and Ortho-helix; is a member of a speakers' bureau or has made paid presentations on behalf of Tornier; serves as a paid consultant to or is an employee of Kinamed and Tornier; serves as an unpaid consultant to Gulf Coast Surgical Services; has received research or institutional support from Tornier; has received nonincome support (such as equipment or services), commercially derived honoraria, or other non–research-related funding (such as paid travel) from Tornier; and serves as a board member, owner, officer, or committee member of the American Shoulder and Elbow Surgeons. Neither Dr. Rodriguez-Santiago nor any immediate family member has received anything of value from or owns stock in a commercial company or institution related directly or indirectly to the subject of this chapter.

Section 2: Shoulder and Elbow

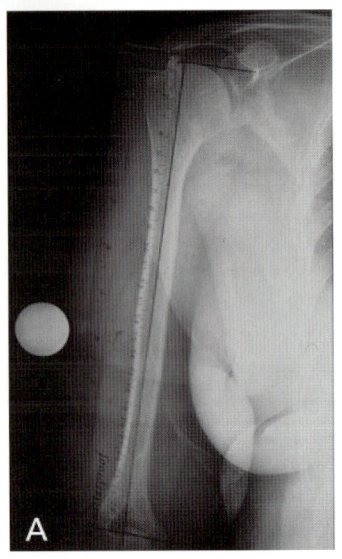

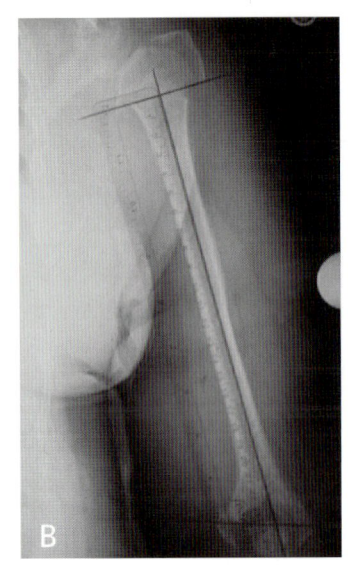

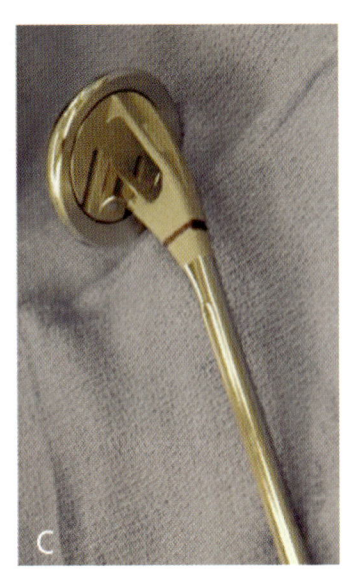

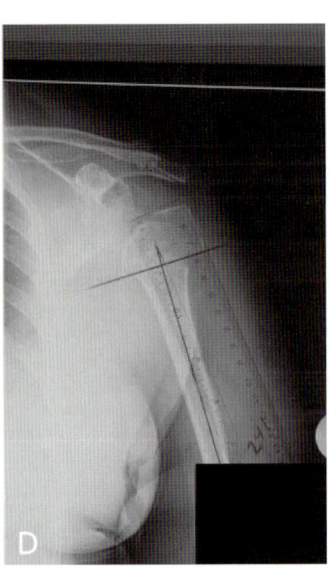

Figure 2 Preoperative planning for the Gothic arch technique of determining proper humeral component position. **A**, From a full-length AP radiograph of the unaffected humerus, the length of the humerus from the superior aspect of the humeral head to the transepicondylar axis is measured and normalized for magnification. **B**, On the AP radiograph of the affected extremity, a line perpendicular to the prosthetic axis is drawn at the level of the fracture medially. The distance between the medial fracture line and the transepicondylar axis (residual humeral length) is measured. The difference between the humeral length measured on the unaffected radiograph and the residual humeral length measured on the affected radiograph is calculated. **C**, This difference is marked on the humeral implant to establish the height at which the humeral stem should be positioned with respect to the medial fracture line. **D**, The length of the greater tuberosity, when available, is used as a checkrein.

The AP humeral radiograph of the affected extremity is used to establish the prosthetic axis and the transepicondylar axis. A line perpendicular to the prosthetic axis is drawn at the level of the fracture medially. The distance between the medial fracture line and the transepicondylar axis (residual humeral length) is measured and corrected for magnification if necessary. In cases in which the greater tuberosity is visible as a single fragment, the length of the greater tuberosity is measured. The difference between the humeral length measured on the radiograph of the unaffected extremity and the residual humeral length measured on the radiograph of the affected extremity is calculated (**Figure 2, B**). This difference is marked on the humeral implant to establish the height at which the humeral stem should be positioned with respect to the medial fracture line (**Figure 2, C**). The length of the greater tuberosity, when available, is used as a checkrein. When the length of the greater tuberosity is added to the length of the residual humerus, the sum should be approximately 3 to 5 mm less than the humeral length measured on the radiograph of the unaffected humerus (**Figure 2, D**).

Procedure

Room Setup/Patient Positioning

Proper patient positioning is crucial during shoulder hemiarthroplasty for fracture. We use a standard operating table with the patient positioned sufficiently to the operative side to allow extension of the arm. A rolled sheet is placed between the scapulae to slightly elevate the shoulder off the operating table and allow proper preparation of the posterior aspect of the shoulder.

The patient is placed in the modified beach-chair position, with the back of the table elevated approximately 45° to 60° relative to the floor. The position of the patient's head and neck is checked to ensure neutral alignment. After the head/neck position is deemed acceptable, the forehead and chin are secured. Care should be taken to pad and protect bony prominences and sites of subcutaneous vulnerable nerves near the elbow (ulnar) and knee (peroneal).

Special Instruments/Equipment/Implants

Instruments used during hemiarthroplasty for proximal humerus fractures are listed in **Table 1**.

Surgical Technique

Surgical Approach and Tuberosity Handling

The area included in the surgical preparation extends medially to the midline, distally to the level of the nipple, and proximally to the level of the mandible and encompasses the entire upper extremity, including the hand. Draping of the patient differs slightly in fracture cases in that the stockinette covers only the forearm so that the elbow and humeral epicondyles are easily accessible to use as reference points in judging prosthetic retroversion.

A standard deltopectoral approach is used for exposure. The skin incision is started at the tip of the coracoid and extends distally and laterally approximately 10 to 15 cm, depending on the size of the patient. A needle-tip electrocautery is used for deep dissection throughout the procedure to minimize blood loss. The interval between the deltoid and the pectoralis major is identified by locating the cephalic vein. If difficulty is encountered in locating the cephalic vein, the deltopectoral interval can be readily detected proximally by identifying a small triangular area devoid of muscle tissue between the proximal portions of the deltoid and pectoralis major muscles. We prefer to retract the cephalic vein laterally with the deltoid because most of the branches of the cephalic vein are based on the deltoid. A self-retaining deltopectoral retractor is placed to maintain exposure during the procedure. The conjoined tendon is identified and traced to its insertion on the coracoid process. The tip of a Hohmann-type retractor is placed behind the base of the coracoid process to provide proximal retraction. With the arm abducted and externally rotated, the apex formed by the insertion of the coracoacromial ligament and the conjoined tendon onto the coracoid process is identified. The conjoined tendon is retracted medially to expose the proximal humerus fracture.

A Cobb elevator is used to perform blunt dissection and begin the process of identification of the tuberosities. In the typical four-part fracture pattern, the lesser tuberosity with the attached subscapularis represents one fragment, the greater tuberosity with the attached posterior superior rotator cuff represents a second fragment, the humeral head represents a third fragment, and the humeral shaft represents the final fragment. A variety of combinations exist; however, the most common fracture pattern for which hemiarthroplasty is indicated involves these major fracture fragments. Control of the lesser tuberosity is achieved by identifying the tuberosity and the subscapularis tendon anteriorly in the shoulder just posterior to the conjoined tendon.

Stay sutures of No. 1 polyester are placed through the subscapularis tendon just medial to its osseous insertion on the lesser tuberosity. One suture is placed superiorly and a second suture inferiorly, if necessary. Sutures are not placed through the lesser tuberosity because it is usually osteopenic and does not support transosseous sutures sufficiently. These sutures will also aid in retracting the lesser tuberosity to gain access to the humeral head fragment.

The humeral head fragment is identified and may be dislocated or split into two or more fragments. The humeral head is removed with locking forceps (Lahey type) and kept on the sterile field for later use as bone graft material. Removal of the humeral head facilitates identification of the greater tuberosity, which is located posteriorly. In elderly patients, in whom these fractures are more common, the greater tuberosity is often a mere thin shell of cortical bone and must be handled with care to avoid further fracture.

Control of the greater tuberosity and the attached postero superior rotator cuff is obtained by passing No. 2 braided permanent suture through the rotator cuff tendons just medial to their insertion on the greater tuberosity (**Figure 3**). A large curved free needle is loaded with two strands of suture and passed through the rotator cuff at the junction of the supraspinatus and infraspinatus. A second free needle loaded with two strands of suture is passed through the rotator cuff at the junction of the infraspinatus and the teres minor. These sutures provide immediate control of the greater tuberosity and are used for later fixation of both the lesser and the greater tuberosity.

Rarely, hemiarthroplasty is indicated in patients in whom the greater or lesser tuberosity remains attached to the humeral head. In these cases, the tuberosities must be detached from the humeral head fragment. A 1-in osteotome is used, leaving as much bone with the tuberosity fragment as possible. The tuberosity is then handled as in a four-part fracture, as described earlier.

Humeral Prosthesis Positioning

After control of both tuberosities is achieved, the humeral shaft is

Table 1 Instruments Used in Hemiarthroplasty for Proximal Humerus Fractures

Instrument (Quantity)	Use
Vascular forceps (2)	Dissection
Ferris-Smith forceps (2)	Dissection
Adson forceps with teeth (1)	Skin closure
Long curved Metzenbaum scissors (1)	Dissection
Long curved Mayo scissors (1)	Dissection
Straight Mayo scissors (1)	Cutting suture
Bandage scissors (1)	Removal of draping
Medium skin rake (2)	Skin retraction
Army-Navy retractor (2)	Deltopectoral retraction
Cerebellar retractor (1)	Deltopectoral retraction
Hohmann retractor (4)	Proximal retraction; humeral retraction
Narrow Richardson retractor (1)	Conjoined tendon retraction
Standard hemostat (6)	Tagging stay sutures
Lahey forceps (1)	Handling of the tuberosities
Battery-powered drill (1)	Humeral drill hole preparation for suture placement
Long No. 3 knife handle (2)	Skin incision, biceps tenotomy
8-in Mayo needle holder (2)	Suture passage
1-in osteotome (1)	Tuberosity osteotomy when required
Mallet (1)	Insertion of implants; tuberosity osteotomy
Freer elevator (1)	Removal of excess cement
Small bone tamp (1)	Impaction of bone graft
Large bone tamp (1)	Impaction of bone graft
Cobb elevator (2)	Blunt dissection; tuberosity identification
No. 0 Vicryl (taper needle)[a] (3)	Hemostasis; wound closure
No. 2 Ethibond (taper needle)[a] (2)	Subscapularis stay suture; biceps tenodesis
No. 2 FiberWire (taper needle)[b] (6)	Tuberosity fixation
2-0 Vicryl[a] (1)	Wound closure
3-0 PDS (polydioxanone suture)[a] (1)	Wound closure
Electrocautery with needle tip (1)	Hemostasis; dissection
Suction tip with tubing (1)	Visualization
Bulb syringe (1)	Irrigation
Catheter-tip 60-mL syringe (1)	Cement application
Bone cement (1)	Humeral implant fixation
Cement restrictor (1)	Humeral implant insertion
Fracture arthroplasty set (1)	Hemiarthroplasty implants and instrumentation

[a] Ethicon.
[b] Arthrex.

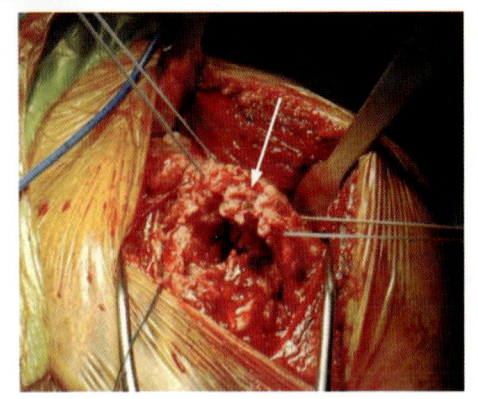

Figure 3 Intraoperative photograph demonstrates mobilization of the greater tuberosity (arrow) with sutures through the posterior rotator cuff.

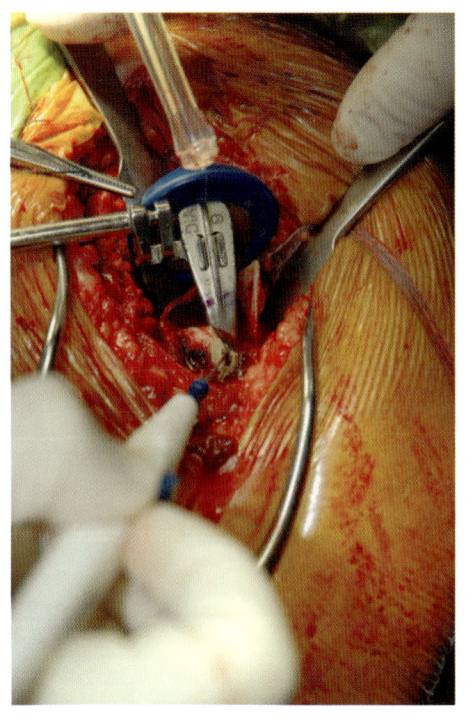

Figure 4 Intraoperative photograph demonstrates insertion of the trial humeral component to the desired level.

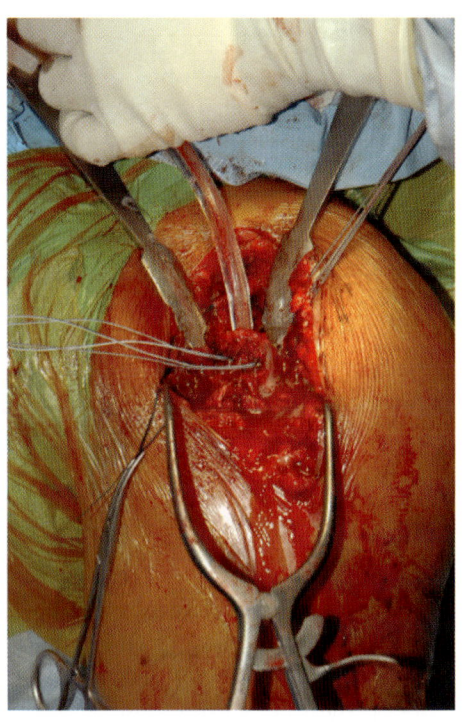

Figure 5 Intraoperative photograph shows placement of the vertical cerclage sutures in the humeral diaphysis before placement of the humeral component.

identified. The humeral shaft is progressively reamed until the size of the reamer that is used corresponds to the diameter of the prosthesis to be implanted. Using the largest diaphyseal reamer that is possible to advance down the humeral canal without difficulty avoids selecting a humeral implant with a diameter that is too small, which can inadvertently be positioned in varus or valgus.

The bicipital groove is located, and two 2-mm holes are drilled to the humeral shaft approximately 1 cm distal to the fracture site, one on each side of the bicipital groove, for use later in tuberosity fixation. The intra-articular portion of the long head of the biceps is excised, and suture tenodesis of the remaining stump to the pectoralis major tendon is performed with No. 1 nonabsorbable braided suture in a figure-of-8 stitch. The trial humeral implant is assembled by selecting a stem with a diameter corresponding to the largest diaphyseal reamer used and a head size corresponding to the size of the removed head fracture fragment. Great care is taken to avoid insertion of a humeral head component that is too large, which can lead to nonunion of the tuberosities.

Prosthesis height is based on preoperative planning, as described earlier, using the Gothic arch technique. With these calculations, the position on the humeral trial implant that should correspond to the position of the medial aspect of the fracture is marked. The trial humeral implant is placed in the humeral canal at the desired height using a prosthesis holder (**Figure 4**). Humeral retroversion is set between 20° and 30° by judging the angle formed by the prosthesis holder and the forearm. After glenohumeral reduction, the humeral head should be directed into the center of the glenoid fossa with the arm held in neutral rotation.

Once proper version is determined, electrocautery is used to mark the position of the prosthesis fin on the humeral diaphysis. An assistant can reduce the tuberosities around the trial implant, thereby further confirming appropriate prosthesis position. Intraoperative fluoroscopy can also be used to help confirm appropriate prosthesis position. Because the plastic trial humeral head is radiolucent, we use the actual humeral implant when judging prosthetic position with fluoroscopy.

A cement restrictor is placed in the humeral canal to create a 1-cm distal cement mantle. Two strands of No. 2 nonabsorbable braided suture are passed in an outside-to-inside direction through one of the previously drilled holes in the humeral shaft adjacent to the bicipital groove. These sutures are then passed from inside to outside through the other hole previously drilled in the humeral shaft adjacent to the bicipital groove (**Figure 5**). The humeral canal is irrigated and dried thoroughly. Bone cement is mixed and introduced into the humeral shaft with a catheter-tip syringe.

The humeral implant attached to the prosthesis holder is introduced into the humeral shaft to the appropriate level marked on the implant and at the version marked on the humeral diaphysis. The position of the prosthesis is continually checked to ensure that no movement occurs as the cement cures.

All excess cement is removed, with special attention to the removal of cement in the fenestration of the prosthesis and at the diaphyseal fracture site. The cement is allowed to fully polymerize, thus completing insertion of the humeral component.

Tuberosity Reduction and Fixation

Tuberosity fixation consists of two major elements: use of a reliable and reproducible suture fixation technique to provide initial fracture stability and use of bone graft to assist in tuberosity healing and provide long-term fracture stability. Autologous bone graft, taken from the humeral head fragment, serves two purposes. First, the bone graft enhances healing between the greater and lesser tuberosities and between the tuberosities and the humeral diaphysis. Second, because the greater tuberosity is often no more than a thin shell of bone, the bone graft acts to position the greater tuberosity laterally in a more anatomic position.

A specially designed bone-graft cutter is used to harvest two bone plugs from the humeral head fragment. The remaining cancellous bone in the humeral head fragment is removed with a large biting rongeur and morcellized. Care is taken to exclude articular cartilage from the bone plugs or the morcellized bone graft. One of the bone-graft plugs is gently impacted into the fenestration of the humeral prosthesis that has previously been cemented into place (**Figure 6**).

Fixation of the tuberosities is achieved with a reproducible suture fixation technique as described by Boileau et al,[3] consisting of four horizontal cerclage sutures (two around the greater tuberosity and two around the greater and lesser tuberosities) and two vertical cerclage sutures (**Figure 7**). The sutures to be used for horizontal cerclage were previously placed when control of the greater tuberosity was initially achieved and consist of two strands of No. 2 braided permanent suture placed through the rotator cuff at the junction of the supraspinatus and the infraspinatus and two strands of No. 2 braided permanent suture placed through the rotator cuff at the junction of the supraspinatus and the teres minor. The vertical cerclage consists of the two strands of No. 2 nonabsorbable braided suture placed in the humeral diaphysis before humeral implant cementation.

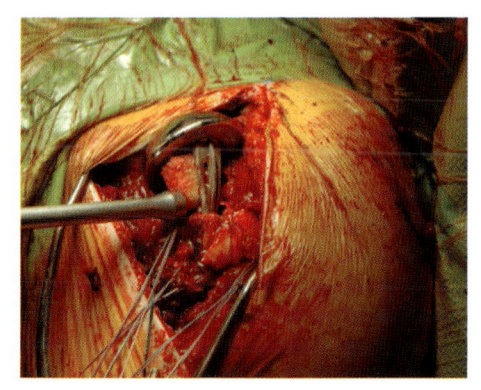

Figure 6 Intraoperative photograph shows impaction of bone graft within the fenestration of the humeral component.

The sutures controlling the greater tuberosity are passed around the smooth-polish medial aspect of the prosthetic neck, and the prosthesis is reduced. The second of the two bone-graft plugs is placed lateral to the neck of the prosthesis to accommodate bone loss in the greater tuberosity and place the greater tuberosity in a more anatomic lateral position. The morcellized bone graft is placed along the diaphyseal fracture line to promote healing of the greater and lesser tuberosities to the humeral shaft.

The greater tuberosity is gently grasped with a Lahey forceps and reduced into position lateral to the second bone-graft plug. Two of the sutures controlling the greater tuberosity, one superior and one inferior, are tied to fixate the greater tuberosity. The remaining two sutures, one superior and one inferior, are passed through the subscapularis tendon just medial to its osseous insertion on the lesser tuberosity. The lesser tuberosity is reduced with the previously placed stay sutures, and the circumferential sutures are tied to secure the tuberosity.

Tuberosity fixation is completed with the two sutures previously placed through drill holes in the humeral diaphysis. One suture is placed through the subscapularis and supraspinatus tendons just medial to their insertion and then tied. The second suture is then passed through the infraspinatus and supraspinatus tendons just medial to their osseous insertion and tied.

The security of the tuberosities must be evaluated by checking the mobility of the shoulder after tuberosity repair. The tuberosities and the humeral head implant should move as one unit. The wound is irrigated thoroughly and closed in layers.

Complications

Intraoperative complications are uncommon during hemiarthroplasty for proximal humerus fractures and are usually related to neurovascular injury or iatrogenic humeral shaft fracture. Many patients with proximal humerus fractures sustain neurapraxic injury to the axillary nerve, and this should be documented on clinical examination before surgery. The treatment of axillary nerve injury is observation, with less than 2% of patients sustaining a permanent axillary nerve deficit.[4] Vascular injuries most often involve injury to the axillary artery. Such injury is usually a consequence of overzealous medial dissection or retraction (or both) combined with vasculature that has been compromised by aging (plaques or calcification).

Most intraoperative humeral shaft fractures occur during reaming of the humeral canal. The diaphyseal cortex in many elderly patients is very thin and hence has an increased risk of diaphyseal penetration. When this complication occurs, it may be unrecognized.

Postoperative complications are much more common than intraoperative complications. Most complications involve the greater or lesser tuberosities (or both) but also may include wound problems (dehiscence, hematoma, glenoid problems, humeral problems, instability, stiffness, and infection).

Nonunion and malunion of the greater and lesser tuberosities are the most common complications after hemiarthroplasty treatment of proximal humerus fractures. When tuberosity complications occur, there is no simple solution that provides a reliable result. Even early recognition and reattachment of the greater

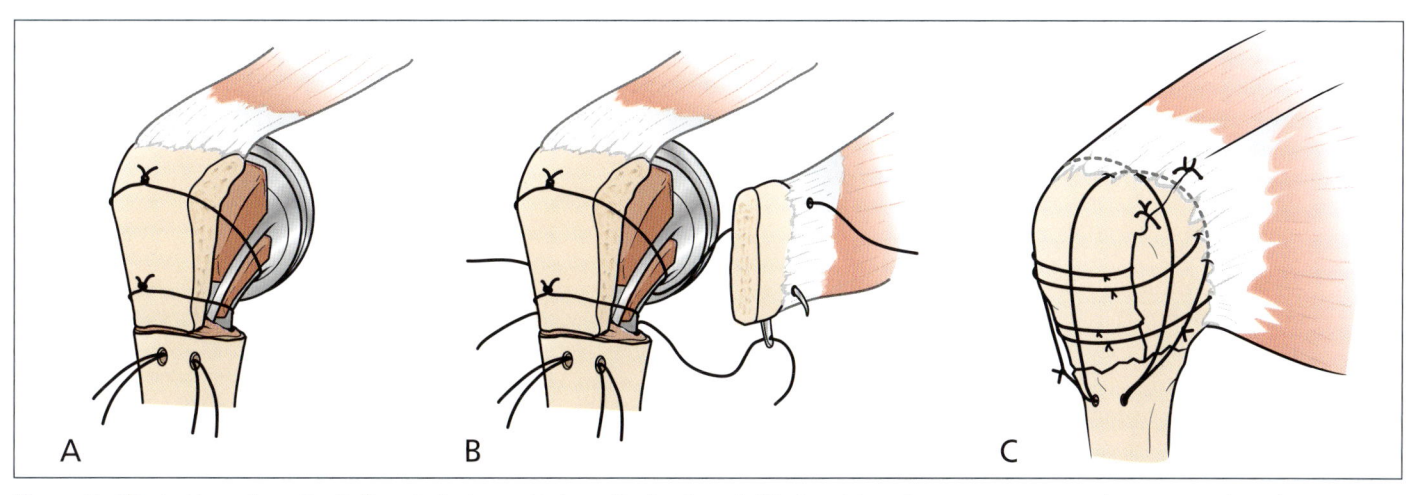

Figure 7 Illustrations show the Boileau technique of tuberosity fixation. **A,** Horizontal cerclage sutures secure the greater tuberosity. **B,** Passage of two additional horizontal cerclage sutures for fixation of the greater and lesser tuberosities. **C,** Completed construct with four horizontal and two vertical cerclage sutures.

tuberosity yields an unsatisfactory result in nearly all cases.[5] Similarly, tuberosity osteotomy produces poor results in cases of malunion.[6,7] The most predictable results are obtained with revision arthroplasty to a reverse prosthesis in these cases.

After hemiarthroplasty for fracture, erosion of the glenoid articular cartilage and the osseous glenoid can occur. Successful treatment of glenoid erosion usually requires revision surgery with resurfacing of the glenoid.

Humeral diaphysis problems are rare and consist of loosening of the humeral component or periprosthetic humerus fracture. Aseptic loosening of the humeral stem occurs more frequently in fracture cases than in nonfracture cases, mainly because of the lack of metaphyseal support of the implant. Use of cement is always indicated in fracture cases to help prevent this potential complication. Whenever the humeral stem loosens, infection must be ruled out. In the rare instance of symptomatic aseptic loosening of the humeral component, treatment is revision of the humeral stem, often with a reverse prosthesis, because this complication is generally accompanied by tuberosity nonunion.

Postoperative periprosthetic humeral fractures are almost always the result of a fall or a similar low-energy trauma. The majority of these fractures occur distal to the tip of the implant and are treated nonsurgically. Our criteria for recommending surgical treatment of periprosthetic fractures (revision surgery) include complete displacement, angulation of greater than 30°, loosening of the humeral component, or failure of nonsurgical treatment.

Instability after hemiarthroplasty for fracture is usually related to tuberosity nonunion or, less commonly, prosthetic malalignment. Tuberosity nonunion may result in static migration of the humerus superiorly or anterosuperiorly, similar to the situation of a patient with cuff tear arthropathy who has undergone hemiarthroplasty. In most cases, reattachment of the tuberosities does not resolve the instability, so we treat these patients with revision to a reverse prosthesis.

Prosthetic malposition may lead to instability despite healing of the tuberosities. The instability is usually caused by version malalignment (excessive retroversion causing posterior instability or excessive anteversion causing anterior instability) or by the humeral stem being implanted at an inappropriate level within the humeral shaft. In this scenario, revision of the humeral stem to change prosthetic positioning is necessary. If prosthetic malalignment has resulted in glenoid cartilage wear, resurfacing of the glenoid must be considered as well.

Glenohumeral stiffness is a common complication after unconstrained shoulder arthroplasty for fracture and is related to capsular contracture or the position of the prosthesis. Prosthetic problems resulting in stiffness are almost always the result of implantation of too large a humeral component or placement in the wrong position. Physical therapy can be attempted in an effort to improve mobility. If no improvement occurs over a 6-month period, revision surgery is indicated, consisting of realignment of the humeral component or downsizing of the humeral head with open release of any capsular contractures that are present.

Patients most at risk for infections are those with systemic illness and those with compromised soft tissues (open fractures). Infections are most commonly caused by *Staphylococcus aureus* or *Propionibacterium acnes*. Infections after shoulder arthroplasty can be divided into perioperative (within 6 weeks of surgery) and late (hematogenous) infections.

Early perioperative infections are initially treated with multiple irrigation and débridement procedures and retention of the humeral component if the tuberosity repair remains intact. At the last planned irrigation and débridement procedure, absorbable antibiotic-impregnated beads are placed in the soft tissues of the shoulder. Consultation with an infectious disease specialist is obtained, and a minimum of 6 weeks of intravenous and oral antibiotics is usually recommended. If this regimen fails or tuberosity repair fails because of infection, the humeral component is removed and treatment is the same as for a late appearing infection. Late-appearing infections are treated by removal of the prosthesis, intravenous antibiotics, and staged revision arthroplasty.

Postoperative Care and Rehabilitation

The postoperative orthosis is placed immediately after the dressing in the operating room and consists of a neutral rotation sling. The sling is maintained for 4 to 6 weeks to protect the tuberosity repair. Patients are allowed to remove the sling for hygiene and rehabilitation exercises. Patients are discouraged from internally rotating or adducting the arm before the postoperative orthosis has been discontinued because of the potential for tuberosity migration. Patients are instructed in hand, wrist, and elbow mobility exercises on postoperative day 1. We use a hydrotherapy-based rehabilitation regimen after shoulder arthroplasty to regain shoulder mobility. For hemiarthroplasty performed for proximal humerus fractures, hydrotherapy is initiated 4 to 6 weeks after surgery.

Pearls

- If difficulty is encountered in locating the cephalic vein, the deltopectoral interval can be readily detected proximally by identifying a small triangular area devoid of muscle tissue between the proximal portions of the deltoid and pectoralis major muscles.
- Using the largest diaphyseal reamer that is possible to advance down the humeral canal without difficulty avoids selecting too small a diameter humeral implant, which can inadvertently be positioned in varus or valgus.
- If the humeral head fragment is between humeral head component head sizes, the smaller size is selected to avoid insertion of too large a component, which can lead to nonunion of the tuberosities.
- After glenohumeral reduction, the humeral head should be directed into the center of the glenoid fossa with the arm held in neutral rotation.
- Autologous bone graft, taken from the humeral head fragment, serves two purposes. First, the bone graft enhances healing between the greater and lesser tuberosities and between the tuberosities and the humeral diaphysis. Second, because the greater tuberosity is often no more than a thin shell of bone, the bone graft acts to position the greater tuberosity laterally in a more anatomic position.
- The tuberosities and the humeral head implant should move as one unit at the termination of the procedure.

References

1. Gartsman GM, Edwards TB: Unconstrained shoulder arthroplasty for fracture, in Gartsman GM, Edwards TB, eds: *Shoulder Arthroplasty*. Philadelphia, PA, Saunders, 2008, pp 163-214.
2. Krishnan SG, Bennion PW, Reineck JR, Burkhead WZ: Hemiarthroplasty for proximal humeral fracture: Restoration of the Gothic arch. *Orthop Clin North Am* 2008;39(4):441-450, vi.

3. Boileau P, Walch G, Krishnan SG: Tuberosity osteosynthesis and hemiarthroplasty for four-part fractures of the humerus. *Tech Shoulder Elbow Surg* 2000;1:96-109.

4. Schild F, Burger B, Williams J: Complications of prostheses for fractures, in Walch G, Boileau P, Molé D, eds: *2000 Prosthèses d'Èpaule. . .Recul de 2 à 10 Ans.* Paris, Sauramps Medical, 2001, pp 539-544.

5. Boileau P, Krishnan SG, Tinsi L, Walch G, Coste JS, Molé D: Tuberosity malposition and migration: Reasons for poor outcomes after hemiarthroplasty for displaced fractures of the proximal humerus. *J Shoulder Elbow Surg* 2002;11(5):401-412.

6. Boileau P, Trojani C, Walch G, Krishnan SG, Romeo A, Sinnerton R: Shoulder arthroplasty for the treatment of the sequelae of fractures of the proximal humerus. *J Shoulder Elbow Surg* 2001;10(4):299-308.

7. Antuña SA, Sperling JW, Sánchez-Sotelo J, Cofield RH: Shoulder arthroplasty for proximal humeral malunions: Long-term results. *J Shoulder Elbow Surg* 2002;11(2):122-129.

Chapter 29
Total Shoulder Arthroplasty for Osteoarthritis

Stephanie H. Hsu, MD   Louis U. Bigliani, MD

Patient Selection

Total shoulder arthroplasty (TSA) is becoming more common, especially with an active aging population. A successful outcome is dependent on several factors, including patient selection, preoperative planning, surgical technique, and postoperative rehabilitation.

The most common etiologies leading to TSA are primary and secondary osteoarthritis, which account for more than 60% of all cases. The pathology of osteoarthritis usually includes osteophyte formation, joint space narrowing with subchondral sclerosis and cyst formation, and posterior glenoid wear in severe cases. Rheumatoid and inflammatory arthritis, as well as osteonecrosis, are also indications for TSA.[1,2]

Contraindications include rotator cuff tear arthropathy, active infection, brachial plexopathy, excessive glenoid bone loss, and Charcot arthropathy. Studies have demonstrated full-thickness rotator cuff tears in only 5% to 10% of patients with osteoarthritis.[3,4] Fortunately, most patients with osteoarthritis have good rotator cuff tissue. A functioning rotator cuff is essential for a successful TSA.

Preoperative Imaging

The preoperative workup includes routine blood tests and medical clearance as indicated. We obtain a series of plain radiographs (**Figure 1, A and B**), including a true AP (Grashey) view in neutral, external rotation, and internal rotation; an axillary view; and a scapular Y view. A CT scan is often obtained, especially for evaluation of the axial cuts (**Figure 1, C**). These help to determine retroversion of the glenoid, depth of the glenoid vault, and wear pattern.[1,5] If there is any history or clinical concern for the rotator cuff integrity, we order MRI to evaluate for a rotator cuff tear, as well as for atrophy of the muscle bellies.

Video 29.1 Total Shoulder Arthroplasty. Louis U. Bigliani, MD; Stephanie H. Hsu, MD; Howard Y. Park, BA (6 min)

Procedure
Room Setup/ Patient Positioning

For anesthesia, we prefer an indwelling regional interscalene catheter block for its safety, effectiveness, and pain control postoperatively. This can be used in conjunction with monitored anesthesia care or a laryngeal mask airway as per anesthesia. General anesthesia may also be considered, especially for a muscular patient who may require paralysis for exposure.

Antibiotics are given within 1 hour of incision and are continued for 24 to 48 hours postoperatively. We prefer cefazolin, or clindamycin if a penicillin allergy is of concern.

We use a beach-chair position, with the head of the bed raised approximately 30° to 40°. A padded head positioner is placed to protect the cervical spine from extension or overrotation. The head is secured gently to the head positioner with a folded towel and tape. A towel "collar" is also placed to protect the interscalene catheter and keep it out of the surgical field. The patient is positioned toward the edge of the table on the surgical side, with the shoulder over the edge laterally, to allow the arm to extend and rotate beyond the bed. Two folded towels are placed under the patient's scapula. A small, short side arm board is placed at the level of the distal humerus, with the ability to slide distally to free the arm for extension and rotation for exposure and humeral work (**Figure 2, A**).

After setup, the range of motion of the surgical side is checked under anesthesia. The surgical shoulder is then prepared and draped in the standard fashion. We prefer not to shave the axilla.

The hand is placed in a stockinette, with self-adherent wrap over the elbow. A small bump is placed under the arm on

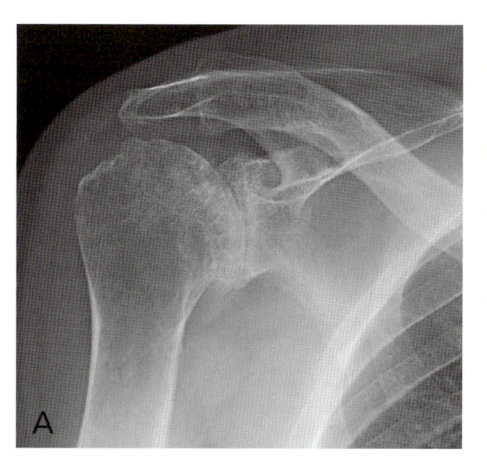

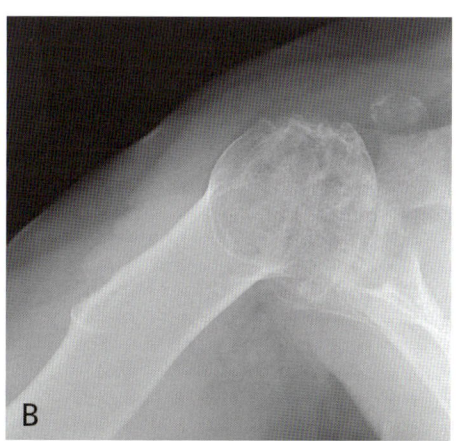

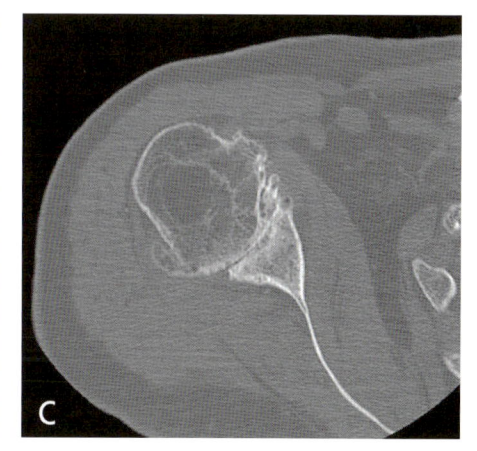

Figure 1 Images obtained before total shoulder arthroplasty for osteoarthritis. **A,** AP radiograph of a right shoulder demonstrates loss of glenohumeral joint space, marginal osteophyte formation, sclerosis, subchondral cysts, and maintenance of acromiohumeral distance, suggesting an intact rotator cuff. **B,** Axillary lateral radiograph demonstrates marginal osteophytes and posterior glenoid wear. **C,** Axial CT cut illustrates posterior wear of the glenoid, with good glenoid vault bone stock and glenoid version.

Dr. Bigliani or an immediate family member has received royalties from Zimmer. Neither Dr. Hsu nor any immediate family member has received anything of value from or owns stock in a commercial company or institution related directly or indirectly to the subject of this chapter.

the short arm board (**Figure 2, B**). Relevant anatomy—usually only the coracoid landmark—and previous incisions are marked. Two full Ioban sheets (3M) are used to create a "sandwich," fully covering the surgical site underneath and above.

Special Instruments/Equipment/Implants
The TSA system of the surgeon's choice is prepared. Additional instruments often used during the case are listed in **Table 1**.

Surgical Technique
Approach
A deltopectoral approach is preferred. An incision starting approximately 2 cm inferior to the clavicle and just lateral to the coracoid continues toward the deltoid insertion, approximately 10 to 12 cm as needed for exposure (**Figure 3, A**). As the deltopectoral fascia is exposed, two large Gelpi retractors are placed at the proximal and distal thirds of the incision for exposure. A needle-tip Bovie is used to raise full-thickness skin flaps medially and laterally, with meticulous hemostasis. Dissection is continued proximally to the level of the clavicle and inferiorly to the midpectoralis level.

The cephalic vein is identified adjacent to a strip of fat in the deltopectoral interval. It is mobilized and usually taken laterally with the deltoid because there are fewer communicating branches from the pectoralis medially. Loop retractors, Richardson retractors, a straight Adson, and a needle-tip Bovie are used to accomplish this. The Richardson retractors can also act as blunt dissectors to expose and clear the clavipectoral fascia.

The clavipectoral fascia is incised with cautery lateral to the conjoined tendon, and blunt dissection is performed underneath so that the strap muscles may be retracted medially with a Richardson retractor. The axillary nerve is palpated under the inferior border of the subscapularis to localize its position. When the arm is externally rotated, the axillary nerve will stay medial and out of the surgical field.

To improve visualization and exposure in the subacromial space, the anterior leading edge of the coracoacromial ligament is excised, along with any "veil" of bursal tissue that may obscure the view superiorly (**Figure 3, B**). Placing the arm in maximal internal rotation, any remaining subacromial bursal tissue is excised. It is important to define subacromial and contiguous subdeltoid space. An elevator is used if there are any adhesions, especially in patients with a history of previous surgery.

Table 1 Instruments Used in Total Shoulder Arthroplasty

Baby Richardson retractors/regular Richardson retractor
Darrach retractors (wide, narrow, and special sharp tip)
Army-Navy retractors
High-speed drill
Drain/Hemovac
No.1 and No.2 nonabsorbable braided nylon sutures
Absorbable monofilament sutures
Needle-tip Bovie
Fukuda posterior glenoid retractor/malleable retractors
Metal finger/elevator
Straight Adson
Flat-blade oscillating saw
Mallet
Gelpi retractors

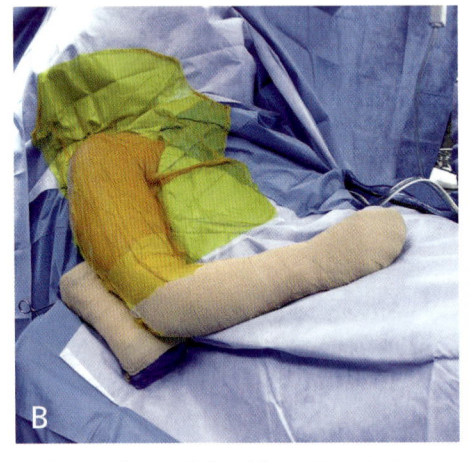

Figure 2 Photographs show patient positioning and setup for total shoulder arthroplasty. **A,** A short arm board is used to support the surgical extremity, and a headrest is used to stabilize the patient's head. **B,** The extremity is draped and a small towel bump is placed beneath the upper arm for support.

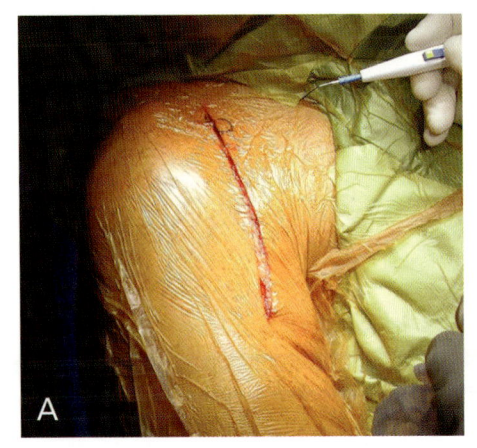

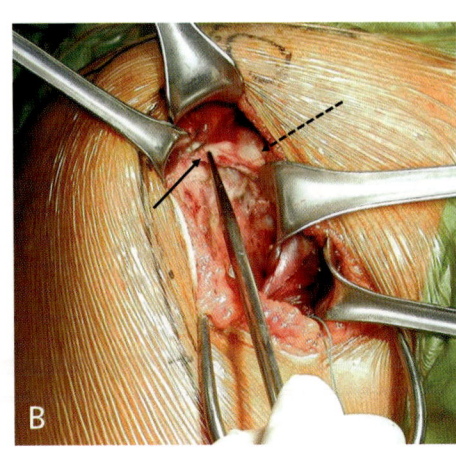

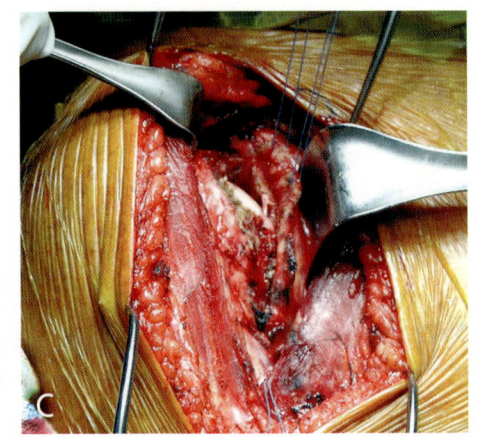

Figure 3 Intraoperative photographs show the deltopectoral approach for total shoulder arthroplasty. **A,** The incision. **B,** The coracoacromial ligament is resected anteriorly for superior exposure. The solid arrow indicates the coracoacromial ligament, and the dashed arrow indicates the coracoid. **C,** The subscapularis tendon is carefully taken down with a needle-tip Bovie, just medial to the bicipital groove, and marked with nonabsorbable heavy suture.

Chapter 29: Total Shoulder Arthroplasty for Osteoarthritis

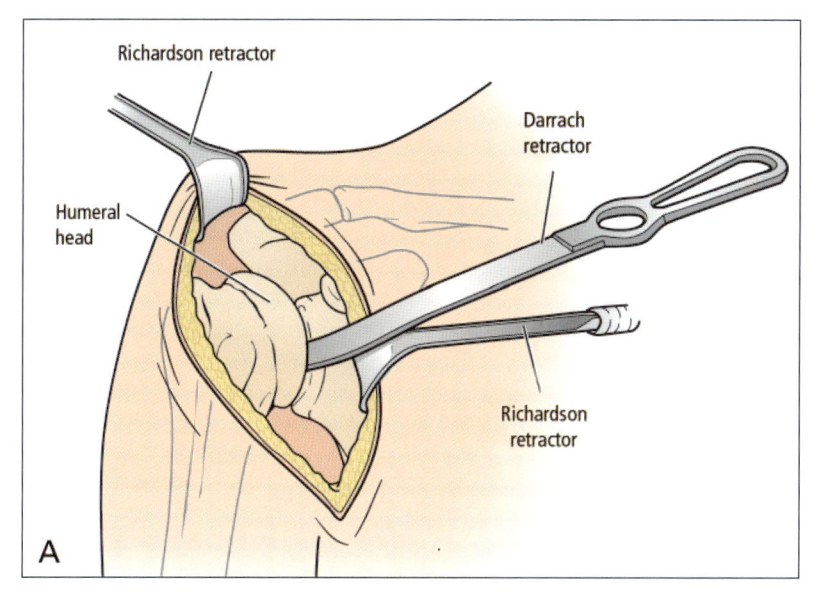

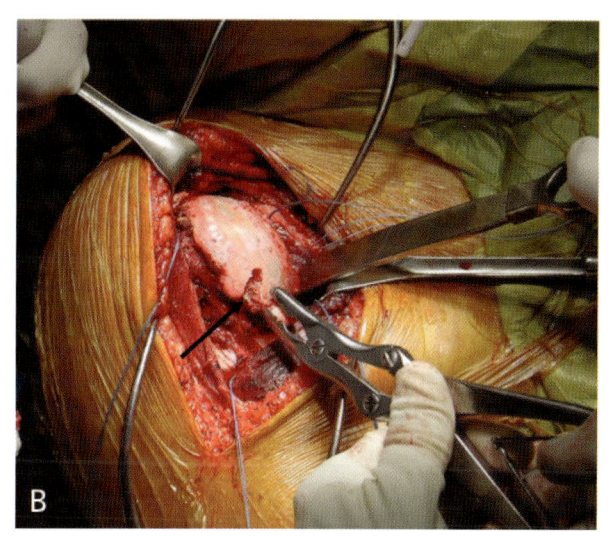

Figure 4 Humeral head exposure for total shoulder arthroplasty. **A,** Illustration shows Richardson retractors used for the soft-tissue retraction and a Darrach retractor used medially to help lever the head out. **B,** Intraoperative photograph shows removal of osteophytes to expose the true anatomic humeral neck (arrow), which is essential to making an accurate humeral head cut.

Inferiorly, the superior third of the pectoralis major insertion on the humerus is released and tagged with a No. 2 braided nylon suture. The inferior subscapularis is exposed by clearing overlying bursa. The anterior circumflex humeral artery and veins are identified near the inferior subscapularis tendon and cauterized to prevent bleeding.

When the superior and inferior borders of the subscapularis tendon are identified, the needle-tip Bovie is used to release the tendon down to bone 1 to 1.5 cm medial to its insertion, just medial to the bicipital groove (**Figure 3, C**). Superiorly, the release continues through the rotator interval toward the coracoid base.

The released subscapularis tendon is tagged with No. 2 braided nylon sutures, the most inferior being a figure-of-8 suture as it passes through a muscular portion. A thorough inferior capsule release is performed while externally rotating the arm. A metal finger or a narrow Darrach retractor may be used around the neck to protect the axillary nerve.

The biceps tendon within the groove is identified and marked for possible later tenodesis. The sheath is entered with a Bovie; then any redundant tissue is excised, and the tendon is marked with a suture and cut proximal to the suture if tenodesis is intended.

Humeral Preparation

The arm is ideally placed in extension, adduction, and external rotation to present the humeral head for preparation. Richardson retractors, a Darrach retractor behind the head, and an elevator or metal finger below the neck are used to create exposure (**Figure 4**). Marginal osteophytes are removed with a rongeur or osteotome to define the true anatomic humeral neck (**Figures 4, B** and **5**). This should start on the anterior superior margin and proceed inferiorly and posteriorly. The arm may be rotated freely to facilitate this.

The starting point for the opening reamer is identified, most often just medial and posterior to the bicipital groove. A short, sharp-tip reamer is used initially and transitioned to long intramedullary reamers with blunt tips, increasing by 1-mm increments until cortical contact is appreciated to the 130-mm mark.

The last appropriately sized reamer is left in the canal, and the humeral head cutting guide is attached (**Figures 6** and **7**). Guide pins are used for alignment at 30°

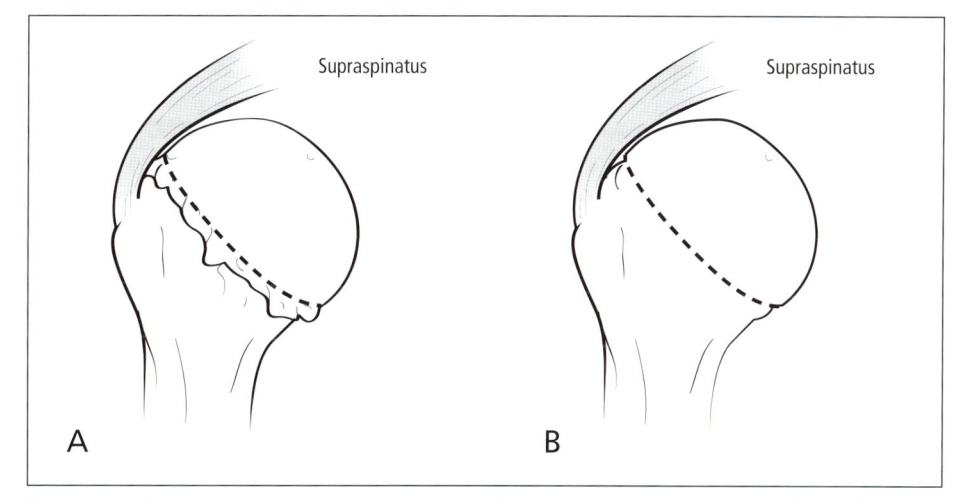

Figure 5 Illustrations show the appearance of the humeral neck before (**A**) and after (**B**) removal of marginal osteophytes. Osteophyte removal allows visualization of the true anatomic humeral neck (dashed line).

of retroversion. The surgeon must ensure that the estimated cut is at the edge of the rotator cuff insertion and the cuff is protected with wings or a metal finger while using the saw. After the saw cut is completed, a proximal reamer is used to open the canal proximally if the trabecular metal press-fit system is used. The trial humeral stem prosthesis is then inserted in the correct amount of retroversion.

The native humeral head is measured against the prosthesis size and offset is aligned appropriately, most often posteriorly. This trial humeral component preparation is then tested with the native glenoid, assuring approximately 30% to 50% posterior subluxation of the head. The trial humeral head is then removed, but the trial humeral stem is left in place to protect the humerus.

© 2013 American Academy of Orthopaedic Surgeons

Section 2: Shoulder and Elbow

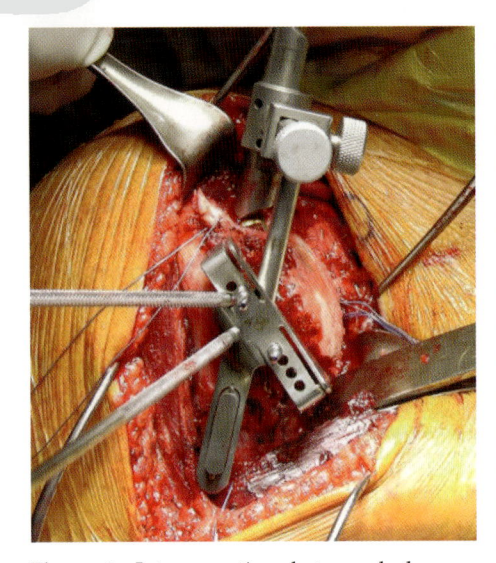

Figure 6 Intraoperative photograph shows placement of the humeral neck cutting guide. The guide is placed over the appropriate trial humeral shaft reamer, making sure to align the cut using the supraspinatus insertion as a guideline for appropriate cut depth. A Richardson or loop retractor is used to protect the rotator cuff, and a Darrach retractor is used to protect tissues medially.

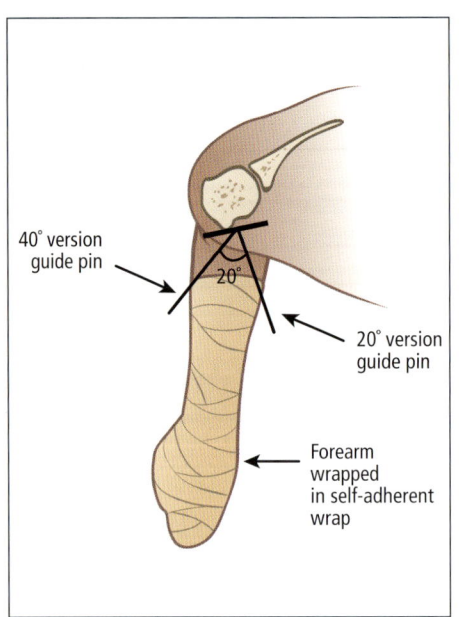

Figure 7 Illustration depicts the preparation of the humerus as viewed from above. Notice the placement of the humeral trial for the cutting guide and setting of 30° of retroversion by placing the forearm directly between the 20° and 40° version guide pins.

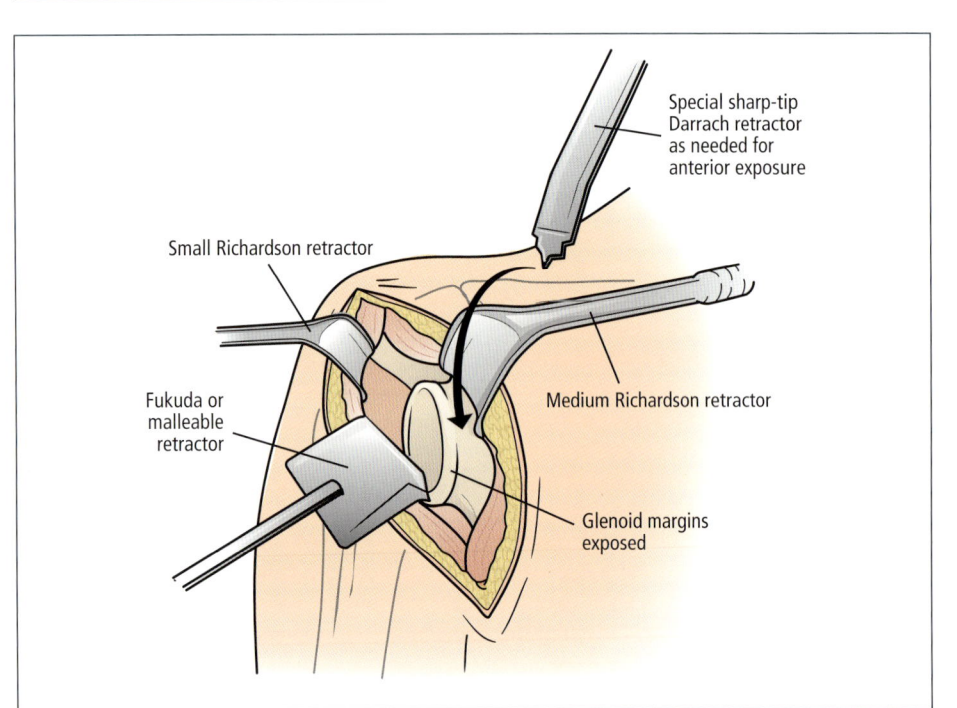

Figure 8 Illustration shows glenoid exposure for total shoulder arthroplasty. Full exposure is attained using Richardson retractors for soft tissue, a malleable or Fukuda retractor posteriorly on the glenoid rim, and a sharp-tip special Darrach retractor if needed anteriorly.

Glenoid Exposure

Glenoid exposure is critical to the successful and correct placement of the glenoid component. With severe eccentric wear and bone loss, exposure can be extremely challenging. Preoperative planning with appropriate axillary radiographs and CT images is essential. It is important to visualize the size of the glenoid vault and the amount of posterior glenoid wear.

A Fukuda retractor or malleable retractor is placed along the posterior glenoid rim to retract the humerus carefully. Richardson retractors are placed for medial and lateral tissue retraction (**Figure 8**). A metal finger may be used at the superior aspect of the glenoid to retract the rotator cuff. A special sharp-tip Darrach retractor is often used along the anterior glenoid rim for improved anterior exposure (**Figure 9, A**). After retractor placement, the needle-tip Bovie is used to release the origin of the biceps, being careful to leave the posterior labrum intact. The rotator interval is checked and released completely to the coracoid.

A partial anterior capsulectomy is performed. It is important to separate the scarred capsule from the labrum and exercise caution not to violate the subscapularis (**Figure 9, B**). The inferior labrum is also carefully removed with the needle-tip Bovie, while the axillary nerve is protected with a metal finger or a narrow Darrach retractor. If the exposure is still inadequate, the capsule can be released from the humerus by removing the Fukuda retractor and then palpating and releasing the tight capsular attachment. A narrow Darrach retractor can be used instead of the Fukuda retractor to improve exposure.

Glenoid Component Placement

It is essential for accurate component placement and good cement technique to make sure the glenoid margins are exposed, residual soft tissue is cleared, and the origin of the long head of the biceps is released if it is limiting exposure.[6] When satisfactory exposure of the glenoid has been achieved, a scraper is used to clean any remaining cartilage off the glenoid face. This is usually anterior. The glenoid centering guide is selected for the appropriate size, estimated for the center of the glenoid—taking into account known glenoid deformity, osteophytes, and version—and marked with cautery (**Figure 10, A**). The guide is removed, and the center point is assessed visually. When correct, the guide is replaced and the center hole is drilled. The hole is deepened with the guide removed. At this stage, it is important to assess the amount of posterior glenoid wear. The corresponding size circular reamer is used to prepare the glenoid face. Usually, more bone is taken off anteriorly. When the surface is conforming, the pegged guide is placed and the superior and inferior holes are drilled and deepened. The pegged punch is used once to ensure the depth of each drill hole and the proper setting of the glenoid component.

The trial glenoid is placed and assessed for positioning against the native glenoid face and stability. Additional reaming can be performed if necessary. The trial is fenestrated to aid in visualization of the glenoid surface (**Figure 10, B**). The trial is removed, irrigation with pulse lavage is performed, and thrombin-soaked

© 2013 American Academy of Orthopaedic Surgeons

sponges are inserted into each drill hole to promote hemostasis while the cement is prepared. The cement is hand mixed and poured into a 60-cm^3 syringe for insertion.

The sponges are removed and the holes are dried for cement placement, which is done with a pressurizing technique. A compressible pad is placed on the impactor, cement is placed in the holes, and the cement is impacted with the device; this is repeated a second time. Care is taken to ensure cement is only within the holes, not on the glenoid face. After the holes are filled with cement the third time, the glenoid component is placed, impacted, and held in place with manual pressure until the cement is hardened (**Figure 10, C**).

The retractors are then removed, exercising caution to expose the humerus without touching the glenoid component.

The head is trialed again and stability checked. The subscapularis is checked for mobility with the arm in 15° to 20° of external rotation. The trial humeral components are then removed.

A high-speed drill is used to create a superior hole in the humeral anatomic neck above the lesser tuberosity. Three drill holes are then placed through the lesser tuberosity for the subscapularis repair. A braided No. 2 nylon suture is passed through each hole as it is drilled (**Figure 11**). The sutures should pass through the stump of the subscapularis and soft tissue above the lesser tuberosity.[7]

A countersink device may be used to make the collar more flush against the humerus. The final humeral component is placed in the appropriate version, generally 30° of retroversion. If there is posterior wear, this may be reduced by 5° to 10°. The use of cement is optional; it is used only if the quality of the bone is poor or the canal is large. The final humeral head prosthesis is placed and impacted. The glenohumeral joint is then reduced and assessed for stability, assuring 50% translation of the head.

Closure

The biceps tendon is tenodesed with nonabsorbable sutures at the bicipital groove with appropriate tension. The subscapularis is then fully mobilized, and a No. 1 braided nylon suture is placed in the lateral aspect of the rotator interval to properly place the superior subscapularis (**Figure 12**). The drill hole sutures are then passed through the subscapularis in a simple fashion while the arm is in 10° to 15° of external rotation. Several soft-tissue sutures are used in addition to the bone sutures. The superior pectoralis major tendon is repaired with No. 1 braided nylon suture as well.

After thorough irrigation, a medium Hemovac drain is placed, exiting just lateral and distal to the acromion. The deltopectoral interval is approximated sparsely with No. 1 braided nylon sutures over the cephalic vein to mark the interval in case of future revision. The dermis and subcutaneous tissue are closed with 3-0 and 4-0 monofilament resorbable suture, respectively. Adhesive skin closure strips and a soft sterile dressing are placed. A well-padded sling is placed with the arm in neutral position. A loose elastic bandage wrap is fashioned as a swathe. A true AP radiograph is taken in the recovery room to check the components and alignment (**Figure 13**).

Complications

Complications such as infection and wound healing are avoided by sterile technique, intraoperative and postoperative antibiotics, drain placement to

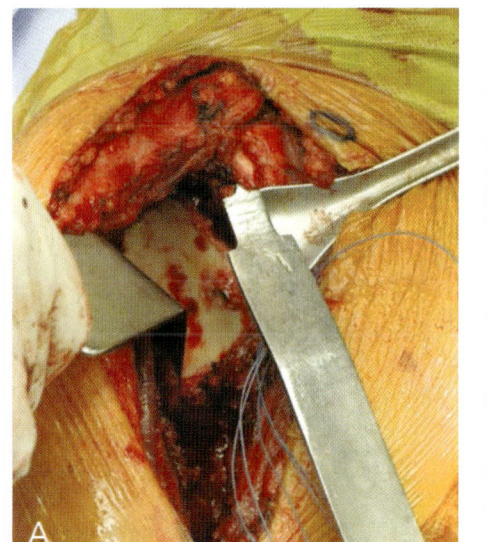

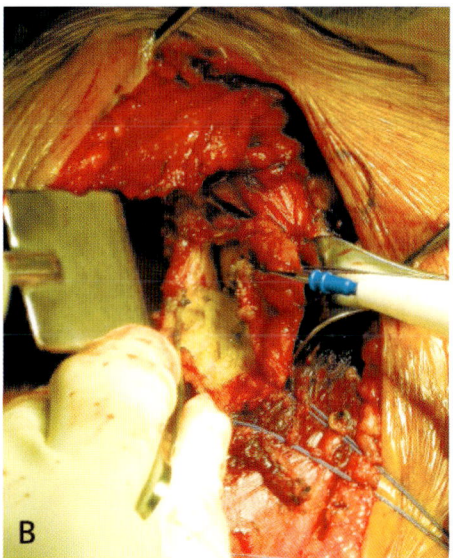

Figure 9 Intraoperative photographs demonstrate glenoid exposure for total shoulder arthroplasty. **A,** The point of a sharp-tip Darrach retractor is placed anterior to the glenoid face to provide stable retraction of tissue and improve exposure. **B,** Partial anterior capsulectomy is performed to assist in the release of the soft-tissue contracture. The scarred capsule is released carefully off the subscapularis, with special attention taken to avoid violating the subscapularis.

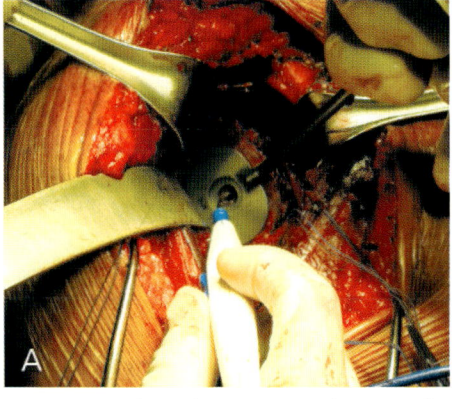

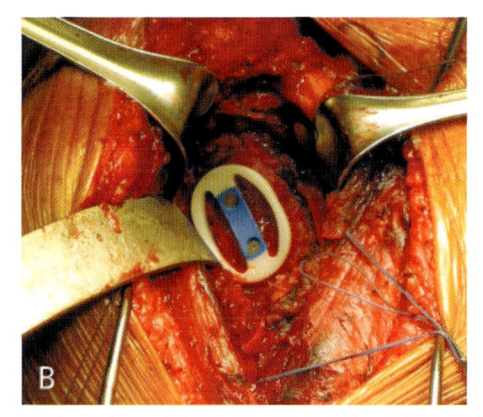

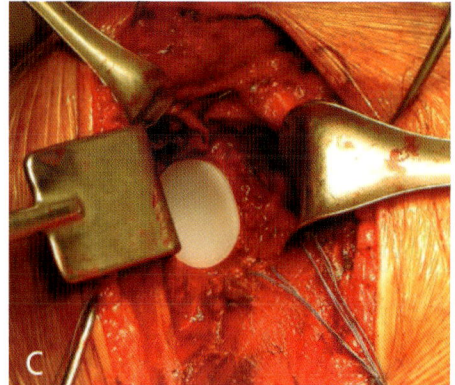

Figure 10 Glenoid component placement for total shoulder arthroplasty. **A,** The glenoid is marked with the centering guide. **B,** A fenestrated trial glenoid is placed, assuring flush seating with the glenoid face and central placement. **C,** The final glenoid is cemented in place.

Section 2: Shoulder and Elbow

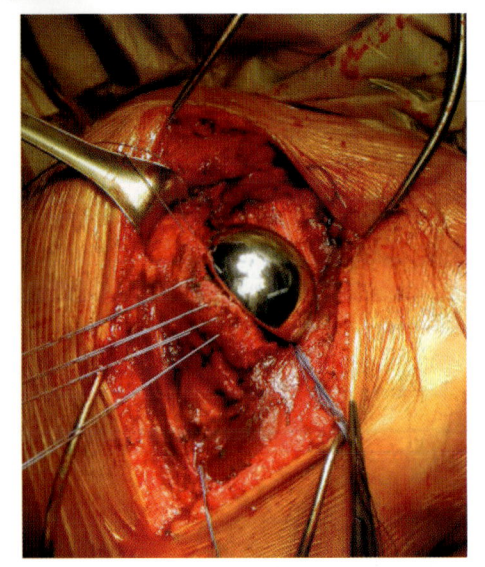

Figure 11 Intraoperative photograph shows the humeral component in place and No. 2 braided nylon suture passed through drill holes, ready for subscapularis repair.

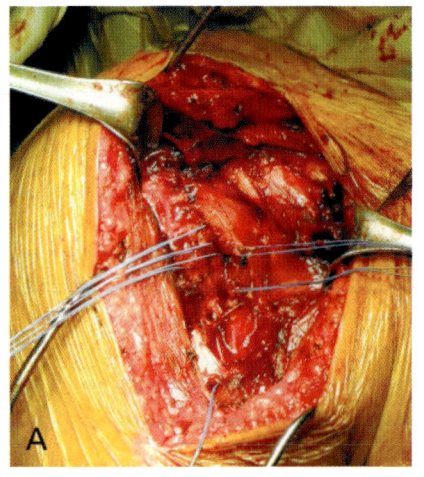

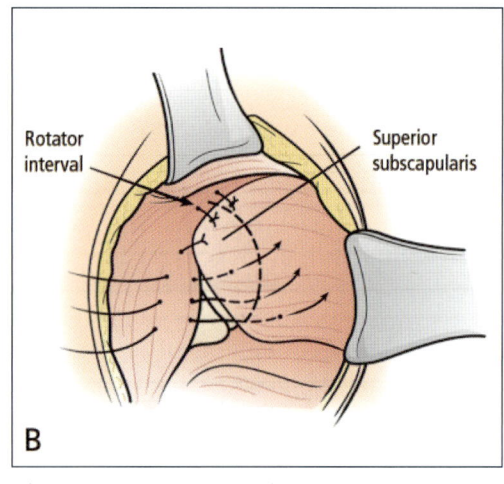

Figure 12 Closure for total shoulder arthroplasty. **A,** Intraoperative photograph shows repair of the rotator interval as well as the superior subscapularis, marking the tension and alignment for the tenotomy repair. **B,** Illustration shows suture placement at the rotator interval and superior subscapularis for tenotomy repair.

prevent hematoma, and careful handling of the soft tissues.

Component-related complications include glenoid loosening, periprosthetic humeral shaft fracture, and dislocation. Although not frequent, these complications are significant. Precise glenoid preparation and cementing techniques are important to prevent glenoid loosening. The use of a pegged component, correct sizing, and, in certain situations, a trabecular metal–backed component may be used to encourage ingrowth and stability. Humeral shaft fracture is avoided by careful sequential reaming at 1-mm increments, with particular attention paid to the feel and direction of reaming and a correct start point. Dislocation is a risk, but with appropriate glenoid placement, correct humeral version, and offset with good tissue tension and subscapularis repair, this risk is minimized.

Postoperative stiffness or failure of the subscapularis repair is possible. To minimize these risks, we follow a passive range-of-motion protocol with limits on external rotation, as detailed in the following section.

Postoperative Care and Rehabilitation

The interscalene catheter is kept in until the afternoon of postoperative day 1. This will minimize postoperative pain and help with passive mobilization. The swathe and abduction pillow are removed on postoperative day 1, as well as the drain. Patients follow an assistive-passive range-of-motion protocol with forward flexion up to 120°, no active internal rotation, and external rotation limited to 10° to 15° for the first 2 weeks to protect subscapularis healing. Exercises are started on postoperative day 1 and continued for 3 to 4 weeks. Patients are routinely discharged on postoperative day 2 and seen in follow-up in 10 to 12 days.

Pearls

- Preoperative planning using an axillary radiograph and CT to evaluate the glenoid vault is essential to a successful surgical outcome.
- Removing the leading edge of the coracoacromial ligament is necessary to release and define the subdeltoid/subacromial space to help with exposure and range of motion.
- Anterior to posterior osteophyte removal from the humeral neck aids in mobilization.
- An anterior capsulectomy is performed to assist with glenoid exposure and subscapularis mobilization.
- Manual pressurization of the cement at the glenoid pegs creates improved bony interdigitation.

References

1. Bigliani LU, Flatow EL: *Shoulder Arthroplasty*. New York, NY: Springer, 2005.
2. Saltzman MD, Mercer DM, Warme WJ, Bertelsen AL, Matsen FA III: Comparison of patients undergoing primary shoulder arthroplasty before and after the age of fifty. *J Bone Joint Surg Am* 2010;92(1):42-47.
3. Edwards TB, Boulahia A, Kempf JF, Boileau P, Nemoz C, Walch G: The influence of rotator cuff disease on the results of shoulder arthroplasty for primary osteoarthritis: Results of a multicenter study. *J Bone Joint Surg Am* 2002;84(12):2240-2248.
4. Norris TR, Iannotti JP: Functional outcome after shoulder arthroplasty for primary osteoarthritis: A multicenter study. *J Shoulder Elbow Surg* 2002;11(2):130-135.
5. Hoenecke HR Jr, Hermida JC, Flores-Hernandez C, D'Lima DD: Accuracy of CT-based measurements of glenoid version for total shoulder arthroplasty. *J Shoulder Elbow Surg* 2010;19(2):166-171.
6. Moen TC, Bigliani LU: Glenoid exposure: Tricks of the trade. *Semin Arthroplasty* 2011;22(1):17-20.
7. Ahmad CS, Wing D, Gardner TR, Levine WN, Bigliani LU: Biomechanical evaluation of subscapularis repair used during shoulder arthroplasty. *J Shoulder Elbow Surg* 2007;16(3, suppl):S59-S64.

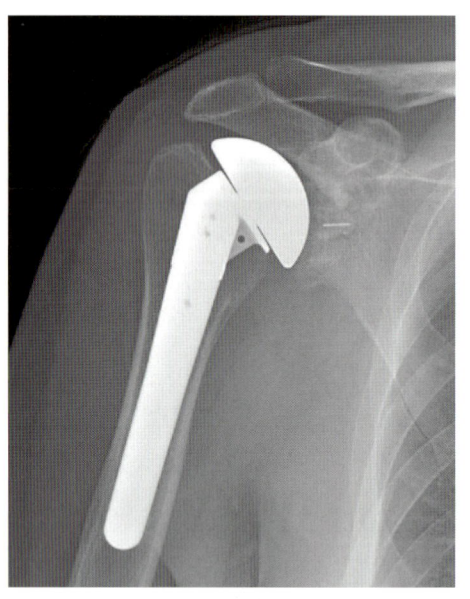

Figure 13 Postoperative AP radiograph of a right shoulder after total shoulder arthroplasty with a press-fit humeral stem and cemented pegged glenoid component.

Chapter 30
Reverse Total Shoulder Arthroplasty for Rotator Cuff Arthropathy

Peter Silvero, MD   Michael A. Wirth, MD

Introduction

Neer first introduced the term *cuff tear arthropathy* in 1977. He published a more detailed description of the clinical findings, pathology, and distinguishing features of the condition in 1983.[1] This entity was described as a relatively rare condition that developed in less than 5% of patients with a complete rotator cuff tear in the absence of other known etiologic factors. Cuff tear arthropathy is characterized by superior migration of the humeral head; erosions of the inferior acromion and superior glenoid; and collapse of the soft, atrophic head in advanced stages. Clinically, patients have long-standing pain that is worse at night and exacerbated by activity. Many patients are unable to elevate the affected arm above 90°, and external rotation is typically weak or absent. Neer et al[1] recommended that these patients be treated with an unconstrained total shoulder arthroplasty with soft-tissue reconstruction followed by "limited goals rehabilitation," noting that results were inferior to patients with an intact rotator cuff.

Introduction of the reverse shoulder prosthesis by Grammont in 1985 provided the first design that restored comfort and function in patients with cuff tear arthropathy. Its unique design featured a lower, more medial center of rotation that lengthened the deltoid lever arm and decreased the shear forces at the implant-glenoid interface. Although a complication rate of 15% was reported in an early midterm study, 96% of patients had no or only minimal pain, with significant improvements in Constant scores and range of motion.[2]

Patient Selection
Indications
Cuff tear arthropathy remains the most common indication for reverse shoulder arthroplasty. Patients older than 65 to 70 years with glenohumeral arthrosis, an irreparable rotator cuff tear, and painful pseudoparesis (active elevation of <90° with normal passive elevation) in whom nonsurgical treatment has failed are the best candidates. A functioning deltoid muscle and adequate glenoid bone stock for secure fixation of the glenoid component are essential.

Contraindications
Absolute contraindications to reverse shoulder arthroplasty include deltoid loss, inadequate glenoid bone stock, and infection. A relative contraindication is age younger than 65 years because functional results and pain tend to worsen after 6 to 8 years. Another relative contraindication is rheumatoid arthritis; patients in this group have been shown to have the highest rate of surgical revisions.[3]

Preoperative Imaging
Plain radiographs are an essential first step in the evaluation of cuff tear arthropathy. They should include an AP, a true AP, and an axillary lateral view (**Figure 1**). Characteristic radiographic findings include (1) an area of collapse of the proximal aspect of the humeral articular surface, (2) a paucity of osteophytes, (3) superior migration and a reduced acromiohumeral distance, (4) rounding of the greater tuberosity (femoralization), and (5) erosion of the undersurface of the acromion (acetabularization).

Many classification systems have been proposed, but we have found the Seebauer classification (**Figure 2**) to be the most useful because it provides a functional and biomechanical radiographic means of assessing cuff tear arthropathy. It focuses on the position and the stability of the center of rotation. In types IA and IB, the center of rotation is not displaced; the humeral head is centered and stable. Type IA exhibits acetabularization of the coracoacromial arch and femoralization of the humeral head. Type IB shows medial erosion of the glenoid. In type IIA and type IIB, the center of rotation is significantly cranially displaced. Type IIA has limited stability provided by the coracoacromial arch, and type IIB is characterized by complete static or dynamic anterosuperior instability. Sometimes it is difficult to differentiate between type IIA and type IIB on a simple static AP radiograph. In this case, a clinical examination with elevation against resistance will show increased superior displacement in type IIB shoulders.[4]

In most patients with cuff tear arthropathy, plain radiographs make the diagnosis clear, and more advanced imaging studies are not required. However, if plain radiographs reveal glenoid erosion, then a CT scan is recommended to evaluate the glenoid bone stock. Advanced imaging

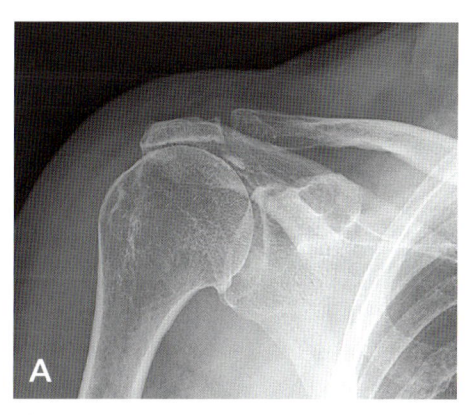

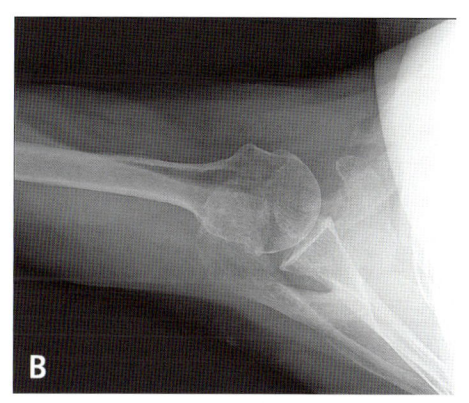

Figure 1 Preoperative AP (**A**) and axillary lateral (**B**) radiographs show the typical changes seen in cuff tear arthropathy. Note the rounding of the greater tuberosity, decreased acromiohumeral distance, and thinning of the acromial arch.

Dr. Wirth has received royalties from DePuy; is a member of a speakers' bureau or has made paid presentations on behalf of DePuy and Tornier; serves as a paid consultant to or is an employee of DePuy and Tornier; owns stock or stock options held in Tornier; and serves as a board member, owner, officer, or committee member of the American Shoulder and Elbow Surgeons. Neither Dr. Silvero nor any immediate family member has received anything of value from or owns stock in a commercial company or institution related directly or indirectly to the subject of this chapter.

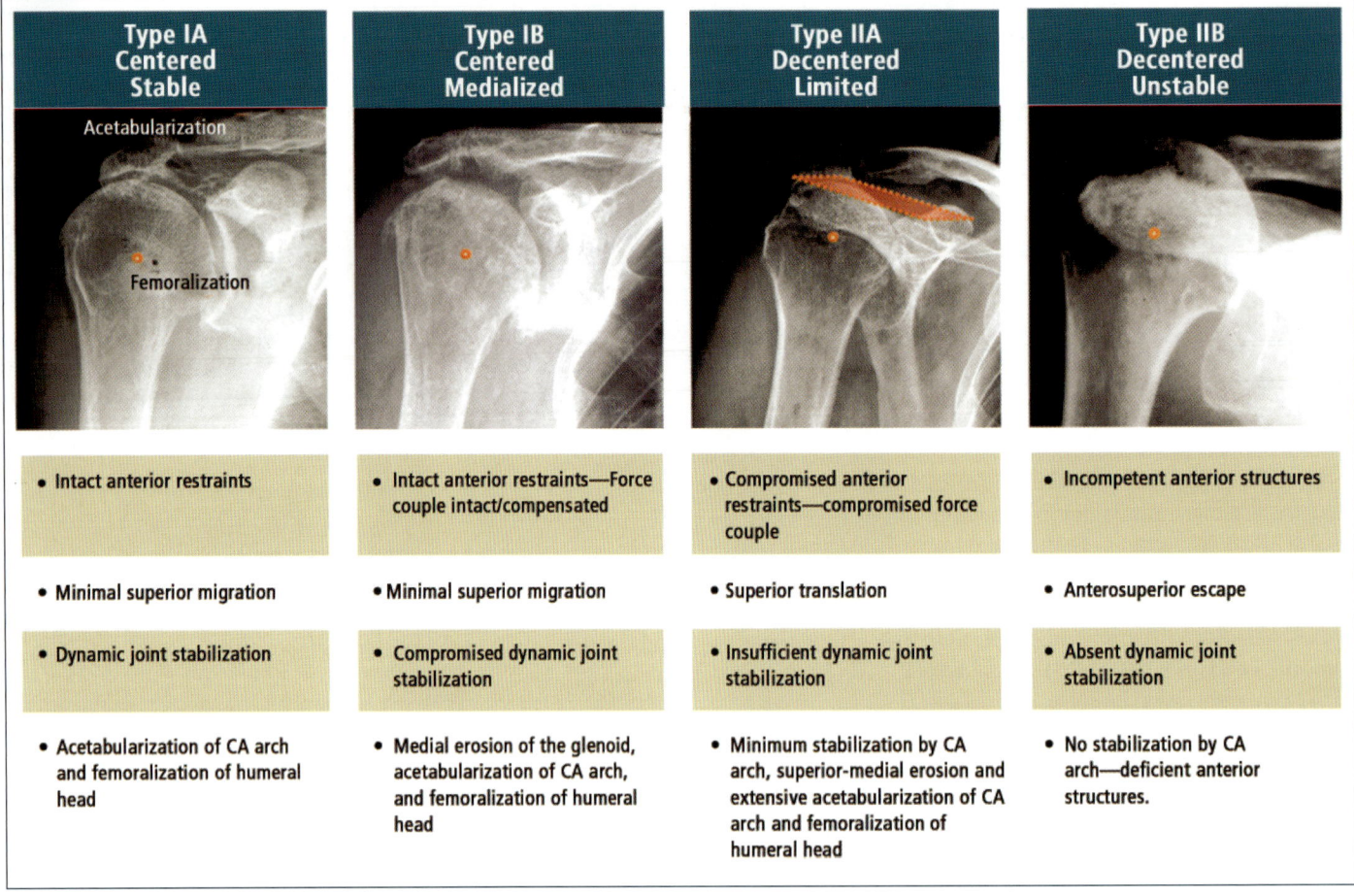

Type IA Centered Stable	Type IB Centered Medialized	Type IIA Decentered Limited	Type IIB Decentered Unstable
• Intact anterior restraints	• Intact anterior restraints—Force couple intact/compensated	• Compromised anterior restraints—compromised force couple	• Incompetent anterior structures
• Minimal superior migration	• Minimal superior migration	• Superior translation	• Anterosuperior escape
• Dynamic joint stabilization	• Compromised dynamic joint stabilization	• Insufficient dynamic joint stabilization	• Absent dynamic joint stabilization
• Acetabularization of CA arch and femoralization of humeral head	• Medial erosion of the glenoid, acetabularization of CA arch, and femoralization of humeral head	• Minimum stabilization by CA arch, superior-medial erosion and extensive acetabularization of CA arch and femoralization of humeral head	• No stabilization by CA arch—deficient anterior structures.

Figure 2 The Seebauer classification of cuff tear arthropathy. CA = coracoacromial. (Adapted with permission from Visotsky JL, Basamania C, Seebauer L, Rockwood CA, Jensen KL: Cuff tear arthropathy: Pathogenesis, classification, and algorithm for treatment. *J Bone Joint Surg Am* 2004;86:35-40.)

studies are also helpful to evaluate the condition of the rotator cuff. The amount of preoperative rotator cuff atrophy and fatty infiltrate is important in discussions of postoperative outcomes. Simovitch et al[5] demonstrated that patients with grade 3 or 4 fatty infiltration of the teres minor can actually lose external rotation after reverse shoulder arthroplasty, and clinical outcomes are significantly inferior to those in patients without advanced fatty infiltration.

Procedure

Room Setup/Patient Positioning

The patient is placed in the semi-Fowler position, with the head on a headrest that allows the patient to be positioned at the edge of the table so that the arm can be freely extended (**Figure 3**). It is best to finalize patient positioning before securing the head to avoid inadvertent extubation or impingement of the cervical spine and, brachial plexus during table and headrest positioning.

After the patient is securely positioned, a true AP view of the shoulder is obtained with C-arm imaging. The position and orientation of the image intensifier is recorded to facilitate reacquisition of this view at the time of surgery for optimal screw placement when fixating the glenoid baseplate.

Surgical Technique

The two primary approaches to the shoulder for a reverse arthroplasty[6] are the anterior deltopectoral and the superior-lateral approach. The deltopectoral approach as described by Neer is our preferred approach. The skin incision is made in a straight line with the arm in 30° of abduction. It extends from the coracoid process distally along the deltopectoral interval for approximately 8 to 10 cm. Subcutaneous flaps are elevated to expose the fatty strip that marks the deltopectoral interval. Dissection should be medial to the cephalic vein and retracted laterally with the deltoid muscle.

The clavipectoral fascia should be incised from the inferior border of the coracoacromial ligament distally to the superior border of the pectoralis tendon. A combination of sharp and blunt dissection is used to free the deep surface of the deltoid from the underlying tissue all the way from its origin to insertion. A key elevator is used to bluntly free any adhesions overlying the subscapularis muscle. At this point, the axillary nerve can be palpated and protected. We typically release the upper 1 cm of the pectoralis insertion with an electrocautery blade to help with exposure.

The anterior humeral circumflex vessels are identified along the inferior subscapularis and cauterized. Next, the subscapularis muscle and underlying capsule are elevated off the lesser tuberosity. The capsule is released along the articular margin down to the anterior inferior neck.

Following capsular release, the humeral head is gently dislocated by externally rotating and extending the humerus. If this proves difficult, then additional release of the inferior capsule may be required.

Next, the starting point for the medullary canal reamer is identified. It should be at the highest point on the humeral head, just posterior to the bicipital groove. We ream sequentially until the reamer begins to bite on the cortical bone

Chapter 30: Reverse Total Shoulder Arthroplasty for Rotator Cuff Arthropathy

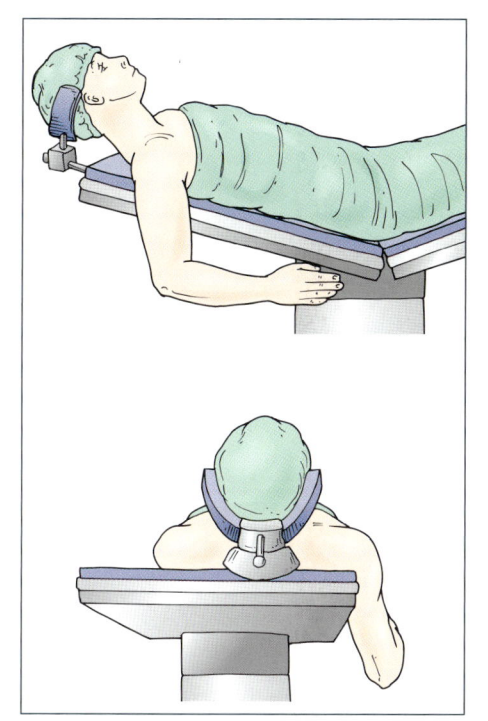

Figure 3 Illustrations show patient in the semi-Fowler position. Proper positioning includes placing the patient at the edge of the table so that the arm can be extended over the side of the table. The head is securely supported on a head holder with the neck in neutral alignment.

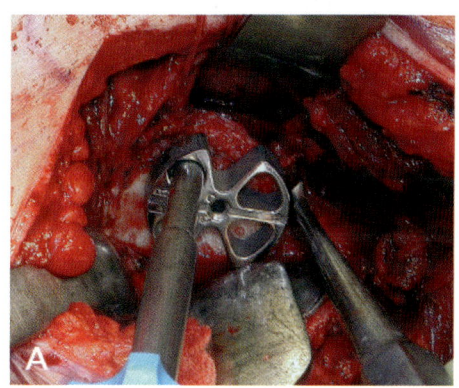

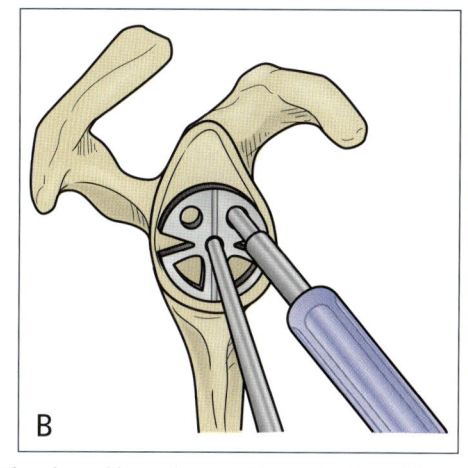

Figure 4 **A,** Intraoperative photograph shows the glenoid baseplate positioner in place. Note the key elevator at the inferior aspect of the glenoid and the positioner placed just above it. **B,** Corresponding diagram of the glenoid baseplate positioner illustrates proper positioning at the inferior glenoid and with the central guide pin in place.

of the canal. The appropriate size cutting assembly is placed down the intramedullary canal. We typically set retroversion at 0°. Excessive retroversion can limit internal rotation and has been recently shown to increase the risk of anterior dislocation in a mechanical model.[7] The cutting handle is rotated to align the orientation pin with the forearm. The cutting plate is slid up or down to adjust the resection level. The normal resection level should be just below the top of the greater tuberosity. A plate is placed over the humeral resection surface to protect it during glenoid exposure. At this point, attention is turned to the glenoid exposure. A moist laparotomy sponge protects the deltoid, and a Darrach or Fukuda retractor is placed along the posterior glenoid and levered down to expose the glenoid.

A 360° release of the subscapularis is then performed. A wide AO elevator is used to release the muscle off the anterior neck of the scapula. The rotator interval is completely released to the base of the coracoid. The inferior capsule should be clearly identified, dissected from the inferior muscle tissue, and excised. A Scofield retractor can be placed inferior to the capsule to protect the axillary nerve. Once the subscapularis muscle has been mobilized, a Bankart retractor is placed over the anterior glenoid. Glenoid exposure continues with removal of any remaining labrum and the biceps stump. The long head of the triceps insertion is released; this allows precise identification of the inferior glenoid rim and removes another potential source of impingement. Once all the soft tissue has been adequately cleared, then a large key elevator can be used to remove any remaining articular cartilage from the glenoid.

Positioning of the glenoid baseplate is crucial to the success of reverse arthroplasty. The position chosen should maximize contact with the glenoid bone and allow secure fixation. The glenoid baseplate positioner should be placed as low as possible so that its border is even with the inferior edge of the native glenoid (**Figure 4**). Some authors have advocated a mild inferior tilt to decrease the risk of notching, but a recent study has shown that inferior tilt is deleterious to intermediate-term results.[8] The guide pin is drilled through the central hole of the positioner to the far cortex of the glenoid, and the positioner is removed.

The reamer should be started at low speed before engaging the glenoid to avoid an inadvertent fracture. Care should be taken to preserve the subchondral bone by not overreaming. The glenoid baseplate is seated in the central hole and rotated so that the inferior screw can be aimed toward the scapular neck. The vertical glenoid baseplate markings should be aligned with the scapular neck inferiorly and with the base of the coracoid superiorly. The glenoid baseplate then undergoes screw fixation. We palpate the scapular neck and aim for good bone, drilling through the subchondral bone to a depth of 10 to 12 mm. Drilling is stopped, and the drill bit is gently pushed to make sure that it is contained in bone. After the surgeon is satisfied that the drill is contained, drilling continues until the cortex is perforated. If there is any question about the location of the inferior drill/guide pin, a C-arm image can be obtained. The superior screw should be directed at the base of the coracoid process and have a slight anterior orientation to avoid the suprascapular nerve.

At this point, the final glenosphere is placed. An inferior overlap of 3 to 5 mm is recommended to avoid impingement on the scapular neck. This overlap can sometimes be achieved with a standard glenosphere. If the glenoid baseplate cannot be placed low enough, then the eccentric glenosphere can provide the needed overlap (**Figure 5**). The real glenosphere is then inserted. For surgeons who are less familiar with the procedure, it is suggested that a trial glenosphere be placed before selecting the final one.

Now attention is directed back to the proximal humerus. We use a plastic skid to protect the glenosphere from the proximal humerus. The humeral component is then prepared based on the specifications of the manufacturer for cemented or uncemented use. A trial reduction should be performed and then joint stability and tension checked. With the arm in a neutral position, longitudinal traction is applied to the arm. The entire shoulder should move before any separation of the components is noted. Next, the arm is adducted with a bump in the axilla. There should be only a small opening of 2 to 3 mm between the lateral cup and the glenosphere. Similarly, if the arm is

© 2013 American Academy of Orthopaedic Surgeons

Section 2: Shoulder and Elbow

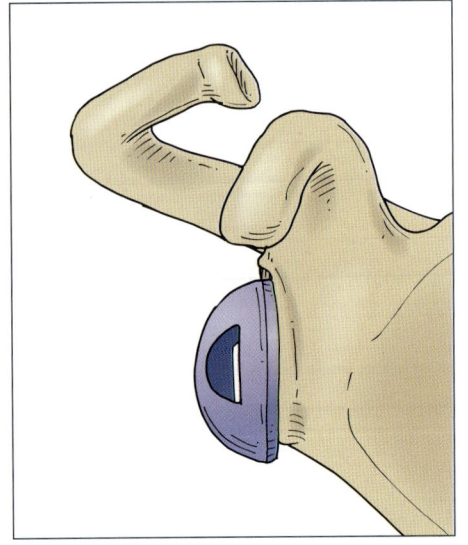

Figure 5 Diagram illustrates the overhang of the glenosphere. Overlap of 3 to 5 mm is recommended to avoid impingement of the proximal humerus on the scapular neck.

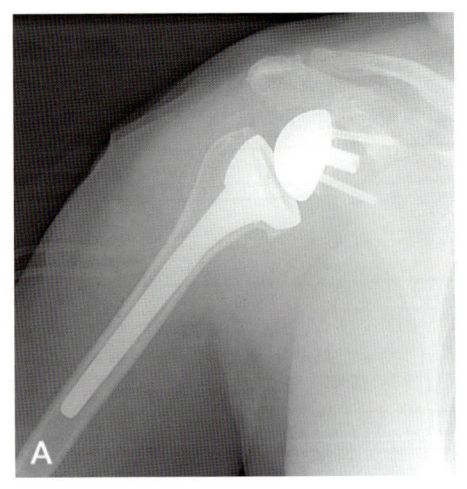

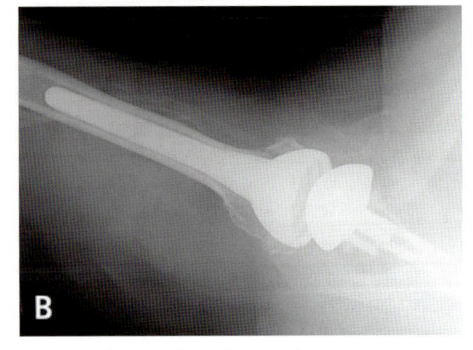

Figure 6 Postoperative AP (**A**) and axillary lateral (**B**) radiographs taken in the operating room.

extended or externally rotated, no more than a 2- to 3-mm gap should exist. Inadequate tension can be resolved with a thicker cup, spacers, or a larger glenosphere. If the joint cannot be reduced, then more bone may be resected from the humerus. If the tension is good, then the final humeral implant may be impacted or cemented into place. Before the final humeral component is placed, two or three nonabsorbable sutures are passed through the proximal humerus near the lesser tuberosity to enable reattachment of the subscapularis.

Once the humeral implant is in, then the final cup is impacted into place. We routinely go up one size in polyethylene thickness from the trial to the final component. The subscapularis is reattached if adequate tendon exists and it is not too tight. The subscapularis should not be closed if the patient's arm cannot be easily placed in at least neutral rotation. The long head of the biceps tendon can be sutured in with repair of the upper portion of the pectoralis major tendon. The wound is irrigated and then closed over a drain. We obtain postoperative AP and axillary lateral radiographs in the operating room (**Figure 6**).

Complications

According to a meta-analysis of reverse total shoulder arthroplasty,[9] the most common complications are scapular notching, hematoma formation, glenoid dissociation, glenohumeral dislocation, acromial and/or scapular spine fracture, infection, humeral component loosening, and nerve injury.

Scapular Notching
The most common radiographic finding associated with reverse shoulder arthroplasty is inferior scapular notching, with a frequency of 44% to 96%.[2,8,10-12] The importance of notching is still somewhat controversial in the literature. Some studies show no correlation with objective or subjective clinical results, complications, Constant scores, or postoperative range of motion.[10,11] In contrast to these findings, Sirveaux et al[2] found inferior scapular notching in 63.6% of their patients and reported that it significantly affected the Constant score when the notch was grade 3 or 4.

Favard et al[12] also found that their patients with no notching had better Constant scores, although in their study, patients with grade 1 or 2 notching had worse scores than patients with grade 3 or 4 notching. In this study, the authors found a much higher percentage of notching in patients who had undergone a superolateral approach.[12]

Another study showed an even greater correlation between scapular notching and outcome. Inferior scapular notching was found in 44% of patients. Patients with inferior scapular notching had a significantly lower Constant score and subjective shoulder value, as well as a more limited range of motion and lower strength compared with those without inferior scapular notching. The height of glenosphere implantation had approximately an eight times greater influence on notching than variation of the prosthetic scapular neck angle.[8]

Hematoma Formation
Hematoma formation has been formally reported as a complication in only one study.[10] Although it occurred in 20.6% of patients in this study and did require a return to the operating room for evacuation in approximately 50% of the patients, it had no overall effect on the final outcome. Suction drains were used in all patients. Early passive and active range of motion was initiated in this series; this may have had some influence on the formation of hematomas. We routinely place drains and delay shoulder motion until the first postoperative visit to avoid this.

Glenoid Loosening
Although one study had a glenoid loosening rate of 11.7%,[13] most other studies show rates of 5% or less.[2,3,10-12] Loosening of the glenoid can occur when the base plate is insecurely anchored because of poor bone quality or with suboptimal positioning. The risk of loosening can be minimized by ensuring that the screws are securely anchored in the best scapular bone available. The placement of the inferior screw is the most critical because it must resist tensile loads applied by the humerus to the inferior aspect of the glenoid component.[14]

Dislocation
Dislocation accounts for up to 40% of all complications and has a reported prevalence of 0% to 9%.[2,3,10-13] Factors associated with an increased risk of dislocation include the number of prior surgeries, the deltopectoral approach, bone deficiency, subscapularis deficiency, component malposition, and trauma.

In a series of patients operated on for cuff tear arthropathy with no prior surgery, Favard et al[12] reported 6 dislocations in 127 patients. All the dislocations in their series occurred with the deltopectoral approach.

© 2013 American Academy of Orthopaedic Surgeons

In a review of results according to etiology, Wall et al[11] reported 15 dislocations in 199 reverse arthroplasties. This complication was associated with more complex cases, such as revision surgery and posttraumatic arthritis. They did not find any correlation between repair of the subscapularis and the occurrence of postoperative complications or dislocations.

In contrast, Edwards et al[15] found that an irreparable subscapularis was a significant risk factor for postoperative dislocation. All dislocations in their series occurred in patients with an irreparable cuff tear. They also noted that dislocations are more likely in patients with complex diagnoses, including proximal humerus nonunion, fixed glenohumeral dislocation, and failed prior arthroplasty.

The effect of component positioning on intrinsic stability was recently investigated.[7] An anterior dislocation force was applied to the reverse prosthesis with varying angles of humeral and glenoid version, ranging from 20° of retroversion to 20° of anteversion. The version of the humeral component was a critical factor, with each 10° of humeral anteversion improving the stability ratio 21% to 27%, depending on arm position. Glenoid version had less of an effect, but retroversion of greater than 10° did lead to a significant drop in stability with the arm in the resting position.

Infection

Infection rates for reverse arthroplasty are higher than for nonconstrained arthroplasty, with a prevalence of up to 10%.[2,3,10-13] Most cases develop in the setting of patient-related immunosuppression secondary to factors such as diabetes, rheumatoid arthritis, previous surgery, and remote sources of infection. Extrinsic causes of infection include chemotherapy, systemic corticosteroid therapy, and repeated intra-articular steroid injections.

Postoperative Care and Rehabilitation

After surgery, the patient is placed in a sling. An abduction cushion may be used to relieve pressure on the deltoid. The morning after surgery, range of motion for the hand, wrist, and elbow is initiated. We typically limit range of motion of the shoulder for the first 2 weeks. After 2 weeks, the patient is started on a physician-directed stretching program. Exercises focus on abduction, forward flexion, and internal/external rotation. Patients are encouraged to use the affected arm to eat and write but are cautioned against using their arm to push behind the back or to raise themselves from a seated position. After 6 weeks, a strengthening program may be added.

Pearls

- Patient positioning: It is important to position the patient's arm completely free of the edge of the table to allow full extension of the arm. Otherwise, it will be difficult to adequately expose the proximal humerus and place guides down the intramedullary canal.
- Avoiding proximal humeral bone loss: Placing a metal plate over the resected proximal humerus will prevent bone loss during glenoid preparation.
- Identification of the axillary nerve: Because a functioning deltoid is crucial for the success of reverse shoulder arthroplasty, it is essential to identify the axillary nerve and protect it throughout the case.
- Adequate glenoid exposure: It is essential to adequately remove soft tissue from around the glenoid. This includes the inferior glenoid, to allow palpation of the inferior glenoid neck and lateral scapular border, and includes soft-tissue releases to remove any capsular contractures. Also, no soft tissue should remain that could be captured between the glenoid baseplate and the glenosphere.
- Proper glenoid positioning and secure glenoid fixation: This requires a good understanding of the glenoid vault and neck morphology, as well as adequate exposure. The glenoid baseplate must be placed low on the glenoid to avoid impingement of the proximal humerus on the lateral scapula and the inferior neck. However, the glenoid baseplate should not be positioned so low that it jeopardizes secure fixation of the inferior screw. With a very horizontal inferior neck, for instance, the glenoid baseplate may have to be moved slightly above the inferior border of the glenoid to allow good fixation of the inferior screw. In this situation, the proximal humerus will be less likely to impinge anyway, and some inferior glenosphere overlap can still be achieved with an eccentric glenosphere.
- Use of a C-arm to confirm position of the inferior glenoid baseplate screw: If there is any question about the position of the inferior screw placement on the glenoid baseplate, an intraoperative radiograph of the glenoid should be obtained.

References

1. Neer CS II, Craig EV, Fukuda H: Cuff-tear arthropathy. *J Bone Joint Surg Am* 1983;65(9):1232-1244.
2. Sirveaux F, Favard L, Oudet D, Huquet D, Walch G, Molé D: Grammont inverted total shoulder arthroplasty in the treatment of glenohumeral osteoarthritis with massive rupture of the cuff. Results of a multicentre study of 80 shoulders. *J Bone Joint Surg Br* 2004;86(3):388-395.
3. Guery J, Favard L, Sirveaux F, Oudet D, Mole D, Walch G: Reverse total shoulder arthroplasty. Survivorship analysis of eighty replacements followed for five to ten years. *J Bone Joint Surg Am* 2006;88(8):1742-1747.
4. Visotsky JL, Basamania C, Seebauer L, Rockwood CA, Jensen KL: Cuff tear arthropathy: Pathogenesis, classification, and algorithm for treatment. *J Bone Joint Surg Am* 2004;86-A(suppl 2):35-40.
5. Simovitch RW, Helmy N, Zumstein MA, Gerber C: Impact of fatty infiltration of the teres minor muscle on the outcome of reverse total shoulder arthroplasty. *J Bone Joint Surg Am* 2007;89(5):934-939.
6. Ekelund A, Seebauer L: Advanced evaluation and management of glenohumeral arthritis in the cuff-deficient shoulder, in Rockwood CA Jr, Matsen FA III, et al, eds: *The Shoulder,* ed 4. Philadelphia, PA, Saunders, 2009, pp 1247-1274.
7. Favre P, Sussmann PS, Gerber C: The effect of component positioning on intrinsic stability of the reverse shoulder arthroplasty. *J Shoulder Elbow Surg* 2010;19(4):550-556.
8. Simovitch RW, Zumstein MA, Lohri E, Helmy N, Gerber C: Predictors of scapular notching in patients managed with the Delta III reverse total shoulder replacement. *J Bone Joint Surg Am* 2007;89(3):588-600.
9. Bohsali KI, Wirth MA, Rockwood CA Jr: Complications of total shoulder arthroplasty. *J Bone Joint Surg Am* 2006;88(10):2279-2292.
10. Werner CM, Steinmann PA, Gilbart M, Gerber C: Treatment of painful pseudoparesis due to irreparable rotator cuff dysfunction with the Delta III reverse-ball-and-socket total shoulder prosthesis. *J Bone Joint Surg Am* 2005;87(7):1476-1486.
11. Wall B, Nové-Josserand L, O'Connor DP, Edwards TB, Walch G: Reverse total shoulder arthroplasty: A review of results according to etiology. *J Bone Joint Surg Am* 2007;89(7):1476-1485.

12. Favard L, Le Du C, Bicknell R, et al: Reverse prosthesis for cuff tear arthritis without previous surgery, in Walch G, Boileau P, Mole D, Favard L, Levigne C, Sirveaux F, eds: *Reverse Shoulder Arthroplasty*. Montpellier, France, Sauramps Medical, 2006, pp 113-123.

13. Frankle M, Siegal S, Pupello D, Saleem A, Mighell M, Vasey M: The Reverse Shoulder Prosthesis for glenohumeral arthritis associated with severe rotator cuff deficiency: A minimum two-year follow-up study of sixty patients. *J Bone Joint Surg Am* 2005;87(8):1697-1705.

14. Chebli C, Huber P, Watling J, Bertelsen A, Bicknell RT, Matsen F III: Factors affecting fixation of the glenoid component of a reverse total shoulder prothesis. *J Shoulder Elbow Surg* 2008;17(2):323-327.

15. Edwards TB, Williams MD, Labriola JE, Elkousy HA, Gartsman GM, O'Connor DP: Subscapularis insufficiency and the risk of shoulder dislocation after reverse shoulder arthroplasty. *J Shoulder Elbow Surg* 2009;18(6):892-896.

Chapter 31
Arthroscopy of the Elbow

Thomas V. Giel III, MD   Larry D. Field, MD   Felix H. Savoie III, MD

Introduction

The arthroscope has proven to be the ideal tool for evaluation of intra-articular pathology about the elbow.[1] However, this has not always been the case. In 1931, Burman[2] described early arthroscopy of the elbow joint with a 3-mm endoscope. He concluded that the elbow is "unsuitable for examination since the joint is so narrow," only to offer a rebuttal the next year. However, it was not until 1985, when Andrews and Carson[3] described their technique, that widespread use of the arthroscope to treat elbow pathology was adopted. Early techniques centered on evaluation of the intra-articular space, synovectomy, excision of osteophytes, débridement of osteochondral lesions, and removal of loose bodies. Recently, this has expanded to include everything from ulnohumeral arthroplasty and the treatment of lateral epicondylitis to the treatment of fractures and autograft replacement for osteochondritis dissecans. It seems as though new applications are being developed constantly.

The potential advantages of treating elbow pathology arthroscopically include reducing iatrogenic insult by decreasing incision size, a more thorough evaluation of the intra-articular compartments of the elbow, and possibly reducing scarring and potential stiffness by limiting disruption of the capsule. The disadvantages center squarely on the technical requirements needed to safely and effectively perform the procedure because of the close proximity of neurovascular structures. A thorough knowledge of the anatomy of the elbow from the arthroscopist's perspective is critical in reducing the chances of neurovascular injury.[4] The purpose of this chapter is to describe the anatomy, portal placement, setup, and technique to perform a safe and thorough arthroscopic evaluation of the elbow.

Anatomy

Prior to performing arthroscopic surgery of the elbow, a thorough understanding of the relevant anatomy must be obtained. Superficial landmarks can be palpated and marked for reference during surgery.[5] Starting posteriorly, the triceps tendon and olecranon can be palpated. Moving medially, the ulnar nerve should be palpated in the groove along the posterior aspect of the medial epicondyle. A subluxable ulnar nerve is present in 16% of the population.[6] The medial epicondyle should be marked. The antecubital fossa is palpated anteriorly. Laterally, the lateral epicondyle, radial head, and tip of the olecranon form a triangle marking the boundaries of the "soft spot" of the elbow.

Superficial nervous structures include the medial and lateral antebrachial cutaneous nerves. The lateral antebrachial cutaneous nerve, the termination of the musculocutaneous nerve, emerges from the distal portion of the biceps and travels laterally across the brachioradialis muscle proximal to the antecubital fossa. As it turns laterally, it branches and provides sensation for the lateral aspect of the forearm. The medial antebrachial cutaneous nerve travels along the medial arm with the basilic vein. It branches well proximal to the elbow joint and provides sensation to the medial aspect of the forearm. Damage to superficial nerves can be avoided by incising skin only and using blunt trocars.[7]

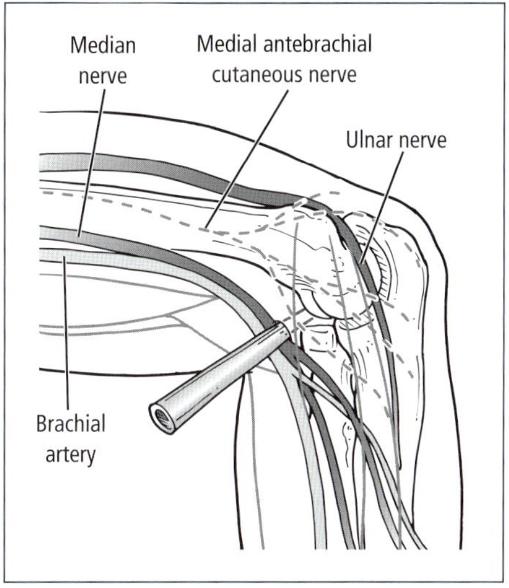

Figure 1 Illustration shows the position of the proximal anteromedial portal, which is approximately 2 cm proximal and 2 cm anterior to the medial epicondyle. The medial antebrachial cutaneous nerve is at risk of injury when this portal is created.

The deeper neurovascular structures include the median, radial, and ulnar nerves and the brachial artery. The brachial artery emerges between the brachialis and biceps muscles lateral to the median nerve (**Figure 1**). It travels just medial to the biceps tendon and deep to the biceps aponeurosis. It bifurcates just distal to the joint at the level of the radial head. The median nerve travels along with the brachial artery along the anterior surface of the brachialis muscle. As it crosses the elbow joint, it is just medial to the brachial artery. As it enters the forearm, it courses just deep to the pronator teres but superficial to the deep head of the pronator. The ulnar nerve travels posterior to the medial intermuscular septum. At the level of the elbow, it courses posterior to the medial epicondyle and can often be palpated in this area. As it enters the forearm, the ulnar nerve travels between the flexor digitorum superficialis and the flexor digitorum profundus. The radial nerve curves posteriorly around the humerus and penetrates the lateral intermuscular septum well proximal to the elbow joint (**Figure 2**). It then travels between the

---

Dr. Field or an immediate family member serves as a paid consultant to or is an employee of Smith & Nephew; has received research or institutional support from Arthrex, Mitek, and Smith & Nephew; and serves as a board member, owner, officer, or committee member of the Arthroscopy Association of North America. Dr. Savoie or an immediate family member serves as a paid consultant to or is an employee of Mitek, Smith & Nephew, and Exactech; serves as an unpaid consultant to Cayenne Medical; has received research or institutional support from Mitek, Smith & Nephew, and Amp Orthopedics; and serves as a board member, owner, officer, or committee member of the Arthroscopy Association of North America, the American Shoulder and Elbow Surgeons, the American Academy of Orthopaedic Surgeons, the American Orthopaedic Society for Sports Medicine, and the International Society of Arthroscopy, Knee Surgery, and Orthopaedic Sports Medicine. Neither Dr. Giel nor any immediate family member has received anything of value from or owns stock in a commercial company or institution related directly or indirectly to the subject of this chapter.

© 2013 American Academy of Orthopaedic Surgeons

Section 2: Shoulder and Elbow

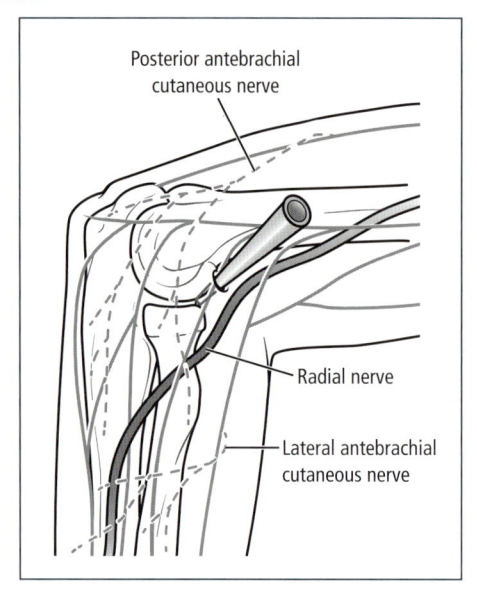

Figure 2 Illustration shows the position of the proximal anterolateral portal. It is approximately 2 cm proximal and 2 cm anterior to the lateral epicondyle. The radial nerve is at risk of injury when this portal is created.

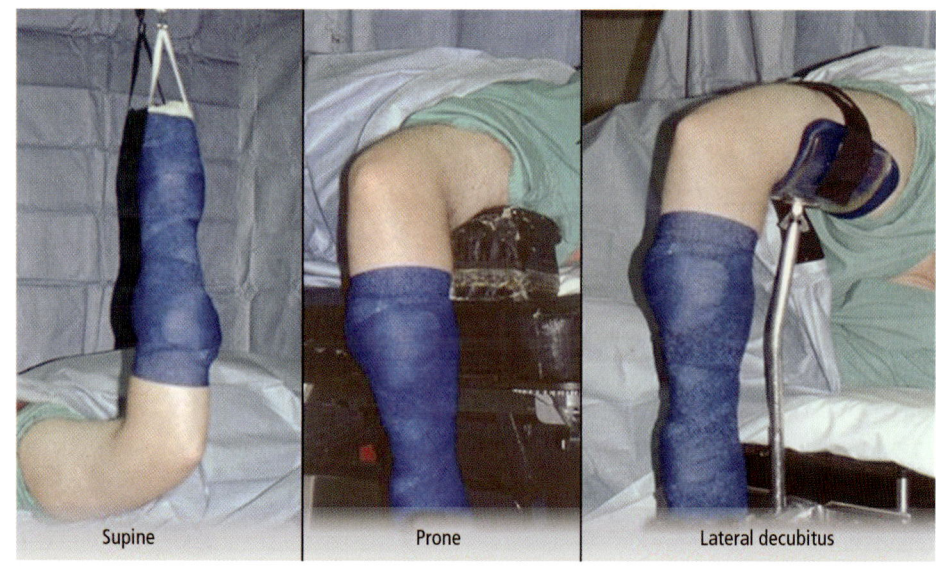

Figure 3 Photographs show three patient positions for elbow arthroscopy. Each position has inherent advantages and disadvantages with respect to anesthesia options, the need for positioning or traction devices, and the ease with which conversion to open procedures can be accomplished.

brachialis and brachioradialis muscles. It branches into the superficial radial nerve and posterior interosseous nerve just proximal to the elbow joint. The superficial radial nerve passes into the forearm just deep to the brachioradialis. The posterior interosseous nerve continues distally and courses into the supinator muscle while curving around the lateral aspect of the radial head.

Patient Selection
Indications
Elbow arthroscopy is a valuable tool in the diagnosis and treatment of several pathologic conditions. Its indications occasionally include diagnostic arthroscopy performed for the evaluation of patients with persistent elbow symptoms, such as pain and/or popping, for whom diagnostic testing and extended nonsurgical measures have been ineffective. More commonly, elbow arthroscopy is indicated and performed for such conditions as elbow arthritis with or without the presence of loose bodies, capsular contracture, osteochondritis dissecans of the capitellum, lateral epicondylitis, synovitis, and certain intra-articular elbow fractures.

Contraindications
Contraindications include patients with gross deformity of the elbow joint that precludes safe access with arthroscopic instruments and patients for whom arthroscopic intervention has a high risk of neurologic or vascular insult. A relative contraindication to elbow arthroscopy is a patient in whom a prior ulnar nerve transposition has been performed, due to the risk of anteromedial portal placement.

Video 31.1 Elbow Arthroscopy: Principles, Portals, and Techniques. Champ L. Baker, Jr, MD, FACS (21 min)

Procedure
A video of this procedure can be seen in the video supplement.

Equipment
In most instances, a standard 4.0-mm, 30° arthroscope can be used. In rare instances, a 70° arthroscope may be used. Metal cannulas without side vents for the arthroscope and inflow as well as plastic cannulas for the instruments can reduce the insult to the capsule.[7,8] Furthermore, cannulas should be changed over a switching stick whenever possible. Blunt trocars should be used to place the cannulas. Mechanical pump or gravity inflow can be used. Switching sticks can also be used as retractors intra-articularly. Most surgeons advocate the use of a tourniquet to assist with hemostasis.

Anesthesia
Anesthesia options range from general anesthesia to regional blocks, local anesthesia, and intravenous blocks. Regional blocks can be safely administered by trained anesthesia personnel and should provide adequate anesthesia for the surgical procedure. However, there is some reasonable concern that they make postoperative assessment of neurologic status difficult.[7] For this reason, many surgeons also choose to avoid using local anesthetics for postoperative pain control. Furthermore, the prone position is poorly tolerated in patients without general anesthesia. Accordingly, many surgeons elect to use general anesthesia when it can be safely tolerated by the patient.[9]

Patient Positioning
The three patient positions for elbow arthroscopy are shown in **Figure 3**.

Supine Position
The supine position for elbow arthroscopy, as first described by Andrews and Carson,[3] has several advantages.[10] For the supine position, the patient's surgical side is placed close to the edge of the operating table. The shoulder is abducted 90°, and the elbow is flexed 90°. After prepping and draping, a traction device is used to maintain joint distraction. This offers several advantages to the surgeon. It allows for ease of setup without having to reposition the patient. It offers the anesthesiologist easy access to the airway. It allows the use of regional blocks if needed. By positioning the extremity in this way, the elbow is placed in a position

Chapter 31: Arthroscopy of the Elbow

that is familiar to the surgeon. Therefore, it facilitates understanding of the intra-articular anatomy. One disadvantage is the need to have the arm fixed in a traction device, which can be difficult to set up and limits the surgeon's ability to manipulate the arm. Another disadvantage is that it makes evaluating the posterior compartment more difficult.

Lateral Decubitus Position
The lateral decubitus position was described by O'Driscoll and Morrey in 1993.[11] For this position, the patient is placed laterally on a beanbag. All bony prominences are well padded, and care is taken to pad the peroneal nerve on the down leg. An axillary roll is used if needed. The surgical extremity is placed up, and the shoulder is flexed to 90° and internally rotated. The elbow is flexed over a bolster or an arm holder, allowing the forearm to hang free. The advantages of this position include that it is fairly easy to position the patient and is better tolerated for regional anesthesia than the prone position. This position affords easy access to the posterior compartment of the elbow, and gravity provides joint distraction. The arm can be manipulated freely to assist with visualization. Furthermore, the lateral decubitus position provides access to the airway for anesthesia. The disadvantages include the need for a specialized arm holder or a padded bolster. Also, if the need for an anterior open procedure should arise, the patient would need to be repositioned.

Prone Position
The prone position was described by Poehling et al in 1989.[12] For the prone position, the patient is rolled onto the operating table after intubation. The chest is padded with chest rolls. The nonsurgical extremity can be positioned out to the side, with the elbow flexed on an arm board or tucked at the patient's side. The surgical extremity is abducted, and the elbow is allowed to flex to 90° with the forearm hanging freely. The extremity is placed over a bolster or a padded arm holder. Advantages to this position are similar to those of the lateral position in that gravity provides traction, and the arm can be taken through a range of motion during the arthroscopy. Furthermore, this can be done without an assistant. It also allows ample access to the posterior compartment. Disadvantages include the need to reposition for an anterior approach if needed and limited access to the airway. For this reason, the prone position is rarely used in conjunction with regional block anesthesia because the patient would have to be repositioned prone should conversion to general anesthesia be needed.

Portal Placement
Enough emphasis cannot be placed on the need for a thorough understanding of the bony and neurovascular anatomy around the elbow before proceeding with elbow arthroscopy. After adequate positioning, prepping, and draping, the landmarks about the elbow should be palpated and marked with a sterile marker. The medial and lateral epicondyles, the olecranon, and the the radial head should be marked. Care should also be taken to palpate the ulnar nerve in its groove. It should be noted whether the nerve is subluxated or subluxatable before portal placement because this could lead to injury of the nerve. Its course should be marked out with the sterile marker as well. It should also be noted that all positions for elbow arthroscopy allow for flexion of the elbow at 90°. This is vital because flexion moves the neurovascular structures anteriorly farther from the joint and provides more space for portal placement.[13]

After the marking of the landmarks, the next step is insufflation of the joint with saline. An 18-gauge needle can be inserted into the joint through the lateral soft spot or from directly posterior into the olecranon fossa (**Figure 4**). Adequate placement into the joint can be confirmed by seeing the expansion of the joint along the medial and lateral joint line, by allowing backflow out of the needle, or by seeing the elbow extend slightly. The joint should accommodate 20 to 30 mL of fluid before providing resistance to flow. Insufflation of the joint has several advantages. Distention allows the cannulas to pass easily through the joint capsule and give confirmation of joint entry with egress of fluid through the cannulas. Furthermore, distention increases the distance from the joint to the neurovascular structures, making cannula placement safer.[14,15]

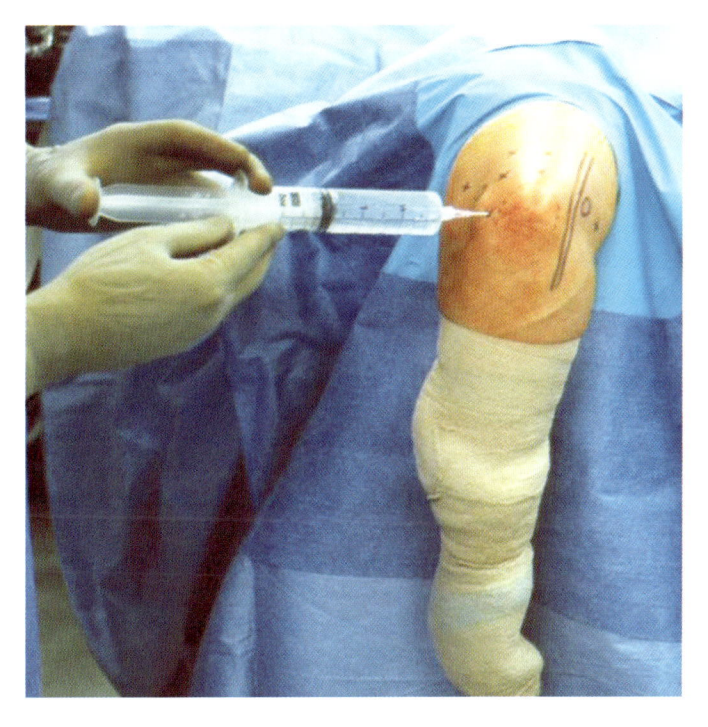

Figure 4 Preoperative photograph of a patient in the prone position shows pertinent landmarks marked for elbow arthroscopy, including the medial and lateral epicondyles (circles), the ulnar nerve (parallel lines), and portal sites (x marks). Insufflation of the joint is demonstrated through the lateral soft spot.

Anteromedial Portal
The anteromedial portal is placed 1 to 2 cm anterior and 2 cm distal to the medial epicondyle.[3] A nick in the skin is made, and the blunt-tip trocar is advanced through the flexor mass, aiming for the radial head and taking care to stay between the humerus and the brachialis. Conversely, a nick-and-spread technique[14] or an inside-out technique with the arthroscope in the lateral portal. This location is 7 to 14 mm from the median nerve as long as the trocar stays posterior to the brachialis muscle. With the trocar anterior to the medial epicondyle and the ulnar nerve in its normal anatomic position, the ulnar nerve should not be at risk. The greatest risk is to the medial antebrachial cutaneous nerve, which passes 1 to 2 mm from the portal site[16] (**Figure 1**). This risk can be minimized by incising skin only and using the blunt trocar for the subcutaneous dissection.[7,14]

Proximal Anteromedial Portal
The proximal anteromedial portal is made 2 cm proximal to the medial epi-

© 2013 American Academy of Orthopaedic Surgeons

Section 2: Shoulder and Elbow

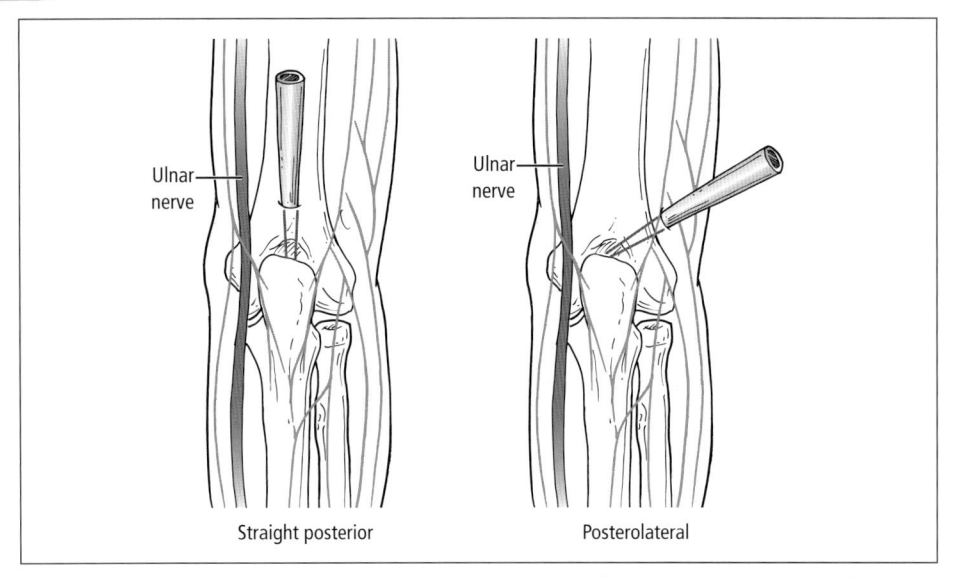

Figure 5 Illustrations show placement of the posterior and posterolateral portals. The posterior portal is established approximately 3 cm proximal to the olecranon tip, and the posterolateral portal is made 3 cm proximal to the olecranon tip and immediately lateral to the triceps tendon. These portals can be used interchangeably for working in the posterior compartment.

condyle and anterior to the intermuscular septum (**Figure 1**). A nick in the skin is made, and the blunt-tip trocar is advanced to the anterior surface of the humerus. The trocar is kept in contact with the anterior cortex and then slid distally to the elbow joint. This technique keeps the trocar posterior to the brachialis muscle and therefore the median nerve and the brachial artery. It also keeps it anterior to the medial intermuscular septum and thus anterior to the ulnar nerve. Once again, the main structure at risk is the medial antebrachial cutaneous nerve, which passes 2 cm from the portal site.[16] Protection of this nerve is performed the same as for the anteromedial portal.

This portal is easily reproducible and provides visualization of the entire anterior compartment from the medial to the lateral gutter. As such, it serves well as the initial portal in elbow arthroscopy. Some authors recommend avoiding the medial portal in the case of ulnar nerve transposition or subluxation.[14,16,17] Others recommend placement with dissection of the ulnar nerve or careful advancement of blunt trocars.

Anterolateral Portal
The anterolateral portal can be placed with an inside-out or an outside-in technique. For the outside-in technique, a portal is made 1 cm anterior and 3 cm distal to the lateral epicondyle. The trocar is advanced toward the joint, entering just proximal to the radial head. For the inside-out technique, the arthroscope in the anteromedial or proximal anteromedial portal is advanced over the radial head and pressed firmly against the joint capsule lateral to the radial head. The camera is exchanged in the cannula for a switching stick, which is advanced through the extensor carpi radialis brevis until it tents the skin. Care must be taken not to place the portal distal to the radial head, because the posterior interosseous nerve courses 1 to 1.5 cm from the radial head around the radial neck. Furthermore, the portal should not be made anterior to the radial head because this too can endanger the radial nerve. The radial nerve passes 5 to 9 mm from this portal site.[14,16,17] This portal provides good access to the radial head and the annular ligament.

Proximal Anterolateral Portal
The proximal anterolateral portal, which was described by Stothers et al[16] and others, can also be used as a primary portal. It is established 2 cm proximal and anterior to the lateral epicondyle (**Figure 2**). The blunt trocar is advanced through the brachioradialis and brachialis muscles into the anterior aspect of the joint. When compared to the standard anterolateral portal, this portal provides greater safe distance to the radial nerve.[16] The radial nerve passes between 10 and 14 mm from this portal when the elbow is flexed to 90°. The lateral antebrachial cutaneous nerve passes 6 mm from this portal site.[16] The proximal anterolateral portal provides adequate visualization of the anterior joint structures from the lateral gutter to the lateral aspect of the ulnohumeral joint. When compared to the standard anterolateral portal, the proximal anterolateral portal provides better visualization of the lateral aspect of the joint.

Direct Lateral Portal
Also known as the soft-spot portal, the direct lateral portal is often used for the initial insufflation of the joint with an 18-gauge needle (**Figure 4**). It is found in the soft spot in the triangle marked by the lateral epicondyle, radial head, and tip of the olecranon. The trocar is advanced directly into the posterolateral gutter. This portal provides visualization of the radiocapitellar joint, the capitellum, the inferior aspect of the radial head, and the posterolateral gutter. This portal is fairly safe with regard to neurologic structures. The biggest risks of this portal are those of fluid extravasation into the soft tissues and postoperative portal drainage.[4,16,17] Because of the risk of soft-tissue extravasation, it is advisable to delay making this portal until near the end of the operation.

Posterior Portal
The straight posterior portal is made in the midline, 3 cm proximal to the olecranon tip, through the triceps tendon[4,12] (**Figure 5**). The skin is incised, and a blunt trocar is then inserted into the olecranon fossa. The joint capsule is very close to the joint in this position with the elbow flexed. Therefore, it is helpful to have an inflow cannula already placed in one of the anterior portals to allow for maximal joint distention. Furthermore, after the trocar is inserted, the edge of the cannula needs to be advanced down to bone. It often helps to turn the cannula as it advances, using the tip like a cutting tool to help penetrate the capsule in this region. If the trocar is removed without advancing the cannula, the tip of the cannula will still be outside the joint capsule because of the length of the trocar tip. Adequate placement can be confirmed by the return of fluid out of the cannula with removal of the trocar, which can happen only if the cannula has been advanced into the joint capsule. This portal provides visualization of the posterior aspect of the ulnohumeral joint, the olecranon fossa, and the medial and lateral gutters.[9] Care should be taken when visualizing or working in the medial gutter because the ulnar nerve lies just superficial to the joint capsule in this region.

Posterolateral Portal

The posterolateral portal is very similar to and is often used interchangeably with the straight posterior portal (**Figure 5**). The portal is made 3 cm proximal to the tip of the olecranon, just lateral to the triceps tendon. The trocar is advanced toward the olecranon fossa, and advancement of the cannula through the capsule must be performed as described previously. However, when making this portal, it is sometimes helpful to bring the elbow to 45° of flexion to relax the triceps and the posterior capsule.[16] This also offers visualization of the ulnohumeral joint as well as the medial and lateral gutters. From this position, the arthroscope can often be advanced into the lateral gutter to visualize the radiocapitellar joint and the posterior aspect of the radial head.

Accessory Posterolateral Portal

The accessory posterolateral portal can be used to instrument the posterior compartment for various arthroscopic techniques. Its location is variable but is typically somewhere between the straight lateral and posterolateral portals. It can be moved proximal and distal as needed. Care should be taken to not place this portal medial to the straight posterior portal because this endangers the ulnar nerve. Exact placement of the portal should be decided by placing a spinal needle into the elbow under arthroscopic visualization. Once the surgeon has confirmed that the pathology can be reached from the selected portal location, the skin is incised and the trocar is advanced as before. The main structures at risk are the triceps tendon and the ulnohumeral articular cartilage, which can be injured with careless instrument placement.

Specific Surgical Techniques
Diagnostic Arthroscopy

After initiating anesthesia and adequate positioning, prepping, and draping, bony landmarks are marked with a sterile marker. Care is taken to palpate the ulnar nerve in its groove, and this is also marked. The arm is exsanguinated, and the tourniquet is inflated. An 18-gauge needle is inserted into the soft-spot portal in the elbow, which is insufflated with sterile saline. The proximal anteromedial portal is made as described previously.

A systematic inspection of the anterior structures can be performed. Starting with the medial aspect of the ulnohumeral articulation and moving laterally,

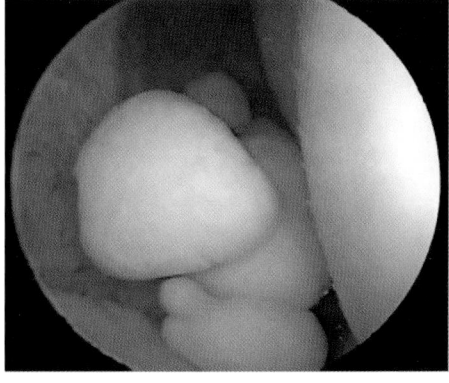

Figure 6 Arthroscopic view shows multiple large osteochondral loose bodies in the anterior compartment of the elbow.

the coronoid process, the trochlea, the lateral aspect of the ulnohumeral articulation, the capitellum, the radiocapitellar joint, and the radial head can be inspected. The forearm can be pronated and supinated to assist with radial head evaluation. The anterior joint line should be carefully inspected for osteophytes, chondral lesions, and loose bodies (**Figure 6**). Continuing laterally, the insertion of the extensor carpi radialis brevis can be seen. Then, by rotating the angle of the arthroscope, the anterior joint capsule can be inspected for synovitis, trapped loose bodies, contracture, and plica. If needed, an anterolateral or proximal anterolateral portal can be made. In the event of prolific synovitis, it may be helpful to insert a switching stick through an anterolateral or proximal anterolateral portal to assist with capsular retraction.

The arthroscope can then be moved into the proximal anterolateral portal using metal cannulas to visualize the medial joint capsule. With the inflow in place, through one of the anterior portals, a posterolateral portal can then be made as described previously. When the arthroscope is introduced, the olecranon fossa will be in view. Turning the angle of the arthroscope to look inferiorly will bring the tip of the olecranon into view. The fossa and the olecranon can be inspected for osteophytes. The elbow can be extended to bring the olecranon tip into contact with the fossa to look for areas of impingement. The ulnohumeral articulation can be followed medially into the medial gutter. Care should be taken when instrumenting the medial gutter because the ulnar nerve lies immediately superficial to the joint capsule in this area.

The arthroscope can be retracted back to the olecranon fossa and then, once again following the ulnohumeral articu-

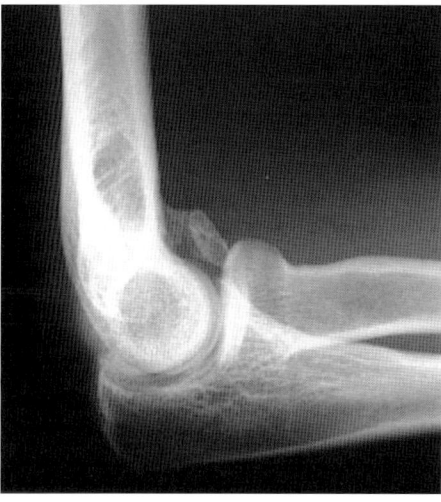

Figure 7 Lateral radiograph shows a large loose body in the anterior compartment of the elbow.

lation, the lateral gutter can be inspected. The arthroscope can be advanced into the lateral gutter, and the angle of the arthroscope can be rotated to look laterally. Doing so will bring the radiocapitellar joint into view, showing the posterior aspect of the radial head. Once again, the forearm can be taken through pronation and supination to inspect the radial head. If needed, an accessory posterolateral portal can be made to address any pathology that is identified.[18]

Loose Bodies

Patients with loose bodies usually present with reports of elbow pain and stiffness and often report catching, snapping, popping, or locking of the joint. Loose bodies do not cause elbow contracture, but they are often present in patients with elbow contracture. Patients with elbow contractures develop loose bodies as a result of the underlying pathologic condition, such as osteochondritis dissecans, posterior impingement, or degenerative arthritis with posterior osteophytes on the olecranon and in the olecranon fossa. On physical examination, patients with loose bodies generally have maintenance of elbow motion but may have mild degrees of flexion and/or extension loss. Also, a mild effusion, best identified in the posterolateral gutter of the elbow, may be present.

Although AP and lateral radiographs of the elbow will often demonstrate loose bodies (**Figure 7**), as many as 30% of loose bodies are not detected on plain radiographs.[1,19,20] Most often, when loose bodies are suspected but not identified on plain radiographs, they will be found in the posterior compartment of the elbow.[21] In addition, loose bodies will often migrate within the elbow and even between compartments, making reliable identification more difficult.

Because loose bodies can often be found in the posterior compartment, it may be best to use the lateral or prone position because they allow for easier visualization of the posterior compartment.

In the arthroscopic treatment of loose bodies, after positioning, prepping, and draping as described previously, the proximal anteromedial portal is made, the arthroscope is introduced, and diagnostic arthroscopy is performed. In the anterior compartment, loose bodies can often be found in the coronoid fossa. Next, a proximal anterolateral portal is made. It is often helpful to use a cannula with a diaphragm in this area to prevent the egress of fluid.

After identifying loose bodies, the surgeon can remove them using a variety of arthroscopic graspers (**Figure 8**). Loose bodies can be surprisingly large and may require a large grasper. In fact, they will often be larger than the plastic cannula used in the procedure. In this instance, options for removal include either breaking the loose body into more easily removable fragments or grasping the loose body with a large grasper and backing the cannula out of the elbow while keeping the loose body in contact with the tip of the cannula. Additionally, the arthroscopic camera can be used to help push the grasped loose body out the opposite side of the elbow. Other tips for removal include "pinning" the loose body with a spinal needle to stabilize it for grasping (**Figure 9**).

Débridement of osteophytes or loose articular fragments and arthroscopic management of other pathologic conditions of the anterior compartment may be necessary at the time of loose body removal. Also, inflammatory tissue and reactive synovitis may be present, and synovectomy should be carefully performed as well. However, using motorized shavers around the anterior capsule can lead to perforation of the capsule and put the neurovascular structures at increased risk for injury.[22-24] Nonetheless, a thorough synovectomy is important to maximize the outcome of arthroscopic treatment and help identify loose bodies that can sometimes be obscured by the presence of this synovial tissue. The supplemental use of arthroscopic retractors is valuable and effective in improving visualization during procedures such as synovectomy and in providing additional protection of the capsule and adjacent neurovascular structures. These retractors can be placed either on the same side as the working portal or opposite that portal, depending on the areas to be assessed. Blunt-tipped switching sticks and smooth Freer elevators can also be used effectively as soft-tissue retractors.

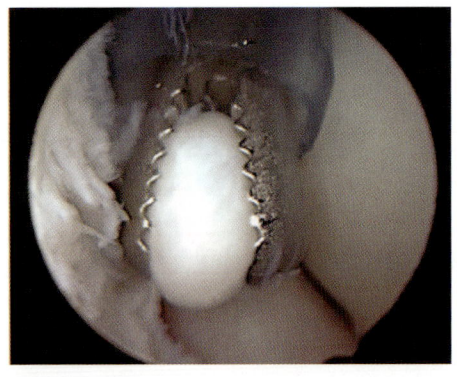

Figure 8 Arthroscopic view shows a grasper used for the removal of a large loose body from the anterior compartment of the elbow.

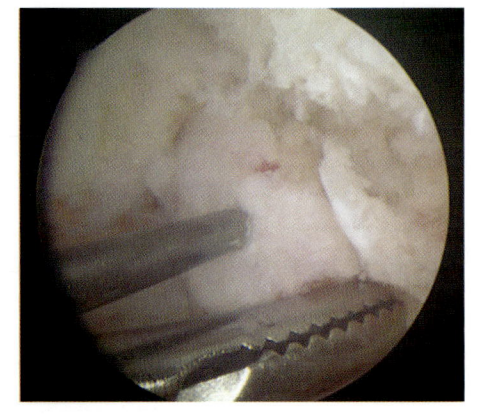

Figure 9 Arthroscopic view shows a spinal needle being used to skewer a large loose body in the posterior compartment of the elbow to facilitate retrieval with a grasper.

Following loose body removal and débridement of the anterior compartment, attention is turned to the posterior compartment. Loose bodies or attached fragments of bone are often present in the olecranon fossa. The direct lateral or posterolateral portals can be used interchangeably as working and viewing portals for the removal of loose bodies. However, when the loose body is too large to fit through the cannula, it should be removed through the posterolateral portal to prevent damage to the triceps tendon. When accessing the posterior portal, it helps to leave the inflow in one of the anterior compartments. This allows for maintenance of insufflation and flushes loose bodies out of the medial and lateral gutters.[25]

After thorough débridement of any loose bodies or osteophytes in the olecranon fossa, attention is turned to the medial gutter. A "milking" maneuver, performed by pressing distally to proximally along the medial and lateral gutters, helps to mobilize loose bodies hidden in these recesses. Attention is then turned to the lateral gutter, and the "milking" maneuver can be repeated. Finally, as is the case for the anterior compartment, débridement and the removal of reactive tissue and prominent osteophytes should be completed at the same time as loose body removal.

Arthroscopic Synovectomy

Synovectomy performed arthroscopically allows access to the anterior and posterior compartments while minimizing the iatrogenic insult of an open approach. It can, however, be difficult to accomplish secondary to thickened reactive synovitis, which limits visualization and can obscure intra-articular structures, such as the articular cartilage and any loose bodies that may also be present. Complete synovectomy is often important to achieve therapeutic goals. The most at-risk areas intra-articularly are the anterolateral inferior capsule and the posteromedial capsule. The posterior interosseous nerve lies just superficial to the anterolateral inferior capsule, and the ulnar nerve is intimately associated with the posteromedial capsule.

Initially, the arthroscope is introduced into the proximal anteromedial portal, and a mechanical shaver is placed through the anterolateral portal. A complete synovectomy of the lateral aspect of the joint is then performed. As much synovium as possible should be removed, taking care to avoid damage to the capsule itself. A supplemental arthroscopic retractor placed through a proximal anterolateral portal can improve visualization and protect the lateral capsule and the posterior interosseous nerve.

The arthroscope is then switched to the lateral portal, and synovectomy of the medial joint is completed with the shaver in the proximal anteromedial portal. Attention can then be turned to the posterior compartment. The arthroscope is placed through the posterior portal, and the shaver is introduced through the posterolateral portal. The olecranon fossa is débrided first. Keeping the scope in the posterior portal, the posterolateral gutter can be débrided as well.

The arthroscope is then moved to the posterolateral portal and the shaver to the posterior portal to allow for débridement of the posteromedial gutter. Extreme care should be taken in the posteromedial gutter to avoid damage to the posteromedial capsule and the overlying ulnar nerve. Limited suction should be used, and the shaver should be kept facing away from the capsule when performing synovectomy in the medial gutter. Arthroscopic retractors can also aid in visualization posteriorly.

Complications

Elbow arthroscopy is performed in immediate proximity to major nerves and vessels and, as a consequence, probably carries the highest risk for serious neurovascular injury. Careful surgical technique along with vigilant maintenance of arthroscopic instrument visualization minimizes the potential for iatrogenic injury. In addition to the risk to neurovascular structures, other potential complications following elbow arthroscopy include the postoperative development of portal infections or even fistulae because of the relative subcutaneous location of the elbow joint. Finally, heterotopic ossification is a rare but potentially serious complication sometimes seen following extensive arthroscopic elbow débridement for arthritis with or without concurrent capsular release.

Pearls

- Elbow arthroscopy is a technically demanding procedure and requires a thorough understanding of the relevant anatomy. Prior to initiation of surgery, careful palpation and marking of superficial landmarks should be performed in every case.
- Great care with meticulous technique should be taken with the placement of arthroscopic portals.
- Palpating the ulnar nerve to confirm that it is present in its groove helps ensure that the nerve is not injured by medial portal placement.
- Joint distention accomplished by injecting saline into the elbow joint makes capsular penetration with blunt trocars more reliably accomplished. Such distention also increases the distance of the neurovascular structures from the arthroscopic instruments in the anterior elbow compartment.
- Relatively proximal anteromedial and anterolateral portals are preferred over more distally placed anterior portals because these more proximal portals are farther from the neurologic structures that span the anterior elbow joint.
- Arthroscopic retractors improve visualization in the elbow joint during arthroscopy and also serve to effectively protect the vital structures.
- Care should be taken during arthroscopic débridement and/or capsular release in the anterior elbow near the radial head because the posterior interosseous nerve is immediately adjacent to the anterior capsule in this location. Likewise, care should also be taken in the posteromedial gutter, because the ulnar nerve lies in close proximity.

References

1. O'Driscoll SW, Morrey BF: Arthroscopy of the elbow: Diagnostic and therapeutic benefits and hazards. *J Bone Joint Surg Am* 1992;74(1):84-94.
2. Burman MS: Arthroscopy for the direct visualization of the joints: An experimental cadaveric study. *J Bone Joint Surg* 1931;13:669-695.
3. Andrews JR, Carson WG: Arthroscopy of the elbow. *Arthroscopy* 1985;1(2):97-107.
4. Poehling GG, Ekman EF, Ruch DS: Elbow arthoscopy: Introduction and overview, in McGinty J, Caspari R, Jackson R, et al, eds: *Operative Arthroscopy*, ed 2. Philadelphia, PA, Lippincott, 1996, pp 821-828.
5. Poehling GG, Ekman EF: Arthroscopy of the elbow. *Instr Course Lect* 1995;44:214-223.
6. Childress HM: Recurrent ulnar-nerve dislocation at the elbow. *Clin Orthop Relat Res* 1975;108:168-173.
7. Baker CL Jr, Jones GL: Arthroscopy of the elbow. *Am J Sports Med* 1999;27(2):251-264.
8. Ramsey ML, Naranja RJ: Diagnostic arthroscopy of the elbow, in Baker CL Jr, Plancher DL, eds: *Operative Treatment of Elbow Injuries*. New York, NY, Springer-Verlag, 2002, pp 162-169.
9. Lyons TR, Field LD, Savoie FH III: Basics of elbow arthoscopy. *Instr Course Lect* 2000;49:239-246.
10. McKenzie PJ: Supine position, in Savoie FH, Field LD, eds: *Arthroscopy of the Elbow*. New York, NY, Churchill Livingstone, 1996, pp 35-39.
11. O'Driscoll SW, Morrey BF: Arthroscopy of the elbow, in Morrey B, ed: *The Elbow and Its Disorders*, ed 2. Philadelphia, PA, Saunders, 1993, pp 120-130.
12. Poehling GG, Whipple TL, Sisco L, Goldman B: Elbow arthroscopy: A new technique. *Arthroscopy* 1989;5(3):222-224.
13. Adolfsson L: Arthroscopy of the elbow joint: A cadaveric study of portal placement. *J Shoulder Elbow Surg* 1994;3:53-61.
14. Lindenfeld TN: Medial approach in elbow arthroscopy. *Am J Sports Med* 1990;18(4):413-417.
15. Lynch GJ, Meyers JF, Whipple TL, Caspari RB: Neurovascular anatomy and elbow arthroscopy: Inherent risks. *Arthroscopy* 1986;2(3):190-197.
16. Stothers K, Day B, Regan WR: Arthroscopy of the elbow: Anatomy, portal sites, and a description of the proximal lateral portal. *Arthroscopy* 1995;11(4):449-457.
17. Plancher KD, Peterson RK, Breezenoff L: Diagnostic arthroscopy of the elbow: Set-up, portals, and technique. *Oper Tech Sports Med* 1998;6:2-10.
18. Savoie FH, Field LD: Basics of elbow arthroscopy. *Tech Orthop* 2000;15(2):138-146.
19. Ogilvie-Harris DJ, Schemitsch E: Arthroscopy of the elbow for removal of loose bodies. *Arthroscopy* 1993;9(1):5-8.
20. Ward WG, Belhobek GH, Anderson TE: Arthroscopic elbow findings: Correlation with preoperative radiographic studies. *Arthroscopy* 1992;8(4):498-502.
21. O'Driscoll SW, Morrey BF: Loose bodies of the elbow: Diagnostic and therapeutic roles of arthroscopy. *J Bone Joint Surg Br* 1992;74(suppl III):290.
22. Lee BP, Morrey BF: Arthroscopic synovectomy of the elbow for rheumatoid arthritis: A prospective study. *J Bone Joint Surg Br* 1997;79(5):770-772.
23. Horiuchi K, Momohara S, Tomatsu T, Inoue K, Toyama Y: Arthroscopic synovectomy of the elbow in rheumatoid arthritis. *J Bone Joint Surg Am* 2002;84(3):342-347.
24. Nemoto K, Arino H, Yoshihara Y, Fujikawa K: Arthroscopic synovectomy for the rheumatoid elbow: A short-term outcome. *J Shoulder Elbow Surg* 2004;13(6):652-655.
25. Savoie FH III, Nunley PD, Field LD: Arthroscopic management of the arthritic elbow: Indications, technique, and results. *J Shoulder Elbow Surg* 1999;8(3):214-219.

Video Reference

31.1 Baker CL Jr: Elbow Arthroscopy: Principles, Portals, and Techniques. Adapted from Baker CL Jr: DVD: *Surgical Techniques in Orthopaedics: Elbow Arthroscopy*. Rosemont, IL, American Academy of Orthopaedic Surgeons, 2005.

Chapter 32
Open Treatment of Radial Head Fractures and Olecranon Fractures

Julie E. Adams, MD, MS   Scott P. Steinmann, MD

Radial Head Fractures
Patient Selection
Radial head fractures may be divided into three types according to the Mason classification (Figure 1). Type I fractures, which are minimally displaced or nondisplaced, have no mechanical block to motion. Appropriate treatment is a sling for comfort for a few days and then early mobilization. In this setting, the hematoma may be aspirated and the joint injected with local analgesic to facilitate pain relief by removing the hematoma and placing local anesthetic to allow early motion. Frequently, these patients present to the office or the emergency department with acute swollen elbow (hemarthrosis) and pain. It may be difficult to assess for any blocked motion because of the hemarthrosis and pain. Therefore, it is reasonable to consider an aspiration of the joint and injection of local analgesics. This may be done through the "soft spot," which is the center of a triangle bordered by the lateral epicondyle, the tip of the olecranon, and the radial head. Alternatively, the anterolateral arthroscopy portal may be used, which is just anterior and distal to the radiocapitellar joint. The hematoma may be extracted using a 19-gauge needle and the syringe then exchanged for 1% lidocaine or other local anesthetic. Following this, the patient generally feels much more comfortable, and the surgeon can assess for any bony block to motion.

Mason type II fractures involve more than 2 mm of displacement and more than one third of the radial head. Mason type III fractures are comminuted, multifragmented fractures that are likely irreparable based on preoperative radiographs.

Options for the management of radial head fractures are fragment excision, if there is a single fragment that is a bony block to motion; open reduction and internal fixation (ORIF); radial head excision; or arthroplasty.

Fragment excision may be considered if elbow stability is not compromised and is best considered for small fragments that are less than 25% of the head; are too small, osteoporotic, or comminuted for fixation; and do not articulate with the proximal radiolnar joint.

Radial head ORIF may be performed using screws or plate-and-screw constructs. Hardware should be placed in the safe zone (or the region that does not articulate with the proximal radiolnar joint), which is identified as the lateral region of the radial head and neck when the forearm is in a neutral position. This area is also bounded by the region between the Lister tubercle distally and the radial styloid.[1-3]

For type III fractures, which preoperative radiographs suggest are irreparable based on the amount of comminution or multifragmentary pieces, replacement arthroplasty or excision may be considered. Excision should be avoided in the setting of instability. In addition, radial head excision is to be avoided in association with longitudinal instability of the forearm, such as an Essex-Lopresti injury.

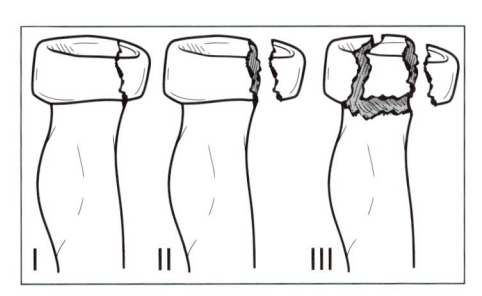

Figure 1 Illustration depicts the Mason classification of radial head fractures.

Preoperative Imaging
Preoperative imaging should include three radiographic views of the elbow (Figure 2). If there has been an associated dislocation, pre- and postreduction images should be reviewed. If there are other complicated bony injuries or suspected injuries, a CT scan with or without three-dimensional reconstructions may be obtained. Radiographs are examined for the presence of other bony injuries, the presence of joint subluxation suggesting instability, the number and size of fracture fragments, and associated osteopenia.

Procedure
Room Setup/Patient Positioning
The patient is positioned supine with an arm table or with the arm over the chest. A tourniquet is used to improve visualization. It is helpful to have a mini C-arm unit available for intraoperative imaging.

Either general or regional anesthesia may be used; however, general anesthesia provides the advantage of patient comfort during the procedure as well as the ability to immediately assess neurovascular status in the postoperative recovery room.

If there are other associated injuries, the surgeon could consider making a single posterior incision to one side of the olecranon tip, raising large full-thickness flaps to obtain deep access to the medial and lateral sides through this single incision. However, this may lead to seroma formation or other wound complications and requires making a larger incision. Generally, a separate lateral incision is preferred, and, if necessary, a separate medial incision can be made to address medial-side pathology.

Special Instruments/Equipment/Implants
In the setting of anticipated ORIF of the radial head, it is prudent to obtain a radial head replacement in the hospital in case fixation is found to be impossible or fails. A variety of small purpose-made implants are available for radial head fixation, including screws, headless screws, and plating systems. When plate fixation is anticipated, it is helpful to discuss with

---

Dr. Adams or an immediate family member has received royalties from DePuy; serves as a paid consultant to or is an employee of Arthrex, DePuy, and Articulinx; serves as an unpaid consultant to Synthes; and serves as a board member, owner, officer, or committee member of the American Association for Hand Surgery, the Minnesota Orthopaedic Society, the American Shoulder and Elbow Surgeons, the American Society for Surgery of the Hand, and the Arthroscopy Association of North America. Dr. Steinmann or an immediate family member has received royalties from DePuy; serves as a paid consultant to or is an employee of Arthrex, DePuy, and Articulinx; serves as an unpaid consultant to Synthes; and serves as a board member, owner, officer, or committee member of the American Association for Hand Surgery, the Minnesota Orthopaedic Society, the American Shoulder and Elbow Surgeons, the American Society for Surgery of the Hand, and the Arthroscopy Association of North America.

Section 2: Shoulder and Elbow

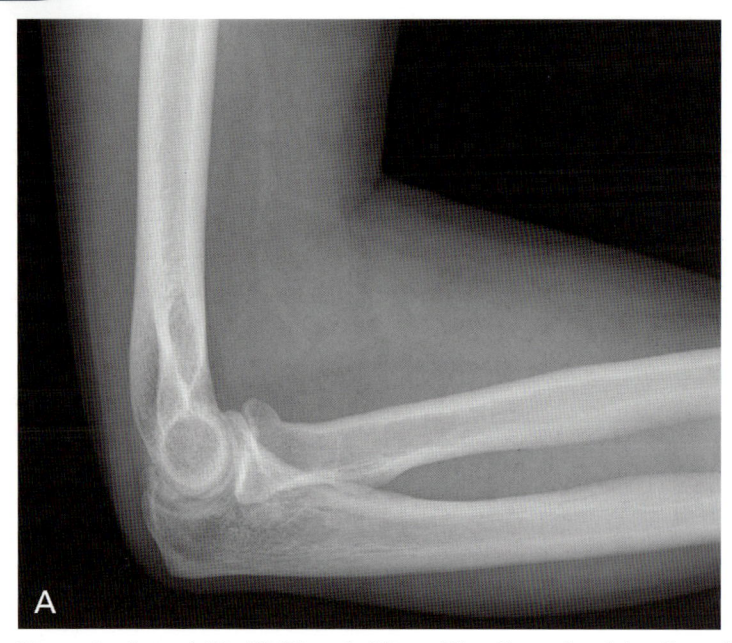

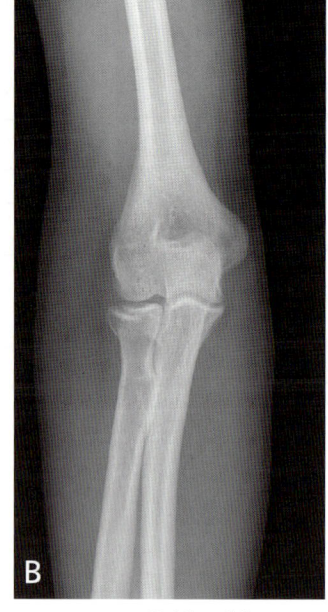

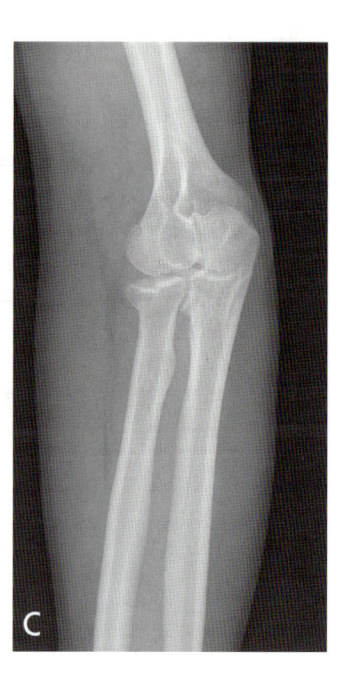

Figure 2 Lateral (**A**), AP (**B**), and oblique (**C**) radiographs of the elbow demonstrate a radial head fracture.

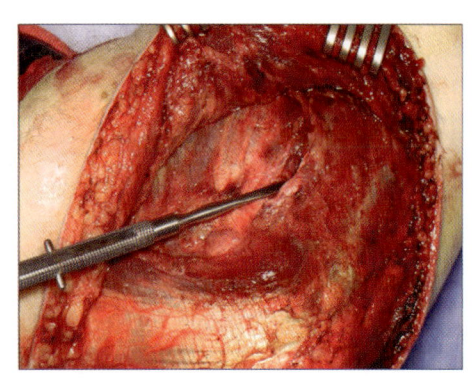

Figure 3 Intraoperative photograph shows the Kocher interval between the extensor carpi ulnaris and the anconeus, which is most useful for exposure in settings in which the radial head is injured in conjunction with an LUCL injury.

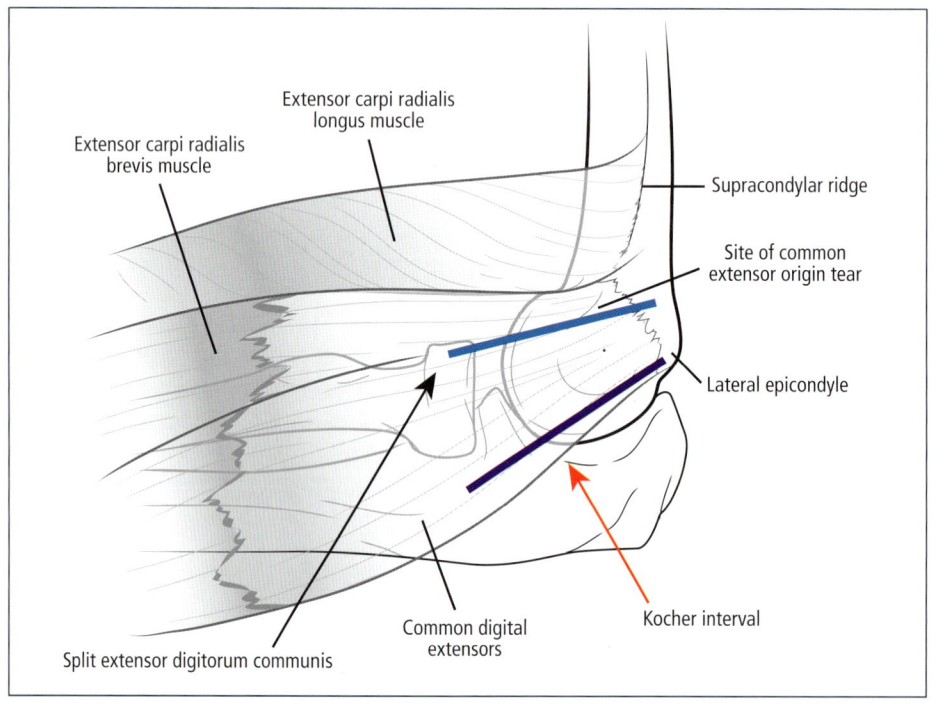

Figure 4 Illustration shows the muscle-splitting approach. The radial head may be easily approached through a split in the tendon origin of the extensor digitorum communis (blue line).

patients that commonly they may experience stiffness postoperatively and may require a second procedure for plate removal and/or manipulation of the elbow following adequate healing of the fracture. Provisional fixation with Kirschner wires (K-wires) is helpful before placing the definitive implants. Suture anchors may be helpful if collateral ligament repair is anticipated.

Surgical Technique

Either a single posterior incision or a separate lateral incision may be made, depending on the pathology to be addressed. In general, a lateral incision is made overlying the epicondyle and extending distally and longitudinally across the radial head. The deep dissection following the creation of full-thickness skin flaps depends on the pathology to be addressed. In the setting of ligamentous instability of the elbow, such as a radial head fracture in conjunction with a dislocation and perhaps a coronoid fracture, such as the terrible triad injury, there may be associated lateral ulnar collateral ligament (LUCL) avulsion, which creates a deep plane amenable for exposure of the radial head as well as for exposure and subsequent repair of the LUCL. In this setting, the avulsion is typically off the humeral epicondyle, and finger dissection will readily reveal a defect that may then be exploited, which is typically in the classic Kocher interval, between the anconeus and the extensor carpi ulnaris tendon (**Figure 3**). This allows for exposure of both the radial head and the LUCL for repair of the latter after the procedure is completed. On the other hand, there may not be any ligamentous injury, in which case a good interval for exposure of the radial head may be using a muscle-splitting approach through the tendinous origin of the extensor digitorum communis (**Figure 4**). This allows for exposure of the radial head without any dissection below the midline of the radial head and does not endanger the LUCL, which lies

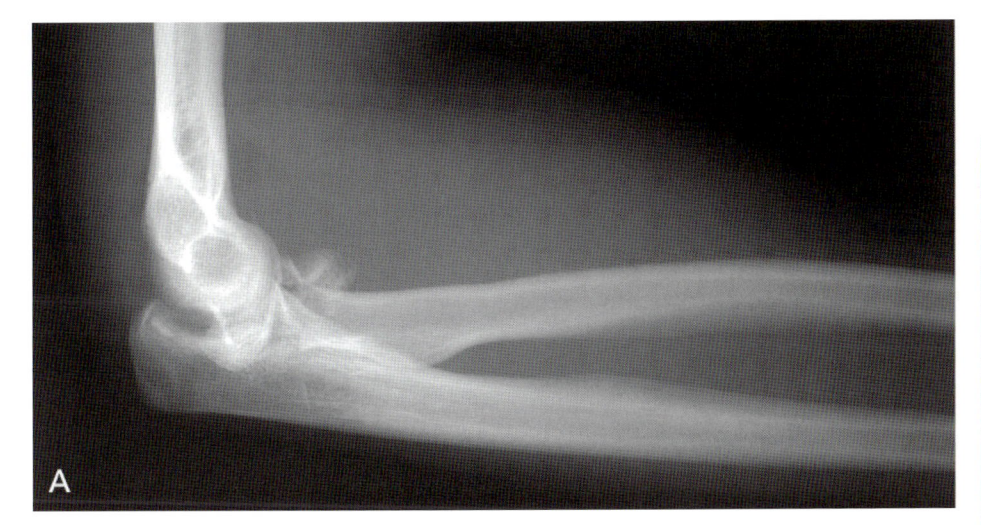

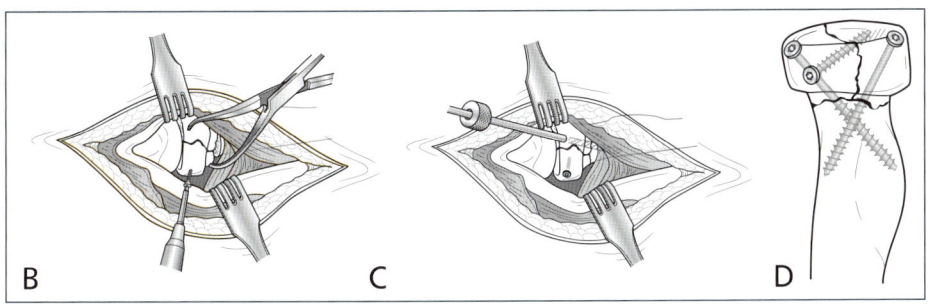

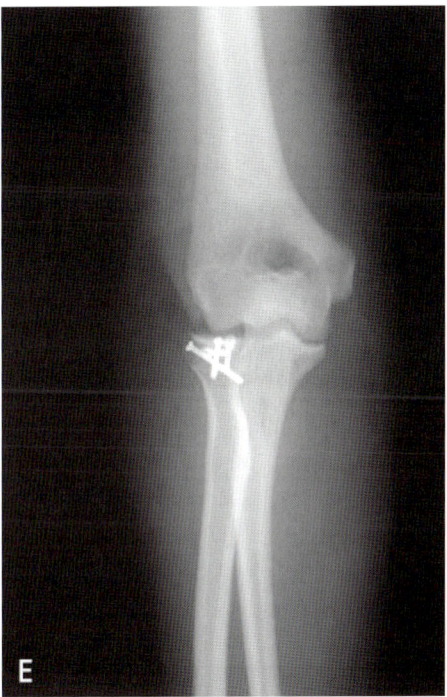

Figure 5 Open reduction and internal fixation of a radial head fracture using screws. **A**, Preoperative lateral radiograph demonstrates the fracture. Illustrations **B** through **D** demonstrate screw fixation. **B**, Provisional reduction and fixation. **C**, Insertion of a second screw for fixation in a crossed-screw fashion. **D**, The final construct. **E**, Postoperative AP radiograph demonstrates screw position.

more posterior to this area. This interval may be incised with the knife or cautery for exposure, and care should be taken distally to place the forearm in pronation to move the posterior interosseous nerve more distal from the surgical site. An arthrotomy is made, and the radial head and neck are exposed. The posterior interosseous nerve is in this region; its location varies from 2.2 to 5.2 cm distal to the radiocapitellar joint, depending on the size of the patient and the position of forearm pronosupination.[4,5]

Following exposure of the radial head and the fracture, a determination is made as to whether the fracture is amenable to excision, ORIF, or radial head replacement. Provisional fixation may be obtained with small K-wires and then headless screws or plates placed. It is preferable to use screws and avoid plating if possible to allow for better motion postoperatively;[6] however, fixation must be secure (**Figure 5**). Moreover, although it may be technically possible to fix a radial head fracture, it may be more advisable to consider replacement. A recent outcomes study suggests a high rate of unsatisfactory results following fixation in type III fractures and many type II fractures. The authors suggest that ORIF for radial head fractures should be restricted to those fractures with minimal comminution and three or fewer fragments and should be avoided in the setting of fracture-dislocations of the elbow.[7]

If fixation is not feasible and cannot be obtained, then the surgeon may consider either excision or radial head replacement. Radial head replacement is available using a wide variety of implants. Such implants can be intentionally loose, smooth-stemmed implants that are intended to act as a smooth spacer; implants that are either cemented or press-fit into the radial head and have an anatomic head; or bipolar-type implants inserted into the radial neck and shaft and having an articulating head-neck junction allowing motion[8] (**Figure 6**). Little information is available regarding the advantages of these implants, and the surgeon should use what he or she feels most comfortable with for the individual patient.

In any case, for placement of the radial head, it is critical not to "overstuff" the joint. Sizing is difficult; however, a few guidelines include using the native resected radial head and its fragments assembled on the back table as a guide to the diameter and thickness of the radial head implant to be placed. Most systems have some element of modularity as well as size variance that allow for this. The dish of the radial head replacement should be approximately the same size as the inner dish of the native radial head surface. In general, there is a tendency to overstuff the joint and place a larger than necessary radial head, which can lead to radiocapitellar arthrosis and maltracking of the elbow. This is particularly problematic in the setting of ligamentous instability, which can be exacerbated by this.

In general, the radial head prosthesis is within 2 mm of the proximal radioulnar joint. On fluoroscopic images obtained in the operating room, the surgeon can assess if there is any asymmetric widening of the joint on the medial or lateral side and narrowing on the other side to see if the implant is too large or too small. If the implant is too large, the medial side of the joint will close down, or narrow—the so-called river delta sign; however, radiographic parameters are relatively insensitive, and overstuffing of up to 6 mm may be undetetected on radiographs. A better determinant is visual inspection for any widening of the lateral ulnohumeral space or an attempt to match the lesser sigmoid notch.[9-14] Most systems have a variety of trial implants that are available to ensure that the appropriate size is chosen before final implantation.

© 2013 American Academy of Orthopaedic Surgeons

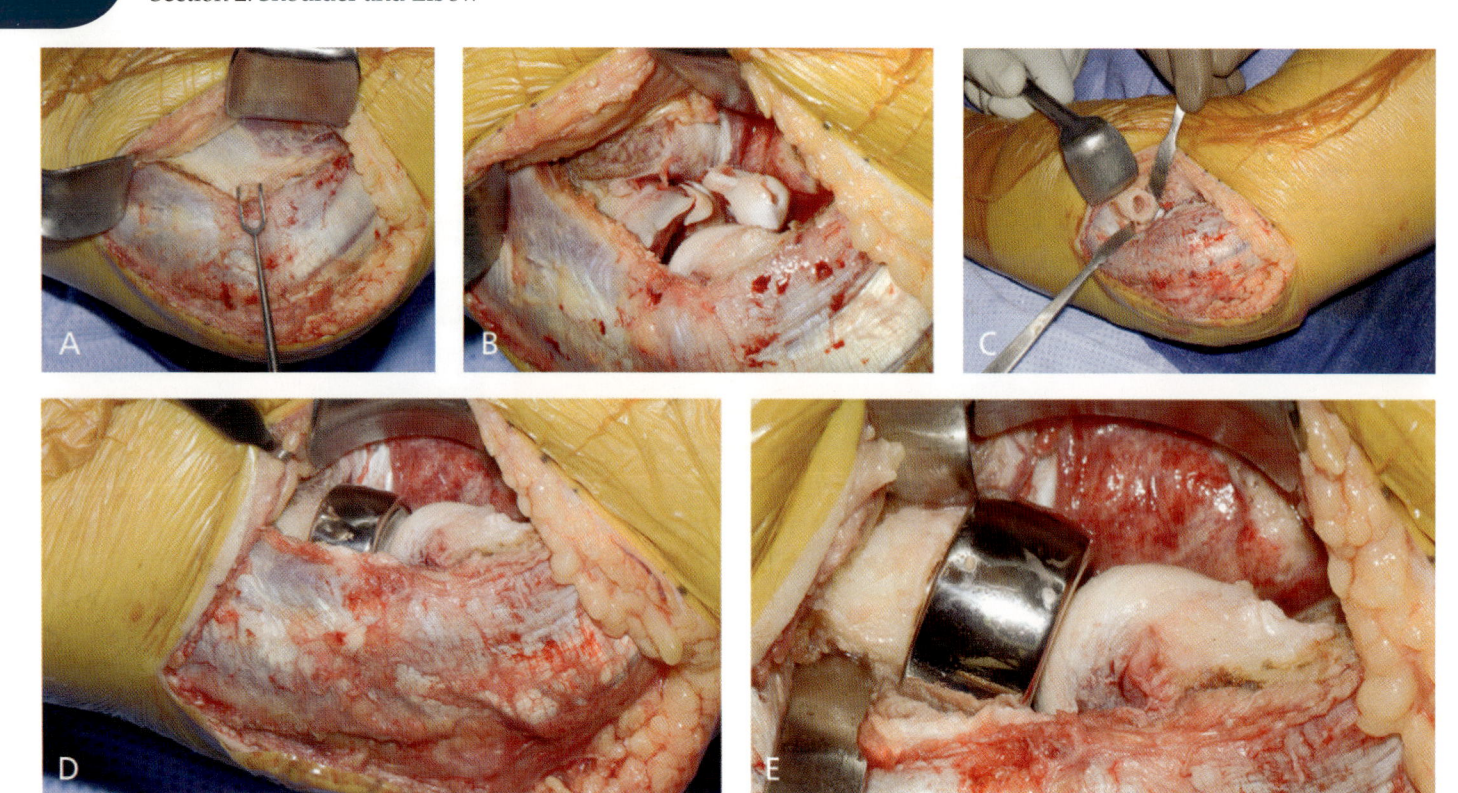

Figure 6 Intraoperative views show the implantation of a radial head prosthesis in an elbow with an irreparable radial head fracture. **A**, The surgical interval. **B**, Exposure. **C**, Excision of the irreparable radial head. **D**, Insertion of the radial head. **E**, Radial head implant of appropriate size in place.

In addition, it is essential to rule out an Essex-Lopresti lesion, or forearm longitudinal instability, particularly if radial head excision is to be entertained. In this situation, the patient may have wrist pain or obvious distal radioulnar joint disruption with ulnar-positive variance; however, this is not always present. One way to assess intraoperatively for competence of the restraints of the longitudinal axis of the forearm is the radial pull test. The stabilizers of the forearm include the radial head, the interosseous membrane (IOM), and the triangular fibrocartilage complex (TFCC). When the radial head is absent, the TFCC and IOM assume a greater role in providing stability to the forearm. Intraoperatively, after the radial head is resected, approximately 90 N of longitudinal traction is applied at the radial neck, and the wrist is examined with fluoroscopy. If migration of the radius is noted by ulnar-positive variance and this variance is more than 3 mm, then the IOM is likely torn. If more than 6 mm of variance is noted, both the IOM and the TFCC are likely torn, and all the restraints to the radial head are gone. In this setting, radial head replacement as well as stabilization of the distal radioulnar joint and the forearm are recommended.[15,16]

Following the intra-articular procedure, the deep structures are repaired with slowly absorbable sutures and, if necessary, the LUCL is reattached to the epicondyle with suture anchors or bony tunnels. The skin and soft tissues are closed in layers, and a sterile dressing is applied.

Complications

Complications following radial head surgery include risk of injury to the posterior interosseous nerve, risk of infection, stiffness, and failure to heal. In addition, patients with residual incongruity of the joint may develop radiocapitellar arthrosis. Alternatively, there may have been an unrecognized or recognized chondral injury to the capitellum that results in radiocapitellar arthrosis even if the joint surface is reduced adequately.

Following a radial head replacement, the long-term implications of metal articulating with a cartilage capitellum are not well understood; however, it is likely that chondral changes will develop. Following ORIF, there may be hardware irritation or prominence requiring a secondary surgery for removal. There may be stiffness and/or heterotopic ossification requiring a second procedure for contracture release with or without hardware removal. In patients with associated ligamentous injuries, residual or recurrent instability may develop. In patients without instability, the surgical exposure may compromise the LUCL if dissection is performed more posterior to the midline of the radial head, and instability may ensue. In the setting of radial head excision or an unrecognized or untreated Essex-Lopresti injury, longitudinal radio-ulnar instability may occur with resultant weakness; forearm, elbow, and wrist pain; and ulnar impaction at the level of the wrist.

Postoperative Care

Postoperative protocols depend on the structures addressed at the time of surgery and those damaged at the time of the injury, as well as stability achieved in the operating room. In the setting of a stably fixed or a replaced radial head without instability, early range of motion is encouraged. The patient may be splinted for a few days for wound healing and swelling purposes and elevation. However, as soon as is feasible, the patient should start early active motion. One of the challenges with elbow surgery is restoring motion; accordingly, a goal is to achieve stable fixation such that early motion may be encouraged for optimal results. If there has been an associated ligamentous injury, such as an LUCL that has been repaired, then the patient is generally immobilized in a splint at 90° in pronation and subsequently allowed to start early flexion-extension motion provided stability permits it, with avoidance of terminal extension and supination. Pronosupination is permitted when the elbow is flexed greater than 90°. At the 6-week mark, if full motion has not yet been achieved, nighttime extension splinting can be considered.

Pearls
- Excision of the radial head without radial head replacement should be avoided in the setting of elbow instability and an Essex-Lopresti injury; radial head replacement or ORIF is preferred in these settings.
- The "safe zone" for hardware placement for the radial head and neck is in the nonarticular region, which is identified as the lateral region of the radial head and neck when the forearm is in a neutral position. This area is also bounded by the region between the Lister tubercle distally and the radial styloid.
- There is a tendency to overstuff the joint and place a larger than necessary radial head. In general, the radial head prosthesis is within 2 mm of the proximal radioulnar joint. On fluoroscopic images obtained in the operating room, the surgeon can assess if there is any asymmetric widening of the joint on the medial or lateral side and narrowing on the other side to see if the implant is too large or too small.

Olecranon Fractures
Patient Selection
The Mayo classification of olecranon fractures (**Figure 7**) includes three types. Type I fractures are nondisplaced and noncomminuted (IA) or comminuted (IB) fractures. Type II fractures are stable displaced fractures and may be noncomminuted (IIA) or comminuted (IIB). Type III fractures are unstable, displaced fractures and may be noncomminuted (IIIA) or comminuted (IIIB). The Mayo classification system does not account for complex olecranon fracture-dislocations, such as those associated with subluxation of the radial head and/or the coronoid process, nor does it classify pure avulsion fractures of the tip of the olecranon.

Type I nondisplaced fractures may be treated with immobilization in midflexion and neutral rotation for 7 to 10 days followed by active range of motion. Active resisted elbow extension and weight bearing should be avoided for 6 to 8 weeks if these fractures are treated

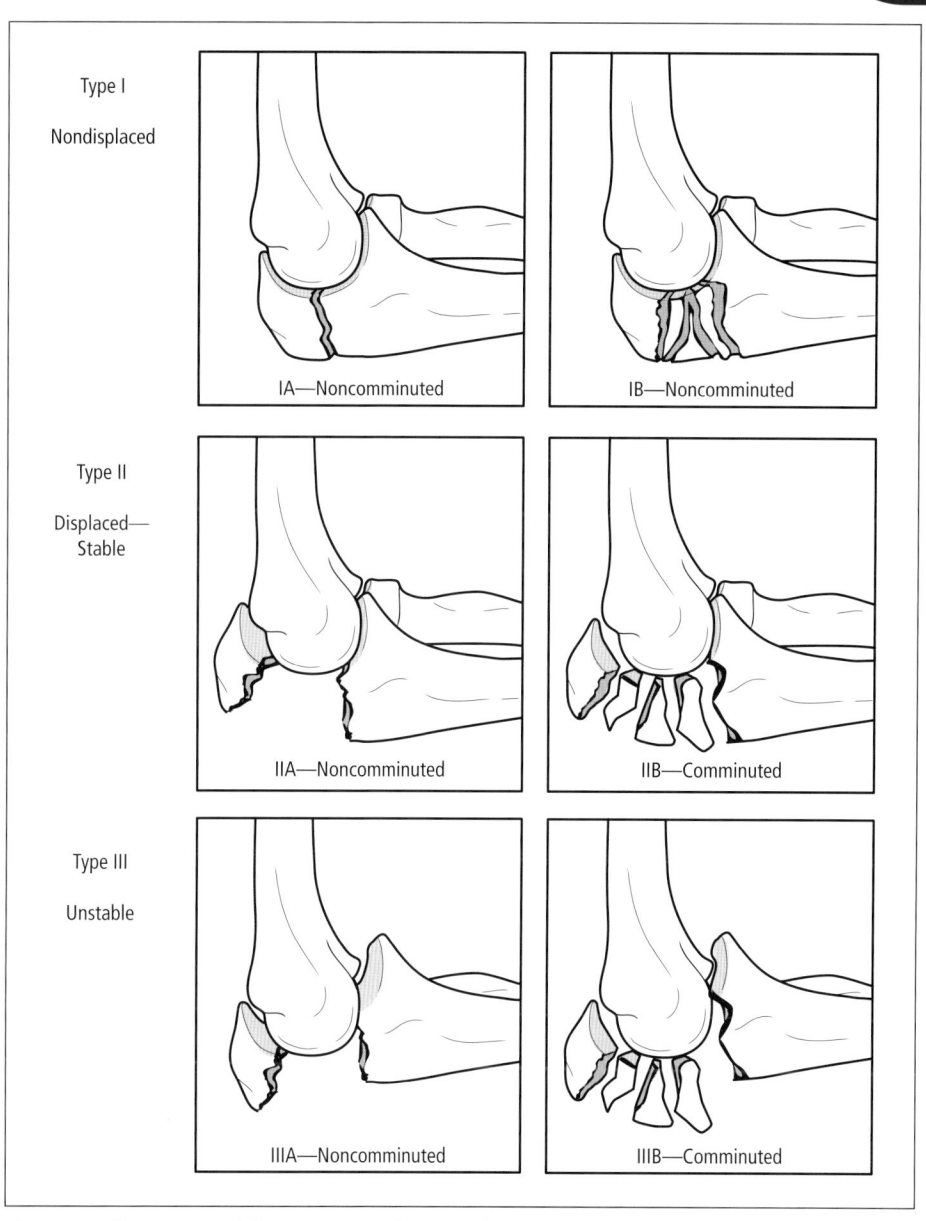

Figure 7 Illustration of the Mayo classification of olecranon fractures.

nonsurgically. In addition, close follow-up with repeat radiographs is essential to ensure that displacement does not occur. Displaced type II and III fractures usually require surgery. The goals of surgery include restoring a congruent joint surface and elbow stability and maintaining extension power by restoring the extensor apparatus. A goal of fixation is to provide stable fixation such that early motion is permitted.

Options for surgery include either excision of the proximal olecranon fracture fragment and advancement and reinsertion of the triceps tendon, or ORIF. Excision of the fracture fragments with advancement and reinsertion of the tendon is most commonly performed in elderly, infirm, or low-demand patients. In addition, it may be used in those who have avulsion-type extra-articular fractures or in those with severe comminution and osteoporosis, which does not permit stable fixation. Likewise, nonunions may be treated in this manner. This treatment technique has an advantage when there is a poor soft-tissue envelope because there will be no hardware to irritate this area. It is contraindicated in the setting of anterior injury of the soft tissues or the coronoid. Up to 30% of the olecranon may be excised without sacrificing stability, although some studies suggest up to 80% or even more may be excised.[17-21]

ORIF is the most common method of treating olecranon fractures and is reliable in restoring extensor power, gaining union, and restoring motion. Plate-and-screw constructs, intramedullary devices, or tension-band wiring fixation may be considered. Plate-and-screw constructs are the optimal fixation technique

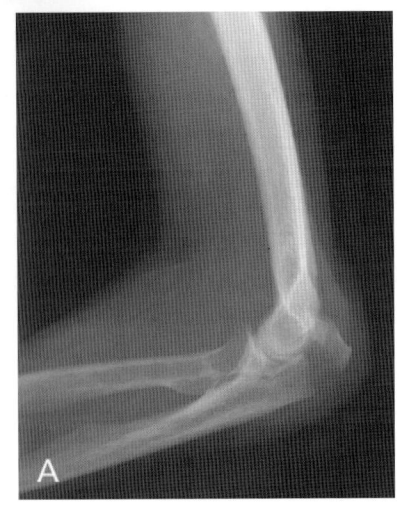

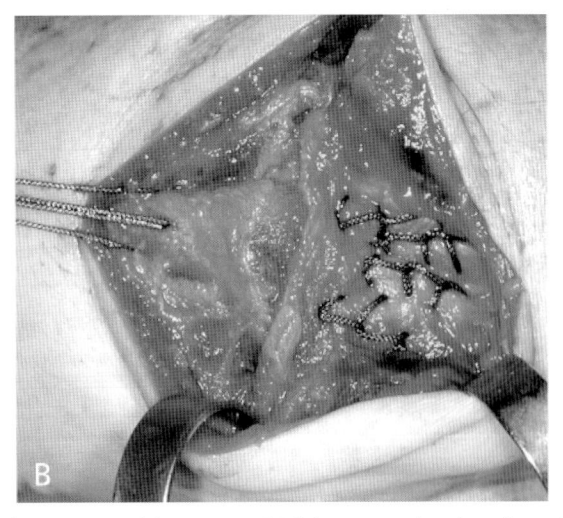

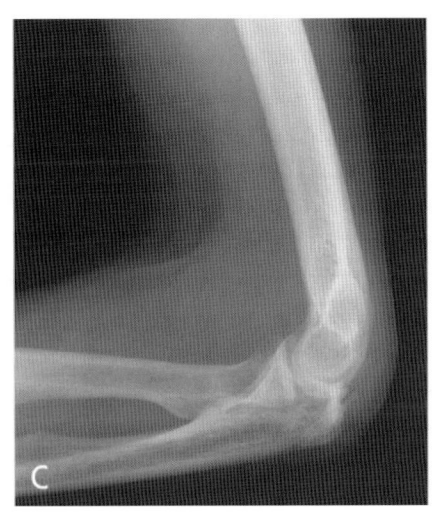

Figure 8 Images demonstrate excision of the proximal fragment, which is appropriate for a few selected olecranon fractures. **A,** Preoperative lateral radiograph demonstrates olecranon fracture. **B,** Intraoperative photograph shows excision and repair of the triceps. **C,** Postoperative lateral radiograph demonstrates a stable elbow following excision of the fracture fragment. (Reproduced with permission from Adams JE, Steinmann SP: Fractures of the olecranon, in Morrey BF, Sanchez-Sotelo J, eds: *The Elbow and Its Disorders.* Philadelphia, PA, WB Saunders, 2009, pp 389-400.)

for fractures in which the fracture line is at or distal to the level of the coronoid.

Preoperative Imaging

Three radiographic views of the elbow are obtained to evaluate the fracture pattern and for preoperative planning. In the setting of complex fracture-dislocations or transolecranon fractures, CT may be helpful, and two- and three-dimensional reconstructions can clarify the position and type of fracture fragments before surgery.

Procedure

Room Setup/Patient Positioning

The patient may be positioned supine with an arm table or with the arm over the chest; alternatively, lateral positioning or prone positioning is favored by some surgeons. A tourniquet is used to improve visualization. It is helpful to have a mini C-arm unit available for intraoperative imaging.

Either general or regional anesthesia may be used; however, general anesthesia provides the advantage of patient comfort during the procedure as well as the ability to immediately assess neurovascular status in the postoperative recovery room.

Special Instruments/Equipment/Implants

A variety of purpose-made, precontoured plating systems are available for olecranon fracture fixation. In addition, intramedullary devices with and without interlocking screws have recently become available; some consist of a simple cancellous screw that may be used in conjunction with tension-band wiring, whereas others are purpose-made devices with interlocking capability. Tension-band fixation with K-wires and fine-gauge wires is a well-established and cost-effective fixation alternative.

If fragment excision is considered, the triceps may be attached to the distal portion of the olecranon with bony tunnels or via suture anchors.

When fixation is anticipated, it is helpful to discuss with the patient that hardware irritation or prominence is a common issue postoperatively and hardware removal may be desired following healing of the fracture.

It is helpful to have a variety of bone reduction clamps, K-wires, 18- to 22-gauge wire, stout needle drivers, and a mini C-arm fluoroscopy unit available for the procedure.

Surgical Technique

The patient is positioned supine and undergoes general anesthesia. Preoperative antibiotics are given. The arm is prepped from the fingertips to the axilla, and a sterile tourniquet is applied. The arm is held over the chest over a bump of towels. A posterior incision is made medial to the tip of the olecranon and dissection proceeds, creating full-thickness flaps. The ulnar nerve is identified, and, if the patient manifested evidence of preoperative ulnar nerve dysfunction, the ulnar nerve can be decompressed. Otherwise, its position is noted so that it may be protected during the procedure. The fracture is identified, and the hematoma is removed in preparation for fixation (or excision).

Excision

The fracture fragments are excised, and the triceps is reattached to the bone with suture anchors or bony tunnels (**Figure 8**). The position of reattachment has been investigated by several authors. Traditionally, it has been suggested that the site of reattachment should be at the level of the articular surface; however, it has been suggested that a more posterior attachment site results in better preservation of extension strength.[21] The elbow is immobilized for 4 to 6 weeks and then motion is allowed.

Open Reduction and Internal Fixation

Plate and screws: A variety of purpose-made plates are now available for fixation of the olecranon and have the advantage of being curved posteriorly to achieve maximal fixation in the proximal fragment. Locking options may be helpful in osteoporotic bone. The fracture site is exposed and provisionally reduced with K-wires or pointed bone reduction clamps. The plate is chosen and applied to bone and then filled with appropriate length screws (**Figure 9**). Recent series have documented a high rate of satisfactory results following treatment with the newer precontoured plating systems, with a low rate of symptomatic hardware.[22-24]

Tension-band wiring: Tension-band wiring is unsuitable for comminuted fractures or those with a component distal to the midpoint of the olecranon. It is also likely to fail in the setting of elbow instability or in association with concomitant fractures of the elbow, such as radial head or coronoid fractures.

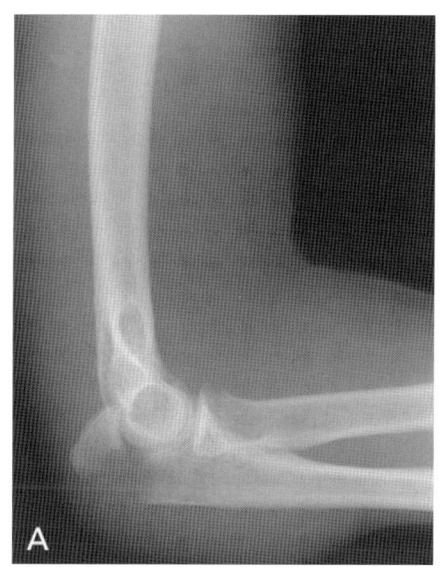

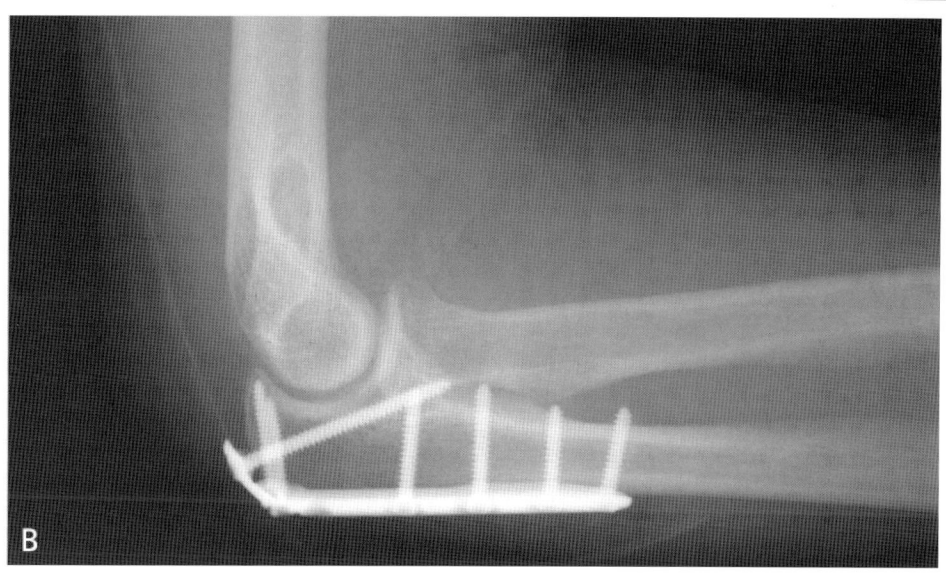

Chapter 32: Open Treatment of Radial Head Fractures and Olecranon Fractures

Figure 9 Radiographs depict an elbow treated with open reduction and internal fixation in which a plate-and-screw construct provides stable fixation. **A,** Preoperative lateral view demonstrates fracture of the olecranon. **B,** Postoperative lateral view demonstrates osteosynthesis with a plate-and-screw construct.

The fracture is exposed and inspected to ensure that it is amenable to tension-band fixation. A bone reduction clamp is helpful to obtain provisional fixation, and the fracture is reduced. Either K-wires or a screw may be used. If K-wires are chosen, two parallel 0.045- or 0.062-in K-wires are driven from the proximal fragment across the fracture site, exiting the cortex distal and anterior to the coronoid. They are then withdrawn 5 to 10 mm in anticipation of subsequent impaction. A transverse hole for the wire is drilled at the region at which the ulna transitions from a flat cortex proximally to the more triangular zone of the diaphysis. A 2.0- or 2.5-mm drill bit is used to create a drill hole at a level sufficiently anterior to the dorsal cortex that there is no danger of fracture through the hole out the dorsal cortex. A single 18- or 20-gauge wire can be used, or two 22-gauge wires may be chosen and passed through separate holes. The wire is passed in a figure-of-8 fashion over the dorsal surface of the ulna, about the K-wires, and through the triceps using a large angiocatheter needle. The wires are tensioned by twisting with large needle drivers on both sides and then cut and impacted into an area such that they will not be prominent. The K-wires are bent to a 180° angle and cut such that the crook of the K-wire captures the tension-band wire. They are then impacted into the triceps and bone with a bone tamp (**Figure 10**). An alternative is to use a large screw, such as a 6.5-mm partially threaded cancellous screw, instead of the K-wires. A high rate of symptomatic hardware is seen with tension-band wiring fixation; hardware removal rates may be as high as 82%.[25-29]

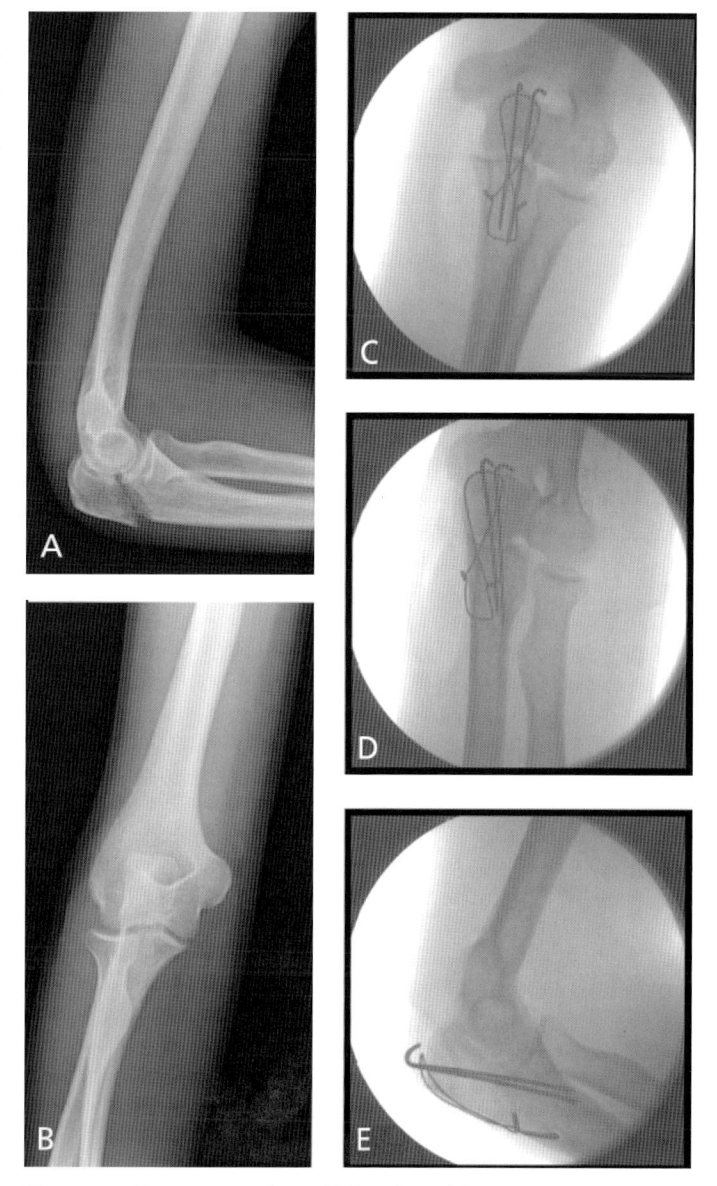

Figure 10 Preoperative lateral (**A**) and AP (**B**) radiographs demonstrate an olecranon fracture amenable to tension-band fixation. Intraoperative PA (**C**), oblique (**D**), and lateral (**E**) fluoroscopic views demonstrate satisfactory open reduction and internal fixation with a tension-band fixation construct.

© 2013 American Academy of Orthopaedic Surgeons

Complications

Prominent hardware is common in the setting of ORIF. Wound complications may plague the surgical site.

Postoperative Care

When ORIF is employed, the elbow should ideally be stable enough that motion may be allowed in the early postoperative period. The elbow may be splinted for a few days to allow for wound healing, but ideally motion is started as soon as is feasible postoperatively. In the setting of proximal fragment excision and triceps advancement, the elbow is casted or splinted for 4 to 6 weeks, and then motion is allowed.

Pearls

- When fixation of olecranon fractures is undertaken, it is advisable to ensure that full-thickness skin flaps are raised to avoid soft-tissue complications over this prominent bone.
- Olecranon fractures are ideally fixed with sufficient stability to enable early active motion.
- Common complications or sequelae following fixation of olecranon fractures include prominent hardware that might require removal and loss of terminal extension of the joint (stiffness).

References

1. Soyer AD, Nowotarski PJ, Kelso TB, Mighell MA: Optimal position for plate fixation of complex fractures of the proximal radius: A cadaver study. *J Orthop Trauma* 1998;12(4):291-293.
2. Caputo AE, Mazzocca AD, Santoro VM: The nonarticulating portion of the radial head: Anatomic and clinical correlations for internal fixation. *J Hand Surg Am* 1998;23(6):1082-1090.
3. Smith GR, Hotchkiss RN: Radial head and neck fractures: Anatomic guidelines for proper placement of internal fixation. *J Shoulder Elbow Surg* 1996;5(2 pt 1):113-117.
4. Diliberti T, Botte MJ, Abrams RA: Anatomical considerations regarding the posterior interosseous nerve during posterolateral approaches to the proximal part of the radius. *J Bone Joint Surg Am* 2000;82(6):809-813.
5. Adams JE, Steinmann SP: Nerve injuries about the elbow. *J Hand Surg Am* 2006;31(2):303-313.
6. Smith AM, Morrey BF, Steinmann SP: Low profile fixation of radial head and neck fractures: Surgical technique and clinical experience. *J Orthop Trauma* 2007;21(10):718-724.
7. Ring D, Quintero J, Jupiter JB: Open reduction and internal fixation of fractures of the radial head. *J Bone Joint Surg Am* 2002;84(10):1811-1815.
8. Adams JE, Steinmann SP: Implant options for elbow arthroplasty, in Lee D, ed: *Total Elbow Arthroplasty*. Rosemont, IL, ASSH Monograph Series, 2009, pp 49-52.
9. Frank SG, Grewal R, Johnson J, Faber KJ, King GJ, Athwal GS: Determination of correct implant size in radial head arthroplasty to avoid overlengthening. *J Bone Joint Surg Am* 2009;91(7):1738-1746.
10. Shors HC, Gannon C, Miller MC, Schmidt CC, Baratz ME: Plain radiographs are inadequate to identify overlengthening with a radial head prosthesis. *J Hand Surg Am* 2008;33(3):335-339.
11. Rowland AS, Athwal GS, MacDermid JC, King GJ: Lateral ulnohumeral joint space widening is not diagnostic of radial head arthroplasty overstuffing. *J Hand Surg Am* 2007;32(5):637-641.
12. van Riet RP, van Glabbeek F, de Weerdt W, Oemar J, Bortier H: Validation of the lesser sigmoid notch of the ulna as a reference point for accurate placement of a prosthesis for the head of the radius: A cadaver study. *J Bone Joint Surg Br* 2007;89(3):413-416.
13. Athwal GS, Frank SG, Grewal R, Faber KJ, Johnson J, King GJ: Determination of correct implant size in radial head arthroplasty to avoid overlengthening: Surgical technique. *J Bone Joint Surg Am* 2010;92(suppl 1, pt 2):250-257.
14. Doornberg JN, Linzel DS, Zurakowski D, Ring D: Reference points for radial head prosthesis size. *J Hand Surg Am* 2006;31(1):53-57.
15. Smith AM, Urbanosky LR, Castle JA, Rushing JT, Ruch DS: Radius pull test: Predictor of longitudinal forearm instability. *J Bone Joint Surg Am* 2002;84(11):1970-1976.
16. Adams JE, Steinmann SP, Osterman AL: Management of injuries to the interosseous membrane. *Hand Clin* 2010;26(4):543-548.
17. McKeever FM, Buck RM: Fracture of the olecranon process of the ulna; treatment by excision of fragment and repair of triceps tendon. *J Am Med Assoc* 1947;135(1):1-5.
18. An KN, Morrey BF, Chao EY: The effect of partial removal of proximal ulna on elbow constraint. *Clin Orthop Relat Res* 1986;209:270-279.
19. Kamineni S, Hirahara H, Pomianowski S, et al: Partial posteromedial olecranon resection: A kinematic study. *J Bone Joint Surg Am* 2003;85(6):1005-1011.
20. Bell TH, Ferreira LM, McDonald CP, Johnson JA, King GJ: Contribution of the olecranon to elbow stability: An in vitro biomechanical study. *J Bone Joint Surg Am* 2010;92(4):949-957.
21. Didonna ML, Fernandez JJ, Lim TH, Hastings H II, Cohen MS: Partial olecranon excision: The relationship between triceps insertion site and extension strength of the elbow. *J Hand Surg Am* 2003;28(1):117-122.
22. Siebenlist S, Torsiglieri T, Kraus T, Burghardt RD, Stöckle U, Lucke M: Comminuted fractures of the proximal ulna: Preliminary results with an anatomically preshaped locking compression plate (LCP) system. *Injury* 2010;41(12):1306-1311.
23. Kloen P, Buijze GA: Treatment of proximal ulna and olecranon fractures by dorsal plating. *Oper Orthop Traumatol* 2009;21(6):571-585.
24. Anderson ML, Larson AN, Merten SM, Steinmann SP: Congruent elbow plate fixation of olecranon fractures. *J Orthop Trauma* 2007;21(6):386-393.
25. Chalidis BE, Sachinis NC, Samoladas EP, Dimitriou CG, Pournaras JD: Is tension band wiring technique the "gold standard" for the treatment of olecranon fractures? A long term functional outcome study. *J Orthop Surg Res* 2008;3:9.
26. Karlsson MK, Hasserius R, Karlsson C, Besjakov J, Josefsson PO: Fractures of the olecranon: A 15- to 25-year followup of 73 patients. *Clin Orthop Relat Res* 2002;403:205-212.
27. Rommens PM, Küchle R, Schneider RU, Reuter M: Olecranon fractures in adults: Factors influencing outcome. *Injury* 2004;35(11):1149-1157.
28. Villanueva P, Osorio F, Commessatti M, Sanchez-Sotelo J: Tension-band wiring for olecranon fractures: Analysis of risk factors for failure. *J Shoulder Elbow Surg* 2006;15(3):351-356.
29. Romero JM, Miran A, Jensen CH: Complications and re-operation rate after tension-band wiring of olecranon fractures. *J Orthop Sci* 2000;5(4):318-320.

Chapter 33
Open Reduction and Internal Fixation of Distal Humerus Fractures

Michael David McKee, MD, FRCSC

Patient Selection

The overall incidence of distal humerus fractures in adults has been reported to be 5.7 per 100,000 people per year.[1] Treatment usually requires surgical fixation, which can be technically demanding. Many issues regarding the management of distal humerus fractures have not been clarified sufficiently to allow surgeon consensus. The optimum surgical approach, plate configuration, indications for arthroplasty, the need for ulnar nerve transposition, and the use of prophylaxis for the prevention of heterotopic ossification (HO) continue to be debated.

The AO/Orthopaedic Trauma Association (AO/OTA) classification for distal humerus fractures is widely used, and is helpful for treatment planning.[2] The classification divides distal humerus fractures into three categories: type A, nonarticular fractures; type B, partial articular fractures; and type C, complete articular fractures.

Paramount features of the treatment goals are to obtain an anatomic reduction with adequate stability to allow early range of motion. Achieving these goals is advantageous for optimizing the patient's recovery time and function. A preoperative discussion about the risks and benefits of surgical versus nonsurgical treatment is key. In particular, outlining that the return of completely normal preinjury range of motion is rarely achieved after such an injury is important. This, combined with informing patients that transient ulnar nerve paresthesias are relatively common secondary to injury and from manipulation of the nerve intraoperatively, can temper expectations to a realistic level.

Indications

Open reduction and internal fixation (ORIF) is appropriate for displaced fractures, open fractures/impending open fractures, fractures with associated vascular injury, ipsilateral upper extremity injury, and pathologic fractures.

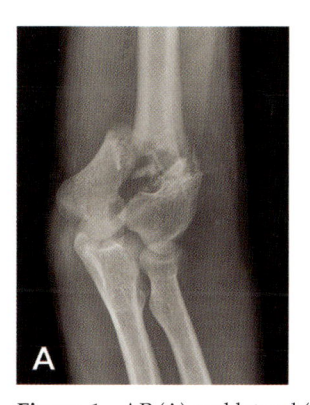

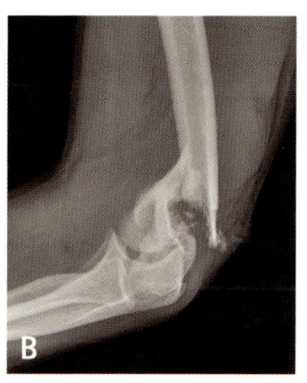

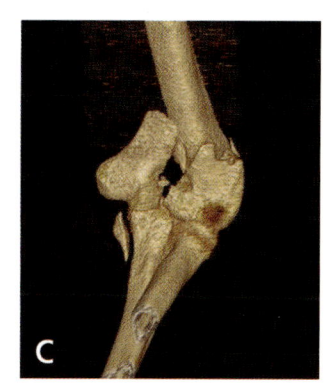

Figure 1 AP (**A**) and lateral (**B**) preoperative radiographs demonstrate an intra-articular distal humerus fracture. Evidence of air is also seen, as this was an open fracture. **C**, CT reconstruction of the same injury. The CT scan was extremely useful in this particular instance because a proximal ulnar fracture was identified that is not readily evident on the radiographs. This fracture was an avulsion of the ulnar insertion of the medial collateral ligament.

Contraindications

Contraindications to ORIF include a patient's poor health precluding the ability to tolerate an operation, active infection, lack of appropriate soft-tissue coverage, poor compliance, and extreme osteoporosis not amenable to stable fixation. In patients older than 70 years with extreme osteoporosis and intra-articular fracture comminution, a linked semi-constrained total elbow arthroplasty is likely the best surgical option.[3]

Nonsurgical treatment is appropriate for stable, nondisplaced fractures and patients with preexisting conditions creating a nonfunctional extremity. Vigilant follow-up is necessary to recognize potential fracture displacement. Institution of early physical therapy will minimize posttraumatic elbow stiffness.

Preoperative Imaging

Imperative investigations include AP, lateral, and oblique radiographs of the elbow and, when indicated, shoulder and wrist radiographs. Traction radiographs and CT scans can be very helpful for preoperative planning and hardware templating[4] (**Figure 1**).

Procedure
Room Setup/Patient Positioning

Room setup should be comfortable for the patient and the surgical team. Positioning should allow access to the surgical site for imaging. There are many described techniques for patient positioning; however, placing the patient in the lateral decubitus position with the affected extremity over an arm bolster provides excellent access to the distal humerus and allows gravity to be a reduction aid (**Figure 2**). Supine positioning of multiple trauma patients, particularly those with chest injuries, is preferable; the affected arm is placed across the chest on a pad or bolster.

Positioning should allow for intraoperative radiographs to be obtained or the use of an image intensifier (mini C-arm). A radiolucent arm bolster is helpful but not a necessity. Although the reduction of fracture fragments can be directly visualized, the fluoroscope can be useful for observing dynamic joint alignment and anterior fragments that can be difficult to directly visualize, as well as to ensure that there is no intra-articular screw penetration.

Special Instruments/Equipment/Implants

Special equipment needed for this procedure includes small-fragment plates

---

Dr. McKee or an immediate family member has received royalties from Stryker; is a member of a speakers' bureau or has made paid presentations on behalf of Synthes and Zimmer; serves as a paid consultant to or is an employee of Synthes and Zimmer; has received research or institutional support from Wright Medical Technology and Zimmer; and serves as a board member, owner, officer, or committee member of the American Shoulder and Elbow Surgeons, the Orthopaedic Trauma Association, and the Canadian Orthopaedic Association.

Section 2: Shoulder and Elbow

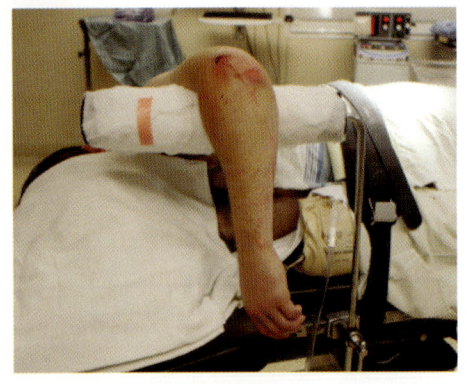

Figure 2 Photograph shows a patient secured in the lateral decubitus position via a beanbag and safety strap, with the affected arm placed over a padded bolster. All bony prominences are padded appropriately. This patient had been transferred from a peripheral facility, where he had undergone an irrigation and débridement of an open distal humeral fracture.

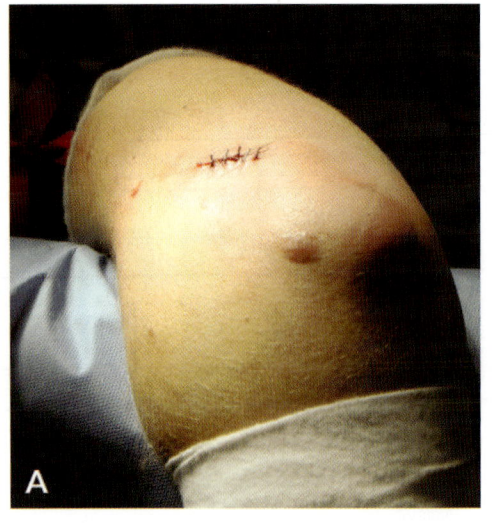

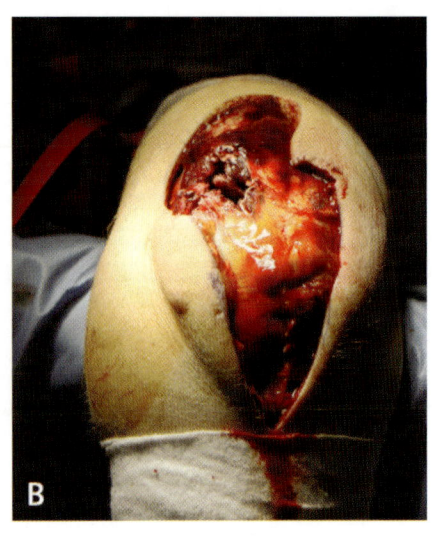

Figure 3 Intraoperative photographs show the straight posterior approach for open reduction and internal fixation of a distal humerus fracture. The patient's open fracture wound (**A**) was incorporated into the incision and the skin edges were excised (**B**). The large rent in the triceps and skin was created by the humeral shaft as it protruded at the time of injury. More than 90% of open wounds in this type of injury are posterior.

(including malleable reconstruction plates or precontoured periarticular plates), mini-fragment plates and screws, Herbert screws, Kirschner wires (K-wires), sterile tourniquet, reduction clamps/osteotomes, oscillating saw (for olecranon osteotomies and bone graft retrieval), wire set (for olecranon osteotomy fixation), bone-graft set, and mini C-arm fluoroscope or plain intraoperative radiography.

Plates must be strong enough to support early range-of-motion exercises following fixation. One third tubular plates are not strong enough and are contraindicated. Although not a necessity, precontoured locking plates have increased the strength of fixation constructs and reduced surgical time dedicated to contouring plates.[5] Plates with variable axis locking holes support capturing small or comminuted distal fragments while avoiding joint penetration and enhancing fixation strength.

Surgical Technique

A complete surgical briefing should be done with the entire surgical team and should include the surgeon initialing the surgical site and reviewing the procedure with the patient and the team, as well as the administration of prophylactic antibiotics, before the induction of anesthesia.

All bony prominences should be padded appropriately to avoid iatrogenic nerve palsy or pressure sores. The patient is placed and secured in the lateral decubitus position with the affected extremity over a padded arm bolster allowing 90° of flexion at the elbow. The posterior iliac crest should be prepared if it is anticipated that bone graft will be required. The upper extremity is prepared beyond the shoulder and draped to allow access to the proximal arm. An extremity stockinette is wrapped to midforearm. A sterile tourniquet is applied to the proximal arm. The extremity is exsanguinated with an Esmarch bandage before the inflation of a pneumatic tourniquet.

Although different approaches have been described, typically a direct posterior incision is used, exposing the triceps as well as the proximal olecranon[6] (**Figure 3**). Some surgeons curve this incision laterally around the olecranon to avoid a scar directly over the olecranon. It is mandatory to identify, protect, and mobilize the ulnar nerve. It should be released sufficiently to allow safe exposure and fixation of the fracture. Flagging the nerve with a Penrose drain/vessel loop serves as a visual reminder of the nerve's position throughout the procedure and facilitates very gentle retraction (**Figure 4**).

Extensor Mechanism

Different options exist for dealing with the extensor mechanism.

Paratricipital Approach

The paratricipital approach allows the surgeon to visualize the fracture on either side of the triceps. Dissection involves freeing the radial and ulnar borders of the triceps and gently elevating the triceps off the humerus and the posterior aspect of the intermuscular septum.[6] The triceps attachment to the olecranon remains undisturbed. Typically this technique is reserved for two situations:

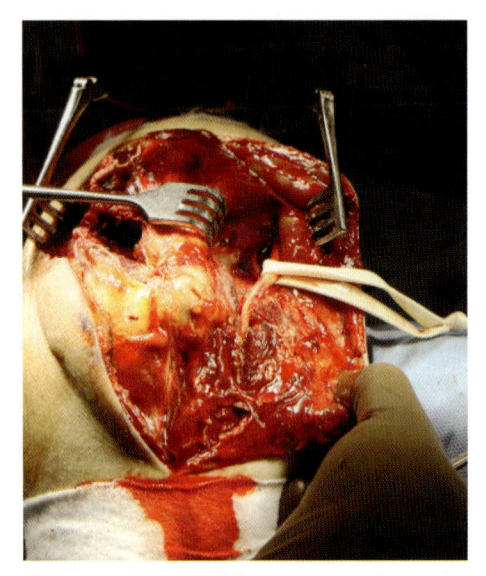

Figure 4 As part of the exposure, the ulnar nerve is identified, and a neurolysis is performed. The nerve is flagged with a Penrose drain throughout the operation.

(1) Elbow arthroplasty in the setting of distal humerus fracture. In this situation, the distal humeral fragments are extracted. The removal of these fragments combined with the paratricipital approach affords a great enough working space to perform an elbow arthroplasty while keeping the triceps attached to the olecranon.[3]

(2) Technically simpler distal humerus fractures (such as extra-articular fractures). In this situation, excellent visualization of the joint is not critical for success. The paratricipital approach will allow exposure to the medial and the lateral column of the humerus, the intended area for plate fixation. Visualization via this technique will allow reduction and

© 2013 American Academy of Orthopaedic Surgeons

stable fixation in such situations but will not allow an optimal view of the joint surface to gauge reduction, which is required for more complex intra-articular fractures.[7]

The paratricipital approach is also needed to allow reflection of an olecranon osteotomy and is a natural transition to this exposure. Switching from a paratricipital approach to a triceps split is not advisable because extensive devitalization of the triceps occurs.

Triceps Split

The triceps spilt allows adequate exposure for most intra-articular fractures and conversion to arthroplasty if needed. It involves a midline split in the triceps, which continues on to the olecranon, reflecting full-thickness flaps of the triceps and its tendon medially and laterally.[8] Anterior coronal shear fractures are not optimally visualized via this technique, and an olecranon osteotomy provides better exposure for such fractures. The triceps split can be combined with removing the proximal tip of the olecranon to improve exposure or, if the need arises, to allow easier insertion of the ulnar component in an elbow arthroplasty.

Employing this approach in open fractures is favorable, because the exposure is partially completed via the rent in the triceps typically created by an open injury (**Figure 5**). The proximal dissection is limited by the radial nerve, which is identified and protected if the surgeon needs greater proximal exposure. Repair of a triceps split involves the use of interrupted transosseous sutures in the proximal olecranon using nonabsorbable braided stitches through drill holes in the olecranon. Reduced pain and better Mayo Elbow Performance and Disabilities of the Arm, Shoulder, and Hand (DASH) scores have been shown with a triceps split versus a transolecranon approach for open fractures.[8]

Olecranon Osteotomy

An olecranon osteotomy provides the best exposure, allowing the proximal olecranon to be reflected while remaining attached to the triceps tendon. The technique involves a chevron-shaped intra-articular osteotomy with the apex pointing distally. A Penrose drain can be placed across the ulnohumeral joint before the osteotomy to help protect the cartilage while the osteotomy is created. Predrilling the ulna in preparation for fixation can be done to ensure anatomic reduction of the osteotomy site. Dissection along the intra-articular bare area of olecranon exposes the osteotomy site. The osteotomy is initiated with a saw and stops subchondrally. The osteotomy is completed using osteotomes to avoid a cartilage kerf.

The disadvantages of this technique include the need for fixation of the osteotomy site—typically tension-band or plate fixation. There is a potential for delayed union and nonunion, and the hardware can be irritating, necessitating an additional operation for removal. Conversion to arthroplasty, although not impossible, is technically challenging and generally requires the removal of some bone on the volar proximal olecranon to accommodate the ulnar component. The osteotomy site is then reduced and secured by plate fixation of the olecranon with screws, avoiding the ulnar stem. The removed bone can serve as bone graft for the osteotomy site. An alternate exposure is preferable if the surgeon suspects that fracture fixation may not be possible, necessitating a conversion to arthroplasty.

Triceps Peel

With the triceps peel, the extensor mechanism is reflected in a full-thickness manner from the olecranon, working from the ulnar to the radial side.[9] The extensor mechanism is not split. This technique allows for excellent exposure and is accommodating for conversion to arthroplasty. Repair involves transosseous olecranon fixation using nonabsorbable suture. Care must be taken not to buttonhole or stray from a full-thickness peel because this can weaken the extensor mechanism.

Reduction and Fixation

The distal humerus has a strong ulnar and radial column that is connected by an articular surface, completing a triangular shape. In a fracture situation, re-creation of this stable triangle is paramount to success. Once full exposure is obtained, the fracture sites are gently cleared of clot, and the fractured fragments are evaluated to confirm that preoperative imaging accurately predicted the shape and size of the articular fragments (**Figure 6**).

The surgeon must determine whether the entire articular surface is present. If gaps are present, structural bone graft may be required to restore the anatomic relationship of the trochlea to the capitellum. This anatomic restoration is critical for normal elbow kinematics. With a deficient articular surface, care must be taken to not overreduce the trochlea. An overreduced trochlea will not allow proper seating of the olecranon, causing an incongruous fit, malalignment, and rapid progression of posttraumatic arthritis.

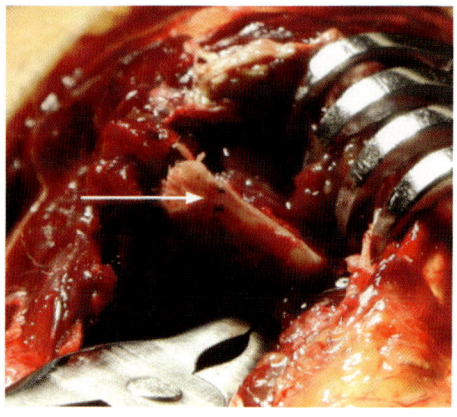

Figure 5 A close-up intraoperative photograph of the fractured humeral shaft through the triceps rent reveals two areas of embedded debris in the bone (arrow). This debris remained despite the fact that this patient had undergone an irrigation and débridement at another facility. This bone was rongeured and discarded as part of the second irrigation and débridement performed. The location of this debris is typical because the humeral shaft is usually responsible for creating the triceps rent and open wound and impacts with the outside environment.

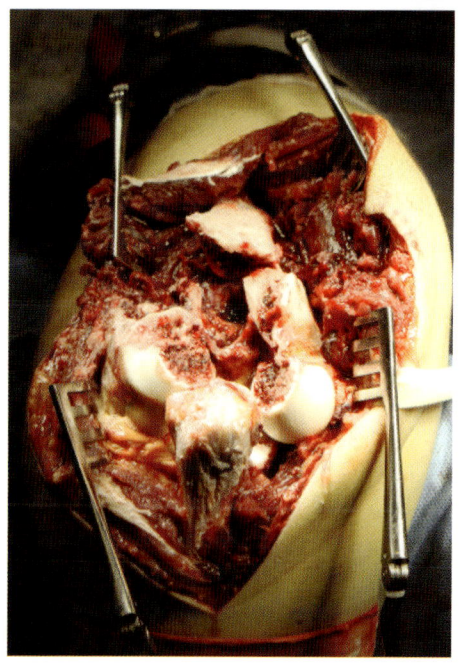

Figure 6 Intraoperative photograph shows a midline triceps split in which the rent in the triceps was débrided and incorporated, exposing the fracture fragments. Preoperative imaging accurately predicted the split into the articular surface with metaphyseal comminution.

Reduction and fixation goals include an anatomic re-creation of the articular surface and then securely fastening it to the humeral shaft in a compressive mode. Often, the temporary placement of plates and fracture reduction are done concurrently. This allows reduction clamps and K-wires to be strategically placed to maintain the reduction and at the same time temporarily hold plates in their correct position. A well-thought-out preoperative plan facilitates K-wire placement to avoid interfering with plate fixation.

Alternatively, a primary reduction maneuver can involve clamping the articular surface with a tenaculum to provide compression of the articular fracture fragments (**Figure 7**). The articular surface of the olecranon can serve as a template to reduction. Some authors feel a free screw not passing through a plate provides inferior stability and takes up limited space in the distal fragments and is therefore not warranted.[10] However, a carefully placed subchondral screw can afford good compression and maintain articular congruity while the surgery progresses, and it causes minimal interference with screws passing through the plate. If articular compression is not possible secondary to comminution, screws should be placed in a noncompressive mode to avoid overreduction.

The goal with distally placed screws through the plate is to traverse as many fracture fragments as possible and gain purchase of fragments on the opposite column. Therefore, the entire joint should be reduced anatomically before definitive screw fixation. Reduction forceps can be used to provide compression across the joint, allowing fully threaded screws through the plate to maintain the fragments in compression. Screws should be as long as possible, and interdigitation of screws originating from opposite sides is favorable to enhance stability.[10] Bony compression, interdigitation of screws, and the ability to use the longest possible screws is easier to achieve with parallel plating than with orthogonal constructs.

Once the articular fragments are reduced and secured to the plates, the plates can be fixed to the shaft via the oblong holes to aid in adjustment of plates, allowing for compression of the articular surface to the metaphysis/shaft (**Figure 8**). Compression of the articular surface to the metaphysis/shaft can be completed by placing a proximal screw through the plate in compressive mode or an obliquely placed reduction clamp capturing the distal fragment and the contralateral metaphysis/shaft. Care must be taken not to translate the fracture when performing this maneuver. The compression of the articular surface to the metaphysis/shaft confers stability to the overall construct. An anatomic reduction can still be obtained if metaphyseal bone is missing on one column. However, if both columns are severely comminuted,

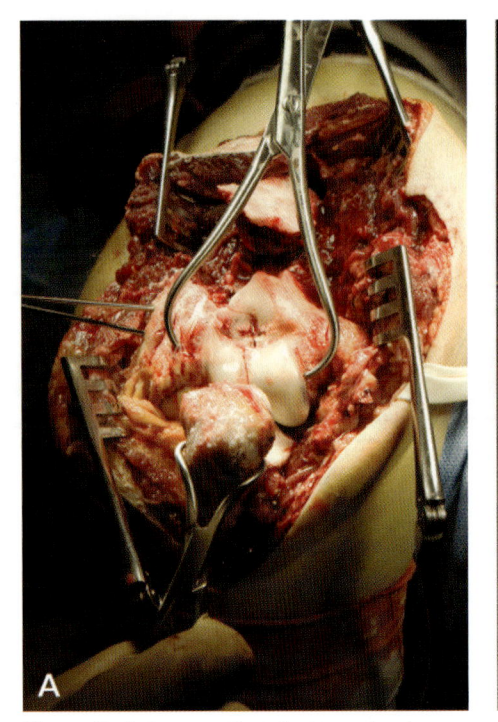

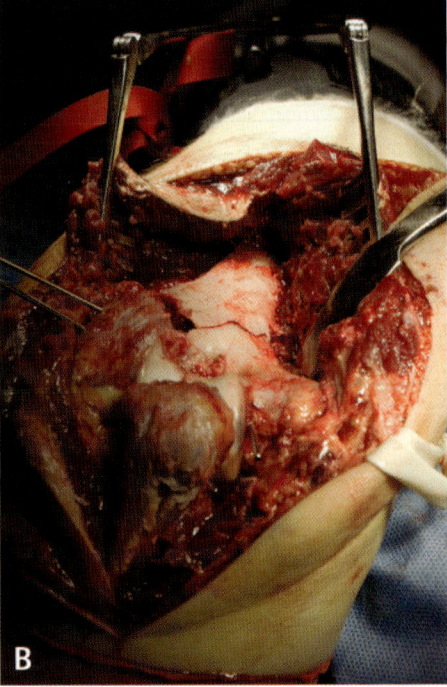

Figure 7 Intraoperative photographs show open reduction and internal fixation of a distal humerus fracture. **A,** With a tenaculum providing compression of the articular fragments, a compression screw is placed in the subchondral region to lag the condyles together. **B,** Kirschner wires are then used to provisionally hold in the assembled articular surface to the metaphysis.

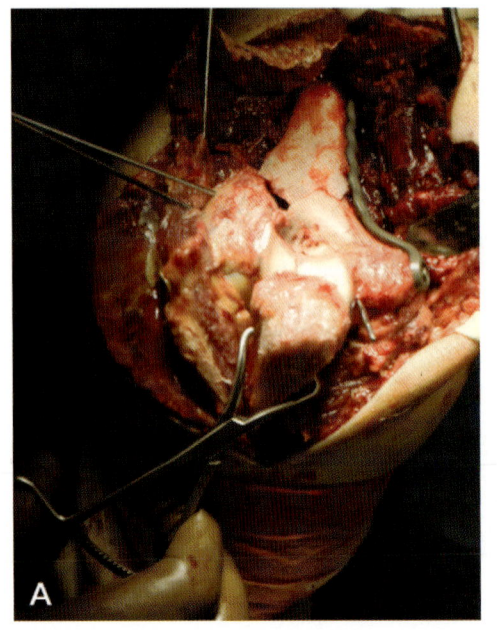

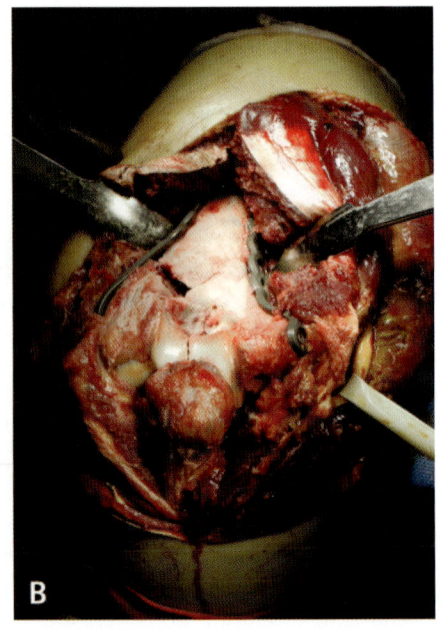

Figure 8 Intraoperative photographs show open reduction and internal fixation of a distal humerus fracture. **A,** Medial and lateral periarticular locking plates secure the articular surface to the metaphysis in a compressive mode. The medial column is anatomically reduced. **B,** Note the metaphyseal comminution and bone loss on the lateral side.

this is best dealt with by shortening the humerus to achieve bony contact and compression. If the humerus is shortened, re-creation of the olecranon fossa by burring away bone may be required to avoid olecranon impingement on the posterior humerus. Gapping without solid bony contact subjects hardware to excessive bending stress, potentially causing hardware failure. Parallel plating in this

Chapter 33: Open Reduction and Internal Fixation of Distal Humerus Fractures

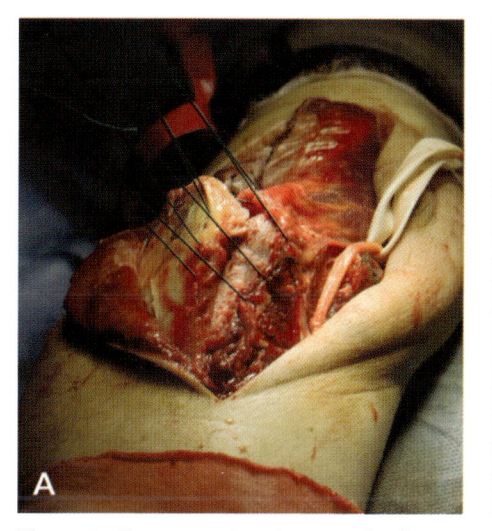

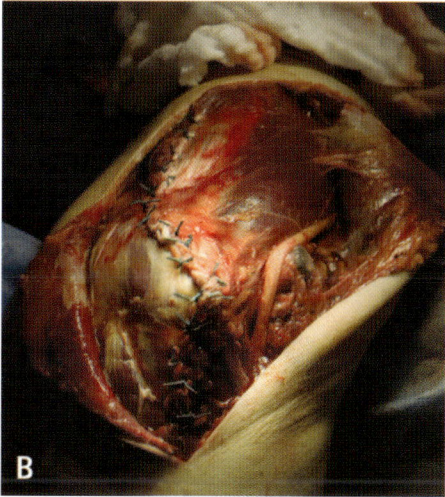

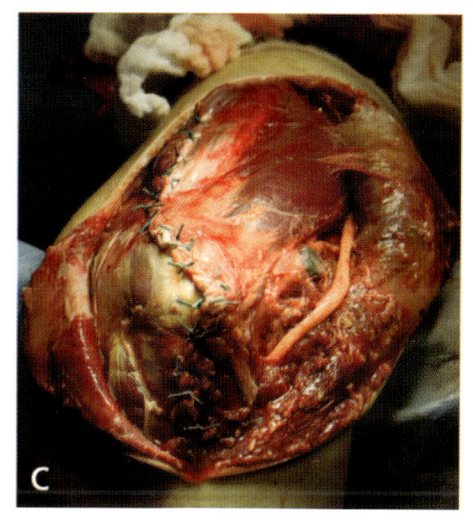

Figure 9 Intraoperative photographs demonstrate transposition of the ulnar nerve. **A,** Transosseous sutures are used to reapproximate the extensor mechanism at the proximal ulna. **B,** The final closure of the midline split of the triceps. **C,** Note the final position of the ulnar nerve.

situation provides superior stability biomechanically.[11]

The plates are then secured to the humeral shaft via bicortical screw fixation using standard technique. A minimum of three screws should be used in each plate for shaft fixation. It is preferable for the plates to be different lengths to decrease stress-riser forces. When working on the radial side, care must be taken to ensure that the proximal aspect of the plate is not entrapping the radial nerve.

Once reduction and fixation is completed, stability and elbow mobility should be assessed. The elbow is put through a passive range of motion, including flexion, extension, pronation, and supination, and tested for coronal plane stability. A full degree of motion is expected under general anesthesia. If this is not achieved, the block to motion must be identified and corrected.

Debate continues concerning the appropriate treatment of the ulnar nerve following surgical fixation of distal humerus fractures. By virtue of mobilizing the nerve, it is decompressed. Some argue that anterior nerve transposition should also be performed. There is some evidence that nerve transposition provides a superior outcome in patients with symptoms of ulnar nerve injury before surgery.[12] I typically transpose the nerve if the patient has clinical preoperative nerve pathology or if the nerve is in direct contact with the hardware (**Figure 9**). Randomized studies are currently in progress to help delineate the risks and benefits of ulnar nerve transposition following distal humerus fracture fixation. If nerve transposition is completed, a detailed record of the resting position of the nerve after transposition in the surgical report is helpful if further operations are required.

The tourniquet can be deflated after the wound is irrigated with normal saline. My practice is to keep pressure on the wound after tourniquet deflation for a minimum of 2 minutes and then examine the wound and achieve hemostasis followed by a standard closure. Drains are not routinely used. Postoperative radiographs are routinely performed.

Complications
Complications after distal humerus fracture fixation include elbow stiffness, hardware failure/irritation, triceps avulsion, nerve injury, infection, nonunion of the olecranon osteotomy or fracture (rarely), and anesthetic issues.

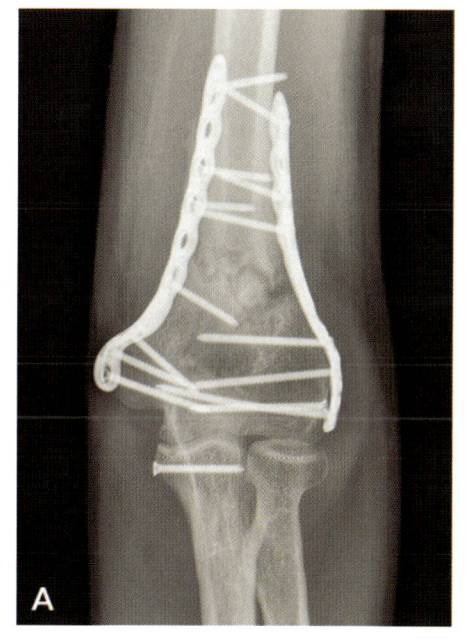

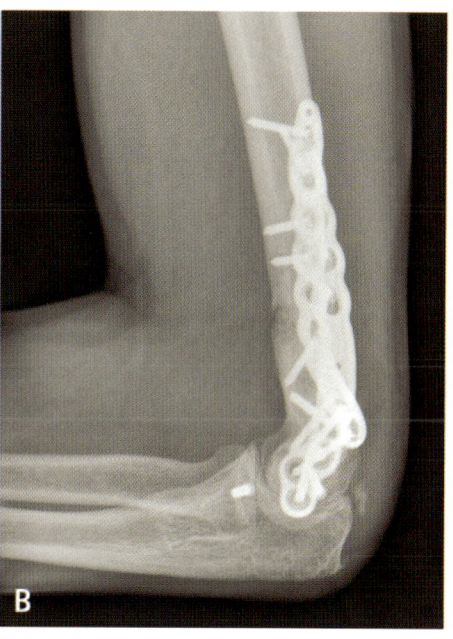

Figure 10 AP (**A**) and lateral (**B**) radiographs after open reduction and internal fixation for a distal humerus fracture. Note the screw in the proximal ulna, which was used to secure an avulsion fracture attached to the medial collateral ligament.

Postoperative Care and Rehabilitation
Usually, patients are splinted in extension with a well-padded plaster splint. The splint is typically removed in 24 to 48 hours so that physical therapy can be initiated. Physical therapy initially consists of active flexion with gravity-assisted extension. If there are concerns about posterior soft-tissue integrity or other injuries, the splint can remain on until the first postoperative follow-up visit about 10 days after surgery. At this visit, a clinical assessment is completed, as well as repeat radiographs (**Figure 10**) and wound staple removal. Prolonged splinting for fear of fixation failure yields poor functional results secondary to elbow stiffness and is not recommended.

© 2013 American Academy of Orthopaedic Surgeons

Some authors advocate routine prophylaxis, typically in the form of indomethacin or radiation, to help prevent or lessen HO. Typically, because of the negative effect prophylaxis has on fracture healing, I reserve HO prophylaxis for high-risk patients, such as patients with head injuries and those necessitating revision surgery for HO resection.

Pearls

- Lateral decubitus patient positioning allows gravity to be a reduction aid.
- If the possibility of converting an ORIF to an arthroplasty exists, an olecranon osteotomy should be avoided.
- Precontoured plates save surgical time dedicated to contouring straight plates.
- Interdigitating screws in the distal fragments contribute to overall construct stability.
- Long screws originating from one column and gaining purchase in the contralateral humeral column are preferable.
- A sterile tourniquet can be removed to allow greater proximal exposure if necessary.
- Institution of early motion after a brief period of splinting (2 to 10 days) optimizes functional results.
- Preoperative discussion with the patient should cover the loss of range of motion that typically occurs with these injuries as well as the chance of ulnar nerve paresthesias.

References

1. Robinson CM, Hill RM, Jacobs N, Dall G, Court-Brown CM: Adult distal humeral metaphyseal fractures: Epidemiology and results of treatment. *J Orthop Trauma* 2003;17(1):38-47.
2. Orthopaedic Trauma Association Committee for Coding and Classification: Fracture and dislocation compendium. *J Orthop Trauma* 1996;10(suppl 1):1-154, v-ix.
3. McKee MD, Veillette CJ, Hall JA, et al: A multicenter, prospective, randomized, controlled trial of open reduction—internal fixation versus total elbow arthroplasty for displaced intra-articular distal humeral fractures in elderly patients. *J Shoulder Elbow Surg* 2009;18(1):3-12.
4. Doornberg J, Lindenhovius A, Kloen P, van Dijk CN, Zurakowski D, Ring D: Two and three-dimensional computed tomography for the classification and management of distal humeral fractures: Evaluation of reliability and diagnostic accuracy. *J Bone Joint Surg Am* 2006;88(8):1795-1801.
5. Korner J, Diederichs G, Arzdorf M, et al: A biomechanical evaluation of methods of distal humerus fracture fixation using locking compression plates versus conventional reconstruction plates. *J Orthop Trauma* 2004;18(5):286-293.
6. Pollock JW, Athwal GS, Steinmann SP: Surgical exposures for distal humerus fractures: A review. *Clin Anat* 2008;21(8):757-768.
7. Erpelding JM, Mailander A, High R, Mormino MA, Fehringer EV: Outcomes following distal humeral fracture fixation with an extensor mechanism-on approach. *J Bone Joint Surg Am* 2012;94(6):548-553.
8. McKee MD, Kim J, Kebaish K, Stephen DJ, Kreder HJ, Schemitsch EH: Functional outcome after open supracondylar fractures of the humerus: The effect of the surgical approach. *J Bone Joint Surg Br* 2000;82(5):646-651.
9. Bryan RS, Morrey BF: Extensive posterior exposure of the elbow: A triceps-sparing approach. *Clin Orthop Relat Res* 1982;166:188-192.
10. Sanchez-Sotelo J, Torchia ME, O'Driscoll SW: Complex distal humeral fractures: Internal fixation with a principle-based parallel-plate technique. Surgical technique. *J Bone Joint Surg Am* 2008; 90(suppl 2 pt 1):31-46.
11. Schemitsch EH, Tencer AF, Henley MB: Biomechanical evaluation of methods of internal fixation of the distal humerus. *J Orthop Trauma* 1994;8(6):468-475.
12. Ruan HJ, Liu JJ, Fan CY, Jiang J, Zeng BF: Incidence, management, and prognosis of early ulnar nerve dysfunction in type C fractures of distal humerus. *J Trauma* 2009;67(6):1397-1401.

Chapter 34
Total Elbow Arthroplasty

Peter Johnston, MD   Matthew L. Ramsey, MD

Introduction

A functional, pain-free elbow joint is dependent on the integrity of the ulnohumeral articulation. Diverse pathology exists that ultimately leads to destruction of the ulnohumeral joint and manifests as painful motion, instability, or ankylosis. The degree of functional limitation is dependent on the severity of bony destruction and the involvement of soft-tissue structures, which vary with the underlying pathology.

Current total elbow arthroplasty (TEA) implant designs are categorized as linked (coupled), unlinked (uncoupled), and hybrid linkable. The decision to use a linked versus an unlinked implant is dependent on the underlying pathology, the adequacy of bone stock, and the integrity of the ligamentous soft-tissue envelope. Unlinked implants require joint stability and bone stock adequate to support the implant, narrowing the indications, but provide a theoretical decrease in stress across the prosthesis and lower loosening rates when compared with a linked joint. Unlinked implants are suitable for pathologies with intact supracondylar columns, minimal subchondral bony deformity, and competence of collateral ligaments. Linked implants are joined by a "sloppy hinge," which allows slight movement in the varus-valgus and axial planes. Indications for linked implants are broader, including ligamentous deficiency and traumatic conditions with severe bone loss, which include acute fractures, established posttraumatic arthrosis, distal humeral nonunion, posttraumatic ankylosis, posttraumatic instability, and revision TEA. Hybrid linkable implants permit implantation in an unlinked fashion, taking advantage of the benefits of an unlinked implant, but can be easily converted to a linked implant if stability cannot be established at initial implantation or if instability becomes an issue remote from the index arthroplasty.

Patient Selection
Indications

The primary indication for total elbow arthroplasty is to treat pain and secondarily to improve function of the elbow joint with disabling disease. TEA is indicated for the treatment of patients with rheumatoid arthritis; posttraumatic arthritis; acute fracture; primary osteoarthritis; and a variety of posttraumatic conditions, such as malunion, nonunion, and recalcitrant instability.

Contraindications

The absolute contraindications to total elbow arthroplasty are infection of the joint as well as lack of motor function necessary to provide active elbow flexion. With regard to relative contraindications, TEA should be avoided in younger patients, particularly in laborers who are better candidates for nonarthroplasty options. TEA in the setting of a neuropathic joint will lead to unpredictable outcomes and a high complication rate. Additionally, TEA should be avoided in patients who are unwilling to live within the activity and weight restrictions that are requirements for implant longevity.

Implant-specific contraindications exist for unlinked implants. These implants should be avoided in situations where the bony architecture or the collateral ligaments will be compromised during surgery or may develop in the postoperative period. These situations, which should be treated with a linked implant, include takedown of an elbow arthrodesis or painless ankylosis, tumor resection of the distal humerus, gross deformity that interferes with soft-tissue balancing, and excision of heterotopic ossification.

Preoperative Imaging

Standard radiographic evaluation of the elbow joint includes AP, lateral, and oblique radiographs (**Figure 1**). These views are usually sufficient to assess bone quality and the degree of bony abnormality, providing the surgeon with information guiding implant selection (linked versus unlinked) and sizing. Additionally, stress radiographs can be taken if there is a suspicion of ligamentous instability.

CT usually is not necessary in the preoperative workup of patients with underlying arthritides, but it can provide the surgeon with additional information on joint or periarticular deformity. CT can be particularly useful in the acute fracture setting, in managing malunion or nonunion, or in cases with heterotopic ossification. MRI has a limited role in the preoperative diagnostic workup for TEA.

Preoperative Evaluation

Prior to surgery, a detailed examination is performed with attention to the status of the overlying skin, prior incisions, contractures, limb alignment, joint stability, and flexion-extension arc. If prior surgery has been performed, the location of the ulnar nerve should be considered as well as the presence of ulnar nerve symptoms.

Preoperative Planning

Preoperative radiographs, any underlying pathology, and surgeon experience should guide the selection of a linked versus an unlinked implant. It is important to recognize that if an unlinked system has been selected, a linked system should be available in case it becomes apparent that an unlinked system will not stabilize the elbow. A linkable system allows easy conversion from an unlinked to a linked arthroplasty.

Procedure
Room Setup/Patient Positioning

The patient is positioned supine on the operating room table with a bump placed beneath the ipsilateral scapula, and the arm is placed on a bolster across the chest (**Figure 2**). The bump allows the arm to be easily draped across the chest throughout the procedure. A well-padded tourniquet

---

Dr. Ramsey or an immediate family member has received royalties from Integra LifeSciences and Zimmer; serves as a paid consultant to or is an employee of Integra LifeSciences and Zimmer; has received research or institutional support from Integra LifeSciences and Zimmer; and serves as a board member, owner, officer, or committee member of the American Academy of Orthopaedic Surgeons, the Philadelphia Orthopaedic Society, the Rothman Institute, and the Rothman Specialty Hospital. Neither Dr. Johnston nor any immediate family member has received anything of value from or has stock or stock options held in a commercial company or institution related directly or indirectly to the subject of this chapter.

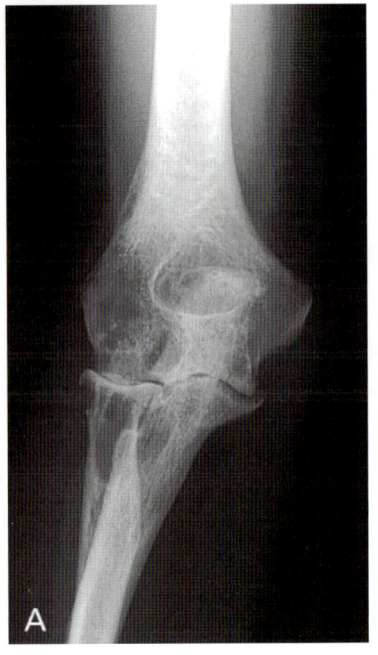

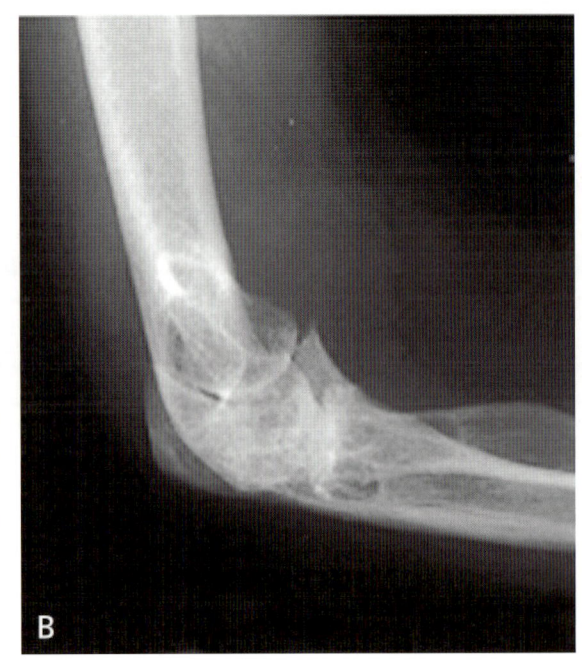

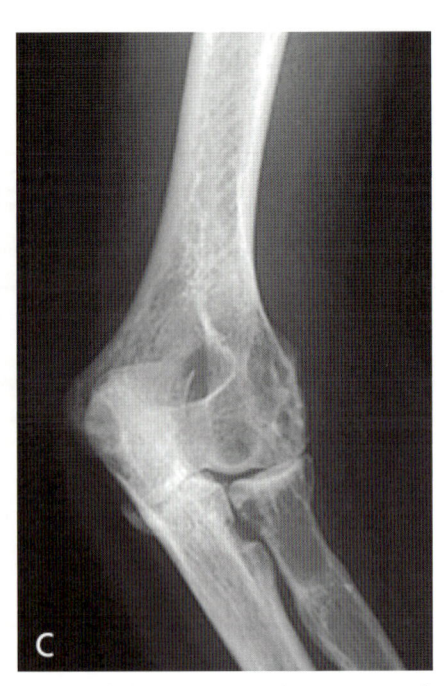

Figure 1 AP (**A**), lateral (**B**), and oblique (**C**) radiographs of the elbow of a patient with rheumatoid arthritis demonstrate joint destruction and cyst formation in the capitellum severe enough to consider total elbow arthroplasty.

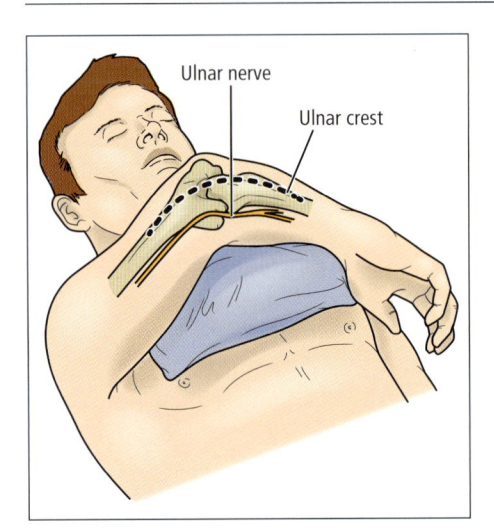

Figure 2 Illustration shows patient positioning for total elbow arthroplasty.

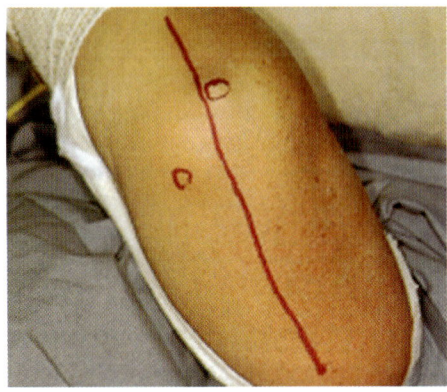

Figure 3 Photograph shows the skin incision for total elbow arthroplasty marked on a left elbow. Note that a straight incision is made just off the medial aspect of the olecranon. (Reproduced with permission from Morrey BM: Semiconstrained total elbow arthroplasty, in Morrey BF, ed: *Master Techniques in Orthopaedic Surgery: The Elbow*. Philadelphia, PA, Lippincott Williams & Wilkins, 2002, p 315.)

Surgical Technique

After the extremity is exsanguinated and the tourniquet is inflated, a straight posterior skin incision is made just off the tip of the olecranon extending approximately 9 cm proximal and 8 cm distal to the olecranon (**Figure 3**). Subcutaneous flaps are elevated but not in excess of what is needed for exposure because elderly patients and those with rheumatoid arthritis are at risk for wound complications. A subcutaneous pocket is created for subcutaneous transposition of the ulnar nerve, which should be performed in all cases. In primary surgery, the ulnar nerve is carefully identified and mobilized from its proximal location at the medial aspect of the triceps (arcade of Struthers) to the first motor branch to the flexor carpi ulnaris (FCU). A Penrose drain or vessel loop is placed around the nerve to facilitate dissection. A 1-cm portion of the distal medial intermuscular septum is excised to prevent nerve constriction as it passes anteriorly for the transposition (**Figure 4**). If the nerve has been previously transposed, its location is identified, but no formal dissection is performed unless necessary for exposure to avoid nerve injury.

Management of the triceps is guided by the underlying pathology, the type of implant to be used, and surgeon preference. Triceps insufficiency is a recognized but underappreciated complication of triceps-reflecting approaches.[1] Therefore, every effort is made to maintain the integrity of the triceps insertion. Several approaches are used in TEA, each with advantages and disadvantages. The traditional Mayo triceps-reflecting approach (Bryan-Morrey) and triceps-on approach will be described in detail.

Bryan-Morrey Triceps-Reflecting Approach

The Bryan-Morrey triceps-reflecting approach is performed by reflecting the triceps tendon, forearm fascia, and periosteum as one unit from medial to lateral off the olecranon.[2] The medial aspect of the triceps is elevated off the posterior humerus to the tip of the olecranon. The superficial fascia between the anconeus and the FCU is incised from the posteromedial border of the ulna distally. The triceps in continuity with the anconeus is subperiosteally elevated from the tip of the olecranon from medial to lateral as a single layer (**Figure 5**). Further lateral elevation of the triceps-anconeus exposes the radiocapitellar joint. The lateral and medial collateral ligaments are released from their origin on the humeral epicondyle. This allows the ulnohumeral joint to be dislocated, exposing the articular surfaces of the elbow. If ligamentous integrity is necessary (unlinked arthroplasty), then the lateral ulnar collateral ligament

Chapter 34: Total Elbow Arthroplasty

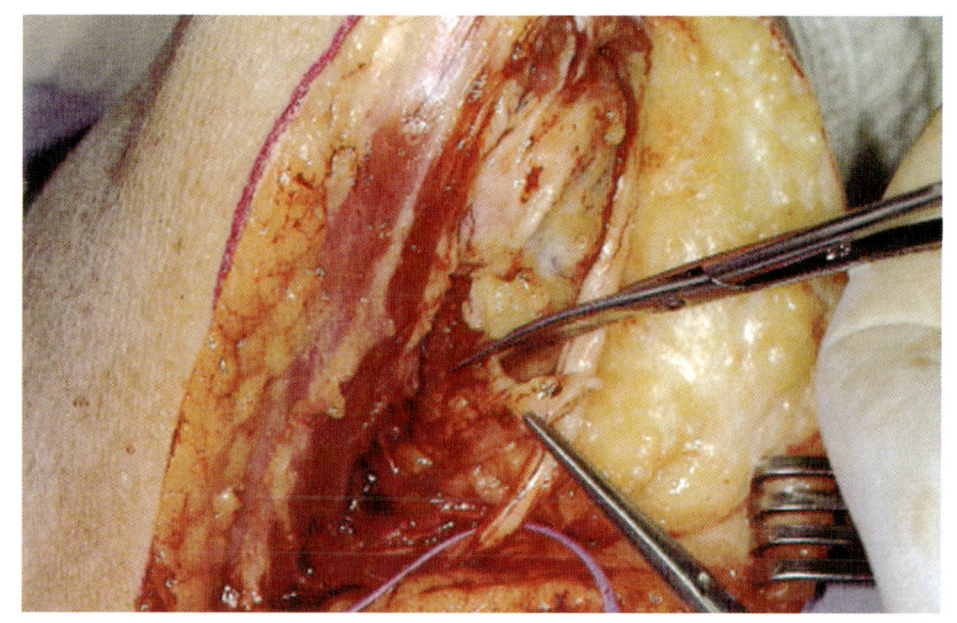

Figure 4 Intraoperative photograph demonstrates resection of the medial intramuscular septum. The ulnar nerve has been transposed into an anterior subcutaneous pocket. (Reproduced with permission from Morrey BF: Semiconstrained total elbow replacement, in Morrey BF, ed: *Master Techniques in Orthopaedic Surgery: The Elbow.* Philadelphia, PA, Lippincott Williams & Wilkins, 2002, p 316.)

and the medial collateral ligament should be tagged so they can be reattached via bone tunnels in the humerus during closure. To improve visualization of the distal humerus, the tip of the olecranon can be removed with a rongeur (**Figure 6**). Finally, the shoulder is externally rotated and the elbow is flexed, allowing the ulna to separate from the humerus.

Triceps-Sparing Approach

The tripceps-sparing (triceps-on) approach is an excellent option for management of acute fracture and cases of humeral nonunion; it is our preferred approach with a linked implant.[3,4] The medial and lateral borders of the triceps are identified, and the triceps is completely mobilized bluntly from the posterior humerus to the proximal ulna (**Figure 7**). The triceps is separated from the underlying joint capsule, which is resected to aid exposure. The flexor-pronator group and the medial collateral ligament are

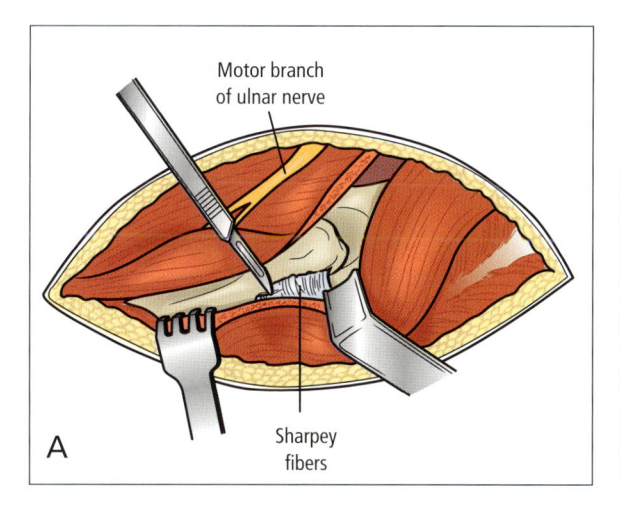

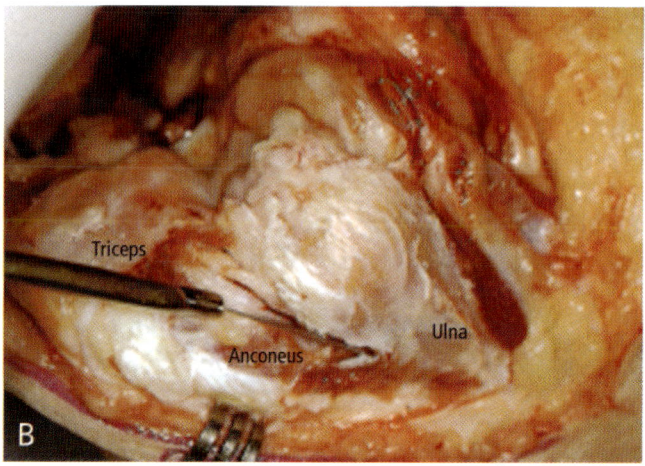

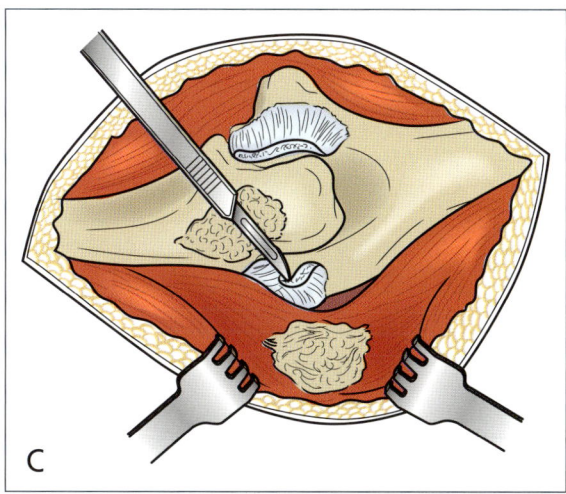

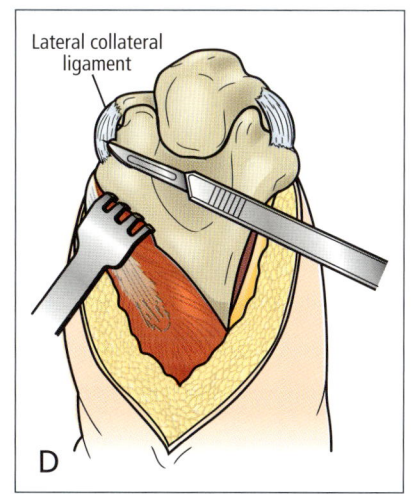

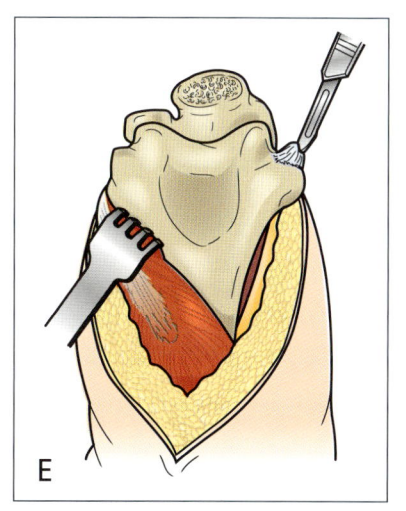

Figure 5 The Bryan-Morrey triceps-reflecting approach. **A,** The triceps in continuity with the anconeus is reflected from the ulna. **B,** Intraoperative photograph demonstrates the Bryan-Morrey approach. **C,** Further elevation laterally allows identification of the radiocapitellar joint. The lateral (**D**) and medial (**E**) collateral ligaments are released, allowing dislocation of the joint. (Panel B adapted with permission from Morrey BM: Semiconstrained total elbow arthroplasty, in Morrey BF, ed: *Master Techniques in Orthopaedic Surgery: The Elbow.* Philadelphia, PA, Lippincott Williams & Wilkins, 2002, p 317.)

© 2013 American Academy of Orthopaedic Surgeons

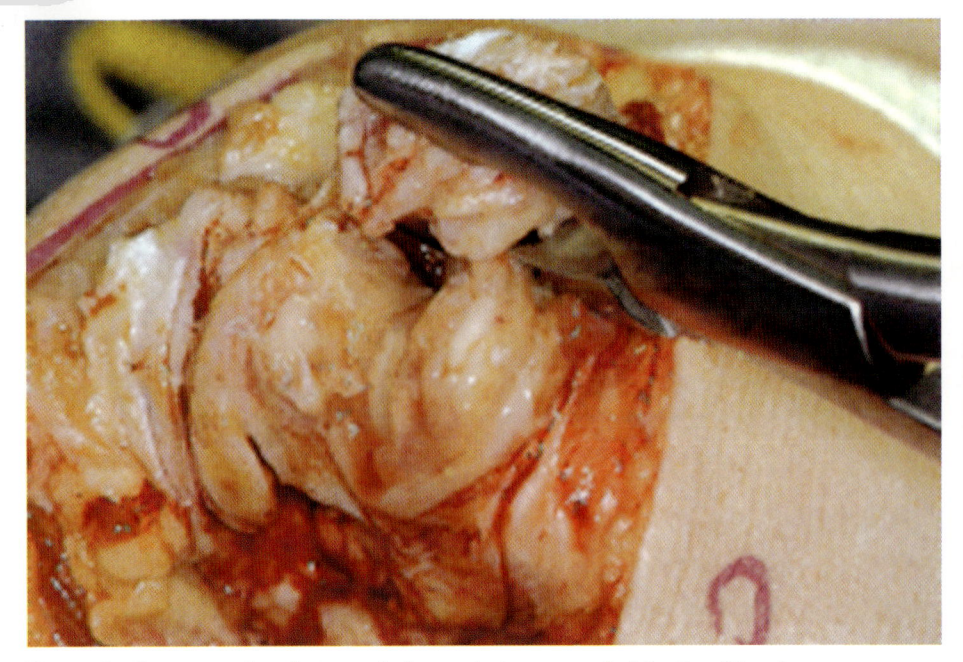

Figure 6 Intraoperative photograph demonstrates removal of the tip of the olecranon. (Reproduced with permission from Morrey BM: Semiconstrained total elbow arthroplasty, in Morrey BF, ed: *Master Techniques in Orthopaedic Surgery: The Elbow*. Philadelphia, PA, Lippincott Williams & Wilkins, 2002, p 318.)

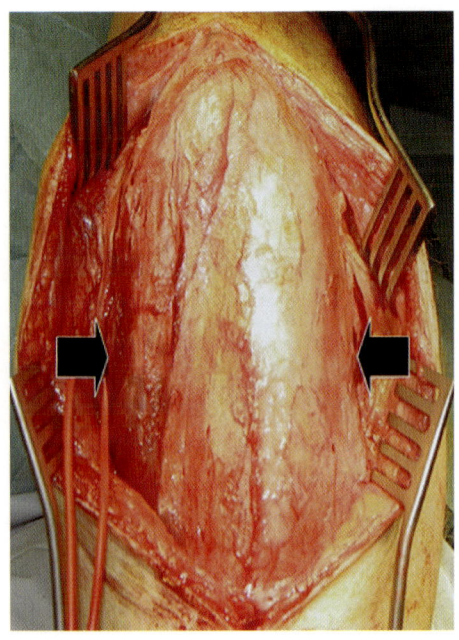

Figure 7 Intraoperative photograph shows the triceps-sparing approach, in which the medial and lateral aspects of the triceps are developed. (Reproduced with permission from Kamineni S: Elbow replacement for acute trauma, in Wiesel SW, ed: *Operative Techniques in Shoulder and Elbow Surgery*. Philadelphia, PA, Lippincott Williams & Wilkins, 2011, p 395.)

subperiosteally dissected from the medial epicondyle. In a similar fashion, the common extensor tendons and the lateral collateral ligament complex are released from the lateral epicondyle. Through the medial and lateral windows, the anterior capsule is released. This completes the circumferential release of the elbow, allowing the joint to be dislocated. The humerus is delivered through the lateral triceps defect to permit bony preparation. Exposure to the ulna for preparation and instrumentation is attained by supinating the forearm, turning the triceps back on itself. This is the most challenging aspect of this approach.

Bone Preparation

Bone preparation is started on the humeral side by removing the central portion of the trochlea. The roof of the olecranon fossa is identified. The intramedullary canal of the humerus is identified by opening a window in the roof of the olecranon fossa (**Figure 8**). Implant-specific cutting jigs are used to guide the resection of the distal humerus. The degree of distal humeral bone resection and cut accuracy is dependent on the implant system that is being used. When an unlinked implant is selected, it is essential to balance the soft tissues with varying degrees of humeral resection and ensure an anatomic fit of the humeral component between the condyles. With excessive bone loss, the posterior flat surface of the supracondylar region is identified because this plane approximates the axis of rotation of the humerus.

The intramedullary canal of the ulna is entered with a high-speed burr at the base of the coronoid (**Figure 9**). The opening of the canal is enlarged to allow unencumbered passage of the ulnar broach. The broaches must be passed parallel to the subcutaneous border of the ulna to ensure proper placement of the prosthesis down the medullary canal and prevent undersizing of the component that occurs by broaching the canal at too steep an angle. Attention to bone quality and the integrity of the medullary canal is essential, particularly in patients with rheumatoid arthritis because it is easy to perforate the thin cortices if the broach is

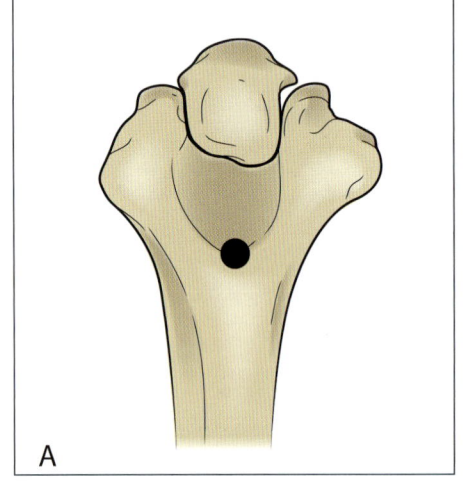

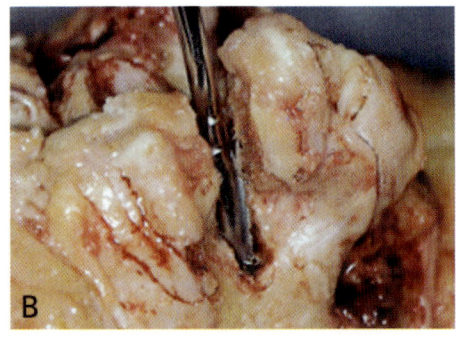

Figure 8 Bone preparation for total elbow arthroplasty. **A,** The intramedullary canal of the humerus is opened by creating a cortical window in the roof of the olecranon fossa. The black dot indicates the entry point to the intramedullary canal. **B,** Intraoperative photograph demonstrates the identification of the intramedullary canal of the humerus through a window created in the roof of the olecranon fossa. (Panel B reproduced with permission from Morrey BM: Semiconstrained total elbow arthroplasty, in Morrey BF, ed: *Master Techniques in Orthopaedic Surgery: The Elbow*. Philadelphia, PA, Lippincott Williams & Wilkins, 2002, p 320.)

not perfectly aligned with the medullary canal.

The radial head is an important stabilizer to both valgus and axial forces, but it can be sacrificed when using a linked implant and with some unlinked designs.

After preparation, trial implants are inserted and a trial reduction is performed to assess alignment, stability, and component tracking. When using a linked implant, full flexion-extension range of motion should be obtained. With an unlinked implant, many surgeons do not aggressively pursue full extension because instability typically occurs near terminal extension. If there is unacceptable limitation of motion, the components should be evaluated for bony impingement, which commonly occurs posteriorly (olecranon impinging on the humerus) or anteriorly (coronoid tip impinging on the humeral component's anterior flange). The soft-tissue elements contributing to contracture need to be fully evaluated and released if necessary. With an unlinked implant, the humeral and ulnar components must align with each other throughout the flexion arc without any pistoning in and out of the bone. If pistoning occurs, the bone preparation and soft-tissue tension must be reexamined and modified to remedy the problem. If stability cannot be obtained, the unlinked implant should be converted to a linked implant.

In the setting of comminuted distal humeral fractures with bone loss or severe contracture with stiffness, up to 2 cm of the distal humerus can be resected without compromising extension strength.[5] Usually, longer stemmed implants are used in this setting to compensate for the loss of bone support in the metaphyseal region.

Cementing is performed with antibiotic-impregnated cement. A long flexible cement nozzle facilitates cement introduction into the intramedullary canal (**Figure 10**). The cement should be a somewhat liquid consistency to flow easily through the nozzle. Methylene blue is added to the cement to facilitate identification of the bone-cement interface if revision surgery is required in the future. Cement restrictors are placed in the humerus and, if possible, the ulna to improve canal pressurization. With a linked implant, the humeral component is seated to re-create the axis of rotation of the distal humerus, and a prepared bone wafer is inserted between the anterior humeral cortex and the flange. The ulnar component is placed to the depth needed to re-create the axis of rotation of the greater sigmoid notch. When using certain linked implants, the components are coupled with an axis pin before the final seating of the humeral component (**Figure 11**). If the components will be inserted unlinked, the humeral component is cemented such that the axis of rotation of the implant coincides with the axis of rotation of the humerus defined at the medial and lateral epicondyles. Similarly, the ulnar component is inserted to reestablish the axis of rotation of the forearm passing through the center of the greater sigmoid notch and the center of the radial head. The previously tagged collateral ligaments are repaired to their anatomic origins on the humerus.

After the cement has hardened, the triceps, if previously reflected, is reattached to the ulna through cruciate tunnels with No. 5 nonabsorbable suture passed through the triceps in a Bunnell fashion. An additional horizontal tunnel allows passage of suture to "cinch" the triceps securely to the olecranon to prevent synovial fluid extravasation behind the repair (**Figure 12**). All knots are tied with the elbow at 90° of flexion, and the knots are oriented to the side to avoid a subcutaneous prominence. The fascia of the

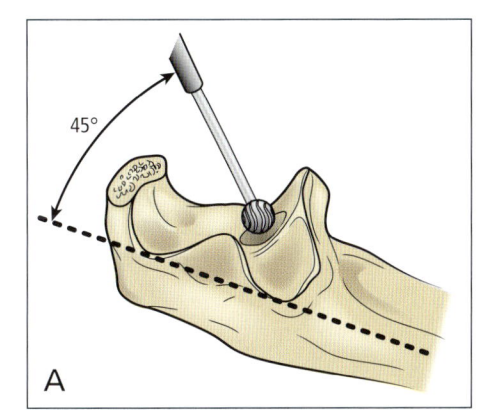

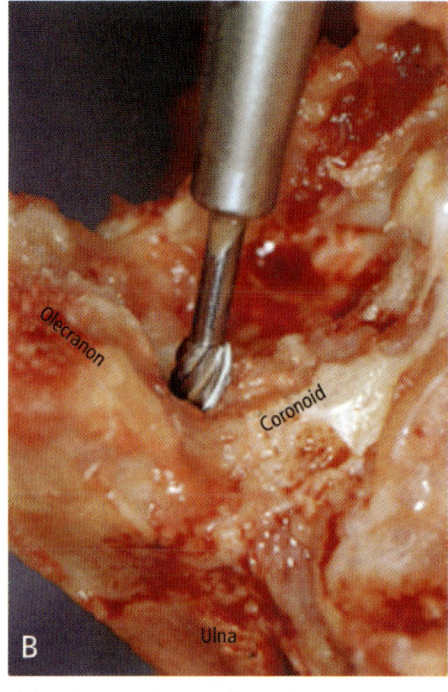

Figure 9 Opening of the intramedullary canal of the ulna. **A,** A cortical window is created at the base of the greater sigmoid notch. **B,** Intraoperative photograph demonstrates the identification of the intramedullary canal of the ulna. (Panel B reproduced with permission from Morrey BM: Semiconstrained total elbow arthroplasty, in Morrey BF, ed: *Master Techniques in Orthopaedic Surgery: The Elbow.* Philadelphia, PA, Lippincott Williams & Wilkins, 2002, p 323.)

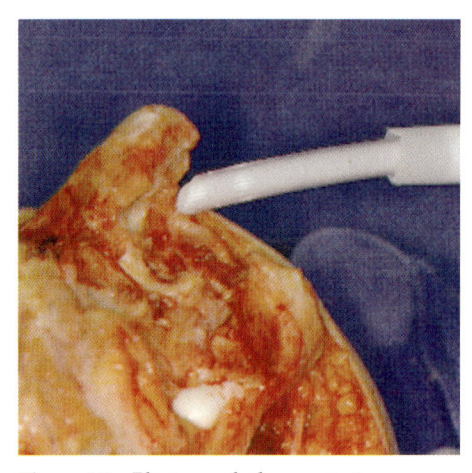

Figure 10 Photograph demonstrates cement introduction into the intramedullary canal with a long flexible cement nozzle. The consistency of the cement needs to be somewhat liquid to flow through the long nozzle. (Reproduced with permission from Morrey BF: Semiconstrained total elbow replacement, in Morrey BF, ed: *Master Techniques in Orthopaedic Surgery: The Elbow.* Philadelphia, PA, Lippincott Williams & Wilkins, 2002, p 327.)

FCU and the anconeus is repaired to surrounding tissue with absorbable suture, and the ulnar nerve is transposed into the prepared subcutaneous pocket. The tourniquet is deflated and hemostasis is obtained, followed by skin closure over a subcutaneous drain.

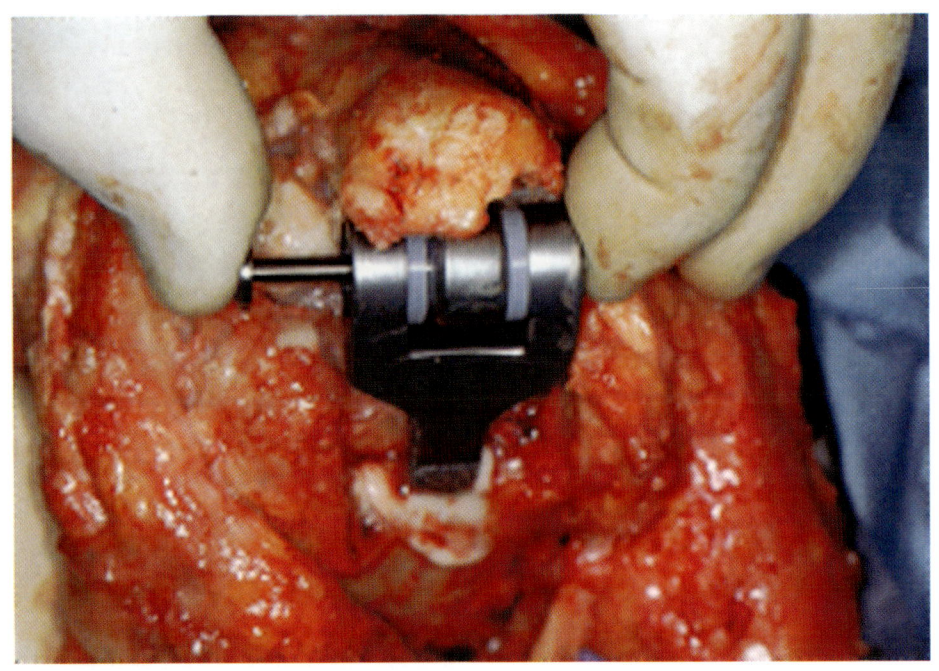

Figure 11 Intraoperative photograph shows articulation of the humeral and ulnar components in a total elbow arthroplasty by placing an axis pin. The humerus is then seated to its final depth. (Reproduced with permission from Morrey BM: Semiconstrained total elbow arthroplasty, in Morrey BF, ed: *Master Techniques in Orthopaedic Surgery: The Elbow.* Philadelphia, PA, Lippincott Williams & Wilkins, 2002, p 329.)

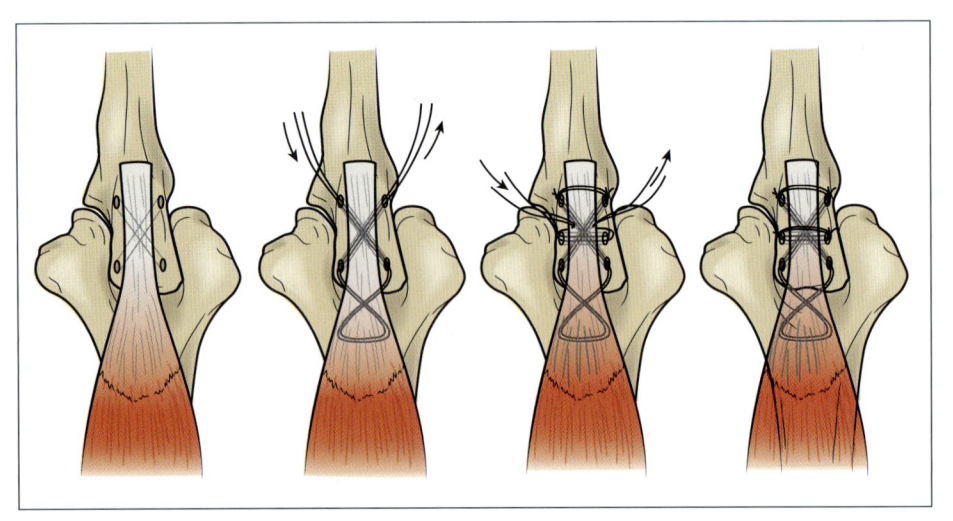

Figure 12 Illustration shows reattachment of the triceps in a total elbow arthroplasty via cruciate drill holes supplemented by a transverse "cinch" suture.

Complications

Deep infection remains the most ominous complication of TEA, with rates reported between 2% and 11%.[6-10] Certain patient groups are at a higher risk. Inflammatory arthritides requiring immunosuppressive therapy and posttraumatic arthritis with multiple previous surgeries have been identified as risk factors for infection. Infection following joint arthroplasty may also be the result of hematogenous seeding from a remote infectious source. Treatment, rarely nonsurgical, depends on the presence of component loosening and the infecting organism. With well-fixed implants, an attempt is made to preserve the implants. Repeated irrigation and débridement is often required to eradicate the infection. The success of eradicating the infection in the face of a well-fixed implant depends on the infecting organism. *Staphylococcus epidermidis* and gram-negative infections often respond poorly to irrigation and débridement alone and may require the removal of components to eradicate the infection.[11] There may be value in attempting irrigation and débridement in these infections, even though the success rate is low because the morbidity of removing well-fixed components is considerable. The physician should discuss with the patient the risks and benefits of irrigation and débridement with component retention versus component removal. Prosthetic infection with gross loosening of the implants is treated with component removal, the placement of an antibiotic spacer, and appropriate intravenous antibiotics, followed by staged reimplantation.

Instability following TEA is almost exclusively associated with unlinked implants.[6,12,13] Instability is classified as immediate, early, or late. Immediate instability occurs during the hospital admission and is usually due to component malposition.[14] Early instability occurs within 6 weeks and, if the implants are in good position, is usually due to attenuation or rupture of soft-tissue stabilizers. Late instability occurs after 6 weeks and usually results from trauma, limb malalignment, component malposition, or polyethylene wear. Instability can be quite obvious, with gross deformity; or it can be difficult to detect, often with a subtle presentation. The rare instances of instability in linked implants are due to disruption of the linking mechanism from polyethylene bushing wear in snap-fit articulations or disengagement of the axis-pin linking system.[15] Immediate and early instability can be prevented with attention to component placement and postoperative limitations to protect soft-tissue repairs. Patient selection and reinforcement of limitations can prevent instability and ultimately improve the implant survival.

Loosening is most commonly associated with linked fully constrained implants, although rates have decreased with the advent of unlinked and semiconstrained designs.[16-18] Improved cementing technique has improved the mechanical pull-out and push-out strength of the implant.[19] Diagnosis is typically based on a history of increasing pain and radiographic evidence of radiolucent lines, component subsidence, fracture of the cement mantle, or a change in position of the implant. It is critical to rule out infection in any prosthesis demonstrating evidence of loosening. Patient age and activity level, the degree of bony involvement, and the ability to restore the axis of the elbow joint guide the surgeon toward revision TEA, arthrodesis, or resection arthroplasty.

Periprosthetic fractures occur either during the procedure (intraoperative) or following the procedure, with rates in some series as high as 23%.[20-22] The surgeon must have a high suspicion for fractures intraoperatively; if not treated, these can lead to early loosening, pain, and dysfunction. Potential sources include stem-canal mismatches and poor exposure in osteopenic bone. Fractures should be managed with plates, strut allografting, and revision with long-stemmed implants. Periprosthetic fractures need to be critically evaluated for component loosening because the integrity of the bone-cement-implant interface and the fracture location guide the treatment. Most periprosthetic fractures are the final manifestation of a loose implant.

Triceps insufficiency is an under-recognized complication of TEA.[1] Tissue quality, which is compromised in inflammatory arthropathy, or the approach used can increase the risk of attenuation or rupture of the triceps tendon. Triceps insufficiency can present as weakness of the elbow during overhead activity and posterior elbow pain. Pierce and Herndon[3] demonstrated that the triceps-sparing approach decreased the incidence of triceps insufficiency when compared with a triceps-reflecting approach.

Ulnar neuropathy is a not uncommon complication of TEA, with rates of permanent deficits reported to be as high as 10% and transient paresthesias in up to 26% of cases.[6,12,23] Ulnar nerve transposition has decreased rates of permanent deficits, and transient deficits usually resolve within 3 to 6 months with observation.

Postoperative wound problems are of particular concern in TEA.[6,23-25] This frustrating complication can be attributed to previous surgery, poor tissue quality, and immunosuppression. Rates have decreased with attention to soft-tissue management, the use of drains, and postoperative immobilization.

Postoperative Care and Rehabilitation

The extremity is placed in a well-padded dressing with a volar splint in full extension to protect the posterior incision. The extremity dressing is taken down at 48 hours for wound inspection; then the elbow is covered with a soft dressing and placed in a sling for comfort.

The wound takes priority over early motion and, if there is any concern over the wound, a period of immobilization and splinting is used. Rehabilitation is only begun when the wound looks healthy and is dictated by the triceps management intraoperatively. If the triceps was reflected, active extension is avoided for 6 weeks, allowing time for healing to the ulna. Gravity-assisted extension and passive extension are permitted. If the triceps is left intact, active motion in all planes is permitted. With each patient visit, the lifetime restrictions of 10 lb in a single event and 5 lb in repetitive lifting are reinforced. No formal physical therapy is prescribed because activities of daily living are usually sufficient.

Pearls

- A careful history, physical examination, and radiographic evaluation should be performed with attention to underlying pathology, associated deformities, previous surgery, and immunosuppressive therapies.
- Patient selection is critical. Success requires compliant patients with realistic expectations and understanding of the postoperative activity limitations.
- Preoperative planning, with critical attention to bone quality/architecture and ligamentous integrity, is key to the selection of an appropriate linked or unlinked implant.
- Careful identification, dissection, and protection of the ulnar nerve throughout the procedure is necessary, with anterior subcutaneous transposition before closure.
- The approach—triceps-reflecting versus triceps sparing—is selected based on surgeon experience and underlying pathology. Careful intraoperative and postoperative management of the triceps will help prevent insufficiency.
- Complete releases of the capsule, excision of scar tissue in the olecranon/coronoid fossa, and release of the triceps from the posterior cortex of the humerus are essential to optimize exposure and range of motion.
- The lateral ulnar collateral ligament and the medial collateral ligament should be tagged for anatomic repair to the humerus for an unlinked implant.
- The use of trial components, with close attention to soft-tissue tensioning, range of motion, and implant stability, is helpful, particularly with an unlinked implant.
- Bony impingement can occur posteriorly between the olecranon and the humerus and anteriorly between the coronoid and the anterior humeral flange of a linked prosthesis.
- Antibiotic cement should be used with intramedullary cement restrictors in the humerus and the ulna.
- Components should be seated to recreate the axis of rotation of the distal humerus and ulna.
- A postoperative extension splint should be used for 48 hours with a subcutaneous drain.
- A conservative postoperative course will reinforce functional limitations.

References

1. Celli A, Arash A, Adams RA, Morrey BF: Triceps insufficiency following total elbow arthroplasty. *J Bone Joint Surg Am* 2005;87(9):1957-1964.
2. Bryan RS, Morrey BF: Extensive posterior exposure of the elbow: A triceps-sparing approach. *Clin Orthop Relat Res* 1982;166:188-192.
3. Pierce TD, Herndon JH: The triceps preserving approach to total elbow arthroplasty. *Clin Orthop Relat Res* 1998;354:144-152.
4. Alonso-Llames M: Bilaterotricipital approach to the elbow: Its application in the osteosynthesis of supracondylar fractures of the humerus in children. *Acta Orthop Scand* 1972;43(6):479-490.
5. Hughes RE, Schneeberger AG, An KN, Morrey BF, O'Driscoll SW: Reduction of triceps muscle force after shortening of the distal humerus: A computational model. *J Shoulder Elbow Surg* 1997;6(5):444-448.
6. Davis RF, Weiland AJ, Hungerford DS, Moore JR, Volenec-Dowling S: Nonconstrained total elbow arthroplasty. *Clin Orthop Relat Res* 1982;171:156-160.
7. Gutow AP, Wolfe SW: Infection following total elbow arthroplasty. *Hand Clin* 1994;10(3):521-529.
8. Morrey BF, Bryan RS: Complications of total elbow arthroplasty. *Clin Orthop Relat Res* 1982;170:204-212.
9. Morrey BF, Bryan RS: Infection after total elbow arthroplasty. *J Bone Joint Surg Am* 1983;65(3):330-338.
10. Wolfe SW, Figgie MP, Inglis AE, Bohn WW, Ranawat CS: Management of infection about total elbow prostheses. *J Bone Joint Surg Am* 1990;72(2):198-212.
11. Yamaguchi K, Adams RA, Morrey BF: Infection after total elbow arthroplasty. *J Bone Joint Surg Am* 1998;80(4):481-491.
12. Trancik T, Wilde AH, Borden LS: Capitellocondylar total elbow arthroplasty: Two- to eight-year experience. *Clin Orthop Relat Res* 1987;223:175-180.

13. Ewald FC, Jacobs MA: Total elbow arthroplasty. *Clin Orthop Relat Res* 1984;182:137-142.

14. King GJ, Itoi E, Niebur GL, Morrey BF, An KN: Motion and laxity of the capitellocondylar total elbow prosthesis. *J Bone Joint Surg Am* 1994;76(7):1000-1008.

15. Wright TW, Hastings H: Total elbow arthroplasty failure due to overuse, C-ring failure, and/or bushing wear. *J Shoulder Elbow Surg* 2005;14(1):65-72.

16. Morrey BF, Bryan RS, Dobyns JH, Linscheid RL: Total elbow arthroplasty: A five-year experience at the Mayo Clinic. *J Bone Joint Surg Am* 1981;63(7):1050-1063.

17. Garrett JC, Ewald FC, Thomas WH, Sledge CB: Loosening associated with G.S.B. hinge total elbow replacement in patients with rheumatoid arthritis. *Clin Orthop Relat Res* 1977;127:170-174.

18. Goldberg VM, Figgie HE III, Inglis AE, Figgie MP: Total elbow arthroplasty. *J Bone Joint Surg Am* 1988;70(5):778-783.

19. Faber KJ, Cordy ME, Milne AD, Chess DG, King GJ, Johnson JA: Advanced cement technique improves fixation in elbow arthroplasty. *Clin Orthop Relat Res* 1997;334:150-156.

20. Carroll EA, Lorich DG, Helfet DL: Surgical management of a periprosthetic fracture between a total elbow and total shoulder prostheses: A case report. *J Shoulder Elbow Surg* 2009;18(3):e9-e12.

21. O'Driscoll SW, Morrey BF: Periprosthetic fractures about the elbow. *Orthop Clin North Am* 1999;30(2):319-325.

22. Sanchez-Sotelo J, O'Driscoll S, Morrey BF: Periprosthetic humeral fractures after total elbow arthroplasty: Treatment with implant revision and strut allograft augmentation. *J Bone Joint Surg Am* 2002;84(9):1642-1650.

23. Ewald FC, Scheinberg RD, Poss R, Thomas WH, Scott RD, Sledge CB: Capitellocondylar total elbow arthroplasty. *J Bone Joint Surg Am* 1980;62(8):1259-1263.

24. Gill DR, Morrey BF: The Coonrad-Morrey total elbow arthroplasty in patients who have rheumatoid arthritis: A ten to fifteen-year follow-up study. *J Bone Joint Surg Am* 1998;80(9):1327-1335.

25. Inglis AE, Pellicci PM: Total elbow replacement. *J Bone Joint Surg Am* 1980;62(8):1252-1258.

Hand and Wrist

Section Editor
Edward Diao, MD

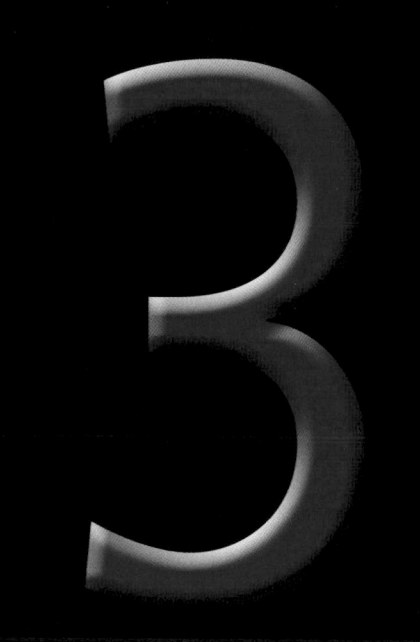

3

35 **Carpal Tunnel Release** 235
Edward Diao, MD

36 **Surgical Treatment of Cubital Tunnel Syndrome** 241
Reimer Hoffmann, MD; John D. Lubahn, MD

37 **First Dorsal Extensor Compartment Release** 247
Aaron I. Venouziou, MD; Filippos S. Giannoulis, MD;
Dean G. Sotereanos, MD

38 **Trigger Finger Release** 253
Randy Bindra, MD; Micah Sinclair, MD

39 **Open Reduction and Internal Fixation of the Distal Radius
With a Volar Locking Plate** 259
Jesse B. Jupiter, MD; David Ring, MD, PhD

40 **External Fixation of Distal Radius Fractures** 263
Michael V. Birman, MD; Jonathan R. Danoff, MD;
Neil J. White, MD; Melvin P. Rosenwasser, MD

41 **Open Reduction and Internal Fixation of Scaphoid Fractures** 269
Kristofer S. Matullo, MD; Alexander Y. Shin, MD

42 **Open Reduction and Internal Fixation of Phalangeal Fractures** 275
William B. Geissler, MD

43 **Surgical Fixation of Metacarpal Fractures** 281
William B. Geissler, MD; Christopher A. Keen, MD

44 **Excision of Ganglion Cysts of the Wrist and Hand** 287
Daniel J. Nagle, MD; Jay V. Kalawadia, MD

45 Surgical Excision of Digital Mucous Cysts 293
Matthew M. Tomaino, MD, MBA

46 Surgical Treatment of Basal Joint Arthritis of the Thumb 295
Edward Diao, MD

47 Partial Palmar Fasciectomy for Dupuytren Disease 305
*Thomas P. Lehman, PT, MD; Steven L. Peterson, MD, DVM;
Ghazi Rayan, MD*

Chapter 35
Carpal Tunnel Release

Edward Diao, MD

Introduction

Carpal tunnel syndrome (CTS) is a common condition, with a 1% to 5% incidence in the adult population. Making an accurate diagnosis of CTS is a critical aspect of successful management and treatment because many other conditions can mimic CTS. The surgeon should not confuse a vague symptom of arm numbness with CTS.

CTS is associated with pain in the distal third of the forearm and the volar wrist area. Characteristic paresthesias occur in the median nerve distribution, involving the thumb, the index finger, the long finger, and the radial portion of the ring finger. However, this anatomic distribution may not occur if there is more proximal nerve compression, multiple nerve compression, or an innervation anomaly such as a Martin-Gruber anastomosis.

The carpal tunnel compression test, in which the examiner exerts finger pressure over the wrist and the median nerve, is useful.[1] A combination of a positive Tinel sign, the Phalen maneuver, and carpal tunnel compression, with appropriate negative aspects of the physical examination to screen for alternative conditions, has been shown to be both sensitive for and specific to CTS, as proved by electrodiagnostic testing.

Once a diagnosis of CTS has been made, nonsurgical treatment is recommended. This may include activity modification, the use of wrist braces, the use of oral nonsteroidal anti-inflammatory drugs or corticosteroids, and a trial of cortisone and local anesthetic injection into the carpal canal.

If nonsurgical treatment fails and the patient presents with significant symptoms, carpal tunnel release (CTR) should be considered. CTR has evolved over the years from a standard open procedure with a long palm and forearm incision to limited incision and endoscopic techniques. These treatments are effective, but there are also reports of complications with all of the treatments. The key objective of the surgery is to completely divide the transverse carpal ligament without injury to the nerve. It is now well established that for index CTS surgery, internal neurolysis is not considered helpful and can be deleterious. Identification and knowledge of the anatomy in this area and the ability to differentiate the median nerve from the palmaris longus and the flexor tendons are key regardless of surgical technique and are based on the surgeon's knowledge and experience with the particular anatomy of the region affected by CTS.[2]

Patient Selection

The diagnosis of CTS is confirmed by a combination of the presence of classic clinical symptoms and signs and positive nerve conduction studies (NCS) and electromyographic (EMG) studies. If the NCS or EMG findings are negative, at least one trial of corticosteroid injection should be given to evaluate the clinical response. The surgeon should confirm that a trial of nonsurgical treatment has been undertaken without a cure and also confirm that differential diagnoses have been considered.

The presence of other conditions will affect the overall results of CTS treatment; this needs to be discussed with the patient before, not after, surgery. In fact, the surgeon should strongly consider delaying CTS treatment to control or improve other conditions that may be amenable to nonsurgical treatment, such as tendinitis of the wrist, forearm, or elbow.

If the above conditions are met, CTR should have good to excellent results in more than 95% of cases.[2] In the case of recurrent CTS, the key to success is patient selection. Although there are scant data to correlate the preoperative evaluation with results, the patient's clinical course and response to nonsurgical treatment along with the interpretation of electrodiagnostic studies and MRI should be carefully considered before revision surgery.

Outcomes

Good or excellent results can be expected in more than 95% of patients.[2] The randomized, double-blinded multicenter study from Trumble et al[2] compared open and single-portal endoscopic CTR and showed statistically significant improvements in the endoscopic group between 6 weeks and 3 months postoperatively in terms of pain and hand strength, compared with that of the open group, and equivalent good results in both groups at 1 year.

Stütz et al[3] reported on a retrospective series of 200 patients who underwent a secondary exploration during a 26-month period at a single institution for persistent or recurrent CTS symptoms after CTR. There were 108 cases of incomplete release of the transverse carpal ligament (TCL). Twelve patients had evidence of median nerve laceration during the index procedure, 46 patients had scarring of the nerve to surrounding tissues, and in 13 patients, the cause of the problem could not be determined.

Varitimidis et al[4] reviewed 22 patients (24 wrists) who underwent revision open CTR after an initial endoscopic CTR and who had persistent CTS. Twenty-two patients had incomplete TCL release. One patient had a partial and another patient a complete median nerve transection. One patient had a Guyon canal release instead of a CTR. Twenty patients returned to work, 15 at the previous level and 5 at lighter duty. The two patients with nerve injuries continued to do poorly, with one requiring a vein-wrapping procedure.

Electrodiagnostic Testing

Electrodiagnostic testing can be helpful in confirming the diagnosis of CTS and potentially eliminating secondary diagnoses. The earliest signs of CTS are generally an increase in sensory and motor latency followed by an increase in distal motor latency. Sometimes, a decrease in amplitude is a soft indicator of peripheral neuropathy. The degree of delay in latency and the degree of decrease in amplitude has some rough correlation with the severity of the neuropathy. Conduction velocity can be a helpful parameter. As the velocity moves from a normal

---

Dr. Diao or an immediate family member serves as a board member, owner, officer, or committee member of the American Society for Surgery of the Hand; is a member of a speakers' bureau or has made paid presentations on behalf of SBI, Stryker, and Auxilium; and has received research or institutional support from the National Institutes of Health (NIAMS & NICHD).

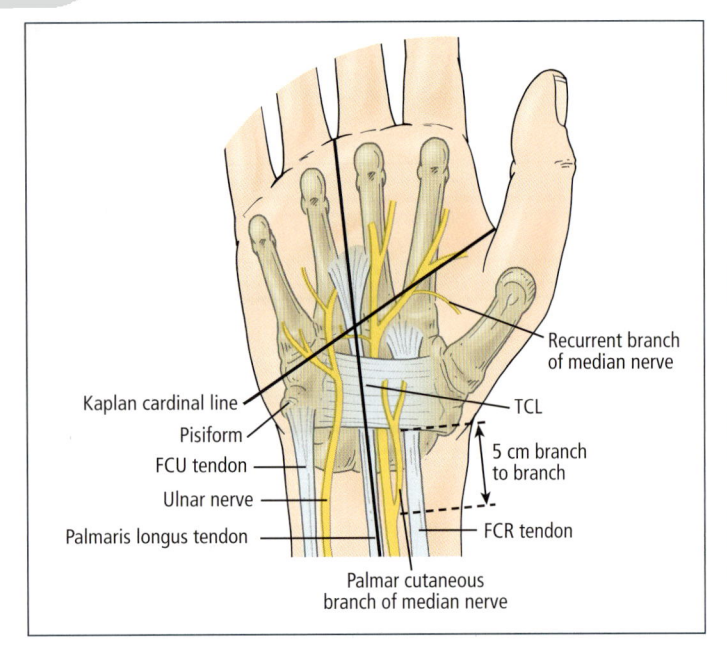

Figure 1 Illustration shows surface landmarks and critical deep structures to be considered when contemplating surgical release of the median nerve. FCR = flexor carpi radialis, FCU = flexor carpi ulnaris, TCL = transverse carpal ligament.

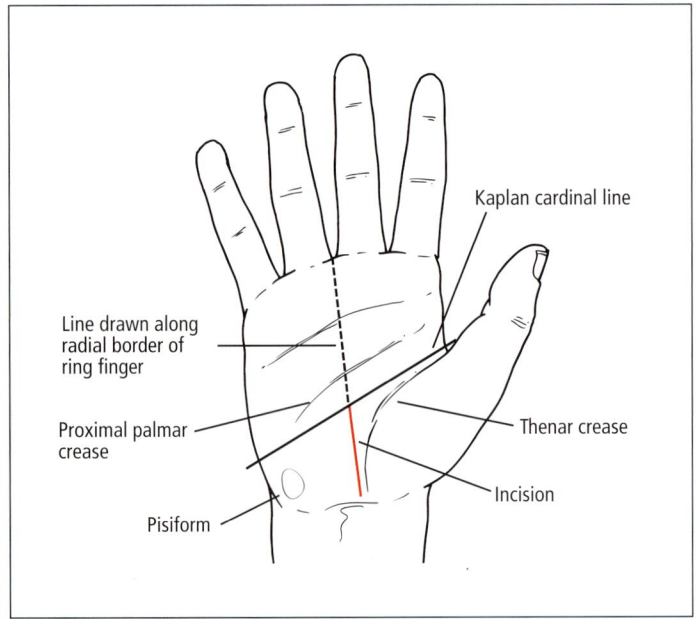

Figure 2 For open carpal tunnel release, the incision (red line) is made 2 mm ulnar to the thenar crease, just proximal to the Kaplan cardinal line (a line drawn from the apex of the interdigital fold between the thumb and index finger, toward the ulnar side of the hand and parallel with the proximal palmar crease, and passing 4 to 5 mm distal to the pisiform bone), and extended 3 to 4 cm proximally toward the distal wrist crease.

conduction velocity of 50 mps (m/s) to 60 mps down toward a conduction velocity of 30 mps, the trend is highly suggestive of peripheral neuropathy.

EMG of median nerve–innervated thenar muscles is helpful in that denervation patterns can be seen in cases of axonal degeneration with positive sharp waves and fibs highly suggestive of a chronic axonal neuropathy. The evaluation of the ulnar nerve at the wrist and the peripheral nerves across the elbow and the forearm can be also performed if there is clinical suspicion of this.

It should be noted that there is disagreement between the electrodiagnostic disciplines and the hand surgery disciplines regarding the sensitivity and the specificity of electrodiagnostic tests. It would be prudent for the physician to not use an NCS and EMG test as an initial screen for diagnosis of CTS. Rather, a careful history and physical examination should take a primary role in the diagnosis of CTS, with electrodiagnostic testing taking a secondary or supportive role in making the diagnosis. The false-positives in NCS- and EMG-diagnosed CTS derive from the fact that many of the conditions noted earlier are not particularly sensitive to electrodiagnostic testing, even if they are screened for. At the same time, there is a population of patients who exhibit all the signs and symptoms of CTS as a discrete diagnosis, but have normal NCS and EMG findings, thus having a false-negative result in electrodiagnostic testing.[5] These patients, whose histories and physical examinations have findings consistent with CTS, should be considered to have the diagnosis of CTS despite the negative electrodiagnostic studies. The surgeon should be careful to reevaluate these patients at multiple intervals if they are being treated nonsurgically and such treatment has failed, particularly if surgical treatment is being contemplated.

Procedure
Patient Positioning
- CTR surgery is performed with the arm outstretched on a hand table.
- Pneumatic tourniquet use facilitates the accurate identification of critical anatomic structures.
- Loupe magnification is recommended.
- Anesthesia can be by general anesthesia or regional anesthesia, such as an axillary block or Bier block.

Video 35.1 Carpal Tunnel Release. Edward Diao, MD (3 min)

Surgical Technique
General Principles
The goal of CTR surgery is to decompress the median nerve at the carpal canal by completely dividing the TCL to allow the carpal tunnel to expand.

Approach
A volar approach is used, but incision position and length vary. The locations of critical deep structures are inferred using superficial landmarks and a line drawn down the axis of the fourth ray and another drawn obliquely across the palm in line with the ulnar border of the abducted thumb (Kaplan cardinal line) (**Figure 1**).

Open CTR
Exposure
The skin incision location is marked, beginning at the intersection of the Kaplan cardinal line and a line drawn along the radial border of the fourth ray and ending at the wrist flexion crease. A longitudinal hypothenar crease is used if available (**Figure 2**).

The incision may be placed anywhere along this mark, depending on the surgeon's preference. I prefer the midpoint of the proximal third of the palm (**Figure 3, A**). The incision should be long enough to allow full access to the proximal to distal extent of the TCL to ensure full TCL division. This generally can be achieved without having the incision extend proximal to the wrist flexion crease.

The line is dissected with the incision using a scalpel or scissors, through the subcutaneous fat and the palmar fascia down to the TCL (**Figure 3, B**). Frequently, the palmaris brevis muscle is encoun-

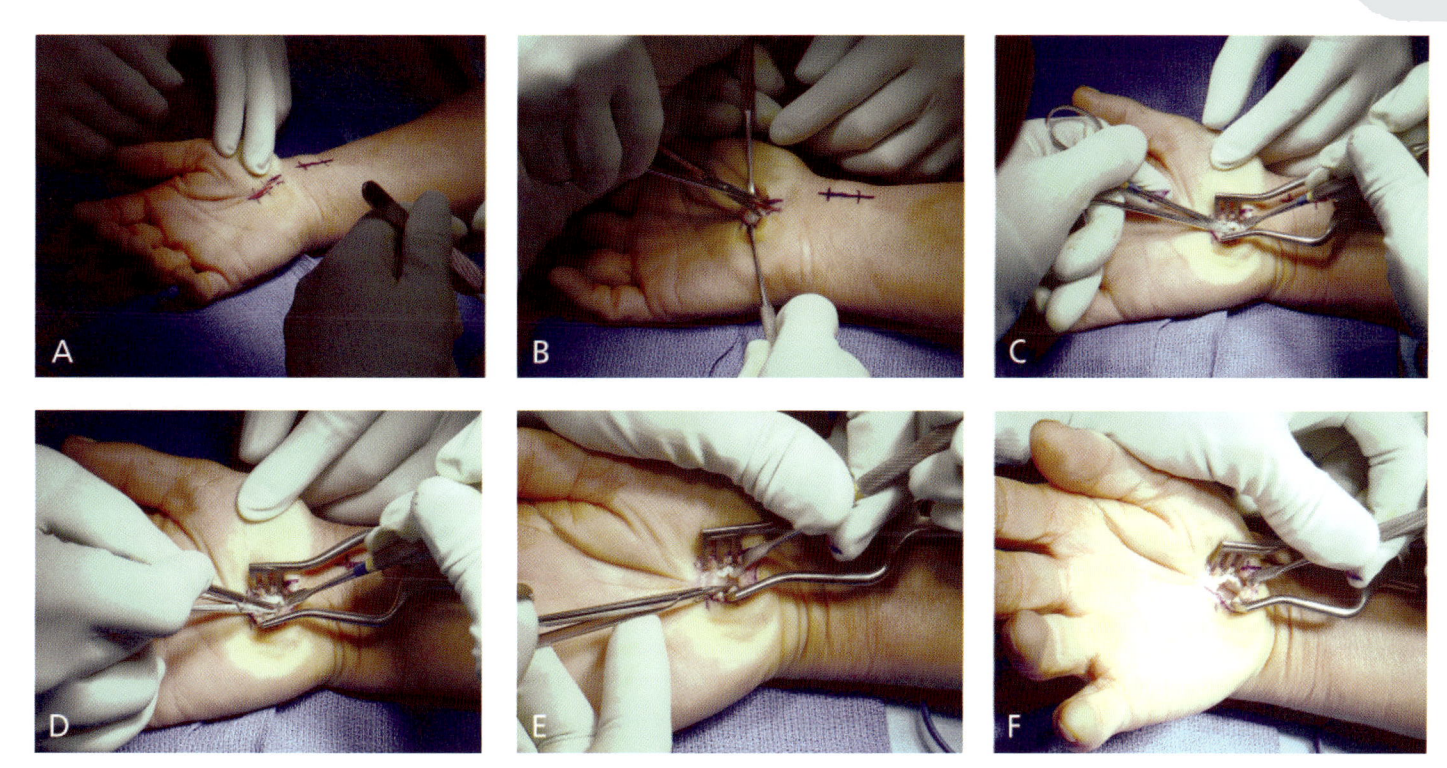

Figure 3 Intraoperative photographs demonstrate open carpal tunnel release. **A,** The incision is made. **B,** Dissection of the palm. **C,** A clamp is placed under the transverse carpal ligament (TCL). **D,** TCL division with a mini-meniscotome blade. **E,** Completion of the TCL division with scissors. **F,** Proximal fascia release.

tered directly superficial to the TCL. It is incised and "feathered" from the ligament to enable adequate visualization of the TCL.

The TCL is incised over a small segment, avoiding injury to deep structures. The contents of the carpal canal will have a characteristic appearance due to the tenosynovium. An instrument such as a mosquito clamp or a Carroll elevator is placed into the carpal canal, just deep to the TCL (**Figure 3, C**). This defines the undersurface of the TCL, the location of the hamate hook, and the proposed direction for release.

The superficial surface of the TCL is visualized along its course, and a right-angle retractor is placed to protect the critical structures located between the skin and the ligament.

TCL Release

The TCL is identified as ulnar as possible in the canal close to the hamate hook and then released under direct vision proximally and distally with a scalpel, scissors, or mini-meniscotome Beaver-type blade (**Figure 3, D**). A radially based TCL leaflet is kept over the median nerve, and the distal forearm fascia is released proximally (**Figure 3, E and F**). This tissue may be a secondary compression site.

The TCL is completely divided, and the median nerve and canal contents are inspected. In rare instances, a space-occupying lesion will require removal (eg, a "billowing" synovium in a patient with rheumatoid arthritis or a ganglion cyst). In primary CTR procedures without systemic disease, there is no role for internal neurolysis or tenosynovectomy.[6-8]

The wound is closed, and sterile dressings are applied. The use of a splint is based on the surgeon's preference, but recent studies have demonstrated superior clinical results if a full-time splint is not used postoperatively.

Single-Incision Endoscopic CTR (Modified Agee Technique)
Exposure

The palmaris longus, the flexor carpi radialis, and the flexor carpi ulnaris are marked out. A transverse 1- to 2-cm incision is made in the wrist flexion crease centered over or just ulnar to the palmaris longus (**Figure 4, A**). If the palmaris longus is not present, the incision is made halfway between the flexor carpi radialis and the flexor carpi ulnaris.

The palmaris longus is exposed and retracted radially with a Ragnell retractor. The flexor retinaculum is identified deep to this structure. The flexor retinaculum is incised, and a distally based U-shaped flap 1 cm wide is created (**Figure 4, B**). The flap is then elevated and retracted. A mosquito clamp can be used on the free edge of the flap to facilitate retraction. On the undersurface of the retinaculum, adherent tenosynovium is frequently seen. The tenosynovium-covered digital flexor tendons and the median nerve should be visible deep to the opening.

Small and large hamate finders are passed down the carpal canal in an antegrade manner to evaluate the space and location of the hamate. The tip of the instruments are palpated as they become subcutaneous distal to the distal edge of the TCL at the Kaplan cardinal line. The surgeon should make sure these instruments are not palpable subcutaneously in the proximal third of the palm, which would indicate incorrect placement superficial to the TCL and the carpal canal and probably within the canal of Guyon.

The tenosynovial elevator is passed proximally and distally a dozen times along the axis of the fourth ray to dissect tenosynovium from the undersurface of the TCL (**Figure 5**).

A "washboard" effect is felt as the instrument passes at right angles to the thick transverse collagen bundles of the TCL.

Device Insertion

The assembled endoscopic CTR device is introduced into the carpal canal, with the endoscope directed palmarly. The undersurface of the TCL, with its characteristic transverse striations, is visible. As the surgeon views the monitor, the instrument is advanced until the distal edge of the TCL is identified. The distal edge

Section 3: Hand and Wrist

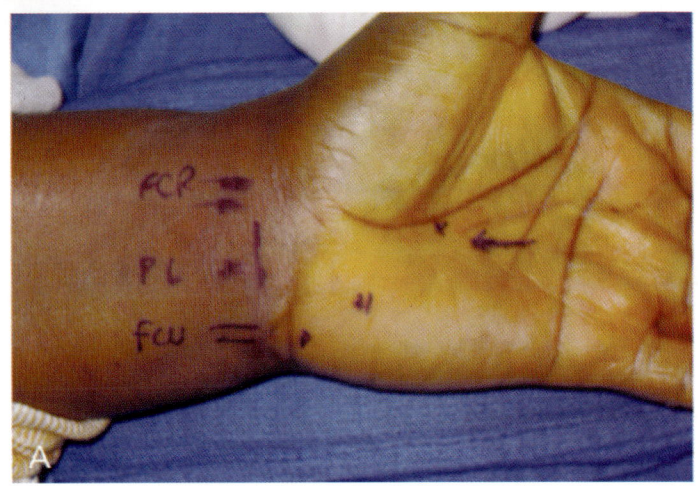

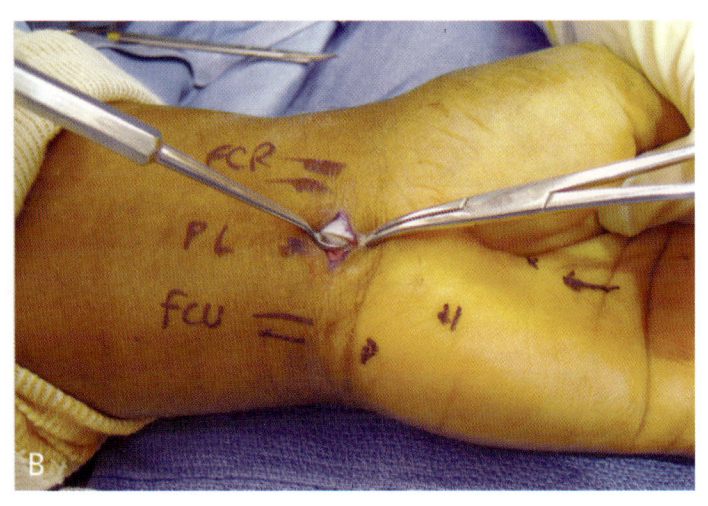

Figure 4 Photographs show single-incision endoscopic carpal tunnel release (CTR). **A,** The key landmarks for endoscopic CTR are shown: the flexor carpi radialis (FCR), the palmaris longus (PL), and the flexor carpi ulnaris (FCU). The arrow indicates the palpated landmark for the distal end of the TCL. The transverse wrist incision is inscribed. **B,** The skin incision has been made, and the fascia has also been incised to create a distally based U-shaped flap held by the clamp.

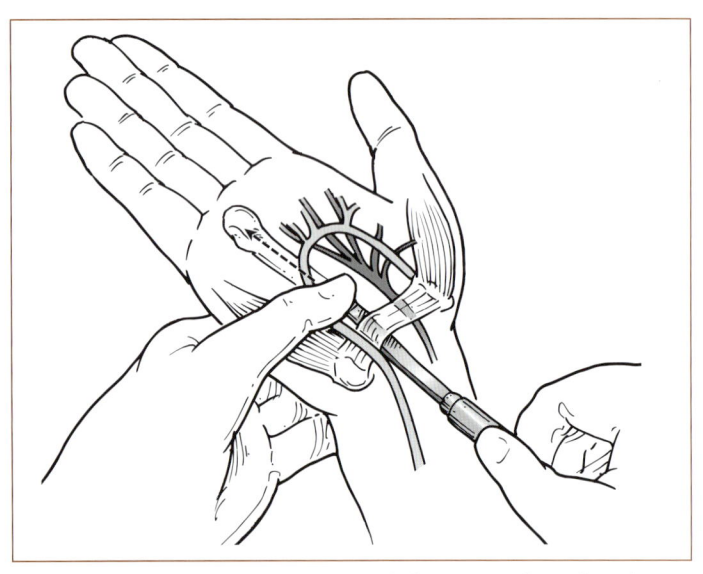

Figure 5 Illustration shows a synovial elevator used to reflect the synovial tissue from the undersurface of the TCL.

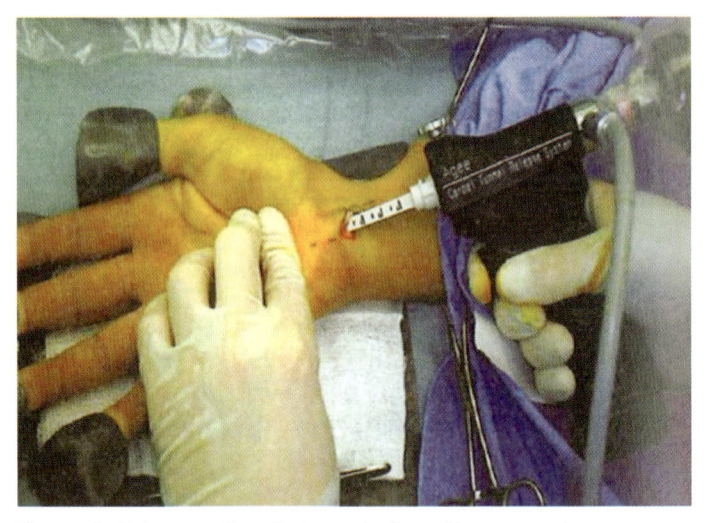

Figure 6 Intraoperative photograph shows the surgeon's nondominant index and long digits palpating the tip of the endoscopic tunnel release device as it emerges into the subcutaneous space just distal to the TCL.

is noted by a transition from the white, transverse fibers of the TCL to the yellow amorphous midpalmar fat, which may contain visible vessels and nerves.

With the surgeon's nondominant hand on the palm, a ballottement maneuver is performed to help distinguish the transition between the midpalmar fat and the distal edge of the TCL while the signal from the endoscope within the carpal canal is viewed on the monitor. In the palm, the tip of the endoscopic CTR device is palpated as it emerges into the subcutaneous space just distal to the TCL (**Figure 6**). The surgeon controls the device with the dominant hand. The transillumination pattern from the endoscopic CTR device light source changes as the device is moved from underneath the TCL to the midpalmar fat.

TCL Release

The blade is elevated and the device is withdrawn slowly, cutting the TCL from distal to proximal. The device is kept pressed up against the undersurface of the TCL so that no structures come between the blade and the TCL; only the TCL is cut (**Figure 7**).

The surgeon should cut only when visualization is excellent. If needed, the device is withdrawn and the undersurface of the TCL is redefined in the manner detailed earlier until visualization is ideal. This step is repeated as needed until there is a full release of the TCL, with good separation of radial and ulnar leaflets from proximal to distal. With a full release, it should not be possible to visualize the radial and ulnar leaflets simultaneously with the endoscopic CTR device up against the palmar tissues. Also, the endocscopic CTR device should be able to be placed within the trough between the radial and ulnar leaflets so that neither leaflet is visible, just the fascia overlying the thenar muscles and the subcutaneous space.

After full TCL release, the endoscopic CTR device is withdrawn. The surgeon confirms the increased volume of the carpal canal by reintroducing the hamate finders down the carpal canal. The proximal antebrachial fascia are divided with long tenotomy scissors under direct vision. Adson forceps help to deliver the tissue for cutting. The incision is then closed, and a soft dressing is applied.

If the surgeon cannot safely visualize the structures with the endoscopic CTR device, conversion to a two-incision or open CTR method is strongly suggested.

Two-Incision Endoscopic CTR (Chow Technique)

The proximal incision is made, and the distally based U-shaped flap of the antebrachial fascia is created in the manner described for the single-incision endoscopic CTR technique.

A clamp, elevator, or trocar is introduced under the TCL, and the instrument is advanced until it is palpable in the palm subcutaneously distal to the TCL. A second small incision is made to expose the tip of the instrument, usually at the junction of the middle and proximal thirds of the palm. The surgeon should take care to identify the superficial arch, the common digital nerves, and the fibers of the distal TCL in the area.

A variety of techniques (open or endoscope-assisted) can be used at this point, including using slotted trocars for a two-incision endoscopic release or a mini-meniscotome blade, scissors, or other cutting instruments with a retractor or an elevator to protect the median nerve and the flexor tendons from the TCL cutting instrument. The wrist must be hyperextended. The complete distal TCL division can be ascertained by direct visualization, also taking note that the vessels and the nerves have not been injured.

A pitfall of the two-incision techniques, aside from the potential injury to the palmar arterial arch and/or the branches of the median or the ulnar nerve, is incomplete release of the TCL distally. Therefore, inspection of the surgical site with magnifying loupes at the distal incision is important.

Revision CTR for Recurrent or Residual CTS

If the recurrent CTS is due to a prior incomplete release, revision surgery can be attempted using an endoscopic CTR technique (**Figure 8**); otherwise, an open release is indicated.

A generous skin incision is used, incorporating previous incisions as needed. The release is performed using a similar technique to that described for primary open CTR. Scarring often requires scalpel dissection, and separation of superficial tissues from the TCL is difficult. The TCL (in the area of its previous division) must be carefully separated from the underlying median nerve. Dense scarring of the median nerve to the TCL is expected and will place the nerve in jeopardy during this exposure. The TCL and the scarred median nerve should be completely released, taking great care to protect the median nerve motor branch. An operating microscope is used to inspect the median nerve for signs of damage or scarring. An external epineurotomy to expose the bands of Fontana on the surface fascicles of the median nerve is recommended in the case of significant nerve scarring.

If there is minimal nerve scarring or damage, the wound can be closed in the usual manner. If nerve injury is dramatic and rescarring seems likely, the damaged nerve should be covered with a hypothenar fat-pad flap, a palmaris brevis muscle flap, vein wrapping, or neural conduit (**Figure 9**). A TCL flap is created through Z-lengthening and tissue arrangement if flexor tendon prolapse or palmar migration of the median nerve seems likely.

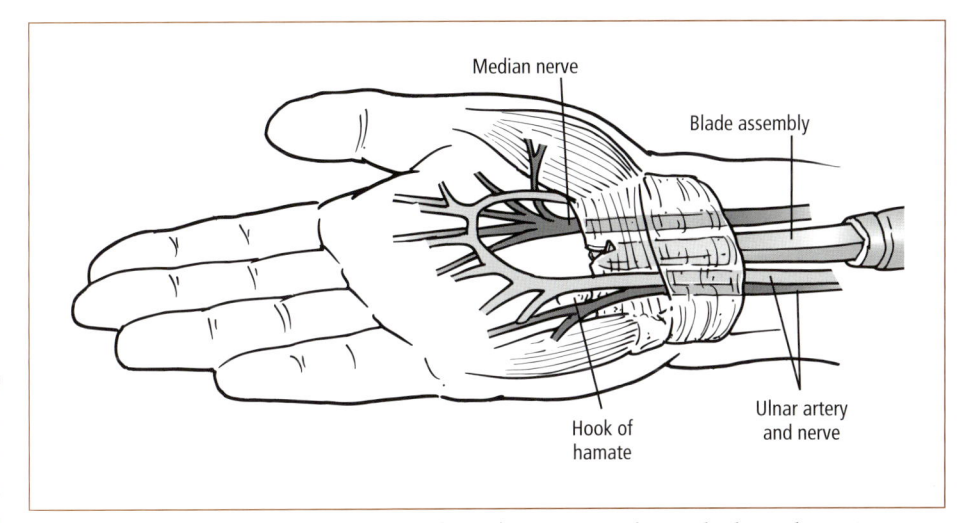

Figure 7 Illustration demonstrates how the endoscopic carpal tunnel release device is inserted into the carpal canal until the distal end of the ligament is visualized.

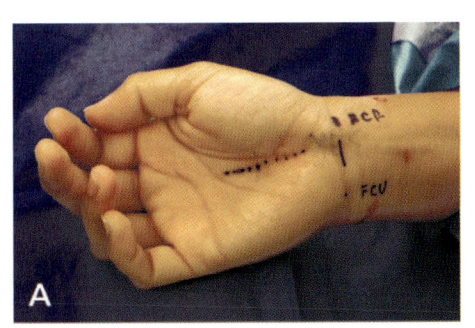

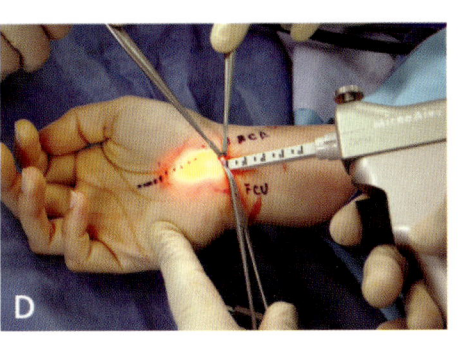

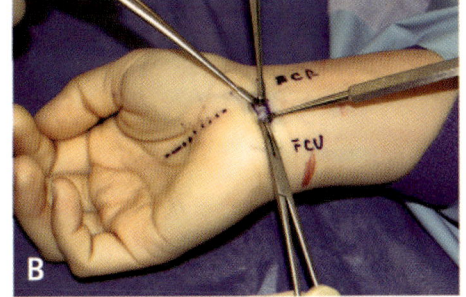

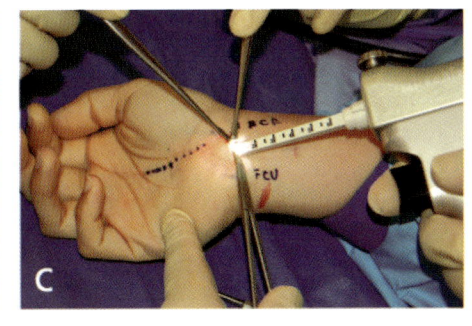

Figure 8 Intraoperative photographs demonstrate revision CTR. **A,** This patient had previous open CTR 1 year prior with recurrent/residual CTS for which a second procedure is being performed. The flexor carpi radialis (FCR) and flexor carpi ulnaris (FCU) are drawn, as is the endoscopic approach (solid line) and the prior open CTR incision (dotted line).
B, A synovial elevator and retractors are used to establish the carpal tunnel space, palpate the undersurface of the TCL, and perform tenosynovectomy so the TCL can be well visualized.
C, Because there are no palpable adhesions between the undersurface of the TCL and the contents of the carpal canal, the endoscopic device is introduced into the incision at the wrist, and the release is performed. The device is introduced. **D,** Post release. Notice the broad pattern of transillumination in the postrelease image.

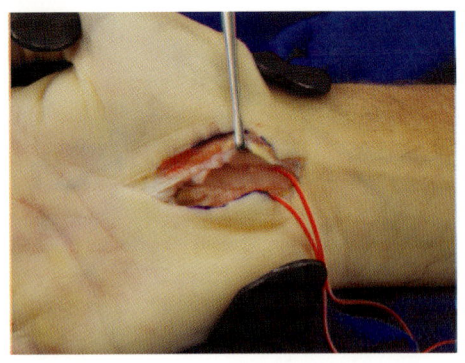

Figure 9 Intraoperative photograph shows revision carpal tunnel release with vessel loop around the scarred branch of the median nerve. This is a candidate for neural wrap to prevent rescarring.

When revision CTR reveals median nerve scarring, surgical tactics to improve the environment around the nerve after the neurolysis and reduce scarring are attractive. The tissue is readily available and has been shown to be of benefit. In a 1996 article, Strickland et al[9] reviewed 62 patients. Results were good based on preoperative and postoperative patient satisfaction scores, with only three transient minor complications.

The fat pad is dissected to the level of the ulnar nerve and artery, and the radial edge is advanced to cover the median nerve. This edge is sewn to the radial flap of the TCL.

Rose et al[10] described the palmaris brevis flap in 1991. The thin palmaris brevis muscle on the ulnar side of the CTR incision is exposed, divided from its insertion in the subcutaneous space, and transposed or rotated into a position covering the median nerve.

Autologous tissues or materials have also been used in cases of nerve scarring. Autologous vein graft can be used, or bioengineered materials as a barrier.

Complications

Complications of CTR include incomplete TCL release, median nerve scarring or damage (especially the common digital nerve to the third web space and the thenar motor branch), ulnar nerve or artery damage, sympathetically mediated pain syndrome, and damage to the palmar arterial arch.

Postoperative Care and Rehabilitation

Traditionally, CTR patients were managed in wrist splints for 1 to 3 weeks after surgery. However, multiple studies have shown that faster recovery occurs when the wrist is not splinted postoperatively. Temporary postoperative splints may still be indicated in specific clinical scenarios, such as open revision surgery.

Hand therapy is helpful in the postoperative period, especially if the patient is having difficulty with full digital active and passive motion. Grip and pinch strength, subjective symptom measures, and functional evaluations are helpful to manage the postoperative course.

Some patients have prolonged periods of tenderness under the TCL or pillar pain on the thenar or hypothenar side of the proximal palm and require extended hand therapy and periods of time to gradually increase hand strength and endurance for hand activities.

Pearls

- A full history and physical examination and contemplation of the entire list of differential diagnoses will help prevent poor patient selection.
- Whatever technique is used, TCL release must be performed in a technically proficient manner. Complete TCL division should be confirmed, especially distally.
- The surgeon must be able to identify the various anatomic structures and distinguish them. The median nerve must be protected during CTR. In techniques where the median nerve is visualized, inspection should be performed after TCL release and before skin closure.

References

1. Kaplan SJ, Glickel SZ, Eaton RG: Predictive factors in the non-surgical treatment of carpal tunnel syndrome. *J Hand Surg Br* 1990;15(1):106-108.
2. Trumble TE, Diao E, Abrams RA, Gilbert-Anderson MM: Single-portal endoscopic carpal tunnel release compared with open release: A prospective, randomized trial. *J Bone Joint Surg Am* 2002;84-A(7):1107-1115.
3. Stütz N, Gohritz A, van Schoonhoven J, Lanz U: Revision surgery after carpal tunnel release—analysis of the pathology in 200 cases during a 2 year period. *J Hand Surg Br* 2006;31(1):68-71.
4. Varitimidis SE, Herndon JH, Sotereanos DG: Failed endoscopic carpal tunnel release: Operative findings and results of open revision surgery. *J Hand Surg Br* 1999;24(4):465-467.
5. Grundberg AB: Carpal tunnel decompression in spite of normal electromyography. *J Hand Surg Am* 1983;8(3):348-349.
6. Gelberman RH, Pfeffer GB, Galbraith RT, Szabo RM, Rydevik B, Dimick M: Results of treatment of severe carpal-tunnel syndrome without internal neurolysis of the median nerve. *J Bone Joint Surg Am* 1987;69(6):896-903.
7. Mackinnon SE, McCabe S, Murray JF, et al: Internal neurolysis fails to improve the results of primary carpal tunnel decompression. *J Hand Surg Am* 1991;16(2):211-218.
8. Rhoades CE, Mowery CA, Gelberman RH: Results of internal neurolysis of the median nerve for severe carpal-tunnel syndrome. *J Bone Joint Surg Am* 1985;67(2):253-256.
9. Strickland JW, Idler RS, Lourie GM, Plancher KD: The hypothenar fat pad flap for management of recalcitrant carpal tunnel syndrome. *J Hand Surg Am* 1996;21(5):840-848.
10. Rose EH, Norris MS, Kowalski TA, Lucas A, Flegler EJ: Palmaris brevis turnover flap as an adjunct to internal neurolysis of the chronically scarred median nerve in recurrent carpal tunnel syndrome. *J Hand Surg Am* 1991;16(2):191-201.

Chapter 36
Surgical Treatment of Cubital Tunnel Syndrome

Reimer Hoffmann, MD   John D. Lubahn, MD

Introduction

Cubital tunnel syndrome is characterized by sensory and/or motor deficiencies of the ulnar nerve. It is the second most common compression syndrome affecting a peripheral nerve, exceeded in prevalence only by carpal tunnel syndrome. Cubital tunnel syndrome occurs at the elbow, where the ulnar nerve passes posterior to the medial epicondyle and beneath the arcuate or Osborne ligament and distal and proximal to the retrocondylar fossa. The syndrome is assumed to be caused by compression that may have one or multiple foci, but the exact cause of the pathology remains unknown. The cause may be traction on the nerve from repetitive or prolonged flexion of the elbow or a combination of traction and compression.

According to the literature, the annual incidence of cubital tunnel syndrome is about one tenth that of carpal tunnel syndrome. Males are affected more often than females, and the left side is affected more often than the right, in contrast to carpal tunnel syndrome. Not infrequently, cubital tunnel syndrome occurs bilaterally.

The cubital tunnel is composed of three parts: (1) The retrocondylar groove, which is partially covered by the humeroulnar arcade; (2) the humeroulnar arcade or Osborne ligament (also known as the arcuate ligament or the epitrochlear anconeus ligament), which passes into the aponeurosis between the two heads of the flexor carpi ulnaris (FCU) muscle and which is also called the cubital tunnel retinaculum; and (3) the deep flexor aponeurosis or flexor-pronator aponeurosis, which contains submuscular bands that may be located at variable distances from the medial epicondyle[1] (**Figure 1, A**). This aponeurosis spreads from 5 to 12 cm distal to the medial epicondyle. The submuscular membrane, described by Matsuzaki et al[2] and Hoffmann and Siemionow,[1,3] covers the nerve in the distal part of the cubital tunnel and is characterized by fibrous bands that may cause or add to compression as far as 9 cm distal to the retrocondylar fossa (**Figure 1, B**). The prevalence of compression distal to the retrocondylar area can only be estimated. According to MRI investigations by Vucic et al,[4] the compression site was in the retrocondylar area in only 38% of their cases.

The role of the arcade of Struthers in compression of the ulnar nerve in the distal part of the humerus proximal to the cubital tunnel is controversial, but it may cause compression on the nerve proximally when the nerve is transposed anterior to the medial epicondyle.

Patient Selection
Physical Examination

The clinical examination includes inspection for muscle atrophy; examination for sensory deficits, including two-point discrimination; examination of ulnar nerve innervated muscles, including the Froment and Wartenberg sign and the crossed-finger test (long over index); measurement of muscle power (M0-M5); measurement of grip strength (Jamar dynamometer); testing for the presence and location of the Tinel sign; palpation of the course of the ulnar nerve for possible complete or partial subluxation of the ulnar nerve from the retrocondylar groove; examination of mobility and stability of the elbow joint; and the elbow flexion test.

Electrodiagnostic Testing

Although ulnar compression at the elbow can be diagnosed clinically, preoperative electrodiagnostic testing is highly recommended to confirm the diagnosis and exclude the possibility of compression at other anatomic sites, quantify the degree of compression, and provide baseline

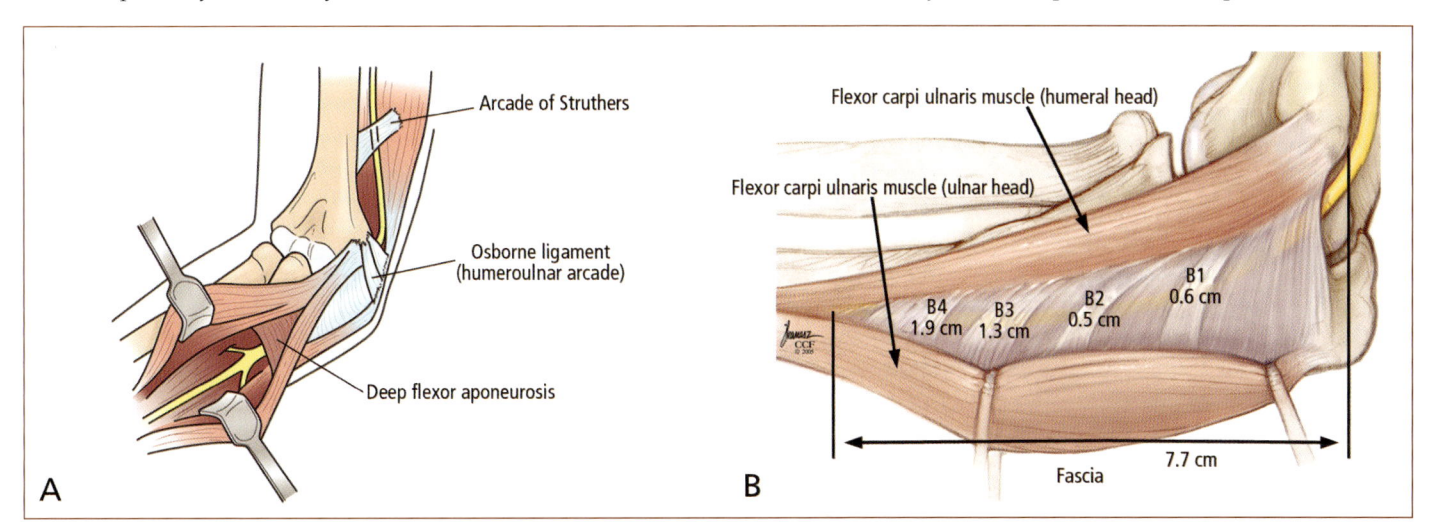

Figure 1 Illustrations depict the anatomy of the cubital tunnel. **A,** The most common sites of ulnar nerve compression are labeled. **B,** Additional potential sites of compression of the ulnar nerve located in the submuscular membrane of the flexor-pronator muscle. (Panel B copyright Joe Kanasz, the Cleveland Clinic Foundation, Cleveland, OH.)

Dr. Lubahn or an immediate family member has received research or institutional support from Auxillium. Neither Dr. Hoffmann nor any immediate family member has received anything of value from or owns stock in a commercial company or institution related directly or indirectly to the subject of this chapter.

numbers against which to compare subsequent studies to document progression or improvement of the condition.

The precision of nerve conduction velocity studies is highly dependent on the examiner and the technique used. Locating the exact point of stimulation distally at the postcondylar groove is difficult, especially in cases of strongly developed muscles in the lower arm or in obese patients. In patients with low skin temperature or gliding of the nerve when the elbow is flexed, wrong measurements may occur.

Preoperative Imaging
Imaging techniques including ultrasonography[5] and MRI[6] have been gaining importance and now are regarded as relevant examination techniques that should be used in addition to electrodiagnostic testing if available. Unlike electrodiagnostic testing, these modalities detect morphologic changes directly and localize them more precisely.

A radiographic examination of the elbow joint in at least two projections, including tangential imaging of the retrocondylar groove, can help to detect anatomic variations. A CT examination is recommended only in exceptional cases of skeletal deformity.

Indications
The goal of the surgical intervention, usually performed in an outpatient center, is the decompression of the ulnar nerve throughout the entire cubital tunnel. There are currently several generally well-accepted surgical procedures for the treatment of cubital tunnel syndrome: (1) in situ decompression; (2) endoscopic decompression (outside-in or inside-out); (3) decompression with subsequent subcutaneous transposition, intramuscular transposition, or submuscular transposition; and (4) in situ decompression in conjunction with medial epicondylectomy. Our preferred technique for the treatment of cubital tunnel syndrome is endoscopic in situ decompression.[7-11]

In cases of a recent onset of intermittent paresthesia and pain that developed over a period of 14 days, it is acceptable to manage symptoms nonsurgically for up to 3 months ("wait and see"). Ongoing neurologic and electrophysiologic surveillance of the patient is recommended, however. If after this period of time the patient shows no signs of improvement or if physical findings such as two-point discrimination and grip strength worsen, surgical intervention should be considered. If electrodiagnostic and ultrasonographic testing remain negative, other neurologic causes have been ruled out, and the patient is unhappy, an operation (preferably in situ and endoscopic) may still be considered.

In situ decompression of the ulnar nerve performed open or endoscopically is the treatment of choice for primary cubital tunnel syndrome.[7,8] In situ decompression is effective in patients with severe compression as well as in patients with milder forms of the syndrome.[8] In situ decompression may also be recommended for cases of ulnar nerve subluxation, although this is one instance where transposition may be indicated if the nerve is snapping back and forth over the medial epicondyle with pain and instability preoperatively. In situ decompression is also effective in cases where the elbow joint is deformed secondary to other posttraumatic changes or where an epitrochlear anconeus muscle or prominent medial triceps are found.

In situ decompression, including endoscopic decompression, also may be chosen in posttraumatic cubital tunnel syndrome because there is currently no evidence to suggest anterior transposition is better.

Contraindications
There are no contraindications to in situ decompression of the ulnar nerve.

In Situ Decompression
Room Setup/Patient Positioning
In situ decompression is almost always performed in an outpatient setting. General anesthesia is preferred, although some patients may prefer local anesthesia with sedation. A bloodless field is an advantage. The patient is positioned supine on the operating table and the arm is abducted 90° at the shoulder, flexed at the elbow, and supinated.

Special Instruments/Equipment/Implants
For the endoscopic decompression described below, a special endoscopy set (Karl Storz Endoscopy) is used. The set includes an illuminated speculum with a blade length of 9 to 11 cm; a 4-mm, 30° endoscope with a shaft length of 15 cm and a blunt dissector on its tip; and an endoscopic bipolar forceps.

Open Decompression
The incision, which is 6 to 8 cm long, is placed in the retrocondylar fossa. In dissecting the ulnar nerve, care is taken not to injure any branches of the medial and posterior cutaneous branches. The nerve is exposed and the Osborne ligament is divided. Distally, the FCU fascia is divided for about 8 cm as well as the raphe between the two heads of the muscle itself and the submuscular membrane (Figure 2). Similarly, the fascia that extends proximally is divided for 6 to 8 cm, looking subcutaneously with the aid of a retractor or speculum for the arcade of Struthers. The arcade does not need to be divided if the nerve is not being transposed, although many surgeons probably do divide the arcade during the dissection proximal to the ulnar nerve. After hemostasis, the skin is closed and a well-padded bandage is applied. A splint is generally not required, and patients are allowed to move their arm early.

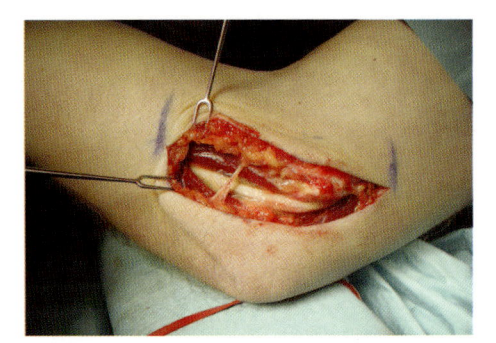

Figure 2 Intraoperative photograph shows open in situ decompression.

Video 36.1 Endoscopic Management of Cubital Tunnel Syndrome. Reimer Hoffmann, MD; John D. Lubahn, MD (7 min)

Endoscopic Decompression (Hoffmann Technique)
Sometimes called "long-distance endoscopic decompression," this technique applies endoscopic technology to the in situ decompression and allows a more complete release of the nerve through a smaller incision. For the Hoffmann technique, the incision is placed posterior to the medial epicondyle and is only 2 to 3 cm in length. The instruments used, however, allow dissection of the nerve for a total of at least 20 cm (10 cm distal and 10 cm proximal to the medial epicondyle). Although the operation can be performed under local anesthesia, we generally recommend general anesthesia. A pneumatic tourniquet is also recommended, as well as exsanguination of the arm with an Esmarch or Martin wrap.

Draping must allow full passive mobility of the elbow.

For the in situ release, the arm is positioned in 90° of abduction on a standard hand table so that the surgeon can flex and turn the arm to face the cubital tunnel area. The hand table should be raised much higher than normal, almost to eye level of the sitting surgeon.

The ulnar nerve can often be palpated in the retrocondylar groove or just proximal to it. Once the ulnar nerve has been located or the surgeon is comfortable with other anatomic landmarks such as the medial epicondyle and the olecranon, a 1.5- to 2.5-cm incision is made in the retrocondylar groove along the natural skin creases, preferably in a longitudinal direction. Dissection is then carried down to the arcuate ligament (Osborne ligament), which forms the roof of the cubital tunnel. We use two-pronged nerve hooks (double hooks) or Senn retractors to expose the nerve. Sometimes adipose tissue or an epitrochlear anconeus muscle makes this step slightly more difficult to perform, although once the adipose tissue has been dissected away from the nerve or the epitrochlear anconeus has been divided, the nerve is easily identified by its appearance and the clearly recognizable vasa nervorum on the surface. The arcuate ligament is then divided under direct vision, keeping the epifascial layer in view so it is not lost in the depth of the incision. A tunneling forceps is introduced into the space between the fascia and subcutaneous tissue (not into the cubital tunnel—ie, not beneath the arcuate ligament, adjacent to the nerve!) and a subcutaneous workspace is created, first distally and then proximally. By spreading the blunt-tipped forceps, a generous cavity is created, which permits the insertion of the instruments required to complete the procedure (**Figure 3, A**). Spreading of the tunneling forceps must be done gently to avoid stretching the cutaneous nerves in this area, specifically the medial antebrachial cutaneous nerve. An illuminated speculum with a blade length of 9 to 11 cm (Karl Storz Endoscopy) is inserted, and the remaining part of the Osborne ligament (sometimes called the cubital tunnel retinaculum) is divided under direct visualization (**Figure 3, B** and **C**). With the use of the speculum alone, the ulnar nerve can be decompressed up to 5 cm distally and proximally from the epicondyle. Routinely, using speculum vision, we incise the fascia until the first muscle fibers of the FCU are seen.

A 4-mm, 30° endoscope (shaft length, 15 cm) with a blunt dissector on its tip (Karl Storz Endoscopy) is introduced and slowly advanced distally. Lifting up the soft-tissue envelope of the forearm with the dissector (like working in a tent) creates a generous space to view the nerve and its surrounding anatomy (**Figure 3, D**). All dissection and cutting is done with blunt-tipped scissors between 17 and 23 cm long (**Figure 3, E**). Under monitor vision, the forearm fascia is divided to a point 10 to 15 cm distal from the epicondyle. Care must be taken not to injure the cutaneous nerve branches or the veins that may cross the fascia (**Figure 3, F**). Once the fascia has been divided, the endoscope is carefully pulled back, and further dissection is performed close to the nerve.

The next step is to divide the two muscular heads of the FCU and to release all fibrous bands crossing the nerve. Distally from the Osborne ligament, the fascia between the two heads of the FCU is divided. At approximately 3 cm distal from the medial epicondyle, the first fibrous arcade can be located and divided. Then the raphe between the two muscular heads of the FCU is transected, and all constricting elements up to a distance of at least 9 cm, but possibly as far distal as 14 cm (measured from the middle of the retrocondylar groove), are divided. The layer between muscle and nerve is the submuscular membrane with three or four fibrous bands crossing the nerve. In the course of this dissection, the submuscular membrane and the fibrous bands are divided, and all muscle branches can be seen and protected (**Figure 3, G**). Only rarely is it necessary to clip or cauterize a vessel. This can be done with a long bipolar forceps or a special endoscopic bipolar forceps, which is part of the instrument set. Lax adipose soft tissue of the forearm, sometimes seen in elderly women, makes the dissection difficult, mainly because the optic needs repeated cleaning and some loose adipose tissue must be removed. The procedure is more difficult in obese arms.

Proximally, the tunnel roof is decompressed in the same fashion. The fascia, but not the intermuscular septum, is divided over a distance of 8 to 14 cm from the retrocondylar groove. No regularly appearing constricting elements have been observed in this area. Sometimes the medial part of the triceps muscle has fibrous elements or arcades that stretch toward the intermuscular septum. These elements are what many authors describe as the arcade of Struthers.

At the end of the operation, a bulky cotton (often called a Robert Jones) compression dressing is applied. Then the tourniquet is deflated.

Postoperative Care and Rehabilitation

Patients are allowed to move the elbow immediately postoperatively but are instructed to avoid resting the arm in flexion for 4 weeks to prevent secondary nerve subluxation. Many patients describe relief of their symptoms immediately after surgery. After 24 to 72 hours, the dressing is removed and an elastic elbow bandage is prescribed for 4 weeks. Normally, postoperative physical therapy is not necessary. Patients with light work (eg, office workers, teachers) can go back to work within days, and heavy workers (eg, builders, carpenters) can return to work after 3 weeks. Many of the self-employed patients we have treated, such as surgeons and dentists, were back at work within 1 week.

Complications are extremely rare. We have seen profuse subcutaneous hematoma that never required surgical removal in 4% to 5% of the cases. The recurrence rate is 1%.[1]

Transposition Techniques and Medial Epicondylectomy

In spite of the fact that recent prospective trials indicate in situ decompression of the ulnar nerve to be as good as, if not somewhat better than, anterior transposition,[7,8] many hand surgeons in the United States continue to recommend anterior transposition in one form or another or medial epicondylectomy. Some authors would argue that although in situ decompression may be successful in moderate cases, it is insufficient for more severe cases. In certain instances where the ulnar nerve subluxates preoperatively (can be palpated or seen to subluxate), a more compelling argument for transposition can be made. Other authors would suggest repositioning the released ulnar nerve in the retrocondylar groove and reconstructing the arcuate ligament when anterior subluxation occurs. (This technique is called neuropexy, which means keeping the ulnar nerve in the anatomic sulcus and preventing subluxation by securing it with a fascial flap taken from the anterior pericondylar area.) Anterior transposition of the ulnar nerve should be considered only in cases with severe posttraumatic or degenerative

Section 3: Hand and Wrist

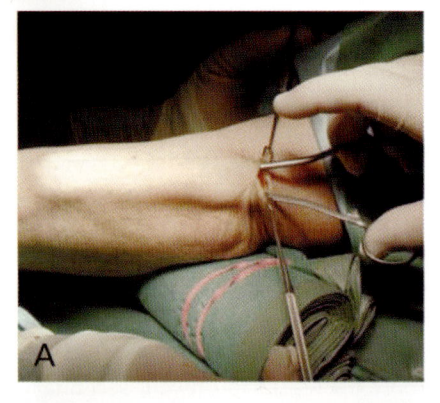

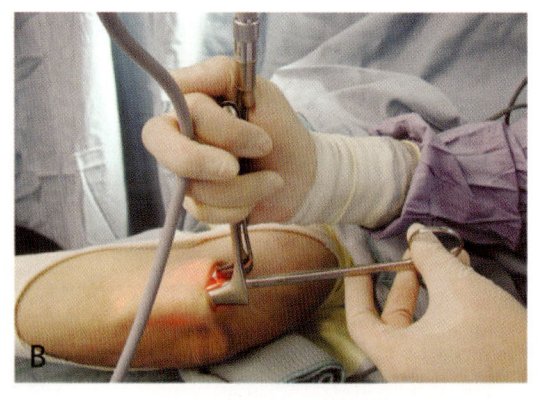

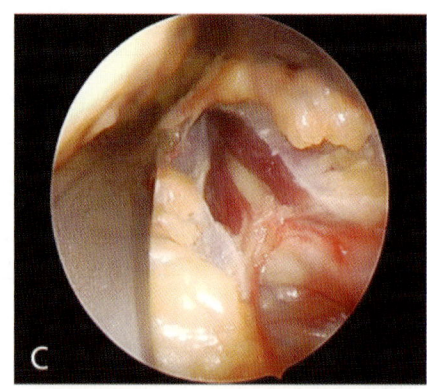

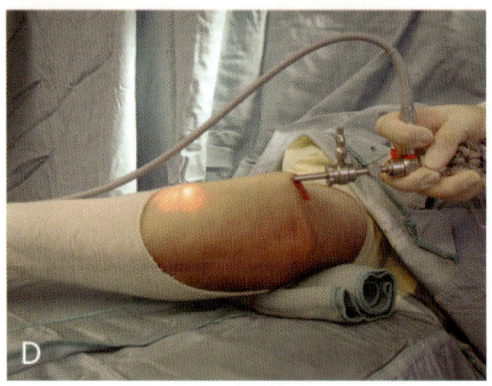

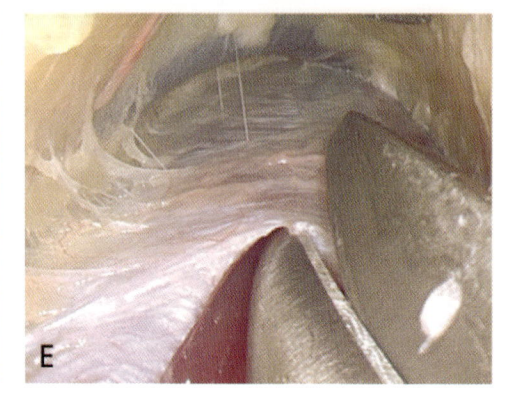

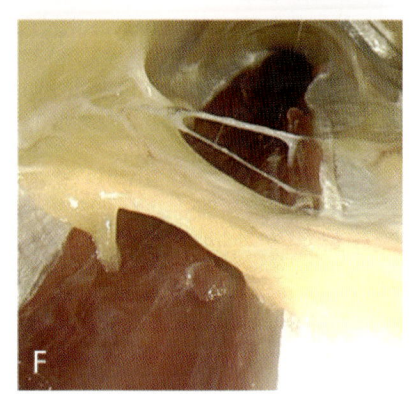

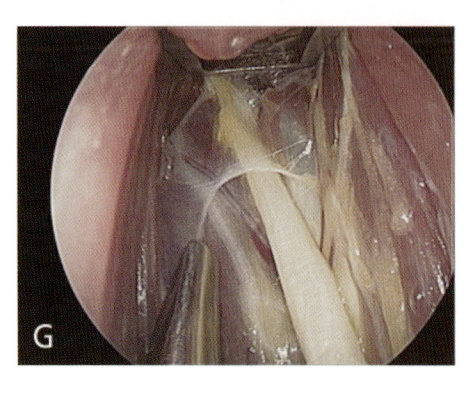

Figure 3 Endoscopic in situ decompression of the ulnar nerve. **A**, Intraoperative photograph shows the creation of a workspace for a soft-tissue endoscope using a specially blunt-tipped tunneling forceps. **B**, Photograph shows release of the flexor carpi ulnaris (FCU) fascia under direct vision through an illuminated speculum. **C**, View down the speculum shows incised fascia, the divided heads of the FCU, and, between them, the submuscular membrane. **D**, Photograph shows the soft-tissue endoscope in use. Note the extent of the dissection 13 cm distal to the medial epicondyle. **E**, Endoscopic view shows the soft-tissue endoscope maintaining a well-visualized workspace while the forearm fascia is released. **F**, Endoscopic view shows the forearm fascia released beneath a crossing branch of the medial antebrachial cutaneous nerve, which must be preserved. **G**, Endoscopic view shows excellent visualization of the muscle branches.

deformations of the elbow joint (cubitus valgus), in cases where the nerve is embedded in scarred tissue, and in cases of ulnar nerve subluxation with elbow flexion.

Open release and anterior transposition has technical challenges and risks of complications. For example, anterior transposition of the ulnar nerve risks local ischemia of the nerve resulting from damage to the vasa nervorum. Therefore, the associated arteries and veins should be left intact during the dissection. This is difficult if not impossible, because 10 to 15 cm of the nerve is being moved from posterior to anterior of the medial epicondyle; thus, some of the vessels must be divided. With recent good results with in situ decompression, anterior transposition should be chosen with very good reason (eg, if after trauma the nerve is scarred in the retrocondylar fossa) and by surgeons familiar with the technique.

Given the ongoing controversy, the following techniques for treatment of cubital tunnel syndrome in addition to endoscopic or in situ decompression are often used.

Subcutaneous Anterior Transposition

Patient preparation and positioning is the same as for in situ decompression, although local anesthesia is generally not adequate for most anterior transposition procedures, so a regional block or general anesthetic is preferred. The incision for subcutaneous anterior transposition is approximately 15 cm in length. As with each of the procedures mentioned, the surgeon should be cognizant of the medial antebrachial cutaneous nerve, which is usually located approximately 3.5 cm distal to the medial epicondyle. Care should be taken to preserve this nerve throughout the course of the dissection.

The ulnar nerve usually can be found by initially locating the medial epicondyle and dissecting directly posterior. Dissection then proceeds proximally to the medial intermuscular septum and its connection to the medial head of the triceps, the so-called arcade of Struthers, which is released to avoid any compression on the nerve when it is transposed anteriorly. The sharp edge of the medial intermuscular septum is incised and resected generously to avoid any kinking after transposition of the nerve. Dissection then proceeds distally releasing the arcuate ligament (Osborne ligament) and continuing distally through the FCU muscle fascia to the first and second branches of the nerve to the FCU (**Figure 4, A**). The nerve is then mobilized from its bed, trying to leave as much of the longitudinal blood supply intact as possible. This is difficult and sometimes impossible to achieve. The nerve is then carefully mobilized anterior to the medial epicondyle (**Figure 4, B**), where it is held in place by a 2-cm flap of flexor forearm fascia that functions as a sling to hold the nerve in position. The flap is sutured loosely over the nerve, with care taken not to cause further compression.

The wound is closed with interrupted sutures, often over a small drain. A splint is worn for 2 to 3 weeks, removing the sutures at 1 week. After removal of the splint, the patient is allowed a very gentle active range of motion, ideally under the supervision of a therapist or occasionally independently, in the case of a trustworthy patient.

Anterior Submuscular Transposition

Some authors recommend anterior submuscular transposition as the procedure of choice for a throwing athlete; however, this technique requires more extensive dissection with detachment of the flexor pronator muscle group, which may weaken the muscles and compromise the throwing mechanism of an athlete. Although the patient's grip strength as well as numbness in the small finger and ulnar side of the ring finger may improve, the weakness of the forearm muscles may have a deleterious effect on the patient's ability to participate in sports and ultimately compromise the final result. Submuscular transposition has also been advocated to salvage any previous failed procedure. The surgeon must be prepared with a backup plan if this procedure fails. In some respects, this procedure "burns all bridges" and leaves little option for salvage other than perhaps neurolysis and/or nerve wraps or local flap coverage.

The patient is positioned supine on the operating table and under general anesthesia. An incision approximately 15 cm in length is designed just posterior to the medial epicondyle. The surgeon should be aware that the medial antebrachial cutaneous nerve will be crossing this incision approximately 3.5 cm distal to the medial epicondyle and should be looking for this structure throughout the course of the dissection. The proximal branch of the same nerve crosses the incision closer to the medial epicondyle and often is found in line with the medial intermuscular septum. The ulnar nerve is identified proximal to the medial epicondyle. Under direct visualization, the arcuate ligament is released and followed more distally through the two heads of the FCU muscle. Distal dissection is carried through this muscle until motor branches can be clearly identified. The nerve is then dissected proximally, releasing any transverse structures but preserving vascularity. The arcade of Struthers is identified running between the medial intermuscular septum and

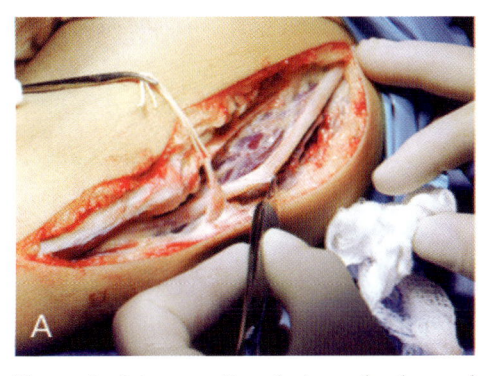

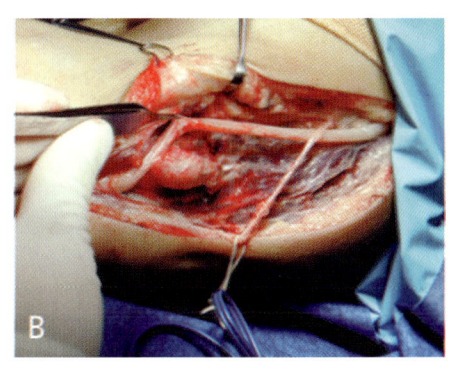

Figure 4 Intraoperative photographs show subcutaneous transposition of the ulnar nerve. **A,** Incision and dissection of the ulnar nerve prior to subcutaneous transposition. **B,** Subcutaneous transposition of the nerve.

the medial head of the triceps; it is usually located approximately 8 cm proximal to the medial epicondyle. The nerve is carefully identified from one end of the incision to the other, and attention is directed to the medial epicondyle, where the flexor pronator is carefully detached from its origin. The flexor pronator origin is then elevated, with dissection proceeding medially until an appropriate bed is created for the nerve. Once the bed is prepared, the mesoneurium is carefully released and dissected to allow the nerve to be moved anteriorly and lie beneath the muscle. This should be done carefully and delicately, touching only the epineurium with small single-tooth forceps and carefully laying the nerve beneath the muscle with no undue tension proximally or distally. The surgeon should also take care to prevent the nerve from being kinked proximally at the arcade of Struthers to make certain that the entire fascial connection between the medial intermuscular septum and the medial head of the triceps is released. Distally, similar care must be taken to be certain that the nerve is not caught in the flexor pronator muscle group.

The flexor pronator origin is reattached to the medial epicondyle with a relatively heavy nonabsorbable stitch. The wound is then closed with a minimal number of interrupted nonabsorbable subcutaneous stitches, care being taken to preserve the cutaneous nerves. A 0.25-in Penrose drain is often placed. The arm is supported in a posterior splint for 3 weeks.

Intramuscular Transposition

The incision for intramuscular transposition is much the same as that described for subcutaneous transposition; however, the surgeon makes an incision in the flexor forearm musculature rather than elevating it or leaving it intact as with the two previous procedures described. The muscle fibers are gently separated to create a well-vascularized muscle bed into which the ulnar nerve is transposed. The fascia is then loosely closed over the nerve for protection. The postoperative protocol for this procedure as described requires 3 weeks of complete immobilization followed by up to 10 weeks of restricted activity.

Medial Epicondylectomy

The surgeon with an appropriate level of experience may also choose to perform a (partial) medial epicondylectomy (in cases of more severe deformation of the medial epicondyle or a valgus deformation). The risk in this technique lies in the potential for instability of the joint if too much of the epicondyle is removed, compromising the medial collateral ligament of the elbow.

The surgical exposure for medial epicondylectomy is identical to that for submuscular, intermuscular, and subcutaneous transposition of the nerve. The ulnar nerve is identified posterior to the medial epicondyle, and the medial epicondyle itself is further exposed with subperiosteal dissection. A small osteotome is used to score the medial epicondyle at the planned depth of resection, which should not exceed 20% of the overall depth of the epicondyle itself. Care is taken throughout the procedure to avoid damage to the anterior medial band of the medial collateral ligament. Care also should be taken to avoid incidental arthrotomy.

After removal of the bone, the edges should be made smooth with a file or rasp. The periosteal flaps are sutured and the wound is closed with 4-0 nylon sutures, usually over a drain. Gentle range of motion is begun in 1 week, but resistance exercises must be avoided for 10 to 12 weeks.

Postoperative Care and Rehabilitation

Generally, early active motion is preferred because it prevents the potential loss of elbow motion and nerve scarring associated with immobilization for 2 or 3 weeks. Increase in work load and strain placed on the elbow is allowed gradually over 4 to 8 weeks. An early onset of motion without the use of force is possible after minimally invasive and endoscopic procedures. Return to work after these procedures is possible for office workers after 3 to 5 days and for heavy laborers at 2 to 3 weeks.

After transposition procedures, time off work usually amounts to 6 to 12 weeks or more. In cases of motor palsy, outpatient therapy under the supervision of a hand therapist is indicated to strengthen the paretic muscles.

Complications

As with any surgical intervention, disturbances in wound healing with or without infections can occur following cubital tunnel release. Therefore, space-occupying hematoma must be removed. Injury to the medial antebrachial cutaneous nerve of the forearm is one of the more common complications that occur with any type of cubital tunnel release and can lead to painful neuroma formation.[12]

Injury to the ulnar nerve itself can occur in difficult dissections and is often seen with severe posttraumatic scar and after epicondylectomy. The nerve can also be kinked in cases of anterior submuscular or subcutaneous transposition when proximal dissection does not extend far enough to release an existing arcade of Struthers. Distal kinking can occur if the deep flexor fascia was not incised properly at the entry of the nerve into the flexor pronator muscles.

Perineural scar formation and insufficient resection of the medial intermuscular septum and the deep flexor fascia have most frequently been the cause for revision surgery. An insufficient transposition of the nerve crossing the medial epicondyle can also lead to increased pain and a bad result or a recurrence. Recurrence is possible after any of the procedures described here, especially after intramuscular transposition. In cases of transposition procedures, treated with immobilization, a joint contraction can occur. Instability of the elbow joint is a serious complication after improper epicondylectomy. Complex regional pain syndrome is a rare complication.

Pearls

- Decompression of the ulnar nerve should be performed from the retrocondylar groove to at least 5 to 7 cm distal and proximal to the medial epicondyle. A circumferential dissection is not necessary and should be avoided because of the risk of provoking subluxation and damaging the blood supply of the nerve.
- An epineurolysis is rarely indicated (eg, in cases of severe fibrosis), and interfascicular neurolysis must be avoided to prevent damage to the delicate plexiform nature of the ulnar nerve at the elbow.
- Sometimes it may be difficult to differentiate a distal (Guyon canal) from a proximal (cubital tunnel) ulnar nerve compression. A safe sign to indicate a proximal lesion is hypoesthesia on the dorsoulnar area of the hand. This area is innervated by the superficial branch of the nerve, which leaves the main nerve stem proximal from the Guyon canal.
- All nerves, large or small, are recognizable by their longitudinal vasa nervorum. Observing this prevents the surgeon from resecting or "buzzing" these nerves.
- In the rare cases in which an anterior ulnar nerve transposition may be indicated, the surgeon should be aware of the option to perform a neuropexy, which carries less risk.
- Quite unlike carpal tunnel problems, patients with cubital tunnel syndrome tend to ignore the onset of symptoms. Likewise, they sometimes ignore improvement following surgery. Accordingly, objective preoperative data (sensory loss with 2-point discrimination, muscular weakness with grading M0-M5, and grip strength) should be documented carefully.
- When a neurologist finds no slowing of nerve conduction, the surgeon should check which muscles were used for the measurement. Sometimes placing the needle into the hypothenar muscles gives a normal reading (and a false-negative result), whereas placing the needle into the first dorsal interosseous muscle gives the suspected pathologic finding.
- When dissecting with scissors, the surgeon should be sure to visualize the entire cutting edge of the scissors to avoid damaging tissue outside the field of vision.

References

1. Hoffmann R, Siemionow M: The endoscopic management of cubital tunnel syndrome. *J Hand Surg Br* 2006;31(1):23-29.
2. Matsuzaki H, Yoshizu T, Maki Y, Tsubokawa N, Yamamoto Y, Toishi S: Long-term clinical and neurologic recovery in the hand after surgery for severe cubital tunnel syndrome. *J Hand Surg Am* 2004;29(3):373-378.
3. Siemionow M, Agaoglu G, Hoffmann R: Anatomic characteristics of a fascia and its bands overlying the ulnar nerve in the proximal forearm: A cadaver study. *J Hand Surg Eur Vol* 2007;32(3):302-307.
4. Vucic S, Cordato DJ, Yiannikas C, Schwartz RS, Shnier RC: Utility of magnetic resonance imaging in diagnosing ulnar neuropathy at the elbow. *Clin Neurophysiol* 2006;117(3):590-595.
5. Wiesler ER, Chloros GD, Cartwright MS, Shin HW, Walker FO: Ultrasound in the diagnosis of ulnar neuropathy at the cubital tunnel. *J Hand Surg Am* 2006;31(7):1088-1093.
6. Bäumer P, Dombert T, Staub F, et al: Ulnar neuropathy at the elbow: MR neurography. Nerve T2 signal increase and caliber. *Radiology* 2011;260(1):199-206.
7. Nabhan A, Ahlhelm F, Kelm J, Reith W, Schwerdtfeger K, Steudel WI: Simple decompression or subcutaneous anterior transposition of the ulnar nerve for cubital tunnel syndrome. *J Hand Surg Br* 2005;30(5):521-524.
8. Gervasio O, Gambardella G, Zaccone C, Branca D: Simple decompression versus anterior submuscular transposition of the ulnar nerve in severe cubital tunnel syndrome: A prospective randomized study. *Neurosurgery* 2005;56(1):108-117, discussion 117.
9. Ahcan U, Zorman P: Endoscopic decompression of the ulnar nerve at the elbow. *J Hand Surg Am* 2007;32(8):1171-1176.
10. Watts AC, Bain GI: Patient-rated outcome of ulnar nerve decompression: A comparison of endoscopic and open in situ decompression. *J Hand Surg Am* 2009;34(8):1492-1498.
11. Zlowodzki M, Chan S, Bhandari M, Kalliainen L, Schubert W: Anterior transposition compared with simple decompression for treatment of cubital tunnel syndrome: A meta-analysis of randomized, controlled trials. *J Bone Joint Surg Am* 2007;89(12):2591-2598.
12. Lowe JB III, Maggi SP, Mackinnon SE: The position of crossing branches of the medial antebrachial cutaneous nerve during cubital tunnel surgery in humans. *Plast Reconstr Surg* 2004;114(3):692-696.

Chapter 37
First Dorsal Extensor Compartment Release

Aaron I. Venouziou, MD   Filippos S. Giannoulis, MD   Dean G. Sotereanos, MD

Introduction

de Quervain syndrome is stenosing tenosynovitis of the first dorsal compartment of the wrist, which contains the abductor pollicis longus (APL) and the extensor pollicis brevis (EPB) tendons. The condition is named for the Swiss surgeon Fritz de Quervain, who described in 1895 a painful condition involving the APL and the EPB tendon sheaths at the radial styloid process. de Quervain recommended simple release of the stenotic extensor retinaculum. In 1927, Finkelstein described the physical examination maneuver that bears his name and recommended excising a portion of the sheath when it is excessively thickened or cartilaginous in nature. Subsequently, authors have recommended various treatment approaches, including splinting, injections, limited retinaculum release, extensive retinaculum release, and retinaculum excision.[1]

Patient Selection

Any patient with de Quervain tenosynovitis in whom nonsurgical treatment of splinting and/or steroid injections has failed would be a candidate for surgical release of the first dorsal compartment. Patients with de Quervain tenosynovitis present with radial-sided wrist pain. The pain is exacerbated by thumb movements, in particular thumb abduction and/or extension, and may radiate distally or proximally along the course of the APL and EPB tendons. Recent epidemiologic studies have demonstrated that risk factors for de Quervain syndrome include female sex (occurs 6 up to 10 times more frequently in females than in males), age greater than 40 years, and black race.[2,3] The condition has also been noted in pregnant and lactating women.

Physical examination often reveals localized swelling and tenderness over the first dorsal compartment, extending 1 to 2 cm proximal to the radial styloid process. In 1930, Finkelstein[4] described a clinical test that is pathognomonic of the disease. The test result is positive when excruciating pain over the styloid tip, is generated by grasping the patient's thumb and quickly abducting the hand ulnarward. Anatomically, the musculotendinous junction of the EPB tendon is close to the first compartment. In the Finkelstein test, when the thumb is in full flexion and the wrist is in ulnar deviation, the EPB muscle belly is pulled into the first compartment, resulting in a bulk effect. The synovial tissue around the EPB and APL tendons also might be stretched in the Finkelstein testing position, causing a tethering effect. Both bulk and tethering effects may induce pain by directly stretching synovial tissue, especially when the synovial tissue is inflamed or fibrotic, as may be the case in de Quervain disease.[5]

Preoperative Imaging

Radiographs consisting of PA and lateral views of the wrist as well as a hyperpronated thumb view, known as a Roberts view (Figure 1), are mandatory to differentiate de Quervain tenosynovitis from other arthritic conditions. Radiographic study should exclude arthritis of the thumb carpometacarpal joint, although this condition may coexist; scaphoid fracture; and arthrosis involving the radiocarpal or intercarpal joints.

Video 37.1 First Dorsal Extensor Compartment Release. Filippos Giannoulis, MD; Douglas S. Musgrave, MD; Alexander H. Payatakes, MD; Dean Sotereanos, MD (3 min)

Procedure

Room Setup/Patient Positioning

The patient is positioned supine with the hand on a table extension. A padded pneumatic tourniquet is applied around the arm, as a bloodless surgical field is essential for the identification of superficial radial sensory nerve branches, and is set to 250 mm Hg. The procedure is performed under general or local anesthesia

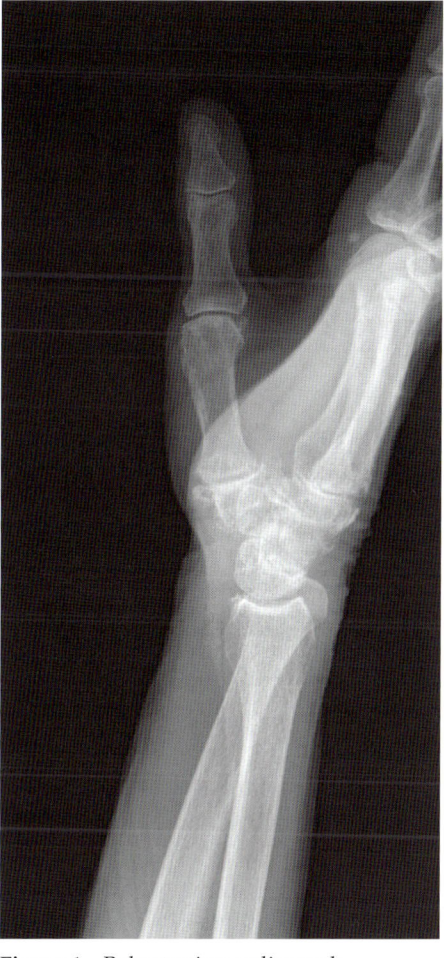

Figure 1 Roberts view radiograph demonstrates thumb basal joint arthritis in a 67-year-old woman with radial-sided wrist pain mimicking de Quervain syndrome.

with intravenous sedation, depending on surgeon and patient preference.

Special Instruments/Equipment/Implants

The procedure is performed under loupe magnification. Magnification is essential to identify and protect the branches of the superficial radial sensory nerve. A soft-tissue set, with fine hand instruments, should be used for this operation.

Surgical Technique

Surgical intervention in de Quervain syndrome must adhere to two principles. The first principle is that care must be taken to protect the superficial radial nerve and its branches. Several branches of the superficial radial sensory nerve lie within

---

None of the following authors nor any immediate family member has received anything of value from or owns stock in a commercial company or institution related directly or indirectly to the subject of this chapter: Dr. Venouziou, Dr. Giannoulis, and Dr. Sotereanos.

© 2013 American Academy of Orthopaedic Surgeons

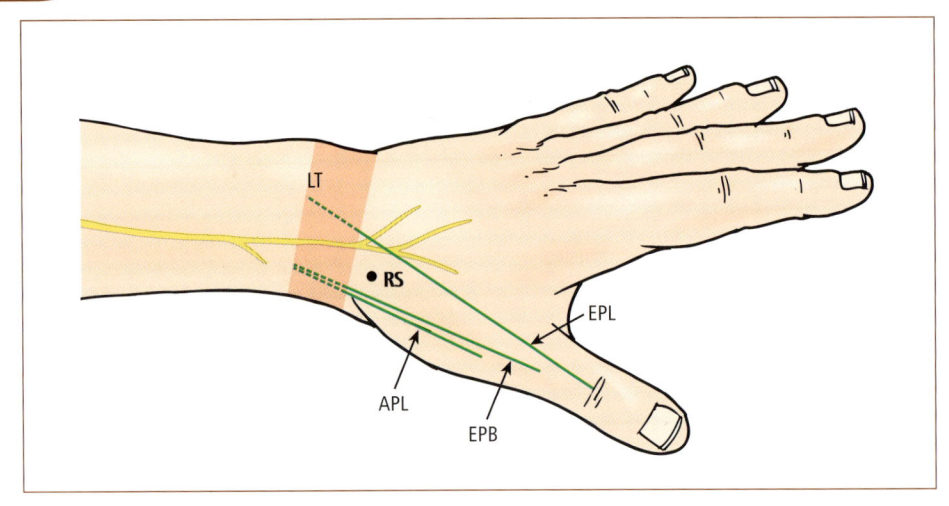

Figure 2 Illustration shows the course of the superficial branch of the radial nerve (SBRN) in the distal forearm. APL = abductor pollicis longus, EPB = extensor pollicis brevis, EPL = extensor pollicis longus, LT = Lister tubercle, RS = radial styloid process.

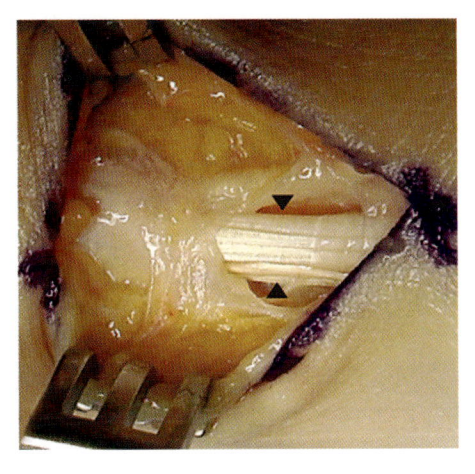

Figure 3 Intraoperative photograph shows the extensor pollicis brevis and abductor pollicis longus tendons (between the black arrowheads).

the subcutaneous fat overlying the first dorsal compartment (Figure 2). The first branch comes off in a radial direction and continues on to the volar aspect of the forearm and innervates the radial aspect of the thumb. The main trunk of the superficial radial sensory nerve continues distally and divides into three to five branches that pass over the extensor pollicis longus tendon. These branches travel in an ulnar direction over the dorsum of the hand, supplying the radial three digits (thumb, index finger, and long finger).[6]

Longitudinal incisions generally lead to fewer superficial nerve injuries than do transverse incisions. For this reason, we use a small longitudinal incision from the tip of the radial styloid distally for approximately 1.5 cm. (The surgical technique can be seen in the video.) Sharp dissection is then carried just through the dermis but not into the subcutaneous fat. After retracting the skin edges, the subcutaneous fat is dissected bluntly with tenotomy scissors down to the retinaculum of the first dorsal compartment. Extreme care is taken to protect the superficial branches of the radial sensory nerve. Excessive dissection and/or retraction can result in neurapraxia or neuroma in continuity. Strict adherence to this principle is important to avoid symptoms secondary to superficial radial sensory nerve injury, which can be far more severe than those due to stenosing tenosynovitis of the first dorsal compartment.

The EPB and APL tendons are identified distal to the stenosing compartment. Correct placement of retractors ensures adequate visualization of the entire sheath, which is usually inflated and sometimes filled with synovial fluid (Figure 3). Then the first dorsal compartment is released on its dorsal margin with tenotomy scissors (Figure 4). Releasing the compartment on its dorsal margin leaves a thick volar-based flap of retinaculum and thus prevents tendon subluxation. In cases where the retinaculum is remarkably thick as a result of inflammation, care must be taken to avoid injury to the EPB tendon while releasing the compartment.

The second principle is to ensure complete release of the stenosing compartment. The first dorsal compartment is subdivided by a septum into two separate fibro-osseous tunnels in 40% to 60% of

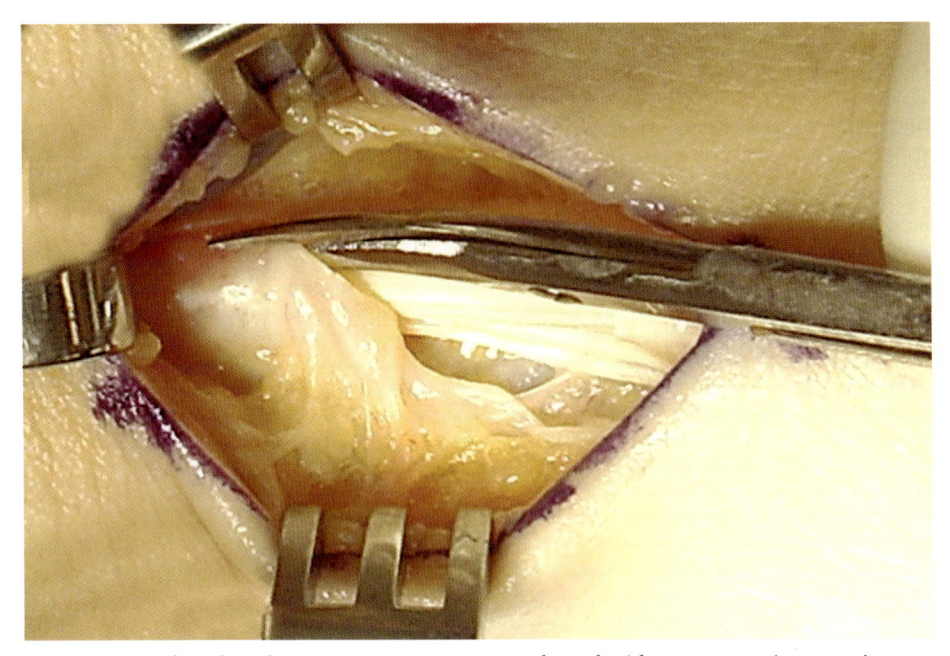

Figure 4 The first dorsal extensor compartment is released with tenotomy scissors on its dorsal margin. Note the thick volar flap of the retinaculum, which prevents volar subluxation on the tendons.

the general population. The ulnar-sided tunnel contains the EPB tendon, and the radial-sided tunnel contains the multiple APL tendon slips (Figure 5). The subcompartment within the first dorsal compartment for the EPB tendon is not always immediately apparent (Figure 6). The most common location for an EPB subcompartment is at the dorsoulnar aspect of the first dorsal compartment. However, a subcompartment can be present within the osseous floor of the first dorsal compartment, or the subcompartment can have a partial septation that does not extend along the entire length of the first dorsal compartment, making it even less

Chapter 37: First Dorsal Extensor Compartment Release

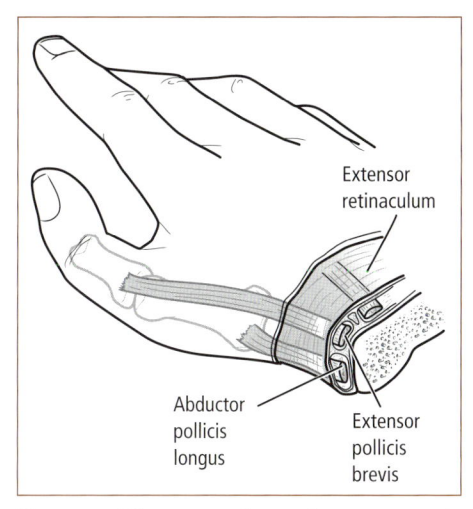

Figure 5 Illustration shows the anatomy of the first dorsal compartment.

evident.[7-9] Any intracompartmental septum should be identified, released, and excised (**Figure 7**).

The floor of the first dorsal compartment should be examined for anomalous tunnels containing aberrant tendons, which must be unroofed. To ensure that complete release of the first dorsal compartment has been achieved, it is imperative to identify the EPB and APL tendons. The EPB tendon is rounder and smaller than the APL tendon and is absent in 5% to 7% of individuals. Muscle fibers, if seen within the first dorsal compartment, usually help identify the EPB tendon as the EPB muscle belly extends further distally.[1,8,9] Gentle traction to the EPB tendon should demonstrate extension of the thumb metacarpophalangeal (MP) joint. If there is no extension of the thumb MP joint, the surgeon should look for a subcompartment.[7]

The APL tendon is then identified. The APL usually has two or more tendon slips (up to five), which may insert onto the trapezium, the volar carpal ligament, the opponens pollicis, or the abductor pollicis brevis in addition to the consistent and functionally important insertion onto the base of the first metacarpal.[8] By pulling the slips of the APL tendon, the surgeon should notice abduction of the thumb.

The wrist is then flexed and extended and any evidence of tendon subluxation is noted. The tourniquet is released, and meticulous hemostasis is performed. The wound is irrigated, and the skin is closed with 4-0 nylon horizontal mattress sutures. To prevent volar subluxation of the tendons, a radial thumb spica splint is applied for 2 weeks, until the skin sutures are removed.

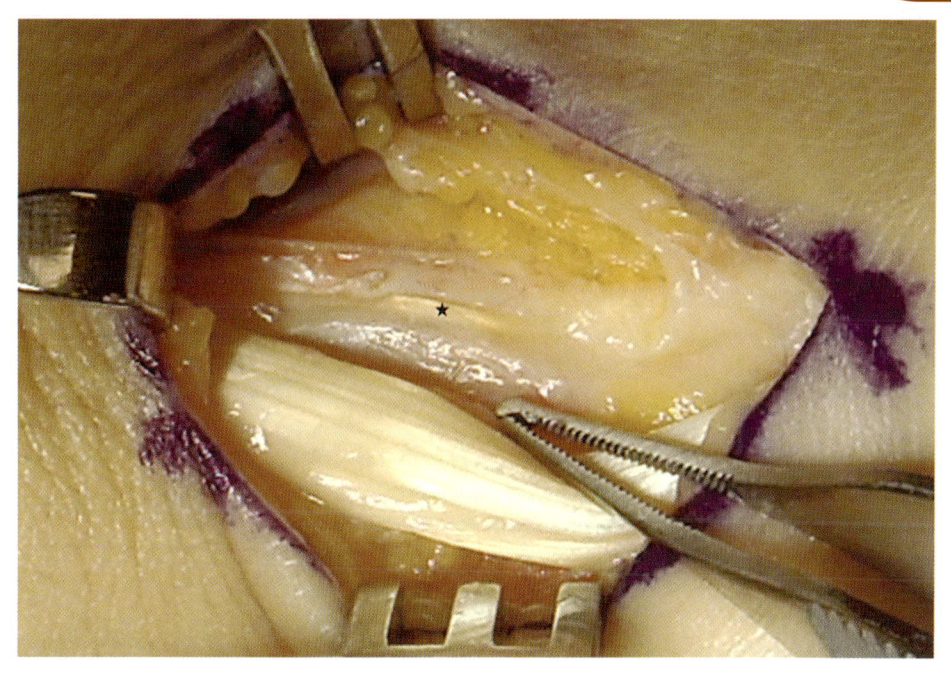

Figure 6 A separate compartment containing the extensor pollicis brevis (EPB) tendon is a common finding in patients with de Quervain syndrome. In this case, the APL tendon is retracted after the release of the first dorsal compartment and a separate compartment of the EPB tendon (star) is seen.

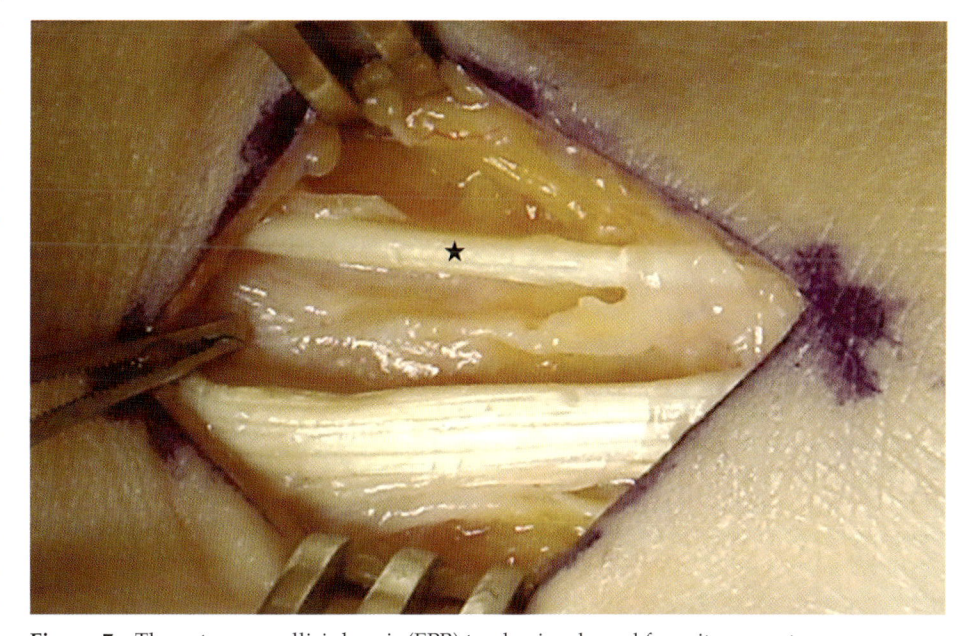

Figure 7 The extensor pollicis brevis (EPB) tendon is released from its separate compartment, and the intracompartmental septum is excised. The EPB tendon (star) is rounder and smaller than the abductor pollicis longus tendon.

Complications

Ninety percent of patients can be expected to have a satisfactory outcome following surgical release of the first dorsal compartment for de Quervain syndrome. The most serious complication of this procedure is iatrogenic injury to the radial sensory nerve, with the subsequent formation of a painful neuroma. Even excessive traction to radial sensory nerve branches can cause prolonged neurapraxia. The treatment depends on the injury to the nerve.

If a neuroma is present, it should be resected and the nerve repaired using microsurgical techniques, to restore sensation to the thumb and index finger. In the case of a neuroma caused by laceration of a terminal sensory branch, a good alternative is to relocate the neuroma. Neuroma relocation consists of neuroma resection and placement of the termi-

© 2013 American Academy of Orthopaedic Surgeons

nal nerve branch into a muscle that is proximal to the level of the nerve lesion and far from the scar.

Fibrosis and adhesion formation after surgical release of the first dorsal compartment can cause compression of the terminal branches of the radial nerve. Symptoms include pain, numbness, and tingling over the dorsal surface of the thumb and index finger. Paresthesias are accentuated by percussion in this area. The treatment in this case is exploration and neurolysis of the scarred nerves. Alternatively, a wrapping technique, with a vein or an off-the-shelf nerve-protecting product, can be used to prevent cicatrix recurrence (**Figure 8**).[10,11]

The anatomy of the first dorsal compartment of the wrist is highly variable. Failure to recognize the anatomic variations, especially multiple APL tendon slips and subdivided first dorsal compartments, can lead to incomplete release of the compartment and thus to persistent pain. A higher incidence of subdivided first dorsal compartments is reported in patients with de Quervain syndrome, suggesting that separate fibro-osseous tunnels may predispose one to developing de Quervain syndrome.[12] Persistent pain after first dorsal compartment release may be due to failure to free the EPB completely from its separate subcompartment.[7-9] Revision surgery to open an unreleased separate compartment should be considered in that case.

Subluxation of released tendons is also problematic. With wrist flexion and extension, the tendons of the first dorsal compartment snap over the radial styloid. This complication is best avoided by releasing the first dorsal compartment at its dorsal margin, leaving a palmar-based flap of retinaculum to prevent tendon subluxation. Symptomatic volar subluxation of the APL and EPB tendons can be addressed with a retinacular sling or a slip of brachioradialis tendon.

Other rare complications of first dorsal compartment release are superficial wound infection, hypertrophic scar formation, and complex regional pain syndrome.

Postoperative Care and Rehabilitation

Postoperatively, a soft bulky dressing and a radial thumb spica splint, allowing movement of the interphalangeal joint, is applied for 10 to 14 days. This will minimize the risk for volar subluxation of the tendons. Motion of the thumb and

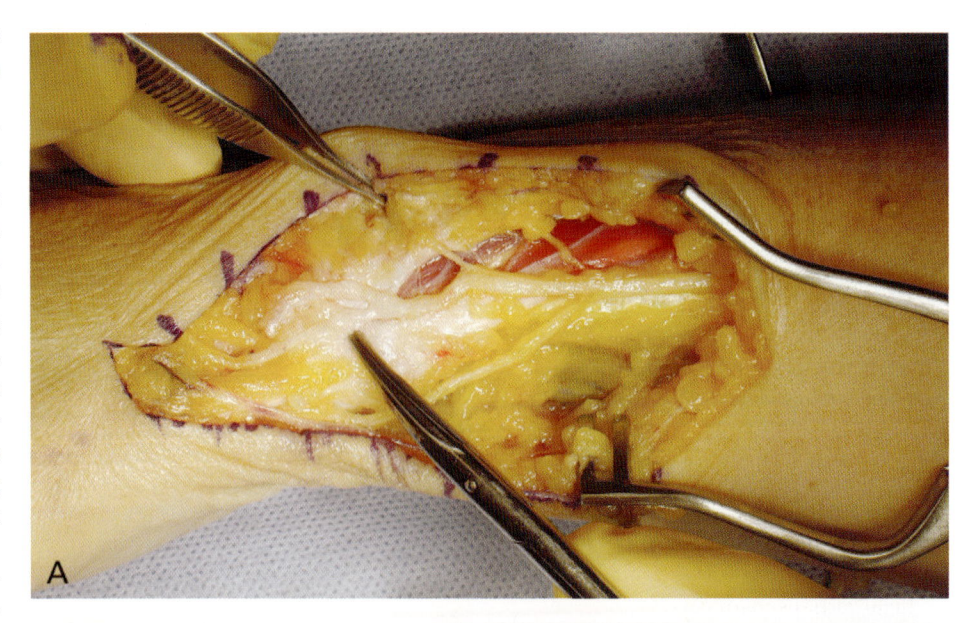

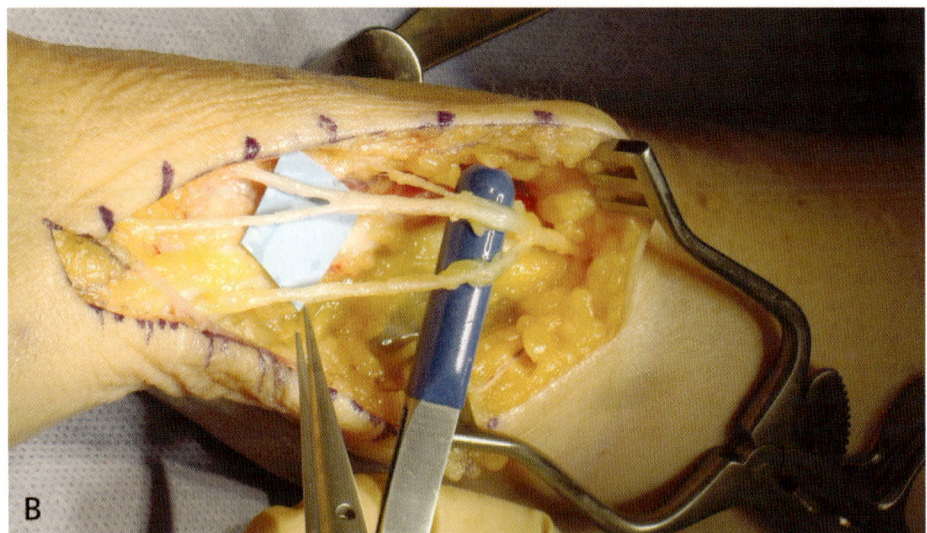

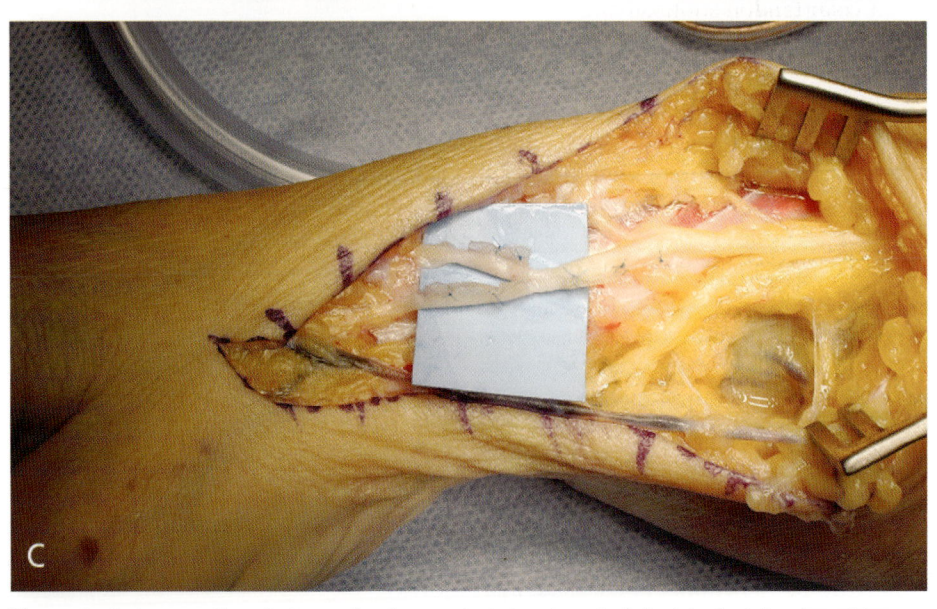

Figure 8 Intraoperative photographs demonstrate treatment of cicatrix that developed in a 62-year-old woman. She had persistent pain and numbness in the thumb and index finger after first dorsal compartment release. **A**, Exploration of the radial sensory nerve, 10 months after the first surgery, revealed extensive cicatrix around its terminal branches. **B**, Neurolysis of the radial sensory nerve was performed, and all branches were freed from cicatrix. **C**, An off-the-shelf nerve protector was wrapped around the terminal branches to prevent recurrence of cicatrix.

hand is immediately encouraged and is increased as tolerated. Skin sutures are removed in 10 to 14 days, at the first postoperative check. Formal hand therapy is rarely necessary.

Localized soreness may persist for 4 to 6 weeks postoperatively and generally responds to wound massage and light use of the hand. We advise patients to avoid heavy mechanical activities for the initial 4 to 6 weeks. Preoperative symptoms lasting greater than 10 months have been reported to adversely affect the prognosis.[1]

Pearls

- A longitudinal incision should be used to help avoid injury to the superficial radial sensory nerve.
- Blunt dissection of the subcutaneous fat should be performed by spreading the blades of the scissors longitudinally, parallel to the radial nerve branches.
- The sheath should be incised on the dorsal margin to prevent tendon subluxation.
- Traction on one of the released tendons must result in extension of the MP joint, indicating release of the EPB tendon. If this does not occur, we inspect for a separate EPB compartment and excise any intracompartmental septa.
- A radial gutter thumb spica is applied for 10 to 14 days to minimize the risk of volar tendon subluxation.

References

1. Giannoulis FS, Musgrave DS, Payatakes AH, Sotereanos DS: Trigger finger, de Quervain's syndrome, and elbow tendinopathy, in Trumble TE, Budoff JE, eds: *Hand Surgery Update*, ed 4. Rosemont, IL, American Society for Surgery of the Hand, 2007, pp 371-388.
2. Wolf JM, Sturdivant RX, Owens BD: Incidence of de Quervain's tenosynovitis in a young, active population. *J Hand Surg Am* 2009;34(1):112-115.
3. Ilyas AM, Ast M, Schaffer AA, Thoder J: De quervain tenosynovitis of the wrist. *J Am Acad Orthop Surg* 2007;15(12):757-764.
4. Finkelstein H: Stenosing tendovaginitis at the radial styloid process. *J Bone Joint Surg Am* 1930;12(3):509-540.
5. Kutsumi K, Amadio PC, Zhao C, Zobitz ME, Tanaka T, An KN: Finkelstein's test: A biomechanical analysis. *J Hand Surg Am* 2005;30(1):130-135.
6. Robson AJ, See MS, Ellis H: Applied anatomy of the superficial branch of the radial nerve. *Clin Anat* 2008;21(1):38-45.
7. Alemohammad AM, Yazaki N, Morris RP, Buford WL, Viegas SF: Thumb interphalangeal joint extension by the extensor pollicis brevis: Association with a subcompartment and de Quervain's disease. *J Hand Surg Am* 2009;34(4):719-723.
8. Kulthanan T, Chareonwat B: Variations in abductor pollicis longus and extensor pollicis brevis tendons in the Quervain syndrome: A surgical and anatomical study. *Scand J Plast Reconstr Surg Hand Surg* 2007;41(1):36-38.
9. Kulshreshtha R, Patel S, Arya AP, Hall S, Compson JP: Variations of the extensor pollicis brevis tendon and its insertion: A study of 44 cadaveric hands. *J Hand Surg Eur Vol* 2007;32(5):550-553.
10. Kokkalis ZT, Pu C, Small GA, Weiser RW, Venouziou AI, Sotereanos DG: Assessment of processed porcine extracellular matrix as a protective barrier in a rabbit nerve wrap model. *J Reconstr Microsurg* 2011;27(1):19-28.
11. Varitimidis SE, Vardakas DG, Goebel F, Sotereanos DG: Treatment of recurrent compressive neuropathy of peripheral nerves in the upper extremity with an autologous vein insulator. *J Hand Surg Am* 2001;26(2):296-302.
12. McAuliffe JA: Tendon disorders of the hand and wrist. *J Hand Surg Am* 2010;35(5):846-853.

Video Reference

37.1 Giannoulis FS, Musgrave DS, Payatakes AH, Sotereanos DG: Video: First dorsal extensor compartment release, in Trumble TE, Budoff JE, eds: *Hand Surgery Update*, ed 4. Rosement, IL, American Society for Surgery of the Hand, 2007.

Chapter 38
Trigger Finger Release

Randy Bindra, MD   Micah Sinclair, MD

Introduction

Trigger finger, also known as stenosing tenosynovitis, is a painful catching of a digit with attempted active extension. This occurs most commonly at the level of the A1 pulley because of a disparity in the size of the flexor tendons and the surrounding tendon sheath, resulting in interference with smooth tendon gliding. The pathologic changes observed with this disorder include stenosis of the fibrous flexor tendon sheath due to chronic inflammation as well as a reactive nodule within the flexor digitorum superficialis tendon.

The highest incidence of trigger finger is seen in patients who are approximately age 60 years; it is more common in females. Although trigger finger is most frequently idiopathic, certain activities that require repetitive finger flexion and diabetes have been independently associated with this condition. The thumb and the ring finger are the most commonly affected digits. A trigger thumb in a child may present as a congenital anomaly.

The diagnosis of trigger finger is a clinical one, based on history and physical examination. Clinical presentation varies with the stage of the disease.[1] In grade 1 (mild), there is a history of catching of the finger that is not reproducible on physical examination, and tenderness over the A1 pulley. In grade 2 (moderate), catching of the digit is observed, but the patient can actively extend the digit. In grade 3 (severe), the flexed digit requires manual passive extension or the patient is unable to flex the digit to the point of triggering. Grade 4 (locked) is characterized by catching with a fixed flexion contracture of the proximal interphalangeal (PIP) joint.

Patient Selection
Special Populations/Situations
Certain populations that present with triggering require special consideration.

Children
Children with trigger thumbs present with an inability to straighten the interphalangeal (IP) joint rather than catching of the digit. The deformity is usually first noted at approximately age 6 months, but late presentation is not uncommon because of the compensatory hyperextension of the metacarpophalangeal (MCP) joint. Spontaneous resolution is possible, and a period of observation for at least 6 months is recommended, especially in children younger than 3 years.[2] Persistent triggering requires surgical release to avoid fixed IP contractures. Trigger fingers are rare in children, accounting for 7% to 14% of all trigger digits in children, and usually indicate underlying aberrant anatomy of the tendon-pulley system that requires more extensive surgical exploration and management.[3]

Patients With Diabetes
Although a steroid injection into the tendon sheath is the appropriate initial treatment for trigger finger, studies have reported a lower success rate of approximately 50% in diabetic patients compared to 86% in nondiabetic patients.[4] Additionally, diabetic patients must be informed of the potential for a hyperglycemic effect with injection that can last up to 5 days.[5] Lastly, residual stiffness of the PIP joint after treatment is common in diabetics, generally leading to less satisfactory outcomes in this group.

Patients With Rheumatoid Arthritis
The primary underlying pathology in rheumatoid arthritis is synovitis within the tendon sheath, not stenosis of the A1 pulley. Not only will pulley release be ineffective in symptom resolution, it may actually cause functional deterioration by contributing to ulnar drift of the fingers. Treatment of these patients should include early surgical intervention with flexor tenosynovectomy to remove the diseased tenosynovium surrounding the tendon.[6] If the condition fails to respond to this treatment or the patient continues to have triggering when evaluated intraoperatively, resection of the ulnar slip of the flexor digitorum superficialis can be performed with reliable results.[7]

Patients With Distal Triggering
Rarely, patients will have triggering related to the A3 pulley at the level of the PIP joint. The report of pain at the PIP joint is consistent with physical examination findings—tenderness palmar to the PIP joint rather than the MCP joint and often a palpable swelling within the flexor tendon adjacent to the PIP joint. These patients characteristically have triggering that occurs when the PIP joint is at or beyond 90° of flexion. The tendon involved is the flexor digitorum profundus, and symptoms can also be found at the distal interphalangeal joint. An A3 pulley excision has been shown to be successful in these patients.[8]

Patients With PIP Contracture
In patients with longstanding and severe disease with inability to straighten the finger, secondary contracture of the PIP palmar plate may develop. In these cases, patients should be advised of the possibility of residual flexion contracture of the digit following release of the A1 pulley.

Indications
Initial treatment of trigger finger should be nonsurgical.[9] In nondiabetic patients, either a single corticosteroid injection or a series of up to three injections have been found to be a successful treatment in 75% of the patients at 6-month follow-up.[4,10,11] Despite the fact that multiple studies have confirmed a lower success rate for corticosteroid injections in patients with diabetes, this should remain the first line of treatment in these patients. In the discussion of a treatment plan with patients with diabetes, they must be informed of the lower success rate of injection as well as the potential for hyperglycemia following injection.[4,5]

Percutaneous release may be considered in selected cases of triggering of

---

Dr. Bindra has received royalties from Tornier; is a member of a speakers' bureau or has made paid presentations on behalf of Auxilium and Integra NeuroSciences; serves as a paid consultant to or is an employee of Acumed and Integra LifeSciences; and serves as a board member, owner, officer, or committee member of the American Association for Hand Surgery and the American Society for Surgery of the Hand. Neither Dr. Sinclair nor any immediate family member has received anything of value from or owns stock in a commercial company or institution related directly or indirectly to the subject of this chapter.

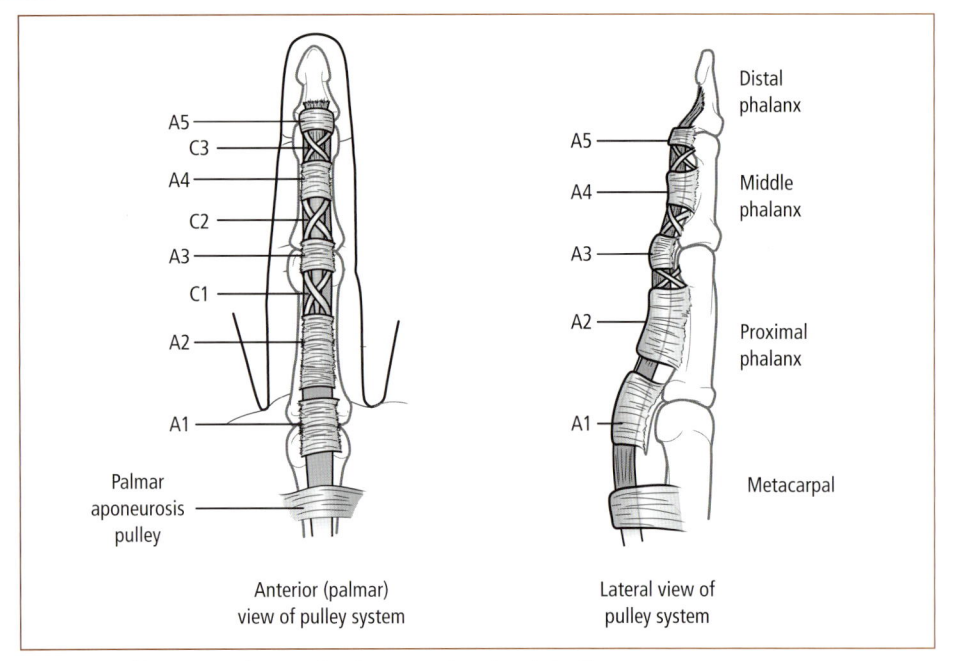

Figure 1 Illustration depicts the flexor tendon sheath/pulley system anatomy.

the long and ring fingers. Performed in the outpatient clinic, the procedure has been reported to be successful in up to 91% of patients.[1,12] Practice in a cadaver model followed by open release using an 18-gauge needle is recommended before performing percutaneous release in the clinic.[12]

Specific indications for open trigger finger release include failed nonsurgical management with steroid injection, failed percutaneous trigger finger release, and long-standing or severe disease.[10,13]

Patient characteristics that contribute to a higher risk of failure of nonsurgical management and likely surgical treatment include younger age, insulin-dependent diabetes mellitus, involvement of multiple digits, and/or a history of other tendinopathies of the upper extremity.[10]

Contraindications

Contraindications to open trigger finger release include rheumatoid arthritis and trigger finger in a pediatric patient. Pediatric patients should be referred to a physician with experience in pediatric hand surgery.

Preoperative Imaging

Investigations such as ultrasound and radiographs are indicated only if other diagnoses, such as arthritis or tumors, are to be considered. Ultrasound can be used to evaluate for thickening of the A1 pulley or to assess any abnormality of the flexor tendon.[14]

Relevant Surgical Anatomy
Surface Anatomy

Traditionally, the surface anatomy of the A1 pulley has been based on the location of palmar creases. The proximal edge of the A1 pulley lies at the level of the distal palmar crease in the ring and small fingers, the proximal palmar crease in the index finger, and halfway between both creases in the long finger. The proximal edge of the A1 pulley of the thumb is at the MCP crease. With recent interest in percutaneous release, the measured distance between the digital palmar crease and the PIP crease has been found to be exactly the same as that from the proximal edge of the A1 pulley to the digital palmar crease. Thus, this measured distance can be used as a landmark for identification of the location of the A1 pulley.[15]

Neurovascular Anatomy

The neurovascular bundles for each digit run parallel to the flexor sheath and are located immediately radial and ulnar to the flexor sheath. If dissection is kept in the midline, these structures are safe.

In the thumb, the radial digital nerve crosses the flexor sheath just proximal to the A1 pulley at the level of the MCP crease and lies very superficial in this location. The radial digital nerve must be identified and carefully preserved during trigger thumb release; percutaneous release is not recommended in the thumb.

Flexor Tendon Sheath Anatomy

The A1 pulley is the most proximal annular thickening of the flexor tendon sheath and measures approximately 10 mm in length (Figure 1). Immediately distal to the A1 pulley lies the A2 pulley. Its function is critical to prevent tendon bowstringing, and it should be preserved during surgery. Anatomic studies have found a nearly 50% incidence of continuity between the A1 and A2 pulleys. The two pulleys can be differentiated by several millimeters of pronounced thinning of the retinacular tissue at the usual site of separation that becomes apparent as release of the A1 pulley is completed at surgery. Immediately proximal to the A1 pulley is the palmar aponeurosis pulley, formed by the distal edge of the palmar fascia. This can be released if thickened or if triggering persists following release of the A1 pulley.[16] In the thumb, the oblique pulley replaces the A2 pulley of the digits and lies at the distal edge of the A1 pulley attached to the shaft of the proximal phalanx. This must be preserved when releasing a trigger thumb.

Video 38.1 Management of Trigger Finger: From Injection to Surgery. Randy R. Bindra, MD (15 min)

Procedure
Surgical Technique
Release of the Central Digits (Ring or Long Finger)

In most cases, surgery can be performed using local anesthesia, with sedation if necessary. The patient is placed in the supine position on the operating room table with the outstretched arm supinated on an arm board. A well-padded tourniquet is placed on the upper arm.

Landmarks are drawn on the skin, including the midline of the finger and the A1 pulley, which begins at the distal palmar crease. The surgical incision is outlined obliquely from the distal palmar crease across the A1 pulley to the digital palmar crease of the finger (Figure 2, A). An oblique incision allows safe exposure of the tendon sheath with the option of extension proximally or distally if required. For a more aesthetic result, the incision can be placed in a skin crease.

Local anesthetic is administered subcutaneously at the incision site. A median nerve block can be performed if the surgical finger is the thumb, the index finger, or the long finger.

Chapter 38: Trigger Finger Release

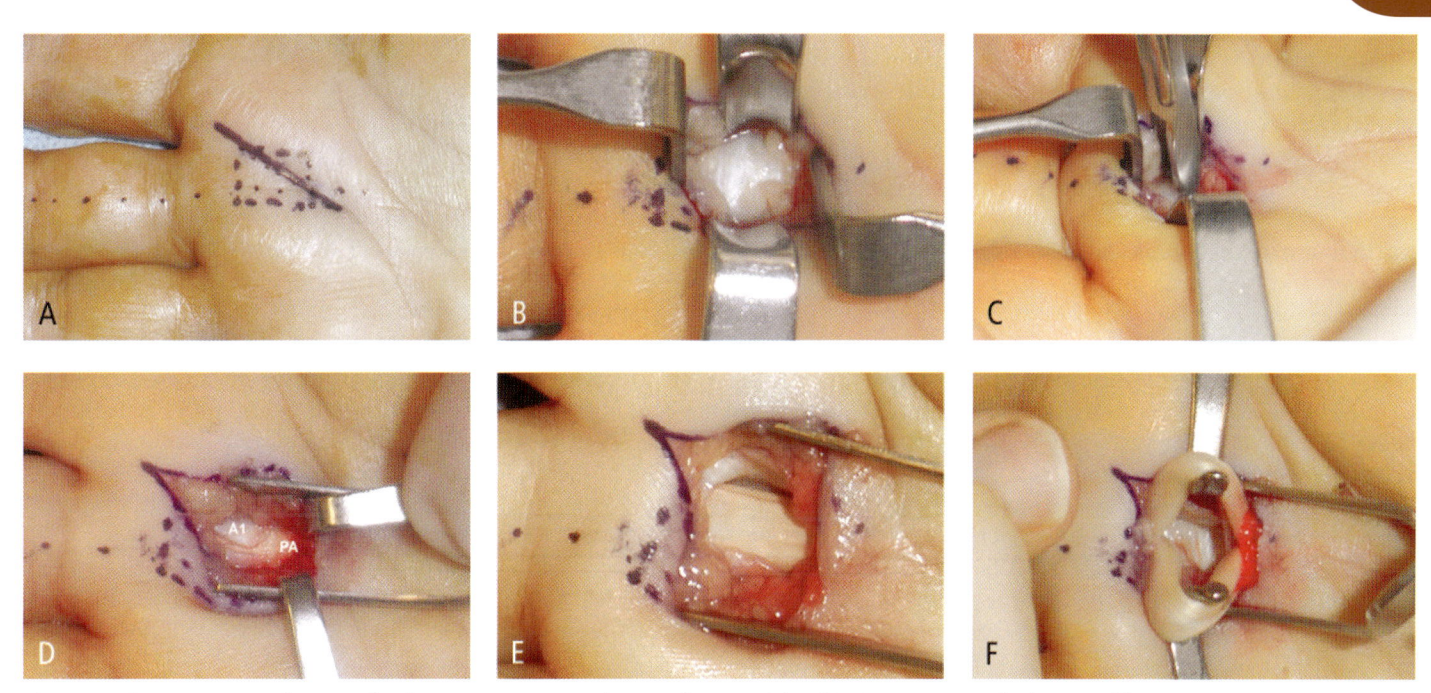

Figure 2 Intraoperative photographs demonstrate trigger finger release. **A,** The skin incision is marked. **B,** A self-retaining retractor is placed. **C,** The incision is made at the center of the A1 pulley. **D,** The anatomic relationship between the A1 pulley, which has been released, and the palmar aponeurosis pulley is visualized. (PA = palmar aponeurosis.) **E,** Complete release of the A1 and palmar aponeurosis pulleys. **F,** The floor of the tendon sheath is visualized. Note the normal appearance of the transverse fibers of the A1 pulley.

After the skin is prepared and draped in sterile fashion, the limb is exsanguinated with an elastic bandage, and the tourniquet is elevated. The skin is carefully incised along the planned incision, and skin hooks are placed initially for retraction on either side of the incision.

The subcutaneous tissues are gently dissected by spreading with tenotomy scissors. Care must be taken to maintain dissection along the midline of the finger to prevent damage to neurovascular structures on either side of the flexor sheath. These may be identified but do not need to be dissected out and isolated.

Next, 90° angled retractors are placed, and spreading dissection is continued in the midline with tenotomy scissors until the flexor tendon sheath is encountered. Once the flexor sheath is adequately exposed, a self-retaining retractor is placed (Figure 2, B). The A1 pulley is identified and, using a sharp No. 15 surgical scalpel, an incision is made at the center of the A1 pulley (Figure 2, C).

The distal and proximal ends of the pulley are then released with the tenotomy scissors. The thickened A1 pulley classically generates a grating sensation when cut. Upon completion of the release of the A1 pulley, the proximal skin edge is retracted and the palmar aponeurosis pulley is exposed. If it is found to be tight or thickened, it can also be released, as it may lead to persistence of triggering[17] (Figure 2, D and E). Adequate release of

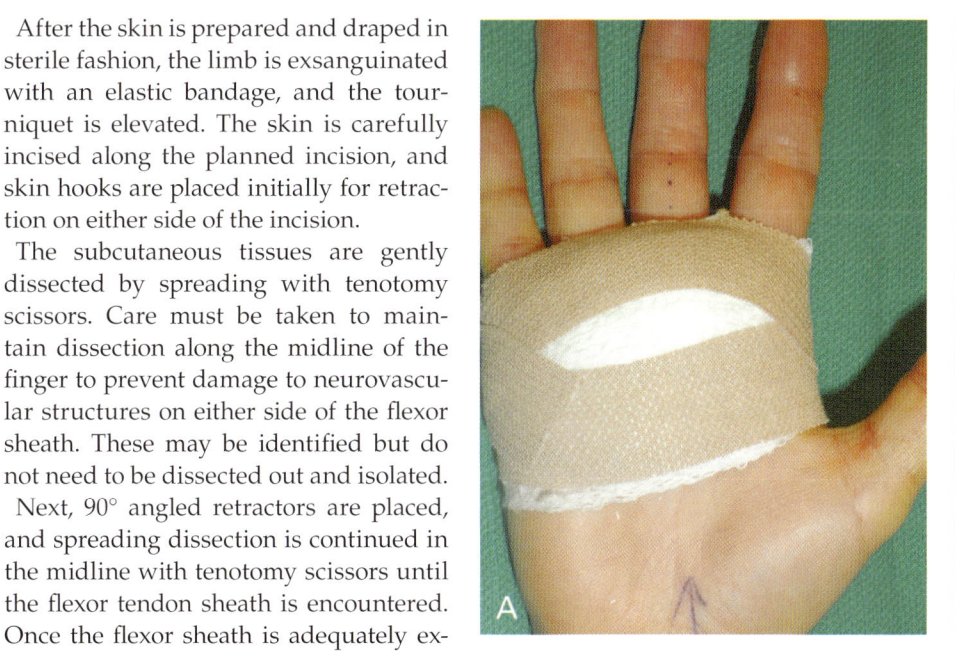

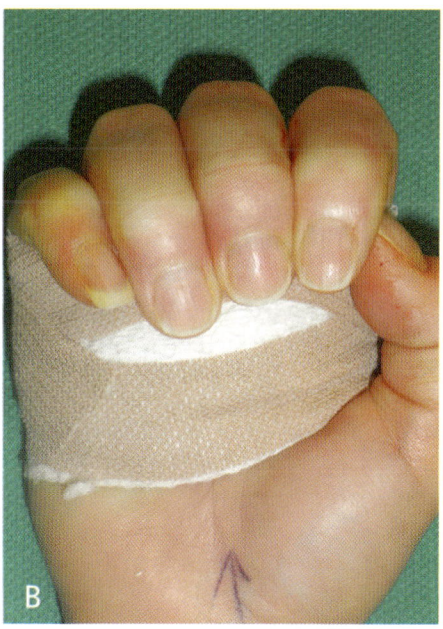

Figure 3 Photographs show the hand of a patient with the fingers extended (**A**) and flexed (**B**) following trigger finger release. The low-profile postoperative dressing allows full range of motion.

the triggering is confirmed by asking the patient to actively and fully flex and extend the finger several times.

It is also possible to deliver both of the flexor tendons into the wound for manual inspection. Retraction of the two tendons to either side, or to the radial and ulnar sides of the pulley will expand the Camper chiasm and allow inspection of the tendons as well as the floor of the tendon sheath for any pathology (Figure 2, F). Débridement or synovectomy of the tendons is not usually necessary but may be required if there is significant synovitis or thickening of the tendon.

The tourniquet is released and hemostasis is secured. Skin edges are approximated with a 4-0 or 5-0 nonabsorbable suture. After placing a nonadherent dressing, a low-profile compression bandage is applied, leaving all digits fully free to mobilize postoperatively (Figure 3).

© 2013 American Academy of Orthopaedic Surgeons

Trigger Thumb Release

Positioning and preparation is similar to trigger release of other digits. The course of the radial and ulnar digital nerves is mapped on the surface. After the skin is prepared and draped in sterile fashion, the limb is exsanguinated with an elastic bandage, and the tourniquet is elevated.

The skin is then incised carefully along an oblique line centered on the MCP crease. The obliquity of the incision runs parallel to the course of the radial digital nerve to avoid inadvertent injury to the nerve as the incision is deepened.

Further dissection of the subcutaneous tissues must be performed carefully using tenotomy scissors and must be maintained parallel to the direction of the neurovascular bundles. Care must be taken to identify and protect the radial digital nerve and its accompanying artery. The radial digital nerve is carefully retracted and protected throughout the procedure.

Once the flexor sheath is identified and clearly visualized, an incision is made sharply with a No. 15 blade in the midline of the A1 pulley at the level of the MCP crease. The remainder of the pulley release is performed using tenotomy scissors by retracting the incision first distally and then proximally. During the proximal retraction, care must again be taken to ensure that the radial digital nerve is protected.

Upon completion of the release of the thickened pulley, the patient is asked to actively move the thumb to demonstrate relief of triggering. The tendon can be retracted into the wound for inspection and débridement if necessary.

After securing hemostasis, the wound is closed in one layer with nonabsorbable sutures. Dressings are applied so as not to obstruct postoperative motion of the finger.

Complications

An understanding of the underlying anatomy, meticulous care during the operation, and adequate postoperative rehabilitation will ensure a successful outcome in all cases of trigger finger release. Common complications and their prevention are highlighted.[11,18]

Incomplete Release

Resolution of triggering should be evaluated intraoperatively by active finger flexion following the release of the A1 pulley and before wound closure. Failure to recognize and release all tight structures can result in persistent triggering or partial release.

Digital Nerve Injury

Digital nerve injury can be avoided by strictly maintaining surgical dissection at the midline over the tendon sheath. In the case of trigger thumb, it is important to identify and protect the radial digital nerve. Neurapraxia of the digital nerve can occur with vigorous retraction and may account for some numbness after surgery. If sensation does not return within 3 months, exploration of the digital nerve should be considered.

Scar Tenderness

Scar tenderness can be minimized by initiation of scar massage and therapy.

Postoperative Stiffness

To avoid stiffness of the operated finger and the rest of the hand, the postoperative dressings must not obstruct digital motion. The patient is instructed to perform gentle active digital exercises upon discharge home. After 2 days, dressings are reduced to allow intensification of digital exercises and the patient is encouraged to use the hand for activities as tolerated while keeping the wound clean and dry. Patients at higher risk of stiffness, such as diabetics and those with preoperative limited range of motion due to severe triggering, should start supervised therapy within the first week after surgery. Consideration may be given to dynamic splinting of the PIP joint for severe flexion contractures.

Bowstringing

Bowstringing may occur if more than 50% of the A2 pulley is inadvertently released.[19] In symptomatic patients, the pulley should be reconstructed using the surgeon's preferred technique.

Postoperative Care and Rehabilitation

The patient is instructed to start actively moving all fingers and using the hand for light activities immediately after surgery. Elevation and ice are used for the first 2 days to prevent edema.

The patient is seen in the outpatient clinic 2 days after surgery. The wound is evaluated, and dressings are reduced to a simple adhesive bandage. Range of motion is evaluated, and active exercises of the fingers and hand are encouraged. Patients are allowed to do their normal daily activities and return to light work if desired.

The patient is seen again in the outpatient clinic 2 weeks following surgery. The sutures are removed, and the patient is instructed in exercises to mobilize and strengthen the hands. The patient is also instructed in scar management, which consists of taping a silicone sheet onto the scar overnight as well as massaging lotion into the scar several times a day for approximately 6 to 10 weeks after surgery. The patient is encouraged to pursue a home exercise program of active finger mobilization, isolating the proximal and distal IP joints. A dynamic splint such as a Capener splint may be used for fingers with persistent flexion contracture of the PIP joint.

Pearls

- Surgery is best performed using local anesthetic when possible to allow intraoperative evaluation of complete release.
- An oblique incision along a skin crease allows safe exposure, easy incision of the tendon sheath, and extension proximally or distally if needed.
- Dissection should be maintained along the midline of the finger to prevent damage to neurovascular structures on either side of the flexor sheath.
- In trigger thumbs, care must be taken to identify and protect the radial digital nerve and its accompanying artery as it crosses the tendon at the proximal aspect of the A1 pulley.
- Following release of the A1 pulley, the patient is asked to actively move the finger to confirm adequate release of triggering.
- If triggering is not completely relieved, consideration should be given to release of the palmar aponeurosis pulley, release of the A3 pulley, reduction flexor tenoplasty,[17] or ulnar superficialis slip resection.[7]

References

1. Eastwood DM, Gupta KJ, Johnson DP: Percutaneous release of the trigger finger: An office procedure. *J Hand Surg Am* 1992;17(1):114-117.
2. Baek GH, Kim JH, Chung MS, Kang SB, Lee YH, Gong HS: The natural history of pediatric trigger thumb. *J Bone Joint Surg Am* 2008;90(5):980-985.
3. Cardon LJ, Ezaki M, Carter PR: Trigger finger in children. *J Hand Surg Am* 1999;24(6):1156-1161.
4. Baumgarten KM, Gerlach D, Boyer MI: Corticosteroid injection in diabetic

patients with trigger finger: A prospective, randomized, controlled double-blinded study. *J Bone Joint Surg Am* 2007;89(12):2604-2611.
5. Wang AA, Hutchinson DT: The effect of corticosteroid injection for trigger finger on blood glucose level in diabetic patients. *J Hand Surg Am* 2006;31(6):979-981.
6. Ferlic DC, Clayton ML: Flexor tenosynovectomy in the rheumatoid finger. *J Hand Surg Am* 1978;3(4):364-367.
7. Le Viet D, Tsionos I, Boulouednine M, Hannouche D: Trigger finger treatment by ulnar superficialis slip resection (U.S.S.R.). *J Hand Surg Br* 2004;29(4):368-373.
8. Rayan GM: Distal stenosing tenosynovitis. *J Hand Surg Am* 1990;15(6):973-975.
9. McAuliffe JA: Tendon disorders of the hand and wrist. *J Hand Surg Am* 2010;35(5):846-853, quiz 853.
10. Rhoades CE, Gelberman RH, Manjarris JF: Stenosing tenosynovitis of the fingers and thumb: Results of a prospective trial of steroid injection and splinting. *Clin Orthop Relat Res* 1984;190:236-238.
11. Turowski GA, Zdankiewicz PD, Thomson JG: The results of surgical treatment of trigger finger. *J Hand Surg Am* 1997;22(1):145-149.
12. Bain GI, Turnbull J, Charles MN, Roth JH, Richards RS: Percutaneous A1 pulley release: A cadaveric study. *J Hand Surg Am* 1995;20(5):781-784, discussion 785-786.
13. Newport ML, Lane LB, Stuchin SA: Treatment of trigger finger by steroid injection. *J Hand Surg Am* 1990;15(5):748-750.
14. Guerini H, Pessis E, Theumann N, et al: Sonographic appearance of trigger fingers. *J Ultrasound Med* 2008;27(10):1407-1413.
15. Wilhelmi BJ, Snyder N IV, Verbesey JE, Ganchi PA, Lee WP: Trigger finger release with hand surface landmark ratios: An anatomic and clinical study. *Plast Reconstr Surg* 2001;108(4):908-915.
16. Sherman PJ, Lane LB: The palmar aponeurosis pulley as a cause of trigger finger: A report of two cases. *J Bone Joint Surg Am* 1996;78(11):1753-1754.
17. Seradge H, Kleinert HE: Reduction flexor tenoplasty: Treatment of stenosing flexor tenosynovitis distal to the first pulley. *J Hand Surg Am* 1981;6(6):543-544.
18. Will R, Lubahn J: Complications of open trigger finger release. *J Hand Surg Am* 2010;35(4):594-596.
19. Tanaka T, Amadio PC, Zhao C, Zobitz ME, An KN: The effect of partial A2 pulley excision on gliding resistance and pulley strength in vitro. *J Hand Surg Am* 2004;29(5):877-883.

Chapter 39

Open Reduction and Internal Fixation of the Distal Radius With a Volar Locking Plate

Jesse B. Jupiter, MD   David Ring, MD, PhD

Patient Selection

Healthy, active patients with an unstable fracture of the distal radius are considered for open reduction and internal fixation (ORIF) with a volar locking plate. Instability is defined as inadequate alignment after manipulative reduction, loss of adequate alignment after manipulative reduction, or a high likelihood of healing with inadequate alignment with cast immobilization alone. The likelihood of losing alignment has been related to several factors, including initial fracture displacement, comminution, and age and functional level (both likely related to osteoporosis).[1,2] Adequate alignment is variably and somewhat arbitrarily defined as more than 10° to 20° of dorsal tilt of the articular surface on a lateral view, more than 3 to 5 mm of ulnar positive variance, and a 2 mm or greater articular step or gap.[2]

Preoperative Imaging

AP and lateral radiographs of the wrist before and after manipulative reduction are usually sufficient to characterize a fracture of the distal radius and inform management decisions. Radiographs with traction applied to the wrist can be helpful, particularly for identifying associated intercarpal ligament injuries. CT can provide additional detail about the number, size, location, and displacement of articular fractures. There is some evidence that three-dimensional reconstructions are easier and more reliable for surgeons to interpret.[3]

Procedure

In this chapter, we describe a patient with a nascent malunion of a volar shearing fracture to illustrate the surgical technique (Figure 1).

Surgical Technique

A longitudinal skin incision is planned over the flexor carpi radialis (FCR). The incision can either end at the transverse wrist creases or cross them obliquely for a thinner scar (Figure 2).

The sheath of the FCR is incised (both volar and dorsal) to access the deeper structures (Figure 3). The radial artery is left undissected in the soft tissues directly radial to the FCR sheath. If the incision is more ulnar than intended, care should be taken to protect the palmar cutaneous branch of the median nerve, which runs between the palmaris longus and FCR tendons.

After sweeping the fat from the space of Parona, the pronator quadratus and the flexor pollicis longus are exposed. The attachment of the flexor pollicis longus to the radial side of the wrist should be mobilized ulnarward. In younger, more active patients, there is often a large vessel to be cauterized in this area (Figure 4).

The pronator quadratus is incised on its radial and distal aspects and elevated subperiosteally from radial to ulnar off the volar surface of the radius. If the surgeon goes to the radial limit of the pro-

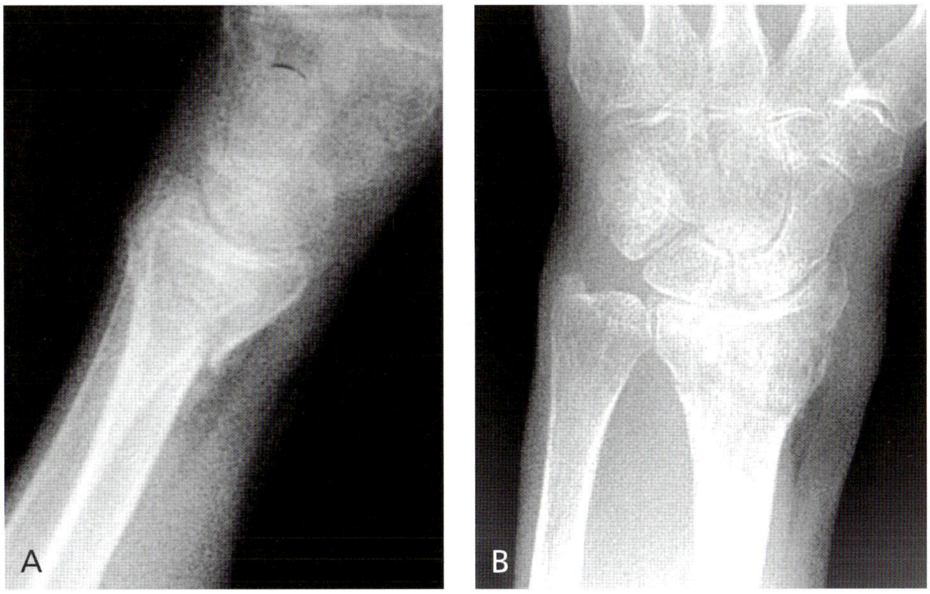

Figure 1 Lateral (**A**) and PA (**B**) image-intensifier views show a fracture of the distal radius.

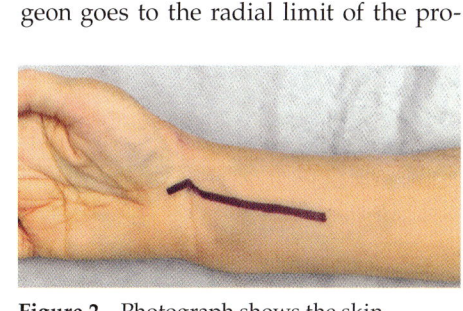

Figure 2 Photograph shows the skin incision for open reduction and internal fixation of a distal radius fracture using a volar locking plate. The incision lies directly over the flexor carpi radialis tendon and zigzags across the transverse wrist creases to limit scar thickness.

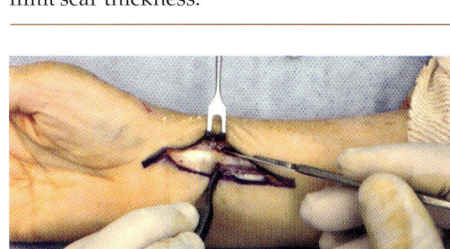

Figure 3 Intraoperative photograph shows the flexor carpi radialis tendon sheath incised to gain deeper exposure.

Dr. Jupiter or an immediate family member serves as a paid consultant to or is an employee of OHK; serves as an unpaid consultant to Synthes Eisomed; has stock or stock options held in OHK; has received research or institutional support from the AO Foundation; and serves as a board member, owner, officer, or committee member of the AAOS International Committee and the American Shoulder and Elbow Surgeons Resident-Fellow Curriculum Committee. Dr. Ring or an immediate family member has received royalties from Wright Medical Technology; serves as a paid consultant to or is an employee of Biomet, Skeletal Dynamics, and Wright Medical Technology; has stock or stock options held in Illuminos; and serves as a board member, owner, officer, or committee member of the American Shoulder and Elbow Surgeons and the American Society for Surgery of the Hand.

Section 3: Hand and Wrist

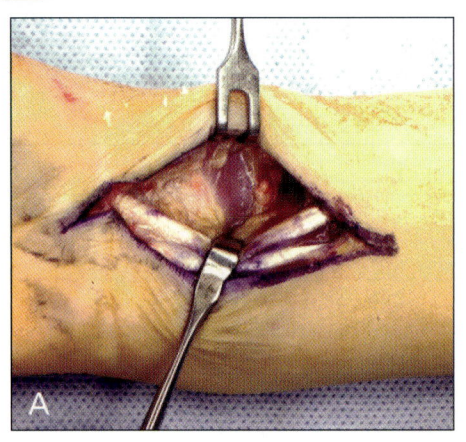

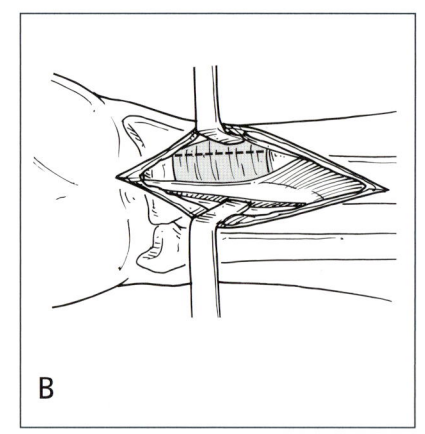

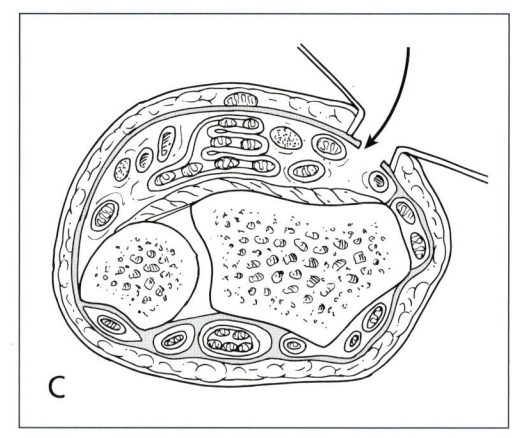

Figure 4 Intraoperative photograph (**A**) and illustration (**B**) show the FCR retracted ulnarward along with the flexor tendons and median nerve, exposing the pronator quadratus. **C,** Illustration shows an axial view of the approach.

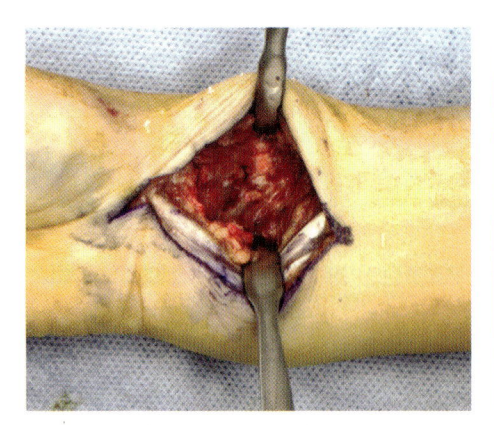

Figure 5 The pronator quadratus is retracted ulnarward.

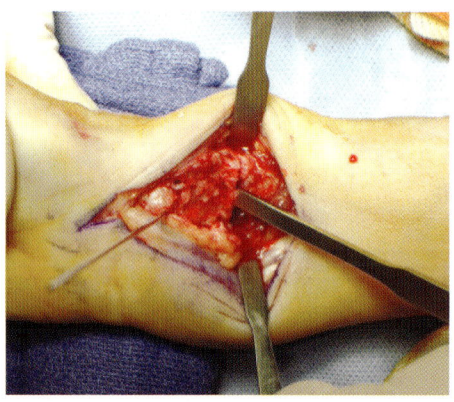

Figure 6 An osteotome is used to help realign the fracture. A wire is used as a landmark in the radiocarpal joint.

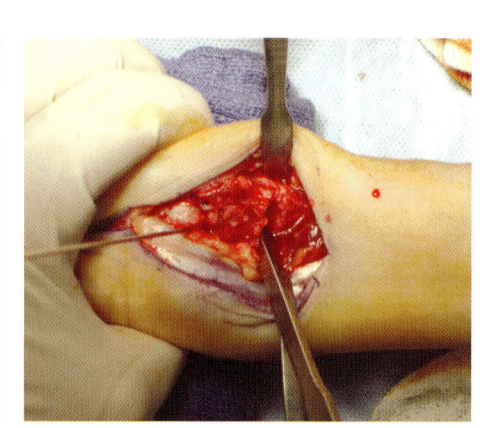

Figure 7 The osteotome is used to lever the fracture.

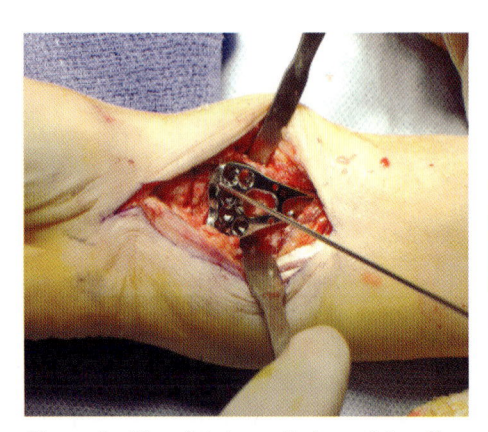

Figure 8 The plate is applied provisionally, and a Kirschner wire is placed to hold the reduction and check alignment on the image intensifier.

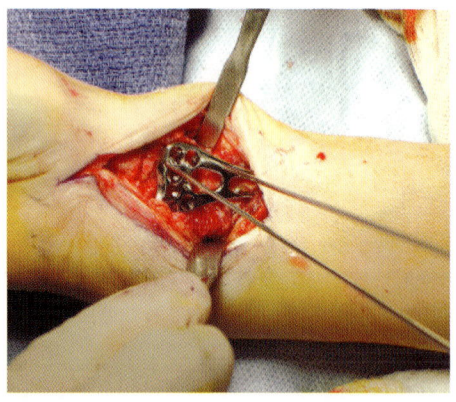

Figure 9 A second Kirschner wire maintains proximal alignment.

nator quadratus, the entire muscle can be elevated, which can facilitate repair back to the brachioradialis tendon at the time of closure (**Figure 5**). The fracture lines are then identified and cleared of muscle, hematoma, and incipient callus (**Figure 6**).

The volar cortex—particularly the volar ulnar corner—is the thickest bone in the metaphysis of the distal radius. In dorsally displaced fractures, there is usually little or no volar comminution. Therefore, it is usually straightforward to realign and stabilize the volar cortex. To reduce the fracture fragments, it can be useful to lever the distal fragments out from under the proximal shaft using an osteotome (**Figure 7**). To limit the possibility of fracturing the proximal fragment during this maneuver, particularly in osteoporotic individuals, the surgeon's thumb can be used as a counterpressure over this bone during the levering maneuver.

Alignment of the radial column can be facilitated by a hook on the brachioradialis. Alternatively, the brachioradialis can be released or Z-lengthened to reduce its deforming force. The reduction can be held provisionally using Kirschner wires (K-wires) either through or adjacent to the plate (**Figure 8**).

The plate should be applied so that it is centered both over the shaft proximally and over the metaphysis distally. Care should be taken to ensure that the plate does not extend more volar than the watershed area of the distal radius, meaning that it is not prominent enough to irritate the flexor tendons.

Provisional K-wires can be placed through some implants to hold provisional reduction (**Figure 9**). Alternatively, one can use a drill bit through a fixed-angle drill guide in the plate to help maintain the reduction. The position of these provisional wires on the image intensifier usually indicates that the screws will not enter the joint when placed, but this varies from plate to plate (**Figure 10**).

The fixed-angle screws are placed distally and standard or locking screws are used proximally, depending on the bone

© 2013 American Academy of Orthopaedic Surgeons

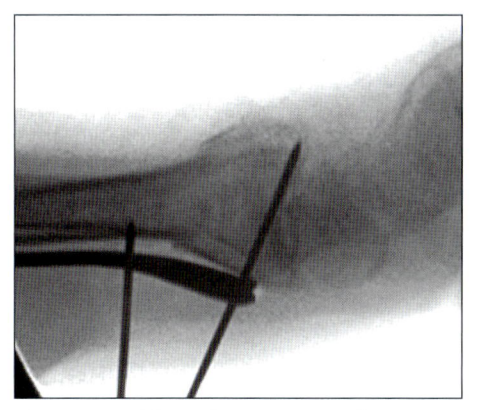

Figure 10 A lateral image-intensifier view verifies alignment and plate position.

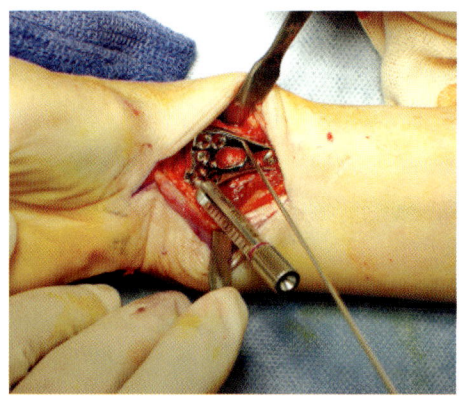

Figure 11 A threaded drill guide is placed in the distal ulnar screw hole. Screws are then applied.

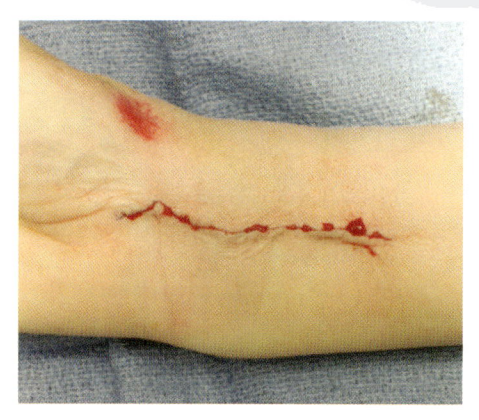

Figure 12 Wound closure.

quality and the surgeon's preferences (**Figure 11**). When possible, the pronator quadratus should be repaired to provide additional protection for the flexor tendons. The surgeon's preferred skin closure is used (**Figure 12**).

The final PA and lateral images of this patient are shown in **Figure 13**.

Complications

Infection, wound problems, and nerve injury are uncommon. Median nerve dysfunction seems related more to the energy of the injury (ie, acute carpal tunnel syndrome) than to the surgical technique.[4] Nonetheless, the median nerve should be handled carefully during exposure. On occasion, a screw tip inadvertantly penetrates the radiocarpal or distal radioulnar joint, and the screw must be removed.[5] Prominent implants can irritate and damage the extensor or flexor tendons. To limit the risk of extensor tendon problems, the surgeon must be aware that the Lister tubercle and other aspects of radius anatomy can hinder visualization of the screw tips on the image intensifier.[6,7] Careful use of the image intensifier may help.[8] Any metal that ends up more prominent than the so-called watershed of the volar surface of the distal radius (defined as the most prominent part) risks tendon irritation and injury. This includes any metal that extends onto the volar lip of the lunate facet (where the flexor digitorum profundus tendons run) or onto the most prominent aspect of the radius on the radial side where the flexor pollicis longus tendon runs.[9] The risk of implant prominance is increased when an adequate reduction is not acheived. To date, flexor pollicis longus rupture is one of the more commonly reported tendon complications of volar plate fixation, but rupture of the flexor digitorum profundus tendon is rare.

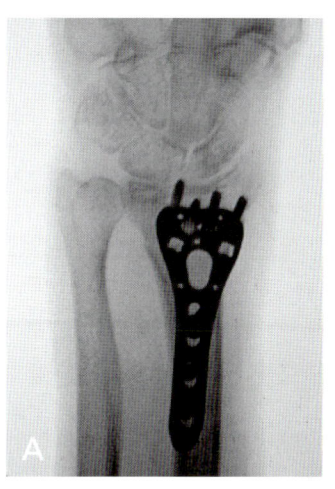

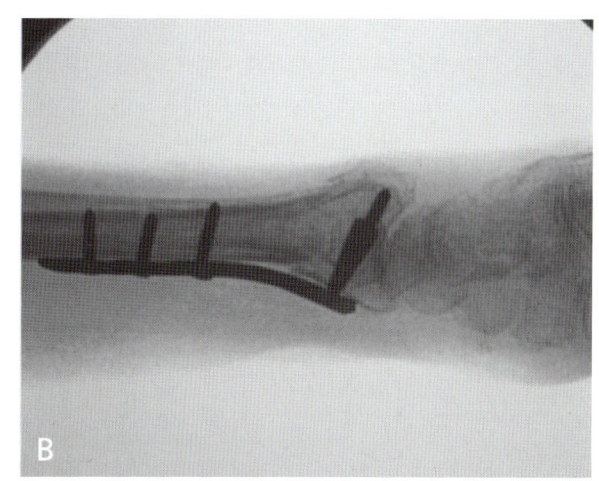

Figure 13 Intraoperative PA (**A**) and lateral (**B**) image-intensifier views show plate position and fracture alignment.

Postoperative Care and Rehabilitation

The priorities for exercise after ORIF with a volar plate are finger motion first, forearm rotation second, and wrist flexion and extension last.[10] Exercises of the fingers and forearm should start right away, but mobilization of the wrist can be delayed for comfort if the patient prefers. Patients can be weaned from the wrist splint when they are ready because the plate provides adequate support for active exercises. Functional use of the hand for light tasks should be encouraged. Patients should be instructed in proper stretching of the fingers, forearm, and wrist to restore as much motion as possible.

The pain associated with injury and surgery will make patients feel protective. It is easy to imagine problems with the plate or an uncertain future ("Will I be able to rely on my hand?") when in pain. Demonstrating empathy and normalizing this part of the recovery process will help ameliorate it. The orthopaedist can help patients change their mind-set from pain as a reminder or evidence of injury to pain as a result of healthy stretching exercise and part of an optimal recovery.

The injured arm can be used for some force at approximately 6 weeks after injury. By 3 months after injury, full activity is reasonable.

Pearls

- The volar ulnar cortex (the strongest bone in the distal radius) should be used to facilitate reduction.
- Once the volar cortex is realigned, the length and ulnarward inclination of the distal radius are restored, so the surgeon needs to work only on the palmar tilt.
- The implants should be kept proximal to the watershed area and monitored for screw prominence dorsally.
- The key to effective exercises after volar plate fixation of the distal radius is not how soon the exercises are started, but rather how confident the patient feels about stretching pain in the setting of illness.

© 2013 American Academy of Orthopaedic Surgeons

References

1. Lafontaine M, Hardy D, Delince PH: Stability assessment of distal radius fractures. *Injury* 1989;20(4):208-210.
2. Mackenney PJ, McQueen MM, Elton R: Prediction of instability in distal radial fractures. *J Bone Joint Surg Am* 2006;88(9):1944-1951.
3. Harness NG, Ring D, Zurakowski D, Harris GJ, Jupiter JB: The influence of three-dimensional computed tomography reconstructions on the characterization and treatment of distal radial fractures. *J Bone Joint Surg Am* 2006;88(6):1315-1323.
4. Dyer G, Lozano-Calderon S, Gannon C, Baratz M, Ring D: Predictors of acute carpal tunnel syndrome associated with fracture of the distal radius. *J Hand Surg Am* 2008;33(8):1309-1313.
5. Soong M, van Leerdam R, Guitton TG, Got C, Katarincic J, Ring D: Fracture of the distal radius: Risk factors for complications after locked volar plate fixation. *J Hand Surg Am* 2011;36(1):3-9.
6. Soong M, Got C, Katarincic J, Akelman E: Fluoroscopic evaluation of intra-articular screw placement during locked volar plating of the distal radius: A cadaveric study. *J Hand Surg Am* 2008;33(10):1720-1723.
7. Thomas AD, Greenberg JA: Use of fluoroscopy in determining screw overshoot in the dorsal distal radius: A cadaveric study. *J Hand Surg Am* 2009;34(2):258-261.
8. Tweet ML, Calfee RP, Stern PJ: Rotational fluoroscopy assists in detection of intra-articular screw penetration during volar plating of the distal radius. *J Hand Surg Am* 2010;35(4):619-627.
9. Soong M, Earp BE, Bishop G, Leung A, Blazar P: Volar locking plate implant prominence and flexor tendon rupture. *J Bone Joint Surg Am* 2011;93(4):328-335.
10. Lozano-Calderón SA, Souer S, Mudgal C, Jupiter JB, Ring D: Wrist mobilization following volar plate fixation of fractures of the distal part of the radius. *J Bone Joint Surg Am* 2008;90(6):1297-1304.

Chapter 40
External Fixation of Distal Radius Fractures

Michael V. Birman, MD   Jonathan R. Danoff, MD   Neil J. White, MD
Melvin P. Rosenwasser, MD

Introduction

External fixators, both spanning (crossing the radiocarpal joint) and nonspanning, have been used successfully for many years in the treatment of distal radius fractures. Over the past decade, with the advent of volar locking plates, there has been widespread interest in open reduction for these injuries. Similarly, new low-profile plates have been designed to buttress displaced facets of the radial and dorsal columns of the distal radius. Despite this shift, recent randomized clinical trials[1,2] have demonstrated equivalent successful patient outcomes with either technique if equivalent fracture reduction is obtained. Certainly, external fixation has been particularly useful in cases of soft-tissue injury in conjunction with fractures, but it has also been useful to neutralize deforming muscle forces with complex fractures, sometimes after internal fixation with modern locking plates. Geographic variation in surgical practice in terms of training, resources, and economics means that this treatment remains a useful one globally.

External fixation of distal radius fractures can consist of spanning and nonspanning constructs. More commonly, spanning external fixation is an adjunctive technique used to help reduce and maintain a reduction that is obtained by manipulative reduction and often includes Kirschner wire (K-wire) fixation, either transradial styloid or via the Kapandji technique. Arthroscopic-assisted articular facet reduction can be combined with spanning external fixation, as can the application of fragment-specific miniplates. In high–kinetic-energy fractures or in severe cases of osteopenia, the metaphyseal void created by impaction requires replacement with either allograft or bone substitutes.[3] This is necessary because the removal of fixators at 6 to 8 weeks does not allow for adequate subchondral support to resist remodeling changes over the ensuing 3 to 6 months, which may allow articular facet subsidence. In short, traction alone will not in most instances adequately reduce articular fractures. Spanning fixators also do not permit by themselves re-creation of physiologic volar tilt because of asymmetric tensioning of the capsular ligaments. Finally, overdistraction with spanning fixators not only fails to reduce displaced and translated fragments but also can actually lead to loss of motion, metacarpophalangeal stiffness, and causalgia or complex regional pain syndrome.[4,5]

A nonspanning external fixator can be a powerful tool to reduce articular facets and allow restoration of a more normal distal radial architecture. It does require an adequate distal radial segment of approximately 10 mm and adequate bone quality to place pins in a subchondral position, which will allow "joystick" reduction and then frame assembly to lock in the position without subsequent loss of fixation. It can also be linked to spanning pins in the second metacarpal shaft so that they can be sequentially deconstructed.

This chapter primarily focuses on the application of spanning external fixators, while also highlighting specific aspects of the use of nonspanning fixators.

Patient Selection

Indications

In general, the indications for the use of external fixation for definitive treatment of a distal radius fracture overlap with those for internal fixation of distal radius fractures. The indications include:

- Failed closed reduction (ie, acceptable closed reduction cannot be achieved). Although small variations exist among various authors, parameters that are generally considered acceptable for closed reduction include restoration of radial length to within 2 to 3 mm of the uninjured wrist, articular tilt at least neutral (but 5° to 10° dorsal tilt may be accepted), and radial inclination greater than 10° (compared to a normal inclination of 22°).
- Unstable distal radius (ie, acceptable closed reduction cannot be maintained). The Lafontaine criteria describe the factors predictive of fracture instability after an initial satisfactory reduction. These criteria include patient age greater than 60 years, dorsal tilt greater than 20°, dorsal cortical comminution, intra-articular extension, and concomitant ulnar fracture.[6] More current studies have reexamined some of these factors. In a more recent analysis, age, metaphyseal comminution, and ulnar variance have been found to be predictors of radiographic outcome.[7]
- Radiocarpal incongruity. Joint congruity should be assessed, step-offs or gaps of greater than 1 to 2 mm require consideration of surgical management for articular reduction.

In addition, at least 1 cm of intact volar cortex—but not dorsal cortex—is required for satisfactory pin purchase of a nonspanning external fixator.[8] Temporary external fixation may also be advantageous in the setting of a high-grade open distal radius fracture or as initial treatment in a multiple trauma setting.[9]

Contraindications

Contraindications for external fixation of distal radius fractures include a skeletally immature patient with open distal radial physes, volar or volar shear (Smith or Barton) displacement patterns, and a dorsal shear displacement pattern.

Additional Considerations

Indication for surgery is not based solely on fracture anatomy but also on patient factors such as hand dominance, occupational requirements, medical comorbidities, and expectations. Emergent presentations with open fractures or evolving neurologic deficits will dictate surgical intervention.

As a caveat to these considerations, recent studies have indicated that in the

---

Dr. Rosenwasser or an immediate family member has received royalties from Biomet; serves as a paid consultant to or is an employee of Biomet and Stryker; and serves as a board member, owner, officer, or committee member of the Foundation for Orthopedic Trauma and the Osteosynthesis and Trauma Care Foundation. None of the following authors or any immediate family member has received anything of value from or owns stock in a commercial company or institution related directly or indirectly to the subject of this chapter: Dr. Birman, Dr. Danoff, and Dr. White.

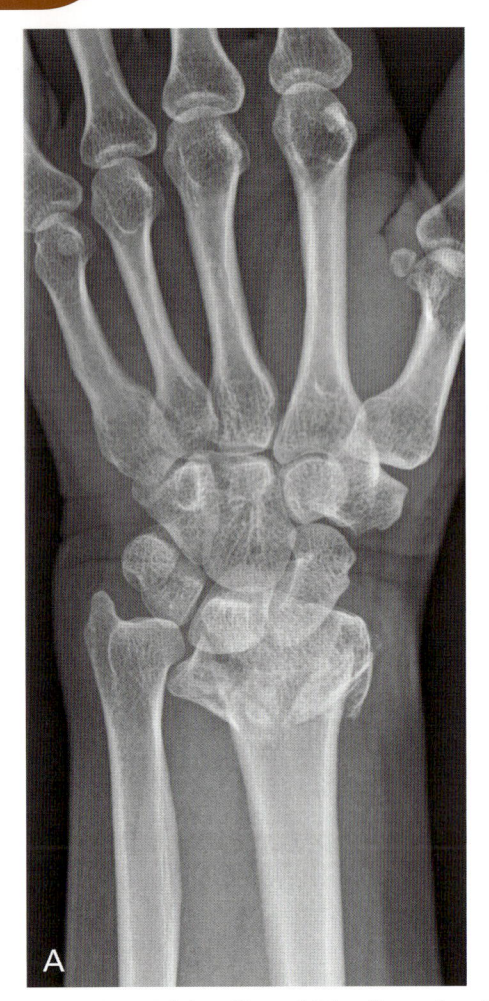

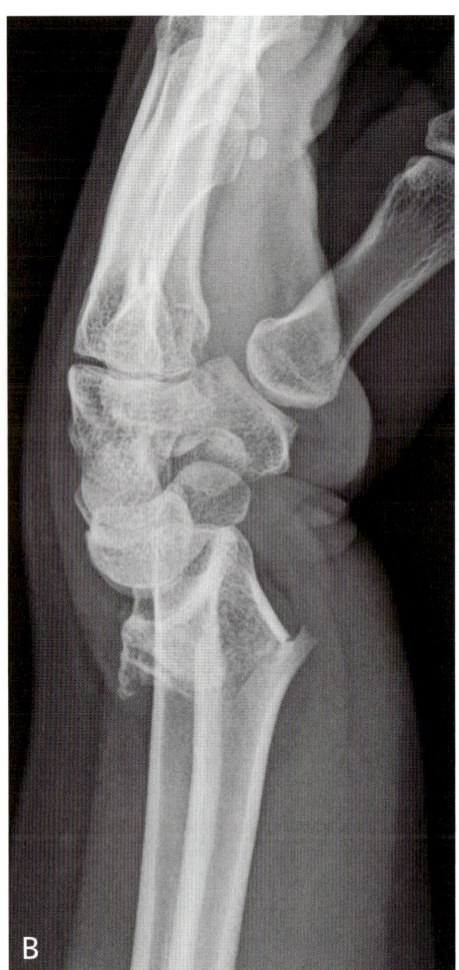

Figure 1 AP (**A**) and lateral (**B**) radiographs of an AO 23-C2.1 distal radius fracture before reduction. (Courtesy of Columbia University Medical Center, New York, NY.)

elderly low-demand patient, distal radius malunion can still result in patient satisfaction. This is in contradistinction to younger high-demand patients, in whom anatomic restoration equates with more predictable clinical outcomes.

Preoperative Imaging
AP, lateral, and oblique radiographs are obtained to evaluate the wrist before (**Figure 1**) and after reduction. Assessment of both of these series is extremely valuable because it allows pattern identification and recognition of articular facet displacement, thereby influencing the surgical approach and implant choice. Radiographs of the uninjured contralateral wrist can be helpful for determining the patient's normal anatomy as an aid to evaluating the quality of reduction. Traction radiographs of the wrist are essential to understand the complexity of fracture fragment displacement and in alerting the surgeon to possible capsuloligamentous injuries in the carpus. These examinations are sometimes performed in the operating room after anesthesia is administered. Combined wrist and forearm patterns, such as Galeazzi, Monteggia, or Essex-Lopresti injuries, must always be considered. CT scans of the distal radius can be helpful to further delineate bony anatomy, but the cost and the fact that they are performed without traction often limit their utility.

Video 40.1 External Fixation of Distal Radius Fractures. Jonathan R. Danoff, MD; Michael V. Birman, MD; Neil J. White, MD, FRCS; Melvin P. Rosenwasser, MD (7 min)

Procedure
After a complete documented examination, the wrist fracture is addressed and splinted in situ if well aligned or after closed reduction with anesthesia. We use intrafracture hematoma block for anesthesia during closed reduction. Complete anesthesia for maximum pain relief during manipulation can be best achieved with a hematoma block when an additional injection is used to anesthetize at the ulnar styloid fracture, when present. This may be supplemented with intravenous narcotics or conscious sedation. If closed reduction is satisfactory by the parameters described previously, then a sugar-tong splint is applied, making sure the metacarpophalangeal joints are free to fully flex. Unstable fractures are then indicated for surgical reduction, either closed or open. Stabilization may then be accomplished with adjunctive fixation techniques, including Kapandji dorsal intrafracture K-wire pinning, radial styloid transosseous pinning, and/or metaphyseal void subchondral allograft, combined with spanning or nonspanning external fixation.

Patient Positioning and Setup
The patient is positioned supine, with the arm on a radiolucent hand table. The procedure may be performed using a regional or a general anesthetic. A nonsterile tourniquet is applied to the upper arm and set to 250 mm Hg. This is useful during limited open pin placement to identify and protect cutaneous nerves. Small or low-radiation fluoroscopy is critical in assessing pin placement depth and the quality of the reduction as well as the stability of the reduction. Prophylactic antibiotics are always given intravenously. The extremity is then prepared and draped to the upper arm in sterile fashion.

Surgical Technique
Closed Reduction and Adjunctive Procedures
Closed reduction is performed; traction alone will not suffice. Manipulation with traction and countertraction is helpful. Usually, the surgeon shakes hands with the injured wrist and manipulates the fracture that is palpated using three point bending principles. After reducing the fracture, the surgeon must decide between the spanning and nonspanning options. If the distal fragment is large enough (10 mm), a nonspanning external fixator may be used. This will allow mechanical advantage for correction of the dorsal tilt of the distal radius. Articular comminution, with splits between the scaphoid and lunate facets, is not necessarily a contraindication, but the halfpins must be centered in those facets.

Spanning external fixation is used for the rest. Adjunctive fixation with K-wires as joysticks will allow for fragment manipulation. Percutaneous or limited open reduction of the fracture can be performed to accomplish initial reduction and correct articular incongruity. Reduction quality and stability are enhanced with K-wires, impaction grafting of the metaphyseal void with allograft bone, or arthroscopy. K-wires through the radial styloid are useful in provisional stabilization and can be placed either subchondrally, to close and support diastasis of the facets, or intramedullarily, for realignment of radial inclination and length. A 3-cm longitudinal dorsal incision (between the third and fourth dorsal compartments) over the fracture will allow elevation of the articular fragments with a blunt elevator, and impaction grafting of the subsequent void will provide excellent stabilization that can then be supplemented by the external fixator.

Wrist arthroscopy may improve fracture reduction in certain fracture patterns, such as transradial styloid perilunate injuries. This will also allow visualization and assessment of intercarpal ligamentous injuries and triangular fibrocartilage complex injuries. With vertical wrist traction through finger traps and a traction tower, the 3-4 portal is initially created to facilitate inspection of the joint. The need for additional portals is guided by the specific case as determined by intraoperative findings. Similarly, after reduction by arthroscopic techniques, using K-wires, screws, or plates, the fracture can be stabilized and then spanned to neutralize deforming forces.

Placement of Proximal Fixator Pins

The first step in the application of the external fixator is to place the proximal pins in the radius approximately 10 cm proximal to the tip of the radial styloid or at least 5 cm outside the zone of injury. The proximal pins can be used with a spanning or nonspanning frame and are placed in the bare area located in the palpable interval between the brachioradialis and the extensor carpi radialis longus muscles. A limited open approach is useful largely to protect the branches of the superficial radial and the lateral antebrachial cutaneous nerves. Two separate mini-incisions may be used, but regardless of approach, it is critical to avoid damage to the nerves to prevent a painful neuroma. The incision also assists in allowing good visualization for placement of the pins in the central axis of the radial shaft. Additionally, the incision(s) must be planned so closure around the pins can be accomplished without significant skin tension. For a spanning frame, optimal pin position is generally at 45° to the long axis of the arm (in the dorsal-radial to volar-ulnar direction); for a nonspanning fixator, dorsal-to-volar pins are placed.

Once the pin location has been determined, a 4-cm incision may be made longitudinally, and blunt dissection is performed through the intermuscular plane. Nerve branches must be identified and protected, as demonstrated in **Figure 2**. Once the periosteum is visualized, using the protection of a soft-tissue sleeve, the holes can be drilled and tapped if necessary, and the half-pins inserted. Many systems now use self-drilling, self-tapping half-pins. A fixator clamp assists in proper spacing of the pins. Pin placement and depth should be checked with fluoroscopy. When drilling for the pins, it is important to avoid drilling across the interosseous membrane to avoid the potential for heterotopic ossification, which limits forearm axis rotation.

Placement of Distal Fixator Pins

The distal fixator pins for the spanning external fixator are placed in the second metacarpal. As in the radius, they are placed into the bone at 45° to the long axis of the shaft. A longitudinal incision is made over the proximal third of the second metacarpal, centered over the bare area between the first dorsal interosseous muscle and the extensor tendon to the index finger. The pins may also be placed through separate longitudinal mini incisions. Both pins should be placed in the proximal 60% of the metacarpal to avoid encroaching on the metacarpophalangeal joint capsule (**Figure 3**). Additionally, the

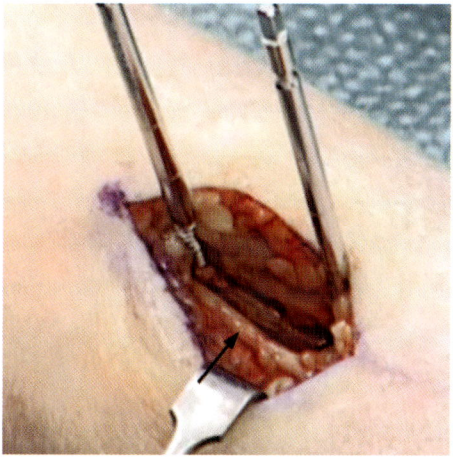

Figure 2 Intraoperative photograph shows incision before pin placement. The radial sensory nerve (arrow) is near the proximal radius pins and is protected via the limited open approach. (Courtesy of Columbia University Medical Center, New York, NY.)

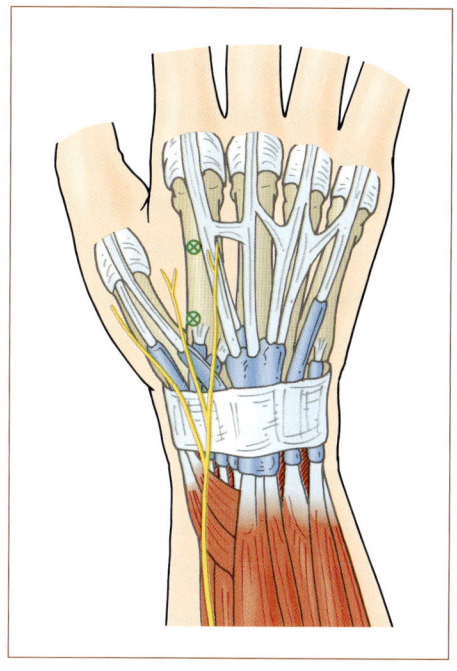

Figure 3 Illustration depicts distal fixator pin placement (green circles).

3-mm half-pins must be placed in the center of the metacarpal shaft to avoid the possibility of stress fracture. The fixator clamp should be used to guide the placement of the distal pin, after placement of the proximal pin. The terminal threads of the half-pins must fully engage the far cortex to gain maximal purchase. Pin placement should be checked with fluoroscopy. The proximal metacarpal half-pin can get four cortices, as it may be passed into the bone of the proximal third metacarpal without violating the interosseous muscles.

The distal fixator pins of a nonspanning external fixator are inserted through 2-cm longitudinal incisions, which are between the dorsal compartments (usually 2-3 and 4-5), rather than percutaneously to protect the cutaneous nerves and tendons (**Figure 4**). Most fractures that have at least 6 mm of cortex (generally, 10 mm is recommended, as noted previously) proximal to the subchondral plate can accept the 3-mm threaded half-pins. Under fluoroscopic guidance, pins are placed on either side of the Lister tubercle. It is important to protect the extensor pollicis longus tendon, use a soft-tissue sleeve, and place the ulnar pin first and parallel to the subchondral surface of the lunate facet. The radial pin need not be parallel if the external fixation pin clamps are modular. The volar cortex must be engaged by the terminal threads when the pins in the fragments are manipulated to ensure that adequate pin-bone interface stability is achieved. The fracture

Section 3: Hand and Wrist

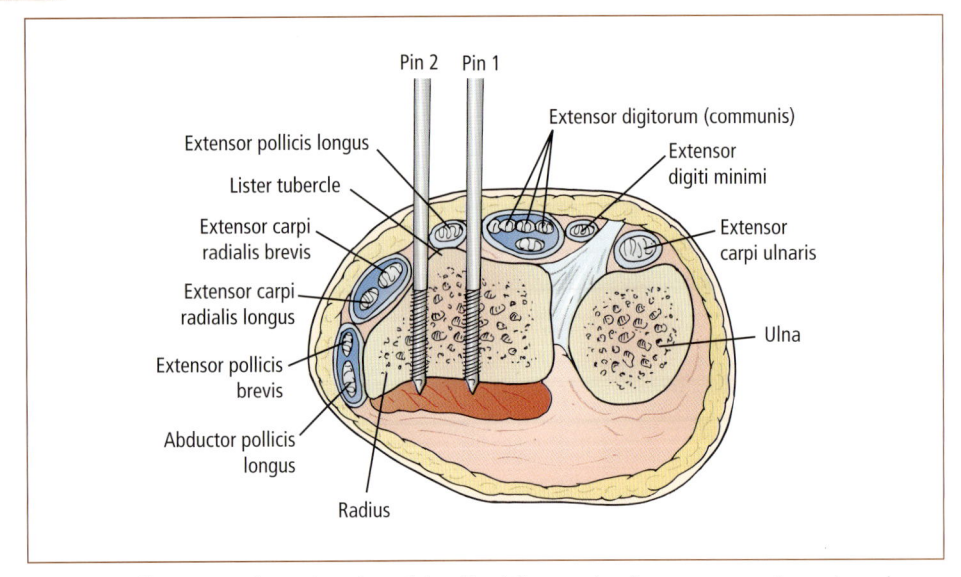

Figure 4 Illustration shows location of the distal fixator pins for a nonspanning external fixator, on either side of the third dorsal compartment.

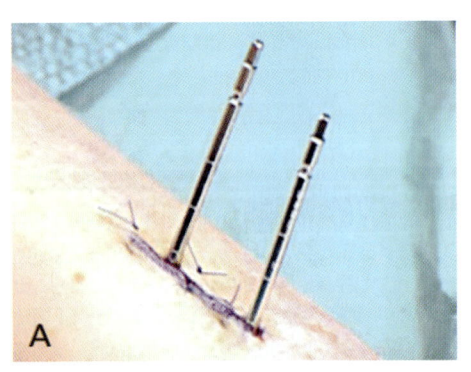

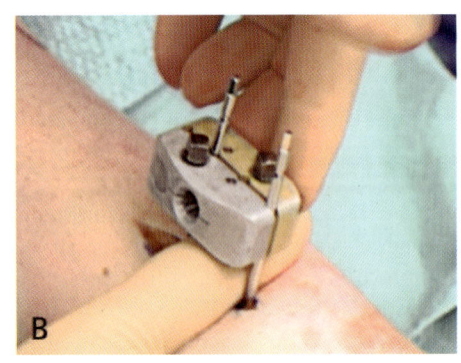

Figure 5 Photographs show assembly of fixator frame. **A,** The skin incision is closed without tension and before attaching the clamp. **B,** The clamp is placed one fingerbreadth away from the skin to allow for dressing application and soft-tissue swelling. (Courtesy of Columbia University Medical Center, New York, NY.)

fragments are reduced, and inclination, length, and tilt are dialed in before locking the frame.

Assembly of Fixator Frame
The skin incisions are closed without tension (**Figure 5, A**). This diminishes the potential for pin-skin interface problems, which may contribute to infection or premature loosening.

Once the proximal and distal pins are placed and verified on fluoroscopy, the frame is applied with pin-to-rod connectors, depending on the fixator system. Clamps are placed one fingerbreadth away from the skin (**Figure 5, B**), and care must be taken to ensure that the thumb and finger (and wrist, if nonspanning, as in **Figure 6**) range of motion is not blocked. The first rod is connected proximally, and after adjustments and fluoroscopic verification, the rod is secured distally. A second rod may be connected to increase the stiffness of the final frame. Only gentle traction is applied during assembly, because other means have been used to hold the reduction in the setting of the spanning frame. Restoration of length, translation, angulation, and rotation are then undertaken. It is important to avoid overpronation of the distal fragment of the fracture, which can lead to loss of supination.

In the case of nonspanning frames, the frame is applied loosely. Reduction is achieved with thumb pressure on the half-pins where they enter the skin. After fluoroscopic assessment of the reduction, the construct can be locked. The pins will be angled slightly distal to proximal, reflecting the restoration of the volar tilt. Caution must be exercised with the reduction technique to avoid overreduction, as well as damage from pin pullout in osteopenic bone.

Final images are obtained, and final tightening is performed. The stability of the distal radioulnar joint is assessed by comparison with the normal contralateral side. If there is increased translation, the surgeon must consider arthroscopic or open repair of the triangular fibrocartilage complex (TFCC) or transosseous K-wire fixation of the distal radioulnar joint.[10]

Complications
Complications of external fixators used for the fixation of distal radius fractures can be grouped into several key areas. These include pin-site infections, nerve injury, nonunion, stiffness, and complex regional pain syndrome (CRPS).

Pin-Site Infections
Most pin-site infections can be treated with oral antibiotics and pin care; rarely, irrigation and débridement and replacement of the pin are required.

Volar interval splinting is recommended[11] to limit the increased skin mobility that predisposes to these infections. Similarly, the pins must remain tight; therefore, any loose pin early in the treatment course should be removed and replaced. In addition, by not tethering the skin during closure of the incisions around the pins, most pin-skin interface problems can be avoided.

Nerve Injury
The branches of the superficial radial and lateral antebrachial cutaneous nerves are vulnerable during placement of the distal radius pins. This can generally be avoided by using a limited open approach for pin placement and protecting the nerve branches.

Avoidance of nerve injury is important, as is early recognition and treatment of evolving carpal tunnel syndrome.

Nonunion
Nonunion may occur secondary to overdistraction of the fracture, which is more likely with use of a spanning external fixator.

Stiffness
Classically, overdistraction through a spanning external fixator has been identified as a factor that may increase the risk of wrist stiffness; however, a recent study, has questioned this association.[12] Nonetheless, finger stiffness is increased by overdistraction and tensioning of the extensor mechanism over the metacarpophalangeal joints.

Complex Regional Pain Syndrome
Although the risk is low, the surgeon must be vigilant for the development of CRPS. An interdisciplinary and multimodal approach is important, in addition

Chapter 40: External Fixation of Distal Radius Fractures

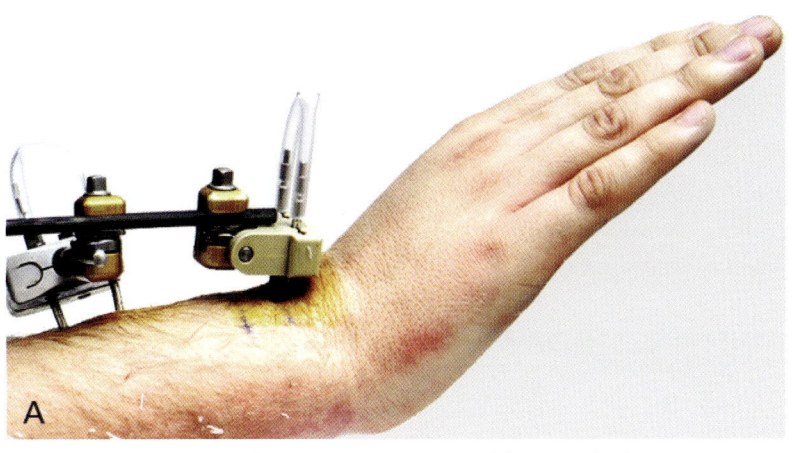

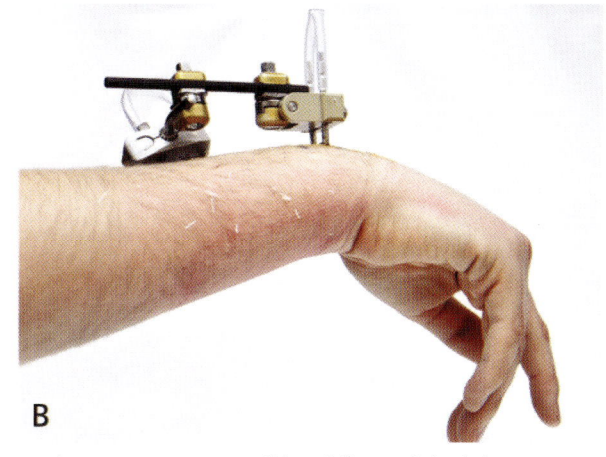

Figure 6 Photographs of a nonspanning external fixator, which permits wrist range of motion in extension (**A**) and flexion (**B**) while maintaining reduction. (Courtesy of Columbia University Medical Center, New York, NY.)

to pain management. Vitamin C, dosed as 500 mg daily for 50 days starting at the time of fracture, has been suggested to decrease the prevalence of CRPS.[13]

Postoperative Care and Rehabilitation

After surgery, these patients are generally admitted overnight (23-hour hospital stay) for pain control. Pin sites are dressed with a petroletum gauze dressing or nonadherent sterile gauze, followed by a bulky dressing. A splint may be used for patient comfort, especially with ulnar styloid/TFCC injuries and for patients in a non–joint-spanning fixator. The patient is instructed on pin-site care the following day, before discharge. Pin-site care is initiated on the first postoperative day and is performed once daily with hydrogen peroxide and a cotton-tipped applicator. The patient is also seen by an occupational therapist on the first postoperative day to instruct finger, elbow, and shoulder range-of-motion exercises. We especially emphasize the importance of making a complete fist as a predictor of successful outcome.

At 10 to 14 days, the sutures are removed and new radiographs are taken (**Figure 7**). A formal supervised or home unsupervised therapy program is then initiated. At each visit, the pin clamp screws should be tightened and the frame inspected. From the time of intraoperative frame application until frame removal, finger motion must be monitored and unrestricted, allowing full finger extension and flexion (**Figure 8**). At union (approximately 6 to 8 weeks), as judged by radiographs and clinical examination with the absence of fracture pain, the fixator and pins are removed under local anesthesia in the office. Hand therapy may be advanced at this time.

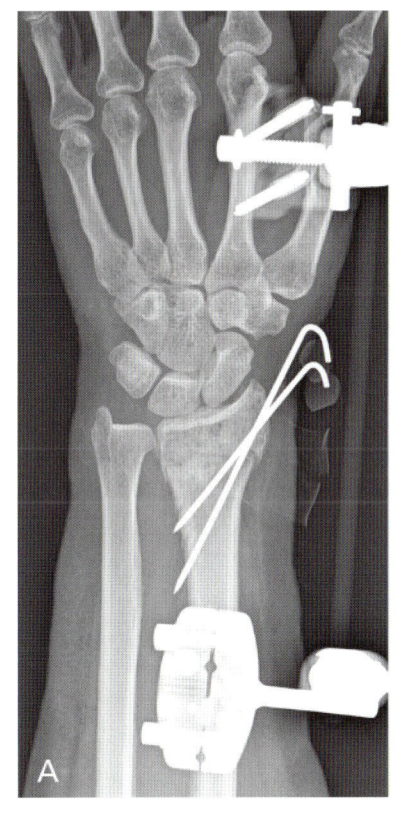

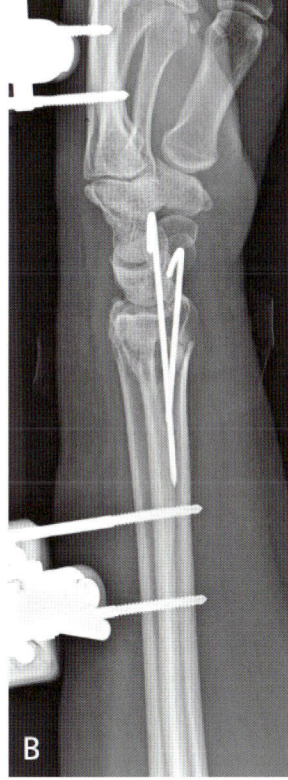

Figure 7 Postoperative AP (**A**) and lateral (**B**) radiographs obtained at 3-week follow-up show the final frame assembled. (Courtesy of Columbia University Medical Center, New York, NY.)

Outcomes

Studies comparing external fixation versus internal fixation or cast immobilization populate the literature; some of these studies are prospective. The general conclusion that arises from examining these studies is that although radiographic parameters, especially volar tilt, may not be restored as well with external fixation as with internal fixation, the clinical results compare favorably.[1,14-17] Most authors in these studies who use a spanning external fixator do so in combination with other techniques, particularly pinning. The limitations of using an external fixator alone without any complementary fixation are highlighted in the study by Arora and Malik,[18] who treated 27 patients with comminuted, displaced intra-articular fractures of the distal radius exclusively by external fixation; they had a 40.7% rate of fair and poor results and a 33% complication rate and reported inadequate restoration of articular congruity in many cases. In general, the decision to use an external fixator is dependent on surgeon experience and preference, patient factors, and available resources. Both external fixation and internal fixation techniques can yield a good long-term outcome based on both subjective and objective parameters, although subjective outcomes may be better early (at 6 weeks) with use of a volar plate versus spanning external fixation.[1,2]

In the most comprehensive prospective comparison of nonspanning external fixation versus spanning external fixa-

© 2013 American Academy of Orthopaedic Surgeons

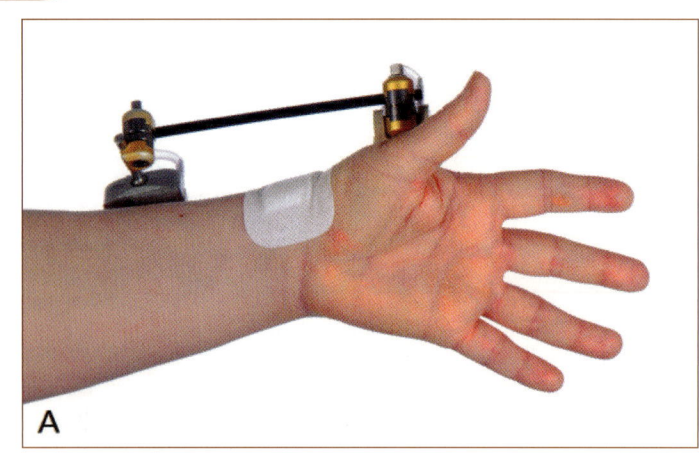

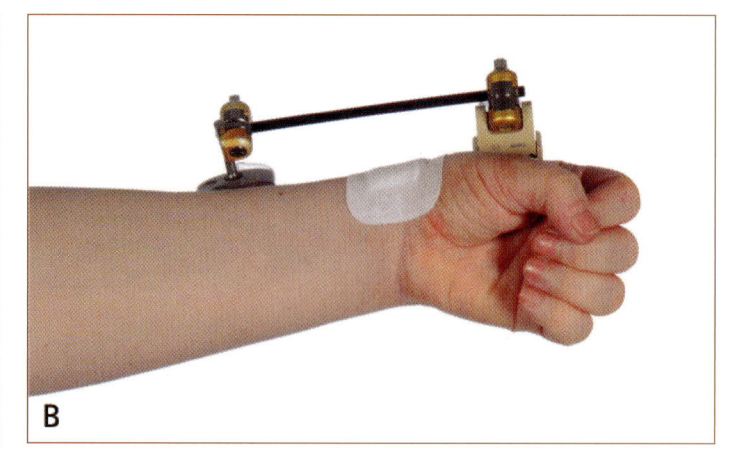

Figure 8 Photographs of a nonspanning external fixation. It is critical to ensure that the extensor tendons are not tethered, permitting finger extension (**A**) and flexion (**B**).

tion, McQueen[8,19] performed a prospective study of 641 patients with unstable fractures of the distal radius treated with external fixation; 378 were treated with nonspanning external fixation. Radiologic results, particularly volar tilt and carpal alignment, as well as functional improvement, were significantly better with nonspanning external fixation throughout the follow-up period. Complication rates were similar between the two groups.[8,19]

Pearls

- The injury, postreduction, and traction radiographs should be assessed in developing the surgical plan.
- Ligamentotaxis (traction) will not achieve and maintain reduction alone, except for the simplest and most stable fractures.
- The sensory nerves must be protected to avoid painful neuromas, which may initiate CRPS.
- A sleeve should always be used when drilling to protect the adjacent soft tissues.
- The distal fragment must not be over-pronated when locking the frame because this can result in loss of supination.
- The terminal threads of the half-pins must fully engage the far cortex to be stable.
- Tensionless closure of the limited incisions will diminish pin-tract complications.
- The stability of the distal radioulnar joint must be assessed before completion of the case with the translation shuck test. If unstable or asymmetric to the other side, the TFCC should be repaired or the distal radioulnar joint pinned extra-articularly.

References

1. Wei DH, Raizman NM, Bottino CJ, Jobin CM, Strauch RJ, Rosenwasser MP: Unstable distal radial fractures treated with external fixation, a radial column plate, or a volar plate: A prospective randomized trial. *J Bone Joint Surg Am* 2009;91(7): 1568-1577.
2. Wei DH, Poolman RW, Bhandari M, Wolfe VM, Rosenwasser MP: External fixation versus internal fixation for unstable distal radius fractures: A systematic review and meta-analysis of comparative clinical trials. *J Orthop Trauma* 2012; 26(7):386-394.
3. Herrera M, Chapman CB, Roh M, Strauch RJ, Rosenwasser MP: Treatment of unstable distal radius fractures with cancellous allograft and external fixation. *J Hand Surg Am* 1999;24(6):1269-1278.
4. Slutsky DJ: Nonbridging external fixation of intra-articular distal radius fractures. *Hand Clin* 2005;21(3):381-394.
5. Slutsky DJ: External fixation of distal radius fractures. *J Hand Surg Am* 2007;32(10):1624-1637.
6. Lafontaine M, Hardy D, Delince P: Stability assessment of distal radius fractures. *Injury* 1989;20(4):208-210.
7. Mackenney PJ, McQueen MM, Elton R: Prediction of instability in distal radial fractures. *J Bone Joint Surg Am* 2006;88(9):1944-1951.
8. McQueen MM: Non-spanning external fixation of the distal radius. *Hand Clin* 2005;21(3):375-380.
9. Bindra RR: Biomechanics and biology of external fixation of distal radius fractures. *Hand Clin* 2005;21(3):363-373.
10. Ruch DS, Lumsden BC, Papadonikolakis A: Distal radius fractures: A comparison of tension band wiring versus ulnar outrigger external fixation for the management of distal radioulnar instability. *J Hand Surg Am* 2005;30(5):969-977.
11. Fischer T, Koch P, Saager C, Kohut GN: The radio-radial external fixator in the treatment of fractures of the distal radius. *J Hand Surg Br* 1999;24(5):604-609.
12. Capo JT, Rossy W, Henry P, Maurer RJ, Naidu S, Chen L: External fixation of distal radius fractures: Effect of distraction and duration. *J Hand Surg Am* 2009;34(9):1605-1611.
13. Zollinger PE, Tuinebreijer WE, Breederveld RS, Kreis RW: Can vitamin C prevent complex regional pain syndrome in patients with wrist fractures? A randomized, controlled, multicenter dose-response study. *J Bone Joint Surg Am* 2007;89(7):1424-1431.
14. Wright TW, Horodyski M, Smith DW: Functional outcome of unstable distal radius fractures: ORIF with a volar fixed-angle tine plate versus external fixation. *J Hand Surg Am* 2005;30(2):289-299.
15. Margaliot Z, Haase SC, Kotsis SV, Kim HM, Chung KC: A meta-analysis of outcomes of external fixation versus plate osteosynthesis for unstable distal radius fractures. *J Hand Surg Am* 2005;30(6): 1185-1199.
16. Westphal T, Piatek S, Schubert S, Winckler S: Outcome after surgery of distal radius fractures: No differences between external fixation and ORIF. *Arch Orthop Trauma Surg* 2005;125(8):507-514.
17. Kreder HJ, Hanel DP, Agel J, et al: Indirect reduction and percutaneous fixation versus open reduction and internal fixation for displaced intra-articular fractures of the distal radius: A randomised, controlled trial. *J Bone Joint Surg Br* 2005;87(6):829-836.
18. Arora J, Malik AC: External fixation in comminuted, displaced intra-articular fractures of the distal radius: Is it sufficient? *Arch Orthop Trauma Surg* 2005;125(8):536-540.
19. McQueen MM: Redisplaced unstable fractures of the distal radius: A randomised, prospective study of bridging versus non-bridging external fixation. *J Bone Joint Surg Br* 1998;80(4):665-669.

Chapter 41
Open Reduction and Internal Fixation of Scaphoid Fractures

Kristofer S. Matullo, MD   Alexander Y. Shin, MD

Introduction

Scaphoid fractures are a clinically significant injury, representing approximately 11% of all hand fractures and 60% of all carpal fractures.[1] They occur most often in men between 20 and 30 years of age and typically follow a traumatic event.[2] The unique anatomy of the scaphoid provides it with articular cartilage over most its surface, with five bony articulations, five ligamentous attachments, and a unique retrograde blood supply.[3] The radial and volar flexed posture of the scaphoid, combined with its unique anatomy, make it vulnerable to trauma when the wrist is positioned in greater than 95° of extension with a force directed over the thenar eminence.[4] The resulting trauma can result in a spectrum of injuries, ranging from an occult fracture (without displacement or initial radiographic findings) to a completely displaced scaphoid fracture with carpal dislocations (transscaphoid perilunar injury). Inadequate treatment of scaphoid fractures can result in chronic pain, weakness, fracture nonunion, and, ultimately, arthritic changes in the wrist. The purpose of this chapter is to describe the basic open surgical approaches to the fractured scaphoid.

Patient Selection

After an appropriate history and physical examination as well as diagnostic studies (multiple view plain radiographs and CT if needed), patients are counseled regarding surgical versus nonsurgical treatment. Fractures that are displaced greater than 1 mm, have significant angulation into the volar or the dorsal plane, exhibit carpal collapse, or are comminuted are indicated for surgical fixation.[5] The radiographs must also be scrutinized for any type of carpal malalignment, associated injuries, or step-off within the scaphocapitate articular surface. The goals of surgical fixation include accurate reduction, restoration of carpal alignment, earlier return to work, and an attempt to decrease time to union.

Nonsurgical treatment is the modality of choice for patients who have no fracture gap or displacement and no comminution in the volar or dorsal plane. The debate on surgical versus nonsurgical treatment of nondisplaced scaphoid fractures is beyond the scope of this chapter. However, careful discussion with the patient should be undertaken to review the benefits and risks of both types of treatment. Distal pole fractures of the scaphoid readily heal given their abundant blood supply and are treated most often with nonsurgical treatment. Comorbidities and the inability to tolerate anesthesia are relative contraindications.

Preoperative Imaging

During the patient's preoperative evaluation, standard PA, lateral, and oblique radiographs should be obtained. A scaphoid view, which is obtained by holding the wrist in approximately 30° of extension and ulnar deviation while pointing the radiographic beam perpendicular to the radial shaft, will show the long axis of the scaphoid and can be used for preoperative templating (**Figure 1**). The amount of extension required for the scaphoid view is often best approximated by having the patient make a clenched fist and rest this on the x-ray cassette. The lateral radiograph should be examined for any type of carpal malalignment, including a DISI or VISI (dorsal or volar intercalated segment instability) deformity, as well as to assess the intrascaphoid angle, which typically is less than 30°. The PA radiograph should be specifically examined for loss of carpal height, any type of intercarpal widening (which may be suggestive of a scapholunate interosseous ligament or lunotriquetral interosseous ligament injury), or any other associated fractures. Fluoroscopy and comparison views of the uninjured views of the uninjured hand can be helpful.

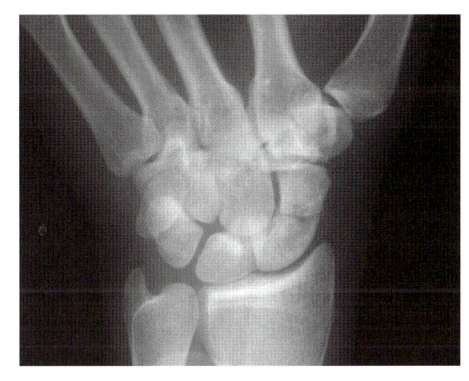

Figure 1 Scaphoid view radiograph, taken with the wrist in extension and ulnar deviation, demonstrates a scaphoid waist fracture.

Initial radiographic imaging can be negative for nondisplaced fractures. When this is the case, and the index of suspicion is high, such as in the patient with significant anatomic snuffbox pain or pain at the distal pole of the scaphoid, the patient must be protected and further imaging obtained to prove or disprove the presence of an occult scaphoid fracture. In the past, patients have been immobilized for approximately 10 to 14 days, with repeat radiographs obtained following this interval to assess for any type of occult fracture once there has been bone resorption along the fracture lines. However, active or working patients often may not be able to tolerate this type of delay and would like more rapid information that can lead to either continuation of immobilization or freedom from the cast and return to activities.

Additional imaging options can be used for scaphoid fractures (**Figure 2**). Technetium MDP (methylene diphosphonate)-99 bone scan has a sensitivity rate of 100% and a positive predictive rate of 93% with a specificity of 98%. However, a minimum delay of 48 to 72 hours after injury is needed for maximal imaging benefit. A bone scan that demonstrates an increased uptake in the area of the scaphoid requires additional studies to verify whether a fracture exists, as was demonstrated in 2005 by Beeres et al,[6] who reported that positive bone scans revealed 15 scaphoid fractures and 23 other fractures in patients with wrist pain.

Dr. Matullo or an immediate family member serves as a paid consultant to or is an employee of Synthes and serves as a board member, owner, officer or committee member of the American Society for Surgery of the Hand. Dr. Shin or an immediate family member has received research or institutional support from the Musculoskeletal Transplant Foundation, Integra LifeSciences, the American Association for Hand Surgery, and Sonoma Orthopedics and serves as a board member, owner, officer, or committee member of the American Society for Surgery of the Hand.

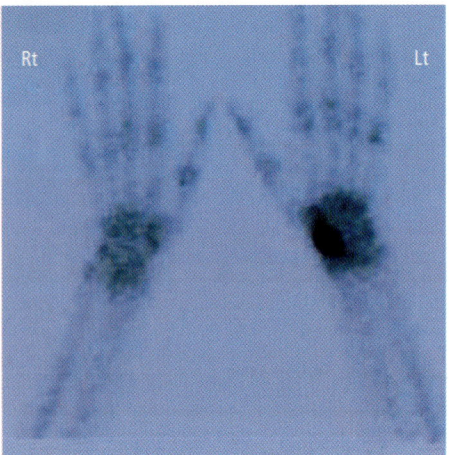

Figure 2 A postinjury bone scan demonstrates increased uptake in the right scaphoid consistent with a scaphoid fracture. (Reproduced with permission from the Mayo Foundation for Medical Education and Research, Rochester, MN.)

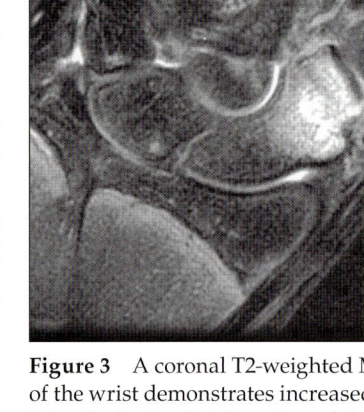

Figure 3 A coronal T2-weighted MRI scan of the wrist demonstrates increased signal intensity in the distal portion of the scaphoid, consistent with an occult fracture.

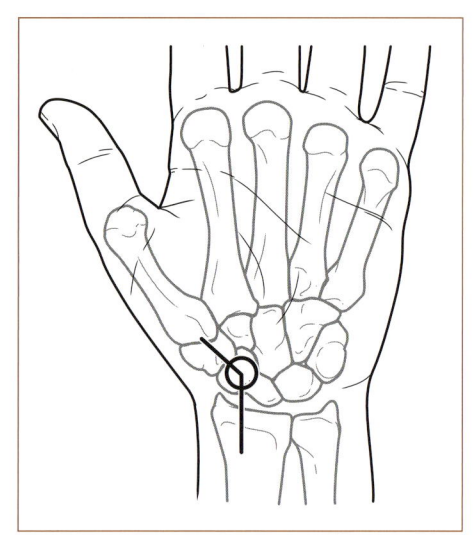

Figure 4 Illustration shows the incision for the volar approach. The incision is hockey-stick–shaped, centered on the distal pole of the scaphoid, extending proximally along the longitudinal axis of the forearm and distally along the longitudinal axis of the thumb metacarpal. (Modified with permission from the Mayo Foundation for Medical Education and Research, Rochester, MN.)

MRI has been reported to have a 100% sensitivity and specificity rate in the diagnosis of acute occult scaphoid fractures (**Figure 3**). MRI can be performed as soon as 24 hours after the injury and is very sensitive in detecting concomitant ligamentous injuries in the wrist. However, false-positive results can occur secondary to marrow edema, which can lead to inappropriately aggressive treatment.[7]

The generally accepted radiographic evaluation is an initial radiographic series including a PA, lateral, oblique, and navicular view. If the fracture is not completely identifiable on the series, the patient is protected in a long arm–thumb spica cast. For patients requiring a quick diagnosis and potential surgical treatment, MRI can be obtained within 24 hours. For patients who have the luxury of time for a diagnosis, 2 weeks of immobilization, followed by a repeat radiographic series, can be undertaken.

For scaphoid fractures that are displaced as defined above, surgical intervention is required.

Video 41.1 Open Reduction and Internal Fixation of Scaphoid Fractures. Kristofer S. Matullo, MD; Alexander Y. Shin, MD (2 min)

Procedure

Room Setup/Patient Positioning

The patient is positioned supine on the operating room table, with a dedicated radiolucent hand table underneath the affected extremity. Appropriate preoperative C-arm images (either mini or standard imaging) are obtained to visualize the fracture and guarantee visualization of the scaphoid during the surgical procedure. A pneumatic brachial tourniquet is placed around the upper extremity to allow for hemostasis during the procedure. Anesthetic choices include either a regional block or general anesthesia with local anesthetic administered at the end of the procedure for postoperative pain relief. Finally, all patients have an iliac crest prepared, for the possibility of bone grafting. In our practice, all patients are consented for this preoperatively as a possibility.

Special Instruments/Equipment/Implants

Besides a standard set of surgical instrumentation, a C-arm will be required for intraoperative radiographic imaging. Many types of implants can be used for scaphoid fracture fixation. Cannulated compression screws are preferred. This screw should be headless, to prevent intra-articular prominence on either the dorsal or the volar articular cartilage. Whichever screw is chosen, it is imperative that the surgeon understand the nuances of the system as well as the instrumentation (in particular, the depth gauge and how it relates to the actual screw length and placement).

Surgical Technique

The two most common approaches to fixation of a scaphoid fracture are the volar and dorsal approaches. Typically, the dorsal approach is used for waist or proximal pole fractures. The volar approach is generally used for waist or distal pole fractures.

Volar Approach

A hockey-stick–shaped incision following the flexor carpi radialis (FCR) tendon and angling at the wrist crease toward the thumb is made. The distal incision is centered over the distal pole of the scaphoid (**Figure 4**). Dissection through the skin and subcutaneous tissues is performed sharply, identifying any branches of the radial artery or volarly encroaching branches of the superficial sensory branch of the radial nerve. The superficial palmar branch of the radial artery is ligated and divided.

The FCR tendon sheath is opened, and the FCR tendon is retracted either radially or ulnarly to allow for exposure of the floor of the sheath. The sheath and volar carpal ligaments are incised sharply in a longitudinal fashion. The long radiolunate and radioscaphocapitate ligaments will be divided with this incision, exposing the waist of the scaphoid (**Figure 5**). In the distal portion of the incision at the scaphotrapezium joint, the capsule is elevated, exposing the distal pole of the scaphoid. Occasionally, improved exposure and access for the guidewire is needed, and a portion of the trapezium may need to be removed using either a sharp osteotome or a surgical rongeur.

Chapter 41: Open Reduction and Internal Fixation of Scaphoid Fractures

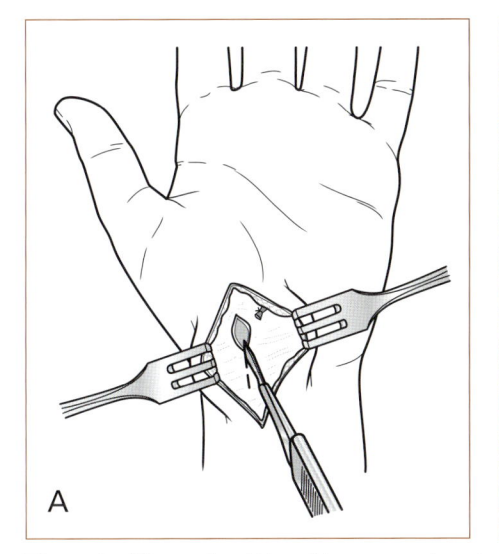

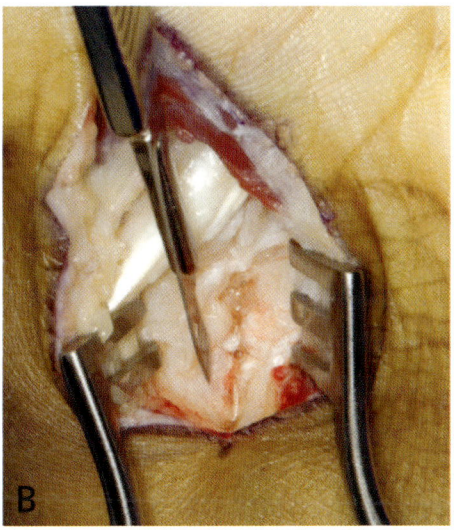

Figure 5 Illustration (**A**) and intraoperative photograph (**B**) demonstrate the division of the volar radiocarpal ligaments. (Modified with permission from the Mayo Foundation for Medical Education and Research, Rochester, MN.)

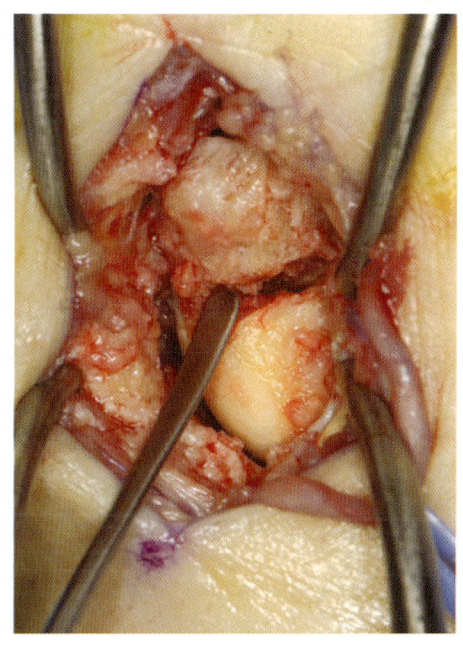

Figure 6 Intraoperative photograph depicts a scaphoid waist fracture as seen through a volar approach. The Freer elevator is located at the fracture site at the scaphoid waist. (Reproduced with permission from the Mayo Foundation for Medical Education and Research, Rochester, MN.)

The wrist can be extended over a bolster to facilitate fracture visualization (**Figure 6**). Typically, the wrist is positioned in extension and ulnar deviation to unlock the scaphotrapeziotrapezoidal joint. If required, two Kirschner wires (K-wires) can be inserted into the proximal and distal fracture fragments as joysticks to aid in reduction. After the fracture has been adequately reduced (as verified by visualization of the midcarpal and radiocarpal portions of the scaphoid), a guidewire (preferably at least a 1.0-mm wire) is inserted down the center axis of the scaphoid from distal to proximal and confirmed by multiple C-arm radiographic views as well as a live rotation view (**Figure 7**). The guidewire is then placed so that it is at the proximal pole articular margin, and the length of screw to be used is measured. Typically, despite the "accurate measurement" of the screw, an additional 4 to 6 mm is subtracted from the measured screw length to prevent articular penetration.

A cannulated drill is used to drill over the wire. It is imperative to recognize that, despite measuring for a shorter screw, the drill depth must be the originally measured depth. Failure to drill to this depth will result in a prominent screw, distraction of the fracture, or even iatrogenic fracture of either the proximal or distal fragment as the screw is inserted. Despite the stop guides on most systems, radiographic visualization is essential to prevent penetration of the dorsal aspect of the wrist. In younger patients or patients with very sclerotic bone, the distal aspect of the scaphoid may need to be overdrilled to allow easier insertion of the cannulated screw without gapping the fracture site. In more comminuted fractures, a second parallel guidewire may need to be inserted before drilling to prevent rotation or displacement of the fracture (**Figure 8**).

Bone grafting should be considered in fractures with comminution, in humpback deformities, or in those that have a defect after reduction. During fixation, if there is significant comminution of the scaphoid resulting in a central void, but the orientation and anatomic axis of the scaphoid are intact, cancellous bone graft is used. Typically, this bone can be obtained from the distal radius or the iliac crest. Distal radius bone graft is obtained through a small incision dorsally overlying the Lister tubercle.

After sharp dissection, the extensor pollicis longus tendon is protected, an osteo-

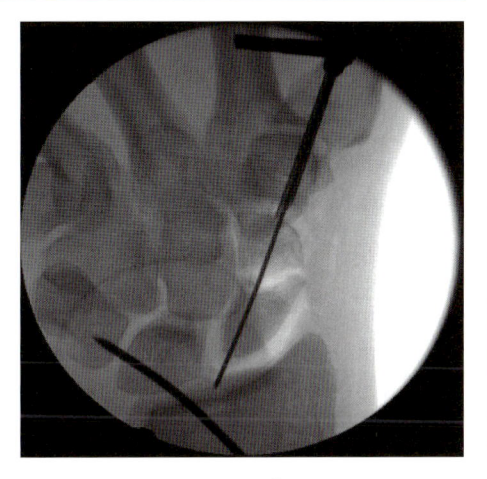

Figure 7 Intraoperative fluoroscopic image demonstrates the guidewire along the central axis of the scaphoid. (Reproduced with permission from the Mayo Foundation for Medical Education and Research, Rochester, MN.)

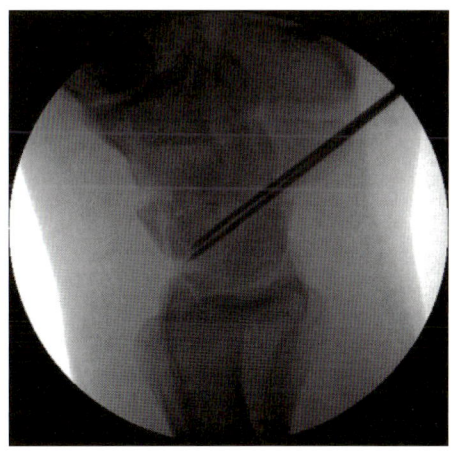

Figure 8 Fluoroscopic image shows parallel K-wires placed in a fracture to prevent rotation during the drilling and screw insertion. (Reproduced with permission from the Mayo Foundation for Medical Education and Research, Rochester, MN.)

tome is used to elevate the tubercle, and cancellous bone is removed from the metaphysis of the radius. If the scaphoid has lost its anatomic alignment, such as in a humpback deformity with an increase of the intrascaphoid angle greater than 30°, a structural bone graft is required. The iliac crest is preferred for harvest of corticocancellous structural graft and the contralateral iliac crest is prepared and draped. Fractures that demonstrate osteonecrosis of the proximal pole typically require vascularized bone grafting, which is beyond the scope of this chapter.

© 2013 American Academy of Orthopaedic Surgeons

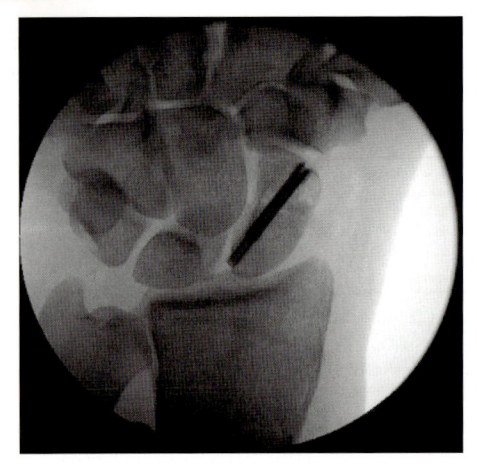

Figure 9 Final fluoroscopic image of a volarly placed scaphoid screw. The screw is located along the central axis of the scaphoid. Even though the screw appears long at the proximal extent, it does not penetrate the articular surface or enter the radiocarpal joint. (Reproduced with permission from the Mayo Foundation for Medical Education and Research, Rochester, MN.)

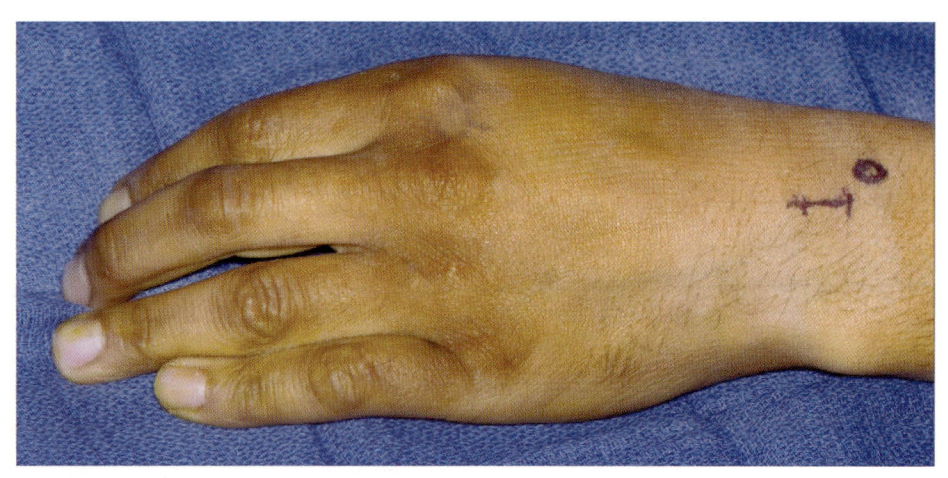

Figure 10 Photograph shows a dorsal incision marked on the skin. It is located just ulnar and distal to the Lister tubercle (represented by the circle). (Reproduced with permission from the Mayo Foundation for Medical Education and Research, Rochester, MN.)

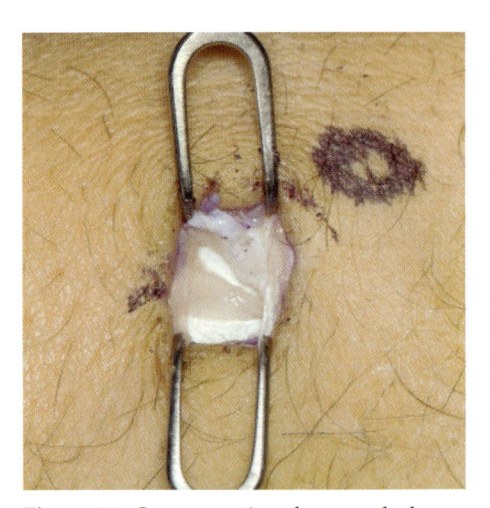

Figure 11 Intraoperative photograph shows the extensor pollicis longus and extensor carpi radialis longus tendons at the base of the wound. (Reproduced with permission from the Mayo Foundation for Medical Education and Research, Rochester, MN.)

After insertion of the screw, with adequate fracture compression as dictated by the instruction manual for the screws, the guidewire is removed and final radiographic images are obtained to guarantee good fracture reduction and placement of the screw without penetration into either the scaphotrapezial or radioscaphoid joint (**Figure 9**).

The wound is then irrigated with sterile saline solution, and the volar radiocarpal ligaments are repaired with a nonabsorbable 2-0 suture. The most superficial portion of the FCR tendon sheath does not need to be repaired, however. The tourniquet is then deflated, and hemostasis is obtained. The skin incision is then closed in standard technique, and sterile dressings are applied. The patient is placed in a well-padded thumb spica splint, awakened from anesthesia, and transferred to the recovery room.

Dorsal Approach

To approach the scaphoid dorsally, a 1- to 2-cm incision is made just ulnar and distal to the Lister tubercle (**Figure 10**). The skin and subcutaneous tissues are dissected sharply, with care taken to preserve the dorsal venous structures. The distal aspect of the extensor retinaculum is incised, and the extensor pollicis longus and the radial wrist extensors are retracted in a radial direction (**Figure 11**). The distal wrist capsule is then opened transversely, with care taken to protect the scapholunate interosseous ligament. Dissection of the capsule must be limited to the level of the scaphoid waist to prevent any injury to blood vessels entering into the scaphoid at the dorsal ridge. The wrist is flexed, pronated, and ulnarly deviated to expose the scaphoid.

A K-wire is inserted at the most proximal aspect of the scaphoid, just radial to the insertion of the scapholunate interosseous ligament (**Figure 12**). The guidewire is advanced along the plane of the thumb, down the center axis of the scaphoid, and confirmed with C-arm imaging. With the dorsal approach, the wrist cannot be extended to obtain adequate radiographs while the K-wire is in position. Therefore, the entire arm must be elevated to obtain a true PA view of the wrist and hand. Once C-arm images confirm the center position of the guidewire and the location of the tip at the subchondral margin, the depth is measured. As with the volar approach, 4 to 6 mm is subtracted from the length to avoid penetration into the scaphotrapezoidal joint and to allow countersinking of the screw head. Once the screw length is determined, the guidewire is advanced distally to avoid inadvertently removing the K-wire while drilling.

A cannulated drill is used to drill over the wire. Despite the stop guides on most systems, radiographic visualization is essential to prevent penetration of the volar aspect of the wrist. In younger patients or patients with very sclerotic bone, the proximal aspect of the scaphoid may need to be overdrilled to allow easier insertion of the cannulated screw without "gapping" the fracture site. In more comminuted fractures, a second parallel guidewire may need to be inserted before drilling to prevent rotation or displacement of the fracture.

After final insertion of the screw, with adequate fracture compression as obtained according to the specific system used, the guidewire is removed, and fluoroscopic imaging is used to confirm placement of the screw and the final reduction of the fracture (**Figure 13**).

The wound is irrigated with sterile saline solution, and the capsule is closed using 2-0 nonabsorbable suture. The tourniquet is deflated, and hemostasis is obtained. The extensor tendons are returned to their previous position, and the extensor retinaculum is repaired. The skin is then closed in standard fashion. Sterile dressings are applied, and the patient is placed in a well-padded, forearm-based thumb spica splint. The patient is then awakened from anesthesia and transferred to the recovery room.

Complications

Complications of open scaphoid fracture fixation are related to either the fracture

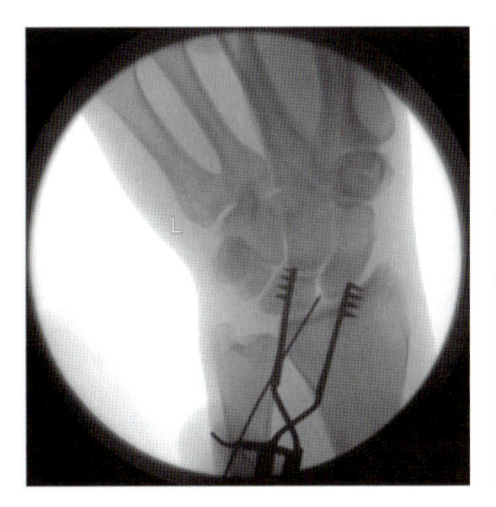

Chapter 41: Open Reduction and Internal Fixation of Scaphoid Fractures

Figure 12 Fluoroscopic image shows the starting point of a dorsal K-wire, just radial to the scapholunate interosseous ligament. The K-wire is aimed up the central axis of the scaphoid. (Reproduced with permission from the Mayo Foundation for Medical Education and Research, Rochester, MN.)

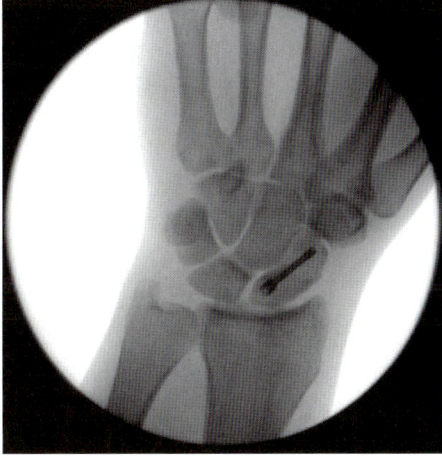

Figure 13 Final fluoroscopic image of a dorsally placed scaphoid screw. (Reproduced with permission from the Mayo Foundation for Medical Education and Research, Rochester, MN.)

pattern itself or the fracture reduction technique. Special attention must be given to the fluoroscopic images to ensure adequate reduction of the scaphoid fracture. The most common area for step-off is located within the scaphocapitate joint. Two separate K-wires, used as joysticks, can help the surgeon obtain adequate reduction of the scaphoid within this articular surface. If this reduction is particularly difficult to obtain, or if the patient has harder bone density, a second, parallel K-wire should be inserted to prevent rotation during drilling and screw insertion. The surgeon must be familiar with the screw insertional technique to obtain compression across the fracture site. Stabilizing the scaphoid with a fracture gap may lead to progression to a delayed union or nonunion.

Another common complication is penetration of the screw into either the radiocarpal joint proximally or the scaphotrapezial joint distally. The guidewire position must be confirmed on multiple fluoroscopic images—typically PA, lateral, navicular, and pronated and supinated oblique—to guarantee subchondral positioning. Once the surgeon is satisfied with the placement of the guidewire, 4 to 6 mm are subtracted from the measured depth of the screw. This allows for fracture compression and subchondral seating of the screw head and prevents penetration of the distal aspect of the screw.

Another common complication is guidewire breakage. This occurs with inaccurate drilling over the guidewire, bent guidewires, or shifting of the scaphoid fragments with motion of the wrist. Once accurate depth is measured, the guidewire should be advanced through the opposite cortex (and subcutaneous, if possible) before drilling. If the wire is accidentally broken, it can be easily retrieved without having to open the scaphoid fracture again.

Other complications include iatrogenic damage to the arterial or neurologic structures during the volar approach or to tendons and venous structures during the dorsal approach. Special care is needed with a dorsal capsulotomy to prevent injury to the scapholunate interosseous ligament. Dissecting distal to the scaphoid waist with a dorsal approach is done meticulously to avoid iatrogenic injury to the dorsal blood supply of the scaphoid. Devascularization may increase the risk of osteonecrosis. The standard rate of osteonecrosis, as well as the potential risk of nonunion, cannot be completely eliminated, however, and must be thoroughly explained to the patient and the patient's family before the beginning of the procedure.

Bone defects should be aggressively bone grafted with autologous cancellous graft to optimize outcome. The need for bone graft (either iliac crest or distal radius) should be discussed with the patient preoperatively.

Postoperative Care and Rehabilitation

The patient is seen in the office 10 to 14 days after the operation. The surgical dressings and sutures are removed, and radiographic images are obtained. The length of immobilization depends on the fracture type, the fixation, and surgeon preference. A minimum of 6 weeks of immobilization is needed to allow the volar carpal ligaments to heal if a volar approach was used. Proximal pole fractures may require up to 12 to 15 weeks of immobilization.[8] With the volar approach, the patient is typically immobilized with a long arm–thumb spica cast for 6 weeks and subsequently placed in a short arm–thumb spica cast until union. The use of a removable splint depends on surgeon preference after the 6 weeks of long-arm casting. Open dorsal approaches can be immobilized for a shorter period of time (2 weeks) if dorsal carpal ligaments are not disrupted.

Once the patient is placed in a thumb spica splint, range of motion, edema management, and scar desensitization exercises are initiated. The splint is expected to be worn continuously, with the exception of personal hygiene and range-of-motion exercises, which should be performed approximately 4 to 5 times a day. The ultimate goal is full wrist and thumb range of motion at the time of fracture union, which typically is 6 to 8 weeks postoperatively. If the surgeon desires, formal hand therapy may be initiated, or the patient may participate in a self-guided exercise program.

The second postoperative visit is 6 to 8 weeks after surgery. Radiographs are taken to determine fracture union. If the fracture is united, strengthening exercises are initiated; however, if the fracture is not united, the splint is continued until fracture union. It may be necessary to obtain a CT scan of the scaphoid to visualize fracture union in some cases.

Once union has been determined, we strongly recommend obtaining a subsequent follow-up radiograph at 4 to 6 weeks to ensure that the fracture union does not resorb.

Pearls

During the volar approach to the wrist, the proximal volar portion of the trapezium is often removed to allow better visualization and access to the distal pole of the scaphoid. This greatly facilitates the placement of the guidewire from a volar direction. We do not hesitate to place K-wires in the proximal and distal aspects of the scaphoid and use these K-wires as joysticks to aid in the reduction of the scaphoid fracture. If this technique is used, the guidewire is often placed in the

© 2013 American Academy of Orthopaedic Surgeons

scaphoid up to the site of the fracture and confirmed to be in good position using radiographic imaging. Once the fracture has been reduced, the guidewire is then advanced across the fracture into the remaining portion of the scaphoid.

The antirotational K-wire must be placed parallel to the guidewire across the fracture site. Placement of this K-wire in a nonparallel fashion will prevent even and uniform compression across the fracture site. With increased divergence of these K-wires, compression across the fracture may even be unobtainable. This second guidewire is placed freehand or with a parallel K-wire guide. Adequate compression of the fracture must be obtained, and if a significant fracture gap exists secondary to comminution, bone grafting should be performed. Autograft can often be taken from the Lister tubercle, and if the dorsal approach has been performed, the incision is extended proximally to allow access to this area. We consent and prepare all patients for iliac crest bone graft harvest. In cases with significant intraoperative comminution or collapse of the scaphoid, the need for structural bone can thus be addressed.

While drilling the path of the screw, care must be taken to maintain the drill collinear to the guide wire. Drilling "off axis" to the K-wire can cause the guidewire to shear intraosseously. To help prevent this complication, the drill is occasionally pulled back during the drilling process to ensure that no binding or difficulty advancing is encountered. If there is any doubt about the integrity of the K-wire, an intraoperative fluoroscopic image is taken, and the K-wire is exchanged.

The compression screw is inserted at least 2 mm below the articular surface of the scaphoid and should be visualized directly at its insertion point. Intraoperative fluoroscopic images do not demonstrate the articular cartilage but only the subchondral bone. The fluoroscopic images may therefore demonstrate that the screw is slightly protuberant into the joint surface when it is buried below the articular cartilage. Multiple fluoroscopic images must be taken to ensure that the distal portion of the screw does not penetrate into the radiocarpal or scaphotrapezial joint surface.

References

1. Larsen CF, Brøndum V, Skov O: Epidemiology of scaphoid fractures in Odense, Denmark. *Acta Orthop Scand* 1992;63(2):216-218.
2. Wolf JM, Dawson L, Mountcastle SB, Owens BD: The incidence of scaphoid fracture in a military population. *Injury* 2009;40(12):1316-1319.
3. Berger RA: The anatomy of the scaphoid. *Hand Clin* 2001;17(4):525-532.
4. Weber ER, Chao EY: An experimental approach to the mechanism of scaphoid waist fractures. *J Hand Surg Am* 1978;3(2):142-148.
5. Cooney WP, Dobyns JH, Linscheid RL: Fractures of the scaphoid: A rational approach to management. *Clin Orthop Relat Res* 1980;149:90-97.
6. Beeres FJ, Hogervorst M, den Hollander P, Rhemrev S: Outcome of routine bone scintigraphy in suspected scaphoid fractures. *Injury* 2005;36(10):1233-1236.
7. Gaebler C, Kukla C, Breitenseher M, Trattnig S, Mittlboeck M, Vécsei V: Magnetic resonance imaging of occult scaphoid fractures. *J Trauma* 1996;41(1):73-76.
8. Rettig ME, Raskin KB: Retrograde compression screw fixation of acute proximal pole scaphoid fractures. *J Hand Surg Am* 1999;24(6):1206-1210.

Video Reference

41.1 Matullo KS, Shin AY: *Open Reduction and Internal Fixation of Scaphoid Fractures.* Rochester, MN, Mayo Foundation for Medical Education and Research, 2005.

Chapter 42
Open Reduction and Internal Fixation of Phalangeal Fractures

William B. Geissler, MD

Introduction

Stable anatomic reduction of a phalangeal fracture with early functional recovery is the goal of internal fixation of hand fractures. Open reduction and internal fixation (ORIF) of hand fractures has become increasingly popular, particularly over the past 3 decades, secondary to improved implant material, designs, surgical technique, radiographic availability, and the demand by the general public for anatomic fracture restoration. ORIF of hand fractures presents a significant challenge to the surgeon, however, because of the difficulty of managing small fracture fragments without causing devascularization. Open reduction without stable fixation increases the risk of adhesions and scarring adjacent to the fracture. Percutaneous techniques offer the advantages of stable fracture fixation and earlier rehabilitation while minimizing the risk of fragment devascularization and surgical scarring. This is particularly true in the proximal and middle phalanx, where the flexor and extensor tendons are close to the bone.

Patient Selection

Most phalangeal fractures are treated nonsurgically. Displaced unstable fractures may require surgical stabilization, however, particularly if the fracture is rotated. In multiple phalangeal or metacarpal fractures or open fractures, stabilization should be considered. "Less is more" in phalangeal fractures because of the high propensity for stiffness from the close association of the flexor and extensor tendons.

Phalangeal Condylar Fractures

Phalangeal condylar fractures were initially classified by London in 1971.[1] Type I fractures were considered stable and nondisplaced, type II fractures were unstable, and type III fractures were bicondylar. London found that bicondylar fractures were common athletic injuries. Stark[2] noted that unicondylar fractures of the proximal phalanx were often missed because the patient can usually bend the finger initially after injury. Affected athletes frequently have a history of a finger dislocation that was reduced by a trainer or coach, and they present to the clinic in a semiacute state; they continue to experience pain and deformity of the finger as the fracture displaces.

Weiss and Hastings[3] noted that unicondylar fractures tend to be common sports injuries that occur when a ball impacts the slightly flexed outstretched digits with high velocity, spreading the digits and resulting in an oblique volar fracture pattern. In their series of 38 patients with unicondylar fractures of the proximal phalanx, they found that the location of an avulsed condylar fracture tends to be the outermost fingers of the hand, and the condyle toward the midline is the most frequently fractured. They also found that when the condyle away from the midline was fractured, either a compressive mechanism (with the finger away from the midline) or a tension mechanism (with the fingers deviating toward the midline) was the most likely cause.

Unicondylar fractures of the phalanges are very unstable. Weiss and Hastings[3] noted that in five of seven patients with nondisplaced condylar fractures managed nonsurgically, the fractures displaced during treatment. They specified that nonsurgical treatment of these fractures requires very close follow-up to reduce the high likelihood of displacement.

At least two Kirschner wires (K-wires) are required for stable fixation of unicondylar fractures of the phalanx. A single K-wire does not provide adequate stability, because K-wires splint and do not compress the fracture site as does screw fixation. Mini-screws provide compression at the fracture site, and a single screw centered in the condylar fragment may provide sufficient stability. K-wires and mini-screws may be used in combination, and two mini-screws may be used in larger fracture fragments. Full recovery of proximal interphalangeal (PIP) joint motion is the exception, not the rule, following unicondylar fractures of the phalanx. Stable fixation does seem to correlate with recovery of motion at the PIP joint. Usually, some loss of extension is present, resulting in a flexion contracture.

In 2006, I presented my technique for percutaneous headless cannulated mini-screw fixation as an option for intra-articular unicondylar fractures and selected bicondylar fractures of the phalanx.[4] The advantage of headless screws is that they fit entirely within the bone fragment, minimizing irritation to the collateral ligament compared with mini-screws with conventional heads. In addition, percutaneous insertion minimizes soft-tissue dissection and scarring, compared with a mini-open approach. This results in less restriction from joint and tendon adhesions and greater range of motion. Insertion of a cannulated screw allows precise placement of the screw over the guidewire and simplifies the procedure.

Surgical Technique

Condylar fractures of the phalanx usually can be treated with closed reduction within 7 to 10 days following injury (**Figure 1**). Under fluoroscopy, a dental pick, K-wire, or hypodermic needle can be used to assist reduction if closed manipulation fails to anatomically reduce the fracture fragment. Once the fracture is reduced, a pointed reduction clamp or a specialized fracture reduction jig may be used to provide provisional fixation (**Figure 2, A**). The fracture reduction is evaluated under fluoroscopy in both the PA and lateral views. The condyles should align concentrically on the lateral view. A displaced condylar fracture that is not anatomically reduced will appear as a double convexity (Touchy sign) when viewed laterally. Once the fracture is anatomically reduced and confirmed under fluoroscopy, one or two K-wires are inserted. One guidewire is placed in the central aspect of the condylar fragment parallel to the articular surface, just distal to the origin of the collateral ligament (**Figure 2, B**). This will be the guidewire used for screw insertion. A second

Dr. Geissler or an immediate family member has received royalties from Acumed, Arthrex, Medartis, and Springer; is a member of a speakers' bureau or has made paid presentations on behalf of Acumed, Arthrex, Medartis, and Ascension; serves as a paid consultant to or is an employee of Acumed and Ascension; and has stock or stock options held in Tornier.

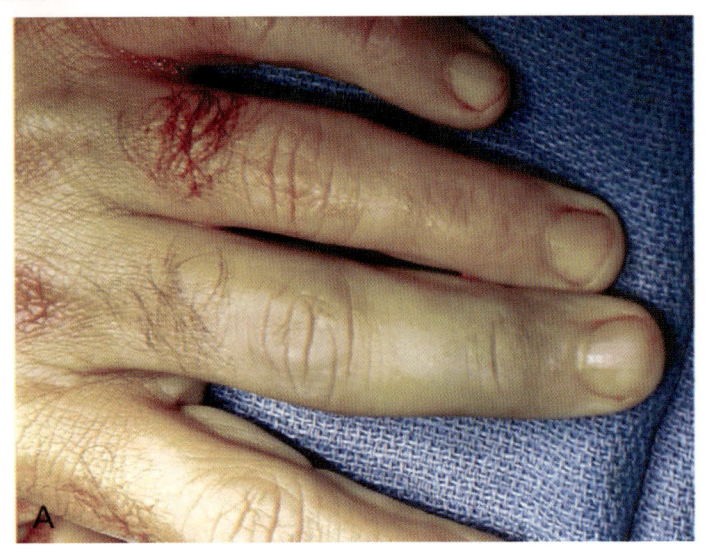

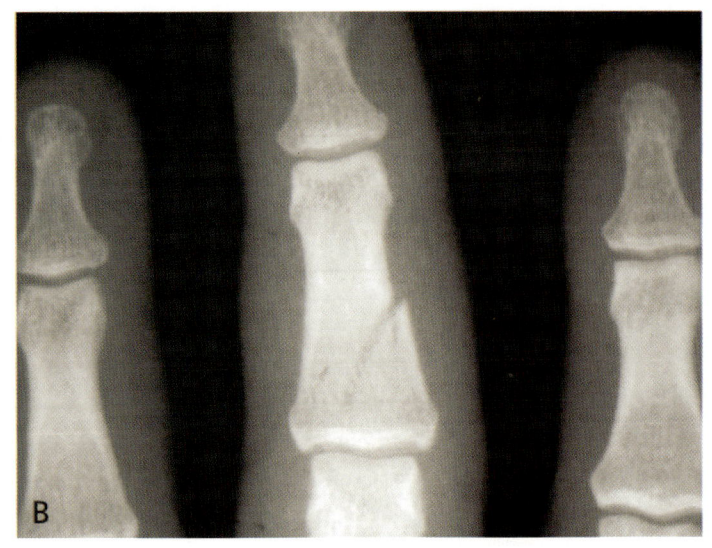

Figure 1 Phalangeal condylar fracture. **A,** Clinical photograph shows a displaced fracture of the middle phalanx of the long finger, resulting in ulnar deviation of the digit. **B,** PA radiograph shows the displaced fracture angulation from the base of the middle phalanx of the long finger.

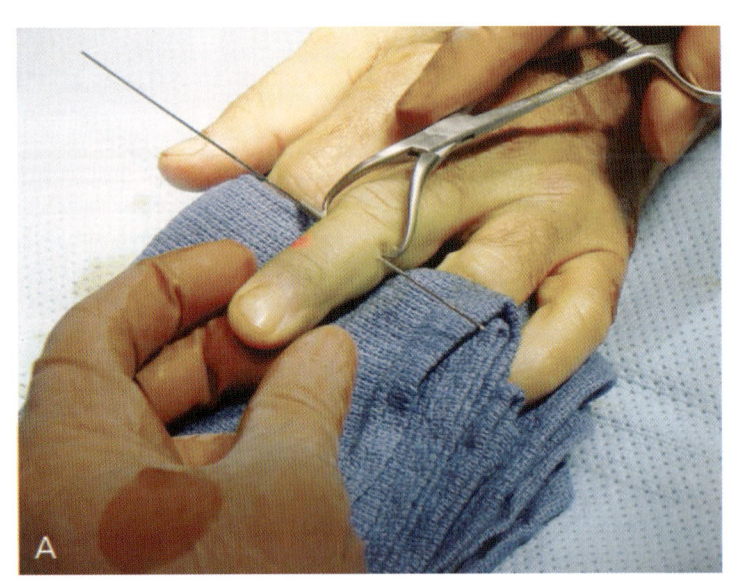

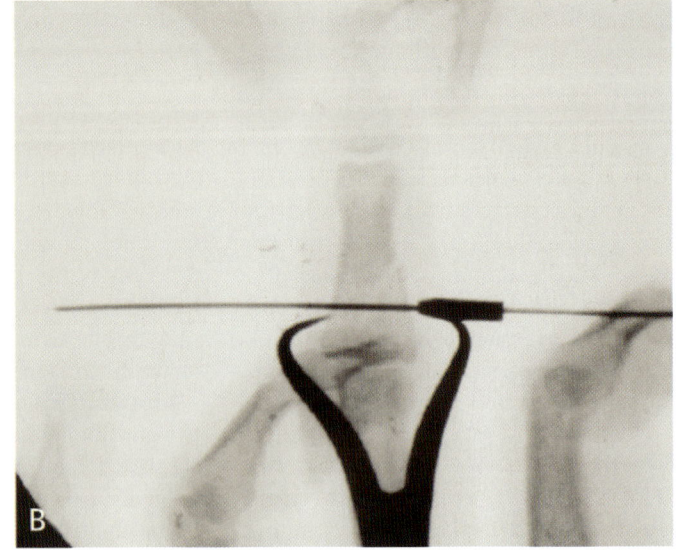

Figure 2 Reduction of a phalangeal condylar fracture. **A,** Photograph demonstrates anatomic reduction of the fracture with closed manipulation. A specialized reduction clamp is used to hold the provisional reduction, and a guidewire is placed for the headless cannulated screw. **B,** PA fluoroscopic view shows the anatomic reduction of the fracture with placement of the guidewire through the reduction clamp.

guidewire is placed eccentrically into the condylar fragment to prevent rotation during drilling and screw insertion. The key is to place both guidewires through the opposite cortex and the skin of the digit so that if the guidewire breaks, it can be easily removed.

The skin is nicked with the tip of a No. 11 blade over the central guidewire (**Figure 3, A**). Then blunt dissection is carried down to the bone surface with a hemostat. In unicondylar fractures, only the near cortex needs to be reamed with a cannulated drill because the metaphyseal bone is relatively soft (**Figure 3, B**). In fractures that have a more proximal or distal extension involving a portion of the diaphysis of the phalanx, both cortices should be drilled, to avoid blow-out of the opposite cortex as the screw is inserted. Typically, the screw length is 8 to 10 mm. The screw is inserted over the guidewire so that it sets entirely inside the bone on both the PA and lateral radiographs (**Figures 3, C** through **F**). A second headless cannulated screw is placed if the fracture line extends toward the diaphysis (**Figures 4** and **5**). The second mini-screw is usually inserted on the opposite side from the initial screw. This allows the smaller-diameter lead portion of the screw to cross the fracture site and engage the smaller remaining cortex of the condylar fragment, decreasing the chance of fragmentation. Following screw placement, the stability of the fracture is judged by performing range of motion of the finger under fluoroscopy. A small adhesive bandage is placed over the insertion site. Usually, no sutures or splint is required.

Postoperative Care and Rehabilitation

Immediate range-of-motion exercises are initiated, and strengthening exercises are typically started 4 to 6 weeks following surgery (**Figure 6**). Athletes typically return to competition within 1 week with the finger buddy taped to the adjacent digit in a skilled player.

Complications

Unicondylar fractures of the phalanges usually have small fragments and involve the joint. Loss of full motion is common following injury and surgery. Weiss and Hastings[3] reported on 38 consecutive

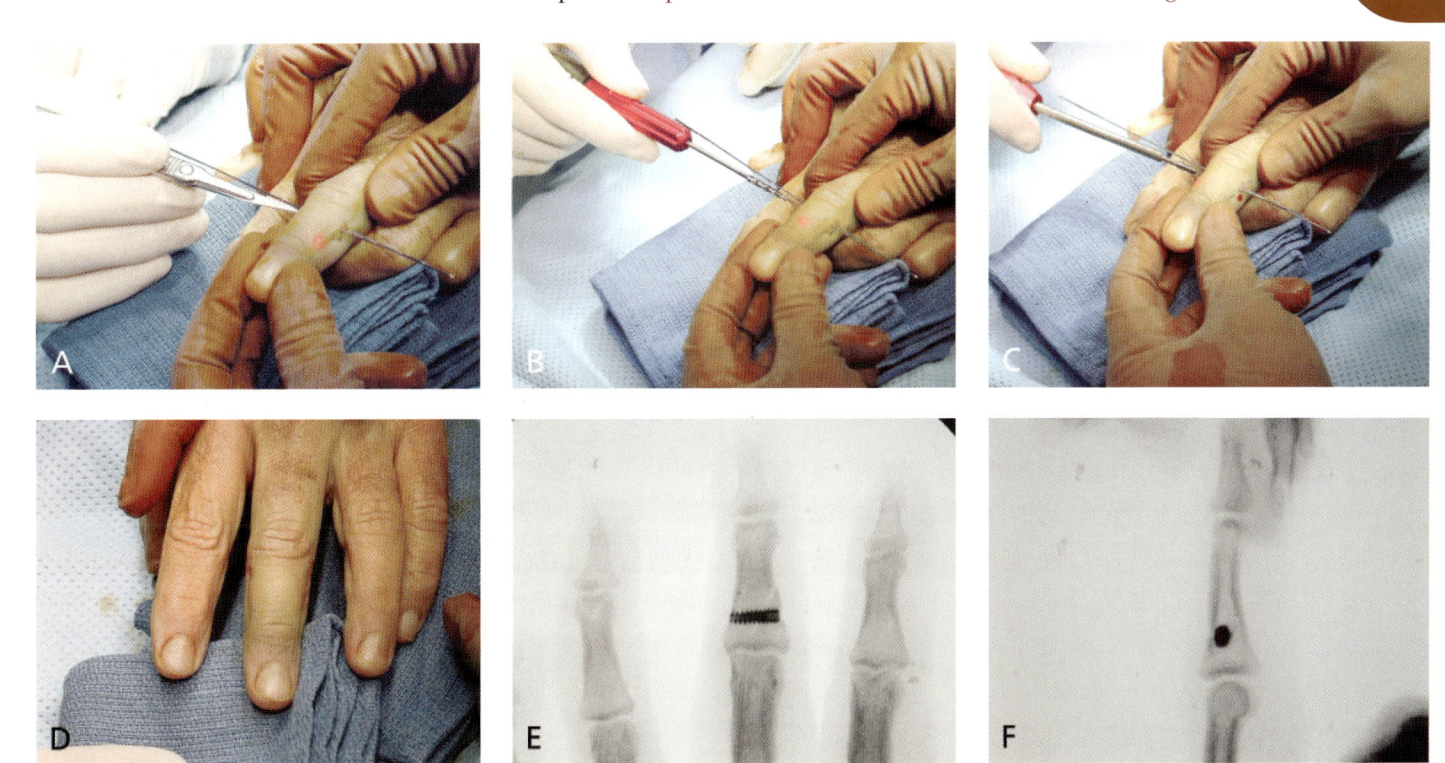

Chapter 42: Open Reduction and Internal Fixation of Phalangeal Fractures

Figure 3 Fixation of a phalangeal condylar fracture. **A,** Intraoperative photograph depicts incision of the skin with the tip of a No. 11 blade over the guidewire. **B,** The guidewire is placed across the finger and exits the opposite cortex and the skin. The near cortex is reamed with a cannulated reamer. **C,** The headless cannulated screw is placed over the guidewire to stabilize the fracture. The fracture is then anatomically reduced and stabilized. **D,** The ulnar deviation of the digit has been corrected. PA (**E**) and lateral (**F**) fluoroscopic views show the placement of the headless cannulated screw within the bone and anatomic restoration of the fracture.

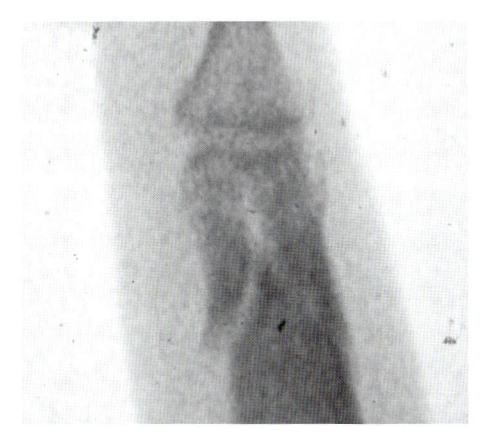

Figure 4 PA radiograph shows a bicondylar fracture of the head of the middle phalanx of the index finger.

unicondylar fractures of the proximal phalanx. The average PIP joint extension lag was 13° (range, 0° to 35°), and the average joint flexion was 85° (range, 60° to 115°). The authors noted that all four patients treated with a single K-wire required a second procedure because of early fracture displacement. They found that multiple K-wire fixation and mini-screw fixation were the most predictable methods for treating fracture reduction and recovery of joint motion for these fractures.

Ford et al[5] reported on a series of 36 patients with fractures of the phalanges who underwent ORIF with Synthes 1.5- and/or 2.0-mm screws. The authors had no excellent results in their series. They noted the tendency for the PIP joint to lose 20° to 30° of extension following

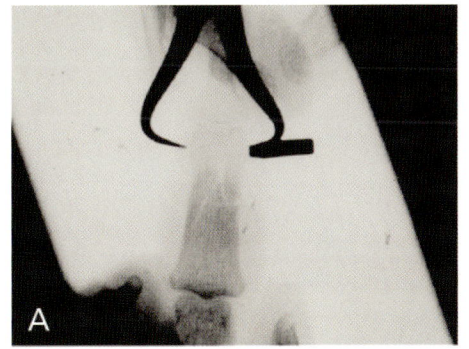

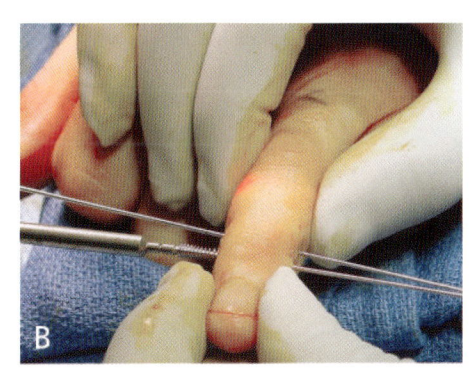

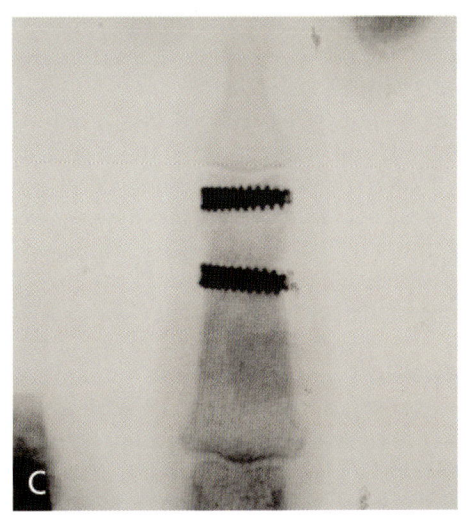

Figure 5 Reduction and fixation of a bicondylar fracture of the middle phalanx. **A,** With traction, the fracture is anatomically reduced and provisionally stabilized with a reduction clamp. **B,** Photograph shows two guidewires placed across the fracture, providing provisional stabilization. **C,** PA radiograph shows two headless cannulated screws placed across the fracture, providing anatomic reduction and stable fixation and enabling the start of early range of motion.

fixation with mini-screws. PIP joint flexion was more reliably restored.

In my series of 25 patients with unicondylar fractures stabilized with percutaneous headless cannulated screw fixation,

© 2013 American Academy of Orthopaedic Surgeons

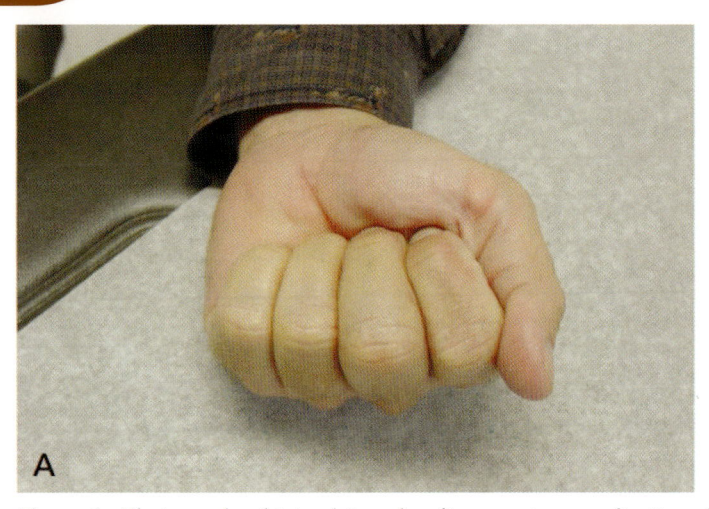

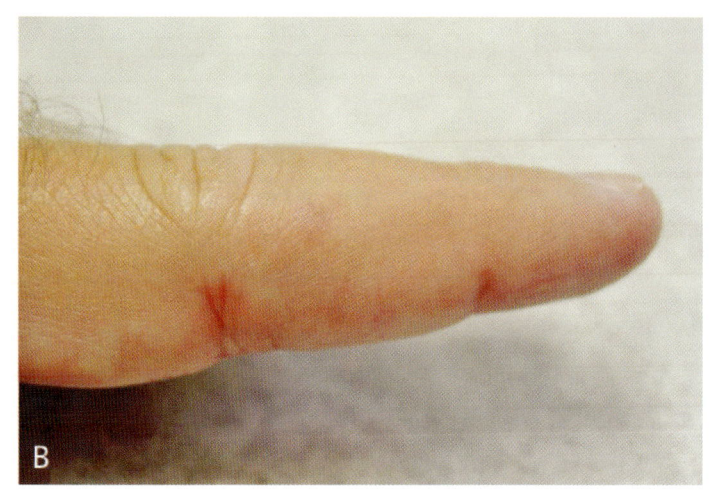

Figure 6 Photographs obtained 4 weeks after percutaneous fixation of a bicondylar fracture of the middle phalanx. **A,** The patient has full flexion and extension of the digits. **B,** The incision site cannot be visualized with the percutaneous cannulated technique.

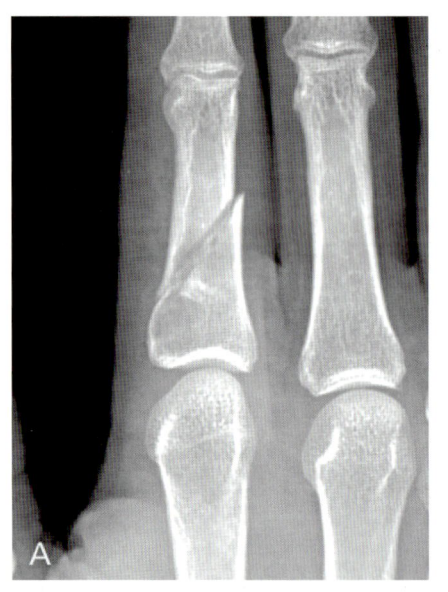

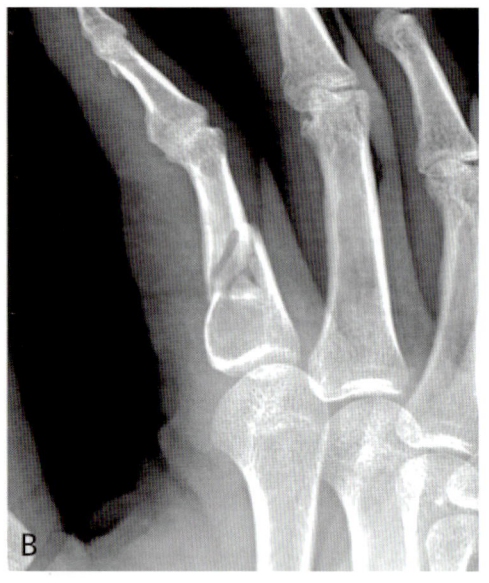

Figure 7 PA (**A**) and lateral (**B**) radiographs show an unstable oblique fracture of the proximal phalanx of the index finger in a college athlete who desired to return to play as soon as possible during the competitive season.

18 had a unicondylar fracture involving the head of the phalanx, 3 had intra-articular displaced fractures at the base of the phalanx, and 4 had intra-articular fractures along the base of the distal phalanx of the thumb.[4] The fractures healed in all patients. No fracture displacement or malunion was present. No patients required metal removal. In condylar phalangeal fractures, the average PIP joint loss of extension was 5° (range, 0° to 10°), and the average PIP joint flexion was 85° (range, 80° to 95°). In the four patients who had an intra-articular fracture involving the base of the thumb, the average interphalangeal joint extension was 15° (range, 10° to 20°), and the average flexion was 60° (range, 50° to 65°). Percutaneous fixation is less traumatic than open stabilization. Percutaneous cannulated mini-screws offer the same advantage as percutaneous K-wires, and they have the additional advantage of compression of the fracture site, which allows more intensive and accelerated rehabilitation. In addition, the headless cannulated screw fits entirely in the bone, resulting in less soft-tissue irritation. Pin-tract infection is eliminated, compared with the use of percutaneous K-wires alone.

Pearls

- Unicondylar phalangeal fractures are inherently unstable and only rarely can be managed by closed treatment.
- A single K-wire has been shown to not provide stable fixation for unicondylar fractures.
- Percutaneous insertion of headless cannulated screws offers some advantages compared with traditional mini-screws or K-wires alone.

Phalangeal Shaft Fractures

Spiral oblique fractures are more common in the proximal phalanx (**Figure 7**), whereas transverse fractures usually are more common in the middle phalanx. Proximal phalangeal fractures typically have apex volar angulation secondary to the proximal fragment being flexed by interosseous muscle insertion. Angulation of middle phalangeal fractures is variable. Phalangeal fractures that are stable and nondisplaced can be effectively managed by buddy taping or splint immobilization. Nonsurgical management of unstable fractures usually will lead to deformity and stiffness.

Surgical management of phalangeal fractures depends on several factors. Fracture patterns that have a potential to rotate, angulate, or shorten are considered unstable. Rotation is best judged by looking for digital overlap while having the patient flex the fingers. Patients who have apex volar angulation of the proximal phalanx present with hyperextension at the metacarpophalangeal (MCP) joint and extensor lag at the PIP joint. Open fractures are usually the result of high-energy trauma, are unstable, and present with associated injuries. Transverse fractures tend to angulate, oblique fractures present with rotational deformities, and comminuted fractures have a tendency to rotate and shorten.

Closed reduction and percutaneous pinning have the advantage of stabilizing the fracture and allowing early range of motion while decreasing surgical scarring and adhesions of the tendons to an implant. Belsky et al[6] described their technique for percutaneous stabilization. The fracture is reduced by flexing the MP joint. An antegrade pin is driven through the metacarpal head across the

Chapter 42: Open Reduction and Internal Fixation of Phalangeal Fractures

MP joint and across the fracture line. The fracture is immobilized for approximately 3 weeks, at which time the K-wire is removed. The authors noted 90% good and excellent results in their series when the patient presented within 5 days of injury. Green and Rowland[7] reported full range of motion in 18 of 22 patients with 26 long oblique fractures of the proximal phalanx treated by closed reduction and stabilization with two or three percutaneous K-wires. The K-wires were placed perpendicular to the fracture line in the midlateral plane.

Freeland[8] described his technique of percutaneous screw fixation for spiral phalangeal fractures. The fracture is provisionally stabilized with a bone tenaculum, and a self-tapping screw is inserted under fluoroscopic guidance through a small incision. His technique has the advantage of minimal soft-tissue dissection and provides more stability with compression of the fracture, compared with K-wires alone.

Percutaneous K-wire fixation or limited open reduction with lag screws is the preferred method of stabilization for unstable phalangeal fractures. Occasionally, plate fixation may be considered in patients who have multiple fractures, comminution to the fracture site, or nonunions/malunions, or in patients who require early return to athletic competition. Plate fixation provides immediate stability and active range of motion to the digits. It also allows immediate return to competition with protective bracing. A plate can be placed on the lateral or dorsal surface of the phalanx. My personal preference is to place the plate on the lateral position of the phalanx. This placement potentially can reduce adhesions from plate fixation secondary to the extensor digitorum communis tendon. In addition, the newer generation low-profile locking plate will further reduce the risk of adhesions and promote early range of motion.

The extensor mechanism covers the phalanges intimately, and scarring of the extensor mechanism can occur from not only trauma from the fracture itself but also the surgical approach required for plate fixation. The potential for complications is high with plate fixation of the phalanges. Tendon gliding may be significantly affected with fixation of the phalanges compared with the metacarpals, where more space is available between the extensor tendons and the bone to accommodate plate fixation. The risk of scarring is decreased, however, when stable fixation is achieved and early range of motion is possible. Particularly in college athletes, for whom a quick return to play is important, access to physical therapy may be available at least once if not twice a day. This easy access to physical therapy allows the option of plate fixation in phalangeal fractures, with a reduced risk of adhesions in certain circumstances.

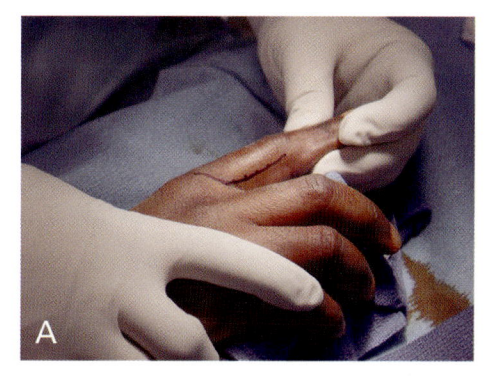

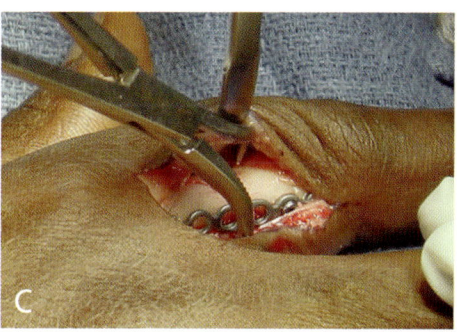

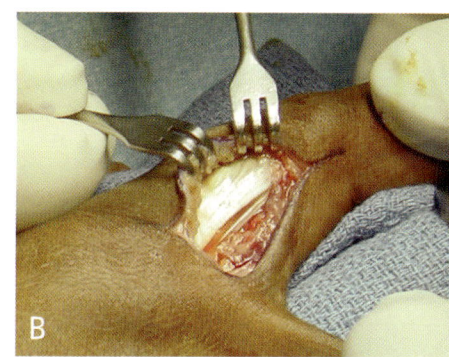

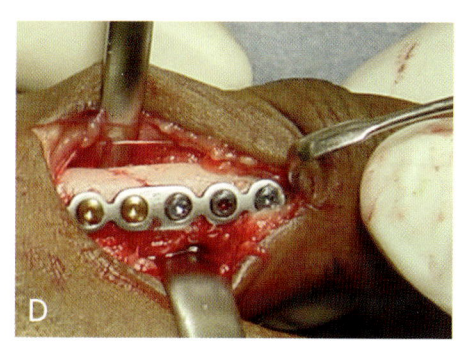

Figure 8 Intraoperative photographs demonstrate the surgical technique for plate fixation of a phalangeal fracture of the index finger. **A,** A lateral approach to the proximal phalanx of the index finger is made along its ulnar aspect. The ulnar-side approach avoids the lumbrical insertion onto the lateral band. **B,** The cutaneous nerves are retracted dorsally. The lateral band is incised along its volar aspect and retracted dorsally to expose the fracture. **C,** The fracture is anatomically reduced, and a plate is placed along the ulnar aspect of the proximal phalanx and provisionally stabilized with a reduction clamp. **D,** A series of locking and nonlocking screws are placed through the plate to stabilize the fracture. Nonlocking screws are placed in lag mode to stabilize the fracture.

Video 42.1 Lateral Approach for Plate Fixation of a Phalangeal Fracture. William B. Geissler, MD (4 min)

Surgical Technique

A demonstration of plate fixation of a phalangeal fracture can be seen in the video supplement.

An incision is made in the midaxial line along the phalanx in the lateral approach (**Figure 8, A**). Blunt dissection is carried down to protect the cutaneous nerves, after they are located on the dorsal aspect of the wound. The volar aspect of the lateral band and the extensor digitorum communis tendon are retracted dorsally. In fractures involving the base of the proximal phalanx, the proximal portion of the lateral band may be excised. The surgeon can approach from either the radial or the ulnar side of the digit, depending on the fracture pattern. The ulnar side is usually preferred, however, because it does not affect the lumbrical insertion into the lateral band, which inserts radially.

The lateral band and the extensor digitorum communis tendon are elevated dorsally, exposing the fracture site (**Figure 8, B**). A low-profile locked plate is placed on the side of the phalanx, and locking and nonlocking screws are inserted (**Figure 8, C**). Initially, nonlocking screws are placed proximal and distal to the fracture to reduce the plate to the bone so that no gap occurs (**Figure 8, D**). Nonlocking screws also may be placed across the fracture site to the plate if the use of a lag screw is possible. Locking screws are placed after the fracture is reduced and the plate lies firmly against the bone surface (**Figure 9**). The wound is then closed in layers.

Occasionally, long oblique fractures (in which the fracture line is twice the diameter of the bone or greater) also may be treated with headless mini-screw fixation. This is an option when immediate return to athletic competition is not an

© 2013 American Academy of Orthopaedic Surgeons

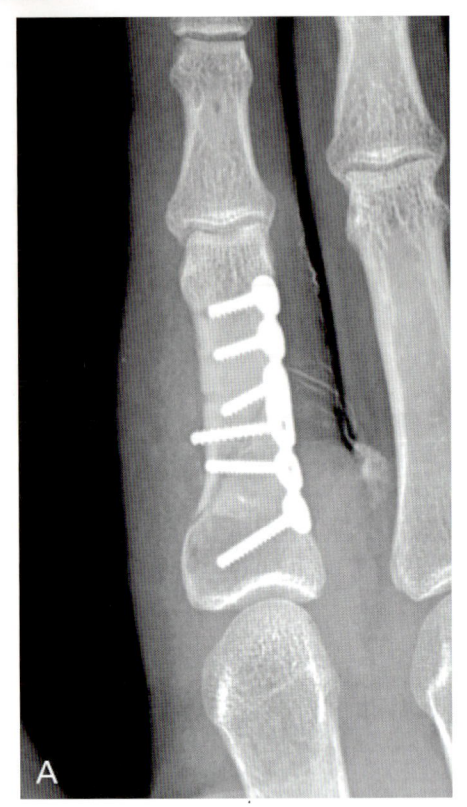

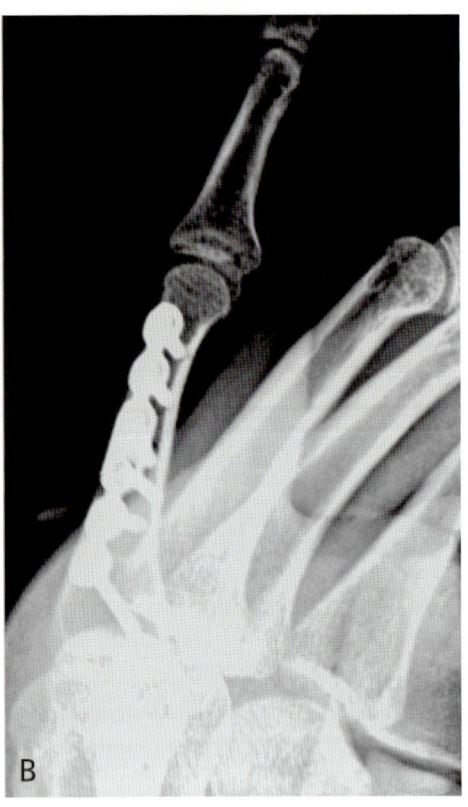

Figure 9 PA (**A**) and lateral (**B**) radiographs show stable fixation of a fracture of the proximal phalanx of the index finger. The fracture has been anatomically restored and stabilized with a series of locking and nonlocking screws.

issue. Pointed reduction forceps provide provisional stabilization after the fracture is anatomically reduced under fluoroscopic control in the PA and lateral views. Guidewires are placed across the fracture fragment and exit the opposite side of the digit. Because the cortical bone is quite rigid compared with soft metaphyseal bone near the joint, the proximal and far cortices are reamed following placement of the guidewires. Headless cannulated screws are inserted to the widest part of the screw, up against and opposite to each other to allow maximum bone purchase.

Complications

Phalangeal fractures treated with ORIF using plate fixation have an inherent tendency to stiffness because of the proximity of the flexor and extensor tendons. Stern[9] reported that only 4 of 37 patients (11%) treated with plate fixation for phalangeal fractures regained a range of motion greater than 220°. Of the patients in his series, 92% had one or more complications, including extensor lag (59.5%), joint contracture (37.8%), delayed union (2.7%), and plate prominence (2.7%).

Dabezies and Schutte[10] reported their results in 22 patients who underwent plate fixation of proximal phalangeal fractures. Full range of motion of the PIP joint was restored in only two cases. The average total active range of motion was 246°.

Bosscha and Snellen[11] noted that six of seven patients treated with ORIF regained motion greater than 220°. Finally, Berman et al[12] noted good to excellent results in 15 of 16 patients (94%) who underwent plate fixation for phalangeal fractures.

Pearls

- Most unstable phalangeal shaft fractures are treated percutaneously with K-wire fixation to minimize scarring.
- Plate fixation is an option in special circumstances. The plate should be placed on the radial or ulnar portion of the phalanx to reduce scarring in the extensor tendon mechanism.

References

1. London PS: Sprains and fractures involving the interphalangeal joints. *Hand* 1971;3(2):155-158.
2. Stark HH: Troublesome fractures and dislocations of the hand. *Instr Course Lect* 1970;19:130-149.
3. Weiss AP, Hastings H II: Distal unicondylar fractures of the proximal phalanx. *J Hand Surg Am* 1993;18(4):594-599.
4. Geissler WB: Cannulated percutaneous fixation of intra-articular hand fractures. *Hand Clin* 2006;22(3):297-305.
5. Ford DJ, Ali MS, Steel WM: Fractures of the fifth metacarpal neck: Is reduction or immobilisation necessary? *J Hand Surg Br* 1989;14(2):165-167.
6. Belsky MR, Eaton RG, Lane LB: Closed reduction and internal fixation of proximal phalangeal fractures. *J Hand Surg Am* 1984;9(5):725-729.
7. Green DP, Rowland SA: Fractures and dislocations in the hand, in Rockwood CA Jr, Green DP, Bucholz RW, eds: *Fractures in Adults*, ed 3. Philadelphia, PA, Lippincott, 1991, pp 441-561.
8. Freeland AE: Phalangeal fractures, in Freeland AE, ed: *Hand Fractures*. New York, NY, Churchill Livingstone, 2000, pp 75-126.
9. Stern PJ: Management of fractures of the hand over the last 25 years. *J Hand Surg Am* 2000;25(5):817-823.
10. Dabezies EJ, Schutte JP: Fixation of metacarpal and phalangeal fractures with miniature plates and screws. *J Hand Surg Am* 1986;11(2):283-288.
11. Bosscha K, Snellen JP: Internal fixation of metacarpal and phalangeal fractures with AO minifragment screws and plates: A prospective study. *Injury* 1993;24(3):166-168.
12. Berman KS, Rothkopf DM, Shufflebarger JV, Silverman R: Internal fixation of phalangeal fractures using titanium miniplates. *Ann Plast Surg* 1999;42(4):408-410.

Chapter 43
Surgical Fixation of Metacarpal Fractures

William B. Geissler, MD   Christopher A. Keen, MD

Introduction

Metacarpal fractures account for as many as one third of all hand fractures.[1,2] The prevalence of metacarpal fractures increases from the radial to the ulnar side of the hand, with fractures of the fifth metacarpal being the most common.[3] Metacarpal neck fractures are the most common; these usually involve the ring and small metacarpals.[3] Fifth metacarpal neck fractures are commonly referred to as boxer's fractures. These fractures are rarely seen in professional boxers, however, occurring most often in amateur boxers who have hit solid objects or in street brawlers.

The metacarpals are long tubular bones with a relatively flat dorsal surface and medial and lateral cortices that converge along the volar aspect, creating a triangular cross section. The metacarpals become quite narrow in the mid-diaphyseal region. The metacarpals have an abundant blood supply, being surrounded by the volar and dorsal interosseous muscles. Although the abundant blood supply from the interosseous muscles may be a blessing, when the musculature is severely disrupted, it initially can result in disabling scarring and intrinsic contractures. The deep transverse intermetacarpal ligament lies at the level of the metacarpal neck, which helps limit deformity with low-energy injuries. When intact, the deep transverse intermetacarpal ligament usually limits shortening to approximately 5 mm. The extensor apparatus surrounds the metacarpophalangeal (MCP) joint. The collateral ligaments originate from the tubercle of the metacarpal head and pass obliquely to the volar aspect of the base of the proximal phalanx. Scar from these ligaments may lead to an extensor contracture at the MCP joint.

Metacarpal fractures are generally the result of one of two mechanisms. The most common mechanism is an axial load transmitted from the MCP joint proximally down the shaft of the metacarpal (**Figure 1**). This results in various common injuries, from fifth metacarpal neck fractures to higher-energy injuries such as metacarpal shaft fractures. A less common mechanism of injury for fractures of the metacarpals is a crush injury. Crush injuries typically involve multiple metacarpal fractures and are also associated with other fractures and significant soft-tissue trauma.

Transverse and short oblique metacarpal fractures tend to angle dorsally because of the deforming forces of the extrinsic flexor tendons and the intrinsic musculature on the distal fragment. Cadaver studies have shown that as much as 7° of extensor lag and 8% loss of grip strength occur for each 2 mm of metacarpal shortening.[4-6] Intrinsic muscle shortening and muscle tension may lead to progressive grip weakness after approximately 30° of dorsal metacarpal angulation.[5] Most metacarpal fractures heal uneventfully and do not require surgery, but spiral fractures, multiple metacarpal fractures, and comminuted fractures are more likely to shorten and rotate, resulting in overlapping of the fingers and tendon imbalance (**Figure 2**). The border (index and small) metacarpals have a tendency to greater shortening compared with the long and ring metacarpals because the former lack the support of the deep metacarpal ligaments. Border metacarpals have a greater tolerance for lateral angulation than do

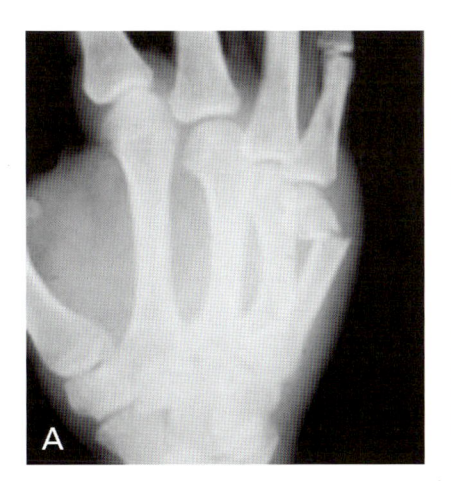

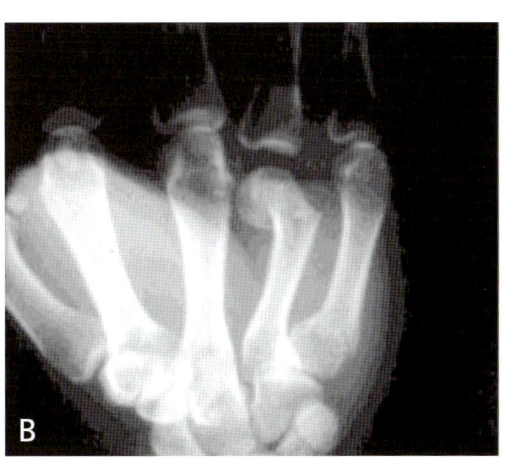

Figure 1 Radiographs show metacarpal fractures. **A,** Oblique view of the hand demonstrates a metacarpal neck fracture of the small finger (boxer's fracture). These fractures typically are seen in a patient who has punched a solid object. **B,** PA view of a different patient demonstrates a fourth metacarpal neck fracture. Concomitant fractures of the ring and small metacarpal neck and/or base are commonly seen as a result of an axial loading mechanism, as seen in **A.**

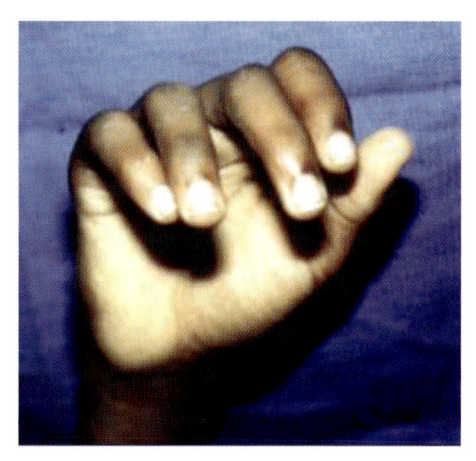

Figure 2 Photograph of the hand of a patient who sustained a spiral fourth metacarpal shaft fracture. Note the rotational deformity of the ring finger and the digital overlap.

Dr. Geissler or an immediate family member has received royalties from Acumed, Arthrex, Medartis, and Springer; is a member of a speakers' bureau or has made paid presentations on behalf of Acumed, Arthrex, Medartis, and Ascension; serves as a paid consultant to or is an employee of Acumed and Ascension; and has stock or stock options held in Tornier. Neither Dr. Keen nor any immediate family member has received anything of value from or owns stock in a commercial company or institution related directly or indirectly to the subject of this chapter.

the long and ring metacarpals because of the greater divergence and because the border fingers have only one adjacent finger. Rotation of the metacarpals is poorly tolerated. Each degree of metacarpal fracture rotation may produce as much as 5° of rotation at the fingertips. Royle[7] demonstrated that approximately 10° of metacarpal rotation resulted in 2 cm of fingertip overlap. Clinical deformity from lateral metacarpal angulation is best observed with the fingers straight, whereas rotational deformity is best observed with the fingers in flexion.

Patient Selection

Most metacarpal fractures are treated nonsurgically. The Jahss maneuver is helpful for reduction of a flexed metacarpal. In this maneuver, a nerve block is performed. The metacarpal shaft is stabilized with the MCP joint flexed to 90°. With the fracture site distracted, upward force is applied to the proximal phalanx metacarpal head to realign the neck and shaft. A splint with three-point molding is applied with dorsal compression at the fracture site and volar support for the metacarpal head and base. Nondisplaced metacarpal fractures are protected in a splint or cast for 3 to 4 weeks, followed by gradual mobilization. The MCP joints should be immobilized in flexion to stretch the MCP joint ligaments to help prevent contracture and to relax the intrinsic musculature to prevent further deformity at the fracture site.

Surgical stabilization is indicated in patients with extensive soft-tissue injuries, multiple metacarpal fractures, or isolated metacarpal fractures with angulation or rotational deformity. Border metacarpal fractures have a tendency to be more unstable than those affecting the central digits because of support from the transverse metacarpal ligament.

Because of the increased motion of the ring and small metacarpals compared with the index and long metacarpals in the anterior-posterior plane, greater angulation is accepted in the ulnar digits. For metacarpal shaft fractures, 5° to 10° of angulation is acceptable in the index and long metacarpals, 20° of angulation in the ring metacarpal, and 30° of angulation in the small metacarpal. Similarly, for metacarpal neck fractures, 10° to 15° of angulation in the index and long metacarpals, 30° to 40° in the ring metacarpal, and 50° to 60° in the small metacarpal neck fracture without pseudoclawing is acceptable.

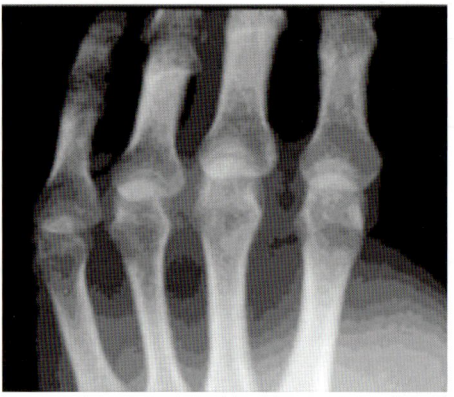

Figure 3 Brewerton view of the metacarpal heads in a normal hand. This view provides excellent visualization of the articular surface.

Preoperative Imaging

Plain radiographs, including AP and lateral oblique views, usually are adequate to assess a metacarpal fracture. Although it is difficult to evaluate a metacarpal fracture on the lateral view, this view is helpful for evaluating subluxation of the MCP or the carpometacarpal joint. The oblique view is particularly useful for measuring flexion deformity at the fracture site. The AP view is especially helpful for evaluating coronal plane angular malalignment, which usually is clinically relevant. The Brewerton view can be used to assess metacarpal head fractures (**Figure 3**). The Brewerton view is obtained by placing the supinated hand on the cassette, with the dorsum of the proximal phalanges flat on the x-ray plate and with the MCP joints flexed to 65° and the x-ray tube positioned 15° ulnar to the midline of the hand.

Metacarpal Neck Fractures

The amount of angulation that is acceptable in metacarpal neck fractures involving the ring and small metacarpals is controversial. Ford et al[8] reviewed 62 fractures of the small metacarpal neck with palmar angulation and concluded that palmar (volar) angulation up to 70° still resulted in good outcomes. In this study, the fracture was not reduced and the hand was immobilized. Eichenholtz and Rizzo[9] considered palmar angulation greater than 40° to require correction. Other authors have recommended surgical intervention when angulation is greater than 30°. If rotation or claw deformity is noted with digital overlap or MCP joint hyperextension and proximal interphalangeal joint flexion, then reduction and stabilization should be considered. Because of the more rigid index and long carpometacarpal joints, angulations

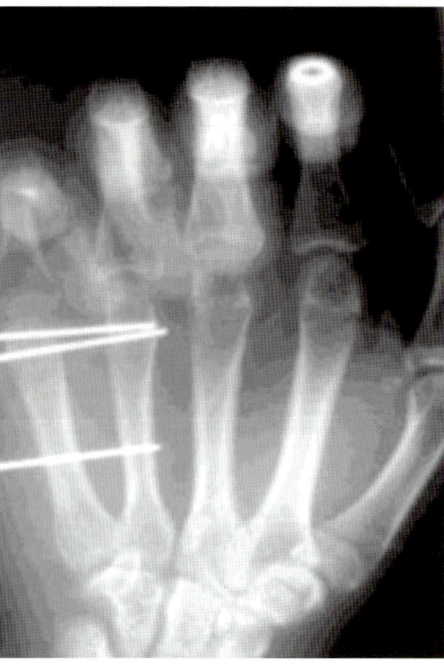

Figure 4 Fluoroscopic PA image shows a fifth metacarpal neck fracture that has been closed reduced and stabilized with crosspinning of the proximal and distal fragments to the fourth metacarpal.

less than 10° for the index finger and less than 15° for the long finger can be tolerated without surgical stabilization. Metacarpal neck fractures with angulation greater than that stated above require reduction and stabilization.

Surgical Technique

Several methods of fixation have been recommended for metacarpal neck fractures. These include transverse pinning of the metacarpal head to the adjacent metacarpal, crossed Kirschner wires (K-wires), and intramedullary pinning. These techniques can result in better cosmesis than plate fixation and may be considered, depending on the clinical scenario and patient expectations.

Several techniques of pin fixation are used. The pins may be placed transversely across the metacarpal neck, particularly for a border fracture (**Figure 4**). Other options are to run the pins from distal to proximal or from proximal to distal. When pinning the metacarpal in a distal to proximal direction, the MCP joint is flexed to gain control of the distal fragment. A smooth 0.045-in K-wire is inserted on the radial and/or ulnar collateral recess, and the ideal placement is confirmed under fluoroscopy. The pin is placed in the deepest cavity of the collateral recess. The wire is then advanced onto the shoulder of the metacarpal and down the intramedullary canal. As the

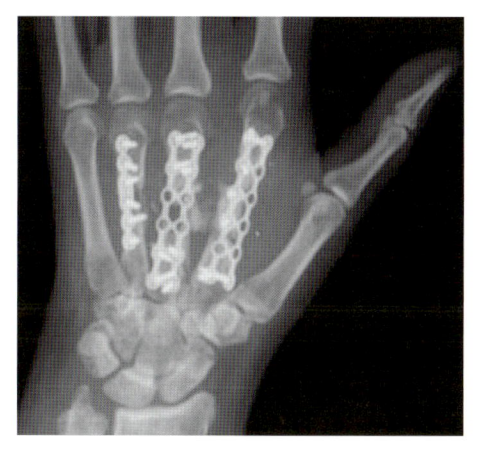

Figure 5 Postoperative PA radiograph shows extensively comminuted fractures of the second, third, and fourth metacarpals that underwent open reduction and internal fixation. The second and third metacarpal fractures have been plated with locking cage plates, which allow additional screw purchase in the proximal and distal fragment to stabilize these fractures.

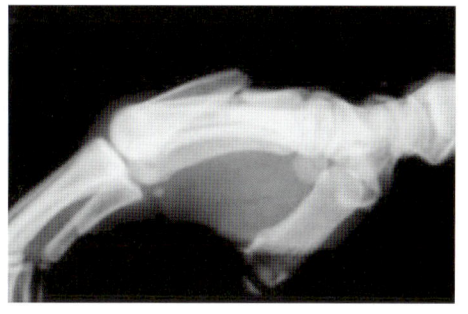

Figure 6 Lateral radiograph shows a transverse fracture of the fourth metacarpal with apex dorsal angulation.

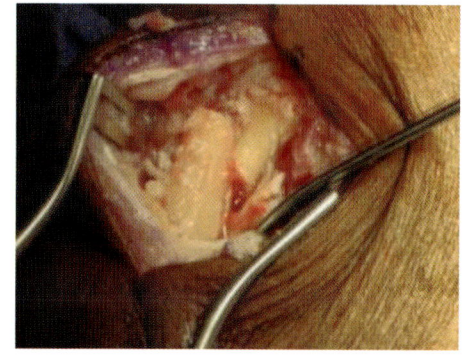

Figure 7 Intraoperative photograph shows an oblique fifth metacarpal shaft fracture with extensive shortening and angulation.

wire approaches the fracture site, the fracture is reduced and the wire is advanced proximally into the base of the metacarpal. Occasionally, it is helpful to advance the wire with a mallet rather than under power so the pin bounces off the far cortex rather than penetrating it.

A bouquet pinning technique can be used for a fracture of the index or small metacarpal. For the index metacarpal, a 2-cm skin incision is made along the radial aspect of the base of the second metacarpal; for the small metacarpal, a similar incision is made on the ulnar side of the metacarpal. The extensor tendon insertion is elevated but not detached. Commercially available pins may be used, or the tip of a 0.045-in K-wire is cut off and the pin is gently bent along its length. Under fluoroscopic imaging, the proximal aspect of the metaphysis is identified. Penetration is made through the canal with a 2-mm drill and may be enlarged to approximately 5 mm. The precontoured 0.045-in K-wire is then placed into the base of the metacarpal and advanced distally across the fracture site. Multiple K-wires may be placed. The goal is to tension the wires off the intact proximal cortex and enter the distal fragment in various locations, creating the so-called bouquet effect.[10]

In fractures with extensive comminution, plate fixation may be considered (**Figure 5**). The dorsal surface of the metacarpal allows for ideal placement of a low-profile locking plate. Plate fixation potentially allows early return to competition or work compared with possibly protruding K-wires. Meticulous dissection is observed at the time of plate fixation, allowing closure of the periosteum over the plate, theoretically decreasing the chance of adhesion and tendon irritation.

Complications

Minimally displaced fractures of the metacarpal neck are treated with cast immobilization, with minimal complications. Hofmeister et al[11] and Poolman et al[12] reviewed various methods of cast immobilization and found no method superior to another. Several authors have compared transverse pinning with intramedullary stabilization to evaluate if either method is complicated by loss of fixation or scarring resulting in decreased motion.[13-15] Winter et al[14] and Schädel-Höpfner et al[15] reported that total active range of motion was greater in the intramedullary group. Wong et al,[13] however, performed a comparison study and found no difference. Ozer et al[16] reported no difference in range of motion when comparing plate fixation with intramedullary pinning, but the authors were concerned about the risk of penetration of the MCP head with pinning.

Metacarpal Shaft Fractures

Most isolated metacarpal shaft fractures are stable and do not require surgical fixation. Border metacarpal fractures are less stable because of a lack of adjacent soft-tissue support. Transverse fractures typically present with apex dorsal angulation because of the volar force of the intrinsic musculature and extrinsic flexor tendons (**Figure 6**). Up to 20° of angulation is acceptable in transverse fractures of the small and ring metacarpals because of the mobility of the hamate saddle joint. Only 5° to 10° of angulation may be acceptable in the index and long metacarpals, however, because of the lack of mobility of the index and long carpometacarpal joint. Most authors suggest surgical intervention for shortening greater than 5 mm.

Surgical Technique

Many internal fixation devices are available for metacarpal shaft fractures, including K-wires, interosseous wires, lag screws when appropriate, and plate fixation. Implant choice is based on the amount of comminution, multiple metacarpal fractures, fracture configuration, and the experience and preference of the surgeon.

When plate fixation is to be used for the metacarpal, 2-mm plates are recommended. Newer generation locking plates are strong and provide multiple-screw fixation in a short distance; they are particularly useful when metacarpal comminution is present.

Oblique metacarpal fractures have a tendency to shorten along the oblique slope of the fracture line. This is particularly true in the index and small metacarpals because of lack of support from the deep transverse metacarpal ligament (**Figure 7**). Frequently, in an oblique fracture pattern, the fracture line is too short for lag screw fixation alone, and a single lag screw needs to be neutralized by a plate. The fracture is compressed by the lag screw and, once fracture stability is achieved, a straight, T-shaped, or L-shaped plate is placed along the dorsal aspect of the metacarpal (**Figure 8**). Appropriate rotational alignment is confirmed with passive wrist flexion and extension.

When considering the use of lag-screw fixation to stabilize bone fragments, the fracture fragment should be at least three times the diameter of the screw. During open reduction, stabilization with a screw is preferable to a K-wire. The

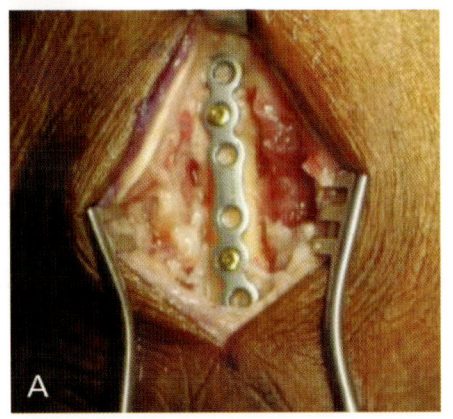

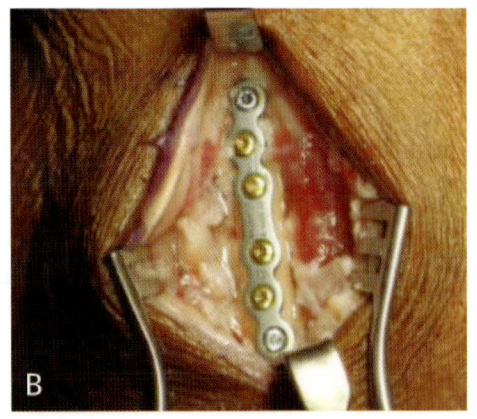

Figure 8 Intraoperative photographs show fixation of a fifth metacarpal shaft fracture. **A,** The fracture has been reduced and initially stabilized with a locking plate and nonlocking screws in the proximal and distal fragments. **B,** After rotational alignment is confirmed, the remaining screw holes are filled with locking and nonlocking screws to enhance fracture stability.

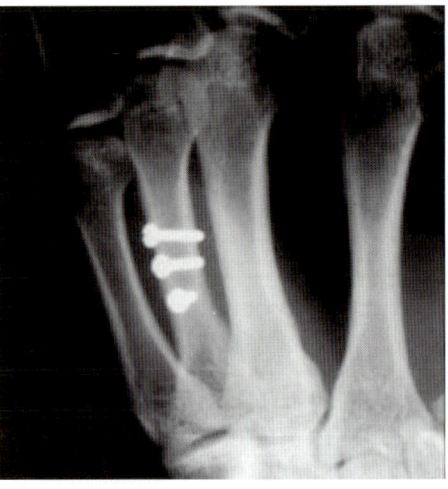

Figure 9 Postoperative oblique radiograph shows a spiral fracture to the fourth metacarpal shaft that has been stabilized with three lag screws.

advantage of a screw is that it can compress the fracture to provide additional stability over a K-wire. If the fragment is large enough to place a K-wire, it is usually large enough to accept a screw for compression and improved stability. A 0.045-in K-wire is equal to the diameter of a 1.1-mm drill bit. Therefore, if a 0.045-in K-wire can be well-placed into a small bone fragment, the surgeon can choose to remove the K-wire, and the hole that remains can accept a 1.5-mm compression screw for superior fixation. Similarly, a 0.065-in K-wire is equal in diameter to a 1.5-mm drill bit, and if the fracture fragment is large enough to support a 0.065-in K-wire, it is usually large enough for fixation with a 2.0-mm screw, which enhances stability.

Lag screws are the recommended implant for spiral fractures of the metacarpals when the fracture line is at least twice the diameter of the bone (**Figure 9**). Lag screw fixation allows reduced soft-tissue dissection and improved fracture stability over K-wire fixation. Lag screw fixation also results in less tendon adhesions and scarring than plate fixation. A minimum of two screws is necessary. One screw may be placed perpendicular to the shaft, which helps with the translation of the fracture, and the second screw is placed perpendicular to the fracture line to compress the fracture site. Alternatively, two screws may be placed by bisecting the angle of the fracture in the shaft. When lag screw fixation is used for a spiral metacarpal fracture, 2.0- or 1.5-mm screws are recommended.[17]

Complications
Dabezies and Schutte[18] reported their results for plating in 27 unstable metacarpal fractures. They had one complication with MCP joint stiffness. They noted that the total active motion of the involved digit was 252°. Bosscha and Snellen[19] reported that 29 of 31 metacarpal fractures treated with open reduction and internal fixation regained total active motion greater than 220°.

Stern et al[20] noted a 34% complication rate with plate fixation of 29 metacarpal fractures. They found stiffness to be the most common complication, and they noted that complications occurred more frequently with associated bone and soft-tissue injuries than with isolated fractures.

The senior author of this chapter (W.B.G.) reviewed his results for open reduction and internal fixation of metacarpal fractures in athletes.[17] In this study, 2.0-mm locking cage plates were used in 8 of 10 patients with fractures of the metacarpal. Two patients underwent lag screw fixation for a spiral fracture of the metacarpal. Patients were allowed to return to work 1 to 2 weeks following fixation. All fractures healed. One patient who underwent lag screw fixation for a spiral fracture to the index metacarpal sustained a refracture to the index metacarpal approximately 1 year following stabilization after sliding into a base during a baseball game. The author concluded that, although lag screws were certainly the implant of choice in spiral metacarpal fractures, plate fixation needs to be considered, particularly in the border digits of metacarpal fractures in contact athletes.

There has been some research on the use of bioabsorbable plates in fractures of the metacarpal. Waris et al[21] compared bioabsorbable plates made of two different copolymers with 1.7- and 2.3-mm titanium plates and 1.25-mm K-wires in 112 cadaver metacarpals. They found that the bioabsorbable plates were stronger than K-wires and equal to or better than 1.7-mm plates but not as rigid as 2.3-mm plates.[21] Dumont et al[22] reported on 14 unstable metacarpal fractures treated with bioabsorbable plates made of a copolymer of poly-lactic and glycolic acid. They noted that the plates provided stable fixation, but there were two implant failures. The authors concluded that bioabsorbable plates, in combination with splinting, are useful for certain metacarpal fractures.[22]

Metacarpal Head Fractures
Metacarpal head fractures are relatively rare. Most metacarpal head fractures occur in the coronal plane; they may be associated with fractures of the neck or shaft.

Surgical Technique
The extensor tendon is split in its midline, and the capsule is longitudinally opened to expose the fracture. The MCP joint is flexed to help facilitate exposure to the fracture site. The fracture is reduced with reduction clamps or provisionally stabilized with a K-wire. Usually, headless cannulated screws are the implant of choice for an intra-articular metacarpal head fracture (**Figure 10**).

Complications
Surgical fixation can significantly improve overall function and alignment following select metacarpal fractures. Complications are possible, however, including rotation deformity, stiffness, tendon irritation, complex regional pain

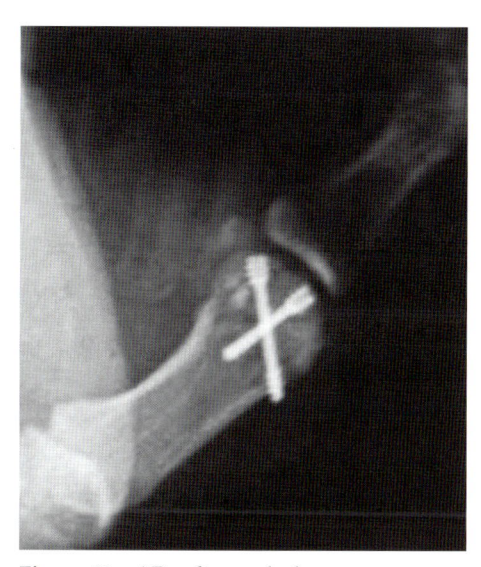

Figure 10 AP radiograph shows a comminuted thumb metacarpal head fracture that has been reduced and stabilized with headless screws.

syndrome, hardware failure, and the possibility of nonunion. To minimize the risk of these complications and optimize the benefits of treatment, surgeons need to be cognizant of the surgical indications for the procedure and aware of their surgical expertise.

Postoperative Care and Rehabilitation

The postoperative protocol following pinning of a metacarpal fracture is to immobilize the hand in the intrinsic (safe) position for 3 weeks, at which time the pins are removed in clinic. The patient is then placed in a removable splint in the safe position, and motion is started. Plate fixation provides the advantage of improved stability; therefore, patients are placed in a soft dressing at the time of surgery, and motion is started immediately. Close follow-up is provided in the postoperative period. If stiffness develops, aggressive hand therapy is started and supplemented with dynamic and static splinting.

Pearls

- K-wire pinning of metacarpal fractures is more cosmetic than plate stabilization.
- Intramedullary stabilization may result in greater range of motion compared with transverse pinning.
- The surgeon should beware of intra-articular penetration of the metacarpal head with intramedullary stabilization.
- Plate fixation of metacarpal fractures is tolerated better in the hand than in the phalanges.
- Plate fixation allows earlier return to athletics and potentially work compared with K-wire fixation.
- Plate fixation is recommended over lag screw stabilization alone in contact athletes because of the risk of refracture.

References

1. Chung KC, Spilson SV: The frequency and epidemiology of hand and forearm fractures in the United States. *J Hand Surg Am* 2001;26(5):908-915.
2. Hove LM: Fractures of the hand: Distribution and relative incidence. *Scand J Plast Reconstr Surg Hand Surg* 1993;27(4):317-319.
3. van Onselen EB, Karim RB, Hage JJ, Ritt MJ: Prevalence and distribution of hand fractures. *J Hand Surg Br* 2003;28(5):491-495.
4. Strauch RJ, Rosenwasser MP, Lunt JG: Metacarpal shaft fractures: The effect of shortening on the extensor tendon mechanism. *J Hand Surg Am* 1998;23(3):519-523.
5. Low CK, Wong HC, Low YP, Wong HP: A cadaver study of the effects of dorsal angulation and shortening of the metacarpal shaft on the extension and flexion force ratios of the index and little fingers. *J Hand Surg Br* 1995;20(5):609-613.
6. Meunier MJ, Hentzen E, Ryan M, Shin AY, Lieber RL: Predicted effects of metacarpal shortening on interosseous muscle function. *J Hand Surg Am* 2004;29(4):689-693.
7. Royle SG: Rotational deformity following metacarpal fracture. *J Hand Surg Br* 1990;15(1):124-125.
8. Ford DJ, Ali MS, Steel WM: Fractures of the fifth metacarpal neck: Is reduction or immobilisation necessary? *J Hand Surg Br* 1989;14(2):165-167.
9. Eichenholtz SN, Rizzo PC III: Fracture of the neck of the fifth metacarpal bone: Is over-treatment justified? *JAMA* 1961;178:425-426.
10. Forthman CL, Graham TJ: Operative treatment of metacarpal fractures, in Wiesel SW ed: *Operative Techniques in Orthopaedic Surgery*. Philadelphia, PA, Lippincott Williams & Wilkins, 2011, vol 3, pp 2365-2377.
11. Hofmeister EP, Kim J, Shin AY: Comparison of 2 methods of immobilization of fifth metacarpal neck fractures: A prospective randomized study. *J Hand Surg Am* 2008;33(8):1362-1368.
12. Poolman RW, Goslings JC, Lee JB, Statius Muller M, Steller EP, Struijs PA: Conservative treatment for closed fifth (small finger) metacarpal neck fractures. *Cochrane Database Syst Rev* 2005;20(3):CD003210.
13. Wong TC, Ip FK, Yeung SH: Comparison between percutaneous transverse fixation and intramedullary K-wires in treating closed fractures of the metacarpal neck of the little finger. *J Hand Surg Br* 2006;31(1):61-65.
14. Winter M, Balaguer T, Bessière C, Carles M, Lebreton E: Surgical treatment of the boxer's fracture: Transverse pinning versus intramedullary pinning. *J Hand Surg Eur Vol* 2007;32(6):709-713.
15. Schädel-Höpfner M, Wild M, Windolf J, Linhart W: Antegrade intramedullary splinting or percutaneous retrograde crossed pinning for displaced neck fractures of the fifth metacarpal? *Arch Orthop Trauma Surg* 2007;127(6):435-440.
16. Ozer K, Gillani S, Williams A, Peterson SL, Morgan S: Comparison of intramedullary nailing versus plate-screw fixation of extra-articular metacarpal fractures. *J Hand Surg Am* 2008;33(10):1724-1731.
17. Geissler WB: Operative fixation of metacarpal and phalangeal fractures in athletes. *Hand Clin* 2009;25(3):409-421.
18. Dabezies EJ, Schutte JP: Fixation of metacarpal and phalangeal fractures with miniature plates and screws. *J Hand Surg Am* 1986;11(2):283-288.
19. Bosscha K, Snellen JP: Internal fixation of metacarpal and phalangeal fractures with AO minifragment screws and plates: A prospective study. *Injury* 1993;24(3):166-168.
20. Stern PJ, Wieser MJ, Reilly DG: Complications of plate fixation in the hand skeleton. *Clin Orthop Relat Res* 1987;214:59-65.
21. Waris E, Ashammakhi N, Happonen H, et al: Bioabsorbable miniplating versus metallic fixation for metacarpal fractures. *Clin Orthop Relat Res* 2003;410:310-319.
22. Dumont C, Fuchs M, Burchhardt H, Appelt D, Bohr S, Stürmer KM: Clinical results of absorbable plates for displaced metacarpal fractures. *J Hand Surg Am* 2007;32(4):491-496.

Chapter 44
Excision of Ganglion Cysts of the Wrist and Hand

Daniel J. Nagle, MD   Jay V. Kalawadia, MD

Introduction

Ganglion cysts are commonly seen by both hand and general orthopaedic surgeons. Although the true etiology of ganglion cysts is unknown, pathologic analysis suggests that some form of mucoid collagen degeneration is responsible for the process.[1] Injection studies suggest that ganglion cysts are created by a rent in the joint capsule, causing synovial fluid to leak into the surrounding tissues. This theory postulates the formation of a one-way valve that leaks joint fluid from the joint space to the cyst via a pedicle. In addition, proponents of this theory believe that underlying joint pathology usually exists and leads to thinning of the capsule, allowing the initial formation of the rent.[2] Other theories postulate that metaplasia of cells derived from connective tissue (ie, ligaments, joint capsules, and tendon sheaths) produces mucin, which coalesces into cysts. In contrast, this theory suggests that the cyst forms initially, followed by the formation of the pedicle.[2,3]

Regardless of etiology, histologic analysis shows that mucin-filled cysts are usually composed of randomly organized collagen fibers without any endothelial lining.[2,4] The viscous material found within the ganglion cysts is composed predominantly of hyaluronic acid, with smaller amounts of glucosamine, globulins, and albumin.[2,5] Ganglions can occur at any joint or over any tendon sheath, but they most often occur in the wrist, followed by the flexor tendon digital sheaths (retinacular cysts) and the distal interphalangeal joints (mucous cysts).[1]

Patient Selection
Patient Presentation

Patients with ganglion cysts present to the clinic for several reasons. Westbrook et al[6] showed that about 28% of patients are worried about malignancy, 38% are bothered cosmetically, 26% are in pain, and 8% are experiencing compromised sensation or function. Ganglion cysts manifest in all age groups. Carpal ganglions most often present in young adults, with women presenting three times more commonly than men. Mucous cysts have an arthritic component and are more common in the elderly.[3] In children younger than 12 years, ganglion cysts occur nearly twice as often in girls as in boys. In the pediatric population, volar ganglion cysts are more common than dorsal cysts (1.2:1); this differs from adults.[7]

Ganglion cysts occurring along the dorsal aspect of the wrist are most common, comprising 60% to 70% of these cysts; they manifest over the scapholunate ligament in 75% of cases[1-3] (**Figure 1**). Ganglion cysts manifest in the volar wrist 13% to 20% of the time.[2] Of volar wrist ganglion cysts, 67% occur over the radioscaphoid joint; the remaining 33% occur over the scaphotrapezial and metacarpotrapezial joints.[1,2] Ganglion cysts can occur at any joint, however, and they often are seen over the ulnocarpal and distal radioulnar joints as well. Retinacular and mucous cysts occur much less frequently, comprising only about 10% of all ganglion cysts each.[2]

A patient's history and physical examination is often the best diagnostic modality. Physical examination will reveal a soft, firm mass with well-circumscribed edges. When masses become large enough, they will transilluminate, which can help differentiate them from solid masses.

Patients generally describe a classic history of waxing and waning of the cyst over months to years. Other symptoms include pain (usually described as an annoyance), tenderness with palpation, and decreased range of motion or grip strength.[2] Small occult dorsal wrist ganglion cysts can be a cause of chronic dorsal wrist pain. Interestingly, the dorsal wrist pain often dissipates once the ganglion becomes palpable or visible. Less commonly, ganglion cysts can cause nerve irritation of the palmar cutaneous nerve, the deep ulnar motor branch, the median nerve within the carpal tunnel,

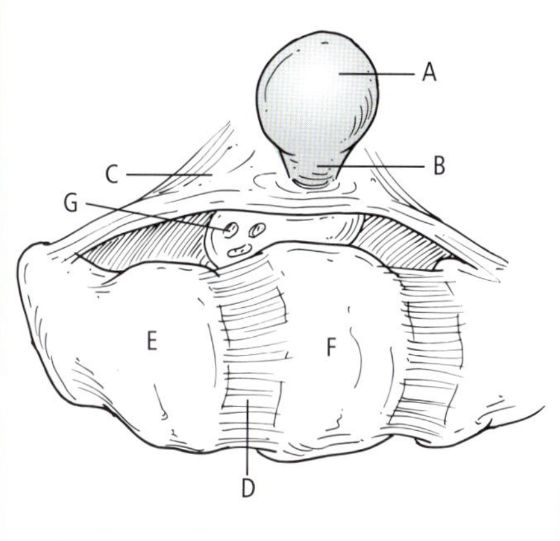

Figure 1 Illustration shows a dorsal ganglion cyst, which typically manifests over the scapholunate ligament. A = cyst, B = stalk of cyst at its confluence with dorsal wrist capsule and scapholunate interosseous ligament, C = dorsal wrist capsule, D = scapholunate interosseous ligament, E = scaphoid, F = lunate, G = capsular microcyst.

or the ulnar nerve within the Guyon canal due to their compressive effects on adjacent nerves. The location and size of the ganglion cyst usually do not correlate with patient symptoms; many people with ganglion cysts are asymptomatic.

Patients with retinacular cysts also may report pain and paresthesias as a result of compression of the digital nerves. In addition to being unsightly, mucous cysts can cause pain, thinning of the overlying skin and irregularities of the nail.[8]

Although ganglion cysts are the most commonly occurring soft-tissue mass in the wrist and hand, accounting for 60% of hand and wrist tumors, a broad differential diagnosis should be considered.[1,3] Other commonly presenting soft-tissue masses in the wrist and hand include vascular aneurysms and malformations, giant cell tumors, brown tumors, tendon sheath fibromas, lipomas, hemangiomas, glomus tumors, osteophytes, and schwannomas. Although rare, synovial cell sarcoma also must be included in the differential diagnosis.

Indications

Patient symptoms and impairment in quality of life generally dictate whether to pursue surgical treatment. From 50% to 79% of ganglion cysts of the wrist re-

---
Neither of the following authors nor any immediate family member has received anything of value from or has stock or stock options held in a commercial company or institution related directly or indirectly to the subject of this chapter: Dr. Nagle and Dr. Kalawadia.

Section 3: Hand and Wrist

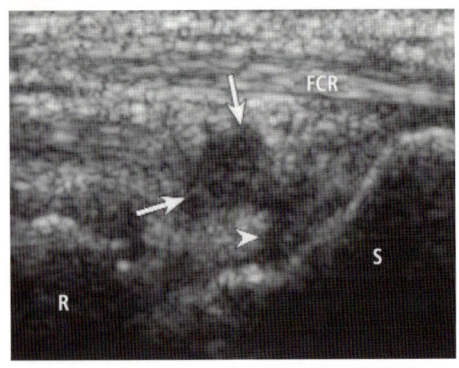

Figure 2 Ultrasonographic image depicts a volar ganglion cyst emanating from the radioscaphoid joint. On ultrasound, the cyst appears as a hypoechoic structure with blurred margins. FCR = flexor carpi radialis, R = radius, S = scaphoid. (Reproduced with permission from Wang G, Jacobson JA, Feng FY, Girish G, Caoili EM, Brandon C: Sonography of wrist ganglion cysts: Variable and noncystic appearances. *J Ultrasound Med* 2007;26[10]:1323-1328; 1330-1331.)

solve spontaneously over 5 years.[2,4,9] Observation is thus a reasonable treatment option in select patients with minimal symptoms. Surgical indications include pain, stiffness, and interference with performance of certain movements of the hand and wrist. Although less frequent, nerve compression or impending overlying skin necrosis, especially from large mucous cysts, are other surgical indications.[3]

Aspiration of the cyst sometimes provides temporary pain relief as well as serving as a diagnostic modality when the viscous mucin is extracted. Recurrence rates are between 13% and 100%, however; thus, aspiration is considered only a temporary solution for carpal ganglion cysts and mucous cysts.[3-5,8] Studies have shown aspiration to be more successful in treating retinacular cysts than carpal ganglion and mucous cysts, leading to recurrence less than 30% of the time.[2,3] In performing aspiration of retinacular cysts, the surgeon should be cautious not to injure the digital nerves. Variations of aspiration, such as using concomitant steroid injection or performing a trephination technique, have shown no benefit and yield similar recurrence rates.[3,9] In addition, postaspiration splinting has shown no benefit.[3]

When aspiration fails or patient symptoms are severe enough to warrant surgical intervention, patients should be made aware that the recurrence rate after surgical excision is between 2% and 39%.[9] Studies have shown that when the entire cystic complex is removed, however, including the pedicle and adjacent joint capsule, the recurrence rate drops to 5%.[3] The recurrence rate after volar ganglionectomy is slightly higher than after dorsal ganglionectomy, with a 7% recurrence rate after excision of the entire cystic complex.[3] Mucous cysts recur at a rate of 10% to 28% with cyst excision alone. The rate drops to 0% to 3.4% with osteophyte débridement in addition to cyst excision.[8] If the primary symptom in a patient with a mucous cyst is pain, the patient should also be made aware that the underlying arthritis may be the etiology, and surgical excision may not relieve their symptoms.

Contraindications
Aspiration should be avoided in the volar wrist because the radial artery, palmar cutaneous nerve, or ulnar nerve can be inadvertently damaged. Corticosteroid injections should not be performed for mucous cysts overlying the distal interphalangeal joint because the overlying skin is thin and can easily become attenuated. If there are overlying signs of infection or if the mass demonstrates irregular properties (eg, abnormal margins), aspiration or excision should not be undertaken until further workup is performed. Pediatric wrist and hand ganglion cysts generally resolve with observation and/or splinting, and surgery can be avoided in most cases.[7]

Preoperative Imaging
Radiographs are of very limited utility in diagnosing ganglion cysts. Obtaining a clenched-fist view and comparing this with the contralateral side can sometimes show widening of the scapholunate joint. Radiographs can also demonstrate arthritis at the distal interphalangeal joint in cases of mucous cysts. Studies have shown, however, that although radiographic abnormalities can be seen in 13% of patients, they rarely change management and thus may not be cost effective.[9,10]

Ultrasonography is a relatively economical diagnostic modality for characterizing a suspected ganglion cyst. Ultrasonography can delineate if a mass is cystic or solid, as well as its vascularity. Ultrasonography is technician dependent, but a well-performed ultrasound can detail the complexity of a cyst, including its walls and tortuous structure emanating from a ligamentous injury (**Figure 2**). This can be helpful in terms of diagnosis and preoperative planning.[11] Ultrasonography has been shown to have 88% sensitivity, 85% specificity, and 87% accuracy, making it a very reasonable diagnostic modality of choice.[9]

MRI can be very helpful when the diagnosis is not absolutely clear, such as in the case of a small dorsal wrist ganglion. MRI can be useful to detect associated wrist pathology (eg, a tear or weakness in one of the wrist ligaments), posterior interosseous neuromas, dorsal impaction syndrome, osteonecrosis of the scaphoid or lunate, tenosynovitis, or other inflammatory arthropathies. In addition, MRI can identify the location of the stalk and the origin of the ganglion, which is particularly important in determining whether an arthroscopically assisted ganglionectomy can be performed. MRI is helpful in elucidating the relationship between the ganglion and adjacent neurovascular structures. Such information is critical to preoperative planning, especially with volar ganglion cysts. Studies have shown that MRI sensitivity for detecting ganglion cysts ranges from 83% to 100%, with a specificity of 50% and an accuracy of 80%.[9] In conclusion, either ultrasonography or MRI is a reasonable option for preoperative planning.

Procedure
Room Setup/Patient Positioning
The patient is placed in the supine position with the affected upper extremity on the radiolucent hand table. A tourniquet is applied.

Instruments/Equipment
- Hand surgery instruments
- Hand holder
- Operating microscope (for open volar ganglionectomy)
- Arthroscopy equipment for arthroscopically assisted ganglionectomy (not discussed in this chapter)

Surgical Technique
Open Dorsal Wrist Ganglionectomy
A Bier block is sufficient for most ganglion cyst excisions. Depending on the magnitude and location of excision, a wrist block can occasionally suffice as well. An axillary block is another alternative.

Prior to incising the skin, the ganglion is filled with a dilute solution of methylene blue (0.1 mL of methylene blue diluted in 5 mL of normal saline). This is accomplished by first placing a 25-gauge venting needle at one side of the ganglion cyst, followed by a very gentle injection of the methylene blue solution using a

25-gauge needle into the opposite side of the ganglion cyst. A 5-mL syringe is used for the injection, and care is taken to not rupture the cyst. Usually, only 1 or 2 mL of methylene blue solution is required.[12]

A transverse incision centered over the ganglion is made following the Langer lines. As dissection is performed through the deeper layers between the second and fourth extensor compartments, the surgeon must be careful not to injure the superficial nerves and the extensor tendons. Dissection is carried deeper following the pedicle, usually to the scapholunate interosseous ligament. The cystic complex is resected from the base in its entirety, taking a small rim of normal ligament in the process. Care must be taken to not weaken the scapholunate ligament. A small rongeur can be used to remove the abnormal tissue, leaving the normal scapholunate ligament intact. Following this step, closure of the rent in the scapholunate ligament with suture or cauterization is not necessary because it has been associated with increased postoperative stiffness.

Closure is performed using a thin, absorbable braided suture for the dermal layers with a buried knot technique. The skin is closed using a running monofilament nonabsorbable suture in a subcuticular fashion. A bulky dressing is applied and reinforced with a dorsal plaster splint holding the wrist in mild flexion to avoid wrist extension contracture. Sutures can be removed anywhere from 2 to 6 weeks after the surgery. Delaying suture removal reduces the tension across the wound and improves cosmesis.[13]

Open Volar Wrist Ganglionectomy

Anesthesia can be conducted in the same fashion as described previously for the open dorsal wrist ganglionectomy.

Prior to an open volar ganglionectomy, the Allen test should be performed. If there is a radial-based ganglion cyst with preexisting occlusion of the ulnar artery, the surgical procedure should commence only if the surgeon is comfortable with the possibility of arterial repair (**Figure 3**). In addition, the operating microscope should be set up in the operating room for most volar ganglionectomies. Prior to incision, the ganglion can be filled carefully with methylene blue to assist with dissection, as described previously for open dorsal wrist ganglionectomy. This optional step should be performed only if the surgeon is confident that the neurovascular structures can be avoided.

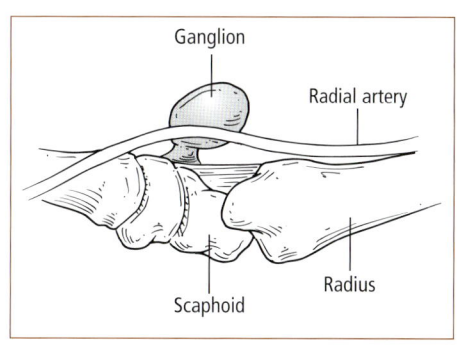

Figure 3 Illustration shows a volar radial-side ganglion cyst. Note the proximity to the radial artery. The cyst can be located adjacent to the radial artery or attached to it. The surgeon must be aware of this possibility and be careful during surgical dissection to avoid injury to the artery.

Radial-Side Ganglionectomy

A radial-side cyst usually lies between the radial artery and the flexor carpi radialis (FCR) tendon. A longitudinal incision is made radial to the FCR tendon. If the wrist needs to be crossed, the exposure can be continued distally over the wrist via a zig-zag incision. For very small ganglion cysts, a small transverse incision usually suffices. As loupe or microscope dissection is carried deeper, branches of the lateral antebrachial cutaneous nerve and the superficial branch of the radial nerve should be protected. Small vessel loops are well suited for this task; retracting the nerves with metal retractors should be avoided. The radial artery should be dissected and mobilized radially; small branches of the radial artery can be tied or cauterized as needed.

If the cyst remains adherent to the radial artery and separation does not seem possible, the remainder of the cystic complex should be removed and the adherent ganglion tissue left on the radial artery. The FCR sheath is opened, and the tendon is mobilized ulnarly. At this step, the surgeon must be aware of the palmar cutaneous nerve, which usually lies ulnarly but can cross the distal aspect of the FCR.[14] Dissection is continued deeper until the carpus is reached (**Figure 4**). The cystic complex should be removed with a cuff of normal capsule. The integrity of the involved ligaments must be protected. As in the dorsal wrist ganglionectomy, a small rongeur can be used to remove the abnormal tissue from the capsule.

Ulnar-Side Ganglionectomy

A longitudinal incision is made just radial to the flexor carpi ulnaris tendon. As dissection proceeds, the ulnar neurovascular bundle is protected and mobilized radially. Loupe or microscope visualization is usually necessary with the dissection. Following that step, the flexor carpi ulnaris tendon should be mobilized ulnarly. In doing so, care is taken not to injure the dorsal sensory branch of the ulnar nerve. If the cyst appears to be originating from the pisotriquetral joint, release of the Guyon canal can provide adequate exposure. Furthermore, after this is done, pisiform excision can be undertaken if there is significant arthritis of the pisotriquetral joint.

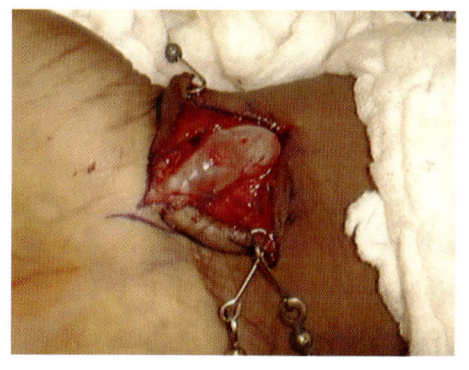

Figure 4 Intraoperative photograph depicts a volar radial-side ganglion cyst located between the radial artery and the flexor carpi radialis tendon.

Wound Closure

Closure for both radial- and ulnar-side volar wrist ganglionectomy is the same as described previously for a dorsal wrist ganglionectomy. A bulky dressing is applied, combined with a volar plaster splint holding the wrist in mild extension. Wrist flexion is avoided because it can lead to a wrist flexion contracture. The suture removal protocol is the same as described previously for the dorsal wrist ganglionectomy.

Arthroscopic Ganglionectomy

The focus of this chapter is on open ganglionectomy techniques. Recent studies have shown, however, that arthroscopic treatment of dorsal wrist ganglions is comparable to open ganglionectomy in terms of recurrence, complication rates, and postoperative function.[15,16]

Retinacular Cyst Excision

Similar to performing a ganglion cystectomy, a proximal brachial tourniquet should be placed. A Bier block, wrist block, or digital block is often sufficient to provide adequate anesthesia.

A transverse volar incision can be made over the ganglion if it lies in the digital or palmar flexion crease. Otherwise, an oblique incision should be centered over

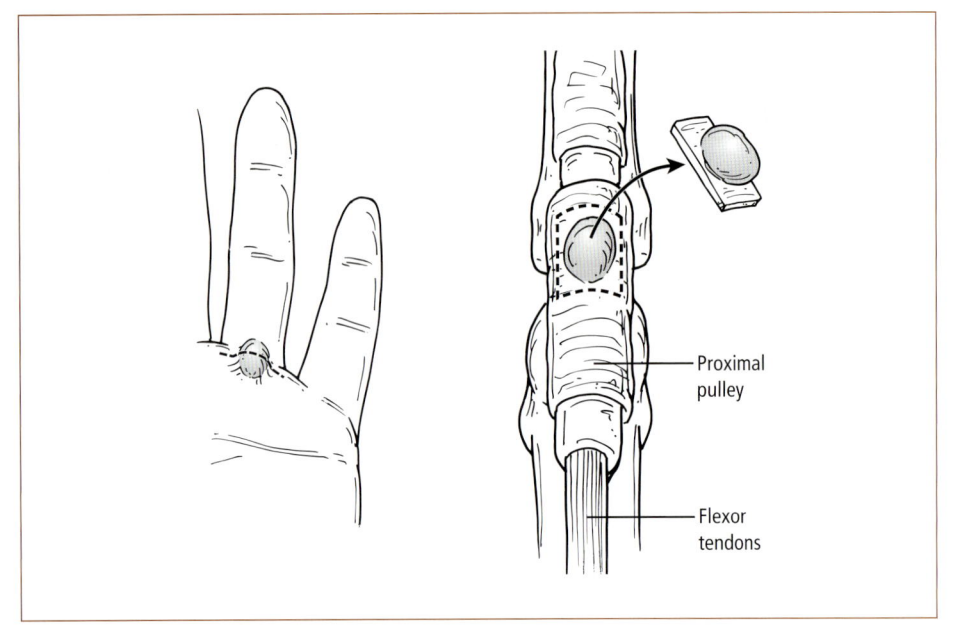

Figure 5 Illustrations show retinacular cysts, which typically are found attached to the tendon sheath. Dissection should be carried out so that the pedicle of the cyst is identified. A cuff of reticular tissue should be excised along with the pedicle, as depicted.

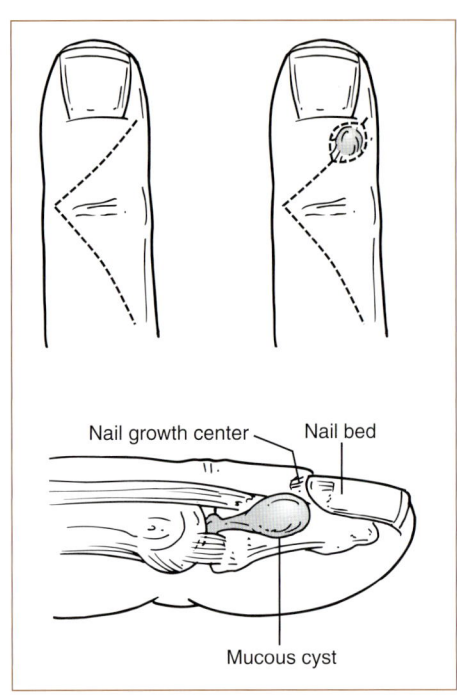

Figure 6 Various incisions can be used for a mucous cyst excision. Illustrations show a dorsal zigzag incision. To minimize the likelihood of a joint contracture, care must be taken to not cross the joint in a linear fashion.

the ganglion and designed such that it can be extended proximally and distally as a Bruner incision. As dissection is continued deeper (loupes should be used), the radial and ulnar digital neurovascular bundles should be protected. The cyst can be sharply excised with a small cuff of tendon sheath. If the ganglion emanates from the A2 pulley, it is often helpful to use a Freer elevator to gently elevate the body of the cyst from the pulley until the pedicle of the ganglion is identified. Only the retinacular tissue immediately adjacent to the pedicle needs to be excised with the cyst. The small defect in the tendon sheath does not require repair (**Figure 5**).

Closure is performed using a nonabsorbable monofilament suture in horizontal mattress technique to approximate the skin edges. A sterile soft dressing can then be applied.

Mucous Cyst Excision

A digital block with a digital tourniquet using a 5/8-in Penrose drain held with a hemostat is often sufficient to provide anesthesia and a bloodless field. Great care must be taken to not apply the Penrose too tightly or for an extended period of time. If these precautions are not taken, a digital nerve neurapraxia can develop.[17]

Various incisions can be used, including H-, T-, L-, or U-shaped patterns (**Figure 6**). Regardless of the technique chosen, the incision should be made over the distal interphalangeal joint and dissection carried down to the joint capsule. Loupe magnification is helpful with this step. Excision should include the origin of the cyst as well as a cuff of the dorsal capsule between the terminal extensor tendon and the collateral ligaments (**Figure 7**). The resultant arthrotomy allows access to the dorsal osteophytes, which can be débrided with a small rongeur. Great care must be taken to avoid injury to the terminal extensor tendon. The terminal extensor should be left in situ to avoid a late mallet deformity.

The use of rotational flaps to close the defect produced by complete excision of the cyst complex is controversial. One study reported that mucous cyst excision with flap coverage can decrease the rate of recurrence from 28% to 8% compared with simple cyst excision.[18] Other authors suggest that excision of the pedicle and the underlying osteophytes is sufficient and advocate leaving the cystic body in situ. This is similar to arthroscopically assisted dorsal wrist ganglionectomy in that only the root of the ganglion and the adjacent dorsal wrist capsule are excised while the cyst body is left. The attenuated dermis covering the cyst will gradually be replaced by normal skin.

Closure is performed using a mattress stitch of nonabsorbable monofilament suture. If a rotation flap is used for closure, care must be taken to close the wound without tension to protect the vascular supply of the flap. Conversely, if the cyst body is left in place, splinting full time with a mallet finger splint for approximately 1 week can aid with soft-tissue healing. During the second postoperative week, the splint can be removed a few times daily for range-of-motion exercises.

Complications

Carpal Ganglionectomy

Wrist stiffness is the most common complication following carpal ganglion excision, seen in about 25% of patients.[2] This often requires occupational therapy to maximize function. Studies have also reported that about 14% of patients report postoperative limited range of motion affecting their ability to perform certain activities.[2] Early (postoperative day 1) range-of-motion exercises and the rapid weaning from splint use can decease the incidence of wrist stiffness. Less common complications include infection, keloid, numbness, neuroma, carpal instability, and scar tenderness.

Dorsal Wrist Ganglionectomy

Care must be taken to avoid injury to the branches of the superficial radial nerve.

Volar Wrist Ganglionectomy

Possible complications include injury to the median nerve or the radial and ulnar arteries (**Figure 8**). More commonly noted complications include scar tenderness and sensory problems over the proximal palm as a result of damage to the palmar cutaneous branch of the median nerve.[2]

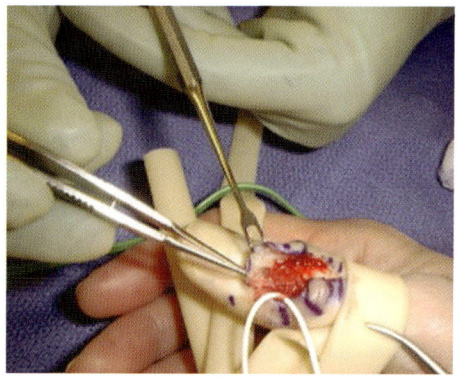

Figure 7 Intraoperative photograph shows a mucous cyst with the pedicle underneath. Once the mucous cyst is excised, the underlying osteophyte should be débrided to minimize the chance of recurrence.

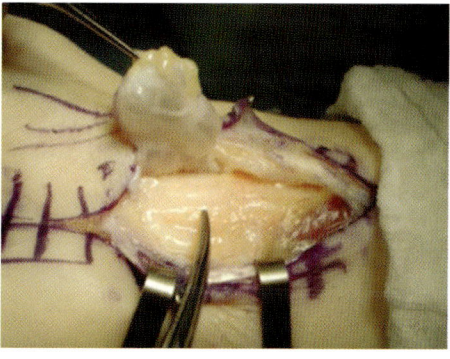

Figure 8 Intraoperative photograph shows a volar radial-side ganglion cyst in a patient with median nerve paresthesias. The cyst was more ulnar than is typically seen and was compressing the median nerve. The cyst was dissected carefully off the median nerve, and the patient's symptoms resolved.

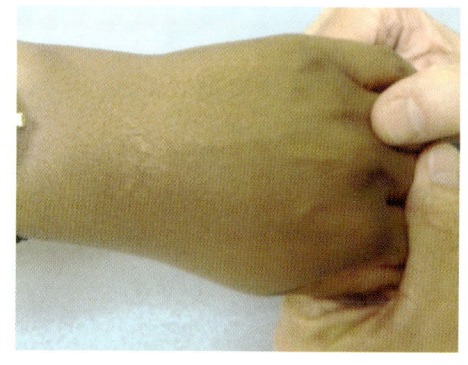

Figure 9 Postoperative photograph shows a well-healed incision following dorsal ganglionectomy.

Digital Mucous Cyst Excision

Mild loss of distal interphalangeal joint extension and nail deformity are the most common complications. Most nail deformities (more than 75%) correct after a year.[8] In addition, iatrogenic injury to the terminal extensor tendon can lead to a mallet deformity. Acceleration of the underlying osteoarthritic process can sometimes occur but is rare.

Postoperative Care and Rehabilitation

For approximately 1 week following surgery, the wrist is placed in slight flexion for a dorsal ganglion cyst excision and in slight extension for a volar ganglion cyst excision. This prevents capsular contracture. Retinacular cysts and mucous cysts can be covered with a soft dressing, which is removed 3 days after surgery (Figure 9).

Pearls

- Although the entire ganglion complex need not be excised, the identification and the excision of the root and the origin of the ganglion is of paramount importance. Failure to remove the root of the ganglion and the adjacent abnormal tissue will likely increase the chance of recurrence.
- Preservation of the cyst by avoiding perforation can help make dissection through superficial and deeper structures easier because the margin is clearer to see.
- Filling the cyst with a dilute solution of methylene blue can help identify the course and the origin of the ganglion.
- After excising the mass, whether to send it to pathology is a matter of surgeon preference. The practice is controversial in routine cases because studies have shown limited cost-effectiveness when the diagnosis is clear both pre- and intraoperatively.[9,19]

References

1. Plate AM, Lee SJ, Steiner G, Posner MA: Tumorlike lesions and benign tumors of the hand and wrist. *J Am Acad Orthop Surg* 2003;11(2):129-141.
2. Gude W, Morelli V: Ganglion cysts of the wrist: Pathophysiology, clinical picture, and management. *Curr Rev Musculoskelet Med* 2008;1(3-4):205-211.
3. Thornburg LE: Ganglions of the hand and wrist. *J Am Acad Orthop Surg* 1999;7(4):231-238.
4. Dias JJ, Dhukaram V, Kumar P: The natural history of untreated dorsal wrist ganglia and patient reported outcome 6 years after intervention. *J Hand Surg Eur Vol* 2007;32(5):502-508.
5. Athanasian EA: Bone and soft-tissue tumors, in Wolfe SW, Hotchkiss R, Pederson W, Kozin S, eds: *Green's Operative Hand Surgery*, ed 6. Philadelphia, PA, Elsevier/Churchill Livingstone, 2011, vol 2, pp 2141-2196.
6. Westbrook AP, Stephen AB, Oni J, Davis TR: Ganglia: The patient's perception. *J Hand Surg Br* 2000;25(6):566-567.
7. Coffey MJ, Rahman MF, Thirkannad SM: Pediatric ganglion cysts of the hand and wrist: An epidemiologic analysis. *Hand (N Y)* 2008;3(4):359-362.
8. Budoff JE: Mucous cysts. *J Hand Surg Am* 2010;35(5):828-830.
9. Gant J, Ruff M, Janz BA: Wrist ganglions. *J Hand Surg Am* 2011;36(3):510-512.
10. Wong AS, Jebson PJ, Murray PM, Trigg SD: The use of routine wrist radiography is not useful in the evaluation of patients with a ganglion cyst of the wrist. *Hand (N Y)* 2007;2(3):117-119.
11. Bajaj S, Pattamapaspong N, Middleton W, Teefey S: Ultrasound of the hand and wrist. *J Hand Surg Am* 2009;34(4):759-760.
12. Lee BJ, Sawyer GA, Dasilva MF: Methylene blue-enhanced arthroscopic resection of dorsal wrist ganglions. *Tech Hand Up Extrem Surg* 2011;15(4):243-246.
13. Elliot D, Mahaffey PJ: The stretched scar: The benefit of prolonged dermal support. *Br J Plast Surg* 1989;42(1):74-78.
14. Nagle DJ, Santiago KJ: Anomalous palmar cutaneous branch of the median nerve in the distal forearm: Case report. *J Hand Surg Am* 2008;33(8):1329-1330.
15. Edwards SG, Johansen JA: Prospective outcomes and associations of wrist ganglion cysts resected arthroscopically. *J Hand Surg Am* 2009;34(3):395-400.
16. Kang L, Akelman E, Weiss AP: Arthroscopic versus open dorsal ganglion excision: A prospective, randomized comparison of rates of recurrence and of residual pain. *J Hand Surg Am* 2008;33(4):471-475.
17. Shaw JA, DeMuth WW, Gillespy AW: Guidelines for the use of digital tourniquets based on physiological pressure measurements. *J Bone Joint Surg Am* 1985;67(7):1086-1090.
18. Crawford RJ, Gupta A, Risitano G, Burke FD: Mucous cyst of the distal interphalangeal joint: Treatment by simple excision or excision and rotation flap. *J Hand Surg Br* 1990;15(1):113-114.
19. Guitton TG, van Leerdam RH, Ring D: Necessity of routine pathological examination after surgical excision of wrist ganglions. *J Hand Surg Am* 2010;35(6):905-908.

Chapter 45
Surgical Excision of Digital Mucous Cysts

Matthew M. Tomaino, MD, MBA

Patient Selection

Indications

In most cases, digital mucous cysts are asymptomatic. They may appear suddenly or develop over a period of months. Grooving of the nail may precede the clinical manifestation of the cyst itself by up to 6 months. Often, osteoarthritis of the small joints is noted at the site of cyst emergence. Intermittent spontaneous discharge of cyst contents can occur, and, in a significant fraction of cases, cysts may disappear spontaneously. Antecedent trauma has been documented in a small minority of cases. As cysts enlarge, pain is an increasingly common symptom (**Figure 1**). Patients are also likely to express concern about the appearance of larger cysts. In short, indications for surgical excision include increasing size, nail grooving, and a painful distal interphalangeal (DIP) joint arthrosis.

Contraindications

There are situations in which surgical excision may be contraindicated. These include inordinate thinning of the skin, after which a higher risk of wound healing complication may occur. In such situations, it may be better to temporize by aspirating the cyst—not as a definitive intervention but to avoid the potential morbidity of a surgical incision. An infection of a mucous cyst is also a contraindication. It is much more advisable to treat the infection and wait for induration to resolve before surgical intervention.

Preoperative Imaging

Plain radiography findings are not diagnostic for digital mucous cysts. In some cases, they will demonstrate a nonspecific soft-tissue density and adjacent bony involvement consistent with osteoarthritic changes. Advanced imaging is not required in most cases, as the diagnosis is most commonly made by history and physical examination. Ultrasonography reveals a rounded or lobulated mass of markedly hypoechoic appearance with smooth, well-defined walls immediately adjacent to the involved synovial compartment. A tapering margin constitutes the "neck" of the cyst. Ultrasonography is faster and better tolerated than MRI, but MRI is less operator dependent. In MRI, homogeneous low-intensity lesions are seen on T1-weighted images, with markedly increased signal intensity and sharp borders on T2-weighted images. Other cyst features include intracystic septa, satellite cysts, cyst pedicles, osteoarthritis of the DIP joint, subungual cysts, and multiple flattened cysts. CT scanning usually demonstrates a well-defined water density mass with normal surrounding soft tissue.[1] Transillumination with a penlight may assist in making the diagnosis and differentiating digital mucous cysts from giant-cell tumors of the tendon sheath.

Procedure

Dermatologic and plastic surgeons have practiced cold-steel surgical excision of digital mucous cysts for several decades. This procedure ranges from simple excision of the cyst to wide, radical excision with possible graft[2] or flap reconstruction. Flaps used for reconstruction have historically been rotation flaps,[3] but rhomboid flaps[4] have been used safely and reliably and may be easier to apply in selected situations. It is key for those caring for these conditions to recognize that these procedures involve opening a direct communication with the DIP joint.

In recent years, excision and débridement of joint osteophytes has been recognized as a necessary adjunct to reduce the risk of recurrence. Some hand surgeons believe that excision and débridement of the marginal osteophyte without removal of the cyst itself may be the best intervention. This results in less postoperative impairment in joint motion and fewer nail deformities because cyst dissection around the germinal matrix potentially may injure the underlying matrix and cause scarring. In general,

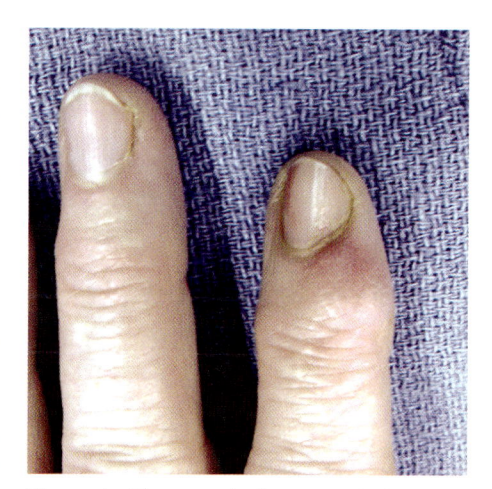

Figure 1 Photograph shows a radial index digital mucous cyst.

more aggressive dissection leads to fewer recurrences and more nail deformities. However, ideally, both the cyst and an osteophyte would be removed; thus, an adequate surgical incision and dissection is advisable.

Overall, significant disagreement exists in the literature regarding optimal treatment approaches, notwithstanding general agreement among hand surgeons. Dermatologists tend to favor nonsurgical treatment, such as multiple needling or aspiration followed by steroid injection. They have reported high success rates and relatively low risks of recurrence.

Hand surgeons have noted success and rare recurrence with osteophyte excision and débridement, but their patient population comprises those for whom other treatments have failed. All of the literature is biased toward the minority of patients who seek medical care for their digital mucous cysts. Asymptomatic cysts and spontaneous regression appear to be common, with several series suggesting that the likelihood of the latter may approximate 50%.

As the aggressiveness of interventions to treat digital mucous cysts increases, the associated costs also increase. Nonsurgical treatments offer the prospect of low cost, low morbidity, and the elimination of disability and time loss related to recovery from surgery. Consequently, a reasonable treatment plan for symptomatic digital mucous cysts may entail initial needling or aspiration and

---

Dr. Tomaino or an immediate family member has received royalties from DePuy and Tornier; is a member of a speakers' bureau or has made paid presentations on behalf of DePuy; and serves as a paid consultant to or is an employee of DePuy.

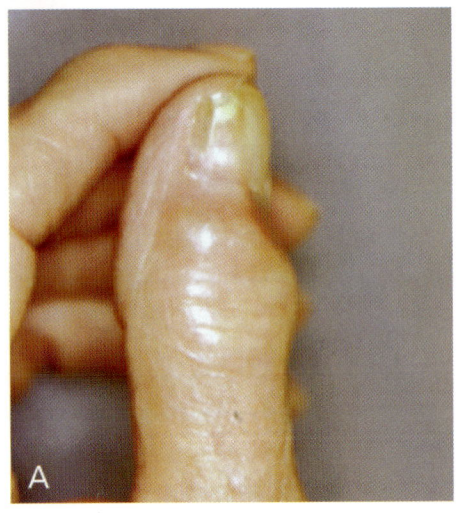

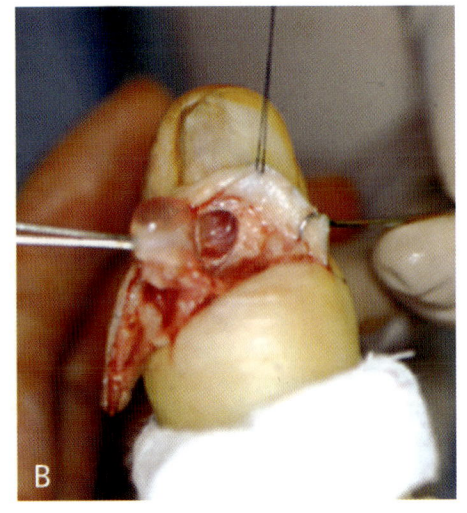

Figure 2 Images depict a digital mucous cyst at the thumb DIP joint. **A,** Preoperative photograph. **B,** Intraoperative photograph.

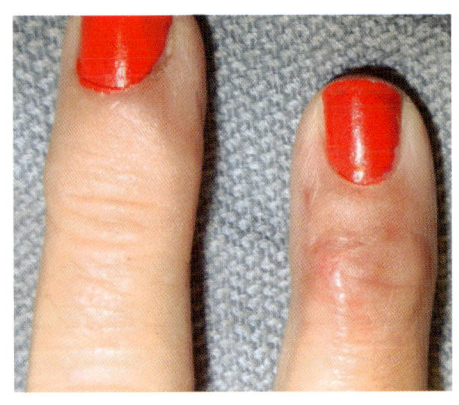

Figure 3 Postoperative photograph of the patient in Figure 1 shows a healed incision 4 weeks after cyst excision.

injection. If these modalities fail repeatedly, patients may be referred to a hand surgeon for more radical surgery but must be forewarned of the increased risk of complications and offered the option of simply deferring treatment of this essentially benign entity.

Surgical Technique
The patient is anesthetized with either a local or a regional anesthetic. The value of the latter is a prolonged period of postoperative pain relief. After insufflation of a tourniquet, subdermal skin flaps are elevated using curvilinear, triradiate, or Bruner-type incisions. The extensor tenson margin is identified, and the cyst is excised (**Figure 2**). It is important to note that the germinal nail matrix begins 1 to 2 mm distal to the extensor enthesis, so care must be taken to avoid injury. If an osteophyte is present, a small rongeur is used to remove it, but care must be taken to avoid injury to the extensor tendon insertion to avoid the development of a mallet deformity.

If an ulcerated skin lesion is removed, a local rotation of skin may be required to afford tension-free wound closure. A compressive dressing is placed, and the wound is checked 3 to 5 days later. Suture removal is delayed for 10 to 14 days. As early as 4 weeks after surgery, wound healing is usually complete (**Figure 3**).

Complications
Digital mucous cysts have a high incidence of recurrence after treatment, typically occurring within 3 months of treatment. Local depigmentation has been reported after steroid injection with triamcinolone. Surgical intervention is associated with many potential complications. Radial or ulnar deviation of the DIP joint with resulting impairment in joint motion can occur. Although some nail deformities may be corrected by surgery, residual nail deformities may persist or be created de novo.[5] Other complications include tendon injury and consequential mallet deformity, superficial infection, DIP joint septic arthritis, increased arthritic symptoms in the joint, and persistent swelling, pain, numbness, and stiffness.

Postoperative Care and Rehabilitation
Little special postoperative care is required as long as wound healing is complete. Sutures should not be removed prematurely. If marginal wound necrosis occurs, this will usually respond to local dressing changes and time.

Pearls
In most cases, digital mucous cysts can be managed nonsurgically. Patients can be reassured of their benign nature. However, if pain, an unsightly appearance, an enlarging cyst, or skin thinning occurs, resection may indeed be indicated. Skillful execution of removal is typically successful and results in high levels of patient satisfaction.[6]

References
1. Drapé JL, Idy-Peretti I, Goettmann S, et al: MR imaging of digital mucoid cysts. *Radiology* 1996;200(2):531-536.
2. Jamnadas-Khoda B, Agarwal R, Harper R, Page RE: Use of Wolfe graft for the treatment of mucous cysts. *J Hand Surg Eur Vol* 2009;34(4):519-521.
3. Blume PA, Moore JC, Novicki DC: Digital mucoid cyst excision by using the bilobed flap technique and arthroplastic resection. *J Foot Ankle Surg* 2005;44(1):44-48.
4. Imran D, Koukkou C, Bainbridge LC: The rhomboid flap: A simple technique to cover the skin defect produced by excision of a mucous cyst of a digit. *J Bone Joint Surg Br* 2003;85(6):860-862.
5. Lin YC, Wu YH, Scher RK: Nail changes and association of osteoarthritis in digital myxoid cyst. *Dermatol Surg* 2008;34(3):364-369.
6. Kasdan ML, Stallings SP, Leis VM, Wolens D: Outcome of surgically treated mucous cysts of the hand. *J Hand Surg Am* 1994;19(3):504-507.

Chapter 46

Surgical Treatment of Basal Joint Arthritis of the Thumb

Edward Diao, MD

Introduction

Arthritis of the basal joint of the thumb is a common debilitating condition; 42% of adult women and 26% of adult men have radiographic evidence of arthritis of this joint. Symptomatic hand osteoarthritis is estimated to occur in 2.4% of all adults, including 26% of women and 13% of men aged 65 years or older;[1,2] radiographic signs of hand osteoarthritis were found in 78% of men and 99% of women in this age group.[3] In a cadaver study, eburnated bone was found in 50% of the female specimens.[4]

Historically, trapezium resection alone or in combination with tissue interposition has been the treatment of symptomatic basal joint arthritis. In the 1970s, Eaton and Littler[5] described the use of the flexor carpi radialis (FCR) tendon to reconstruct the volar beak ligament of the symptomatic hypermobile trapeziometacarpal (TMC) joint. This procedure appeared to work best for symptomatic basal joints without significant arthritis (Eaton stage I). In 1987, Carroll[6] advocated fashioning the FCR tendon into a ball, or "anchovy," to replace the excised trapezium as part of his reconstruction. Alternative procedures using hemiresection of the trapezium and adaptations of this original FCR technique also have been described by Eaton et al.[7]

Based on the previous work of Eaton and Littler,[5] Burton[8] described ligament reconstruction tendon interposition (LRTI) arthroplasty in the 1980s and reported long-term follow-up in 1995.[9] In Burton's method, the surgeon harvests half the FCR and places drill holes first at the center of the articular surface of the thumb metacarpal base and then at the dorsal metaphysis of the metacarpal, approximately 1 cm proximal to the articular surface. These drill holes are connected to form a bone tunnel through which the free end of the FCR is passed in an antegrade direction to support the base of the thumb metacarpal. The surgeon then brings the free end or tail of the tendon around from the dorsal exit of the bone tunnel back under the articular surface and sutures it to itself, providing further support for the base of the thumb metacarpal. The remaining tendon is fabricated to form an interposition much like Carroll's "anchovy." It is then sutured together and placed in the arthroplasty space resulting after trapezium resection.

In the early 1980s, Thompson[10] described a technique for reconstruction of the arthritic basal joint using a bone tunnel similar to that used in LRTI arthroplasty in the metacarpal base. Thompson's and Burton's methods can be distinguished by differences in the tendon graft; in Thompson's technique, the donor is the abductor pollicis longus (APL) tendon; in Burton's, it is the FCR. Thompson's technique requires the surgeon to harvest and detach half the APL at the musculotendinous junction, leaving its insertion at the dorsal base of the thumb metacarpal intact. Using the same two bone holes and creating a bone tunnel similar to that in the LRTI procedure, the surgeon passes the free end of the APL retrograde through the dorsal metacarpal hole to emerge from the articular surface hole. At this point, Thompson devises an oblique bone tunnel from the trapezial facet of the proximal index metacarpal, exiting in a dorsal-ulnar orientation from the dorsum of the index metacarpal. The APL tendon passes through the second bone tunnel and is woven into the extensor carpi radialis brevis (ECRB) tendon for stability. This technique was first devised as a means to salvage failed reconstructions with silicone implants, but subsequently it became a primary procedure for the treatment of osteoarthritis.

Part of the appeal of this procedure is the ability to directly provide tension in the ligament reconstruction by applying tension on the free end of the APL tendon graft that emerges from the dorsum of the index metacarpal. Tension can be transmitted through the weave to the ECRB and secured with sutures.

Since 1989, I have been using a variation of Thompson's APL suspensionplasty.[11] In this modification, the harvesting of the APL and the creation of the bone tunnel in the thumb metacarpal follow the methods described. The variation lies in the index metacarpal bone tunnel. Instead of creating this tunnel obliquely at the original trapezial/first metacarpal facet joint in the proximal portion of the index metacarpal, a bone hole is made in the palmar portion of the metaphyseal-diaphyseal junction of the index metacarpal. The drill or awl is then directed dorsally, allowing it to emerge from the dorsum of the proximal index metacarpal. This variation results in a more desirable placement of the bone tunnel, with stronger cortical bone at the tunnel's borders and, most importantly, a more distal suspension point for the APL ligament reconstruction. The APL is anchored through a tendon weave with the ECRB.

Patient Selection

As in any surgical procedure, patient selection is important. Candidates for this surgery include patients who have been diagnosed with Eaton stage II, III, or IV basal joint arthritis and in whom symptoms have not been relieved by nonsurgical management with splints, NSAIDs, cortisone injections, or activity modifications.

Preoperative Imaging

Radiographic staging is a useful tool in preoperative assessment and surgical planning. The radiographic stage correlates poorly with the patient's symptoms, however; essentially, the sole indication for surgical reconstruction of the arthritic basal joint is pain.[9] Furthermore, plain radiographs accurately predict involvement of the scaphotrapezial (ST) joint only two thirds of the time.[12] If the surgeon does different procedures for stage III and IV disease, final determination of which procedure to use should be reserved until intraoperative assessment of

Dr. Diao or an immediate family member is a member of a speakers' bureau or has made paid presentations on behalf of SBI, Stryker, and Auxilium; has received research or institutional support from the National Institutes of Health (NIAMS and NICHD); and serves as a board member, owner, officer, or committee member of the American Society for Surgery of the Hand.

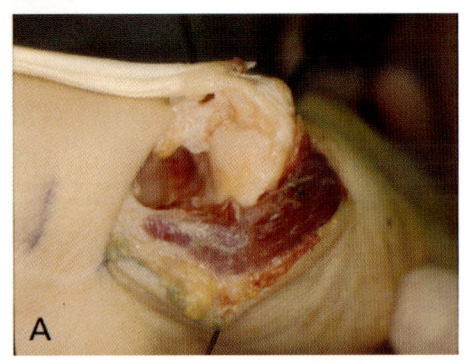

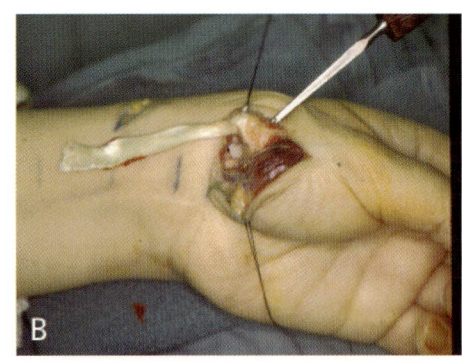

Figure 1 Intraoperative photographs show initial steps in abductor pollicis longus (APL) suspensionplasty. **A,** The base of the thumb metacarpal is seen with the APL having been separated at its musculotendinous junction but remaining attached to its insertion on the dorsal base of the thumb metacarpal. **B,** The thumb metacarpal is shown with an elevator within the bone tunnel through which the APL will be passed in a dorsal-to-palmar direction.

the ST joint is made by arthrotomy and direct visualization and palpation with a blunt instrument such as a dental probe.

Procedure
Surgical Technique: APL Suspensionplasty

The thumb is exposed during surgery using a Wagner incision. In this approach, the junction of the glabrous skin along the radial border of the thumb metacarpal marks the line of the distal incision. The incision should be curved so that at its most proximal point, it lies transversely over the FCR tendon. Skin and subcutaneous tissue flaps are raised, and branches of the radial sensory nerve should be easily identifiable and preserved. Skin retraction sutures of 3-0 silk are placed on either side of the incision. The dorsal flap is elevated, and a dorsal dissection is performed to expose the extensor mechanism on the dorsum of the thumb metacarpal. The APL insertion is exposed at the base of the thumb metacarpal, and distally the extensor pollicis brevis (EPB) and extensor pollicis longus (EPL) are identified. A subperiosteal dissection between the EPL and EPB is made approximately 1 cm distal to the insertion of the APL.

The thenar muscles are reflected off the radial aspect of the thumb metacarpal. Generally, there is an accessory slip of the APL that inserts into the thenar muscles. The accessory APL and thenar muscles can be reflected in continuity and repositioned at the end of the procedure, or the surgeon can detach the accessory APL from its insertion on the thenar muscles, to be repaired later. After this exposure, the ST and TMC joints can be exposed with gentle thumb distraction. The trapezium bone is exposed using subperiosteal dissection. It is desirable to remove the trapezium piecemeal with an osteotome, dividing the trapezium longitudinally in line with the fibers of the FCR, which lies deep to the trapezium. The trapezium can then be split transversely and the four quadrants of bone removed. The trapezium in an arthritic thumb is generally deformed with some sclerosis at the TMC joint; if a medial osteophyte is present, it should be removed completely from the surrounding joint capsule with a rongeur and/or a curet.

Once the trapezium has been removed completely, the base of the thumb metacarpal should be exposed to facilitate formation of the bone tunnel (**Figure 1, A**). A Carroll elevator is helpful to position the thumb metacarpal in the wound by elevating the proximal metacarpal and exposing the articular surface. The center of the articular surface is pierced with a bone awl, a small Kirschner wire (K-wire), or a drill. A second hole is made in the dorsum of the metacarpal approximately 1 cm distal to the articular surface and perpendicular to the plane of the thumbnail. These holes are expanded perpendicular to the surface of the bone so the two holes will meet in the medullary canal of the metacarpal. Using a small curet, these holes are carefully expanded so that an oblique bone tunnel results (**Figure 1, B**). Caution should be exercised not to fracture the bone dorsal to these bone holes because this would significantly compromise the stability of the reconstructed ligament. Once the bone tunnels are created, the APL can be harvested. Originally, this was performed through a separate incision near the musculotendinous junction; the APL can, however, be harvested with a large tendon stripper similar to those used in reconstructive knee surgery. The surgeon places the tendon stripper around the APL, taking care upon lifting the proximal skin flap that the radial sensory nerves are kept away from the tendon stripper. Then, using a rotating action while holding the tendon stripper, the APL can be divided at its musculotendinous junction. The distally based tendon is delivered into the Wagner incision. Normally, some trimming of the free end of the tendon graft is required to remove residual muscle.

The APL is then passed retrograde first through the dorsal metacarpal hole, then through the tunnel, to emerge from the articular surface hole. This can be done using a tendon-passing instrument or a small-gauge stainless wire tied in a loop around the free end to prevent fraying the tendon as it is passed through the bone tunnel, as shown in **Figure 2, A and B,** and **Figure 3**.

The ST joint should be inspected. If there is significant wear in the distal scaphoid or proximal trapezoid, a curet should be used to expand the involved area, removing any abnormal cartilage and the subchondral bone. The base of the index metacarpal is exposed by retracting the radial flap containing the thenar muscles. The index metacarpal base should be palpated by the surgeon as well as visualized. The junction of the metaphysis is flared, whereas the diaphysis is more cylindrical in shape. At the junction of the metaphysis and diaphysis, the surgeon should create a palmar bone hole. The bone is relatively soft and will easily accept a bone awl under manual pressure. The awl is then passed directly dorsally to create a bone tunnel, as shown in **Figure 2, C**. The end of the awl will be palpable subcutaneously on the dorsum of the hand. A 2-cm longitudinal incision is made over the awl, and the subcutaneous tissue is dissected to expose it.

The index metacarpal bone tunnel is expanded using handheld instruments (such as a curet or gouge) of a caliber large enough to accept the tendon graft. The tendon graft is then passed in a palmar-to-dorsal direction through the index metacarpal.

At this point, the efficacy of the ligament reconstruction can be assessed. With one hand, the surgeon applies tension to the tendon graft, maintaining manual tension on the free end of the APL now emerging from the dorsum of the hand. With his or her free hand, the surgeon can assess the stability of the thumb metacarpal by performing a displacement ma-

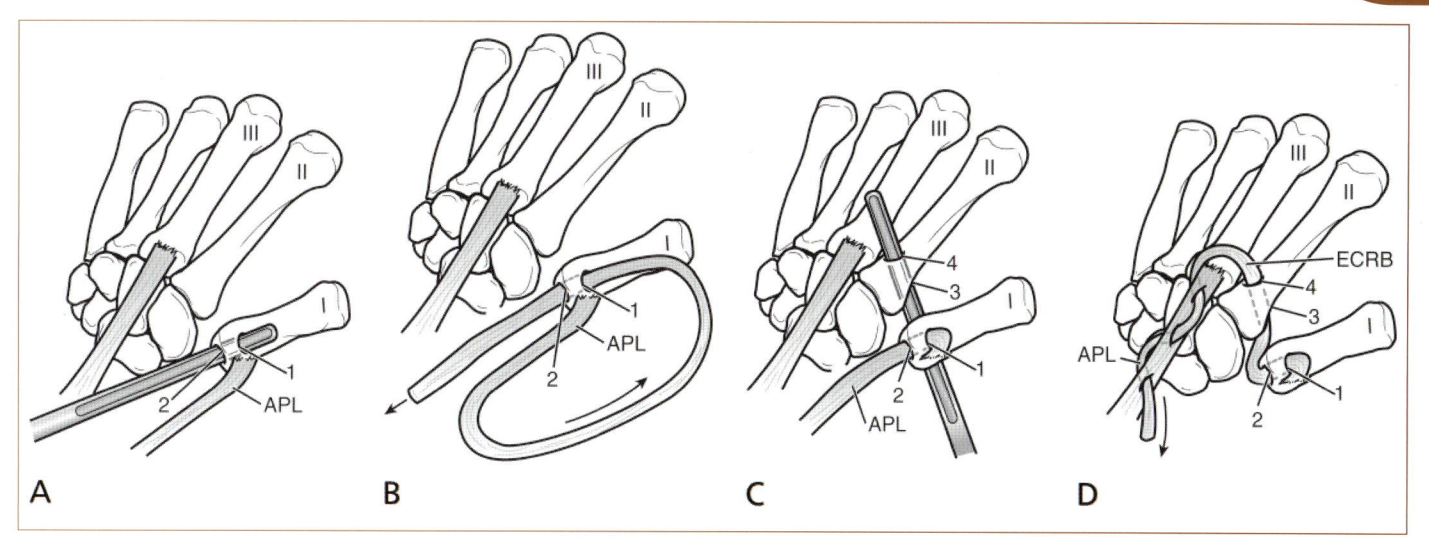

Chapter 46: Surgical Treatment of Basal Joint Arthritis of the Thumb

Figure 2 Illustrations demonstrate the surgical technique for abductor pollicis longus (APL) suspensionplasty. **A,** Creation of a bone tunnel in the thumb metacarpal. The bone tunnel is carefully created to connect hole 2, which is located in the articular center of the metacarpal base, and hole 1, which is located at the dorsal surface of the proximal metacarpal metaphysis 1 cm distal to the articular surface. **B,** After division of the APL at the proximal musculotendinous junction, the free end of the APL tendon is passed through the bone tunnel from hole 1 to hole 2. **C,** A bone tunnel is created from palmar (3) to dorsal (4) in the index metacarpal at the metaphyseal-diaphyseal junction. **D,** The APL tendon is passed through both bone tunnels at the thumb and index metacarpal (from 1 through 2 and from 3 through 4), emerging dorsally from the index metacarpal tunnel with a weave through the extensor carpi radialis brevis (ECRB) tendon to anchor the ligament reconstruction and tension the tendon transfer. I = thumb metacarpal, II = index finger metacarpal, III = long finger metacarpal.

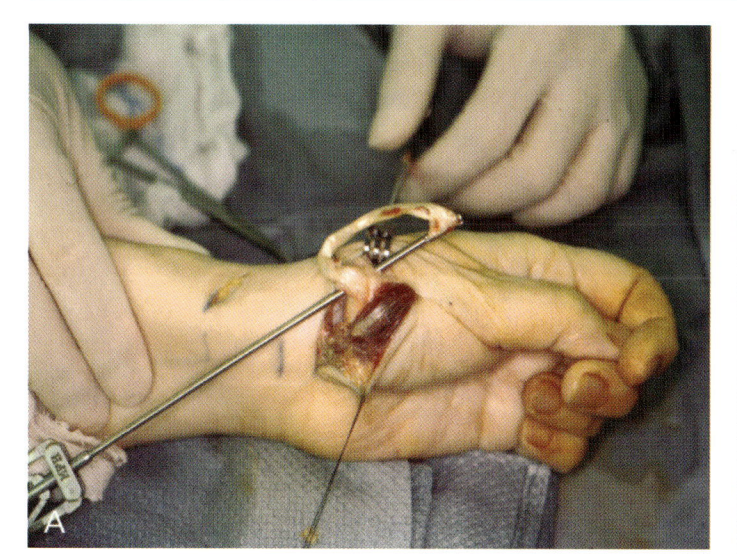

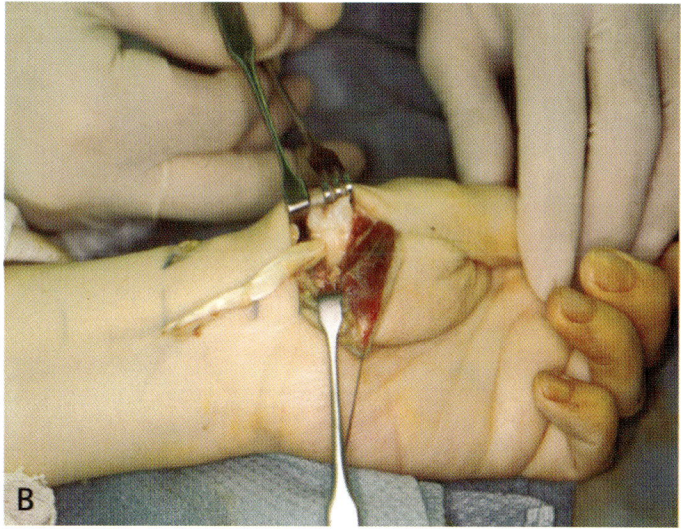

Figure 3 Intraoperative photographs show passage of the graft in APL suspensionplasty. **A,** A tendon retriever is passed in a palmar-to-dorsal direction through the bone tunnel at the thumb metacarpal base. The instrument is grasping the free end of the APL after it has been separated from the muscle more proximally. **B,** Once the APL has been passed through the thumb metacarpal base bone tunnel in a dorsal-to-palmar direction, the APL serves as a tendon transfer/ligament reconstruction, emerging from the articular base of the thumb metacarpal. This can now be used to position the base of the thumb metacarpal in terms of a "suspensionplasty."

neuver. Resistance to proximal migration should be felt when tension is placed on the free end of the APL tendon (**Figure 4**).

Once the efficacy of the ligament reconstruction is ascertained, the APL is fixed to the dorsum of the hand. Scissor dissection with division of some transverse fascial fibers will expose the ECRB just ulnar to the dorsal bone tunnel in the index metacarpal. The extensor carpi radialis longus inserts on the radial aspect of the index metacarpal, whereas the ECRB inserts at the radial aspect and dorsum of the third metacarpal.[13]

Using a tendon weaver, the ECRB is pierced and the free end of the APL is passed through the hole. With tension on the end of the APL, the juncture is secured with a 4-0 nonabsorbable synthetic suture. This process should be done three times, with sutures placed at each juncture, as seen in **Figure 2, D**. After the three tendon weaves have been performed, any remnant of the APL should be removed. The thumb is tested again to ensure that it can resist migration in all directions. When the full APL is used in ligament reconstruction, no tendon interposition is necessary.

In my earlier cases, when only half the APL was used, a transfixing 0.045-in K-wire was used to hold the thumb metacarpal in a distracted position. In the new procedure using the entire APL, no transfixing pin is used.

The thenar muscles are reattached using 4-0 Vicryl suture (Ethicon). If the accessory APL has been detached from the thenar musculature, this can be repaired with the same suture. The skin is closed with 5-0 plain absorbable suture, and sterile dressings are applied with a

© 2013 American Academy of Orthopaedic Surgeons

Section 3: Hand and Wrist

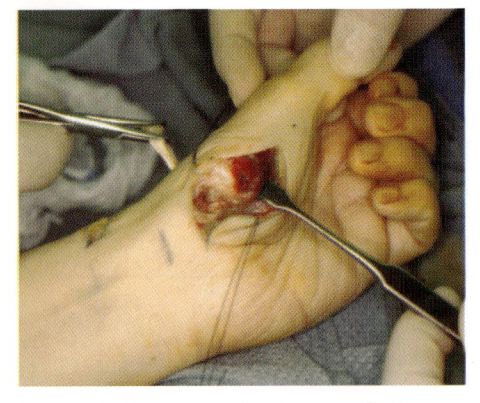

Figure 4 Intraoperative photograph shows assessment of the ligamentous reconstruction in APL suspensionplasty. The APL has been passed through the second bone tunnel, which is a palmar-to-dorsal transverse bone tunnel at the metaphyseal-diaphyseal junction of the proximal index metacarpal. The tendon is being tensioned by the clamp on the upper left. By applying this tension, the thumb is suspended into a position that maintains the space that the trapezium had once occupied and maintains overall thumb ray length.

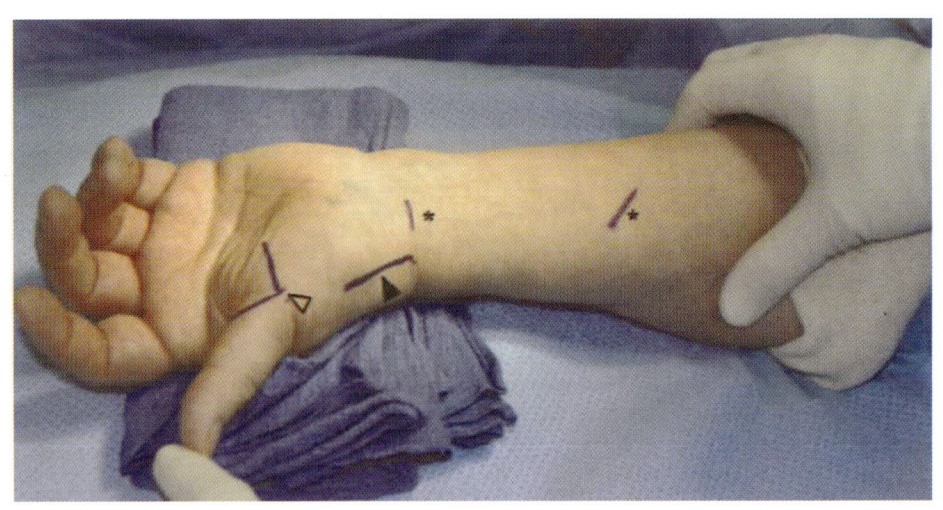

Figure 5 Photograph shows skin markings for surgical incisions for ligament reconstruction tendon interposition (LRTI) arthroplasty. A straight longitudinal incision in the interval between the volar glabrous and dorsal nonglabrous skin is indicated by the solid arrowhead. A zigzag incision over the thumb metacarpophalangeal joint (open arrowhead) facilitates exposure to perform a volar capsulodesis if adaptive hyperextension is present. Incisions at the radial wrist crease and proximally at the musculotendinous junction of the flexor carpi radialis (FCR) (asterisks) facilitate the harvest of the FCR tendon.

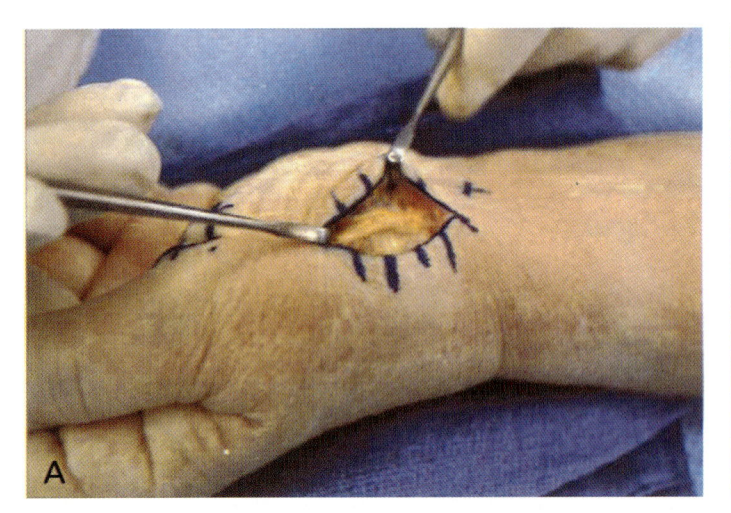

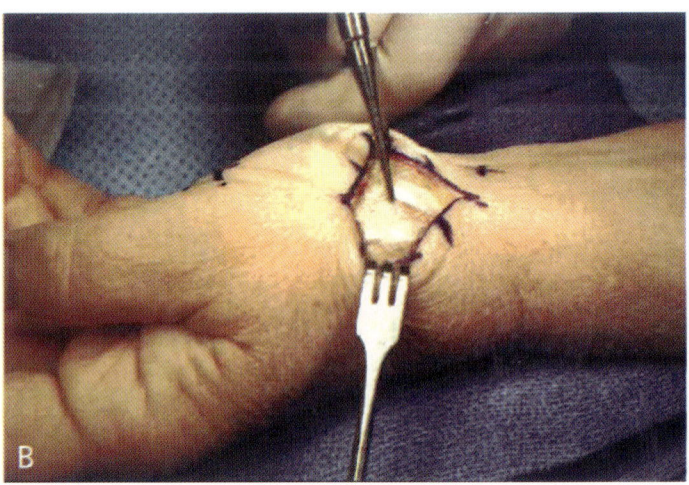

Figure 6 Intraoperative photographs show initial steps in LRTI arthroplasty. **A,** The distal branch of the superficial branch of the radial sensory nerve is seen in the wound. **B,** The plane between the extensor pollicis longus (EPL) and extensor pollicis brevis (EPB) tendons is developed to expose the underlying capsule of the trapeziometacarpal (TMC) joint. The probe is placed in the TMC joint; the EPB is seen volarly adjacent to the probe, and the EPL is seen dorsal to the probe.

radial gutter splint. With experience, the procedure can be performed in less than 1 hour of tourniquet time under regional or general anesthesia. Postoperative management includes 2 to 4 weeks of immobilization in the postoperative dressing, allowing some interphalangeal joint motion. After the initial dressing and splint are removed, a removable long opponens splint is provided, and the patient is given active range-of-motion exercises, with full abduction allowed as tolerated. After 2 months of postoperative care, grip strengthening exercises are initiated.

Surgical Technique: LRTI Arthroplasty

In their original description of the LRTI procedure, Burton and Pellegrini used a triradiate incision to expose the trapezium and TMC joint. I prefer to use a Wagner incision interval between the volar glabrous and dorsal nonglabrous skin (**Figure 5**). This approach obviates the need for elevating the thenar musculature. A branch of the superficial branch of the radial sensory nerve invariably crosses the surgical field (**Figure 6, A**), and it should be identified, mobilized, and carefully retracted, taking care to avoid traction on the nerve. The plane between the EPL and EPB tendons is developed to expose the underlying capsule of the TMC joint and periosteum of the trapezium (**Figure 6, B**).

The base of the thumb metacarpal and the TMC joints are identified. A longitudinal arthrotomy is made perpendicular to the long axis of the TMC joint and parallel to the long axis of the trapezium at approximately its midline. The incision is carried proximally across the ST joint. The periosteum is elevated circumferentially using a scalpel and periosteal eleva-

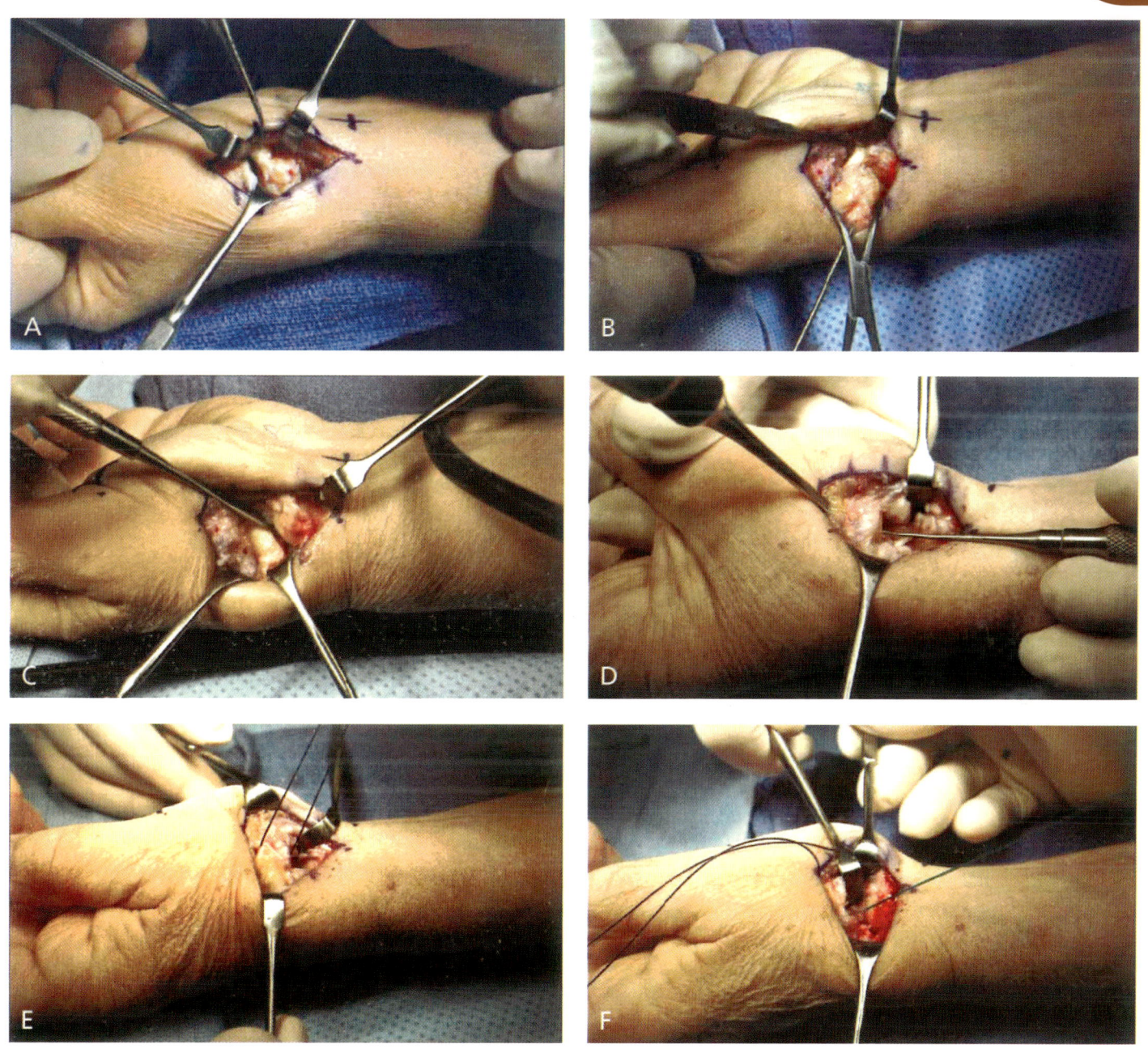

Chapter 46: Surgical Treatment of Basal Joint Arthritis of the Thumb

Figure 7 Intraoperative photographs show steps in LRTI arthroplasty. **A,** Trapezium exposure. The trapezium is exposed after the capsule is incised and the periosteum is elevated. The probe demonstrates a large osteophyte off the trapezium. **B,** The trapezium is removed in toto. The probe marks the underlying flexor carpi radialis (FCR) tendon, which should be protected. A Kirschner wire has been placed into the trapezium to function as a joystick for manipulation to liberate this bone from its soft-tissue attachments. **C,** Visualization of the scaphotrapezial (ST) joint. The Freer elevator is placed in the ST joint; if it is found to be arthritic, the articulating facet of the trapezoid is removed. **D,** Creation of the oblique tunnel for ligament reconstruction. A gouge is seen here with an entry point about 1 cm distal to the metacarpal base and perpendicular to the thumbnail. The exit point is through the base of the thumb metacarpal just volar to the center point of the articular surface, demonstrated by the probe. **E,** Preparation for FCR graft passage. After the oblique hole is created through the base of the thumb metacarpal, a Prolene suture (Ethicon) is placed through the hole for later passage of the FCR. **F,** Capsular suture passage for interposition. A double-armed 3-0 Ethibond suture (Ethicon) is placed in the capsule at the base of the arthroplasty space created by the trapeziectomy. This will later be used to secure the interposed FCR tendon.

tor (**Figure 7, A**). Frequently, peripheral osteophytes of the metacarpal base and a large medial osteophyte of the trapezium are present; these should be removed with a rongeur and/or curets before or during the trapeziectomy. Trapezial resection should be performed piecemeal. Care must be taken to avoid injury to the underlying FCR tendon, which is to be used later in the procedure for the ligament reconstruction (**Figure 7, B**). The FCR tendon runs obliquely from ulnar to radial just underneath the volar cortex of the trapezium. The ST is visualized. If it is arthritic, an approximately 0.4-cm wafer of the articulating facet of the trapezoid is removed with a rongeur or sagittal saw (**Figure 7, C**).

An oblique tunnel is made in the base of the thumb metacarpal using handheld gouges, a high-speed burr, or a drill. Gouges are preferred because they provide excellent control and avoid the possibility of wrapping up adjacent tissue. The hole is begun approximately 1 cm distal to the articular surface of the metacarpal base, perpendicular to the plane of the thumbnail. The tunnel is directed toward the base of the thumb metacarpal, just volar to the center point of the articular surface (**Figure 7, D**). It is better to err on the side of the exit point of the tunnel being more volar than dorsal both because it is

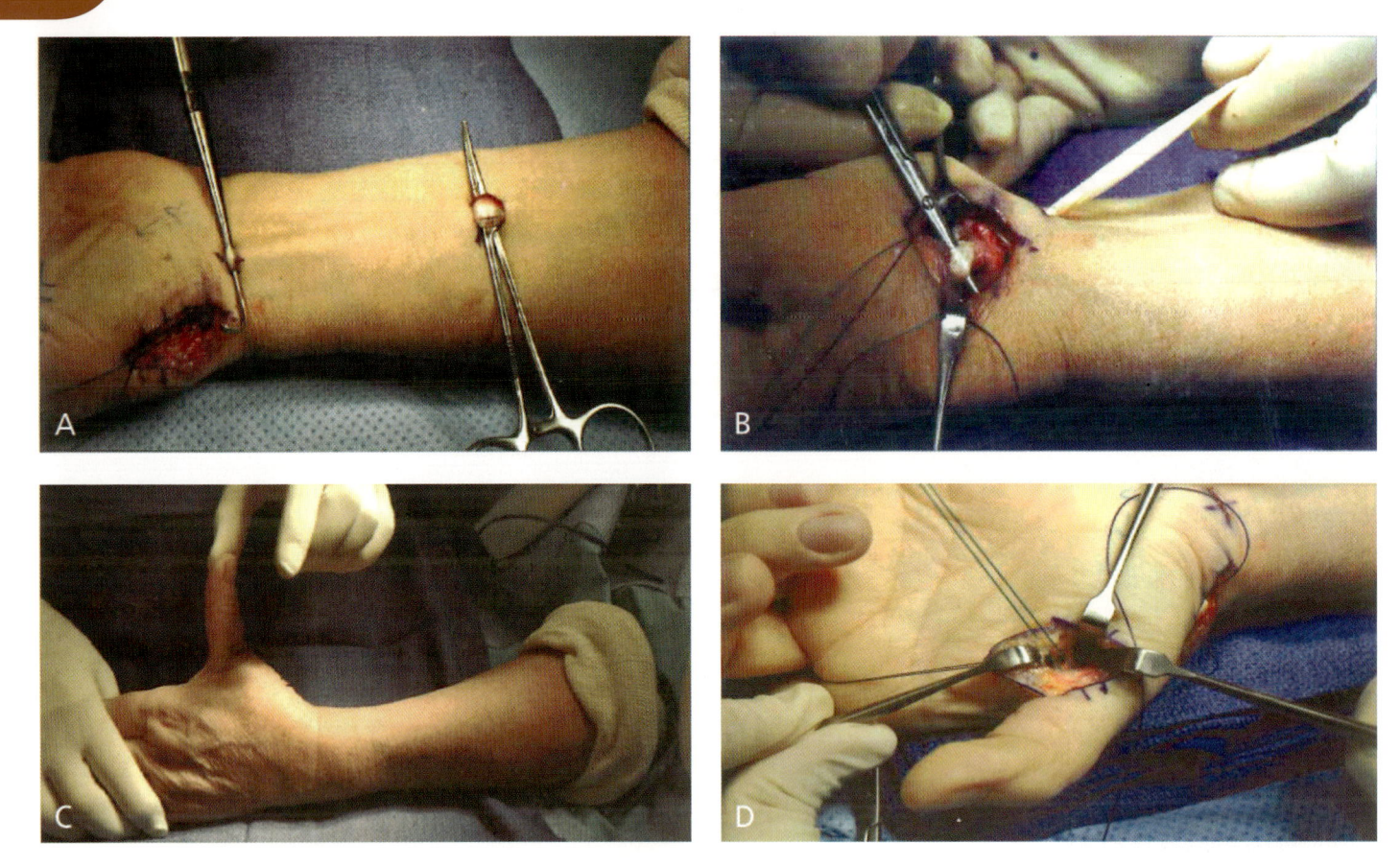

Figure 8 Intraoperative photographs show tendon harvest and delivery and capsulodesis in LRTI arthroplasty. **A,** Flexor carpi radialis (FCR) tendon harvest. The FCR tendon is harvested by incising its sheath and mobilizing the tendon at the distal and proximal incisions. A hemostat or retractor is placed completely around the tendon at both locations. **B,** Delivery of the FCR tendon. A hemostat or Littler scissors are used to withdraw the tendon into the arthroplasty space. **C,** Adaptive hyperextension of the metacarpophalangeal (MP) joint. If extreme hyperextension is present, I advocate a volar capsulodesis or arthrodesis if arthrosis is present. **D,** Volar capsulodesis of the MP joint. The proximal edge of the volar plate is recessed proximally in the retrocondylar fossa of the metacarpal head using a suture anchor with nonabsorbable suture, shown in green.

more physiologic and because it diminishes the likelihood of cracking the bony bridge between the entry and exit point of the hole. The gouges allow progressive enlargement of the hole. If half of the FCR is used for the reconstruction, the medium gouge sometimes makes a hole that is sufficiently large to accommodate the tendon slip. If the entire FCR is used, the hole must be enlarged with the large gouge. As the procedure was initially described, half the width of the tendon was used for reconstruction. Over time, the trend shifted to using the entire tendon, which provides more tissue to interpose in the arthroplasty space.

A 28-gauge stainless steel wire or a 0 Prolene suture (Ethicon) is placed through the hole for later passage of the tendon slip (**Figure 7, E**). A double-armed 3-0 braided synthetic (eg, Ethibond [Ethicon]) figure-of-8 suture is placed in the capsule or other soft tissue at the base of the arthroplasty space created by the trapeziectomy (**Figure 7, F**). This will be used to secure the interposed tendon.

The FCR tendon can be harvested through two small transverse incisions (**Figure 5**). The distal incision is at the level of the distal wrist crease, and the proximal incision is over the musculotendinous junction in the mid forearm. One half of the FCR tendon or the entire tendon is harvested by incising the sheath and mobilizing it in the distal incision. A hemostat is placed deep to the tendon. The proximal incision is made over the musculotendinous junction where the FCR is dissected circumferentially and divided (**Figure 8, A**). The FCR tendon is delivered into the distal wound by putting traction on the tendon. The FCR is then identified in the base of the arthroplasty space, and a hemostat is placed around it. The hemostat is used to withdraw the tendon into the arthroplasty space (**Figure 8, B**).

If hyperextension of the metacarpophalangeal (MP) joint is present, it is addressed at this point in the procedure (**Figure 8, C**). If the MP joint is not arthritic, a volar capsulodesis is preferred, in which the proximal edge of the volar plate is recessed proximally in the retrocondylar fossa, where it is secured with a 2-0 Ethibond suture with or without bone anchor (**Figure 8, D**). If the joint is arthritic, arthrodesis is done with a K-wire, screw, or tension-band technique.

A 0.045-in K-wire is placed down the medullary canal of the metacarpal. It can be started in the metacarpal head and used to keep the MP joint flexed at the end of the procedure, particularly if a volar capsulodesis of the MP joint is done in combination with the basal joint arthroplasty. Alternatively, the K-wire can be placed from the midshaft of the metacarpal obliquely down the medullary canal, where it is left until the end of the procedure when it is used for fixation of the metacarpal to the scaphoid (**Figure 9, A**). Some surgeons prefer not to use K-wire fixation of the joint. The advantage of a pin is primarily to ensure that the metacarpal is extended and abducted, which may not be as predictable with a splint or cast.

The previously placed 28-gauge stainless steel wire or 0 Prolene suture is secured to the cut end of the tendon. The tendon is drawn through the hole in the metacarpal base from proximal to distal, emerging on the dorsum of the meta-

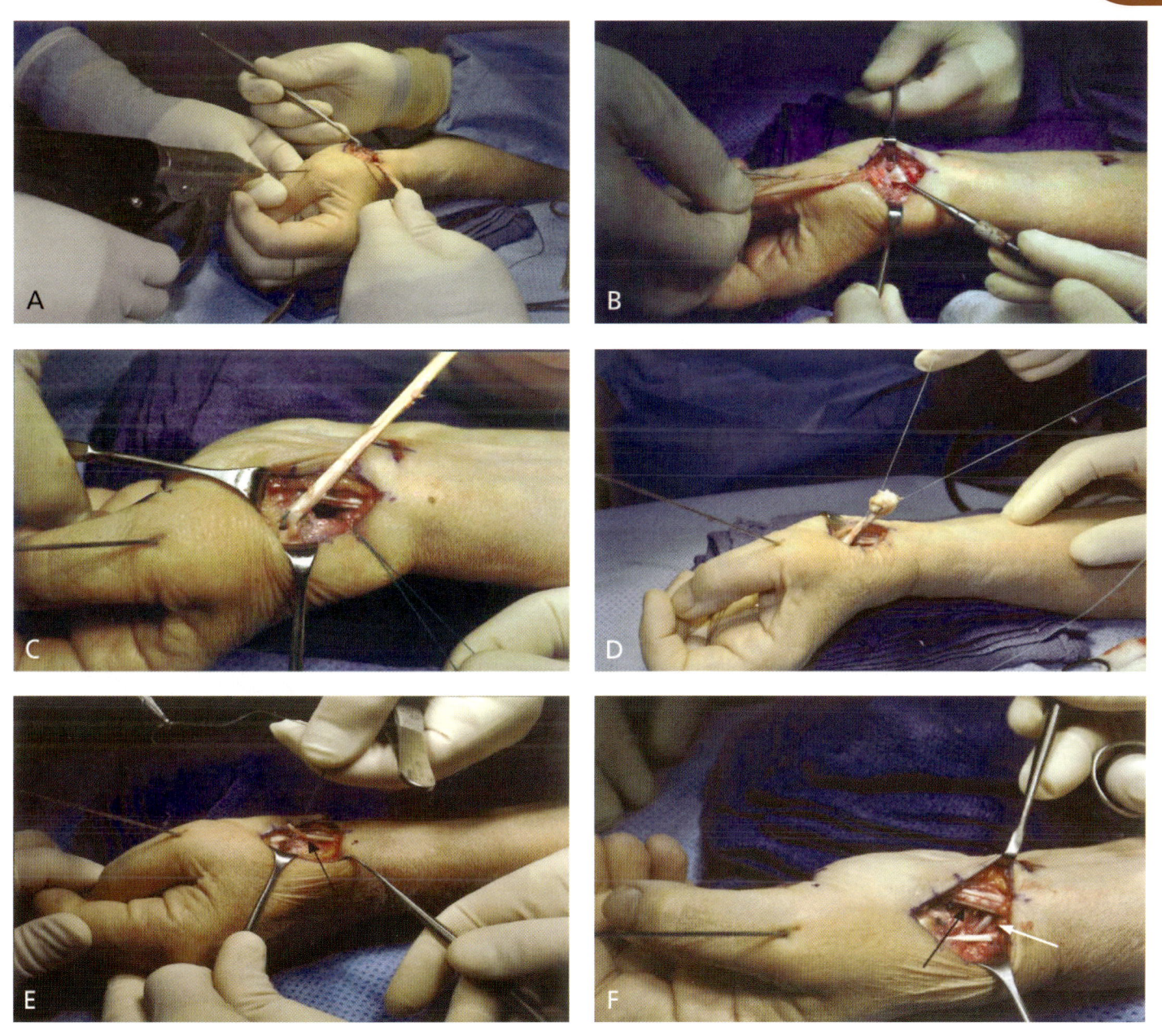

Chapter 46: Surgical Treatment of Basal Joint Arthritis of the Thumb

Figure 9 Intraoperative photographs show final steps in LRTI arthroplasty. **A,** A 0.045-in Kirschner wire is placed through the metacarpal head and down the medullary canal to position the metacarpal. This wire can be left in place until the end of the procedure, when it is used for fixation of the metacarpal to the scaphoid. **B,** Passage of the flexor carpi radialis (FCR) tendon. The FCR tendon is drawn through the hole in the metacarpal base from proximal to distal, emerging on the dorsum of the metacarpal. The probe is placed in the arthroplasty space. **C,** Thumb metacarpal positioning. The metacarpal is positioned in extension and abduction with traction placed on the FCR. The tension of the reconstruction is fixed by suturing the FCR to the adjacent periosteum with two mattress or figure-of-8 nonabsorbable sutures. **D,** Interposition of the FCR tendon into the arthroplasty space. The "anchovy" created is shuttled, interposed, and secured into the arthroplasty space with the previously placed double-armed suture. **E,** The EPB tendon is divided distally (arrow), and the cut end is transferred and sutured to the periosteum at the base of the metacarpal. **F,** The transferred EPB is shown (black arrow), along with the terminal branch of the radial artery seen within the snuffbox (white arrow).

carpal (Figure 9, B). The metacarpal is positioned in extension and abduction, and traction is placed on the FCR tendon slip. The metacarpal is placed in its normal anatomic position when the tension of the reconstruction is set and the tendon is sutured to the adjacent periosteum with two mattress or figure-of-8 sutures of 3-0 braided synthetic suture (Figure 9, C). The remainder of the graft is rolled around a hemostat and sutured at each end with absorbable sutures to keep it from unraveling. This creates an "anchovy," which is interposed into the arthroplasty space and secured with the previously placed double-armed Ethibond suture over which the interposition is slid into the arthroplasty space (Figure 9, D). The previously placed K-wire is driven into the scaphoid or, occasionally, the trapezoid, and the position is checked with the image intensifier. The capsule is closed over the graft. The APL tendon insertion with a mattress suture will increase abduction force. The EPB tendon is divided distally, and the cut end is sutured to the periosteum at the base of the metacarpal (Figure 9, E and F). The skin is sutured with a 5-0 absorbable suture that obviates the need to change the cast and remove sutures at 2 weeks postoperatively. A hand dressing and thumb spica cast are applied (Figure 10).

Surgical Technique: Thumb TMC Arthroscopy

The preferred technique for thumb TMC arthroscopy has been described by Culp and Rekant.[14] Either regional or general

© 2013 American Academy of Orthopaedic Surgeons

Section 3: Hand and Wrist

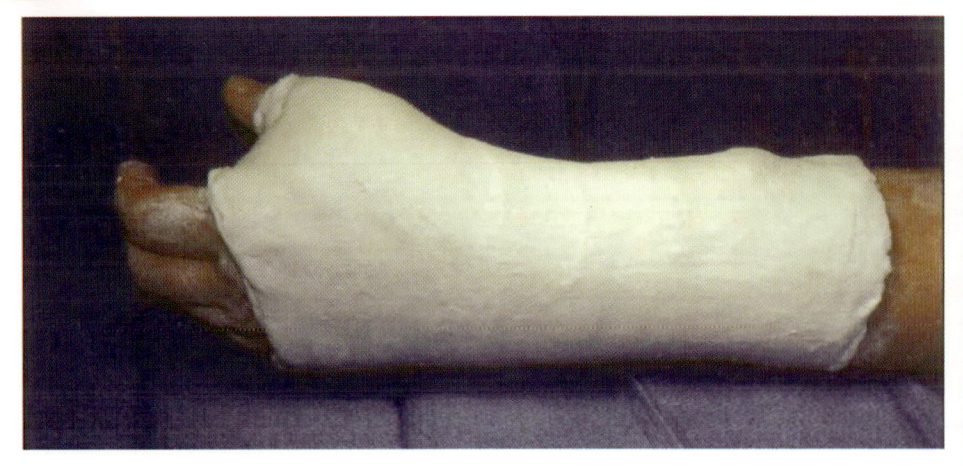

Figure 10 Photograph shows immobilization in a thumb spica cast following LRTI arthroplasty.

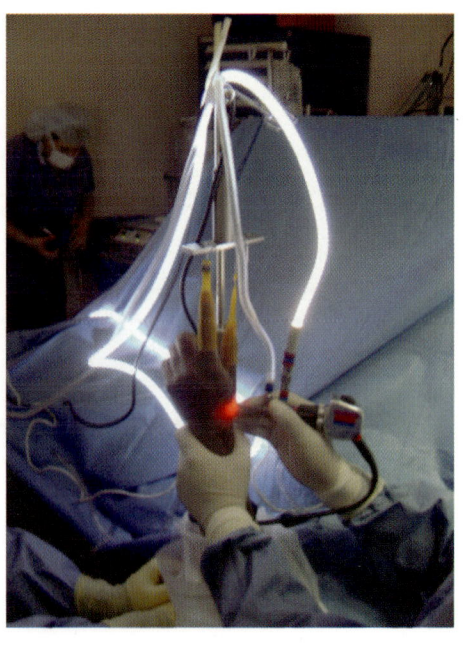

Figure 11 Intraoperative photograph shows the standard arthroscopy setup for thumb trapeziometacarpal arthroscopy with a traction tower and finger traps on the thumb and index fingers. A small-joint arthroscope is introduced into the basal joint space.

anesthesia may be used. A single dose of preoperative antibiotics is administered. With the patient lying supine and the surgical extremity on an arm table, a pneumatic tourniquet is applied and preset to 250 mm Hg. Standard sterile preparation and draping is performed.

The surgical limb is placed in a vertical traction tower, with a Chinese fingertrap placed on the thumb to apply 5 lb of longitudinal traction. An assistant holds the forearm in pronation. Anatomic landmarks are identified by palpation to assist with placement of the standard 1-R (radial) and 1-U (ulnar) portals. A palpable depression at the base of the thumb metacarpal indicates the level of the TMC joint. The APL, EPB, and EPL tendons and the radial artery are palpated. The expected course of the superficial radial nerve is noted.

At the level of the TMC joint, the 1-R portal is marked just radial to the APL tendon. The 1-U portal is marked just ulnar to the EPB tendon. The extremity is then exsanguinated and the pneumatic tourniquet is inflated to 250 mm Hg.

An alternative thenar portal has been described by Orellana and Chow.[15] This portal is located just distal to the oblique ridge of the trapezium, following a line referencing the radial edge of the FCR tendon. Better visualization of the TMC articulation has been reported using the thenar portal because it lies 90° from the 1-U portal. In a cadaver study, Walsh et al[16] found the thenar portal to be "potentially a safer and easier portal."

I routinely establish the 1-U portal first. A 20-gauge needle is advanced into the joint at the previously marked site to confirm placement and appropriate entry angle. Two milliliters of normal saline is injected to distend the joint capsule. The skin is incised with a No. 11 blade. Care is taken to raise the skin to the blade to avoid incising too deeply, which could injure the radial artery or branches of the superficial radial nerve. A small hemostat is passed bluntly through subcutaneous tissues down to the capsule, penetrating the joint bluntly.

A 1.9-mm arthroscope is then introduced into the joint (**Figure 11**). The working portal is established under direct visualization in a similar fashion. A diagnostic arthroscopy is then performed. The base of the first metacarpal is identified by moving the thumb at the carpometacarpal joint. The joint is systematically inspected for evidence of synovitis, ligamentous laxity, and articular cartilage loss. Initially, a 2.0-mm synovial resector may be used to débride the synovium. This aids visualization of the trapezium, which is inspected from ulnar to radial, noting any marginal osteophytes or articular eburnation. The articular cartilage of the metacarpal base is evaluated in a similar manner.

The integrity of the superficial and deep anterior oblique ligaments is then tested with a probe in the radial portal and the scope in the ulnar portal. Portals are then switched to inspect the dorsoradial ligament and posterior oblique ligament. The ulnar collateral ligament can be visualized and probed from either portal.

If early changes are identified with no significant cartilage loss, a 2.0-mm full-radius shaver is introduced to perform a synovectomy and débridement. The thumb metacarpal base is manipulated, and joint capsule and ligamentous structures are evaluated. If ligamentous laxity is identified, electrothermal capsular shrinkage is performed. I have used both monopolar and bipolar probes with success. Care is taken to intermittently apply the electrothermal source to achieve a "striping" or "dotting" effect to set the appropriate tension in the affected ligaments and collagenous capsule. Copious irrigation should be used.

If most of the trapezial articular surface is eburnated, at least one half of the distal trapezium is resected with a 2.0-mm burr. If scaphotrapeziotrapezoid joint arthritis is visualized through the midcarpal portal, then a complete trapeziectomy is performed. Fluoroscopic evaluation is used throughout the resection to identify the position of the burr and the location of remaining trapezial bone. The arthroscope is reintroduced, and final arthroscopic and fluoroscopic images are obtained, confirming appropriate bony resection and osteophyte removal.

If a hemitrapeziectomy has been performed, I prefer to proceed with interposition of a polyurethaneurea spacer, a biodegradable, biocompatible material made of polyglycolic acid and polyurethane urea that serves as a resurfacing scaffold (**Figure 12**). The dorsal wings of the spacer are trimmed off or folded back onto the spacer and the spacer is inserted through a transverse incision incorporating both arthroscopic portals. It is then laid down on the prepared trapezial surface, using a probe. Careful trimming of the material may be required to cover the joint surface optimally. Generally, the metacarpal base is kept intact during

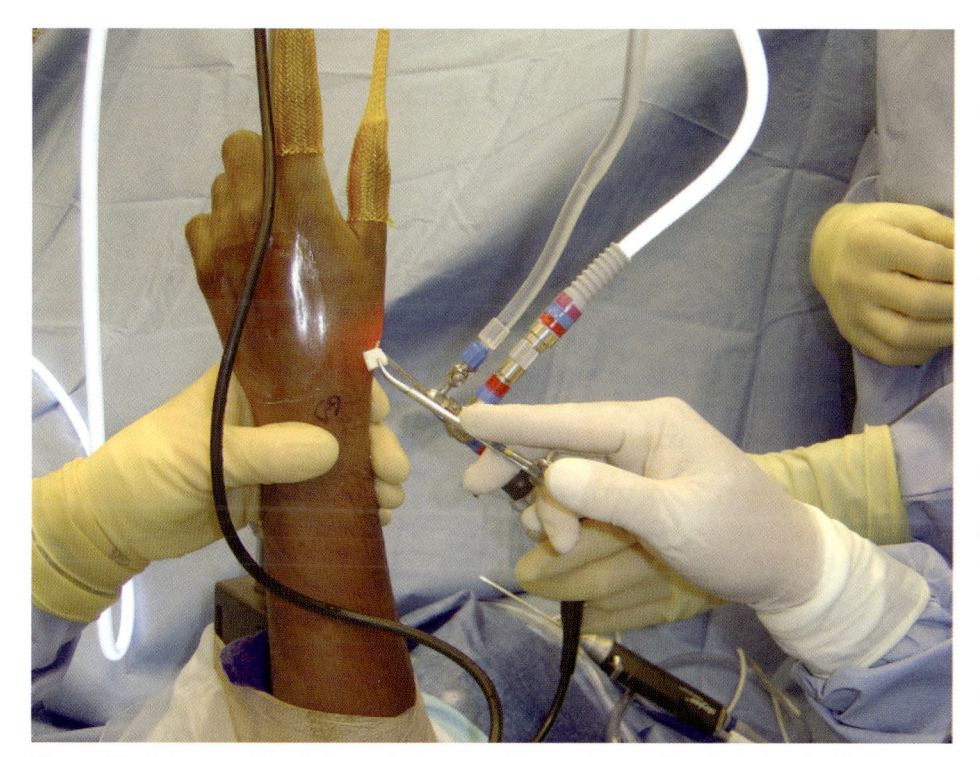

Figure 12 Intraoperative photograph shows an interposition arthroplasty implant being placed in the basal joint in a thumb trapeziometacarpal arthroplasty procedure.

trapezial resection. With complete trapeziectomy, I prefer to pin the joint under fluoroscopic guidance with a 0.045-in K-wire. After complete or hemitrapeziectomy, an electrothermal capsuloligamentous shrinkage can be performed as described previously to establish appropriate tension.

Complications

Myriad techniques for basal joint arthroplasty have been described by myriad experts; therefore, it can be deduced that not all techniques work in all cases. In my experience with both APL suspensionplasty with complete trapezial excision and arthroscopic débridement with interposition of bioengineered materials, 90% good to excellent results represents an acceptable success rate. Although some authors have reported even higher success rates, these are generally difficult to reproduce. The primary pitfall is a failure to adequately diagnose the patient. Clinical examination and imaging are generally sufficient to identify symptomatic basal joint arthritis; however, concurrent conditions (eg, carpal tunnel syndrome, flexor tendon or extensor tendon stenosis) and misidentification of scaphotrapeziotrapezoid arthritis as carpometacarpal arthritis are pitfalls that can be avoided by appropriate preoperative planning.

Some major complications can be avoided with careful technical execution. For example, in creating the bone tunnels for both the LRTI and the APL suspensionplasty, care must be exercised not to "fracture" the bone tunnel with breakthrough of the bony bridge. When this happens, the biomechanical constraints of the operation are clearly altered. The use of temporary pin fixation in these cases is mandatory, and revision surgery may be necessary in the future.

Obtaining appropriate tension and interposition in the LRTI operation are other important technical concerns. The APL suspensionplasty is, in my opinion, more easily tensioned, but care also must be exercised during this step.

Residual ST joint changes can sometimes be the cause of complication or failure, and this area should be evaluated preoperatively and, if possible, inspected intraoperatively. A curettage of this small joint is possible with LRTI and APL suspensionplasty operations.

Postoperative Care and Rehabilitation

Patients are initially immobilized in a thumb spica splint. At the first postoperative visit, they are transitioned to a removable custom splint. If hemitrapeziectomy and polyurethaneurea spacer insertion was performed, hand therapy is initiated at 4 weeks for active range-of-motion exercises. The custom splint is initially worn full time when the patient is not in therapy and then weaned as tolerated after the sixth postoperative week. Strengthening exercises commence at 8 weeks postoperatively, and patients are then advanced as tolerated. If a pin was placed for total trapeziectomy, it is removed at 6 weeks. These patients begin therapy for active range of motion at 6 weeks and strengthening at 8 weeks.

The terms of postoperative care and the period of immobilization required vary somewhat. With experience, I have found a 2-week period of immobilization is adequate to obtain consistent clinical success.

Pearls

- Patients with basal joint arthritis must be clearly identified and given the opportunity to try nonsurgical treatment first.
- Whatever technique is selected, the surgery must be performed in a technically competent manner.
- For open technique, trapezial restriction should be performed piecemeal to protect surrounding soft-tissue structures.
- For arthroscopic techniques, distal trapezial preparation with resection of medial osteophytes is critical to success.
- Fluoroscopy should be used in all cases to facilitate an accurate and thorough operation.
- The postoperative time period should be tailored to intraoperative findings, technical aspects of the completed operation, and patient compliance.
- Although 90% good to excellent results can be achieved, patients should be aware that revision surgery is sometimes necessary.

References

1. Armstrong AL, Hunter JB, Davis TR: The prevalence of degenerative arthritis of the base of the thumb in post-menopausal women. *J Hand Surg Br* 1994;19(3):340-341.
2. Oliveria SA, Felson DT, Reed JI, Cirillo PA, Walker AM: Incidence of symptomatic hand, hip, and knee osteoarthritis among patients in a health maintenance organization. *Arthritis Rheum* 1995;38(8):1134-1141.
3. Chaisson CE, Zhang Y, McAlindon TE, et al: Radiographic hand osteoarthritis: Incidence, patterns, and influence of pre-existing disease in a population based sample. *J Rheumatol* 1997;24(7):1337-1343.
4. Bhatia A, Pisoh T, Touam C, Oberlin C: Incidence and distribution of scaphotrapezotrapezoidal arthritis in 73 fresh

cadaveric wrists. *Ann Chir Main Memb Super* 1996;15(4):220-225.

5. Eaton RG, Littler JW: Ligament reconstruction for the painful thumb carpometacarpal joint. *J Bone Joint Surg Am* 1973;55(8):1655-1666.

6. Carroll RE: Arthrodesis of the carpometacarpal joint of the thumb: A review of patients with a long postoperative period. *Clin Orthop Relat Res* 1987;220:106-110.

7. Eaton RG, Glickel SZ, Littler JW: Tendon interposition arthroplasty for degenerative arthritis of the trapeziometacarpal joint of the thumb. *J Hand Surg Am* 1985;10(5):645-654.

8. Burton RI: Basal joint implant arthroplasty in osteoarthritis: Indications, techniques, pitfalls, and problems. *Hand Clin* 1987;3(4):473-487.

9. Tomaino MM, Pellegrini VD Jr, Burton RI: Arthroplasty of the basal joint of the thumb: Long-term follow-up after ligament reconstruction with tendon interposition. *J Bone Joint Surg Am* 1995;77(3):346-355.

10. Thompson JS: Complications and salvage of trapeziometacarpal arthroplasties. *Instr Course Lect* 1989;38:3-13.

11. Thompson JS: Suspensionplasty technique. *Atlas Han Clin* 1997;2:2.

12. Glickel SZ, Kornstein AN, Eaton RG: Long-term follow-up of trapeziometacarpal arthroplasty with coexisting scaphotrapezial disease. *J Hand Surg Am* 1992;17(4):612-620.

13. Imaeda T, An KN, Cooney WP III, Linscheid R: Anatomy of trapeziometacarpal ligaments. *J Hand Surg Am* 1993;18(2):226-231.

14. Culp RW, Rekant MS: The role of arthroscopy in evaluating and treating trapeziometacarpal disease. *Hand Clin* 2001;17(2):315-319, x-xi.

15. Orellana MA, Chow JC: Arthroscopic visualization of the thumb carpometacarpal joint: Introduction and evaluation of a new radial portal. *Arthroscopy* 2003;19(6):583-591.

16. Walsh EF, Akelman E, Fleming BC, DaSilva MF: Thumb carpometacarpal arthroscopy: A topographic, anatomic study of the thenar portal. *J Hand Surg Am* 2005;30(2):373-379.

Chapter 47
Partial Palmar Fasciectomy for Dupuytren Disease

Thomas P. Lehman, PT, MD   Steven L. Peterson, MD, DVM   Ghazi Rayan, MD

Introduction

Dupuytren disease (also called Dupuytren contracture) is a benign fibroproliferative disorder of the palmar fascial complex that leads to the development of pathologic tissue that may extend from the palm to any digit. In its early stages, Dupuytren disease leads to the formation of nodules and cords; in its advanced stage, flexion contracture of the digits may develop. The presentation of the disease varies, depending on its severity and whether palmar or digital fascial structures are affected.

It is important to differentiate between two clinical types of palmar fascial proliferation: Dupuytren disease and non–Dupuytren disease. A patient with typical Dupuytren disease is usually a Caucasian male of Northern European ancestry, approximately 50 years of age, with bilateral progressive digital contracture with more than one hand or digit involved, and a positive family history with or without ectopic disease. In contrast, non–Dupuytren disease is a clinical entity in which the patient has palmar fascial proliferation that usually occurs following trauma or surgery to the hand. The patient can be of any age, sex, or race and may be diabetic with no family history of Dupuytren disease. The condition is unilateral and nonprogressive, and usually affects only one hand without digital involvement or contracture.[1]

Patient Selection and Alternative Treatments

Variations of open fasciectomy—total or subtotal—have been used to treat Dupuytren disease. However, less invasive techniques have been revisited recently as alternatives to fasciectomy. These include needle fasciotomy and enzymatic lysis of the cords.

Needle aponeurotomy presents a less invasive surgical option to limited fasciectomy that may be performed as an office procedure with local anesthetic. This technique may be used independently or as an adjunct to partially correct a severely contracted finger before fasciectomy. In this procedure, the contracture-producing cord or cords are released by cutting the fibers with a needle inserted percutaneously. Careful consideration of the pathoanatomy of the abnormal cords is essential to avoid injury to adjacent neurovascular structures. For cords proximal to the metacarpophalangeal (MCP) joints, it is safer to initially release the deeper portion, followed by more superficial release. For cords distal to the MCP joints over the proximal phalanx, it is safest to approach the cord laterally to weaken the deeper, more dorsal portion of the cord while avoiding the palmarly displaced neurovascular structures. Cords are weakened by multiple passes of a 25-gauge needle mounted on a 10-mL syringe. Usually, more than one site is needled along the palpable course of the cord. Needle passages are performed with the cords under tension by passive extension of the involved digit. Often the cord will rupture during the course of therapy; however, if this does not occur and sufficient sites have been addressed, rupture can be achieved by more forceful extension. Following rupture, standard maneuvers are performed to ensure independently intact flexor digitorum superficialis and flexor digitorum profundus tendons. A soft dressing is applied, and nighttime extension splinting is performed for the next 4 to 6 weeks.

The second technique involves weakening the cord enzymatically by injecting collagenase 24 hours before rupturing the cord manually. Preliminary data indicate that these techniques may have more efficacy than the numerous alternatives previously proposed, including splinting, ultrasonic therapy, radiotherapy, topical application of vitamins A and E and gamma interferon, and steroid or dimethylsulfoxide injection.[2-4] Partial fasciectomy remains the standard treatment for severe and recurrent cases of Dupuytren disease.

Indications

Although absolute indications for surgical treatment of Dupuytren disease have not been objectively established, some guidelines are generally accepted. Surgery is recommended for patients whose disease limits function, with MCP joint contracture of at least 30° and/or proximal interphalangeal (PIP) joint contracture of 15°. Prominent cords or nodules that do not restrict motion may also require excision if they interfere with hand function because of their location.

Contraindications

Contraindications for treatment include non-Dupuytren disease, open hand wounds, and infection. Additionally, some patients may be physiologically unable to undergo a major surgical procedure or may have low functional demands and would not benefit from surgery. A subset of these patients may, however, be candidates for the less invasive techniques mentioned earlier that can be performed in an office setting. Patients who are on chronic anticoagulation therapy that cannot be temporarily discontinued should be approached with caution, as hematoma formation in the hand can lead to adverse outcomes regardless of the technique used for treatment.

Preoperative Imaging

Preoperative imaging is not routinely performed. However, in patients with underlying degenerative disease that may affect the reestablishment of joint motion, plain radiographs of the hand may be indicated.

Procedure

Room Setup/Patient Positioning

The patient should be positioned supine with the upper extremity abducted at the shoulder and the hand resting comfortably on a surgical hand table. Some older patients with Dupuytren disease may have degenerative changes that limit shoulder range of motion. When this situation exists, care must be taken to en-

---

Dr. Peterson serves as a board member, owner, officer, or committee member of the American Society for Surgery of the Hand. Dr. Rayan serves as a board member, owner, officer, or committee member of the American Society for Surgery of the Hand Ethics and Professionalism Committee. Neither Dr. Lehman nor any immediate family member has received anything of value from or owns stock in a commercial company or institution related directly or indirectly to the subject of this chapter.

Section 3: Hand and Wrist

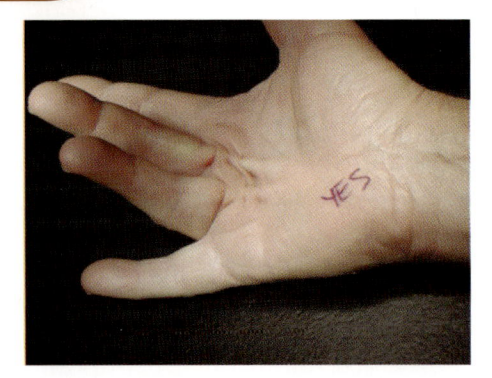

Figure 1 Photograph depicts metacarpophalangeal joint flexion contracture due to pretendinous cords in the palm.

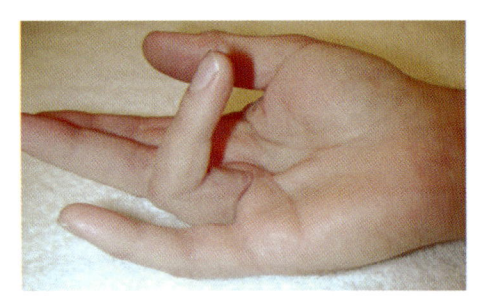

Figure 3 Photograph shows flexion contracture of the metacarpophalangeal and proximal interphalangeal joints due to an affected spiral cord.

sure that the extremity is not placed in a position that will aggravate underlying shoulder disease. A padded pneumatic tourniquet is placed on the brachium. In the presence of severe deformity, it may be difficult to place the digits in a lead hand or similar device that maintains the desired position during the procedure.

Full-thickness skin grafts are sometimes necessary to complete wound closure. These are most often harvested from the volar wrist, but the proximal forearm can provide a larger graft for more extensive skin shortage. The surgeon must also be prepared to use flap coverage if vital structures such as tendons and neurovascular structures are exposed after reapproximation of the skin edges. The patient should be positioned and prepared so that the donor site of choice is readily available if grafts are needed. Alternatively, wounds can be left open if vital structures are not exposed, to heal by secondary intention.

Special Instruments/Equipment
Partial fasciectomy can be completed with basic instrumentation appropriate for surgery of the hand. A No. 15C Bard-Parker surgical blade can be extremely valuable for dissecting adherent diseased tissue from dermis. Small Beaver blade scalpels may be of value.

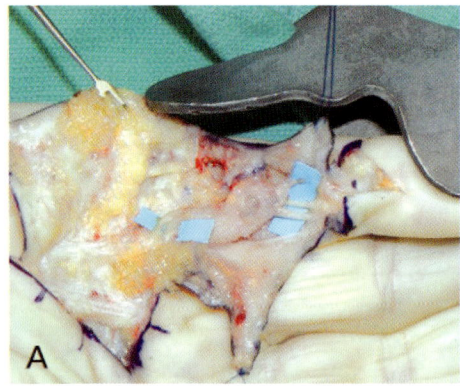

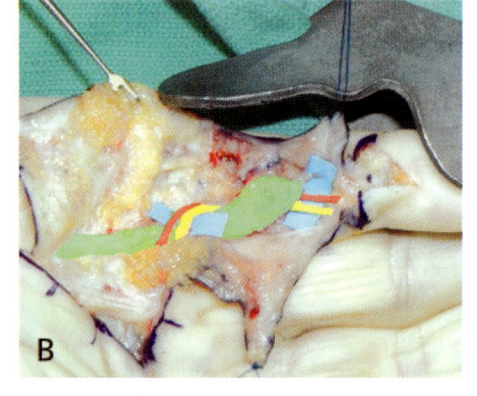

Figure 2 Intraoperative photographs of palmar fasciectomy for Dupuytren disease. **A,** The small finger radial digital artery and nerve are identified proximally where they pass over the spiral cord superficially. The neurovascular structures then pass beneath the cord and emerge on the radial side of the digit distally. Blue background material is present beneath the neurovascular structures proximally and distally. **B,** The spiral cord has been colored green, the digital artery red, and the digital nerve yellow to improve visual contrast.

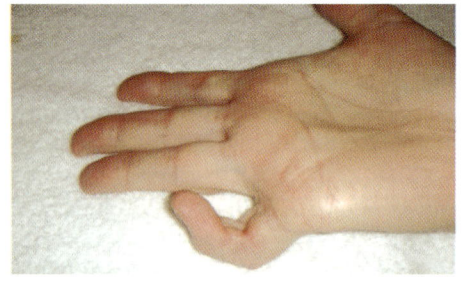

Figure 4 A pathologic abductor digiti minimi cord results in flexion and abduction of the small finger.

Limited fasciectomy does not require an operating microscope or microsurgical instruments. These items should be available, however, because injury to nerves and arteries are known risks associated with the surgical treatment of Dupuytren disease. If a nerve or vessel injury occurs at the time of fasciectomy, it should be immediately repaired.

Surgical Technique
Preoperative Planning
Fasciectomy for Dupuytren disease involves selective removal of the diseased tissue that is contributing to digital joint contracture. This tissue may distort the anatomy and displace digital nerves and vessels. Therefore, a thorough understanding of the normal palmar fascial anatomy and Dupuytren disease pathology is essential for the execution of a successful fasciectomy. Several anatomically distinct pathologic cords have been described in Dupuytren disease, and more than one cord may be present in the same hand/digit.

Dupuytren Cords
Pretendinous Cord
The pretendinous cord arises from the pretendinous band and is the most commonly encountered cord in the hand. Contracture of this cord results in flexion deformity of the MCP joint (**Figure 1**). This cord does not typically displace neurovascular structures.

Spiral Cord
The spiral cord arises from the pretendinous band proximally and continues distally to involve the spiral band, the lateral digital sheet, and the Grayson ligament. As these diseased structures coalesce and shorten, the adjacent digital neurovascular bundle spirals around the cord, which takes a straight-line course (**Figure 2**). This frequently results in flexion deformity of the MCP joint as well as the PIP joint (**Figure 3**).

Lateral Cord
The lateral cord is the diseased lateral digital sheet and may result in contracture of the proximal and occasionally the distal interphalangeal joints. It does not result in displacement of the neurovascular bundle, except by its bulk.

Central Cord
The central cord is the diseased central terminal fibers of the split pretendinous bands in the distal palm and proximal digits. It is the distal continuation of the pretendinous band into the digit and leads to PIP joint contracture in addition to MCP joint flexion deformity.

Abductor Digiti Minimi Cord
The abductor digiti minimi cord is also known as an isolated digital cord and is analogous to the spiral cord but without the pretendinous component. It is located on the ulnar side of the small finger (**Figure 4**). This cord arises from the abductor

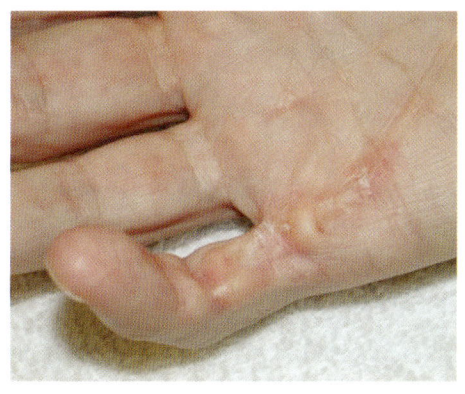

Figure 5 Recurrent flexion contracture of the small finger proximal interphalangeal joint with adherent overlying skin may require dermofasciectomy.

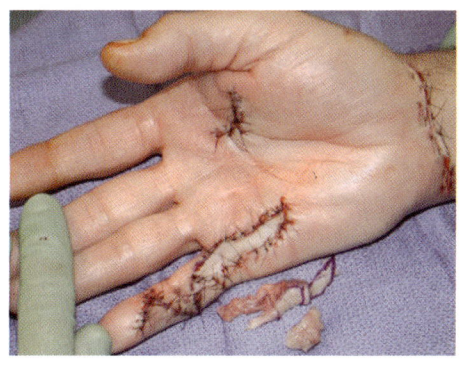

Figure 6 Following dermofasciectomy, the resulting skin defect in the palm is addressed with full-thickness skin graft harvested from the palmar aspect of the wrist.

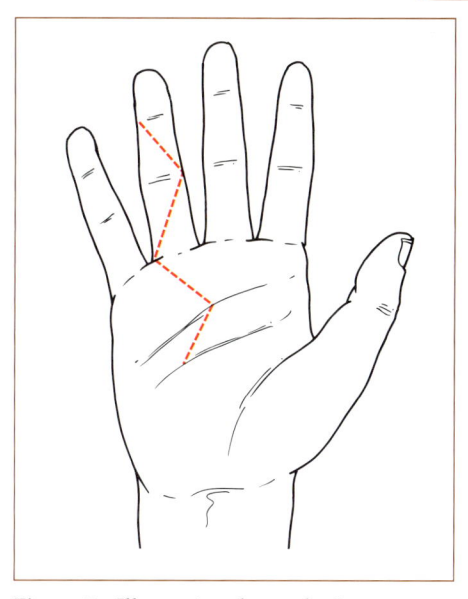

Figure 7 Illustration shows the Bruner incision (dashed line) for fasciectomy of the ring finger and palm.

digiti minimi tendon and often results in displacement of the ulnar digital nerve.

Natatory Cord
The natatory cord arises from the natatory ligament in the digital web space. It causes digital web-space contracture and does not result in displacement of the neurovascular structures.

Proximal and Distal Commissural Cords
The proximal and distal commissural cords are the diseased proximal and distal commissural ligaments of the thumb-index web space. They lead to first web-space contracture.

Fasciectomy Types
Fasciectomy may be divided into limited (regional), extensive, radical (total), and dermofasciectomy. Limited fasciectomy involves selective removal of only the diseased fascia and is the most frequently performed procedure. Extensive fasciectomy is reserved for patients with more widespread disease, where the removal of multiple cords in more than one digit is done while sparing any normal-appearing tissue. The goal of radical fasciectomy, in contrast, is to remove the entire palmar fascia, including normal tissue. This procedure is associated with considerable morbidity and complications and is no longer recommended. Dermofasciectomy involves the removal of diseased fascia and the very adherent overlying diseased and/or scarred skin from prior surgery. The resulting skin deficit must be replaced with a full-thickness skin graft. This is often indicated for recurrent cases but also for some primary cases, when skin is very adherent to underlying pathologic tissue (Figures 5 and 6).

During the excision of well-defined cords, other areas of the palmar fascial complex must be inspected for additional diseased tissue that should be addressed as well. Attempts should be made to remove all diseased fascia with minimal trauma to normal tissue. Surgical planning must take into account that neurovascular structures may be displaced. This cannot be accurately predicted preoperatively, but flexion contracture of the PIP joint, especially in the small finger, should raise suspicion that this will be the case.

Incisions
No universal surgical approach can be used for all fasciectomy procedures. The most frequently used approach is through a Bruner incision placed in the palm, which can be extended into the digit (Figure 7). An alternative is placing a longitudinal midline incision in the digit that is closed with multiple Z-plasties. This will provide the necessary extra skin for closure without a graft and prevent scar contracture across flexion creases. Both of these incisions may be combined with transverse palmar incisions, which may be primarily closed, skin grafted, or left open to heal by secondary intention.

Initial Dissection
Bruner skin flaps are dissected carefully from the often-adherent diseased tissue, elevated, and retracted. Atraumatic technique should be used. Neurovascular structures displaced by the cords can often be located more superficially or toward the midline.

Skin may be thin and adherent to the underlying diseased tissue. Careful dissection will allow separation of the skin from the fascia without leaving diseased tissue behind or thinning of the flaps. Buttonholing the flap, especially near the base, will compromise its viability. Small perforations of the skin away from the base should not jeopardize flap survival. If the skin flaps cannot be safely elevated, consideration should be given to dermofasciectomy and skin grafting.

Skin flaps can be retracted by placing a stay suture in the flap tip held with a small surgical hemostat.

Digital arteries and nerves are identified, carefully dissected from the diseased tissue, and protected during the entire procedure.

Initial dissection may be especially difficult in patients with severe digital flexion contracture. Division of the proximal portion of the cord in the palm by needle fasciotomy or limited fasciectomy may allow sufficient extension of the digit to improve visualization for completion of the dissection and the formal fasciectomy. In these cases, neurovascular structures are more likely to be injured, and they should be dissected carefully.

Tissue Excision
The excision of diseased tissue should not be done until the important neurovascular structures are identified and protected. The resection of diseased tissue is initiated proximally and carefully advanced distally. Sometimes it is helpful to proceed with proximal and distal dissections simultaneously toward the most affected region, where dissection is most tedious.

Limited fasciectomy and the removal of diseased tissue that contributes to contracture should be sufficient. In patients with multiple cords, more extensive fasciectomy may be necessary. The diseased portion of

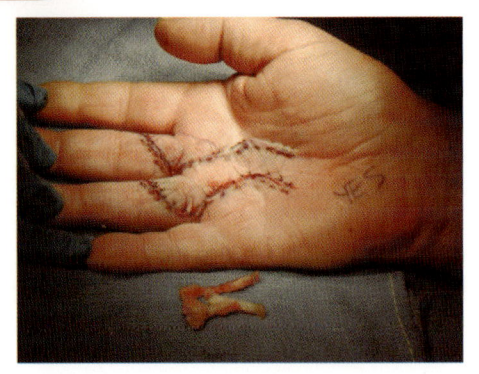

Figure 8 In most cases, Bruner incisions can be closed primarily.

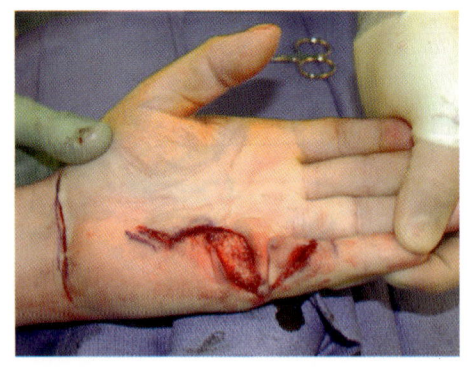

Figure 9 After correction of the flexion deformity, a skin deficit may be present in the palm.

the palmar fascia may be resected en bloc, or each cord may be excised individually. Skin is preserved whenever possible, however, when it is densely adherent to the underlying diseased tissue; when the skin is scarred from previous surgery, dermatofasciectomy should be considered.

The anatomic area where injury of the neurovascular structures is most likely is the palmodigital region. Hence, special attention must be given to preventing their damage.

Addressing Joint Contracture

Complete resection of all diseased tissue should correct all joint contracture, in particular the MCP and distal interphalangeal joints. If these digits cannot be fully extended, residual diseased tissue should be suspected and addressed. If PIP joint contracture remains, gentle manipulation usually improves or corrects the residual deformity. Residual PIP flexion contracture greater than 30° that cannot be corrected by manipulation requires the release of the checkrein ligaments' component of the palmar plate and, if necessary, a portion of the collateral ligaments.

After achieving the desired correction of joint deformity, the digital neurovascular bundle should be inspected for signs of excessive tension during digital extension. In some cases, full extension of all digital joints, in particular the PIP joint, may not be possible without inflicting undue tension on these important structures. In these situations, postoperative splinting of the hand should be done in some flexion to relieve any tension on the neurovascular bundle.

Prior to wound closure, the tourniquet is deflated, and hemostasis is obtained with bipolar cautery. Care must be taken to avoid thermal injury to the neurovascular structures while using the cautery. Gentle pressure on the wound for a few minutes can achieve hemostasis in many cases.

It is important to ensure that there is adequate circulation to all digits. Vascular compromise is evidenced by loss of the normal capillary refill following deflation of the tourniquet. This may be due to arterial laceration or, more often, spasm from manipulation or tension. Arterial spasm can be corrected by using topical vasodilators such as lidocaine, whereas arterial laceration should be addressed by direct repair or vein grafting. If the vessels are intact, the digit should be slightly flexed, and the hand warmed with warm saline.

Wound Closure

Bruner incisions are closed primarily when possible (**Figure 8**). If necessary, the corners may be closed in a Y-V fashion to allow skin approximation. If a midline longitudinal incision was used, it should be closed with multiple Z-plasty flaps to prevent scar contracture.

Closure should not leave any hematoma that may accumulate beneath the skin flaps, which could produce sufficient pressure on the skin to result in necrosis.

If dermofasciectomy was performed, full-thickness skin graft should be harvested, defatted, and applied to the resulting defect. The most accessible donor site is the volar wrist; however, other potential areas are the antecubital fossa, glabrous skin of the foot, and, less often, the groin. In long-standing cases with severe deformity, skin shortage may be present at the conclusion of the procedure even if no skin was resected (**Figure 9**).

Closure of the palmar wounds is not always required. All or part of the palm may be allowed to heal secondarily, as in the open palm method of McCash.[5]

Complications

Infection

Postoperative wound infection is infrequently reported following surgery for Dupuytren disease. The use of prophylactic antibiotics in lengthy or complicated cases and careful attention to sterile technique can help to minimize this risk.

Hematoma and Skin Necrosis

Hematoma and skin necrosis are frequently encountered complications after Dupuytren disease surgery. The accumulation of hematoma beneath the skin flap may result in pain, excessive scar formation, and stiffness, as well as an increased risk of infection. It can also contribute to compromise of flap circulation and necrosis of the overlying skin, along with failure of skin grafts. Adequate hemostasis must be achieved before wound closure. Leaving the wound open or retaining a drain in the wound is advised if a hematoma is expected to develop, such as following extensive dissection. If a hematoma develops in the early postoperative period, it should be evacuated immediately.

Poorly designed skin incisions may also contribute to skin necrosis. Skin flaps that are excessively long or narrow are at risk, as are areas of adherent skin that were thinned during elevation. Multiple incisions placed in proximity can also contribute to skin necrosis. During fasciectomy of multiple digits, the incisions must be carefully planned to minimize this risk.

Full-thickness skin necrosis usually occurs in the margins of flaps and small isolated areas. Often, the resulting eschar can be left in place as a biologic dressing and allowed to slough as reepithelialization occurs. The presence of small areas of necrosis should not delay rehabilitation. Occasionally, skin necrosis may involve large areas, which will require treatment with skin grafting or local flap coverage.

Neurovascular Injury

Patients may experience numbness in the surgical digits following surgery due to neurapraxia of the digital nerves caused by nerve retraction, dissection, or mobilization. This typically resolves within days or weeks. Laceration of digital nerves may occur in recurrent cases and those associated with severe contracture and, if encountered, should be repaired immediately.

Slow or absent capillary refill in a digit following tourniquet deflation is usually due to arterial spasm caused by excessive stretching and gaining extension and often responds to repositioning and warming of the hand. Arterial lacerations are rare, but if encountered should be immediately repaired or reconstructed using microvascular technique.

Complex Regional Pain Syndrome
Complex regional pain syndrome has been reported following partial palmar fasciectomy. There is controversy about potentially increased risk of this pain disorder if fasciectomy is performed concurrently with carpal tunnel release. This concept has been challenged in clinical studies, which showed that no such association exists.[6] Doing extensive Dupuytren disease surgery along with any other procedure can predispose the patient to have pain out of proportion to the norm. Early recognition and treatment of this complication can help minimize the long-term effects, namely stiffness.

Recurrence and Extension of Disease
Dupuytren disease is a progressive condition, and fasciectomy does not eliminate the underlying physiologic tendency for contracture of other digits. Recurrence of disease in the same location of surgery is relatively common and is related to the patient's underlying predisposition or diathesis. Extension of disease refers to the development of contracture in previously uninvolved parts of the hand that were not previously treated surgically. There are no known measures that can limit Dupuytren disease recurrence or extension.

Stiffness
Permanent loss of motion following surgical treatment may be functionally significant. The loss of digital extension may be related to the recurrence of disease or persistent contracture of the PIP joint following surgery. The loss of digital flexion is often transient, due to postoperative edema. Failure to relieve swelling in a timely manner will result in permanent residual flexion with greater functional impairment than flexion contracture.

Postoperative Care and Rehabilitation
Following skin closure, the hand should be dressed in a bulky dressing and placed in a splint with the digits in extension. It is important to ensure that the digits are not extended to a degree that causes vasospasm. The tips of the digits should be visible so that their circulation can be monitored in the early postoperative period. If vascular embarrassment occurs, the splint should be removed and the digits gently flexed until normal color and circulation are restored.

The hand is maintained in the splint and evaluated for 7 to 10 days. The sutures are removed 10 to 15 days after surgery. Depending on the severity of the initial contracture, the splint may be discontinued at 2 weeks or used for another 2 weeks, especially at night. During this period, the patient is allowed to remove the splint two or three times a day for active and gentle passive range-of-motion exercises if the condition of the soft tissues allows. At 4 weeks after surgery, the patient discontinues the use of the splint during the day but maintains nocturnal splinting (**Figure 10**). If severe PIP joint contracture was corrected at surgery, further splinting may be necessary to prevent recurrence (**Figure 11**). Formal hand therapy may be necessary for residual flexion deformity and scar mobilization.

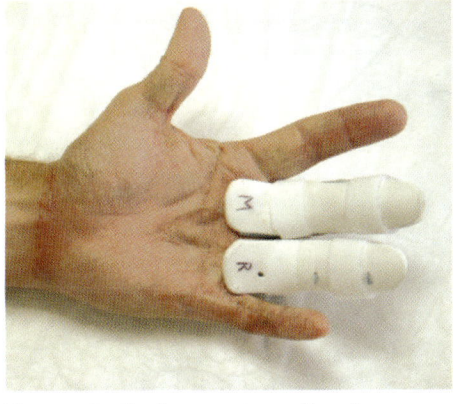

Figure 10 Static extension splints for the metacarpophalangeal and proximal interphalangeal joints may be used during sleep for several weeks postoperatively.

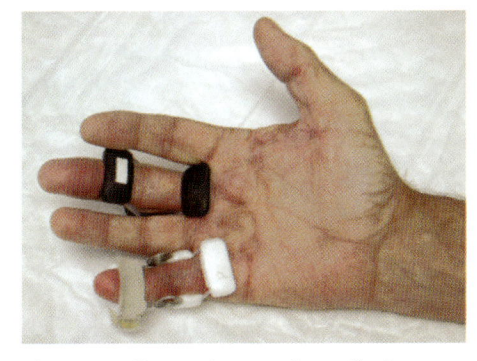

Figure 11 Dynamic extension splinting of the proximal interphalangeal joints can minimize recurrent flexion contracture of the involved joints, although it does not prevent recurrence of the underlying disease.

Pearls
- If the skin flaps cannot be safely elevated, consideration should be given to dermofasciectomy and skin grafting.
- Digital arteries and nerves must be identified, carefully dissected from the diseased tissue, and protected during the entire procedure.
- In patients with severe digital flexion contracture, division of the proximal portion of the cord in the palm by needle fasciotomy or limited fasciectomy may allow sufficient extension of the digit to improve visualization for completion of the dissection and formal fasciectomy.
- In addressing joint contracture, residual PIP flexion contracture greater than 30° that cannot be corrected by manipulation requires release of the checkrein ligaments' component of the palmar plate and, if necessary, a portion of the collateral ligaments.
- Following fasciectomy, circulation to all digits should be confirmed. Flexion and warming of the digits or topical vasodilators should be considered if circulation is not adequate. If vessels are lacerated, primary repair or grafting should be performed.
- Hemostasis must be obtained prior to wound closure to minimize the risk of hematoma formation and subsequent flap necrosis.

References
1. Rayan GM, Moore J: Non-Dupuytren's disease of the palmar fascia. *J Hand Surg Br* 2005;30(6):551-556.
2. Rayan GM: Nonoperative treatment of Dupuytren's disease. *J Hand Surg Am* 2008;33(7):1208-1210.
3. van Rijssen AL, Gerbrandy FS, Ter Linden H, Klip H, Werker PM: A comparison of the direct outcomes of percutaneous needle fasciotomy and limited fasciectomy for Dupuytren's disease: A 6-week follow-up study. *J Hand Surg Am* 2006;31(5):717-725.
4. Hurst LC, Badalamente MA, Hentz VR, et al; CORD I Study Group: Injectable collagenase clostridium histolyticum for Dupuytren's contracture. *N Engl J Med* 2009;361(10):968-979.
5. McCash CR: The open palm technique in Dupuytren's contracture. *Br J Plast Surg* 1964;17:271-280.
6. Lilly SI, Stern PJ: Simultaneous carpal tunnel release and Dupuytren's fasciectomy. *J Hand Surg Am* 2010;35(5):754-759.

Adult Reconstruction

Section Editor
William Macaulay, MD

48   **Hip Arthroplasty via Small-Incision Enhanced Posterior Soft-Tissue Repair** 313
Jonathan H. Lee, MD; William Macaulay, MD; Brett Rebal, BA

49   **Hip Arthroplasty via a Direct Lateral Approach** 319
Tahir Mahmud, BSc (Hons), MBBS, FRCS (Tr & Orth);
Robert B. Bourne, MD, FRCSC

50   **Direct Anterior Approach for Hip Arthroplasty** 325
Gregory K. Deirmengian, MD; William J. Hozack, MD

51   **Revision Total Hip Arthroplasty via Extended Trochanteric Osteotomy** 333
Scott M. Sporer, MD, MS; Wayne G. Paprosky, MD, FACS

52   **Total Knee Arthroplasty via the Medial Parapatellar Approach** 341
Stephen J. Incavo, MD; Michael R. Dayton, MD;
Jesse James F. Exaltacion, MD

53   **Total Knee Arthroplasty via Small-Incision Midvastus Approach** 345
Steven B. Haas, MD, MPH; Stephen Kim, MD

54   **Total Knee Arthroplasty via the Mini-Subvastus Approach** 351
William C. Schroer, MD

55   **Revision Total Knee Arthroplasty via Quadriceps Snip** 359
Ari Seidenstein, MD; Scott Scuderi, BS; Giles R. Scuderi, MD

56   **Revision Total Knee Arthroplasty via Tibial Tubercle Osteotomy** 363
Jeffrey A. Geller, MD

Chapter 48

Hip Arthroplasty via Small-Incision Enhanced Posterior Soft-Tissue Repair

Jonathan H. Lee, MD   William Macaulay, MD   Brett Rebal, BA

Introduction

Total hip arthroplasty (THA) and hemiarthroplasty can be performed successfully through a variety of approaches. The choice of approach depends largely on the training and preference of the surgeon, whose comfort with the exposure and familiarity with any approach are the most important factors in achieving a successful clinical result and avoiding complications. The posterior approach to the hip remains a very commonly performed technique despite having been shunned by some surgeons, who cited a higher risk of posterior dislocation. The balance of the literature has determined that this risk of dislocation is obviated, however, when the posterior soft tissues are formally repaired in a way that reconstructs the native soft-tissue anatomy.[1] In this chapter, we review our preferred approach and outline a small-incision[2] version of the enhanced posterior soft-tissue repair technique.[3] This is an evolution from the standard posterior, posterolateral Moore, or Southern approach. The small-incision enhanced posterior soft-tissue repair (SIEPSTR) technique has also been modified for use in metal-on-metal hip resurfacing.[4] Although we do not favor the term "minimally invasive," we do strive to make our well-placed incision small so that excessive prolonged retraction pressure on the soft tissues is unnecessary.

Patient Selection
Indications

One of the great benefits of the SIEPSTR technique is that it can be used in almost every clinical scenario in which THA is performed, regardless of the size of the patient, the complexity of the anatomy (including altered anatomy and the existence of hardware in place in conversion or revision surgeries), and the difficulty of the exposure because of muscle girth or stiff or fused hip contractures. The small-incision aspect of the technique can be abandoned at any time simply by making the incision longer, because it is easily expansile.

Contraindications

Although a hip surgeon may be more likely to avoid this approach in certain clinical scenarios such as a patient with Parkinson disease or with previous anterior incisions, no absolute contraindications exist for the SIEPSTR technique, which distinguishes it from many of the other surgical approaches to the hip.

Preoperative Imaging and Planning

We routinely obtain low AP pelvis, AP hip, and cross-table lateral hip radiographs and rely on a combination of preoperative templating and clinical examination in determining the plan for leg length. The preoperative low AP pelvis radiograph is crucial for templating purposes. A standard radiologic marker, such as a 25-mm marker ball, is essential to determine the degree of magnification and is especially important for digital radiography. Conventional low AP pelvis radiographs, which typically have a magnification of 15% to 25%, can be used with a manufacturer's cellophane templating overlay. We use the measurement from the lesser trochanter to the center of the femoral head as our guide to reestablishing the appropriate leg lengths. A similar measurement, from the center of the femoral head to the tip of the greater trochanter, can be used to plan offset. Of course, these are rough measurements that may need to be fine-tuned during surgery based on intraoperative measurements and soft-tissue assessments during trialing.

Video 48.1 Cementless Total Hip Arthroplasty via a Posterior Approach Using Enhanced Posterior Soft-Tissue Repair. William Macaulay, MD (16 min)

Procedure
Room Setup/Patient Positioning

The patient, preferably under hypotensive regional anesthesia, is positioned in the lateral position with all bony prominences well padded. Our preferred operating room table is one that has been modified by the manufacturer specifically for posterior approach THA to allow ease of positioning, stable fixation of the patient's pelvis with adjustable anterior and posterior padded pelvic holders, and the ability to "airplane" the table, tilting the posterior aspect of the patient down approximately 30° toward the surgeon, who is standing posteriorly during acetabular preparation.[5] Care must be taken to ensure appropriate padding, especially in the axillary region and the region of the peroneal nerve on the nonsurgical leg. A surgeon and two assistants are helpful for efficient execution of this technique. Three assistants, not including the isolation-suited scrub technician, can be accommodated when education is part of the mission.

Special Instruments/Equipment

The operating room table mentioned previously is very useful for this procedure but is not essential. Likewise, the instruments mentioned in the following discussion are our preference, but other similar instruments can be substituted.

Surgical Technique: THA
Preparation, Draping, and Incision

The leg is prepared and draped free in the usual sterile manner—we prefer a colored chlorhexidine prep stick covered when dry with an iodine-impregnated plastic wrap—by a surgical team in which each member is clad in an isolation suit. A bump is placed under the knee of the surgical leg to position the femur parallel to the floor, and the tip of the greater trochanter is palpated and marked. The anterior and posterior aspects of the

---

Dr. Lee or an immediate family member has received nonincome support (such as equipment or services), commercially derived honoraria, or other non–research-related funding (such as paid travel) from Aesculap/B. Braun. Dr. Macaulay or an immediate family member has received research or institutional support from Pfizer and Wright Medical Technology and serves as a board member, owner, officer, or committee member of the American Association of Hip and Knee Surgeons. Neither Mr. Rebal nor any immediate family member has received anything of value from or has stock or stock options held in a commercial company or institution related directly or indirectly to the subject of this chapter.

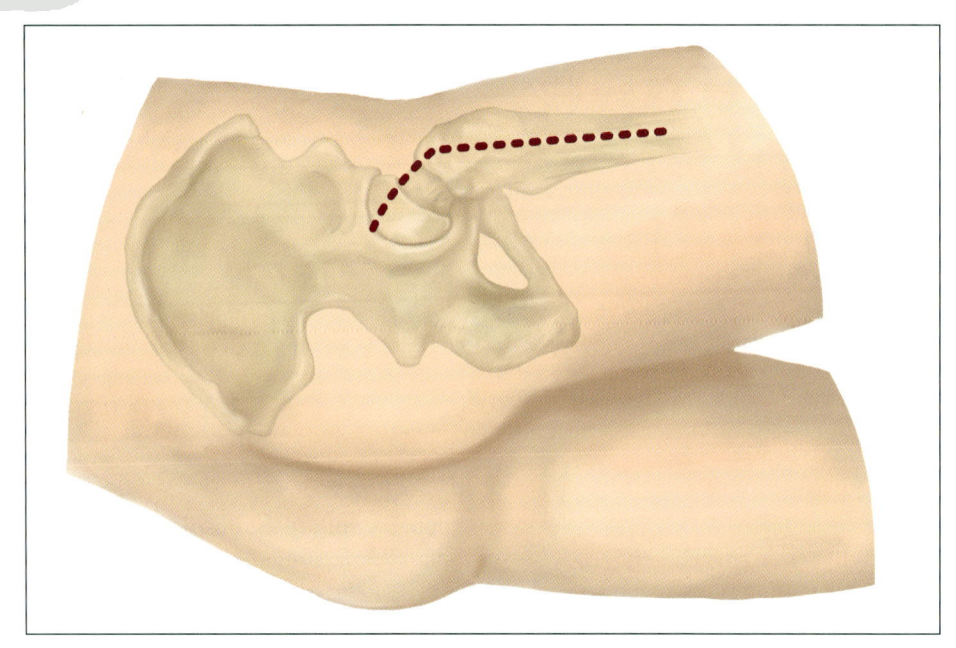

Figure 1 Illustration shows the position of the planned incision for hip arthroplasty using the small-incision enhanced posterior soft-tissue repair (SIEPSTR) approach.

femur also are palpated and marked. The resulting inverted U serves as a reference point for the position of the femur and subsequent placement of the incision. We also palpate the vastus ridge routinely and place this point near the distal end of the curvilinear incision. A longer incision is indicated when the patient is large or when a thick adipose layer or excessive local musculature is present. Distally, the incision is centered over the lateral aspect of the femur and, as the tip of the trochanter is approached, the incision is curved posteriorly, roughly in line with the fibers of the gluteus maximus. The goal is to have two thirds of the incision distal to the greater trochanter and one third proximal to the greater trochanter (**Figure 1**). This approach also can be performed successfully with a straight incision.

Exposure

Sharp dissection is performed to the level of the fascia. Retractors or self-retainers can be used to facilitate fascial exposure. When the fascia is identified clearly, a new blade is used to penetrate the fascia sharply (a 2-cm–long slit) over the most prominent lateral aspect of the greater trochanter. If the fascia is incised too posteriorly, anterior exposure will be compromised during the THA, and the gluteus maximus muscle will be visible. If the fascia is incised too anteriorly, tensor fascia lata muscle will be encountered and divided. Distally, this fascial slit is divided further with curved Mayo scissors and carried slightly distal to the end of the incision to enhance deeper exposure, but not so far as to make reapproximation difficult at the start of closure. More proximally, care should be taken to incise only the fascia over the gluteus maximus without sharply cutting the muscle fibers themselves. The muscle is finger divided bluntly between fibers; therefore, essentially no trauma occurs to this large muscle. The superior portion of the gluteus maximus tendon, seen distally in the wound on the posterior aspect of the femur, is released using electrocautery. The amount of gluteus maximus tendon to be released depends on several factors, such as the degree of preoperative hip contracture, the thickness of the hip capsule, the amount of lower limb lengthening to be provided (if any), the existence of preoperative lumbar spine disease, and the size of the muscles, especially the gluteus maximus. A Charnley retractor can be placed at this point to facilitate exposure; however, if two or three assistants are at the table, the surgeon may choose to avoid the use of this large self-retaining retractor, which may require undertensioning or repositioning to avoid damage to adipose tissue and muscle.

The short external rotators should soon be visible beneath the bursa and fat. Electrocautery can be used to penetrate the bursa carefully, and a thin bent Hohmann retractor can be placed in a posterior-to-anterior direction above the piriformis, between the gluteus minimus and the gluteus medius; this elevates the gluteus medius gently to better expose the short external rotators. An Aufranc retractor is used to sweep the bursa, fat, and inferior short external rotators from superior to inferior. The tip of the Aufranc retractor is hooked between the inferior aspect of the hip capsule overlying the inferior neck of the femur and the quadratus femoris muscle. Excellent visualization of the piriformis and conjoined tendon is now achieved.

An anterior assistant internally rotates the leg slightly to stretch the short external rotators. The piriformis (which was already released on its superior edge from the underlying minimus muscle) and conjoined tendon are then released as close to their femoral insertions as possible. Bending the electrocautery tip and aiming as anteriorly as possible helps to ensure that the tendons are resected as close to the bone as possible. If the tendons are cut short, the posterior soft-tissue repair might not reach back to the femur, thus compromising the eventual posterior soft-tissue repair. During this step, care is taken to not violate the hip capsule because synovial fluid released at this time may hinder progress. Hip capsule violation can be prevented if the surgeon carefully watches the longitudinal fibers of the tendon fall away as they are resected with the electrocautery. As the last fibers of the tendons fall away, the white capsule becomes visible. It also should be noted that the piriformis and the conjoined tendon become confluent close to their insertion on the femur. Therefore, it is not unusual if only one large, wide tendon is seen at this step. In fact, this is encouraging because it suggests that the resection of the tendons was quite close to their insertion points on the femur. The tendons are tagged with two No. 2 nonabsorbable colored braided sutures, and the short sutures are clamped. These sutures are cut relatively short (approximately 15 cm) to differentiate them from the capsular sutures (**Figure 2**).

A Cobb-type elevator is used to sweep the gluteus minimus off the capsule and develop the plane superiorly between the capsule and the gluteus minimus; if this raphe is difficult to see at first, the electrocautery tip may be useful in identifying this raphe along the outer aspect of the posterosuperior hip capsule. The thin bent Hohmann retractor is repositioned so that it is aimed more anterior than superior in this interval. At this part of the approach, the technique begins to deviate more distinctly, depending on whether THA or hemiarthroplasty is being performed.

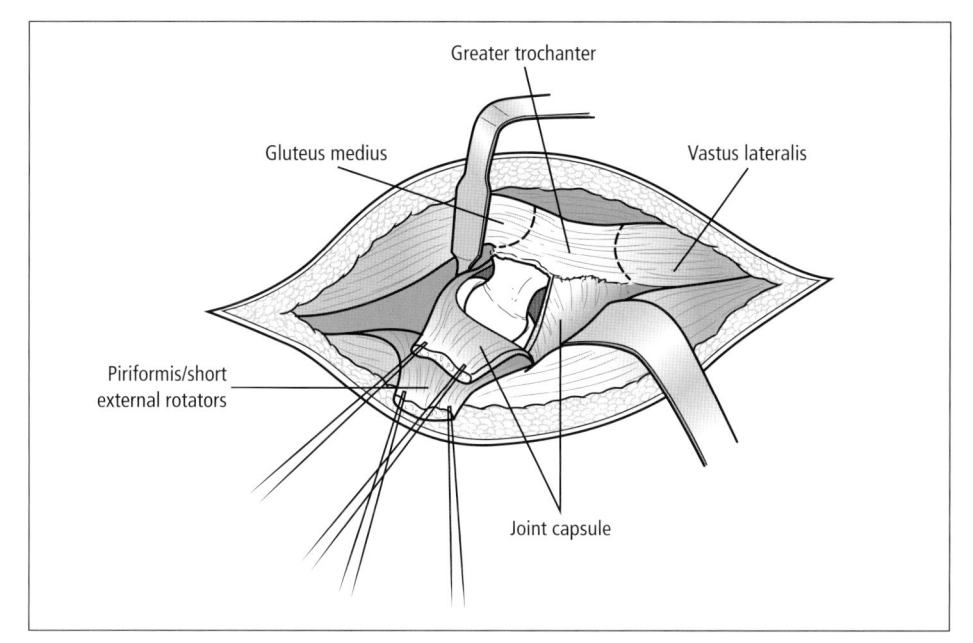

Figure 2 Illustration shows exposure for total hip arthroplasty using the small-incision enhanced posterior soft-tissue repair (SIEPSTR) approach. The piriformis tendon and the conjoined tendons, which have been detached as a tendinous sleeve from their insertions, are tagged superiorly and inferiorly using nonabsorbable sutures and then reflected posteriorly. Arthrotomy of the posterior capsule has created a posteriorly based trapezoid-shaped capsular sleeve that is likewise tagged twice with sutures and reflected posteriorly.

For THA, the capsulotomy should start posterosuperiorly, just proximal to the labrum, and extend anteriorly (roughly along the path that the inferior aspect of the gluteus minimus followed on the capsule) along the superior aspect of the femoral neck, stopping near the trochanteric fossa as the capsule is lifted off the femur. The capsule is tagged using a Mason-Allen–like stitch, cut long, and grouped (with a Kelly clamp) with the more cephalad of the two short No. 2 nonabsorbable sutures. Tension applied to this capsular suture allows the surgeon to put the capsule under more tension and use the long-handled scalpel to remove the capsule directly from the trochanteric crest. The final braided suture is placed through the edge of the hip capsule in a similar fashion, approximately 1.5 cm below the cephalad suture. This braided capsular suture is cut long to differentiate it from the sutures attached to the tagged short external rotators. The superior tags of the capsule and rotators (clamped with a Kelly clamp) are grouped together, and the inferior tags also are bundled (tagged with a mosquito clamp) for ease of later use (**Figure 2**). The Aufranc retractor is repositioned inside the capsule, and the superior aspect of the quadratus femoris muscle is ligated using electrocautery to reveal the superior aspect of the lesser trochanter. With all retractors removed, the femoral head is dislocated gently from the acetabulum by flexing, adducting, and internally rotating the leg. Once dislocated, the femoral head is rested on the outer superolateral aspect of the acetabulum and labrum. This is best done with the hip held in 0° of flexion, 0° of adduction, and 90° of internal rotation, and the knee in 90° of flexion. A slight proximally directed force vector on the knee will keep the femoral head from relocating back within the acetabulum. We prefer to use a single-sided reciprocating saw blade, with the blade directed away from the saw handle, to perform the femoral neck cut at the templated distance above the lesser trochanter. The femoral head is removed, and the leg is brought to the neutral position. We prepare the acetabulum first and the femur second.

Acetabular Preparation

The table is airplaned toward the surgeon posteriorly about 30°, which is the limit of the table. Acetabular 360° exposure is established by first placing a C retractor anteriorly (at the 3-o'clock position for a right hip, outside the labrum but piercing the anterior hip capsule and hooked over the anterior wall of the acetabulum). Next, after releasing the inferior aspect of the capsule sharply down to the posterior aspect of the transverse acetabular ligament (TAL), a sharp tipped, wide bent Hohmann retractor is impacted posteroinferiorly into the ischium inside the capsule, but outside the labrum. Care is taken to have the tip come to rest firmly in bone approximately 1 cm posterior to the greatest extent of posterior acetabular reaming. A smooth Steinmann pin is slid under the gluteus minimus and then superiorly (roughly to the 12:30 or 1-o'clock position for the right hip, approximately 1 cm from the superiormost point of acetabular reaming) and impacted directly toward the ground. This keeps the gluteus minimus and medius retracted anteriorly. The Steinmann pin is placed last; it is not required if exposure is already adequate. If necessary, an Aufranc retractor can be placed inferiorly (inside the TAL and under the teardrop) to help expose the inferior socket as soft tissue is removed from the socket before acetabular reaming. The Aufranc retractor is removed before acetabular reaming starts.

The soft tissue of the acetabulum is removed sharply with a scalpel and a Kocher clamp. The TAL is preserved as a guide for acetabular orientation. Reaming begins when the soft tissue is removed and the surgeon can identify the cortical bone in the deep portion of the acetabular fossa. We start reaming 8 mm below the templated prediction, carefully moving medially to the medial wall before redirecting the reamer into the appropriate amount of abduction (inclination) and anteversion (generally 40° and 20°, respectively). We ream evenly, with an incremental increase in reamer sizes until three blushes are visible: iliac, pubic, and ischial. An elevator can be used to palpate the pubis if needed. Being mindful of osteophytes, the surgeon should consider marking the anterior acetabular margin with electrocautery and the TAL with a marking pen. The trial is placed, lining it up with the anterior rim and the TAL, and the rim fit is assessed. The trial should be snug but not too tight. If it is too tight, the last reamer (one size larger than the last reamer used) is used to open the mouth of the superficial aspect of the acetabulum. The trial cup is removed, and the actual acetabular implant is placed in the same position. Some experienced surgeons elect to skip the acetabular trialing step, but the correct position of the socket must be verified. The liner is then placed, and the locking mechanism is engaged appropriately. Any impinging osteophytes can now be removed. Next, all retractors are removed and the operating room table is returned to the level position, parallel to the floor.

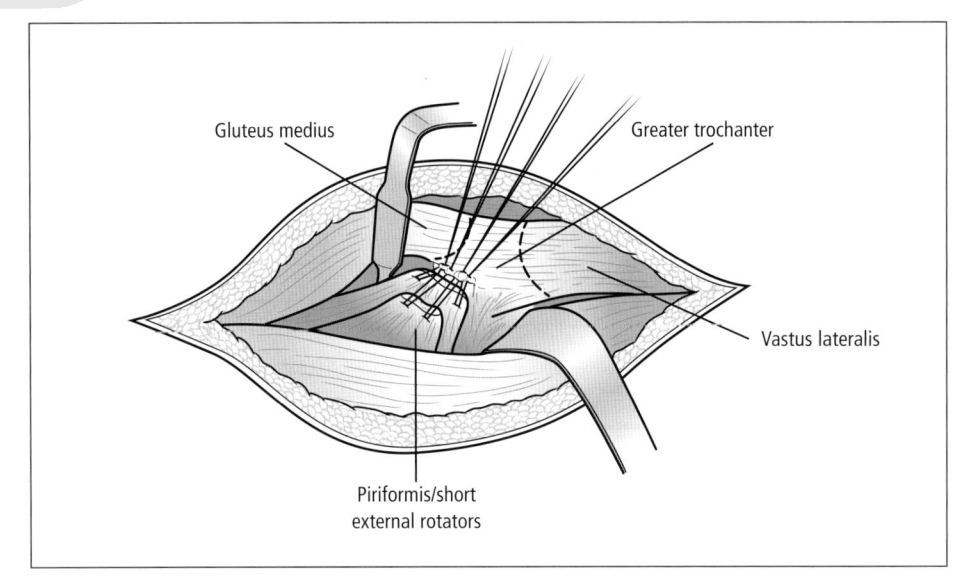

Figure 3 Illustration shows the reapproximation of the muscles and the hip capsule following implant placement for total hip arthroplasty using the small-incision enhanced posterior soft-tissue repair (SIEPSTR) approach. The longer superior and inferior capsular sutures are tied together first. Then the shorter external rotator sutures are tied together to restore the posterior soft-tissue envelope.

Femoral Preparation

The proximal femur is exposed again by placing the corner of a moist lap pad in the cup, internally rotating the hip, and placing a femoral elevator on the anterior aspect of the femur, an Aufranc retractor on this elevator near the calcar area, and a thin bent Hohmann retractor laterally, anterior to the abductor hooked on the cortex of the anterior greater trochanter. The neck cut is revised at this time if necessary. Remnants of the short external rotators are removed, and a slightly anteverted box osteotome is used to enter the femoral canal as posterolaterally as possible. Next, the Charnley awl is passed. Depending on the implant system, the femur is prepared with a reamer and broaches or with broaches alone. After an appropriate fit is obtained, a calcar planer can be used to fine-tune the femoral neck cut, but this usually is not necessary if the saw was used correctly for the neck osteotomy. With the trial broach, neck, and head in place, we check the lesser trochanter–to-center-of-head distance with a 6-in metal ruler, comparing this distance with the preoperative template and adjusting as needed.

Trialing and Final Implant Placement

At this point, the hip should be reduced and the construct should be trialed for stability. Care should be taken to make sure no intervening soft tissue gains access to the socket as the trial femoral head is relocated. The Ranawat combined anteversion is checked by retracting the soft tissues (so that the hip joint can be visualized) and repositioning the leg. When the head is coplanar with the liner, the angle of the tibia with the floor is the combined anteversion. The combined lateral opening can be assessed as well. In general, we aim for 35° to 45° of combined anteversion. With the articulation exposed, we flex the hip up to 90° and then internally rotate the hip. We aim for at least 60° of stable internal rotation. Next, the leg is brought to full extension, and the knee is flexed to check for overly tight anterior musculature. It is useful to test this before the surgery begins to appreciate what the tension was like preoperatively. The surgeon can also check for posterior impingement by externally rotating the leg with the leg in full extension while keeping one finger between the greater trochanter and the ischium. The surgeon should be able to just feel the trochanter with his or her finger at maximal external rotation. If the anterior capsule is too tight, the surgeon will not feel the trochanter. If the reconstruction is too loose, the surgeon's finger will be squeezed, indicating impingement and the need for increased offset or less combined anteversion.

When trialing is complete, we dislocate the hip carefully and remove the provisional trial implants. The surgeon must be careful of the greater trochanter, especially when removing the broaches, and, if cementless fixation is to be used, should consider performing a little more lateral hand rasping if the porous coating of the implant may make the final implant sit proud compared with the trial. Next, the actual femoral component is placed in the same position as the trial. The implant is malleted down carefully until it engages the bone and is stable. Usually this will be accompanied by a pitch change. The lesser trochanter–to-center-of-head distance and offset are measured to make sure they are the same as the trial. If the actual stem sits up higher than the trial, the surgeon should consider using a modular femoral head with a shorter neck length. We then reduce and recheck stability and component position.

The SIEPSTR is initiated by drilling two holes in the posterior aspect of the greater trochanter approximately 1.5 cm apart—the same distance that the braided sutures in the capsule were placed. The proximal sutures are passed through the superior hole, and the distal sutures are passed through the distal hole (**Figure 3**). The leg is placed in a neutral position, and the sutures are tied. The long sutures are tied to each other first because they are attached to the deeper capsular structure. Great care should be taken to tension the capsule, and the surgeon should be able to palpate the edge of the capsule, reaching the posterior aspect of the femur. The shorter sutures are tied to each other in a similar fashion. The rotators also should be palpated at the level of the femur.

Closure

The wound is irrigated copiously with pulsatile lavage. Depending on surgeon preference, subfascial drains can be placed at this point. The fascia is closed and the wound is again irrigated copiously. The closure is completed according to surgeon preference. A sterile dressing is applied. Our current preference is a sealed impervious waterproof silver dressing that allows the patient to shower. A triangular abduction pillow is placed between the legs, and the patient is transferred to the recovery room and then to the floor.

Surgical Technique: Hemiarthroplasty

The SIEPSTR approach can also be used for hemiarthroplasty. As noted previously, the procedure essentially diverges at the moment of capsulotomy. The same positioning and initial exposure steps are used as described previously for THA. Arthrotomy is performed in a similar manner as described for THA, starting posterosuperiorly and extending anteriorly. It is critically important, however, to keep the labrum intact throughout the procedure. The labrum is most at risk during capsulotomy.

Before entering the capsule, we prefer to palpate the posterosuperior aspect of the intact capsule along the line where the posteroinferior border of the gluteus minimus muscle had been attached to the capsule. The surgeon often can feel the junction at which the femoral head meets the posterior wall of the acetabulum beneath the capsule because the anatomy of the acetabulum often is pristine when hemiarthroplasty is being performed. The labrum sits at this junction. The labrum often is difficult to palpate, but it is assumed to lie at the junction of the femoral head with the rim of the posterior wall of the acetabulum. Instead of using electrocautery for this capsular incision (with the hip internally rotated), we prefer to use a scalpel because the hematoma within the socket often causes the electrocautery to work less effectively. Care is taken to stay more than 10 mm from the palpated edge of the acetabulum; this will protect the labrum adequately. With the capsular incision taken to the posterior aspect of the greater trochanter (the trochanteric crest), the superior capsular tagging suture is placed so it can be used to further retract the capsule and further remove it sharply from its attachment more distal to the trochanteric crest. The inferior tagging suture is placed using a Mason-Allen stitch through the edge of the capsule about 1.5 cm distal to the first suture. The capsule is retracted posteriorly, revealing the fractured femoral neck within the hip capsule, and the capsule is incised posteroinferiorly, down toward the posterior aspect of the TAL. The next step is to remove the femoral head and all bony fragments from the acetabulum.

For stable femoral neck fracture patterns, the femoral head may be removed from the socket simply by manipulating the leg as described previously for THA. Usually, however, internal rotation, flexion, and adduction of the hip will not accomplish this. Our preferred method to expose the femoral head for removal is to place the C retractor anteriorly over the anterior wall of the acetabulum (outside the labrum, as with THA). This is done by placing the retractor directly through the fracture site in the femoral neck, which may be easier with the hip internally rotated. For subcapital fractures, a femoral neck osteotomy that is performed with the reciprocating saw the same way as for THA can be done before head removal. This creates space between the head and neck as the intervening segment of bone is removed and facilitates access to the femoral head for removal. If the femoral head does not come out of the acetabulum easily when the edge of the femoral head is grabbed inferiorly with a Kocher clamp, we prefer to use a corkscrew-like device. Once the femoral head is engaged deeply, taking care to avoid screwing through the head, the head may begin to rotate unimpeded by detachment of the ligamentum teres. Care should be taken to not fragment the femoral head or lever unnecessarily on the soft tissues; the surgeon should interpose the palm of his or her contralateral hand and lever on it instead. Fragmentation of the femoral head could make proper measurement of the diameter of the femoral head, which determines the size of the prosthetic femoral head to be used, more challenging. Once the acetabulum is inspected and the surgeon is assured that the acetabulum and labrum are free of cartilage damage and all bony fragments are removed, the socket can be trialed and attention turned to the femoral side of the reconstruction. If any damage to the acetabular cartilage is present, the procedure should be converted to a THA. The surgeon should keep in mind that an undersized head may lead to early acetabular cartilage degeneration due to increased contact pressures. The pulvinar should be left intact. The neck cut can be revised at this time if necessary. Femoral preparation should proceed in the same manner as described previously, using the specific method recommended for the chosen hemiarthroplasty system.

Complications

Complications specific to the posterior approach are minimal. Periprosthetic fractures are extremely rare. A recent analysis of 1,883 THAs demonstrated that the posterior approach is an independent predictor of accurate positioning of the cup. Acetabular components positioned using the posterior approach were 20% more likely than components positioned with any other approach to fall within the window of acceptable abduction and version angles.[6] With the SIEPSTR technique, the superiority of the posterior approach is compounded by the addition of the enhanced soft-tissue repair. As Pellicci et al[3] reported in 1998, the addition of the enhanced soft-tissue repair dropped the dislocation rate from 26 in 555 to 1 in 519, a statistically significant improvement.

Postoperative Care and Rehabilitation

We typically keep our THA patients in the hospital for 2 or 3 days postoperatively. Patients begin weight bearing as tolerated immediately, getting out of bed with assistance at least three times daily, for two physical therapy sessions and one occupational therapy session. Multimodal deep venous thrombosis prophylaxis is used, consisting of early mobilization, lower extremity compression devices, and pharmacologic prophylaxis (aspirin, low-molecular-weight heparin, or warfarin). Pain control is tailored to each patient and consists of short-term intravenous narcotics via patient-controlled analgesia (typically discontinued on postoperative day 1) or oral analgesics with parenteral administration only for breakthrough pain. Patients are discharged to an acute or subacute rehabilitation center or return home, where services typically include home physical therapy and nursing visits. The duration of time spent in the rehabilitation center is variable but usually is 1 to 3 weeks. Depending on the patient's progress, physical therapy continues for approximately 6 to 12 weeks after the surgery.

Pearls

- After positioning the patient on the operating table but before preparing and draping the patient, be sure that full hip range of motion can be achieved.
- A bolster under the knee can help relax the lateral structures and can make the exposure easier.
- Internally rotating the leg prior to removing the piriformis and short external rotators will allow removal of the tendons as close as possible to their insertion points.
- "Airplaning" the table toward the surgeon during acetabular preparation facilitates exposure.
- After the acetabular retractors are in place, flexing the hip slightly will allow further access to the acetabulum and prevent the shaft of the reamer from impinging on the proximal femur.
- Reaming should be done concentrically because there is a tendency with this approach to preferentially ream the posterior wall. The thickness of the posterior wall should be checked by palpation.
- Clear visualization of the inferior neck should always be maintained

when broaching the femur to observe if any fracture has occurred.
- A bone hook is used to dislocate the hip when trialing. This is particularly important in osteoporotic bone.

References

1. Kwon MS, Kuskowski M, Mulhall KJ, Macaulay W, Brown TE, Saleh KJ: Does surgical approach affect total hip arthroplasty dislocation rates? *Clin Orthop Relat Res* 2006;447:34-38.

2. Sculco TP, Jordan LC, Walter WL: Minimally invasive total hip arthroplasty: The Hospital for Special Surgery experience. *Orthop Clin North Am* 2004;35(2):137-142.

3. Pellicci PM, Bostrom M, Poss R: Posterior approach to total hip replacement using enhanced posterior soft tissue repair. *Clin Orthop Relat Res* 1998;355:224-228.

4. Macaulay W, Colacchio ND, Fink LA: Modified enhanced posterior soft tissue repair results in a negligible dislocation rate after hip resurfacing. *Oper Tech Orthop* 2009;19(3):163-168.

5. Macaulay W, Salvati EA: Primary total hip arthroplasty, in Fitzgerald RH, Kaufer H, Malkani AL, eds: *Orthopaedics*. Philadelphia, PA, Elsevier Health Sciences, 2002, pp 900-910.

6. Callanan MC, Jarrett B, Bragdon CR, et al: Risk factors for cup malpositioning: Quality improvement through a joint registry at a tertiary hospital. *Clin Orthop Relat Res* 2011;469(2):319-329.

Chapter 49
Hip Arthroplasty via a Direct Lateral Approach

Tahir Mahmud, BSc (Hons), MBBS, FRCS (Tr & Orth)   Robert B. Bourne, MD, FRCSC

Patient Selection
Indications
The direct lateral approach to the hip, also called the modified Harding[1] or anterolateral approach, can be used for primary and revision total hip arthroplasty (THA). This approach also can be used for the treatment of femoral neck fractures requiring hip arthroplasty. The direct lateral approach preserves the posterior hip capsule and short external rotators, thereby reducing the risk of dislocation in patients who have risk factors for postoperative instability (eg, neuromuscular disorders, dementia, alcoholism).[2-4] Another advantage of this approach is that it avoids direct exposure of the sciatic nerve.[5]

Contraindications
The direct lateral approach may not provide adequate exposure if access to the posterior wall is required for bone grafting or removal of internal fixation devices. Procedures requiring extensive exposure of the superior acetabulum, such as reconstructions involving high hip centers and degenerative dysplasia of the hip, might result in damage to the terminal branch of the superior gluteal nerve (SGN). Therefore, an alternative surgical approach might be considered.[6,7]

Preoperative Imaging
AP radiographs of the pelvis and AP and lateral radiographs of the affected hip are recommended. The radiographs should be templated to determine component size and position and to ensure that leg length and offset are restored. CT can be used in patients with abnormal anatomy (eg, dysplasia, bone loss, subchondral cysts).

Video 49.1 Total Hip Arthroplasty via a Direct Lateral Approach. Tahir Mahmud, BSc (Hons), MBBS, FRCS (Tr & Orth); Robert B. Bourne, MD, FRCSC (3 min)

Procedure
Room Setup/Patient Positioning
The patient is placed in the lateral decubitus position and secured to the operating table using a device with padded pubic and sacral supports. It is important to firmly secure the patient to prevent shifting of position during the procedure.[2] The contralateral leg must be well padded to prevent damage to the common peroneal nerve. A sterile drape bag is placed on the anterior aspect of the patient to keep the ipsilateral leg sterile upon hip dislocation (**Figure 1**).

Special Instruments/Equipment
Using a blunt Hohmann retractor, which has a smooth curve on the end that is inserted into the patient, helps to avoid iatrogenic injury to the neurovascular bundle that sits anterior to the hip joint. The sharp Hohmann retractor, which has a sharp, pointed tip, works well to slip posterior to the acetabulum, between the bone and capsule, to help retract the femur posteriorly.

Surgical Technique: THA
Surgical Approach
A small skin incision is centered over the tip of the greater trochanter and runs slightly oblique from anterodistal to posteroproximal (**Figure 2**). The length of the incision varies from 10 to 15 cm, depending on the size of the patient, but we do not hesitate to lengthen the incision if excessive retraction is required for the visualization needed to perform the THA as safely as possible. The incision is carried down through the subcutaneous tissue and onto the fascia lata, with electrocautery used to ensure hemostasis along the way. An incision is made in the fascia lata distally using a knife. The incision is extended proximally in the interval between the gluteus maximus and the tensor fascia muscle using cutting diathermy. Care should be taken to not extend the fascia lata incision too far posterior, as this will result in splitting of the gluteus maximus muscle too far posteriorly, making retraction of the larger anterior part difficult. A Charnley retractor can be inserted to aid access (**Figure 3**). The trochanteric bursa may then be incised longitudinally.

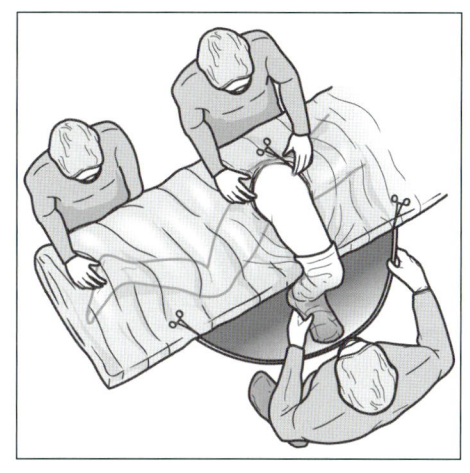

Figure 1 Illustration shows the use of a sterile drape bag to keep the ipsilateral leg sterile during hip arthroplasty via a direct lateral approach.

Exposing the Hip Joint
The muscle fibers of the gluteus medius are bluntly split at the junction of the anterior one third and posterior two thirds of the muscle belly. An anterior sleeve, consisting of the gluteus medius and minimus conjoined tendons and the anterior capsule, are then reflected off the anterior aspect of the greater trochanter and femoral neck down to bone (**Figure 4, A**). The split is carried distally into the vastus lateralis muscle in an omega (Ω)–like fashion (**Figure 4, B**).

Distally, a blunt Hohmann retractor may be placed medially just proximal to the lesser trochanter to facilitate retraction of the soft-tissue sleeve anteriorly, aiding its release off the femoral neck and intertrochanteric line. Care must be taken to not extend the split in the gluteus medius more than 5 cm proximal to the tip of the trochanter. Doing so may result

---

Dr. Bourne or an immediate family member has received royalties from Smith & Nephew; serves as a paid consultant to or is an employee of Smith & Nephew; and serves as a board member, owner, officer, or committee member of the Canadian Joint Replacement Registry and The Knee Society. Neither Dr. Mahmud nor any immediate family member has received anything of value from or has stock or stock options held in a commercial company or institution related directly or indirectly to the subject of this chapter.

Section 4: Adult Reconstruction

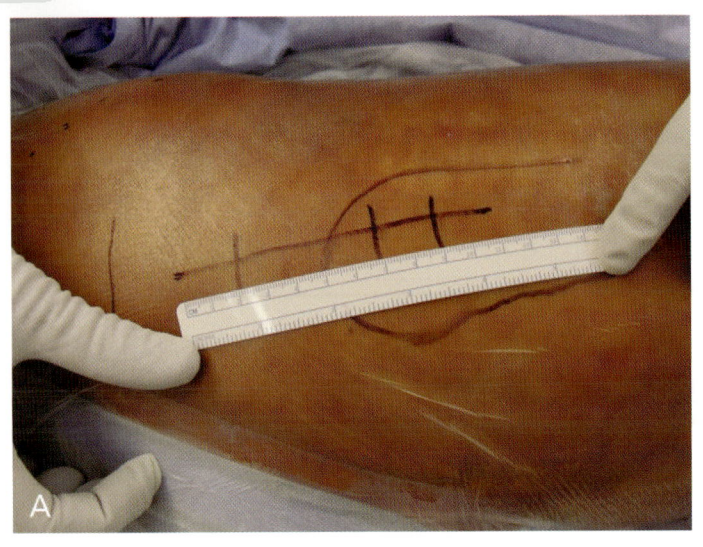

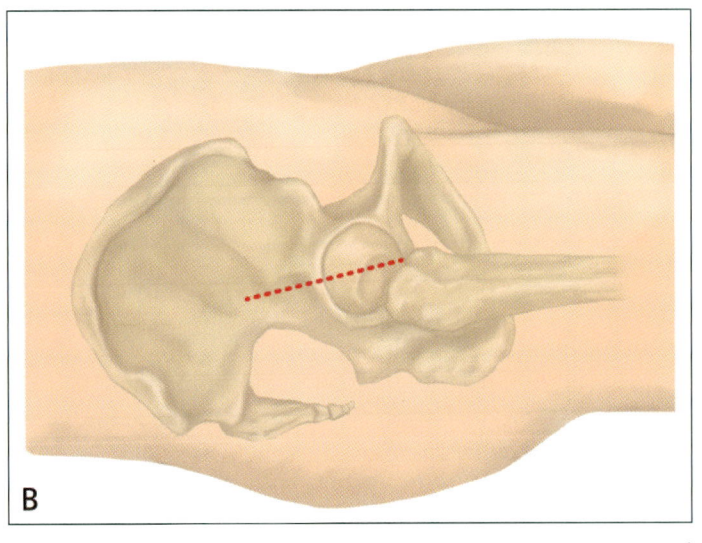

Figure 2 Photograph (**A**) and illustration (**B**) show the skin incision for the direct lateral approach for hip arthroplasty. The incision is centered over the tip of the greater trochanter.

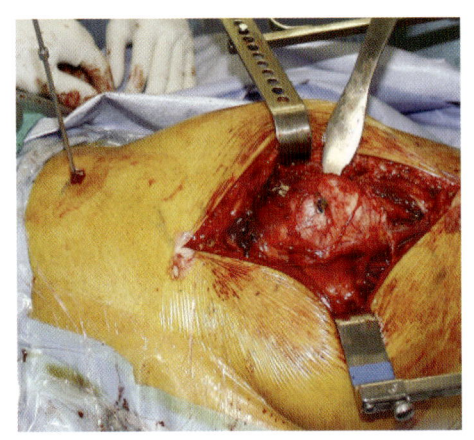

Figure 3 Intraoperative photograph shows a Charnley retractor used to aid exposure for total hip arthroplasty.

in paralysis of part of the gluteus medius and tensor fascia muscles, resulting in a limp and possibly instability.

A Cobb elevator may be used to help sweep away the fat proximally to protect the SGN. The gluteus minimus tendon and underlying capsule are now incised in line with the femoral neck. The incision is taken down to bone, allowing the anterior soft-tissue sleeve, including the gluteus medius, gluteus minimus, and capsule, to be retracted anteriorly. A retractor with a deeper blade can now be inserted to aid in retracting the anterior soft-tissue sleeve.

Prior to dislocating the hip, a femoral offset/leg-length guide is inserted and a reference point on the femur is marked (**Figure 5**). The femoral head is dislocated by flexing and externally rotating the adducted femur carefully. The leg is placed in a leg bag with the tibia perpendicular to the floor. The femoral neck is then osteotomized using an oscillating saw. The level and angle of resection can vary, depending on the type of femoral implant used (**Figure 6**).

Acetabular Preparation

An anterior capsular incision is made with capsular scissors, and a blunt Hohmann retractor is inserted over the anterior rim of the acetabulum (at the 9-o'clock position) to retract the anterior flap of the gluteus medius and the vastus lateralis. Acetabular exposure is achieved by retracting the femur posteriorly with a carefully placed sharp curved Hohmann retractor over the posterior lip of the acetabulum (in the 4-o'clock position for a left hip). Further retraction of the femur is possible following division of the inferior capsule. Exposure of the acetabulum may be further enhanced, if necessary, by placing a sharp Hohmann retractor superiorly to retract the gluteus medius and minimus muscles.

Following excision of the labrum, the acetabulum is sequentially reamed for insertion of the appropriate acetabular component (**Figure 7**). Osteophytes are then removed.

Femoral Preparation

The femur must be readily accessible so it can be reamed and/or broached. Access is improved by placing a blunt curved Hohmann retractor under the posterior greater trochanter. Care must be taken to not trap the sciatic nerve between the retractor and the bone. The femur is then flexed and externally rotated so that the leg is perpendicular to the floor. An additional curved thin Hohmann retractor is placed under the posteromedial neck. The two retractors are used to deliver the femur out of the wound (**Figure 8**).

The overhanging trochanter and the gluteus medius tendon can push the femoral component into a position of flexion and varus. A thin Hohmann retractor can be placed between the trochanter and the gluteus medius tendon to retract it laterally. This retractor also serves to protect the gluteus medius tendon. Following preparation of the femur, a trial reduction and an inspection of the components are essential to ensure that no impingement or instability is present in extension and external rotation and flexion, internal rotation, and adduction.

Wound Closure

The wound is closed in layers. We prefer to use a suture that retains its strength for 4 to 6 weeks, such as a monofilament absorbable suture. The capsule should be repaired if a capsulotomy was performed. The vertical split in the gluteus minimus tendon is reapproximated first with a running suture. The key to a good repair is reapproximating the conjoined gluteus medius and gluteus minimus tendons plus the capsule to the cuff of the tendon insertion left on the anterior aspect of the trochanter.

A strong tendon-to-tendon repair of the gluteus medius and the vastus lateralis with interrupted sutures is vital. A weak repair may result in failure of the repair, resulting in pain, a limp, or instability. The fascia lata and subcutaneous fat layers can be closed with interrupted sutures. The skin may be closed with a subcuticular stitch or with staples.

© 2013 American Academy of Orthopaedic Surgeons

Chapter 49: Hip Arthroplasty via a Direct Lateral Approach

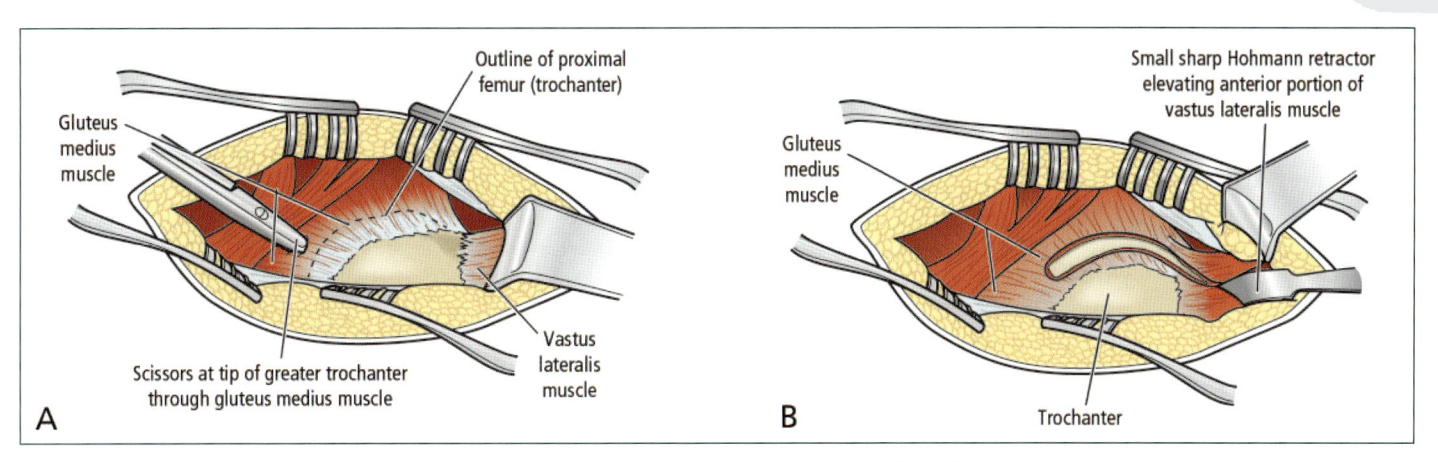

Figure 4 Illustrations demonstrate exposure of the hip joint for total hip arthroplasty. **A,** The gluteus medius muscle is split carefully. **B,** An anterior sleeve consisting of the gluteus medius and minimus conjoined tendons is mobilized anteriorly.

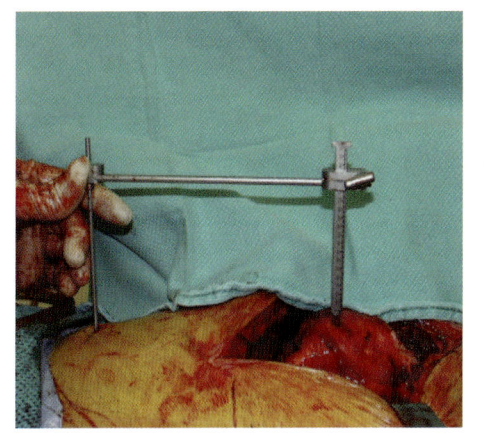

Figure 5 Intraoperative photograph shows the leg-length and offset guide with pin in situ.

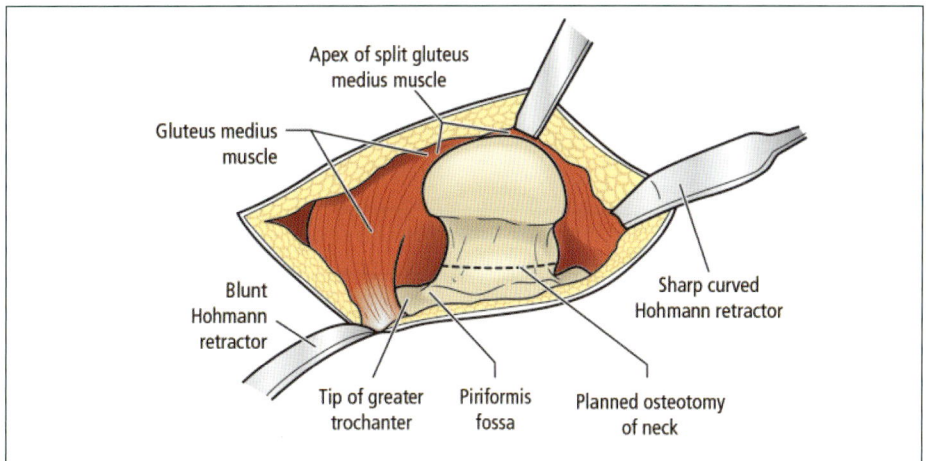

Figure 6 Illustration demonstrates femoral neck osteotomy for total hip arthroplasty.

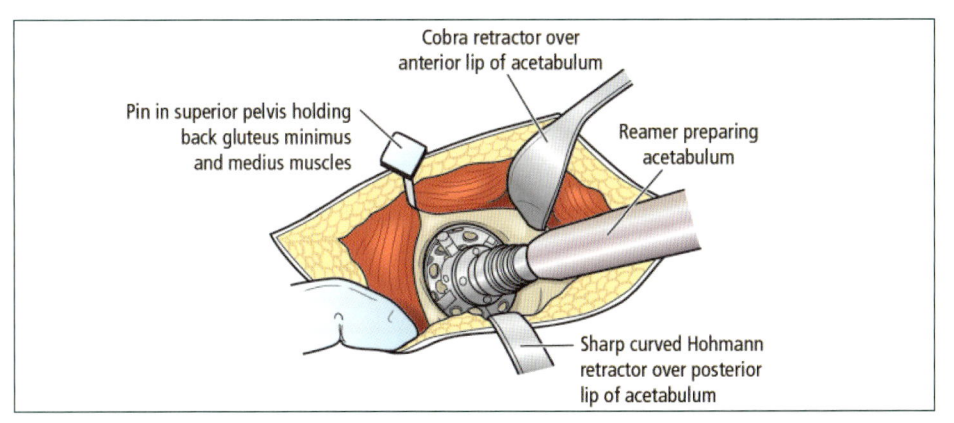

Figure 7 Illustration shows the exposure of the acetabulum to facilitate reaming in a total hip arthroplasty.

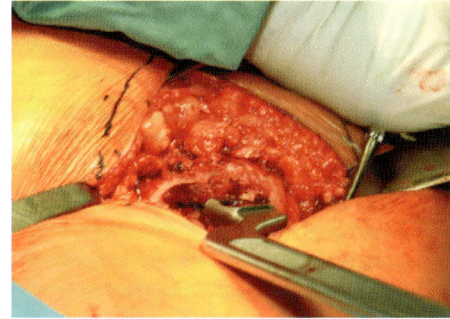

Figure 8 Intraoperative photograph demonstrates the exposure and preparation of the proximal femur for total hip arthroplasty.

Surgical Technique: Hemiarthroplasty

The direct lateral approach also can be used for hemiarthroplasty. The same positioning and initial exposure steps described previously are used. Arthrotomy is performed in a similar manner as described for THA; however, it is critical to keep the labrum intact throughout the procedure. The labrum is most at risk during capsulotomy. Care is taken to stay more than 10 mm from the palpated edge of the acetabulum; this will protect the labrum adequately.

The capsule is retracted anteriorly, revealing the fractured femoral neck within the hip capsule. A deeper anterior Charnley retractor blade can be inserted to aid in retracting the anterior soft-tissue sleeve. The next step is to perform the femoral neck osteotomy to the desired resection level using a reciprocating saw (per the preoperative plan). This is performed with the leg in the leg bag and with the tibia perpendicular to the floor (as described previously for THA). Performing the femoral neck osteotomy creates space between the head and neck as the intervening segment of bone is

© 2013 American Academy of Orthopaedic Surgeons

removed and facilitates access to the femoral head for removal.

The next step is to remove the femoral head (and all bony fragments) from the acetabulum. This is best performed with the leg back on the operating table. Acetabular exposure is achieved by retracting the femur posteriorly with a carefully placed Langenbeck retractor around the medial calcar. Gentle longitudinal traction on the leg may help to improve acetabular exposure. We prefer to use a corkscrew-like device for femoral head extraction. Once the femoral head is engaged deeply (screwing through the head should be avoided), the head may begin to rotate unimpeded by detachment of the ligamentum teres. Care should be taken to not fragment the femoral head or lever unnecessarily on the soft tissues. We recommend that the surgeon interpose the palm of the contralateral hand and lever on the hand instead. Fragmentation of the femoral head could make proper measurement of the diameter of the femoral head—which determines the size of the prosthetic femoral head to be used—more challenging.

Once the acetabulum is inspected (and the surgeon is assured that the acetabulum and labrum are free of cartilage damage) and all bony fragments are removed, the socket can be trialed and attention can be turned to the femoral side of the reconstruction. If any damage to the acetabular cartilage is present, the procedure should be converted to a THA. The surgeon must keep in mind that an undersized head may lead to early acetabular cartilage degeneration due to increased contact pressures. The pulvinar should be left intact. The neck cut can be revised at this time if necessary. Femoral preparation should proceed in the same manner as described previously, using the specific method for the chosen hemiarthroplasty system.

Complications

General postoperative complications include wound infection, deep hip sepsis, thromboembolic events, bleeding, heterotopic ossification, limb-length discrepancy, hip dislocation, sciatic nerve injury, and periprosthetic fracture.[8]

Approach-specific complications include nerve injury (eg, neurapraxia, axonotmesis, neurotmesis) to the terminal branch of the SGN with denervation of the abductor muscles (rare), dehiscence of the surgical repair (rare), fracture of the greater trochanter, limp, and trochanteric bursitis. To avoid a postoperative limp, care must be taken to avoid injury to the SGN while splitting the gluteus medius muscle proximally and to ensure a strong repair of the gluteus medius tendon.

Postoperative Care and Rehabilitation

Our preference is to allow weight bearing as tolerated, progressing from crutches, to a single crutch, to a cane, and then to independent ambulation. Resisted ab-

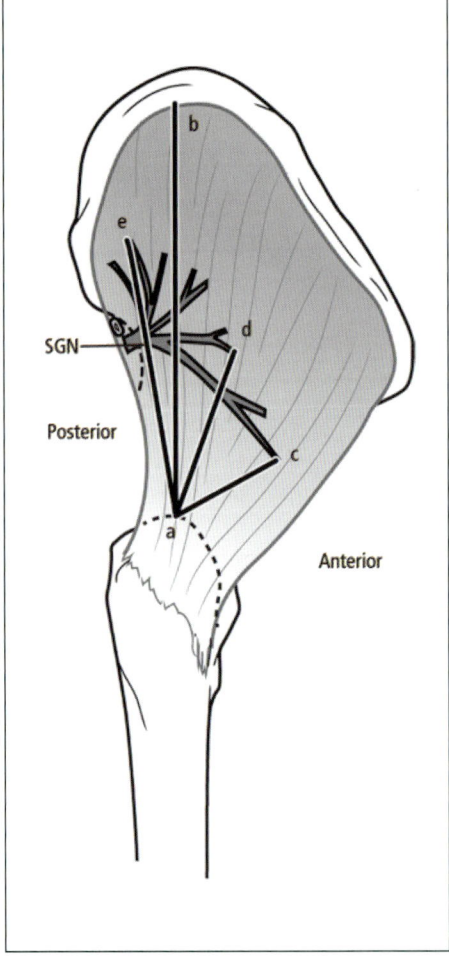

Figure 9 Illustration depicts the relationship of the superior gluteal nerve (SGN) to the greater trochanter. a = tip of the greater trochanter; b = gluteal ridge; c = inferior branch of the SGN; d = middle branch of the SGN; e = superior branch of the SGN.

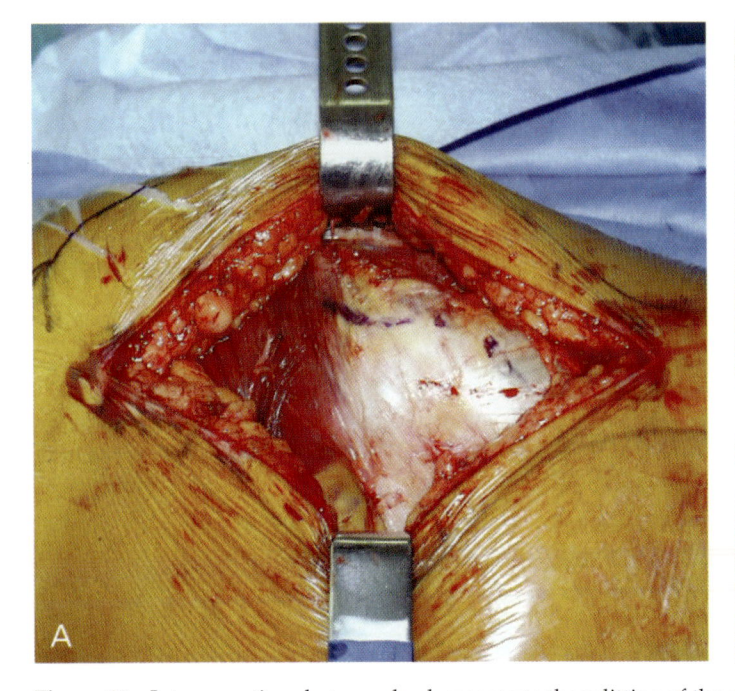

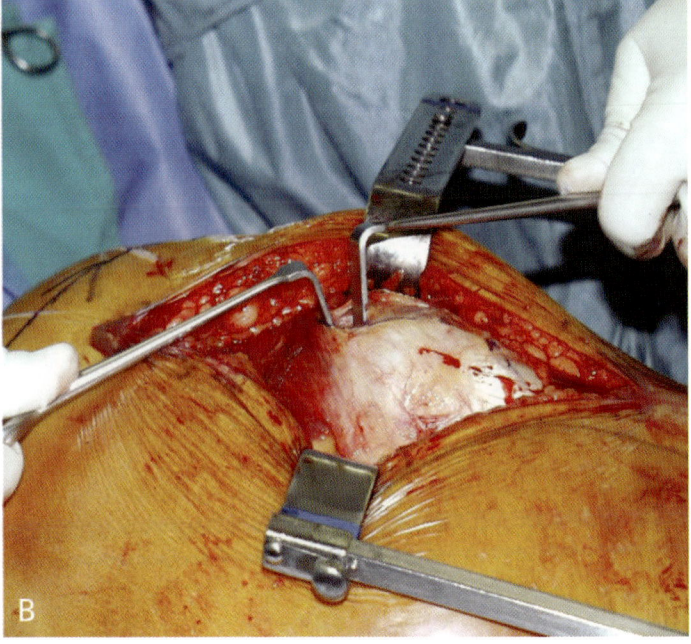

Figure 10 Intraoperative photographs demonstrate the splitting of the gluteus medius muscle at the tendinous junction in total hip arthroplasty. **A,** The gluteus medius musculotendinous insertion onto the greater trochanter is shown. **B,** The gluteus medius muscle is split at the level of the greater trochanter.

ductor strengthening exercises are deferred for the first 6 weeks.

Pearls

- To prevent damage to the SGN, the height of the split in the gluteus medius muscle should be limited. The terminal branch of the SGN runs obliquely in a thin layer of fat between the gluteus medius and minimus tendons, coursing 9 cm proximal to the posterior aspect of the greater trochanter and 5 cm proximal to the anterior aspect of the greater trochanter (**Figure 9**). The SGN can be protected by gentle retraction of the nerve superiorly.
- To ensure a strong abductor repair,[9] the gluteus medius muscle should be split at the tendinous junction, just anterior to the greater trochanter, leaving a cuff of tendon on both sides of the split (**Figure 10**).

References

1. Hardinge K: The direct lateral approach to the hip. *J Bone Joint Surg Br* 1982;64(1):17-19.
2. Masonis JL, Bourne RB: Surgical approach, abductor function, and total hip arthroplasty dislocation. *Clin Orthop Relat Res* 2002;405:46-53.
3. Demos HA, Rorabeck CH, Bourne RB, MacDonald SJ, McCalden RW: Instability in primary total hip arthroplasty with the direct lateral approach. *Clin Orthop Relat Res* 2001;393:168-180.
4. Kwon MS, Kuskowski M, Mulhall KJ, Macaulay W, Brown TE, Saleh KJ: Does surgical approach affect total hip arthroplasty dislocation rates? *Clin Orthop Relat Res* 2006;447:34-38.
5. Ritter MA, Harty LD, Keating ME, Faris PM, Meding JB: A clinical comparison of the anterolateral and posterolateral approaches to the hip. *Clin Orthop Relat Res* 2001;385:95-99.
6. Jacobs LG, Buxton RA: The course of the superior gluteal nerve in the lateral approach to the hip. *J Bone Joint Surg Am* 1989;71(8):1239-1243.
7. Picado CH, Garcia FL, Marques W Jr: Damage to the superior gluteal nerve after direct lateral approach to the hip. *Clin Orthop Relat Res* 2007;455:209-211.
8. Mulliken BD, Rorabeck CH, Bourne RB, Nayak N: A modified direct lateral approach in total hip arthroplasty: A comprehensive review. *J Arthroplasty* 1998;13(7):737-747.
9. Vaz MD, Kramer JF, Rorabeck CH, Bourne RB: Isometric hip abductor strength following total hip replacement and its relationship to functional assessments. *J Orthop Sports Phys Ther* 1993;18(4):526-531.

Chapter 50
Direct Anterior Approach for Hip Arthroplasty

Gregory K. Deirmengian, MD William J. Hozack, MD

Introduction

Total hip arthroplasty (THA) is one of the most successful surgical procedures in modern medicine. The procedure reliably relieves pain, restores function, and improves quality of life for most patients with debilitating hip arthritis. Successful achievement of the technical goals of THA requires surgical exposure of the acetabulum and proximal femur. This may be achieved through one of many well-described and commonly used approaches, each with its own advantages and disadvantages.

The long-term success of THA has been well established. Recent attention has been placed on early outcomes and the achievement of a rapid recovery. It appears that this goal may be attained through the integration of a combination of tactics, including patient education and preconditioning, anesthesia, surgical technique, aggressive postoperative physical therapy, and modern approaches to pain management.[1-3] The literature has placed considerable focus on elements of surgical technique that may influence the speed of recovery.

The most common approaches for THA include the posterior approach and the modified Hardinge (also called direct lateral) approaches. Attempts to minimize the invasiveness of these approaches have involved limiting the size of the skin incision and the extent of the corresponding deep dissection. Several studies have shown, however, that the size of the skin incision does not influence the speed of recovery.[4] Furthermore, in inexperienced hands, small-incision surgery may lead to inadequate exposure, resulting in technical errors that may compromise the long-term outcome of the procedure.[5]

The direct anterior approach is a modification of the classic Smith Petersen approach and was first described for use in THA by Judet in 1947.[6] Recently, the direct anterior approach has become popular for THA because of its unique potential for achieving the goals of the procedure while minimizing the splitting or detaching of muscles or tendons. Careful technique leads to minimization of soft-tissue trauma, which is known to affect rapid recovery. As with any approach to the hip, proper exposure is the most important factor in achieving proper component sizing and positioning. This chapter describes our method of achieving appropriate exposure and minimizing soft-tissue trauma with the direct anterior approach.

Patient Selection
Indications
The direct anterior approach may be used in almost any patient.

Contraindications
Proficiency in THA through a direct anterior approach is like any other surgical procedure in that it involves a learning curve.[7] Careful patient selection is critical during the time when the surgeon is becoming comfortable with the approach. As with any other hip approach, the direct anterior approach is more challenging in patients who are obese or muscular, or in whom the femoral neck is short and varus (**Figure 1**). In addition, more complicated cases, such as those involving dysplasia, deformity, or prior surgery, should be avoided until the surgeon and other members of the surgical team achieve proficiency in the approach.

Obesity that involves excessive soft-tissue folds that override the area of the skin incision is a relative contraindication to the direct anterior approach. Although such soft-tissue folds may be retracted during surgery, they raise the risk of wound healing complications in the postoperative period. Also, although the direct anterior approach is extensile, cases that require more extensive femoral exposure, such as those involving femoral deformity or femoral revision arthroplasty, are likely better served with an alternative approach.

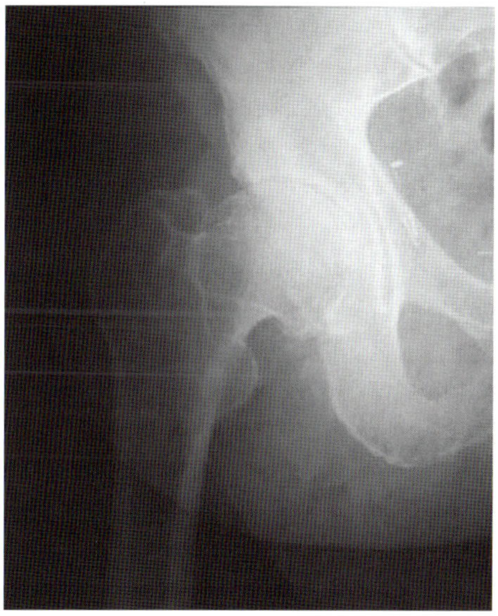

Figure 1 AP radiograph of the hip demonstrates a short, varus femoral neck. This anatomic pattern is associated with a difficult reconstruction.

Preoperative Imaging
Radiographic evaluation is standard for all hip approaches. AP radiographs of the pelvis and hip and a lateral radiograph of the hip are obtained and reviewed. The radiographs also are used for templating with standard overlay templates or with a digital templating system. Preoperative prediction of the appropriate component sizes may provide important clues in the intraoperative setting. For example, if the femoral trial broach is several sizes smaller than the size predicted with templating, then the surgeon may have inadequately lateralized the broach in preparing the femur.

Video 50.1 Direct Anterior Approach for Total Hip Arthroplasty. Gregory K. Deirmengian, MD; William J. Hozack, MD (23 min)

Procedure
Room Setup/Patient Positioning
Many surgeons who perform this procedure use a specialized table that facilitates

---

Dr. Deirmengian or an immediate family member is a member of a speakers' bureau or has made paid presentations on behalf of Angiotech; serves as a paid consultant to or is an employee of Synthes, Angiotech, Zimmer, and Biomet; and has stock or stock options held in CD Diagnostics. Dr. Hozack or an immediate family member has received royalties from Stryker; serves as a paid consultant to or is an employee of Stryker; has received research or institutional support from Stryker; and serves as a board member, owner, officer, or committee member of The Hip Society.

Section 4: Adult Reconstruction

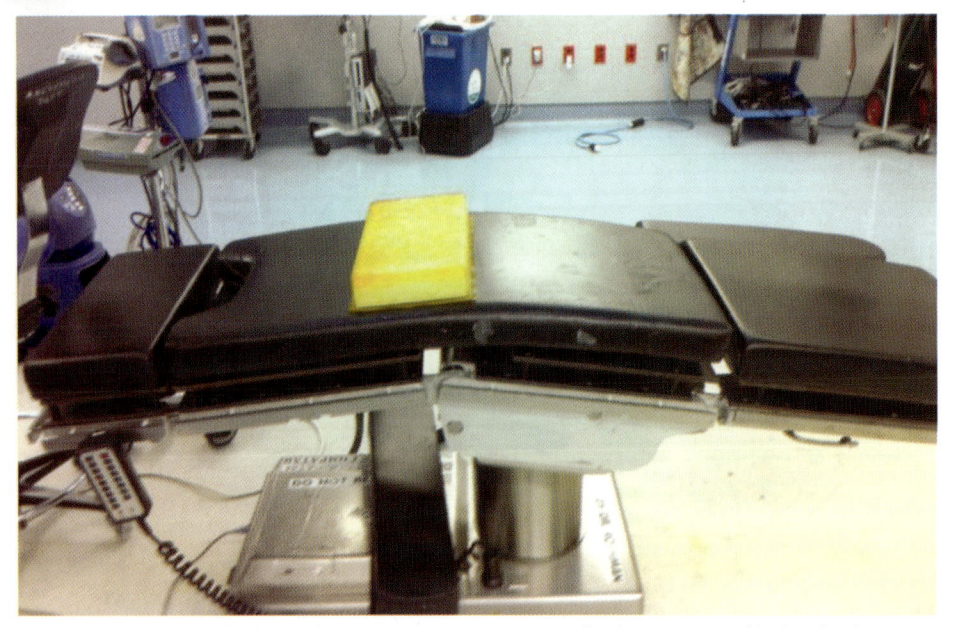

Figure 2 Photograph shows the room setup using a standard operating table for the direct anterior approach for total hip arthroplasty. The gel bump, 30° of table flexion, and the distal arm board on the nonsurgical side of the table facilitate the extension and adduction of the surgical lower extremity necessary for femoral exposure.

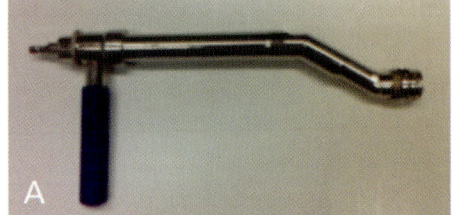

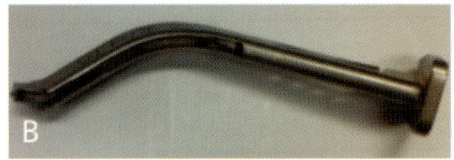

Figure 3 Photographs depict the specialized angled and offset acetabular (**A**) and femoral (**B**) instruments that are essential for the direct anterior approach for total hip arthroplasty.

the positioning of the surgical extremity in a manner that optimizes proximal femoral exposure. Our preference is to perform the procedure with the patient in the supine position on a standard table. We achieve the flexion, adduction, and external rotation of the surgical hip that is required for adequate exposure to ensure safe and effective femoral preparation as follows: Hip flexion is achieved by placing a gel bump under the patient's pelvis and by flexing the table approximately 30° at the time of femoral exposure (**Figure 2**). During patient setup, the gel bump is placed just proximal to the break of the operating table to allow for extension of the hip as the operating table is flexed. Adduction is achieved with the use of an arm board attached to the distal aspect of the nonsurgical side of the table. At the time of femoral exposure, the nonsurgical leg is placed on the arm board, opening space on the table for placement of the surgical extremity in an adducted position. External rotation is achieved by gentle manipulation by an assistant. We typically perform the procedure with six team members: the surgeon and first assistant on the operating side of the table, a second assistant on the nonsurgical side of the table, a surgical technician at the foot of the bed, the anesthesia team member at the head of the table, and a circulating nurse.

Using a standard table for the direct anterior approach has several advantages and avoids some of the disadvantages associated with specialized tables. Standard tables are familiar to all operating room staff members, are used for most other orthopaedic procedures, and are associated with time and cost savings. Using a standard table allows faster patient setup, draping, and room turnover. It also allows more controlled manipulation of the extremity during femoral exposure and preparation. As a result, the increased risk of ankle and trochanteric fracture that has been associated with the use of specialized tables is minimized. Lastly, with a standard table, the surgical extremity is draped free, allowing better assessment of motion, stability, and leg length.

Special Instruments/ Equipment/Implants

The direct anterior approach does not dictate or limit the components used for reconstruction, but it is of utmost importance that the chosen system has the specially designed curved, angled, or offset instrumentation available for acetabular and femoral preparation and component implantation (**Figure 3**). The use of standard instrumentation may lead to inadequate or inappropriate access to the femur and acetabulum, which may result in technical errors and/or undue soft-tissue damage. In addition, certain femoral component design features, such as a reduced lateral shoulder and contoured distal tip, facilitate femoral reconstruction with the direct anterior approach.

Surgical Technique: THA
Incision Planning and Superficial Dissection

Careful planning of the skin incision is one of the most critical aspects of the direct anterior approach. The superior, inferior, and medial borders of the anterior superior iliac spine (ASIS) are palpated and marked. The superior aspect of the incision starts 2 to 3 cm distal and 2 to 3 cm posterior to the inferomedial aspect of the ASIS. The incision is continued distally with a gentle posterior angle (**Figure 4, A**). In slender individuals, the borders of the tensor fascia lata (TFL) are palpable. The incision should be located in the mid-aspect of the TFL, following its course from proximal to distal. The incision length is typically 8 to 10 cm, but it is critical that the surgeon err on the side of enlarging the incision when necessary to improve the exposure, relax the soft tissues, and avoid undue soft-tissue injury.

The skin and subcutaneous tissue are incised, and subcutaneous bleeders are carefully cauterized. Below the subcutaneous tissue, a thin fascia layer is encountered and incised (**Figure 4, B**). Underneath the fascia lies a thin layer of fat that is bluntly swept to expose the TFL. Careful planning of the incision of the thin fascia that encases the TFL is critical. Typically, the mid-aspect of the TFL muscle can be visualized through the thin fascia. Laterally, the fascia becomes thicker, obscuring visualization of the muscle. Medially, a fat stripe often is visible deep to the fascia at the medial border of the TFL. Lastly, small vessels

Chapter 50: Direct Anterior Approach for Hip Arthroplasty

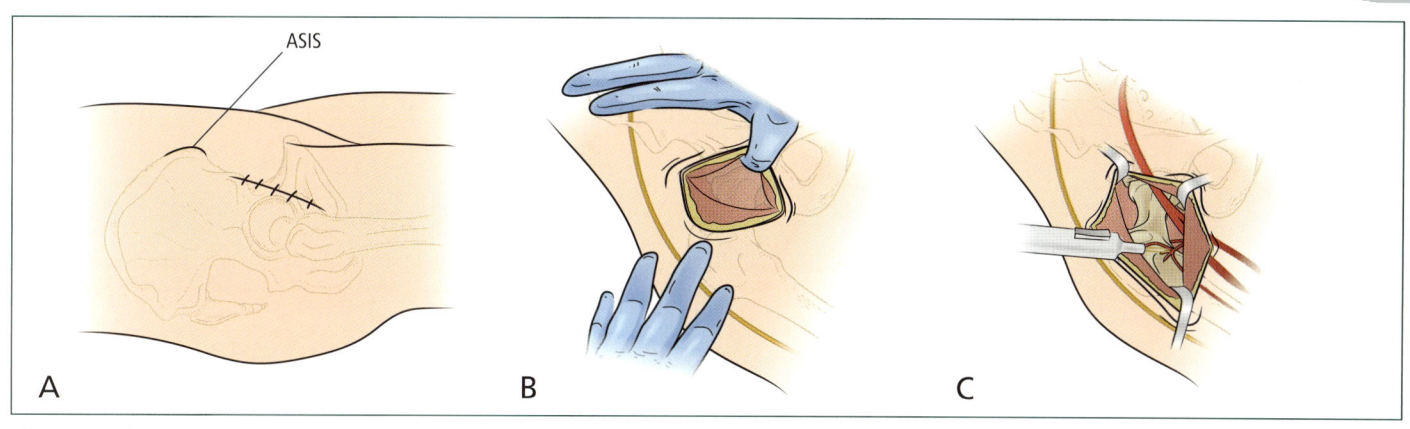

Figure 4 Illustrations demonstrate incision planning, dissection, and exposure for total hip arthroplasty using the direct anterior approach. **A,** The anterior superior iliac spine (ASIS) is marked as a landmark. The marking for the incision starts 2 to 3 cm distal and 2 to 3 cm lateral to the inferomedial corner of the ASIS and proceeds distally 8 to 10 cm with a gentle lateral angle. **B,** Superficial exposure. After the skin and subcutaneous tissue are incised, a thin layer of fascia (Scarpa fascia) is encountered. The fascia is partially incised for demonstration purposes. **C,** The lateral femoral circumflex vessels and their branches are cauterized.

often perforate the thin fascia at the mid-aspect of the TFL; the number, pattern, and location of these vessels vary. After these combined landmarks are used to define the anatomy, the thin fascia is sharply incised at the mid-aspect of the TFL in line with the skin incision. Care is taken to avoid damaging the underlying muscle with the scalpel. Next, the medial border of the incised fascia is dissected free of the TFL muscle, and this path is followed until the medial border of the muscle is encountered. The stripe of fat within the Smith Petersen interval is visualized when the medial border of the TFL is encountered.

With blunt dissection in a posterior direction around the medial aspect of the TFL, the surgeon's finger encounters the anterior capsule over the femoral neck. With continued blunt dissection posterolaterally, the surgeon's finger passes into the space between the abductor musculature and the capsule overlying the lateral femoral neck. A blunt angled Hohmann retractor is placed in this space. Next, a sharp angled Hohmann retractor is placed on the vastus ridge, retracting the TFL laterally. These retractors expose a thin layer of fascia overlying the vastus lateralis and anterior femoral neck. From distal to proximal, this layer is incised, exposing the lateral femoral circumflex vasculature. These vessels are carefully and thoroughly cauterized (**Figure 4, C**).

Next, blunt dissection is undertaken to gain access to the space adjacent to the capsule over the medial femoral neck, where a blunt angled Hohmann retractor is placed. The anterior pericapsular fat is then removed. At this point, the entire anterior capsule overlying the femoral neck should be cleanly exposed, with the superior blunt Hohmann retractor exposing the lateral capsule and the inferior blunt Hohmann retractor exposing the medial capsule. Next, the capsule over the femoral head and anterior acetabular lip is exposed. A Cobb elevator is used to develop the space between this region of the capsule and the rectus femoris muscle. A sharp Hohmann retractor with a light source is placed over the capsule covering the anterior acetabular lip, retracting the rectus femoris muscle. At this point, the entire anterior hip capsule should be cleanly exposed (**Figure 5**).

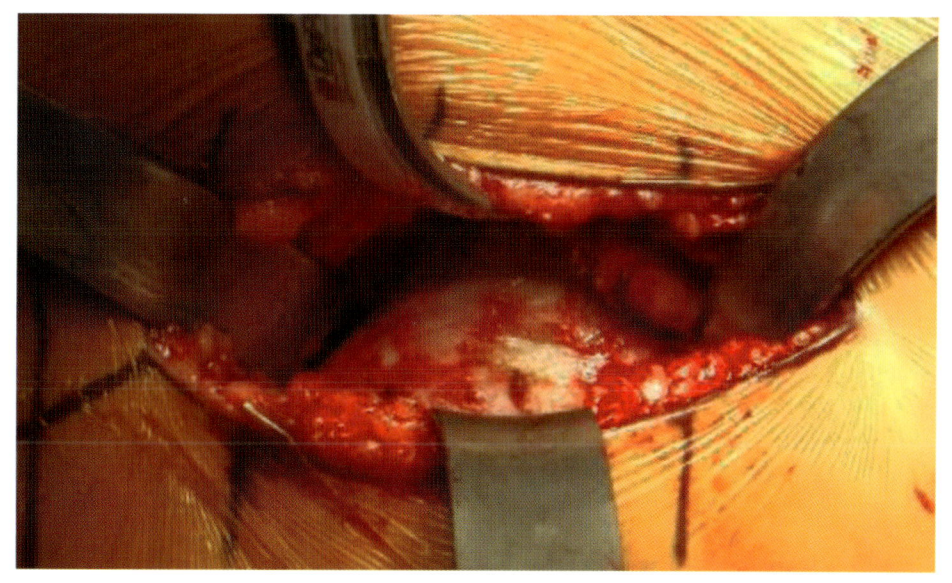

Figure 5 Intraoperative photograph shows the full exposure of the anterior capsule of the hip for total hip arthroplasty using the direct anterior approach.

Acetabular Exposure

We prefer to excise the anterior capsule; in our experience, this technique has no appreciable negative clinical consequence. The capsule is first incised in line with the planned femoral neck cut. This incision starts at the point of origin of the anterior fibers of the vastus lateralis and proceeds inferomedially at a 45° angle. Care is taken to identify the saddle of the femoral neck, which is to be used as a landmark for the femoral neck cut. The second incision is made perpendicular to the first incision, starting at the level of the anterior acetabular lip and proceeding inferolaterally until it intersects the middle of the first incision. The medial and lateral capsular flaps that result from these incisions are then excised. Next, the blunt retractors that contain the femoral neck are repositioned within the capsule (**Figure 6, A**).

The femoral neck is osteotomized with an oscillating saw at two sites, and a 1- to 2-cm wafer of bone is removed. This

© 2013 American Academy of Orthopaedic Surgeons

Section 4: Adult Reconstruction

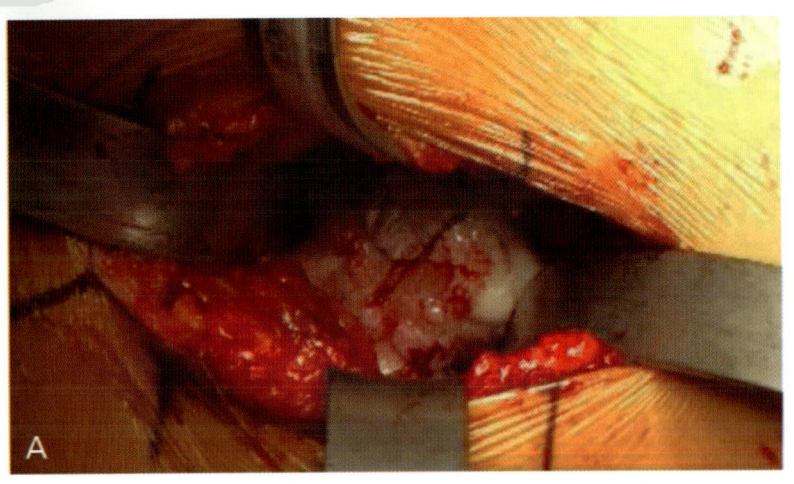

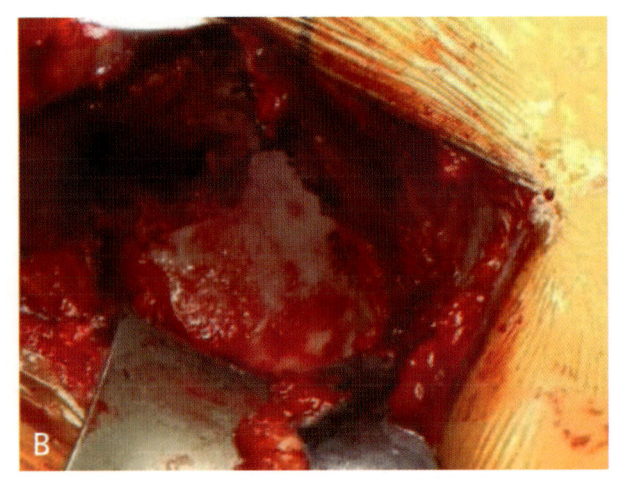

Figure 6 Intraoperative photographs demonstrate acetabular exposure for total hip arthroplasty using the direct anterior approach. **A**, Exposure of the intact femoral head and neck within the acetabulum after the anterior hip capsule has been incised. **B**, Exposure of the acetabulum after the retractors have been placed, the obscuring soft tissues have been excised, and osteophytes have been removed. Full exposure of all anatomic landmarks, including the entire rim of the acetabulum, is critical.

technique improves access to the femoral head and aids in its removal in an atraumatic manner. The first osteotomy is performed at the level of the femoral head-neck junction, perpendicular to the femoral neck. After completing the cut, an osteotome is inserted and twisted to further mobilize the femoral head from its soft-tissue attachments. The second osteotomy begins at the saddle of the femoral neck and proceeds in an inferomedial direction at an angle that matches the geometry of the femoral component. The osteotome is inserted into this cut and twisted, mobilizing the femoral neck wafer, which is then carefully removed. Using the space that results from removal of the femoral neck wafer, a corkscrew is driven into the femoral head, and the corkscrew and the attached femoral head are carefully removed from the wound.

The sharp angled retractor that is attached to the light source is then moved into an intercapsular position. Next, a sharp double-angle or Muller-type retractor is placed behind the posteroinferior acetabular lip, retracting the femur posteriorly. The medial capsule is visualized, and a small capsulotomy is performed just inferior to the acetabular teardrop. The tip of an angled blunt Hohmann retractor is placed within the capsulotomy site, and then the tip of the retractor is advanced and placed inferior to the teardrop. After placement of the acetabular retractors, the bony acetabular anatomy is clearly exposed and identified. The acetabular labrum and periacetabular osteophytes are completely removed. Osteophytes and soft tissues that obscure the acetabular teardrop must be obtained also are removed. A complete 360° view of the acetabular rim and the medial teardrop must be obtained before proceeding with acetabular reaming (**Figure 6, B**).

Acetabular Preparation and Component Implantation

For initial acetabular reaming, a small reamer and a straight reamer handle are used. With initial acetabular preparation to a hemispherical shape, the planned position of the final component is envisioned. Larger reamers are then progressively placed in this position and used to ream the remaining cartilage to a bed of bleeding subchondral bone. During reaming, care must be taken to avoid eccentric anterior, posterior, or lateral reaming. These errors are typically the result of soft tissues misdirecting the reamer handle and can be prevented by using offset reamer handles (**Figure 3**). In addition, the sharp reamer edges may cause undue soft-tissue damage with insertion and removal through the wound. Such trauma can be avoided by carefully maneuvering the larger reamer through the wound and then attaching the offset reamer handle once the reamer is positioned within the acetabulum. Once the reaming is completed, the handle is detached from the reamer within the acetabulum, and then the free reamer is carefully maneuvered out of the wound.

After reaming is completed to the appropriate size, the final component is placed. An offset acetabular component insertion handle should be used because a straight insertion handle may lead to inappropriate component positioning due to misdirection induced by the soft tissue. Once the final component is impacted, complete seating is verified through the insertion hole. If necessary, one or more screws may be placed to augment the initial component fixation. The space around the rim of the cup is then inspected to ensure that the component is completely contained within the acetabulum and that all overhanging osteophytes have been removed. The liner is then inserted into the wound and impacted to lock it within the acetabular component.

Femoral Exposure

Femoral exposure is often the most challenging aspect of the direct anterior approach. Without proper exposure, accurate femoral preparation with minimal soft-tissue injury is impossible. With a series of steps involving retractor placement, leg positioning, and soft-tissue releases, the proximal femur is maneuvered around the acetabulum and delivered to the wound. After inserting the acetabular component, the inferior and posterior retractors are removed, but the anterior lighted retractor is left in place. At this point, the bed is flexed approximately 30°, the nonsurgical leg is shifted to the arm board, and the surgical leg is gently held in an adducted and externally rotated position by an assistant. A sharp angled retractor is placed on the vastus ridge, retracting the TFL. These maneuvers expose the cut surface of the femoral neck and the surrounding soft tissues.

Next, a Muller-type retractor is placed in the plane between the remaining lateral capsule and the abductor musculature. This interval typically can be identified by palpation, with the capsule feeling firm and the muscle feeling soft. With the retractor protecting the abductor musculature, the lateral capsule is excised

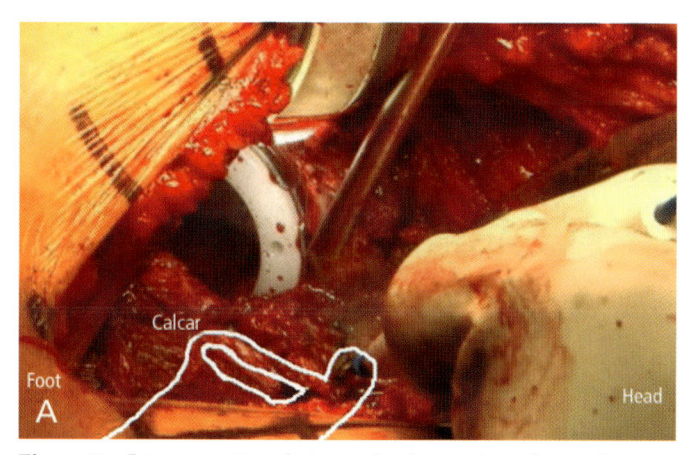

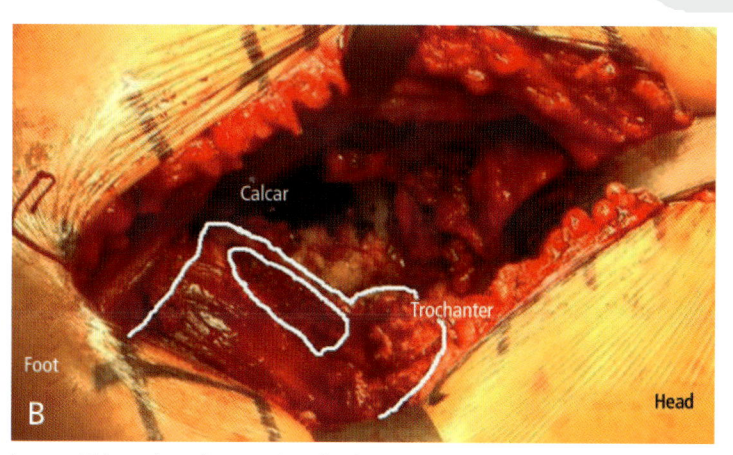

Figure 7 Intraoperative photographs demonstrate femoral exposure for total hip arthroplasty using the direct anterior approach. The superior aspect of the wound is shown, with the proximal femoral bony anatomy outlined in white. **A,** The anterior retractor attached to the light source rests on the anterior aspect of the acetabulum. An electrocautery instrument releases soft tissues to allow femoral elevation. **B,** A Muller-type retractor rests posterior to the trochanter, maintaining its elevated state. A second Muller-type retractor rests on the posteromedial aspect of the calcar.

from the saddle of the femoral neck to the rim of the acetabulum. After the lateral capsule is removed, the Muller-type retractor is placed between the tip of the greater trochanter and the abductor musculature. The purpose of this retractor is to retract the abductor musculature and to maintain the elevated position of the proximal femur once this is achieved. A bone hook is placed into the cut surface of the femoral neck and gentle pressure is applied, placing tension on the posterolateral soft tissues. These tissues are carefully incised (**Figure 7, B**), leading to the delivery of the proximal femur into the wound. The anterior retractor with a light source is removed from the anterior acetabulum and replaced by a second Muller-type retractor placed along the posterior cortex of the remaining femoral neck (**Figure 7, B**).

Femoral Preparation, Trialing, and Component Implantation

Several technical tips facilitate accurate femoral preparation while minimizing unnecessary soft-tissue trauma. First, adequate proximal femoral exposure must be maintained. One assistant maintains the extended, adducted, and externally rotated position of the surgical extremity while the other maintains the elevated position of the proximal femur with the Muller-type retractor. Second, a femoral system that provides broach handles with offset must be used.[8] With a straight broach handle, the soft tissues misdirect the broaching and become damaged in the process. Lastly, a femoral system with certain important features, including a reduced lateral shoulder, facilitates insertion and removal of the broaches into the femoral canal with minimal soft-tissue trauma.

Proximal femoral preparation begins with removal of lateral bone with a box osteotome and/or a rasp, which helps avoid inappropriate varus stem positioning. A curved curet is then used as a canal finder. Next, broaching proceeds. The size of the final broach is determined by preoperative templating and intraoperative assessment. The tendency to direct the broach in an anterior-to-posterior direction must be avoided. The trial neck and head are placed on the broach, the retractors are removed, and the hip is reduced with gentle traction of the extremity and pressure applied to the trial in a posterior direction.

Next, soft-tissue balancing and leg length are assessed. Soft-tissue balancing is determined by evaluating the tension with reduction of the hip, the stability when taking the hip through a complete range of motion, and the amount of ball and liner separation that occurs with manual traction of the extremity. The leg length is easily determined by palpating the level of the medial malleoli and/or heels. Trial heads and necks are exchanged until appropriate soft-tissue balance and leg length are achieved. The hip is dislocated with manual traction of the extremity combined with an anterolateral force on the proximal femur provided by the surgeon's finger or a bone hook.

After removal of the trial head, neck, and broach, the final stem is inserted. The stem is first inserted manually and advanced completely. Next, the insertion handle is applied (but not attached) to the stem and then gently impacted. Angling the insertion handle posteroinferiorly with impaction allows the stem to slide into its appropriate position and relieves stress from the calcar. These techniques facilitate correct positioning and orientation of the stem while minimizing the risk of fracture. The final head is impacted onto the trunion, and the hip is reduced. The operating table is then reset into its normal position.

Closure

After thorough irrigation, the lateral circumflex vessels are reexposed and recauterized as necessary. These vessels should be reevaluated because they often begin to bleed when the soft tissues around them are manipulated during the procedure. The fascia of the TFL is carefully closed. Grasping only a few millimeters of the cuff of fascia medially prevents incarceration of branches of the lateral femoral cutaneous nerve. A tapered suture needle helps maintain the integrity of the thin fascia of the TFL. Next, the deep fat layer is closed. Remaining superficial in closing this layer also prevents incarceration of branches of the lateral femoral cutaneous nerve. The subcutaneous tissue and skin are closed in a standard manner, and a sterile dressing is applied.

Surgical Technique: Hemiarthroplasty

With the following modifications, the anterior approach may be used for hemiarthroplasty, possibly decreasing the incidence of postoperative periprosthetic instability. The surgical setup, incision planning, and surgical exposure to the level of the anterior capsule are identical to that described previously for THA. In performing the capsulotomy, it is essential to avoid transection of the anterior labrum. As in THA, the surgeon should first incise the capsule in line with the planned femoral neck cut at the level of the base of the femoral neck. Rather than starting the perpendicular capsular incision at the level of the acetabular lip, which would lead to labral damage, the surgeon should make the perpendicular capsular incision from inferior to superior. When approaching the anterior acetabular lip with this incision, tension is placed on the anterior capsule to facilitate its elevation, which exposes and allows for the protection of the underlying labrum. Careful exposure in this manner allows the surgeon to incise the capsule independently of the labrum. The remainder of the capsulectomy is carried out in a manner similar to that used for THA, again taking care to protect the acetabular labrum in the process.

The technique for removal of the femoral head also differs from that used for THA. For THA, the femoral neck is cut in two segments with the hip in the reduced position. For hemiarthroplasty, the fracture line may substitute for the superior femoral neck cut in THA. After femoral neck exposure is completed, the inferior osteotomy is initiated at the saddle of the femoral neck and proceeds in an inferomedial direction at an angle that matches the geometry of the femoral component. The osteotome is inserted into this cut and twisted, mobilizing the femoral neck wafer, which is then carefully removed. To create more space and aid in the removal of the femoral head, it may be useful to use a rongeur to resect a portion of the femoral neck that remains attached to the femoral head. Next, a corkscrew is driven into the femoral head, and the corkscrew and the attached femoral head are carefully removed from the wound.

After sizing the native acetabulum for the closest-matching prosthetic femoral head size, attention is turned to the femur. It is critical that the surgeon take great care in exposing the proximal femur and elevating it for preparation. In the setting of a hemiarthroplasty for femoral neck fracture, the surgeon should expect poor bone quality in the proximal femur, which places it at risk for iatrogenic fracture. For exposure and elevation of the femur, the surgeon should follow the same general technique as for THA. The use of force should be avoided when elevating the proximal femur with the bone hook. If resistance is met, the surgeon should advance the posterolateral release in an inferior direction to the level of the piriformis tendon. Use of force, rather than soft-tissue releases, may result in trochanteric fracture. The remainder of the surgical technique mimics the technique used for THA. With gentle, complete exposure, it is feasible to use a cementless proximally fitting stem, a cemented stem, or a cementless distally fitting stem.

Complications

As with any approach, component malpositioning must be avoided with the direct anterior approach because it will increase the likelihood of impingement and instability and threaten the long-term success of the procedure. Surgeons accustomed to performing THA through a lateral incision with the patient in the lateral decubitus position may be confused by the view that is provided by the direct anterior approach, which could lead to errors in component positioning in the early stages of learning the technique.

Additionally, if care is not taken, soft tissues may misdirect the tools used to prepare the acetabulum and proximal femur and insert the components. The tendency is for the reamer handle to be misdirected anteriorly, causing excessive anterior reaming. In addition, the acetabular component insertion handle often is directed into excessive anteversion. During femoral preparation and component insertion, the soft tissues tend to misguide the instruments into excessive varus positioning and into an extended position, risking perforation of the posterior cortex. Awareness of these tendencies, achieving complete exposure, and using the appropriate instruments help to avoid these errors.

Trochanteric fracture is another potential complication of particular concern with the direct anterior approach. This complication most often occurs when the surgeon attempts to elevate the proximal femur to deliver it to the wound. This error can be avoided by applying gentle traction with the bone hook while releasing the posterolateral soft tissues in a graduated manner. A careful and controlled soft-tissue release facilitates an atraumatic femoral exposure. If a fracture occurs, the treatment is dictated by its location. Most fractures that occur at the tip of the greater trochanter should not be treated. Attempts to expose the fragment devascularize and destabilize it, and fixation often is difficult to achieve and maintain. Fractures that occur below the level of the vastus ridge threaten the stability of a proximally fitting stem; accordingly, a component that achieves distal fixation should be used (**Figure 8**). Fixation of the

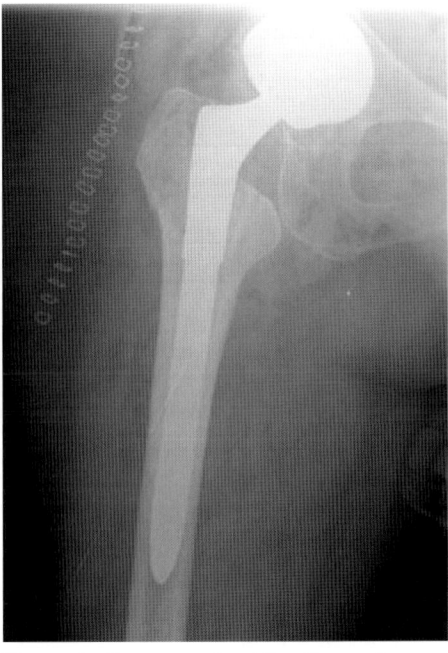

Figure 8 Postoperative AP radiograph of the hip of a patient who sustained a trochanteric fracture below the level of the vastus ridge shows a component that achieves distal fixation, which was required for secure fixation.

fragment is often unnecessary because the soft tissues that attach to the fracture fragment help maintain appropriate reduction.

Neurovascular structures at increased risk of injury during the direct anterior approach include the femoral nerve, the femoral artery, and the lateral femoral cutaneous nerve. Injury to the femoral neurovascular structures can be avoided by careful exposure of the anterior acetabulum and careful retractor placement. Damage to the main trunk of the cutaneous nerve may result in numbness or dysesthesia (meralgia paresthetica) and sometimes pain in the lateral distal thigh area.[9] Damage to the more lateral branches of the nerve may result in numbness lateral to the incision, which is common with any approach. Damage to the lateral femoral cutaneous nerve can be avoided by careful incision placement and careful technique during the approach and closure, as described previously.

Postoperative Care and Rehabilitation

Rapid recovery depends on several factors that are implemented in the postoperative period. Effective pain management and control of medication-related side effects are prerequisites for patient participation in aggressive rehabilitation programs. We have had success with using combinations of several classes of pain medications, avoiding narcotics as much as possible, providing medications on a scheduled basis, and administering premedication to patients in the preoperative and intraoperative periods.[10]

Aggressive physical therapy is another important element of a rapid recovery program. Patients are mobilized on the day of surgery and encouraged to ambulate as much as tolerated. On the first postoperative day, therapy goals are aggressively pursued. To achieve these goals, patients should be educated before surgery to set appropriate expectations.[11] In addition, monitoring devices and tubes should be removed from the patients on the morning of the first postoperative day. Patients are discharged as soon as all therapy goals are met, typically within the first 2 postoperative days.

We do not find it necessary to implement hip precautions in the postoperative period. Frequently, patients are able to discontinue assistive devices in the first postoperative week. We often encourage patients to continue using a cane during the first month to promote appropriate soft-tissue healing and bony ingrowth into the prosthetic components.

Pearls

- Careful incision placement, deep dissection, and meticulous closure avoid undue damage to the main branch of the lateral femoral cutaneous nerve.
- Careful patient positioning, specialized instrumentation, and the use of the flex feature of standard tables obviate the need for specialized operating tables for the anterior approach.
- A two-step approach to cutting the femoral neck, with removal of a wafer segment, facilitates removal of the femoral head without dislocating the hip.
- Femoral exposure prior to broaching is often the most difficult aspect of the anterior approach. Safe and complete exposure depends on careful positioning of the lower extremity, the use of the flex feature of a standard table, specialized instrumentation, and stepwise soft-tissue releases.
- Rapid recovery after the direct anterior approach depends on early and frequent mobilization with physical therapy and effective pain management.

References

1. Yoon RS, Nellans KW, Geller JA, Kim AD, Jacobs MR, Macaulay W: Patient education before hip or knee arthroplasty lowers length of stay. *J Arthroplasty* 2010;25(4):547-551.
2. Wang AW, Gilbey HJ, Ackland TR: Perioperative exercise programs improve early return of ambulatory function after total hip arthroplasty: A randomized, controlled trial. *Am J Phys Med Rehabil* 2002;81(11):801-806.
3. Hu S, Zhang ZY, Hua YQ, Li J, Cai ZD: A comparison of regional and general anaesthesia for total replacement of the hip or knee: A meta-analysis. *J Bone Joint Surg Br* 2009;91(7):935-942.
4. Ciminiello M, Parvizi J, Sharkey PF, Eslampour A, Rothman RH: Total hip arthroplasty: Is small incision better? *J Arthroplasty* 2006;21(4):484-488.
5. Hungerford DS: Minimally invasive total hip arthroplasty: In opposition. *J Arthroplasty* 2004;19(4, suppl 1)81-82.
6. Judet R, Judet J: Technique and results with the acrylic femoral head prosthesis. *J Bone Joint Surg Br* 1952;34:173-180.
7. Woolson ST, Pouliot MA, Huddleston JI: Primary total hip arthroplasty using an anterior approach and a fracture table: Short-term results from a community hospital. *J Arthroplasty* 2009;24(7):999-1005.
8. Nogler M, Krismer M, Hozack WJ, Merritt P, Rachbauer F, Mayr E: A double offset broach handle for preparation of the femoral cavity in minimally invasive direct anterior total hip arthroplasty. *J Arthroplasty* 2006;21(8):1206-1208.
9. Grothaus MC, Holt M, Mekhail AO, Ebraheim NA, Yeasting RA: Lateral femoral cutaneous nerve: An anatomic study. *Clin Orthop Relat Res* 2005;437:164-168.
10. Post ZD, Restrepo C, Kahl LK, van de Leur T, Purtill JJ, Hozack WJ: A prospective evaluation of 2 different pain management protocols for total hip arthroplasty. *J Arthroplasty* 2010;25(3):410-415.
11. Pour AE, Parvizi J, Sharkey PF, Hozack WJ, Rothman RH: Minimally invasive hip arthroplasty: What role does patient preconditioning play? *J Bone Joint Surg Am* 2007;89(9):1920-1927.

Chapter 51
Revision Total Hip Arthroplasty via Extended Trochanteric Osteotomy

Scott M. Sporer, MD, MS   Wayne G. Paprosky, MD, FACS

Introduction

Total hip arthroplasty (THA) predictably provides pain relief and improved function in patients with degenerative hip arthritis. Despite the overwhelming success of THA, several situations necessitate the revision of the femoral component. The extended trochanteric osteotomy (ETO) is an essential surgical tool for the revision arthroplasty surgeon. To obtain a successful surgical result during femoral revision, the femoral stem must be removed with minimal bone loss, the remaining host bone must be prepared without inadvertent perforation, and a femoral implant must be inserted concentrically with adequate axial and rotational stability. The ETO, which allows exposure of the proximal femur through a controlled cortical fracture, can facilitate these goals by allowing (1) improved access to the implant-bone or implant-cement interface, (2) concentric reaming of the distal femur in patients with proximal femoral deformity, (3) appropriate abductor tensioning, (4) improved acetabular visualization, and (5) predictable healing of the osteotomy. In general, an ETO should be performed if it is being considered as an option, because this technique often will minimize surgical time and surgical complications and ultimately will minimize undersizing of the femoral components, improve initial implant stability, and minimize the risk of cortical perforation. Familiarity with the ETO technique is crucial for surgeons who frequently perform revision THA or primary THA in patients with proximal femoral deformity.

Patient Selection
Indications

The most common indications for ETO include removal of a well-fixed femoral component, removal of retained distal cement, insertion of a femoral component in patients with proximal femoral remodeling, and the need for improved surgical exposure.[1]

Removal of a well-fixed cemented, proximally coated, or extensively coated femoral implant can be very challenging. Indications for removing a well-fixed femoral implant may include sepsis; recurrent dislocation due to femoral component malposition, inadequate offset, or both; an implant with damage from or a poor track record of excessive corrosion or fatigue failure; and the need to improve acetabular exposure.[2] Extensive bone damage can occur while attempting to remove a well-fixed implant because of inability to disrupt the bone-prosthesis interface distally with proximal exposure alone. Although a cortical window can be helpful, this technique will weaken the remaining host bone and require a longer stem to bypass the stress riser (**Figure 1**).

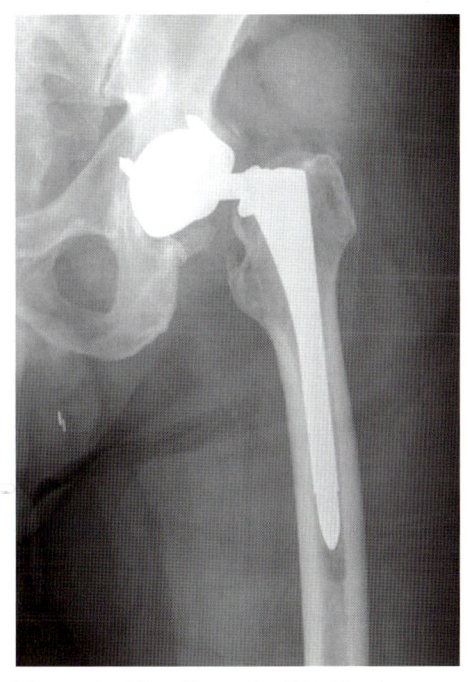

Figure 1 AP radiograph of the hip shows a well-fixed femoral implant with a fracture of the proximal modular neck.

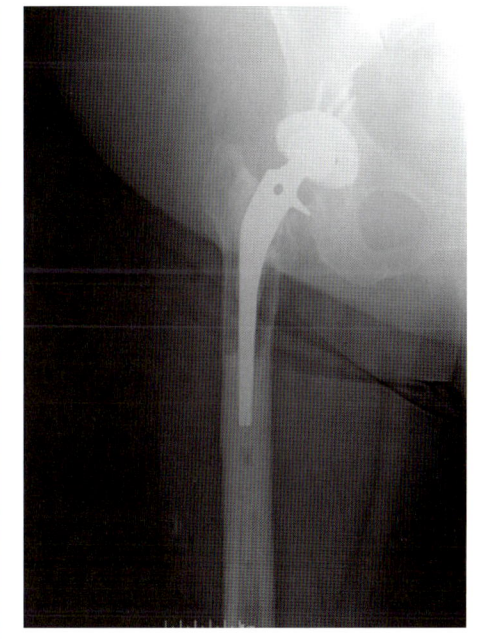

Figure 2 AP radiograph of the hip depicts a loose femoral component with severe femoral osteolysis. Note the large amount of well-fixed distal cement.

The removal of well-fixed distal cement is equally challenging, especially when proximal femoral remodeling has occurred or the previous implant was cemented into a varus position. Proximal exposure alone (with the femoral canal intact) has been shown to result in a higher prevalence of cortical perforation when removal of distal cement is attempted in such instances. The length of the ETO can be planned to allow easy visual access to the distal cement plug so that standard drills, taps, and curets can be used to disrupt the bone-cement interface and facilitate the removal of retained cement (**Figure 2**).

Proximal femoral varus remodeling is observed in up to 30% of patients with a loose femoral stem. Although component extraction may be relatively easy in these patients, the subsequent surgical reconstruction often is challenging because of the deformed proximal bone. An ETO will allow concentric reaming of the femoral canal. Attempts to obtain distal fixation in a femur with proximal deformity will result in a high likelihood of cortical perforation, undersizing of the femoral component, or varus malposition[3,4] (**Figure 3**).

Dr. Sporer or an immediate family member serves as a paid consultant to or is an employee of Smith & Nephew and Zimmer and has received research or institutional support from Central DuPage Hospital. Dr. Paprosky or an immediate family member has received royalties from Wright Medical Technology and Zimmer; is a member of a speakers' bureau or has made paid presentations on behalf of Zimmer; serves as a paid consultant to or is an employee of Biomet and Zimmer; and serves as a board member, owner, officer, or committee member of The Hip Society.

© 2013 American Academy of Orthopaedic Surgeons

Section 4: Adult Reconstruction

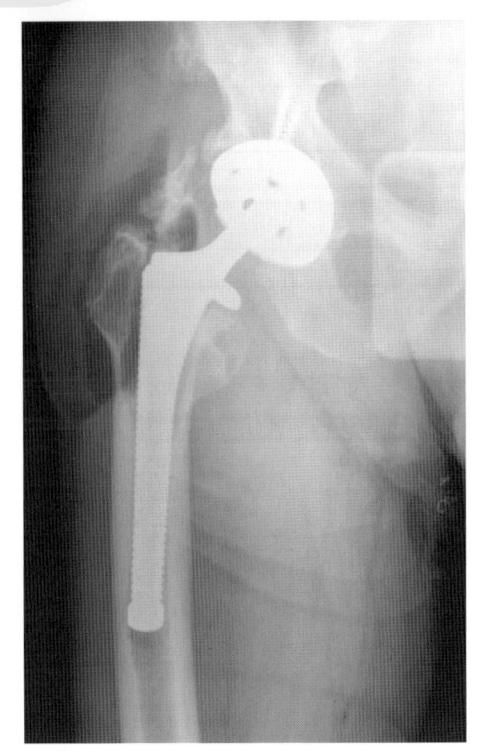

Figure 3 Intraoperative AP radiograph demonstrates varus proximal femoral remodeling. An extended trochanteric osteotomy at the apex of the deformity is required to allow concentric placement of a distally fixed implant.

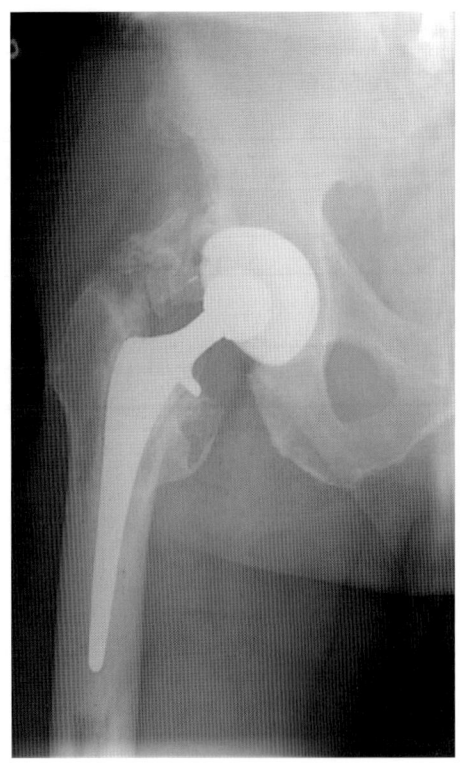

Figure 4 AP radiograph of a hip following total hip arthroplasty shows severe heterotopic bone formation.

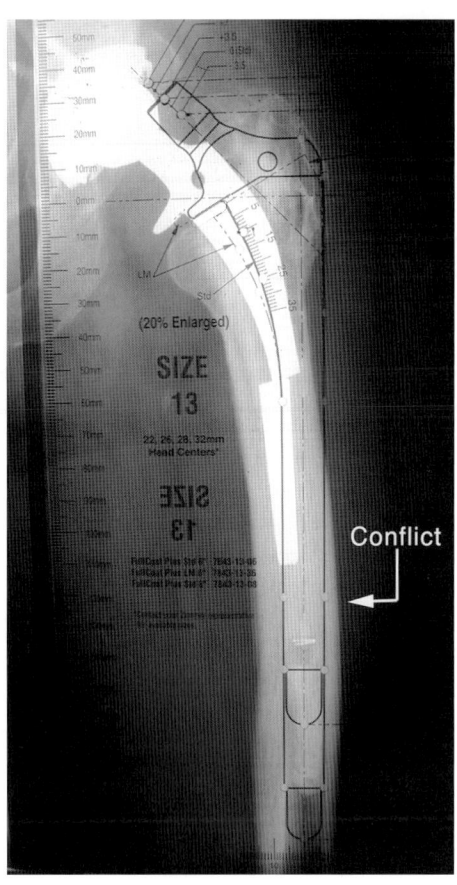

Figure 5 AP radiograph of a hip with a cemented total hip arthroplasty shows mechanical failure with associated proximal femoral varus remodeling, causing a "conflict." An extended trochanteric osteotomy is required for correction of the proximal deformity, as well as distal cement extraction. Note the conflict.

Additional relative indications for an ETO include the need for improved acetabular exposure because of heterotopic bone formation (**Figure 4**) or the need to visualize both the anterior and posterior columns. An ETO also may be helpful during femoral revision in patients with severe trochanteric osteolysis, to minimize inadvertent fracture. Rarely, an ETO may be used in the primary setting in the patient with a prior osteotomy, malunion, or proximal femoral deformity due to congenital dysplasia.[5]

Contraindications

Essentially, no absolute contraindications to ETO exist. Nonetheless, the rare clinical scenario may be encountered in which the surgeon decides that impaction bone grafting inside an ectatic femoral shaft is preferable to cementless femoral fixation because of poor bone quality in the area where femoral fixation is to be obtained.

Preoperative Imaging

Standard AP pelvis radiographs and AP and lateral radiographs of the femur are required for preoperative planning of an ETO. The AP pelvis radiograph can be used to estimate the limb-length discrepancy, and the AP radiograph of the femur can be used to determine the apex of the deformity in a varus-remodeled femur.[6]

Video 51.1 Revision Total Hip Arthroplasty via Extended Trochanteric Osteotomy. Scott M. Sporer, MD, MS; Wayne G. Paprosky, MD, FACS (6 min)

Procedure

Preoperative Planning

The length of the proposed osteotomy will depend on the surgical indication. Varus remodeling of the proximal femur occurs in up to 30% of femoral revisions and is most frequently observed at the tip of a loose femoral stem. Because of the remodeling, neutral component alignment cannot be achieved in these situations from a proximal starting position. The inability to place a femoral component in neutral position because of varus remodeling is termed a "conflict" (**Figure 5**). In these situations, the length of the ETO should extend at least to the apex of the deformity. Failure to reach the level of the deformity will necessitate the femoral preparation remaining in a varus alignment.

When the ETO is performed for removal of retained distal cement, the length of the ETO needs to be within a few centimeters of the distal cement plug (**Figure 6**). A shorter osteotomy can be performed if the indication is to improve surgical exposure or the distal cement mantle is loose; however, a sufficient length of cortical bone below the lesser trochanter is required to securely reattach the osteotomy fragment at the completion of the procedure. At least two cables are required to fix the trochanteric fragment securely at the completion of the procedure. In general, an ETO should be located a minimum of 14 cm below the tip of the greater trochanter.

The length of the osteotomy also depends on the implant chosen for the reconstruction. Preoperative templates are essential in determining the length of the osteotomy required to obtain a stable implant. If an extensively porous-coated stem is used, a minimum of 4 to 5 cm of "scratch-fit" will be required to obtain sufficient axial and rotational stability[7] (**Figure 7**). If a tapered stem is chosen, it is important that the osteotomy does not extend past the distal metaphyseal/diaphyseal flare. Once the position of the osteotomy is determined, the location of the transverse limb is measured from a fixed bony landmark, such as the tip of the greater trochanter or the lesser trochanter.

Special Instruments/Equipment/Implants

Instrumentation that should be available in the operating room when considering an ETO include a small oscillating sagittal saw with a narrow blade for the longitudinal limb of the osteotomy and a pencil-tip high-speed burr for the transverse limb. Several wide osteotomes are required to distribute stress along the trochanteric fragment while the osteotomy is being completed. Depending on the indication for the osteotomy, a metal cutting burr may be required to section a well-fixed extensively porous-coated stem before a Gigli saw can be used to remove the proximal portion of the stem and cylindrical trephines to remove the distal portion of the stem. Reverse hooks, cement drills, and osteotomes will be required to remove well-fixed distal cement. A minimum of two cerclage wires or cables are required to fix the osteotomy fragment securely upon completion of the procedure.

Exposure

The surgical approach in the revision setting may be directed by previous surgical incisions. A posterior approach to the hip is the most common surgical approach for an ETO; however, several authors describe a similar technique performed through a direct lateral approach.[8] A posterolateral approach allows both proximal and distal extension and provides excellent visualization of both the femur and the acetabulum.

The patient is placed in the lateral decubitus position, taking care to stabilize the pelvis with positioners along the sacrum and pubic symphysis. A lateral surgical skin incision is made in line with the femur over the posterior one third of the greater trochanter (**Figure 8**). The tensor fascia lata and the fascia of the gluteus maximus are split in line with the surgical incision and retracted with a Charnley bow. The posterior border of the gluteus medius tendon is identified and retracted anteriorly. The posterior pseudocapsule and the short external rotators then are elevated as a posteriorly based flap. Elevating these structures as a flap will allow a posterior capsular repair at the completion of the surgery. The anterior and proximal portion of the gluteus maximus insertion is released to allow mobilization of the femur (**Figure 9, A**). The femoral head is dislocated posteriorly when the hip is placed in flexion and internal rotation. The knee remains flexed to reduce tension on the sciatic nerve.

The soft tissue surrounding the proximal portion of the femoral stem is removed, and the stability of the femoral component is assessed. If the stem is grossly loose and the greater trochanter is not preventing extrication, the component is removed. If the greater trochanter is preventing component removal or if the stem is well fixed, however, an in situ ETO should be performed. An in situ osteotomy also should be considered if hip dislocation is difficult due to severe acetabular protrusio or extensive heterotopic bone formation.

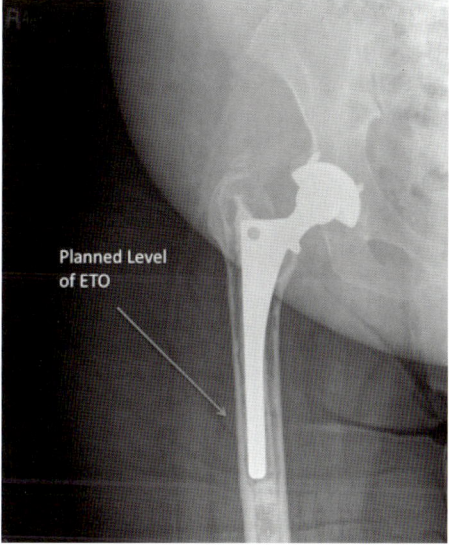

Figure 6 AP radiograph of a hip requiring revision total hip arthroplasty with an extended trochanteric osteotomy (ETO) shows the planned level of the ETO. The length of the osteotomy is determined by the surgical indication. The osteotomy should be as short as possible, yet long enough to correct the deformity, remove well-fixed cement, and allow at least two cables distal to the lesser trochanter.

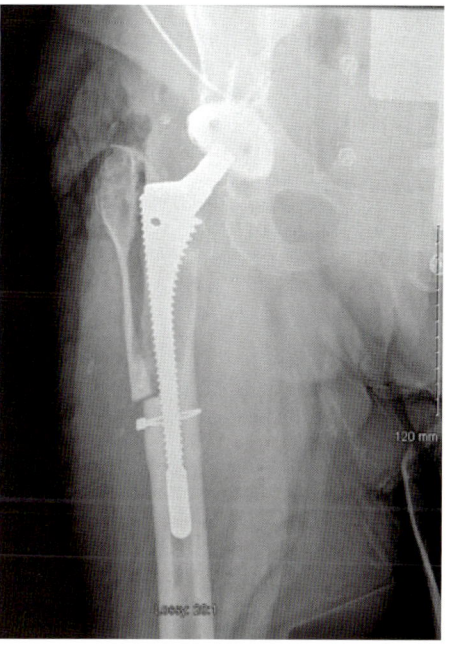

Figure 7 AP radiograph of a hip with a periprosthetic fracture. When determining the length of the osteotomy, it is important to consider the future femoral reconstruction. A minimum of 4 to 5 cm of scratch-fit is required for extensively coated implants to obtain axial and rotational stability.

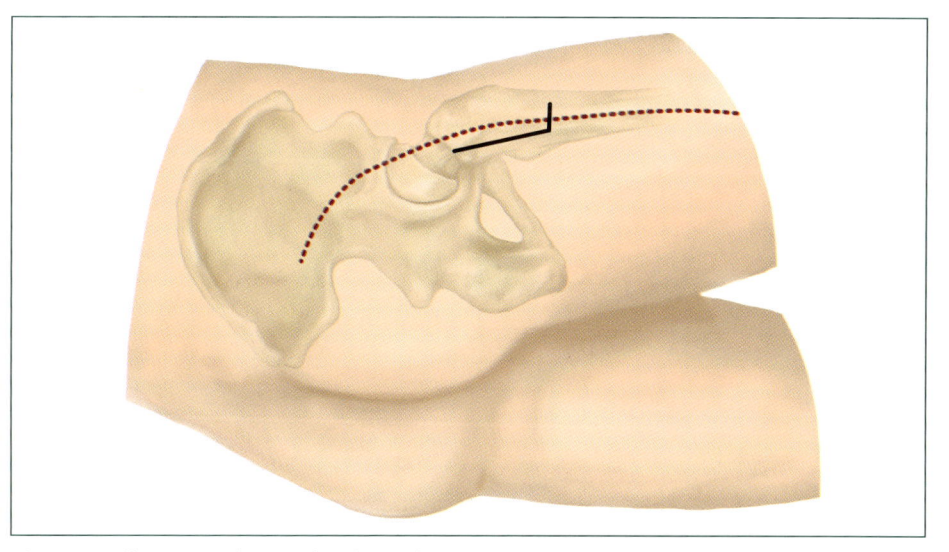

Figure 8 Illustration depicts the planned incision (dashed line) for a posterior approach to the hip, which allows excellent visualization of the posterolateral aspect of the proximal femur and will facilitate anterior mobilization of the vastus lateralis. The solid black line indicates the location for an extended trochanteric osteotomy.

Osteotomy

During the ETO, the hip is placed in extension and internal rotation with the knee flexed. This position minimizes

Section 4: Adult Reconstruction

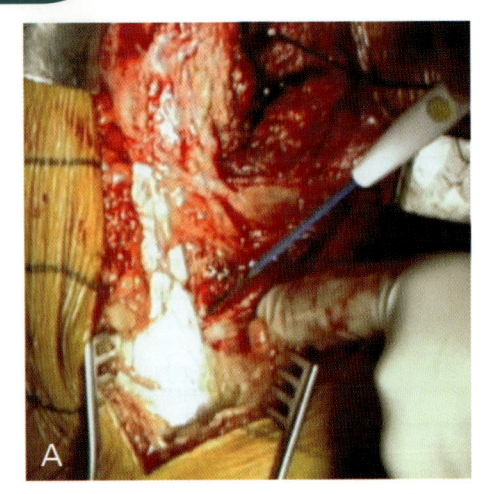

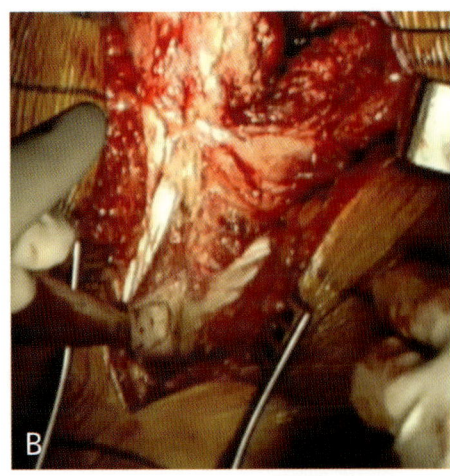

Figure 9 Intraoperative photographs demonstrate initial steps in exposure for an extended trochanteric osteotomy of a left hip. **A,** The proximal and anterior portion of the gluteus maximus insertion is released to allow mobilization of the femur. Distally, the tendon remains intact unless additional exposure is required. **B,** A Hohmann retractor is placed deep to the vastus lateralis to expose the underlying femoral shaft at the level of the proposed osteotomy.

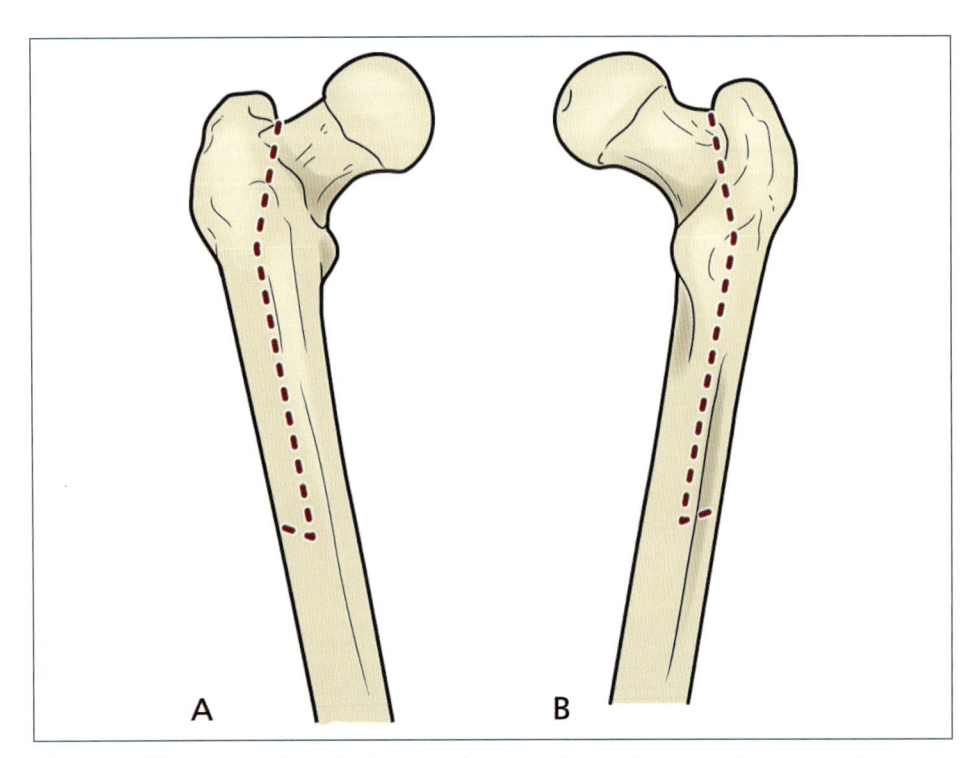

Figure 10 Illustrations show the location of an extended trochanteric osteotomy on the anterior (**A**) and posterior (**B**) aspects of the femur. The length of the osteotomy is measured from the tip of the greater trochanter. Depending on the indication for the osteotomy, the trochanteric fragment should allow placement of a minimum of two cerclage wires and generally should be 15 to 16 cm in length.

the risk of a traction injury to the sciatic nerve yet allows exposure of the posterior aspect of the femur. The posterior margin of the vastus lateralis is identified, and the muscle belly is mobilized anteriorly off the lateral femur, with care taken to minimize soft-tissue stripping. A Chandler or Hohmann retractor is placed around the femoral shaft at the desired length of the osteotomy, exposing the underlying periosteum (**Figure 9, B**). The distal and posterior portion of the gluteus maximus insertion is preserved unless release is required to mobilize the femur for visualization.[9]

The position of the proposed osteotomy is marked with electrocautery or a pen (**Figure 10**). The tip of the greater trochanter can be used as a landmark; alternatively, if the femoral stem has been removed, it can be used to determine the length of the osteotomy (**Figure 11, A**). With the femur remaining in full extension and internal rotation, a sagittal saw is directed from posterolateral to anterolateral beginning anterior to the linea aspera (**Figure 11, B**). Ideally, the osteotomy fragment should encompass the posterolateral third of the proximal femur and should be oriented perpendicular to the anteversion of the hip. If the femoral component had been extracted previously, the oscillating saw then can be guided toward the far anterolateral cortex, where the cortical bone can be "etched" to facilitate a greenstick-type fracture. If the femoral component is retained, the oscillating saw must be angled anterolaterally to maximize the width of the osteotomy yet avoid hitting the retained femoral component. Proximally, the saw is angled posteromedially so that the entire greater trochanter is released with the osteotomy.

The distal transverse limb of the osteotomy is made with a pencil-tip burr. The corners of the osteotomy are rounded to eliminate a stress riser and reduce the risk of propagating a distal fracture. An oscillating saw or the pencil-tip burr can be used to initiate the distal anterior limb of the osteotomy.

Multiple wide osteotomes are used to lever the osteotomy site gently from posterior to anterior (**Figure 11, C**). The entire osteotomy fragment should be moved as a unit to avoid fracture at the level of the vastus ridge. Once the anterior limb of the osteotomy has been initiated, the trochanteric fragment can be retracted anteriorly with the attached abductors and vastus lateralis. The tight pseudocapsule along the anterior aspect of the greater trochanter must be released while mobilizing the osteotomy fragment to avoid inadvertent fracture of the greater trochanter (**Figure 11, D**). Because the blood supply and innervation to the vastus lateralis enter anteriorly, it is important to minimize dissection along the anterolateral limb of the osteotomy.

If the femoral component had been extracted before the osteotomy, the pseudomembrane within the femur can now be removed. If cement had been used previously, a high-speed burr and cement splitters can be used to remove the retained cement and the distal plug. Cement remaining on the trochanteric fragment is retained until the end of the procedure to strengthen the often compromised trochanteric bone during surgical retraction. If an osteotomy was required to remove a well-fixed proximally coated implant, a pencil-tip burr can be used to expose the implant-bone interface around most of the implant. A Gigli saw then can be placed

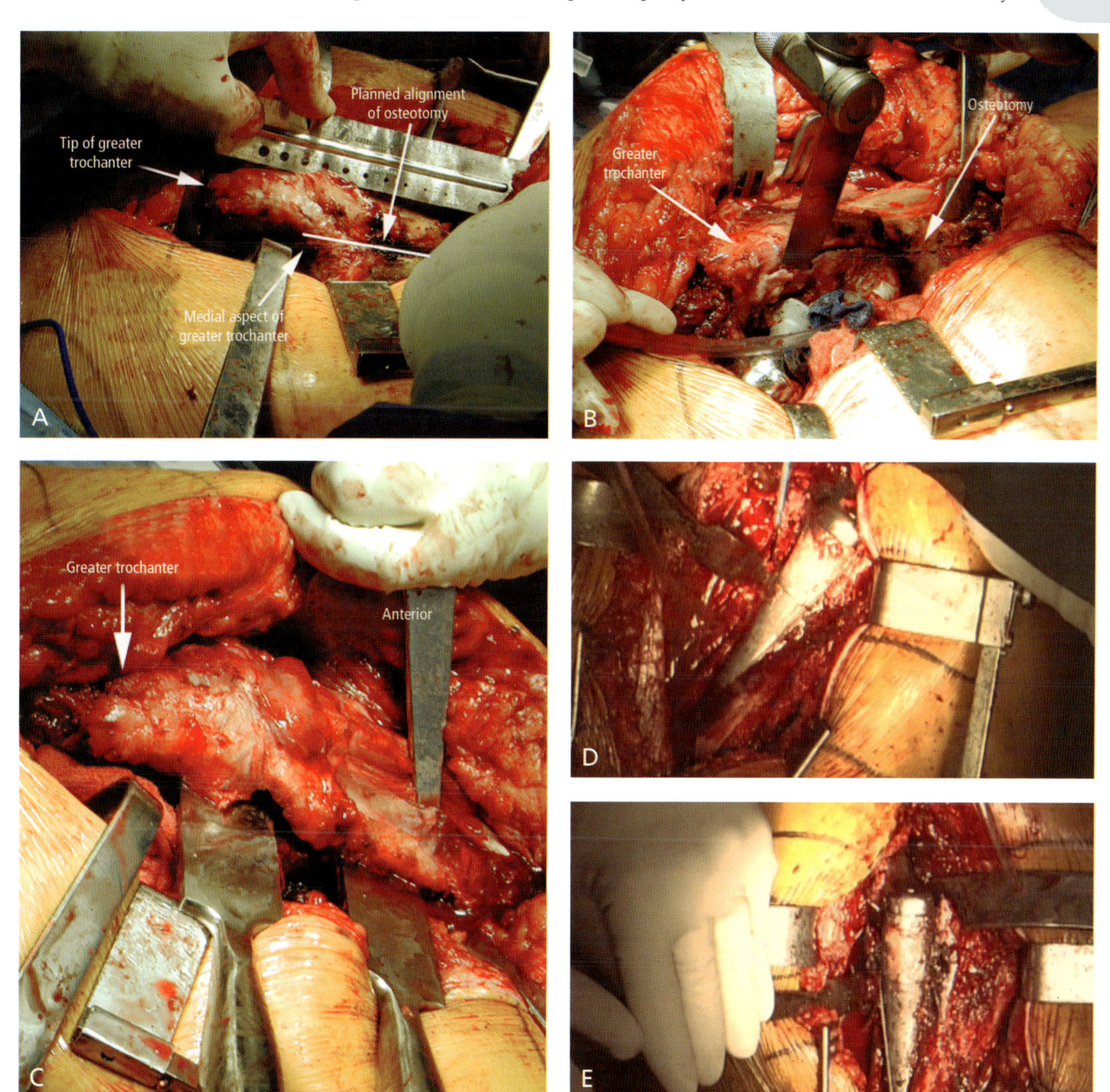

Chapter 51: Revision Total Hip Arthroplasty via Extended Trochanteric Osteotomy

Figure 11 Intraoperative photographs demonstrate an extended trochanteric osteotomy. **A,** The length of the osteotomy can be determined from the length of the explanted component or, as shown here, from a fixed landmark on the femur such as the greater trochanter. **B,** An oscillating saw with a thin blade is directed from posterior to anteromedial. Approximately one third of the lateral femur, along with the entire greater trochanter, should be elevated. **C,** Multiple broad osteotomes are used to lever the osteotomy fragment anteriorly. Great care must be taken to avoid fracture at the level of the vastus ridge. **D,** The soft tissue along the proximal-anterior aspect of the osteotomy must be excised once the trochanteric fragment is elevated to minimize fracture of the greater trochanter. This step should be performed before attempts are made to remove the femoral component. **E,** A Gigli saw can be used to disrupt the medial interface between the prosthesis and the host bone.

around the proximal femur and used to disrupt the bone-prosthesis interface before component removal (**Figure 11, E**).

If the osteotomy was required to remove a well-fixed extensively coated stem, the stem can now be transected with a metal cutting burr at the junction between the tapered and cylindrical portion of the implant. The proximal portion of the implant can be removed as described previously, whereas the remaining distal cylindrical portion of the stem can be removed using a trephine 0.5 mm larger than the implanted stem.

Bone Preparation

Once the previous femoral component has been removed successfully, any remaining pseudomembrane or cement should be removed with a reverse hook to minimize the risk of inadvertent femoral fracture during femoral preparation. A distal pedestal often is observed in loose cementless implants; it also should be removed to allow concentric femoral reaming.

Most femoral revisions are performed using a cementless implant that relies on distal fixation. Depending on the pattern of bone loss, the patient's anatomy, and the length of the osteotomy, a bowed or straight extensively coated stem or a distally tapered stem may be chosen.

© 2013 American Academy of Orthopaedic Surgeons

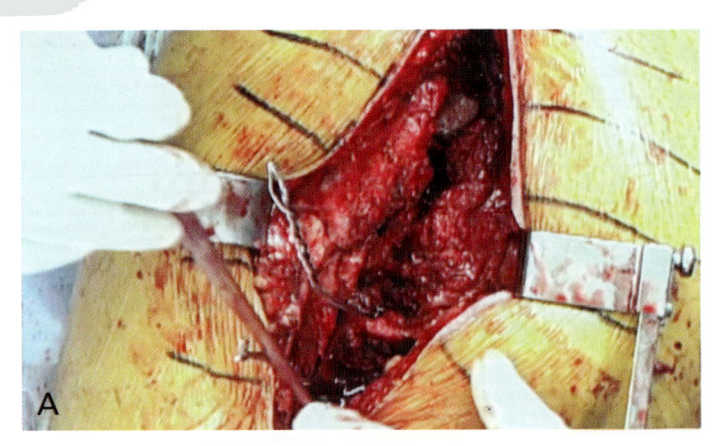

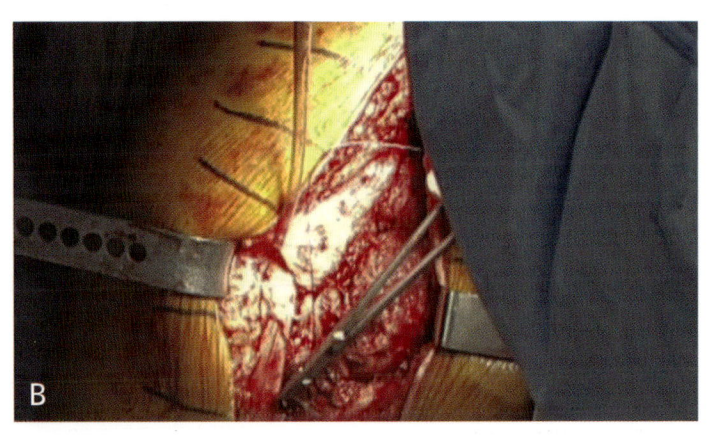

Figure 12 Intraoperative photographs demonstrate finals steps in an extended trochanteric osteotomy. **A,** A minimum of two cables or cerclage wires are required to secure the trochanteric fragment to the host bone. The osteotomy should be advanced distally and posteriorly along the femoral shaft. **B,** The proximal aspect of the gluteus maximus insertion is repaired.

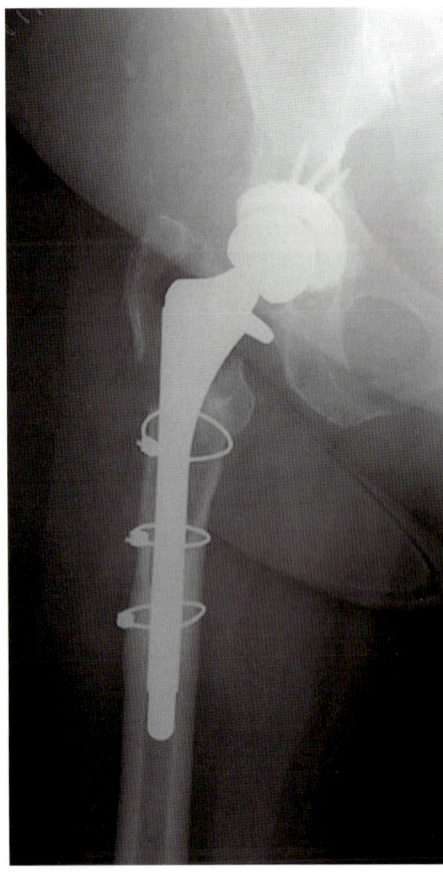

Figure 13 AP radiograph depicts a fracture of the osteotomy fragment at the greater trochanter following an extended trochanteric osteotomy. Such a fracture can occur during the postoperative period, frequently at the vastus ridge.

Wound Closure

Any cement adherent to the trochanteric fragment should be removed once the femoral stem is seated fully. The leg is placed in slight abduction and internal rotation during reattachment of the osteotomy fragment. A minimum of two cables or wires are needed to secure the greater trochanteric fragment to the remaining femoral shaft (**Figure 12, A**). A high-speed barrel burr may be required to shape the medial aspect of the trochanteric fragment, to allow the osteotomy to rest against the lateral shoulder of the prosthesis, and to maximize bony apposition to the femoral shaft. The trochanteric fragment may not be able to achieve bone apposition both anteriorly and posteriorly in situations in which the ETO was performed for varus femoral remodeling. In these situations, the osteotomy should be advanced slightly distally and posteriorly to improve stability and minimize impingement during internal rotation. The cables around the osteotomy are tightened from distal to proximal with a decreasing amount of force.

Care must be taken to avoid a trochanteric fracture at the level of the vastus ridge. Bone grafting of the osteotomy site is not performed routinely unless host bone from the reamings of the acetabulum or femur are available. We prefer to repair the posterior capsule and short external rotators to the posterior aspect of the gluteus medius. The gluteus maximus fascia and the iliotibial band are closed over a drain with a nonabsorbable No. 1 suture, and the subcutaneous tissue is closed with an absorbable 2.0 suture (**Figure 12, B**).

Complications

Potential complications from an ETO include proximal migration, nonunion or malunion of the osteotomy fragment, fracture, and recalcitrant trochanteric bursitis. From 1992 to 1996, we performed 142 consecutive hip revisions via an ETO; 122 patients were available for follow-up at a mean of 2.6 years.[10] No nonunions of the osteotomized fragments and no cases of proximal migration greater than 2 mm occurred. Radiographically, all cases demonstrated bony union by 3 months.[10] This cohort of patients was re-evaluated with additional patients from 1992 to 1998. At a mean 3.9-year follow-up, two nonunions (1.2%) and one malunion (0.6%) were seen. The remaining osteotomies achieved bony union. Other surgeons have seen similar clinical results with an ETO. Chen et al[11] reported a 98% union rate in 46 hips when an ETO was used during revision surgery.

Proximal migration of the osteotomy fragment is rarely a problem because the vastus lateralis prevents significant proximal migration. Similarly, nonunion of the osteotomy rarely is a problem clinically because dense fibrous tissue forms. A fracture of the osteotomy fragment at the greater trochanter (**Figure 13**) can be problematic, leading to trochanteric escape and subsequent abductor weakness. Most of these fractures can be treated nonsurgically because of the distal pull of the vastus lateralis.

Postoperative Care and Rehabilitation

Patients who have undergone a femoral revision may be treated with an abduction orthosis for 6 to 8 weeks postoperatively to minimize the risk of instability. During this time, they are allowed 30% weight bearing on the surgical leg using a walker or crutch for ambulation. At the end of 6 weeks, patients are converted to a cane and weight bearing is advanced as tolerated. Patients are instructed to avoid active abduction for 6 to 12 weeks, until radiographic evidence of healing at the osteotomy site is present.

Pearls

- An ETO should be considered for the removal of well-fixed implants, the re-

moval of retained distal cement, and in patients with varus femoral remodeling.
- The length of the ETO should be minimized to use the shortest femoral revision stem possible yet should be long enough to bypass the apex of the femoral remodeling, facilitate component and cement removal, and allow at least two cerclage cables to be placed around the osteotomy.
- When levering the osteotomy anteriorly, multiple wide osteotomes should be used simultaneously to distribute the stress along the greatest distance.
- A prophylactic cerclage cable can be placed distal to the osteotomy before femoral preparation and stem insertion to minimize the risk of fracture.
- Any cement along the osteotomy fragment should be retained until the time of reattachment to provide additional structural support.
- The osteotomy fragment should be advanced distally and posteriorly before securing it to the remaining shaft of the femur. This will provide appropriate abductor tension and minimize the risk of impingement.

References

1. Archibeck MJ, Rosenberg AG, Berger RA, Silverton CD: Trochanteric osteotomy and fixation during total hip arthroplasty. *J Am Acad Orthop Surg* 2003;11(3):163-173.
2. Glassman AH: Exposure for revision: Total hip replacement. *Clin Orthop Relat Res* 2004;420:39-47.
3. Egan KJ, Di Cesare PE: Intraoperative complications of revision hip arthroplasty using a fully porous-coated straight cobalt-chrome femoral stem. *J Arthroplasty* 1995;10(suppl):S45-S51.
4. Meek RM, Garbuz DS, Masri BA, Greidanus NV, Duncan CP: Intraoperative fracture of the femur in revision total hip arthroplasty with a diaphyseal fitting stem. *J Bone Joint Surg Am* 2004;86(3):480-485.
5. Della Valle CJ, Berger RA, Rosenberg AG, Jacobs JJ, Sheinkop MB, Paprosky WG: Extended trochanteric osteotomy in complex primary total hip arthroplasty: A brief note. *J Bone Joint Surg Am* 2003;85(12):2385-2390.
6. Meek RM, Greidanus NV, Garbuz DS, Masri BA, Duncan CP: Extended trochanteric osteotomy: Planning, surgical technique, and pitfalls. *Instr Course Lect* 2004;53:119-130.
7. Aribindi R, Paprosky W, Nourbash P, Kronick J, Barba M: Extended proximal femoral osteotomy. *Instr Course Lect* 1999;48:19-26.
8. MacDonald SJ, Cole C, Guerin J, Rorabeck CH, Bourne RB, McCalden RW: Extended trochanteric osteotomy via the direct lateral approach in revision hip arthroplasty. *Clin Orthop Relat Res* 2003;417:210-216.
9. Younger TI, Bradford MS, Magnus RE, Paprosky WG: Extended proximal femoral osteotomy: A new technique for femoral revision arthroplasty. *J Arthroplasty* 1995;10(3):329-338.
10. Paprosky WG, Sporer SM: Controlled femoral fracture: Easy in. *J Arthroplasty* 2003;18(3, suppl 1):91-93.
11. Chen WM, McAuley JP, Engh CA Jr, Hopper RH Jr, Engh CA: Extended slide trochanteric osteotomy for revision total hip arthroplasty. *J Bone Joint Surg Am* 2000;82(9):1215-1219.

Chapter 52
Total Knee Arthroplasty via the Medial Parapatellar Approach

Stephen J. Incavo, MD   Michael R. Dayton, MD   Jesse James F. Exaltacion, MD

Patient Selection
Indications
Many methods of surgical exposure allow successful total knee arthroplasty (TKA).[1-9] Regardless of the method used, exposure that is sufficient to allow consistently successful total knee implant placement and alignment should be a primary concern. A standard anterior midline skin incision with a medial parapatellar arthrotomy continues to be the most widely used method of exposure for TKA.[10] The extensor mechanism of the knee—composed of the quadriceps muscle and tendon, patella, and patellar tendon—comprises biomechanically and anatomically complex, interacting structures that work together to provide effective knee function. Proper preservation of the extensor mechanism is vital to successful recovery following TKA. The main advantage of the anterior approach to the knee is that it provides excellent visualization and access to the distal femur, proximal tibia, and patella. Although not extensile in the classic sense, it is more extensile than most TKA approaches.

The medial parapatellar approach is used for both primary and revision TKA. Variations in pathologic morphology may include varus or valgus deformity, patella alta or patella infera, and previous tibial or femoral osteotomy. The approach can be used regardless of preoperative range of motion. Patients of short stature, obese patients, and patients with muscular lower extremities are ideal candidates for this approach. The tissue along the medial course of the patella and knee capsule is sufficiently thick to provide a satisfactory closure following TKA. The approach is straightforward to perform and exposes the knee joint efficiently.

Additional indications for the medial parapatellar arthrotomy include the situation when lateral patellar subluxation is required, because this approach allows medial imbrication (advancement) of the arthrotomy. Furthermore, should the patellar tendon be excessively thin or compromised by the approach, a side-to-side repair of this structure can be achieved. In the setting of revision or a profoundly ankylosed knee, a modified anterior exposure may be necessary. Quadriceps snip, V-Y quadricepsplasty, and tibial tubercle osteotomy have all been used in conjunction with the medial parapatellar approach to enhance safe exposure.

The medial parapatellar approach has evolved over the past decade, largely due to the popularization of minimally invasive surgical techniques. In general, incisions have decreased in length from the traditional incision, which was made from one handbreadth proximal to the patella and extended distally past the tibial tubercle. Excellent exposure usually can be achieved by a shorter incision, from 4 cm proximal to the superior pole of the patella to 1 cm proximal to the tibial tubercle. Lateral eversion of the patella is no longer considered necessary in all cases of TKA and has been replaced frequently by simple lateral subluxation of the patella. Enthusiasm for minimally invasive approaches to the knee has decreased considerably because of the belief that the limited surgical exposure achieved may result in less-than-optimal component placement or inadvertent soft-tissue damage.[11]

Contraindications
Previous skin incisions oriented longitudinally and lateral to the line through which a medial parapatellar approach would be performed are a relative contraindication. Narrow skin bridges pose a considerable risk of skin necrosis; therefore, incisions 4 cm or less from a previous incision should be avoided. If skin bridges of 4 cm or less must be used for the TKA, close attention to wound healing is mandatory. If skin necrosis develops, soft-tissue coverage should be obtained expeditiously, before wound breakdown. The blood supply to the skin overlying the knee is supplied by perforating arteries located just superficial to the deep fascia. To minimize disruption of these vessels (and the skin blood supply), dissection of medial and lateral soft tissues should be deep to the fascia (**Figure 1**).

Specific circumstances may require alternative approaches to the medial parapatellar arthrotomy. Previous surgery using a lateral approach may compromise the blood supply to the patella. The patella is supplied by the midpatellar vessels in the middle third of the anterior surface. These vessels enter the patellar apex behind the tendon. Specifically, the upper half of the patella is supplied only by the midpatellar vessels. Cadaver studies have shown absence of vascular filling after medial arthrotomies done too close to the patella and also after radical fat pad excision, lateral release too close to the patella, and cautery of the prepatellar vessels. Although osteonecrosis of the patella is uncommon after a medial parapatellar surgical approach, unnecessary vascular disruption should be avoided.

This chapter adapted from Incavo SJ, Dayton MR, Exaltacion JJF: Total knee arthroplasty via the medial parapatellar approach, in Lieberman JR, Berry DJ, Azar FM, eds: Advanced Reconstruction: Knee. Rosemont, IL, American Academy of Orthopaedic Surgeons, 2011, pp 3-9.

Dr. Incavo or an immediate family member has received royalties from Exactech; serves as a paid consultant to or is an employee of Stryker and Wright Medical; has stock or stock options held in Otismed; has received research or institutional support from Stryker; has received nonincome support (such as equipment or services), commercially derived honoraria, or other non–research-related funding (such as paid travel) from Nimbic Systems; and serves as a board member, owner, officer, or committee member of The Knee Society, the American Association of Hip and Knee Surgeons, the American Association of Orthopaedic Surgeons, and the Texas State Orthopaedic Society. Dr. Dayton or an immediate family member is a member of a speakers' bureau or has made paid presentations on behalf of Smith & Nephew; serves as a paid consultant to or is an employee of Smith & Nephew; serves as an unpaid consultant to Smith & Nephew and DePuy; and has received research or institutional support from Exactech, DePuy, Stryker, and Smith & Nephew. Neither Dr. Exaltacion nor any immediate family member has received anything of value from or has stock or stock options held in a commercial company or institution related directly or indirectly to the subject of this chapter.

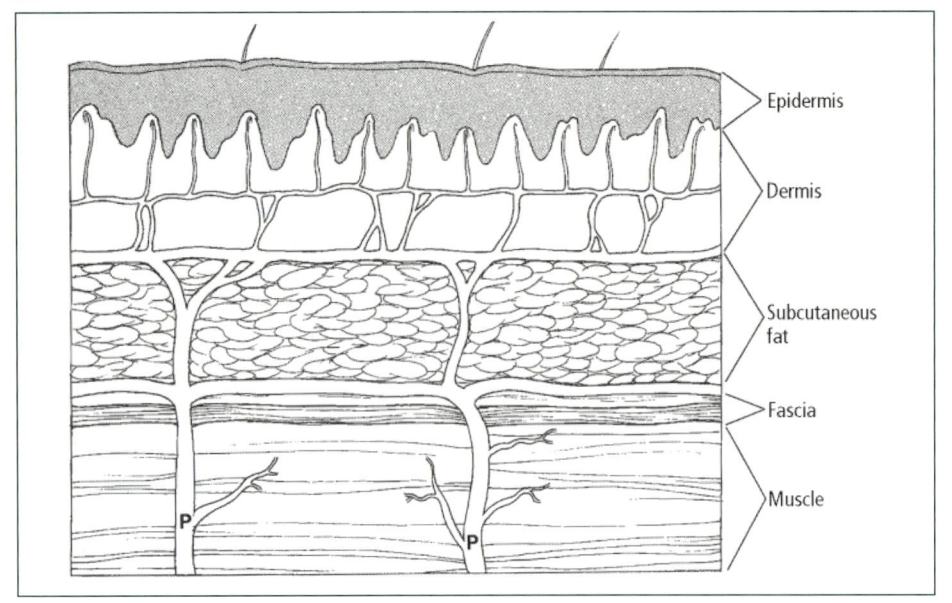

Figure 1 Illustration depicts soft-tissue microvascular anatomy. Note that the vessels just superficial to the deep fascia form a vascular anastomosis, which provides the skin's blood supply. Perforating arteries just superficial to the deep fascia supply this anastomosis. Because of this, dissection of the soft tissue just into the deep fascia is more protective of the skin blood supply than dissection of the dermis and subcutaneous fat from the deep fascia. *P* = perforating artery. (Reproduced from Younger AS, Duncan CD, Masri BA: Surgical exposures in revision total knee arthroplasty. *J Am Acad Orthop Surg* 1998;6[1]:55-64.)

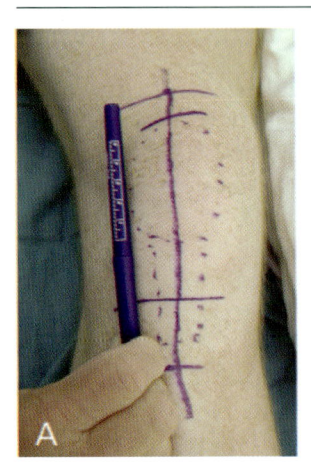

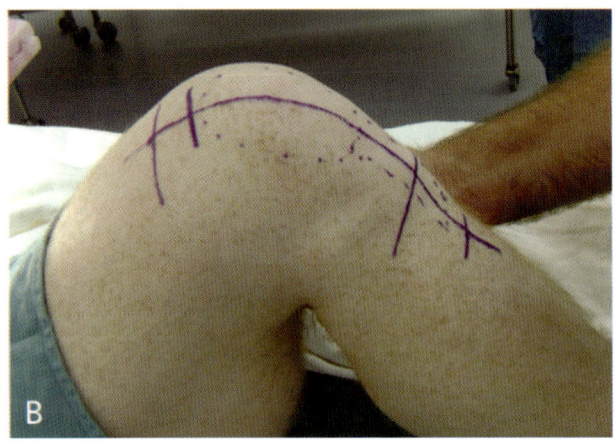

Figure 2 Photographs show skin incision for the medial parapatellar approach. **A,** The incision has been marked from 4 cm proximal to the superior pole of the patella to 2 cm distal to the tibial tubercle. The incision initially begins from the superior pole of the patella to 1 cm proximal to the tibial tubercle and is extended as needed to prevent skin tension during exposure. **B,** With the knee flexed, the incision stretches longitudinally to provide additional exposure without additional soft-tissue tension. This also aids in the dissection of the medial and lateral flaps deep to the muscular fascia.

Extensive scarring of the extensor mechanism prohibits a simple medial parapatellar approach. In patients with quadriceps contracture and limited flexion, modification of the standard medial parapatellar approach may be necessary to avoid compromise of the extensor mechanism and facilitate proper flexion and exposure for TKA.

Procedure

Room Setup/Patient Positioning

The patient is placed supine, with a bump under the affected hip if excessive lower extremity external rotation is present. A device to hold the foot alternately in flexion and extension is helpful. Application of a proximal thigh tourniquet is standard, and routine preparation and draping should allow full exposure of relevant anatomy and landmarks, including the tibial tubercle, patella, and distal quadriceps.

Special Instruments/Equipment/Implants

The medial parapatellar approach generally does not require specific instrumentation or equipment. Some retraction tools, however, may be very helpful. A bent Hohmann retractor is useful for lateral tissue distraction whether or not the patella is everted. A marking tool may be helpful to note the extent of the arthrotomy from the medial side of the quadriceps tendon, along the medial border of the patella (ensuring at least 5 mm from the medial patellar edge), distally to the medial border of the patellar tendon. This is to ensure reapproximation at identical points. In cases of a tight extensor mechanism, a pin through the patellar tendon and into the proximal tibia may be helpful to avoid avulsion of the former from its attachment into the tibial tubercle. If the extensor mechanism is extremely tight, however, the surgeon should not hesitate to decrease patellar ligament tension by using a quadriceps snip or tibial tubercle osteotomy.

Surgical Technique

With the knee in extension, the anterior skin incision is marked from 4 cm proximal to the patella to 1 cm distal to the tibial tubercle (**Figure 2, A**). The knee is placed in the flexed position for the skin incision (**Figure 2, B**). Often, the entire length of the marked skin incision is not needed because of the stretching of the skin with the knee flexed. The incision should be extended far enough proximally to provide exposure of at least 2 to 3 cm of the quadriceps tendon. The dissection should occur through the fat just deep to the muscle fascia to minimize disruption to the skin blood supply. Full-thickness skin flaps, one medial flap and one smaller lateral flap, are developed. The arthrotomy is then started 2 cm proximal to the patella, curving along the medial patella and then parallel to the patellar ligament to the tibial tubercle. The arthrotomy should maintain a 5-mm cuff of soft tissue lateral to the vastus medialis insertion and medial to the patella and patellar ligament (**Figure 3**).

The knee is then extended, and the proximal medial tibia is exposed. In most knees, this is done by elevating the medial capsular flap and deep medial collateral ligament from the bone to the midcoronal plane (**Figure 4**). If more medial release is required, this can be continued farther, to the posteromedial corner of the knee joint. In the case of a valgus knee with possible medial collateral ligament laxity, the medial capsular dissection should initially be limited and not carried all the way to the midcoronal plane. This can be released farther if needed later in the procedure. The anterolateral tibia is ex-

Chapter 52: Total Knee Arthroplasty via the Medial Parapatellar Approach

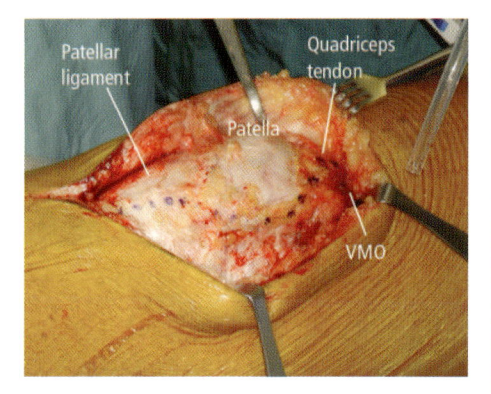

Figure 3 Intraoperative photograph shows a medial patellar arthrotomy. This should leave a 5-mm cuff of soft-tissue attachment medial to the patella and to the patellar ligament. VMO = vastus medialis obliquus.

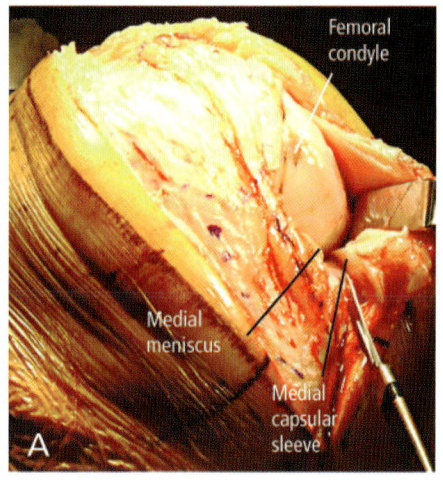

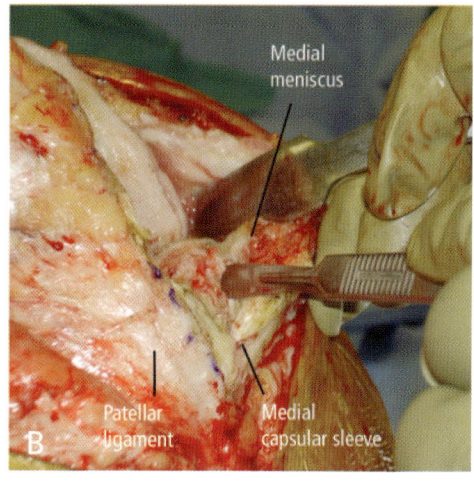

Figure 4 Intraoperative photographs show deep dissection of the medial capsule and deep medial collateral ligament tissue. **A,** Initial release. **B,** Farther release to the midcoronal plane. In cases of severe deformity and difficult exposure, this release can be performed farther to release the posteromedial capsule.

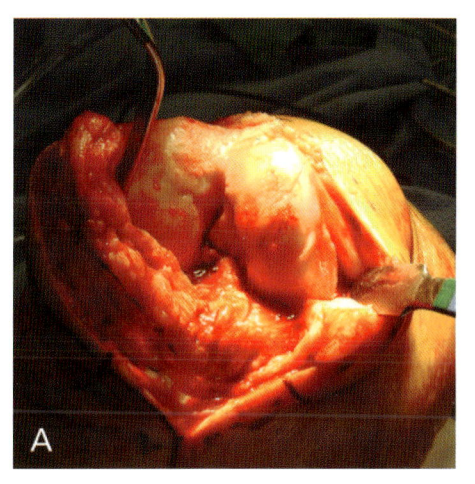

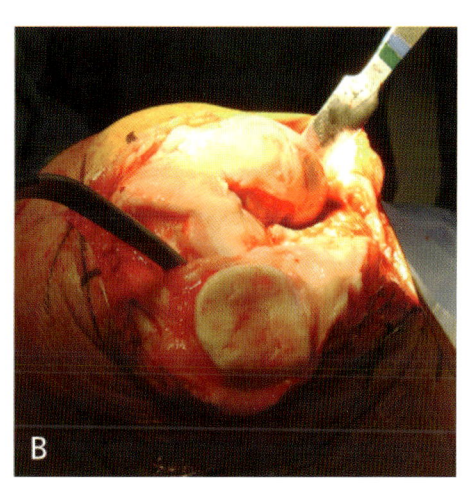

Figure 5 Intraoperative photographs show exposure with the medial parapatellar approach. **A,** Exposure with lateral patellar subluxation. **B,** Additional exposure with eversion of the patella.

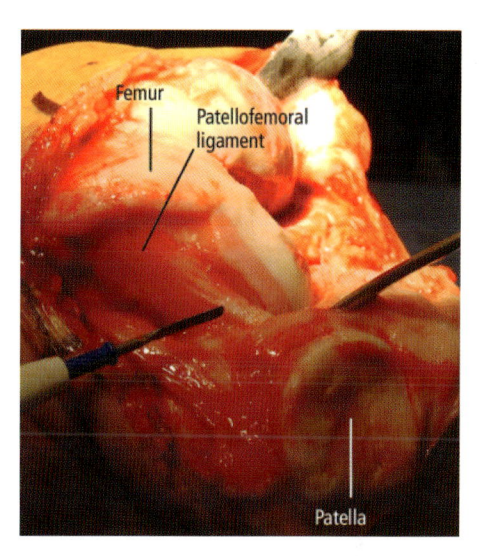

Figure 6 Intraoperative photograph shows release of the patellofemoral ligament for additional exposure. This is best performed with the patella everted, to place this structure in stretch.

posed by retracting the patellar ligament anteriorly. The patella can then be subluxated laterally (**Figure 5, A**) or everted (**Figure 5, B**) when the knee is flexed, with care being taken to not place undue tension on the patellar tendon insertion. A Hohmann retractor is placed under the lateral meniscus after the anterior portion has been cut. If additional lateral exposure is desired after patellar eversion, the patellofemoral ligament can be cut in its midsubstance, which is facilitated by gentle retraction with the lateral retractor (**Figure 6**). With retractors in place, the areas of the patellar fat pad that are limiting lateral visualization can be carefully resected.

The distal femoral or proximal tibial bone cuts can now be performed. With the knee manually flexed, a small posterior retractor is placed anterior to the posterior cruciate ligament to subluxate the tibia anteriorly to aid in instrumentation and resection of the proximal tibia (**Figure 7**). Proper tibial component rotation is critical to a successful TKA. After all bone cuts are made, the proximal tibia can be visualized completely by using a posterior retractor. We prefer a large posterior retractor for optimal visualization, but this can be difficult to place in an obese patient. A smaller posterior retractor can be used in this case (**Figure 8**).

Side-to-side closure of the medial parapatellar arthrotomy is achieved by first securing the arthrotomy at the superior and inferior aspects of the patella. Once this is done, the wound can be closed further with interrupted or running absorbable sutures in a single layer (**Figure 9**). If medial advancement of the arthrotomy is desired, this can be performed in a "pants-over-vest" fashion; once this is secured and stable with the knee in 90° of flexion, the free edge of the medial capsule can be oversewn. Care should be taken to realign the arthrotomy correctly to avoid advancing the patella inferiorly. Large suture knots should be avoided, even if using absorbable suture, particularly in patients with thin subcutaneous tissue or skin within overlying soft tissue, as dermal irritation may occur.

Variations

Although there is general consensus on the utility of the anterior midline incision, variations of the arthrotomy bear consideration. The most common variations include making the proximal limb of the arthrotomy 5 mm medial to the VMO insertion (von Langenbeck) or making the patellar portion of the arthrotomy in a straight line directly over the medial patellar bone (Insall). These

© 2013 American Academy of Orthopaedic Surgeons

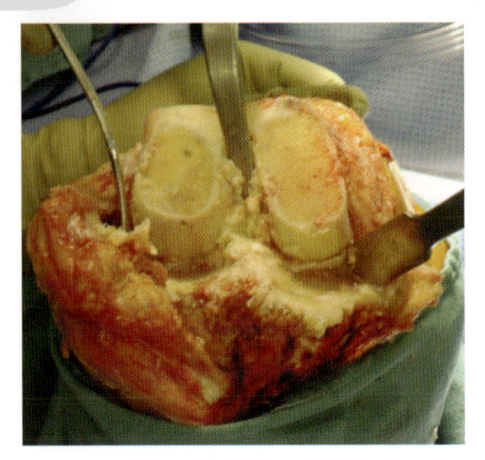

Figure 7 Intraoperative photograph shows the knee after the distal femoral bone cut has been made. The tibia is subluxated anteriorly with maximal knee flexion, and a small retractor is placed just anterior to the posterior cruciate ligament.

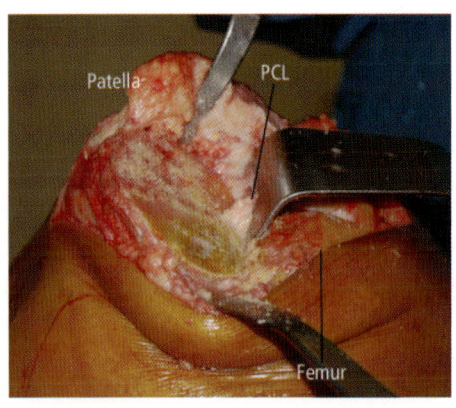

Figure 8 Intraoperative photograph shows the knee after all bone cuts have been made. The proximal tibia is completely visualized by using a large posterior retractor. This greatly facilitates tibial component placement. PCL = posterior cruciate ligament.

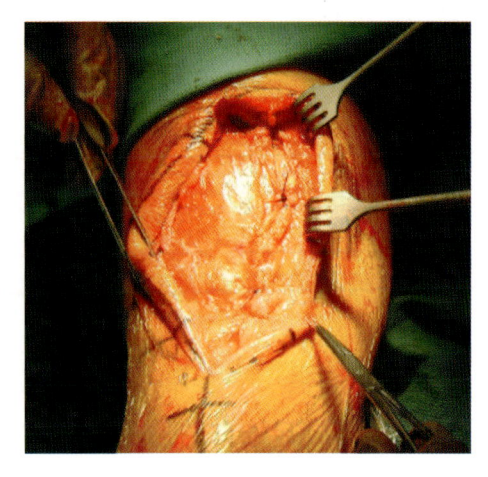

Figure 9 Intraoperative photograph shows closure of the arthrotomy. Note that it was not necessary to use the full extent of the planned skin incision.

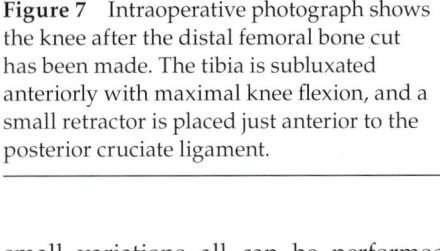

small variations all can be performed using a standard anterior skin incision. For a true extensile approach to the distal femur and knee joint for a tumor-style prosthesis, a lateral knee arthrotomy (Kocher) continued proximally and laterally below the vastus lateralis is advisable.

Instead of an anterior skin incision, a medial parapatellar skin incision may be used. Although this incision has been shown to be better oriented in relation to cleavage lines about the knee and to be subject to less tension during flexion of the knee, it is not commonly used at present.

Complications

The surgeon should avoid malalignment in extensor mechanism closure, a situation that may lead to patellar maltracking, pain, and poor range of motion. Inaccurate closure also may induce patella infera, with similar consequences. Excessive patellar eversion without proximal release may encourage tendon avulsion, particularly in revision TKA and patella infera. Surgical approaches, particularly those minimizing incision length, that limit full visualization of relevant anatomy may defeat the purpose of minimally invasive surgery. This can lead to a protracted recovery at best, and, at worst, revision of poorly aligned implants or extensor mechanism failure.

Postoperative Care and Rehabilitation

Full weight bearing is permissible postoperatively, with early range of motion. In cases in which tight capsular closure is not achieved, a drain may be preferable to avoid hematoma communication between the joint and superficial structures.

Pearls

- Narrow skin bridges pose a considerable risk of skin necrosis; therefore, incisions 4 cm or less from a previous incision should be avoided.
- In cases of a tight extensor mechanism, a pin through the patellar tendon and into the proximal tibia may be helpful to avoid avulsion of the former from its attachment into the tibial tubercle.
- If the extensor mechanism is extremely tight, the surgeon should not hesitate to decrease patellar ligament tension by using a quadriceps snip or tibial tubercle osteotomy.
- In the case of a valgus knee with possible medial collateral ligament laxity, the medial capsular dissection should initially be limited and not carried all the way to the midcoronal plane.
- We prefer a large posterior retractor for optimal visualization, but this can be difficult to place in an obese patient. A smaller posterior retractor can be used in this case.
- Care should be taken to realign the arthrotomy correctly to avoid advancing the patella inferiorly.

References

1. Dalury DF, Jiranek WA: A comparison of the midvastus and paramedian approaches for total knee arthroplasty. *J Arthroplasty* 1999;14(1):33-37.
2. Engh GA, Holt BT, Parks NL: A midvastus muscle-splitting approach for total knee arthroplasty. *J Arthroplasty* 1997;12(3):322-331.
3. Hofmann AA, Plaster RL, Murdock LE: Subvastus (Southern) approach for primary total knee arthroplasty. *Clin Orthop Relat Res* 1991;269:70-77.
4. Lin WP, Lin J, Horng LC, Chang SM, Jiang CC: Quadriceps-sparing, minimal-incision total knee arthroplasty: A comparative study. *J Arthroplasty* 2009;24(7):1024-1032.
5. Matsueda M, Gustilo RB: Subvastus and medial parapatellar approaches in total knee arthroplasty. *Clin Orthop Relat Res* 2000;371:161-168.
6. Parentis MA, Rumi MN, Deol GS, Kothari M, Parrish WM, Pellegrini VD Jr: A comparison of the vastus splitting and median parapatellar approaches in total knee arthroplasty. *Clin Orthop Relat Res* 1999;367:107-116.
7. Scott RD: Primary total knee arthroplasty, in Scott RD, ed: *Surgical Technique in Total Knee Arthroplasty*. Philadelphia, PA, Saunders Elsevier, 2006, pp 20-38.
8. Stern SH: Surgical exposure in total knee arthroplasty, in Barrack RL, Booth RE Jr, Lonner JH, McCarthy JC, Mont MA, Rubash HE, eds: *Orthopaedic Knowledge Update: Hip & Knee Reconstruction* 3. Rosemont, IL, American Academy of Orthopaedic Surgeons, 2006, pp 3-15.
9. White RE Jr, Allman JK, Trauger JA, Dales BH: Clinical comparison of the midvastus and medial parapatellar surgical approaches. *Clin Orthop Relat Res* 1999;367:117-122.
10. Johnson DP, Houghton TA, Radford P: Anterior midline or medial parapatellar incision for arthroplasty of the knee: A comparative study. *J Bone Joint Surg Br* 1986;68(5):812-814.
11. Dalury DF, Dennis DA: Mini-incision total knee arthroplasty can increase risk of component malalignment. *Clin Orthop Relat Res* 2005;440:77-81.

Chapter 53
Total Knee Arthroplasty via Small-Incision Midvastus Approach

Steven B. Haas, MD, MPH   Stephen Kim, MD

Introduction

Total knee arthroplasty (TKA) is a commonly implemented and highly successful treatment of symptomatic end-stage arthritis of the knee when nonsurgical management has failed.[1,2] Although TKA has traditionally been performed through a standard medial parapatellar arthrotomy with eversion of the patella, the development of new surgical techniques and instrument design has facilitated TKA using smaller incisions with less disruption of the extensor mechanism.[3-5] One such method is the small-incision midvastus approach, which avoids eversion of the patella.[3,5] The potential benefits of this approach include earlier return of quadriceps function, earlier return of motion, improved flexion, decreased postoperative narcotic use, and improved cosmesis.[5-10]

The safe and accurate application of the small-incision midvastus approach is predicated on a proper understanding of the principles of minimally invasive surgery, which include (1) a complete understanding of anatomy, (2) gentle handling of the soft tissues, (3) positioning of the extremity in coordination with accurately placed and tensioned retractors to fully use the mobile window, and (4) the use of instrumentation and equipment designed for minimally invasive surgery.[5] In cases where these principles are compromised, a more standard approach may be preferable. If used appropriately, a small-incision midvastus approach can result in less surgical insult to the soft tissues and allow for an earlier return to function without increasing the rate of complications.[5-7]

Patient Selection
Indications
The indications for surgery using the small-incision midvastus approach are the same as those for a standard TKA: a patient with significant disability arising from an underlying arthritic condition of the knee that is refractory to nonsurgical measures. Prior to considering surgery, patients should attempt a course of activity modification, anti-inflammatory medication, physical therapy, and weight reduction if appropriate.

Contraindications
Although there are no absolute contraindications to use the small-incision midvastus approach, the relative contraindications are generally patient related[11,12] (**Table 1**). Surgical considerations and expectations must be discussed preoperatively with the patient. Patients should be aware that although there are potential benefits with a small-incision approach, these benefits are outweighed by the need for the placement of well-aligned components in a knee with balanced ligament restraints. Thus, patients should be aware that if there is any compromise in surgical safety or quality due to a limited exposure, the incision and the dissection will be increased as needed.

Preoperative Imaging
Planning proceeds as for standard knee arthroplasty. We obtain weight-bearing AP, lateral, 45° flexed PA, and Merchant view radiographs. Full-length views are not obtained unless otherwise indicated by the history or the physical examination. Radiographs are interpreted for deformity, bone loss, the presence of patellar baja, and overall bone quality. In cases of deformity, anticipating an appropriate distal femoral cut angle and the height of tibial resection can be useful.

Video 53.1 Mini-Midvastus Approach. Steven B. Haas, MD, MPH; Stephen Kim, MD (16 min)

Table 1 Relative Contraindications to the Small-Incision Midvastus Approach

- Substantial quadriceps muscle mass in men
- Significant obesity (body mass index >40 kg/m²)
- Severe coronal plane deformity
- Flexion contracture >25°
- Passive flexion <80°
- Severe patella baja
- Significant scarring of the quadriceps mechanism
- Revision surgery

Procedure
Patient Positioning
The patient's body is positioned in the same way as for a standard TKA. However, appropriate leg positioning is crucial when performing minimally invasive TKA. A bolstered sandbag is placed under the drapes at the level of the opposite ankle so that the knee can sit flexed at approximately 70° to 90° (**Figure 1**). Most of the procedure is done with the leg in this position. Hyperflexion is required only to prepare the proximal tibia and insert the definitive tibial tray. A lateral support is used so that the leg sits without being held by an assistant.

Special Instruments
Specialized instrumentation is critical in performing a small-incision midvastus approach TKA. Most systems today have made appropriate instrument modifications for a minimally invasive TKA to be performed. Cutting blocks and guides have been made smaller, with rounded edges that can be accommodated through smaller incisions. Additionally, side-specific instruments and cutting guides have been developed so that placement is not impeded by the extensor mechanism. A rigid saw blade with a narrow body that fans out at the distal tip to facilitate bone cuts is also helpful.

Some systems have also developed specific implants for use with a minimally invasive technique. These im-

---

Dr. Haas or an immediate family member has received royalties from Smith & Nephew and Innovative Medical Products; is a member of a speakers' bureau or has made paid presentations on behalf of Smith & Nephew; serves as a paid consultant to or is an employee of Smith & Nephew; has stock or stock options held in Ortho.Secure; and has received research or institutional support from Smith & Nephew. Neither Dr. Kim nor any immediate family member has received anything of value from or has stock or stock options held in a commercial company or institution related directly or indirectly to the subject of this chapter.

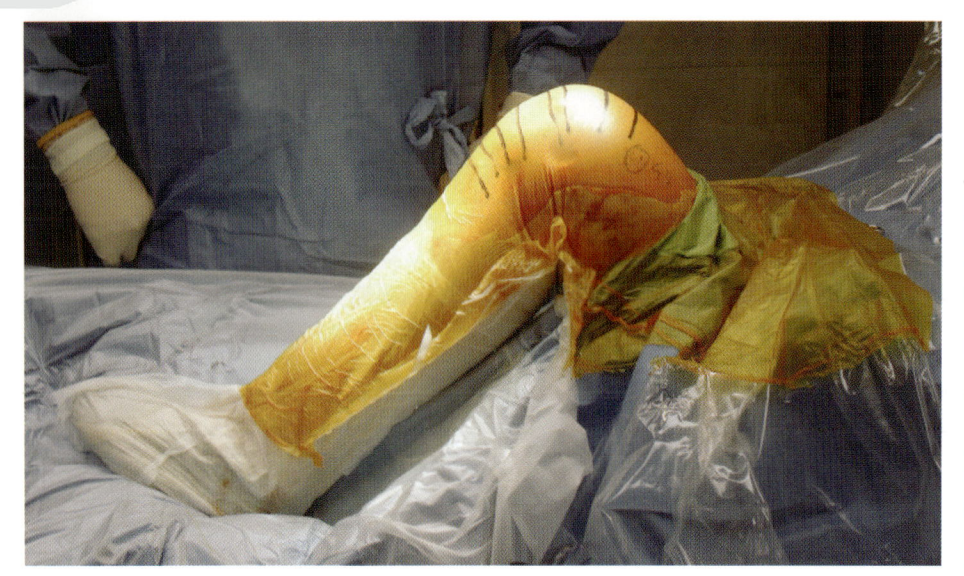

Figure 1 Photograph shows a patient positioned on the operating table with a bump placed across from the opposite ankle to hold the leg at 70° to 90°.

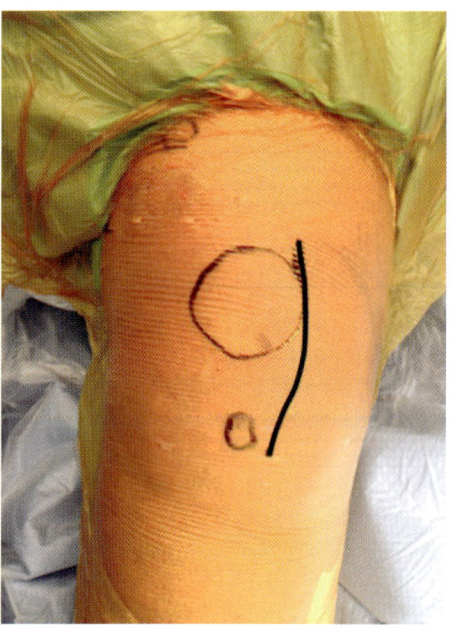

Figure 2 Photograph shows the incision for the small-incision midvastus approach for total knee arthroplasty. The incision extends from 1 cm above the superior pole of the patella to the proximal half of the tibial tubercle on its medial side.

plants have shape modifications, such as a short keel on the tibial component or modular stems. We have found that standard side-specific tibial base plates with an asymmetric tibial tray facilitate accurate insertion through a limited exposure.

Surgical Technique

Anesthesia

Unless contraindicated, we prefer that all patients receive a combined spinal/epidural anesthetic with an indwelling epidural patient-controlled anesthesia that is continued for 48 hours. Patients also receive a bupivacaine femoral nerve block, which we have found aids significantly in postoperative pain control. Intravenous cefazolin is our antibiotic of choice. Patients with significant allergies to penicillin are given vancomycin.

Exposure

Once the patient is appropriately anesthetized and preoperative prophylactic antibiotics have been administered, the leg is prepped and draped in standard fashion for surgery. The leg is exsanguinated with an Esmarch bandage, and the above-knee tourniquet is inflated to 250 to 350 mm Hg, depending on the morphology of the leg. In an obese leg, a higher pressure may be required on the tourniquet.

Landmarks for the skin incision are the borders of the patella and the tibial tubercle (**Figure 2**). These are marked and then a longitudinal incision line is drawn at the junction of the middle and medial thirds of the patella. The incision extends from 1 cm medial to the proximal half of the tibial tubercle on its medial side. The length of the incision depends on the size of the patient but is typically between 8.5 and 12 cm. Regardless of the length, the surgeon should not hesitate to extend the incision at any stage if there appears to be undue tension, especially at the distal apex.

A medial arthrotomy is performed, extending from the superior pole of the patella to the level of the tibial tubercle. A 5-mm cuff of tissue adjacent to the tubercle is preserved to aid in closure. The vastus medialis obliquus (VMO) is identified, and an oblique split is made in the muscle in the line of its fibers at the level of the superior pole of the patella (**Figure 3**).

The first centimeter of the muscle split is initiated sharply, but the remainder is completed using blunt finger dissection to separate the muscle fibers. Performing the split completely by sharp dissection places the distal innervation of the vastus musculature at risk. The muscle split is generally between 2 and 4 cm in length. Once the split is made using this technique, there is usually no further propagation throughout the case. The suprapatellar pouch is preserved except in cases of severe inflammatory disease.

With the knee extended, a subperiosteal dissection is carried around the medial pretibial border, releasing the meniscotibial attachments. The patella is then retracted laterally, and a partial excision of the infrapatellar fat pad is performed. This excision is necessary to allow adequate mobility of the patella. It is important that the patella is subluxated laterally rather than everted, because eversion can place undue tension on the extensor mechanism in this approach. The medial fat pad can also be removed at this stage. The tibial attachments of the anterior cruciate ligament and the anterior horn of the lateral meniscus are released. This allows placement of a thin bent Hohmann retractor laterally to hold the patella in a subluxated position. A small synovial window is made over the anterolateral femoral cortex to aid in the initial anterior femoral resection.

In patients with large or tight extensor mechanisms, large patellae, or an abundance of patellar osteophytes, the patella can be cut first to facilitate subluxation. This is more frequently necessary in men. Initial patellar resection is usually not required in small- to medium-sized females and should be avoided in older osteoporotic patients because of the risk of iatrogenic crushing of the patella from retractors.

Distal Femoral Resection

The distal femur cut is performed first to relax the extension space. This is done with the knee in 70° to 90° of flexion. Limiting knee flexion to this range allows the soft-tissue window to be mobile and thus enables visualization of the distal and anterior femur through the minimal incision. Full visualization of the anterior femoral cortex is necessary for accurate

Chapter 53: Total Knee Arthroplasty via Small-Incision Midvastus Approach

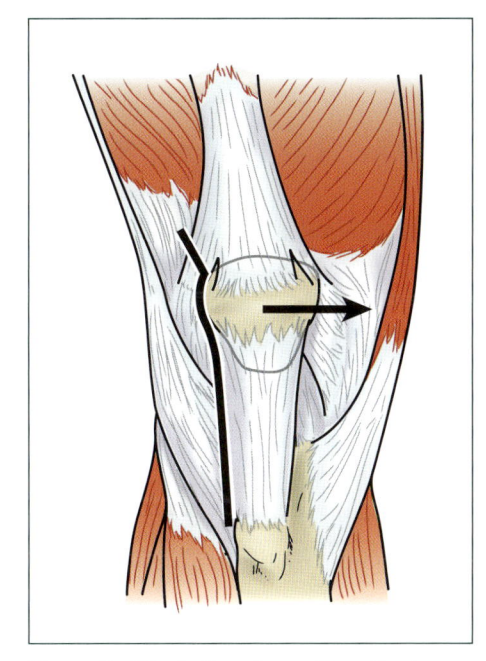

Figure 3 Illustration shows the arthrotomy with the mini-midvastus approach, which extends from the tibial tubercle to the superior patella and then to the muscle of the vastus medialis obliquus. The muscle fibers are not cut. The arrow indicates lateral subluxation of the patella.

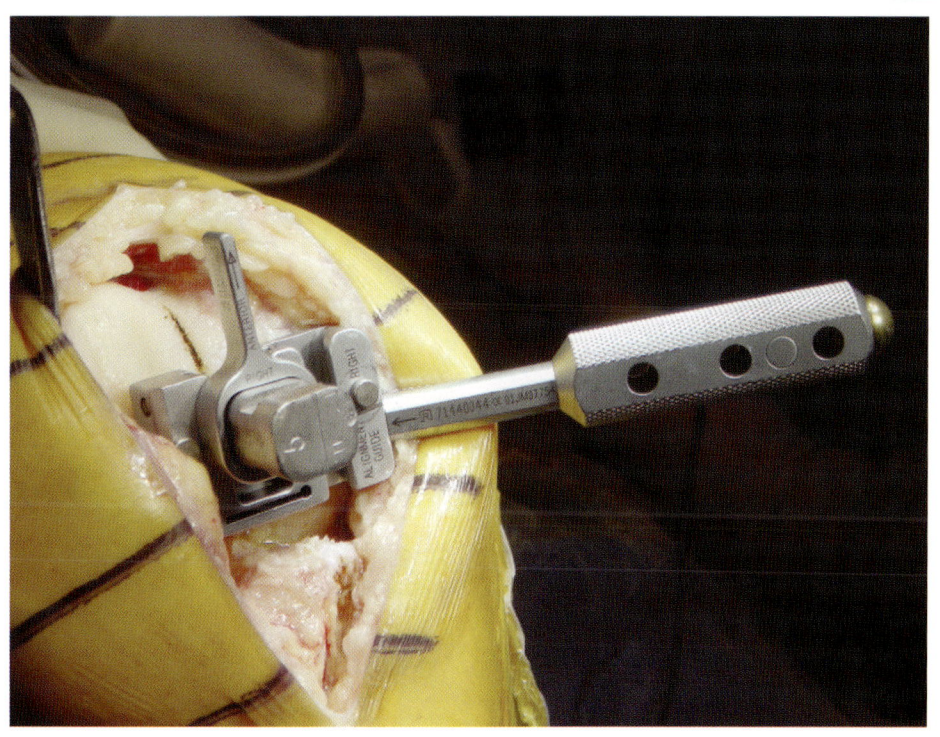

Figure 4 Intraoperative photograph demonstrates the use of an intramedullary alignment guide in the femur. Alignment is determined using the intramedullary guide with the appropriate valgus angle bushing. Rotation is set by aligning the guide with the anterior-posterior or epicondylar axis.

and safe femoral preparation. Hyperflexion should be avoided because this will excessively tighten the extensor mechanism and limit exposure.

For exposure in flexion, a thin bent Hohmann retractor is placed laterally to retract the patella. This retractor is most easily placed with the knee in extension because the extensor mechanism is most relaxed in this position. Once the retractor is placed at the posterior third of the lateral tibia, the retractor and the patella are held in place as the knee is brought into flexion. Once the knee is in flexion, a second thin bent Hohmann retractor can be placed medially for full exposure. The retractors should not be pulled with excessive force because this restricts the mobile window, compromises the viability of the skin edges, and risks avulsion of the extensor mechanism.

The anterior-posterior (A-P) axis (Whiteside line) is marked on the distal femur and is used as the major landmark for establishing component rotation. The posterior condylar axis is used as a secondary reference in varus knees where it is most reproducible. The transepicondylar axis is more difficult to assess with this approach because it requires excessive retraction of the patella laterally.

A 9.5-mm drill is used to enter the femoral canal at a starting point in the notch just anterior to the posterior cruciate ligament insertion on the femur. The canal is then suctioned of its marrow contents to reduce the risk of fat embolization. An intramedullary alignment guide set at 5° of valgus relative to the anatomic axis is inserted, with rotation of the guide determined by the Whiteside line (**Figure 4**). Posterior paddles can be added to the alignment guide for additional posterior referencing of femoral rotation. Once the appropriate rotation is confirmed, the guide is secured in place with pins.

A preliminary anterior resection cutting guide with a stylus is then inserted under the quadriceps mechanism and set for an appropriate anterior cut (**Figure 5**). This guide is secured in place once the stylus makes contact with the anterolateral femoral cortex, which usually represents the highest point. Visualization of stylus contact with the femur is important to avoid anterior femoral notching. The preliminary anterior femoral cut is then performed with careful protection of the proximal skin and soft tissues with right-angle retractors. Alternatively, distal-cut–first instrumentation may be used (**Figure 6**).

The distal femoral cutting guide is then secured in place with pins. After the intramedullary rod and the alignment guide are removed, the level of distal femoral resection is assessed. If there are any concerns regarding block position, this can be reassessed before the distal femoral cut with an extramedullary rod that should be parallel with the mechanical axis of the femur. After the surgeon is satisfied with the position of the guide, the cut is made with careful protection of the patella and the soft tissues. Attention is then directed to the tibia.

Tibial Preparation

The proximal tibial resection is performed. Either extramedullary or intramedullary referencing cutting guides can be used with this technique. However, if extramedullary guides are used, they must be designed for a minimally invasive approach, with side specificity to allow accurate positioning through the limited exposure.

The knee is placed in approximately 90° of flexion. Excessive external rotation, which is often used in the standard approach, must be avoided because this decreases visualization of the lateral compartment by rotating the lateral tibial plateau under the femur. A thin bent Hohmann retractor is then placed medially and laterally, to once again protect the medial collateral ligament and the extensor mechanism. Any overhanging anteromedial osteophytes are removed at this stage so that the tibial resection guide can sit in direct contact with the margin

Section 4: Adult Reconstruction

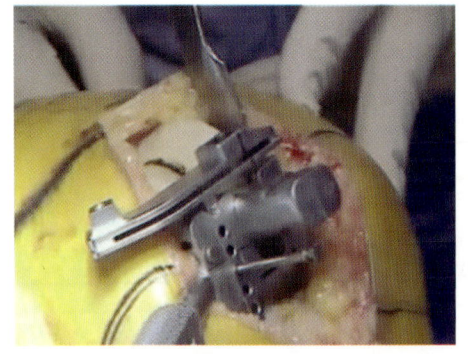

Figure 5 Intraoperative photograph shows the use of a cutting guide on the femur. A preliminary anterior resection is made to place the implant flush with the anterior cortex. This resection also aligns the implant rotation.

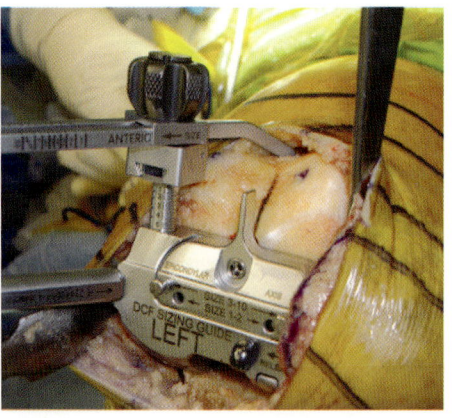

Figure 6 Intraoperative photograph shows the use of a distal-cut–first instrument. This guide measures implant size and rotation. Rotation can be set by the anterior-posterior axis, the posterior condyles, or the epicondylar axis.

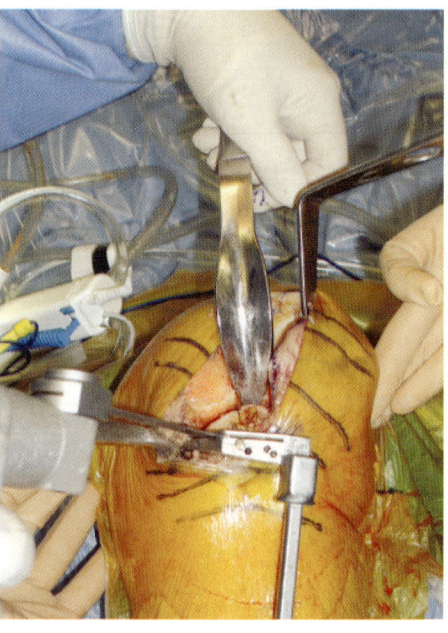

Figure 7 Intraoperative photograph shows an Aufranc retractor being placed in the midline posteriorly to protect the neurovascular structures and hold the tibia in an anteriorly subluxated position. The tibia cutting guide is placed on the anteromedial tibia.

of the tibia. The tibial guide is placed parallel to the tibial crest proximally, with appropriate rotational alignment. The tibialis anterior tendon over the ankle and the second metatarsal are used as distal reference points. The posterior slope is then adjusted in standard fashion, and the appropriate measured resection level is determined. The amount of desired resection is determined by the implant system used as well as the preoperative deformity and bone loss. Once well aligned, the guide is pinned in place. An Aufranc retractor is placed posteriorly to protect the posterior neurovascular structures during the cut without changing the position of the knee (**Figure 7**).

The proximal tibial resection is then performed. Once the saw blade is embedded in the bone, the medial resection can be safely completed by directing the blade in an anterior to posterior direction under direct visualization. The blade is then directed laterally to complete the resection. With this minimally invasive approach, it is preferable to leave a small rim of bone on the posterolateral cortex to avoid damaging the ligaments and the posterior neurovascular bundle with the blind saw blade. The tibial cut surface is then removed, with the remaining rim of bone left in place for later removal. The alignment of the tibial cut is then rechecked using an alignment rod connected to a spacer block.

The knee is then placed into full extension, and the extension gap is opened using a laminar spreader. With this maneuver, combined with lateral retraction of the patella, there is clear visualization of the entire tibial cut surface. The remaining rim of posterior bone can be safely removed at this time. The extension gap and extension ligament balance can also be checked at this time.

Femoral Sizing and Anterior-Posterior Resection

The femoral component size is then determined. When using distal-cut–first instrumentation, rotation is set at this time. The anterior-posterior axis and posterior condyles are used to set rotation. The appropriately sized femoral finishing guide is then pinned in place. At this point, the transepicondylar axis is clearly identified without excessive retraction of the extensor mechanism, and thus the position of the femoral finishing guide can be referenced to this landmark for a final confirmation before making any cuts. If there is any concern for malrotation, the finishing guide can be adjusted. The posterior condylar, posterior and anterior chamfer, and anterior femoral cuts are then made. It is critical that thin bent Hohmann retractors are placed deep to both collateral ligaments during these cuts for protection.

The knee is then placed in 90° of flexion. Using laminar spreaders, we assess the posterior condyles for any retained osteophytes. These are removed with a curved osteotome. The meniscal remnants are also excised at this stage, along with the posterior cruciate ligament if a posterior stabilized system is being used.

Sized spacer blocks are then inserted in full extension and at 90° of flexion to assess the extension and flexion spaces. The knee should be well balanced on the medial and lateral sides in both flexion and extension with the correct-sized block. If asymmetric gaps are present, appropriate soft-tissue releases or bony resections should be performed in the same sequence as a standard approach TKA to achieve full balance.

Patellar Preparation

The patella is prepared after the femur and tibia have been cut but before the trial implants are placed. Preparation of the patella can be done at this stage with either a freehand cut or milled technique. Once the patella is sized and drilled, a trial patellar component can be inserted. If there are remaining osteophytes or large portions of remaining uncovered patella, especially on the lateral side, these can be removed to minimize the chance of impingement.

Final Preparation

Once balanced, the knee is flexed to 120° and the tibia is again exposed with the medial and lateral retractors (**Figure 8**). An additional posterior retractor is inserted to anteriorly subluxate the tibia. The proximal tibia is then sized with trial trays, with the correct size maximizing coverage without component overhang. Good visualization of the entire tibia is necessary for appropriate sizing. Once sized, the tibial trial component is then pinned in place. The proximal tibia is then reamed and broached to accept the definitive prosthesis. Any remaining overhanging tibial osteophytes, which

© 2013 American Academy of Orthopaedic Surgeons

are most commonly found posteromedially, can be removed at this time.

The final femoral preparation is then performed with the knee in 90° of flexion. Once the femoral trial component is aligned with appropriate medial-lateral positioning, the posterior-stabilized box is prepared by reaming through the trial with the guide, and the box/cam trial is inserted (if a posterior stabilized component is used).

The knee is then placed in hyperflexion to allow insertion of the appropriately-sized trial liner. This is reduced into place as the knee is then brought to full extension. The stability of the trials in the coronal plane is then assessed in both extension and 90° of flexion. If multiple trial liner designs are available, the design with the least constraint should be used to allow full assessment of ligamentous stability and balancing. Any additional soft-tissue releases or bony resections can be made at this time if necessary to achieve a well-balanced knee.

After the surgeon is satisfied with the femur and the tibia, the patella can be assessed. Patellar tracking is assessed through a range of motion. If maltracking is present and the components are well aligned, the patella can be rechecked with the tourniquet deflated. If the tracking remains suboptimal, a lateral retinacular release can be performed at this time.

Component Insertion

We prefer to use cemented implants. However, uncemented devices may also be used with a small-incision approach without any additional difficulty. Once the trial components are removed, the bone surfaces are cleaned using pulsatile lavage to achieve a bloodless and dry bone bed. A bone plug is fashioned and impacted into the hole on the distal femur. If sclerotic bone is present, a 2.5-mm drill can be used to make multiple perforations to allow cement interdigitation.

The tibial component is inserted first. Exposure is obtained using an identical technique to that employed when inserting the trial component. Once the cement is mixed, the final tibia is impacted into place, and the excess cement is removed. Careful attention must be paid to ensure appropriate rotation of the component during insertion. If permitted by the type of implant used, an asymmetric tibal component is preferable with the minimally invasive technique because this design allows easier tibial insertion with the more limited exposure.

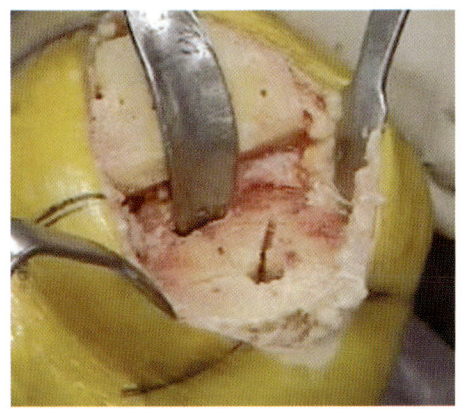

Figure 8 The tibia is exposed by placing an Aufranc retractor posteriorly and thin bent Hohmann retractors medially and laterally.

Once the tibial component is implanted, the knee is placed into the 90° flexed position for insertion of the femoral component (**Figure 9**). Once the femur is firmly impacted into place and the excess cement is removed, an appropriately sized trial liner is inserted, and the knee is reduced into full extension to allow further cement compression. With the knee in extension, the patellar component is cemented into place. Also in the extended position, the mobile window is used to remove any additional cement from the suprapatellar pouch and gutters.

After cement curing is complete, the trial liner is removed and the knee is again positioned in hyperextension to fully expose the tibia. The tibial tray locking mechanism is cleared of debris, and the posterior knee is thoroughly irrigated and cleared of remaining cement. Lastly, the final polyethylene liner is inserted into place with engagement of the locking mechanism. The knee is then reduced into extension and taken through a full range of motion.

Closure

The tourniquet is deflated at this stage, and bleeding is controlled. The knee is copiously lavaged with normal saline solution, and two deep drains are inserted. The capsular layer is closed by placing 0-Vicryl sutures (Ethicon) into the VMO tendon and the perimuscular fascia. Three to five sutures will usually suffice in this area. The remainder of the arthrotomy and the subcutaneous tissues are closed with interrupted sutures. We prefer to use 0-Vicryl sutures for the capsular layer and deep fat and 3/0 Vicryl for the subcutaneous layers. Clips are used to oppose the skin edges. A sterile dressing is then placed, and the leg is wrapped with a bulky Jones dressing.

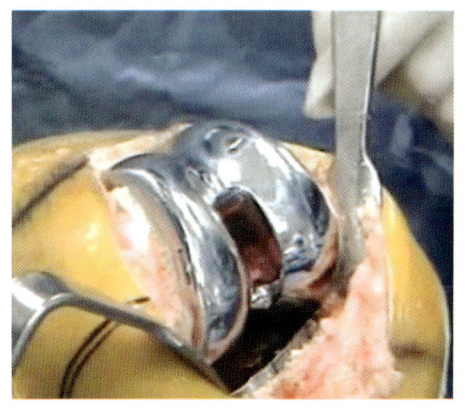

Figure 9 The femoral component is cemented with the knee at 90° of flexion. Avoiding hyperflexion keeps the extensor tendons relaxed, allowing easier lateral cement removal.

Complications

The potential for soft-tissue trauma exists in any small-incision approach. Skin tearing and trauma to muscle and/or adipose tissue are avoided by extending the incision proximally or distally at any time during the procedure deemed necessary. General surgical principles dictate that the risk of infection is kept lowest by minimizing soft-tissue trauma.

The smaller incision described here also highlights the need for very carefully placed retractors, especially during performance of the tibial cut. The laterally placed thin bent Hohmann retractor helps protect the patellar tendon from direct damage from the saw blade, and the posteriorly placed Aufranc retractor further protects the posterior neurovascular structures.

Tension on the extensor mechanism and the sequence of bony cuts suggested above during this procedure place the patella itself at more risk of damage than in standard TKA approaches. This risk can be mitigated by extending the incision when necessary, optimal lateral retractor placement, changing the sequence of bony cuts when necessary, and keeping the patellar trial in place for patients with osteopenic bone.

Postoperative Care and Rehabilitation

All patients are started on a continuous passive motion machine in the recovery room, and flexion is increased as pain allows. Weight bearing is commenced on the first postoperative day. Thromboembolic prophylaxis, including foot compression devices and mobilization, can be started immediately. Chemoprophylaxis can be started as soon as the surgeon and the anesthesiologist feel comfortable, depending on the type of anticoagulation and anesthetic used. All attempts should be made to provide adequate pain control without causing oversedation, to allow aggressive early range of motion and therapy.

Pearls

- To decrease the formation of local heterotopic ossification and fibrosis in the quadriceps, dissection in the suprapatellar pouch is minimized. After first taking care to preserve the quadriceps tendon above the patella and the synovium, a small window is created in the anterior distal femoral synovium/adipose tissue to expose the high point on the anterolateral femoral cortex and place the stylus to judge the extent of the anterior bony resection. This can prevent the development of arthrofibrosis and the resultant poor flexion.
- Preparing the patella prior to cutting the tibia enhances exposure, enabling the surgeon to properly place retractors and protect the vital anatomic structures mentioned in the chapter. However, care must be taken to avoid damaging the patella, which is weakened by the cut.
- If a posterior-stabilized TKA design is to be used, cutting the box later in the procedure is more efficient than doing so immediately after anterior, posterior, and chamfer cuts are made.

References

1. Font-Rodriguez DE, Scuderi GR, Insall JN: Survivorship of cemented total knee arthroplasty. *Clin Orthop Relat Res* 1997;345:79-86.
2. Kelly MA, Clarke HD: Long-term results of posterior cruciate-substituting total knee arthroplasty. *Clin Orthop Relat Res* 2002;404:51-57.
3. Laskin RS: Minimally invasive total knee arthroplasty: The results justify its use. *Clin Orthop Relat Res* 2005;440:54-59.
4. Engh GA, Holt BT, Parks NL: A midvastus muscle-splitting approach for total knee arthroplasty. *J Arthroplasty* 1997;12(3):322-331.
5. Haas SB, Manitta MA, Burdick P: Minimally invasive total knee arthroplasty: The mini midvastus approach. *Clin Orthop Relat Res* 2006;452:112-116.
6. Watanabe T, Muneta T, Ishizuki M: Is a minimally invasive approach superior to a conventional approach for total knee arthroplasty? Early outcome and 2- to 4-year follow-up. *J Orthop Sci* 2009;14(5):589-595.
7. McAllister CM, Stepanian JD: The impact of minimally invasive surgical techniques on early range of motion after primary total knee arthroplasty. *J Arthroplasty* 2008;23(1):10-18.
8. Flören M, Davis J, Peterson MG, Laskin RS: A mini-midvastus capsular approach with patellar displacement decreases the prevalence of patella baja. *J Arthroplasty* 2007;22(6, suppl 2):51-57.
9. Walter F, Haynes MB, Markel DC: A randomized prospective study evaluating the effect of patellar eversion on the early functional outcomes in primary total knee arthroplasty. *J Arthroplasty* 2007;22(4):509-514.
10. Karachalios TH, Giotikas D, Roidis N, Poultsides L, Bargiotas K, Malizos KN: Total knee replacement performed with either a mini-midvastus or a standard approach: A prospective randomised clinical and radiological trial. *J Bone Joint Surg Br* 2008;90(5):584-591.
11. Laskin RS: Surgical exposure for total knee arthroplasty: For everything there is a season. *J Arthroplasty* 2007;22(4, suppl 1):12-14.
12. Tenholder M, Clarke HD, Scuderi GR: Minimal-incision total knee arthroplasty: The early clinical experience. *Clin Orthop Relat Res* 2005;440:67-76.

Video Reference

53.1 Stuchin SA: DVD: *Surgical Techniques in Orthopaedics: Minimally Invasive Total Knee Arthroplasty*. Rosemont, IL, American Academy of Orthopaedic Surgeons, 2005.

Chapter 54
Total Knee Arthroplasty via the Mini-Subvastus Approach

William C. Schroer, MD

Introduction

The mini-subvastus approach for total knee arthroplasty (TKA) described in this chapter uses an anterior incision and is an evolution of Hofmann's subvastus technique.[1-4] The incision length is generally shorter than what has been used traditionally in a medial parapatellar approach, but the length of the incision does not define the mini-subvastus approach or guarantee a different recovery pattern for the TKA patient. The mini-subvastus approach attempts to improve functional recovery from TKA by avoiding both a quadriceps arthrotomy and patellar eversion.

The mini-subvastus approach follows a standard surgical sequence. The surgical guides are scaled-down versions of traditional TKA instruments. The same surgical steps—bone preparation, trialing, cleanup, and final implantation—are performed, with only slight adjustments. Familiarity with the surgical sequence, the traditional instruments, and the anatomy of the anterior approach will enable the surgeon to rapidly and safely put this surgical technique into practice. Although a learning curve requiring additional surgical time has been described for the mini-subvastus technique, a more rapid recovery without an increased risk of complication has been seen in the first patients who underwent the procedure.[5,6]

Patient Selection
Indications

Although many authors have described selection criteria that limit the application of minimally invasive surgery (MIS) TKA techniques, the mini-subvastus technique as described here can be applied to nearly all primary TKA patients.[7,8] Even in obese and muscular patients, in whom MIS procedures frequently are avoided, the mini-subvastus exposure permits extension of the subvastus release to improve surgical visualization without increasing quadriceps damage or compromising quadriceps recovery.

Dr. Schroer or an immediate family member has received research or institutional support from Biomet and Pfizer.

Contraindications

The mini-subvastus approach is contraindicated in knees requiring the removal of significant hardware from previous fracture fixation; the exposure afforded with this technique is not adequate for this purpose. The surgeon who is learning this technique should avoid using it in knees requiring augments or stems because of severe deformity.[8]

Procedure

The following describes my surgical technique for the mini-subvastus approach.

Room Setup/Patient Positioning

The patient is placed supine on the operating table. For patients with significant external hip rotation, the table can be tilted away from the surgical side. A mechanical leg holder generally is used throughout the procedure. If a beanbag is preferred for maintaining knee flexion, it must be secured more distally than is usual in traditional TKA techniques because the knee usually will be flexed and held at only 90° rather than in the hyperflexed position used with traditional TKA.

Although a traditional TKA can be performed routinely with a single surgical assistant, an additional set of hands is suggested for the additional retractors needed to perform the mini-subvastus technique. With the mini-subvastus technique, retractors are used not only to retract but also to protect the soft tissues. A tourniquet is used in all but those few patients with a history of vascular surgery on the involved lower extremity. The tourniquet usually is deflated following final bone preparation, and significant bleeding vessels are cauterized; then the tourniquet is reinflated before implant cementation.

Special Instruments/Equipment/Implants

MIS instruments, which are smaller and lower profile versions of standard TKA instruments, are used for the mini-subvastus approach (**Figure 1**). To improve the accuracy of cutting guide positioning, drill pins should be used rather than push pins hammered into the bone. The use of full-thickness retractors with a fulcrum off the bone minimizes skin trauma. Rakes and retractors that pull directly on the skin should be avoided because they can lead to more wound damage. Thin retractors that require little space are preferred; they can be used during the operation to protect the skin and ligaments from saw blades and osteotomes.

Video 54.1 Total Knee Arthroplasty via the Mini-Subvastus Approach. William C. Schroer, MD (12 min)

Surgical Technique
Incision and Arthrotomy

A midline incision is made from the superior pole of the patella to the tibial tubercle. The incision can range from 10 to 16 cm depending on patient size, the presence of any previous incisions, and surgeon experience. Again, the length of the incision is not critical to the patient's

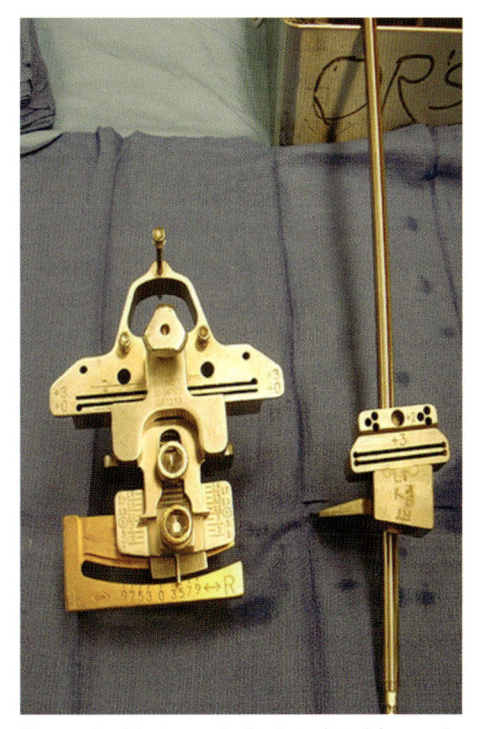

Figure 1 Photograph depicts distal femoral cutting guides for total knee arthroplasty. The large instrument is used for traditional total knee arthroplasty, and the smaller one is used in minimally invasive surgery.

© 2013 *American Academy of Orthopaedic Surgeons*

recovery and should be optimized to facilitate a safe and accurate surgical procedure (**Figure 2**). Subcutaneous mobilization is required both medially and superiorly to allow patellar mobility. A horizontal arthrotomy is made along the inferior aspect of the vastus medialis obliquus (VMO), leaving a cuff of retinaculum on the VMO for closure (**Figure 3, A**). The arthrotomy is completed in a standard manner along the medial patellar tendon. The reflected retinaculum, which contains the medial patellofemoral ligament, is tagged for identification, protection, and retraction (**Figure 3, B**). To facilitate exposure, I create a subcutaneous mobile window, through which different parts of the knee joint can be visualized depending on the position of the knee but the entire joint is not visualized at any one time. For example, with the knee placed in the figure-of-4 position, the posterolateral aspect of the knee is well visualized.

Patellar Mobilization

The extensor mechanism is mobilized to allow patellar subluxation. The patella and VMO are tethered medially and released through a series of three steps. First, unlike a true subvastus exposure, in which the VMO is released from the intermuscular septum up to the Hunter canal to allow patellar eversion, the mini-subvastus arthrotomy incises just through the retinacular cuff of the VMO on its medial border (**Figure 4, A** and **B**). This allows significant lateral mobility of the VMO. In large, muscular patients, the VMO often will "self-release" a few centimeters above the joint line along the intermuscular septum. Next, the synovial capsular reflection underneath the VMO is released (**Figure 4, C** and **D**). Depending on the amount and thickness of the synovium, a limited synovectomy can be done at this time. Finally, the patellar tendon fat pad is excised (**Figure 4, E** and **F**). These three steps allow the patella to be subluxated laterally.

A Z retractor is placed under the VMO laterally, and the knee is flexed to 90°. It should be emphasized that the knee is flexed to only 90°, leaving it in an in situ position; much of the operation is performed with the knee at this angle. This avoids the hyperflexed knee position routinely described in traditional TKA techniques, in which the tibia is dislocated forward, damaging the posterior knee capsule.

Femoral and Tibial Preparation

A 9-mm drill is used to open the intramedullary canals of the distal femur and the proximal tibia. An intramedullary distal femoral alignment guide is positioned on the anteromedial surface of the femur. Two parallel threaded pins are drilled into the femur. The distal resection is checked with an angel wing, and the final position of the guide is adjusted to ensure adequate distal femur resection. A third pin is then drilled in a different plane to provide secure fixation of the cutting guide. This distal femoral cutting guide arcs around the femur from anterior to medial, allowing an initial cut of the medial femoral condyle from anterior to posterior. Then the saw can be angled from more medial to lateral to complete the distal femoral cut.

Tibial preparation is next. An intramedullary cutting guide is used to make the tibial cut. Although both intramedullary and extramedullary guides are available, the intramedullary tibial guide requires fewer soft-tissue landmarks for orientation and is thought to provide a more accurate tibial resection. Once the tibial cut is made, the knee is brought into full extension. The cut tibia is grasped on its anteromedial surface and rotated out,

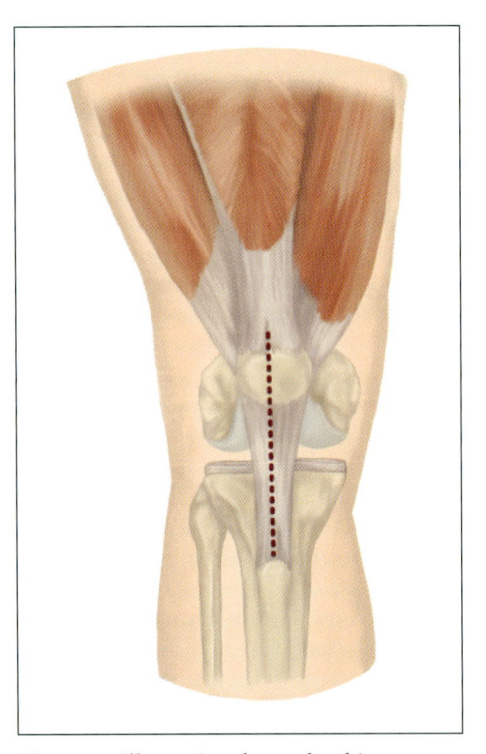

Figure 2 Illustration shows the skin incision (dashed line) for the mini-subvastus approach for total knee arthroplasty.

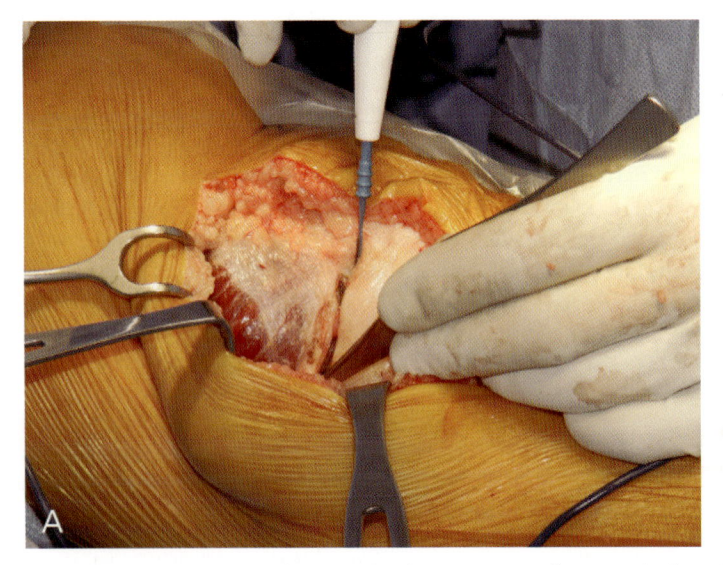

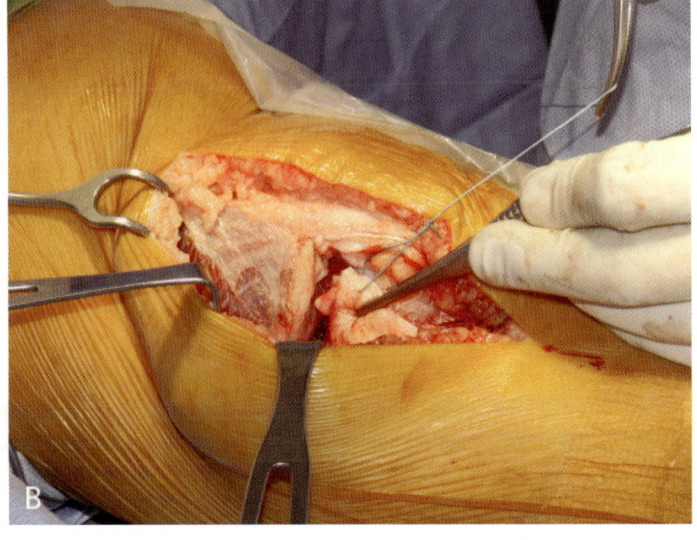

Figure 3 Intraoperative photographs demonstrate arthrotomy in the mini-subvastus approach. **A**, A horizontal arthrotomy is made along the vastus medialis obliquus (VMO). Note the small cuff of retinaculum left on the VMO. **B**, The completed arthrotomy with tagged retinaculum is shown. Note that the VMO is still tethered medially.

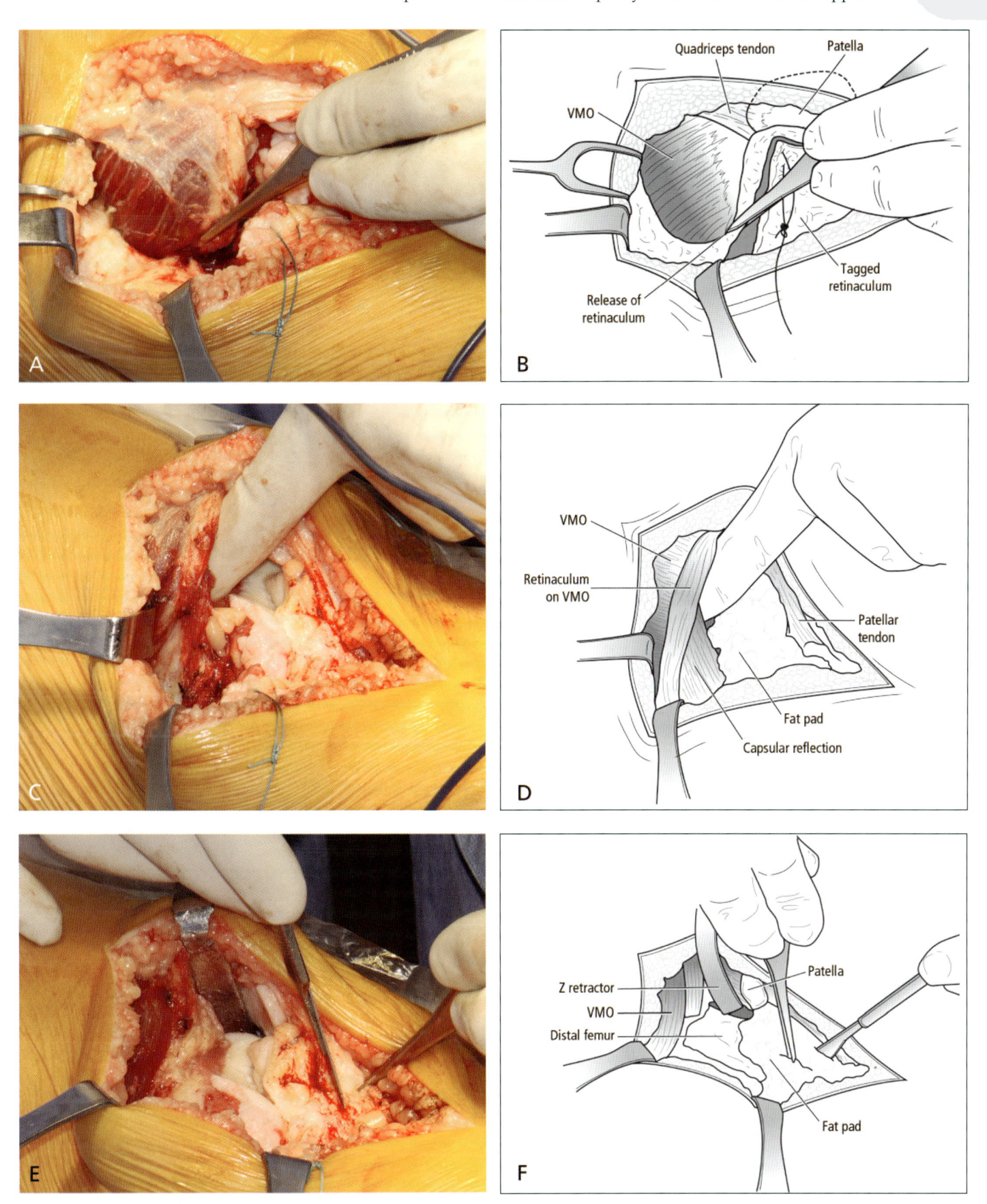

Figure 4 Subvastus release and patellar mobilization in total knee arthroplasty via the mini-subvastus approach. **A,** Intraoperative photograph shows the vastus medialis obliquus (VMO) released through the retinacular cuff. The forceps are grabbing the recently released retinacular cuff. Note that the patella has started to move laterally. **B,** Illustration shows the same procedure shown in panel A. **C,** In this intraoperative photograph, the surgeon's index finger is under the capsular reflection. Note that the VMO is releasing laterally. **D,** Illustration shows the same procedure shown in panel C. **E,** In this intraoperative photograph, a Z retractor has subluxated the patella laterally. Note that the entire anterior distal femur is well visualized. Excision of the fat pad as shown completes the mobilization of the patella. **F,** Illustration shows the same procedure shown in panel E.

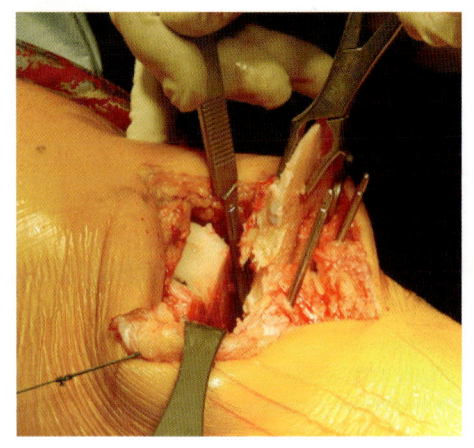

Figure 5 Intraoperative photograph shows tibial preparation for total knee arthroplasty via the mini-subvastus approach. The tibia is rotated out, medial side first. The cut bone is released from the medial meniscus, the posterior cruciate ligament, and the lateral meniscus.

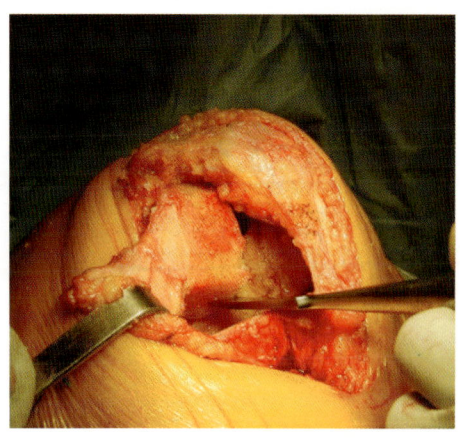

Figure 6 Intraoperative photograph shows posteromedial femoral osteophytes visualized through the mobile window, which affords a medial view for posterior cleanout. A view of the lateral side is obscured here but can be obtained in a subsequent step. Everything can be well visualized with the mini-subvastus surgical technique, although unlike a medial patellar tendon approach, not everything can be seen at once.

medial side first (**Figure 5**). As the tibia rotates out, the medial meniscus, posterior cruciate ligament, and lateral meniscal attachments are released sharply off the cut tibia with a knife. With the knee still in full extension, the meniscal remnants are removed from the posterior capsule with electrocautery, and the extension gap is checked to ensure that adequate bone has been resected for final implants.

The knee is brought back into a 90° flexed position. The distal femur is measured with a posterior reference guide, femoral rotation is determined, and the low-profile distal femoral four-in-one cutting block is positioned on the distal femur. Saw cuts are made and bone fragments are removed. If a posterior stabilized implant is being used, the femoral notch cut is made at this time. The patella is allowed to subluxate back into an anatomic position, and the knee is flexed again to 90°. With posterior pressure placed on the proximal tibia, the posteromedial osteophytes are visible through the mobile window and can be removed with a curved osteotome (**Figure 6**). Then the patella is subluxated laterally again with a Z retractor, the knee is brought into a figure-of-4 position, bringing the posterolateral aspect of the knee into view through the mobile window, and the posterolateral osteophytes are removed with a curved osteotome.

Trialing, Balancing, and Final Preparation

Trial femoral and tibial tray components are positioned, and a trial reduction is performed. Collateral ligament balancing may occur during several steps of the procedure, but final balancing is performed and confirmed at this time. Patellar tracking and tibial rotation are determined. After the trial components are removed, the knee is placed in extension and the patella is tilted onto its side and prepared for a cemented patellar button. The laxity provided by the distal femur and proximal tibial cuts allows access to the patella with little tension on the quadriceps. Concern over damaging or fracturing a previously prepared patella is reduced by preparing the patella last.

The knee is brought back into a 90° flexed position. Medial and lateral retractors are positioned, and a posterior retractor is used to subluxate the tibia forward. This step is the only point of the procedure in which the knee is taken out of an anatomic position. The tibia is finished for the final tibial component using previously determined rotation from the trial reduction. The cut bony surfaces then are cleaned with pulsatile irrigation in preparation for final component implantation. The tibial and femoral components are cemented into position, excess cement is removed, and a trial tibial polyethylene component is placed to allow the cement to cure under compression. The patellar component is then cemented with the knee in extension. Appropriate polyethylene thickness is determined, and final soft-tissue balancing checks are made throughout flexion and extension. Prior to the final polyethylene component insertion, a final check for bone and cement debris is made with the knee in full extension. Once the polyethylene component is positioned and patellar tracking is confirmed, the angle of the arthrotomy is closed, followed by the VMO and patellar tendon arms of the arthrotomy. A single figure-of-8 nonabsorbable suture is positioned at the apex of the arthrotomy, and a double-armed running suture is used to close the remainder of the capsule.

Postoperative Care and Rehabilitation

Multimodal Pain Management

Possibly no changes to TKA care over the past decade have been more significant than the adoption of multimodal pain management strategies. On the day of surgery, multimodal pain management addresses pain before anesthesia is initiated, and it continues throughout the surgical procedure, through the postanesthesia care unit, and onto the joint arthroplasty care unit. Prior to surgery, a cyclooxygenase-2 (COX-2) inhibitor is given to block the formation of prostaglandins that develop in response to the surgical trauma of the soft tissues. A long-acting narcotic is given to desensitize the afferent nerve pathways before pain stimulation and acetaminophen is given, which can slow the intrathecal pain pathways. Intraoperatively, a regional block minimizes stimulation of the efferent pathways, and intraoperative infiltration of the soft tissues around the knee with a long-acting local anesthetic decreases pain formation. Postoperatively, the multimodal pain management strategy uses a combination of COX-2 inhibitors, oral narcotics, and cryotherapy to prevent large spikes in pain. Intravenous narcotics are minimized because of their association with nausea, and antiemetics are delivered on a scheduled basis through the first 24 hours. COX-2 inhibitors are continued, when medically appropriate, for 6 weeks after surgery.[9]

Mobilization

Adequate management of pain and nausea is imperative for rapid recovery after TKA. If pain is not controlled effectively, the patient will have difficulty mobilizing. Following a mini-subvastus TKA, patients routinely are seen by physical therapy on the day of surgery, assisted up to a chair, encouraged to use the bathroom rather than bedside commodes or bedpans, and instructed in the proper use of a walker. Patients are allowed to bear weight as tolerated and are encouraged to perform quad sets while in bed and gravity-assisted knee flexion when sitting up in a chair. Formal physical therapy continues twice daily during the second and, if needed, the third day of hospitalization. Instruction focuses on patient safety, stair management, and progressive knee range of motion. Although epidurals and femoral nerve blocks provide variable benefits in pain management, they are used only rarely because their use significantly slows the patient's ability to mobilize. Similarly, continuous passive motion machines rarely have demonstrated significant benefit and are not used because they slow patient mobilization by keeping the patient in bed for several hours a day.

Following hospital discharge to home on the second or third day after surgery, home health care is scheduled for 2 or 3 weeks to oversee physical therapy and wound management. A consistent therapy message to optimize knee range of motion is taught to the patient and their families. Using a stationary bicycle in several short sessions per day is encouraged to promote knee flexion and proprioception. Patients are progressed from a walker to a cane and subsequently to independent ambulation with guidance from the home therapist. Patients are seen in the surgeon's office 3 weeks after surgery, at which time surgical wounds and knee motion are assessed.

Since 2003, I have applied the mini-subvastus technique to more than 4,500 primary TKA cases. Wound concerns requiring additional outpatient visits or prescription of oral antibiotics have occurred in less than 5% of patients; knee flexion at 3 weeks has been greater than 100° in more than 95% of patients; and formal outpatient physical therapy has been required in less than 5% of patients.

Pearls

- In the mini-subvastus technique, skin incision length is not as important as the avoidance of quadriceps violation and patellar eversion.
- To improve the accuracy of cutting guide positioning, drill pins should be used rather than push pins that are hammered into the bone. Push pins tend to deflect off the underlying bone and may not be immediately identified. Cutting guides are held more securely if a third pin is positioned through the guide in a separate plane from the first two drill pins.
- Using full-thickness retractors with a fulcrum off the bone minimizes skin trauma. Rakes and retractors that pull directly on the skin can lead to more wound damage. Thin retractors that require little space are preferred; they can be used during the operation to protect the skin and ligaments from saw blades and osteotomes.
- MIS is really about minimizing soft-tissue damage. Throughout the operation, efforts should be made to avoid excessive and unneeded retraction. Anterior displacement of the tibia on the femur damages the posterior capsule. Efforts should be made to avoid dislocating the knee; instead, the joint should be maintained in an anatomic position whenever possible.
- The surgeon needs to know when and where soft tissue is at risk and should protect the soft tissue from the saw blade with a retractor. For example, the patellar tendon is at risk during the tibial cut (**Figure 7**) and during the four-in-one femoral cuts. An additional retractor, positioned perpendicularly to the oscillating blade, will protect the tendon during these steps.

Concerns About Minimally Invasive TKA

Several concerns have been raised regarding MIS TKA techniques. These concerns are well outlined in the physician advisory statement from the American Association of Hip and Knee Surgeons, titled "Minimally Invasive and Small Incision Joint Replacement Surgery: What Surgeons Should Consider." This statement outlines several areas of concern, including (1) the applicability of MIS TKA techniques, (2) the learning curve associated with MIS TKA, and (3) the increased risk of complications associated with MIS TKA. As with any new surgical technique, these concerns are appropriate. The mini-subvastus technique needs to be fully investigated and these three concerns addressed.

Applicability

Several studies have described superior functional results with MIS TKA compared with conventional medial parapatellar arthrotomy TKA techniques.[1-3] Shorter hospital stays, improved early knee motion, and quicker return of quadriceps strength have been reported with each minimally invasive approach. Many early reports have listed selection criteria for MIS TKA. Patient weight, body mass index, knee deformity, age, previous surgery, and preoperative knee range of motion all have been reported as selection criteria that limit which patients should undergo an MIS procedure. Although improved functional recovery has been described following MIS TKA, most studies fail to disclose the percentage of primary TKAs performed using the MIS technique. Limiting the application of a technique to optimal patients raises the concern that positive clinical outcomes are a result of patient selection rather than surgical technique.

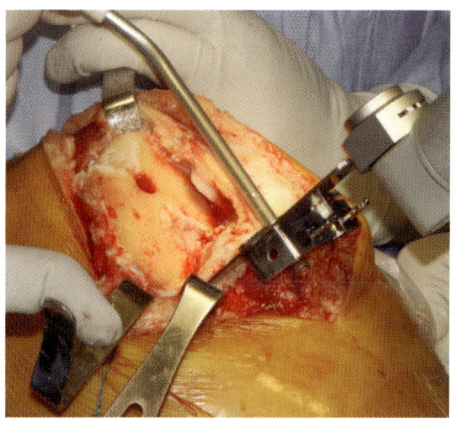

Figure 7 Intraoperative photograph demonstrates retractors used as safeguards for the soft tissue. Note that the retractor is guarding the medial soft tissues as bone cuts are made.

Recent studies on the mini-subvastus technique have demonstrated nearly universal application of this MIS TKA technique. Pagnano and Meneghini[7] reported that the mini-subvastus technique was applied to more than 100 consecutive primary TKA cases. The authors reported earlier return of quadriceps strength, increased knee range of motion, and shorter hospital stays compared with their results using a medial parapatellar arthrotomy in traditional TKA. My prospective evaluation of the mini-subvastus technique demonstrated similar clinical results, with an applicability rate greater than 99% in 732 consecutive primary TKA cases.[8] This high applicability rate obviates concerns that positive clinical outcomes are a result of patient selection rather than surgical technique. Although this study demonstrated the successful use of the mini-subvastus technique in patients who are obese, muscular, or have a large knee deformity, it also demonstrated that the mini-subvastus technique should be avoided when significant hardware removal is required or when the use of augments and stems is anticipated. Routine use of the mini-subvastus technique would, therefore, be discouraged in revision TKA surgery. Surgeons may still wish to avoid patellar eversion. Improved quadriceps recovery after TKA has been demonstrated by avoiding patellar eversion alone.[10]

Learning Curve
A learning curve exists whenever a surgeon is developing expertise with new surgical techniques or instruments. The concern with MIS TKA techniques is that this stage of surgical skill development may be too severe, leading to increased complications, or too prolonged, such that an average-volume surgeon may not be able to develop proficiency in a reasonable time. MIS total hip arthroplasty (THA) studies have demonstrated a steep learning curve, with significantly increased complications during a surgeon's first 50 MIS THA cases.[11,12] Only a few reports on the learning curve associated with MIS TKA are available.[5,6]

In a review of my first 600 MIS TKA cases using the mini-subvastus technique, the learning curve was evaluated by assessing surgical time, clinical outcomes, and complications as surgical experience with the mini-subvastus technique progressed.[6] When compared with my traditional medial parapatellar approach experience, the mean surgical duration increased significantly, from 74 minutes for a traditional TKA to 82 minutes for the first 100 mini-subvastus TKAs (P = 0.034). During this learning curve of approximately 100 surgical cases, new surgical instruments, a modified surgical sequence, and alterations in retractor placement and knee positioning were developed. Essentially, the mini-subvastus technique as described in this chapter was developed. The mean surgical time of the next 100 mini-subvastus TKA cases was equivalent to that of my traditional control group, and then actually decreased significantly to 65 minutes for the last 400 MIS procedures (P = 0.024). With respect to surgery duration, a learning curve existed through the first 100 TKA cases using the mini-subvastus technique.

Knee flexion at 1 year following my first 50 MIS procedures increased when compared with knee flexion in the traditional medial parapatellar arthrotomy control group (P < 0.0001). No further increase in knee flexion occurred as experience with the MIS procedure increased. Patients in this study benefited from the MIS technique independent of the learning curve. During an initial learning curve of approximately 100 mini-subvastus TKA cases as determined by mean surgical time, clinical results improved despite the learning curve.[6] Similarly, King et al[5] demonstrated an increased surgical time through an initial 50 MIS TKA cases while demonstrating a more rapid recovery.

Complications
The principal concern with MIS techniques is that limited exposure will lead to increased complications. Increased wound complications may develop as a result of excessive pull of retractors on the skin. Saw cuts made under poor visualization may lead to an increased risk of ligament, tendon, or neurovascular injury. Increased soft-tissue damage as well as increased surgical time also may lead to an increased perioperative infection rate. Finally, because of limited visualization, the risk of inaccurate positioning of the implant may increase, leading to inferior long-term results.[13,14] Early clinical results that showed increased complications following MIS THA compared with conventional THA have supported these concerns.[11,12]

Few MIS TKA studies have reported complications in detail. My colleagues and I previously reported the complication rate following the first 600 TKAs performed with the mini-subvastus technique with a minimum 2-year follow-up.[6] In this study, no increase in the complication rate occurred when compared with our historical controls and with large published series of traditional TKA.[15,16] This previously published cohort has been expanded to the first 875 mini-subvastus TKA patients, who are now a mean 5.5 years postoperative (range, 48 to 90 months). Twenty-three knees (2.6%) required additional procedures in this group of 875 MIS TKAs. Sixteen knees (1.8%) required revision, 6 for infection and 10 (1.1%) for aseptic loosening. Seven knees (0.8%) required nonrevision knee surgery. This major complication rate of 2.6% is consistent with results reported by Vessely et al,[15] who found equal rates of further knee surgery for septic failure, aseptic failure, and non-implant–related complications. All non-implant–related procedures in my series were performed to address complications that previously have been described in the TKA literature.

In the study of the first 600 TKAs performed with the mini-subvastus technique, my colleagues and I reported that 16 failed and required component revision.[6] This 0.33% annualized failure rate through 5.5 years compares favorably with other large TKA series. In a review of more than 2,000 posterior stabilized TKAs with a 14-year follow-up, Font-Rodriguez et al[16] determined an annualized failure rate of up to 0.51%. The rate of septic failure (0.7%) was less than that reported in large TKA series.[17] Although other reports have suggested that an increased rate of failure will occur when using MIS TKA techniques, my own experience with the mini-subvastus TKA technique has demonstrated no increased risk of failure, with a 1.8% aseptic revision rate over a minimum of 4 years of follow-up. Although longer follow-up is certainly required, previous reports on the mechanism of aseptic failures have demonstrated an early failure rate of nearly 5% during the first 5 years following traditional TKA.

My mini-subvastus TKA cohort is still only at midterm follow-up. Continued follow-up is ongoing to monitor the outcomes. Previous knee studies, however, have demonstrated that most failures tend to occur in the first few years after TKA. More than half of all failures leading to revision TKA have been shown to occur in the first 2 years postoperatively.[17]

Conclusions
The efficacy and safety of the mini-subvastus TKA technique will continue to be monitored and discussed. As with several primary TKA issues, proponents and critics of MIS techniques will continue to argue at meetings and in journals for several years to come. This chapter describes the mini-subvastus TKA technique that has been used for the past 9 years in more than 4,000 cases of primary TKA, and the results demonstrate a rapid functional recovery without an increase in early or late complications. Outcome variability is certain between different MIS techniques, and, within the same MIS technique, even greater outcome variation is expected among different surgeons, just as variable outcomes have been demonstrated by different surgeons using traditional TKA techniques for the past several decades. TKA results can be poor with either MIS or traditional surgical techniques.

Critics of MIS TKA target only short-term improvements that diminish rapidly within a few weeks after surgery. Proponents of MIS TKA demonstrate functional differences several months after surgery. What is indisputable is the impact of MIS thinking. All surgeons, regardless of their preferences in surgical technique, have become much more aware of the soft-tissue envelope around the knee. For example, few surgeons still cut the skin and quadriceps tendon "one handbreadth above to one handbreadth below" the patella, as most were taught in orthopaedic residency training. This amount of soft-tissue invasion is simply not necessary to perform a primary TKA. Just as importantly, surgeons have become aware of the need to optimize their patients' recovery after TKA, leading to a variety of multimodal pain management strategies.

In summary, the mini-subvastus technique can be applied to nearly all primary cases of TKA, has complication rates comparable to several large traditional TKA series, and has both subjective and objective measures of improved functional recovery.

References

1. Laskin RS: New techniques and concepts in total knee replacement. *Clin Orthop Relat Res* 2003;416:151-153.
2. Bonutti PM, Mont MA, McMahon M, Ragland PS, Kester M: Minimally invasive total knee arthroplasty. *J Bone Joint Surg Am* 2004;86(suppl 2):26-32.
3. Tria AJ Jr, Coon TM: Minimal incision total knee arthroplasty: Early experience. *Clin Orthop Relat Res* 2003;416:185-190.
4. Hofmann AA, Plaster RL, Murdock LE: Subvastus (Southern) approach for primary total knee arthroplasty. *Clin Orthop Relat Res* 1991;269:70-77.
5. King J, Stamper DL, Schaad DC, Leopold SS: Minimally invasive total knee arthroplasty compared with traditional total knee arthroplasty: Assessment of the learning curve and the postoperative recuperative period. *J Bone Joint Surg Am* 2007;89(7):1497-1503.
6. Schroer WC, Diesfeld PJ, Reedy ME, LeMarr AR: Evaluation of complications associated with six hundred mini-subvastus total knee arthroplasties. *J Bone Joint Surg Am* 2007;89(Suppl 3):76-81.
7. Pagnano MW, Meneghini RM: Minimally invasive total knee arthroplasty with an optimized subvastus approach. *J Arthroplasty* 2006;21(4, suppl 1):22-26.
8. Schroer WC, Diesfeld PJ, LeMarr A, Reedy ME: Applicability of the mini-subvastus total knee arthroplasty technique: An analysis of 725 cases with mean 2-year follow-up. *J Surg Orthop Adv* 2007;16(3):131-137.
9. Schroer WC, Diesfeld PJ, LeMarr AR, Reedy ME: Benefits of prolonged postoperative cyclooxygenase-2 inhibitor administration on total knee arthroplasty recovery: A double-blind, placebo-controlled study. *J Arthroplasty* 2011;26(6, suppl):2-7.
10. Walter F, Haynes MB, Markel DC: A randomized prospective study evaluating the effect of patellar eversion on the early functional outcomes in primary total knee arthroplasty. *J Arthroplasty* 2007;22(4):509-514.
11. Bal BS, Haltom D, Aleto T, Barrett M: Early complications of primary total hip replacement performed with a two-incision minimally invasive technique. *J Bone Joint Surg Am* 2005;87(11):2432-2438.
12. Archibeck MJ, White RE Jr: Learning curve for the two-incision total hip replacement. *Clin Orthop Relat Res* 2004;429:232-238.
13. Barrack RL, Barnes CL, Burnett RS, Miller D, Clohisy JC, Maloney WJ: Minimal incision surgery as a risk factor for early failure of total knee arthroplasty. *J Arthroplasty* 2009;24(4):489-498.
14. Dalury DF, Dennis DA: Mini-incision total knee arthroplasty can increase risk of component malalignment. *Clin Orthop Relat Res* 2005;440:77-81.
15. Vessely MB, Whaley AL, Harmsen WS, Schleck CD, Berry DJ: Long-term survivorship and failure modes of 1000 cemented condylar total knee arthroplasties. *Clin Orthop Relat Res* 2006;452:28-34.
16. Font-Rodriguez DE, Scuderi GR, Insall JN: Survivorship of cemented total knee arthroplasty. *Clin Orthop Relat Res* 1997;345:79-86.
17. Sharkey PF, Hozack WJ, Rothman RH, Shastri S, Jacoby SM: Why are total knee arthroplasties failing today? *Clin Orthop Relat Res* 2002;404:7-13.

Video Credit

54.1 Adapted from Schroer WC: Video: *Total Knee Arthroplasty via the Mini Subvastus Approach.* Copyright Video Journal of Orthopaedics, Santa Barbara, CA, 2010.

Chapter 55
Revision Total Knee Arthroplasty via Quadriceps Snip

Ari Seidenstein, MD   Scott Scuderi, BS   Giles R. Scuderi, MD

Introduction

The quadriceps snip has evolved from more traditional surgical techniques, such as the V-Y quadriceps turndown described by Coonse and Adams and Insall's patellar turndown.[1-3] In 1988, Insall discovered that by extending the medial arthrotomy proximally and transecting the quadriceps tendon laterally, greater exposure was achieved. This observation led to the use of the quadriceps snip (**Figure 1**) as a means of exposing the tight knee in primary and revision total knee arthroplasty (TKA).[1,4]

Patient Selection
Indications

The quadriceps snip should be the first-line workhorse approach for revision TKA because it allows exposure of the tight knee without risking avulsion of the tibial tubercle or patellar tendon rupture.[1] (The quadriceps snip can also be used for difficult exposures in primary TKA.) After arthrotomy via a standard medial parapatellar approach, the knee should be passively flexed and lateral subluxation of the patella attempted. If the exposure is insufficient or an inordinate amount of tension is placed on the patellar tendon, the quadriceps snip is indicated and should be performed at this point in the procedure.

Contraindications

If the knee can be flexed more than 90° with the patella subluxated laterally, with minimal tension on the patellar tendon, then the standard medial parapatellar retinacular incision need not be carried superolaterally and thus converted to the quadriceps snip.

Procedure
Room Setup/Patient Positioning

The quadriceps snip does not typically require special attention to room setup or

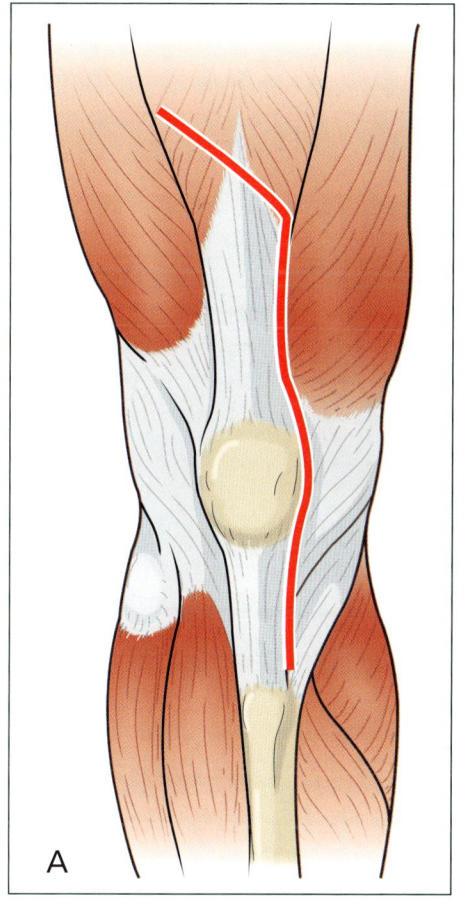

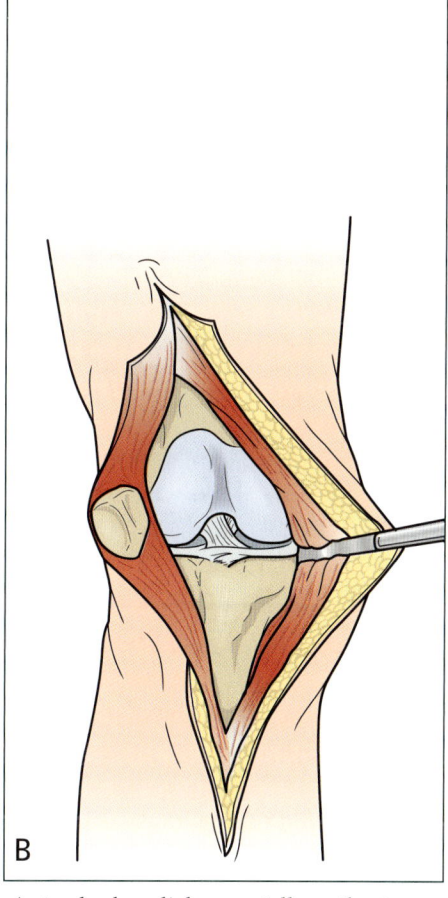

Figure 1 Illustrations of the quadriceps snip. **A,** A standard medial parapatellar arthrotomy with proximal transection of the quadriceps tendon in an oblique fashion into the fibers of the vastus lateralis. **B,** With release of the quadriceps tendon proximally, the patella is subluxated laterally, and the joint is exposed.

Video 55.1 Exposure for Revision Total Knee Arthroplasty via Quadriceps Snip. Ari Seidenstein, MD; Scott Scuderi, BS; Giles R. Scuderi, MD (1 min)

patient positioning beyond what is done for a primary TKA. For an exceptionally short patient with a high body mass index, consideration should be given to the use of a sterile tourniquet. Of course, if a tourniquet is to be used, it should be placed as high on the thigh as possible.

Special Instruments/Equipment/Implants

The quadriceps snip does not typically require special equipment or implants. The snip itself can be performed safely with curved Mayo scissors or a scalpel blade.

Surgical Technique

Adequate exposure is one of the most common difficulties encountered in revision TKA. A well-performed arthroplasty can easily be complicated by inadequate exposure and damage to the extensor

---

Mr. Scott Scuderi or an immediate family member is a member of a speakers' bureau or has made paid presentations on behalf of Zimmer and Salient Surgical; serves as a paid consultant to or is an employee of Zimmer and Medtronic; and serves as a board member, owner, officer, or committee member of The Knee Society. Dr. Giles R. Scuderi or an immediate family member has received royalties from Zimmer and Medtronic; is a member of a speakers' bureau or has made paid presentations on behalf of Zimmer and Medtronic; serves as a paid consultant to or is an employee of Zimmer and Medtronic; and serves as a board member, owner, officer, or committee member of The Knee Society and the International Congress for Joint Reconstruction. Neither Dr. Seidenstein nor any immediate family member has received anything of value from or has stock or stock options held in a commercial company or institution related directly or indirectly to the subject of this chapter.

mechanism. Preoperative stiffness with limited range of motion requires careful planning for not only implant selection, position, and alignment but also the method of surgical approach. A well-planned case with consideration of all surgical options avoids complications.[5]

With revision TKA surgery (because patient positioning, tourniquet placement, and performance of the snip do not require special consideration), planning begins with the skin incision and then the arthrotomy. There are general principles to follow when selecting the skin incision that should help avoid wound complications, such as delayed healing and marginal skin necrosis. When possible, prior skin incisions should be used and incorporated into the planned new incision. In most cases, a prior midline skin incision exists and should be used. Initially, it is useful to start the midline incision more proximally than the previous incision to establish normal tissue planes proximal to the extensor mechanism.[6-8] However, a situation might present itself in which a new incision is required. When a new skin incision is anticipated, attention must be paid to details. Previous incisions that do not allow proper access to the joint may determine which incision is chosen.[9,10] Close parallel incisions and narrow skin bridges must be avoided to minimize the risks of vascular compromise and skin necrosis. Transverse scars should be crossed in a perpendicular manner with minimal compromise to the junction zone. If the vascular integrity of the skin surrounding the knee is at all questionable, a plastic surgeon should be consulted, and the use of soft-tissue expanders should be considered.[10]

Following the skin incision, the deep fascia is incised and medial and lateral flaps are developed to expose the extensor mechanism. In a complex primary TKA or a revision TKA, where there is known limited motion and foreseen difficulty in exposing the joint, it is best to visualize the entire extensor mechanism, including the quadriceps tendon, the patella, and the patellar tendon.

Initial exposure begins with a long medial parapatellar arthrotomy (**Figure 2**). Once the arthrotomy is performed, the exposure should be extended to allow access to the medial and lateral femoral gutters. Frequently, the medial parapatellar arthrotomy alone will not allow enough flexion to adequately expose the joint.[7,11] At this point, it is helpful to clear the medial and lateral femoral gutters

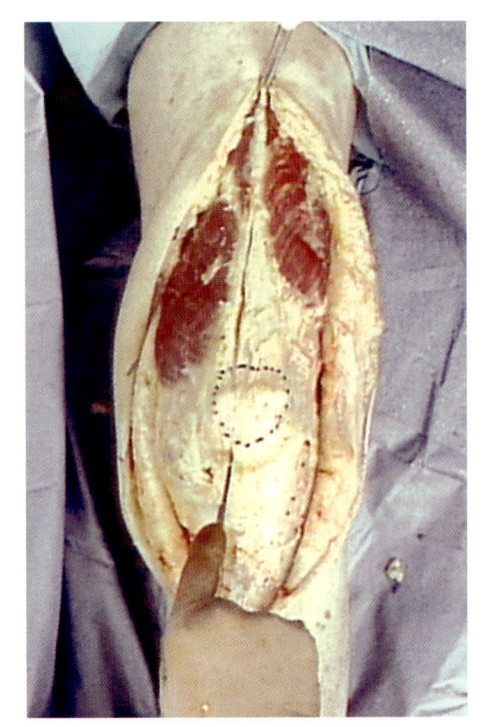

Figure 2 The standard medial parapatellar arthrotomy, which is performed to the apex of the quadriceps tendon, is shown in a cadaver specimen. The patella is outlined with blue dots.

and excise any excessive synovium overlying the distal femur in the suprapatellar pouch. In cases with patella infera or a fibrotic fat pad, it is helpful to longitudinally split or excise the infrapatellar fat and release the fibrous scar tissue from the anterolateral tibia between the patellar tendon and the lateral tibial plateau. Another maneuver is to perform a subperiosteal medial soft-tissue release from the proximal tibia, releasing the deep medial collateral ligament and the semimembranosus insertion posteriorly. This will allow external rotation and anterior translation of the tibia, relaxing tension on the patellar tendon attachment at the tibial tubercle and decreasing the risk of patellar tendon avulsion. The lateral patellofemoral ligament, which extends from the lateral epicondyle to the lateral border of the patella, is also released. This assists in patellar dislocation and allows easier lateral retraction of the patella, thus improving exposure.[12,13]

After these maneuvers, the knee can be passively flexed and subluxation of the patella can be attempted. Special attention must be paid to the patellar tendon insertion at the tibial tubercle. If the knee can be flexed more than 90° with the patella subluxated laterally, with minimal tension on the patellar tendon, the surgery can be continued. However, if the

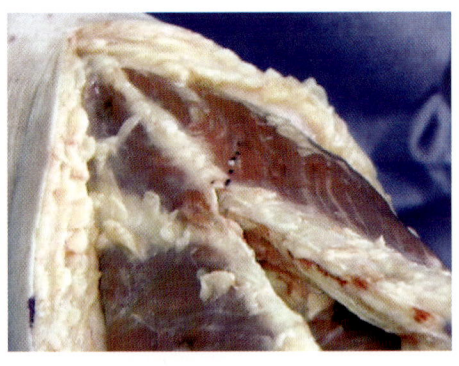

Figure 3 A close-up view of the apex of the quadriceps tendon in a cadaver specimen shows the tendon transected in an oblique fashion (blue dots) in line with the fibers of the vastus lateralis.

exposure is insufficient or an inordinate amount of tension is placed on the patellar tendon, the quadriceps snip is indicated and should be performed at this point in the procedure so as to not risk avulsion of the tibial tubercle or patellar tendon rupture.[1]

The quadriceps snip is easily incorporated as a proximal extension of the medial parapatellar arthrotomy (see the video supplement). Attention is first directed to the proximal end of the quadriceps tendon. Beginning at the apex of the medial arthrotomy, the quadriceps tendon is incised in a lateral oblique fashion from distal to proximal at a 45° angle, splitting the vastus lateralis muscle fibers (**Figure 3**). This enhances lateral patellar subluxation, knee flexion, and exposure of the lateral compartment of the knee. The oblique incision has the advantage that it is directed in line with the vastus lateralis muscle and away from the superior geniculate artery and the vastus lateralis tendon (**Figures 4** and **5**). The quadriceps snip should exit the quadriceps tendon distal to the musculotendinous junction of the rectus femoris muscle. Proximal extension of the arthrotomy beyond the tendon before the oblique snip will lead to transection of a portion of the rectus femoris fibers and should be avoided. If adequate exposure still cannot be achieved and the patella cannot be dislocated, all hypertrophic scar, capsule, and fibrotic peripatellar tissues should be excised.[1,6] If after performing a quadriceps snip and lateral retinacular release the exposure is still unsatisfactory, a tibial tubercle osteotomy is indicated and should be performed.[3,14]

At the completion of the procedure, the vertical and oblique portions of the quadriceps tendon are repaired in a typical side-to-side fashion.

Complications
This extensile approach should be the workhorse for revision TKA, in part because it is relatively devoid of potential complications. Proximal extension of the arthrotomy beyond the quadriceps tendon before the oblique snip will lead to transection of a portion of the rectus femoris fibers and should be avoided.

Postoperative Care and Rehabilitation
When a quadriceps snip is performed during the TKA, postoperative physical therapy can begin without delay and is not altered because of the surgical exposure. Patients are allowed unrestricted passive and active range of motion. Continuous passive motion can be initiated immediately postoperatively. Full weight bearing may progress as tolerated unless it is contraindicated because of the complex nature of the joint reconstruction.[1,4]

Clinical Results
The outcome of a TKA should not be compromised by an injury to the extensor mechanism. The quadriceps snip is an excellent method for gaining adequate exposure to the stiff, tight knee without injury to the extensor mechanism. Clinical results have shown that performing this approach does not interfere with the final outcome.[1]

In one of the first reports on the quadriceps snip, Garvin et al[4] found that this enhanced exposure technique caused no change in functional outcome or any adverse complications. In this initial study of 16 patients, 10 patients were rated excellent, and 6 rated good using the Hospital for Special Surgery knee score. No patients had a postoperative extensor lag, and dynamometer testing showed no difference in muscle performance when compared to knees that underwent a medial parapatellar arthrotomy.[4]

Barrack et al,[12] in a comparison study of the medial parapatellar arthrotomy, quadriceps snip, V-Y quadriceps turndown, and tibial tubercle osteotomy, reported a discernible difference between the various approaches. However, in this review of 123 revision TKAs with 2- to 4-year follow-up, there was no discernible disadvantage when comparing the 31 TKAs performed with a quadriceps snip to the 63 TKAs performed with a standard medial parapatellar approach in every parameter measured, including range of motion, extensor lag, patellofemoral symptoms, Knee Society scores, and patient satisfaction. The patients in the study who had a quadriceps turndown or a tibial tubercle osteotomy had equivalent scores postoperatively, but both were significantly lower than the standard and quadriceps snip groups.[12,13]

Meek et al,[15] in a study of 107 patients who underwent revision TKA with a minimum of 2 years of follow-up, reported no statistically significant difference with regard to Western Ontario and McMaster Universities Osteoarthritis Index function, pain, stiffness, and satisfaction scores between the 57 knees that underwent a standard approach and the 50 knees with a revision performed via a quadriceps snip.

Other authors have reported that the quadriceps snip is effective only for knees with mild to moderate stiffness and that more extensive procedures are necessary for very stiff knees. In this scenario, the quadriceps snip can be combined with an osteotomy of the tibial tubercle or converted to a patellar turndown.[3,6,8,9,14]

Pearls
- The quadriceps snip is indicated when insufficient exposure is achieved via a standard medial parapatellar approach and the patella cannot be laterally subluxated with the knee in at least 90° of flexion.
- We clear synovium from the lateral and medial femoral gutters, perform a medial subperiosteal tibial soft-tissue release to externally rotate the tibia, and release the lateral patellofemoral ligament before deciding whether a quadriceps snip is necessary.
- Beginning at the apex of the medial arthrotomy, the quadriceps tendon is incised in a lateral oblique fashion from distal to proximal at a 45° angle, splitting the vastus lateralis muscle fibers.
- If necessary, a lateral retinacular release may be performed to facilitate patellar tracking.
- Postoperative physical therapy can begin without delay and is not altered because of the surgical exposure.

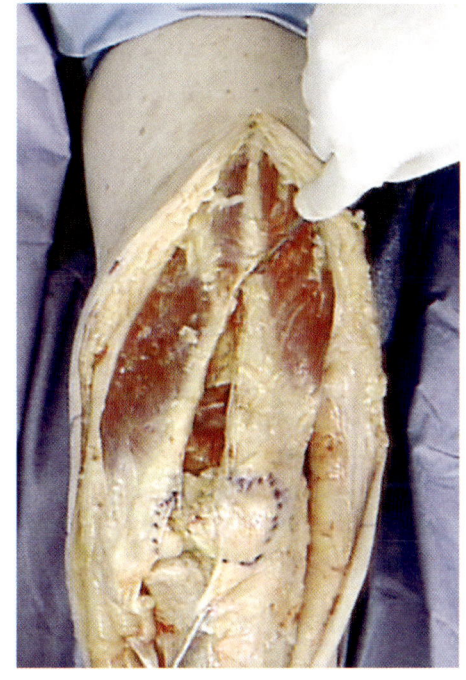

Figure 4 The quadriceps snip is performed at the apex of the quadriceps tendon shown in a cadaver specimen.

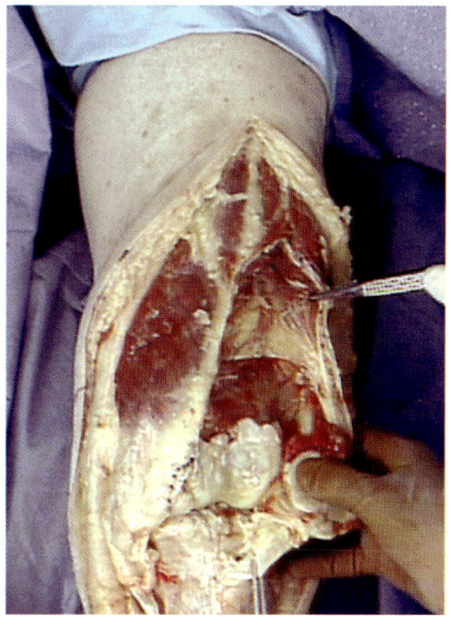

Figure 5 Following the quadriceps snip, the patella is subluxated laterally, exposing the knee joint and preserving the attachment of the patellar tendon at the tibial tubercle (shown in a cadaver specimen).

References
1. Arsht SJ, Scuderi GR: The quadriceps snip for exposing the stiff knee. *J Knee Surg* 2003;16(1):55-57.
2. Coonse K, Adams JD: A new operative approach to the knee joint. *Surg Gynecol Obstet* 1943;77:344-347.
3. Trousdale RT, Hanssen AD, Rand JA, Cahalan TD: V-Y quadricepsplasty in total knee arthroplasty. *Clin Orthop Relat Res* 1993;286:48-55.
4. Garvin KL, Scuderi GS, Insall JN: Evolution of the quadriceps snip. *Clin Orthop Relat Res* 1995;321:131-137.
5. Clarke HD, Scuderi GR: Revision total knee arthroplasty: Planning, management, controversies, and surgical approaches. *Instr Course Lect* 2001;50:359-365.

6. Jacofsky DJ, Della Valle CJ, Meneghini RM, Sporer SM, Cercek RM; American Academy of Orthopaedic Surgeons: Revision total knee arthroplasty: What the practicing orthopaedic surgeon needs to know. *J Bone Joint Surg Am* 2010;92(5):1282-1292.

7. Scuderi GR: Surgical approaches to the knee, in Scott WN, ed: *Surgery of the Knee*, ed 4. New York, NY, Churchill Livingstone, pp 120-141.

8. Younger AS, Duncan CP, Masri BA: Surgical exposures in revision total knee arthroplasty. *J Am Acad Orthop Surg* 1998;6(1):55-64.

9. Dennis DA, Berry DJ, Engh G, et al: Revision total knee arthroplasty. *J Am Acad Orthop Surg* 2008;16(8):442-454.

10. Manifold SG, Cushner FD, Craig-Scott S, Scott WN: Long-term results of total knee arthroplasty after the use of soft tissue expanders. *Clin Orthop Relat Res* 2000;380:133-139.

11. Kelly MA, Clarke HD: Stiffness and ankylosis in primary total knee arthroplasty. *Clin Orthop Relat Res* 2003;416:68-73.

12. Barrack RL, Smith P, Munn B, Engh G, Rorabeck C: The Ranawat Award: Comparison of surgical approaches in total knee arthroplasty *Clin Orthop Relat Res* 1998;356:16-21.

13. Barrack RL: Specialized surgical exposure for revision total knee: Quadriceps snip and patellar turndown. *Instr Course Lect* 1999;48:149-152.

14. Whiteside LA: Exposure in difficult total knee arthroplasty using tibial tubercle osteotomy. *Clin Orthop Relat Res* 1995;321:32-35.

15. Meek RM, Greidanus NV, McGraw RW, Masri BA: The extensile rectus snip exposure in revision of total knee arthroplasty. *J Bone Joint Surg Br* 2003;85(8):1120-1122.

Chapter 56
Revision Total Knee Arthroplasty via Tibial Tubercle Osteotomy

Jeffrey A. Geller, MD

Patient Selection

Total knee arthroplasty (TKA) is a well-proven intervention that relieves pain and improves the quality of life in individuals with advanced degenerative joint disease of the knee. The number of TKA surgeries performed annually in the United States has increased steadily over the past 20 years and is anticipated to reach approximately 3.5 million by the year 2030. It also has been estimated that approximately 268,000 revision TKAs will be performed per year by 2030.[1] Some of these revisions will be performed because of a painful and stiff knee, but most will be required because of aseptic loosening.

Several techniques have been developed to improve exposure to the knee during a difficult revision. Although the quadriceps snip should be the workhorse procedure, tibial tubercle osteotomy (TTO) is an important procedure for the knee arthroplasty surgeon to have in his or her armamentarium.[2] The TTO was initially described by Whiteside.[3] This technique can be used to improve exposure for both revision TKA and complex primary TKA. Before the surgeon enters the operating room, it is important to know whether the patient will require a more extensive surgical approach. In most patients, a quadriceps snip procedure will provide sufficient exposure, but opting for the TTO early may be judicious, to avoid being forced to resort to secondary TTO if the quadriceps snip fails to provide appropriate exposure.

Indications

The primary indication for TTO is a severe, rigid lack of range of motion (ROM). TTO should be strongly considered when ROM is less than 90° of flexion, especially when accompanied by a severe fibrous block in motion, as demonstrated by passive ROM testing under anesthesia. These patients often have a flexion contracture that further complicates the surgical exposure, which should be an early indication that a more extensile procedure is necessary to avoid extensor mechanism avulsion. Such scenarios are common when revision TKA requires a two-stage procedure because of infection; where there may be further stiffness caused by heterotopic bone formation; when revision TKA is performed to treat a stiff and painful primary TKA; or when the aseptically loosened TKA has been neglected for a long time, leading to progressive stiffness.

Contraindications

The main contraindication to TTO is extremely poor bone stock in the proximal tibia. This may be due to infection, extreme osteolysis, or a poor fibrous union from a prior TTO, although this is extremely rare. In general, this scenario can be overcome by extending the osteotomized segment farther distally into the diaphyseal portion of the tibia, where there is better bone stock that can be repaired at the conclusion of the procedure.

Preoperative Imaging

The recommended preoperative images are the standard radiographs that are obtained in the routine workup of a patient, including AP weight-bearing, lateral, and sunrise views (**Figure 1**). More relevant is the physical examination of the patient, specifically the preoperative ROM assessment.

Procedure

Room Setup/Patient Positioning

Patient positioning for revision TKA via TTO is the standard supine positioning for TKA, although a padded bolster placed under the ipsilateral hip is essential to keep the lower extremity from excessive external rotation.

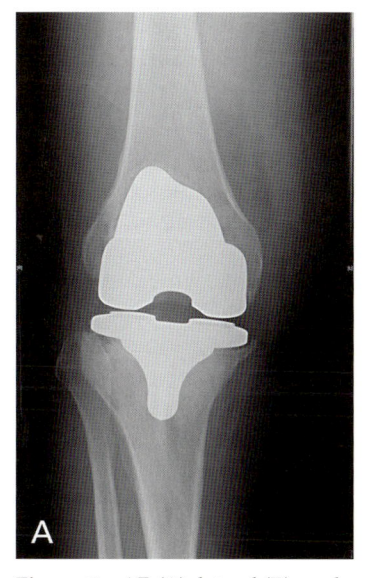

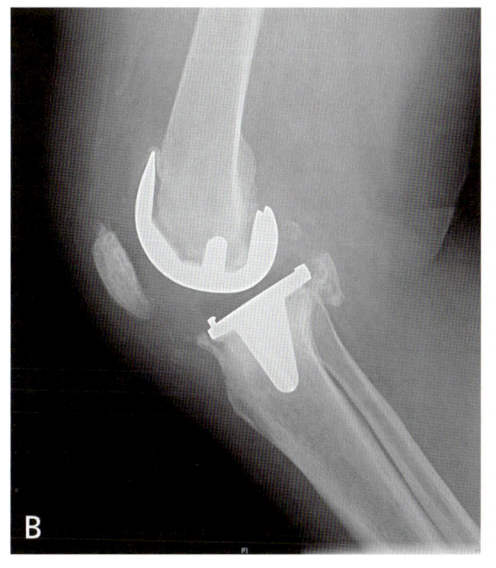

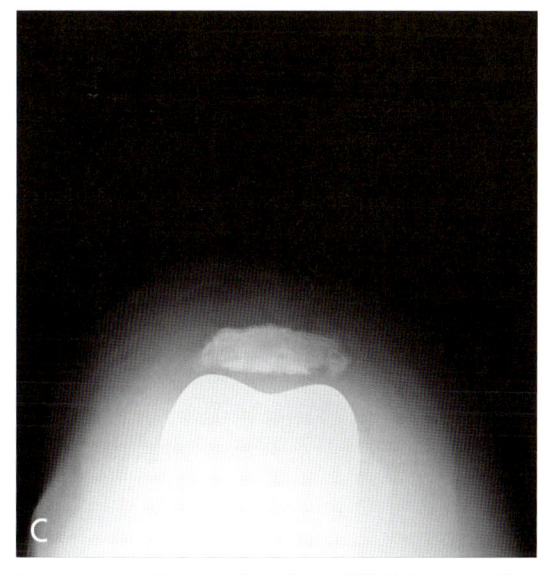

Figure 1 AP (**A**), lateral (**B**), and sunrise (**C**) radiographs of the knee of a patient who underwent a total knee arthroplasty (TKA) 1 year earlier. The TKA was revised for pain and stiffness.

Dr. Geller or an immediate family member serves as a board member, owner, officer, or committee member of the American Association of Hip and Knee Surgeons and the American Association of Orthopaedic Surgeons.

Section 4: Adult Reconstruction

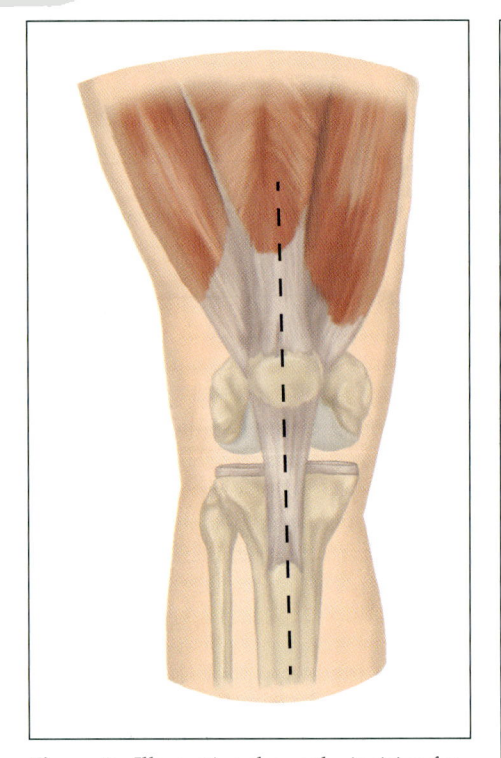

Figure 2 Illustration shows the incision for a revision total knee arthroplasty via tibial tubercle osteotomy.

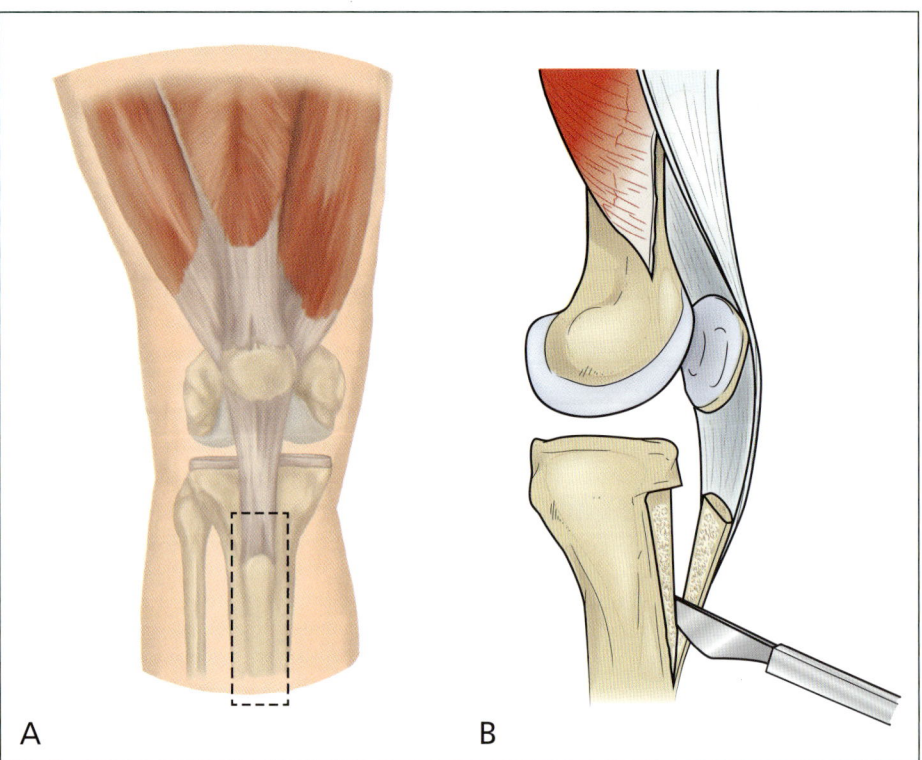

Figure 3 Illustrations show the location of the cuts for a tibial tubercle osteotomy. **A,** Anterior view. **B,** Lateral view.

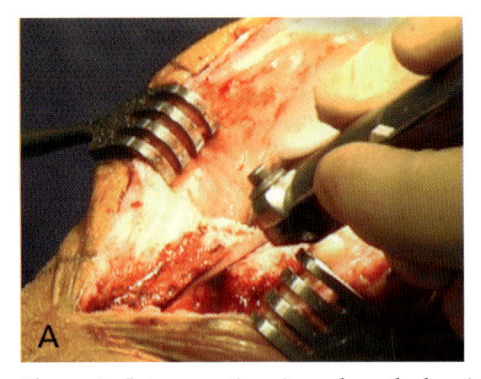

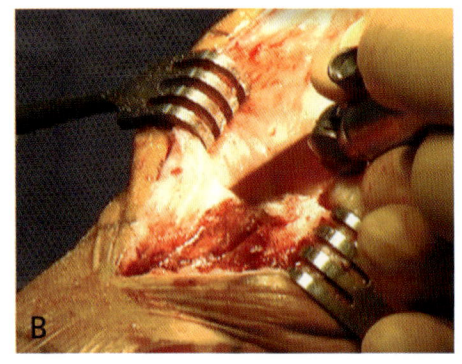

Figure 4 Intraoperative views show the longitudinal osteotomy cut (**A**) and proximal transverse step cut (**B**) for a tibial tubercle osteotomy.

Special Instruments/Equipment/Implants

The tools needed to successfully perform a TTO are found in most operating rooms. It is necessary to have a full set of straight and curved osteotomes and a motorized microsagittal saw. Repair of the TTO has been described using either wires or screws. The instruments needed depend on the surgeon's preferred method. When wires are used to repair the TTO, a standard 2.7-mm drill bit and 18-gauge stainless steel wire are needed. A wire tightener is also helpful to facilitate the twisting and securing of the wires; several modifications of this device are available. If screws are preferred, 6.5-mm cannulated screws can be used.[4] My preference is to use wires because they have a lower profile and are less likely to fracture the osteotomized fragment than are screws.

Surgical Technique

The surgical approach for a TTO is similar to the standard extensile approach to the knee for a revision TKA. The skin incision should follow the prior skin incision, although it should be adequately extended to improve visualization and identify normal tissue at the ends of the old incisions. The distal aspect of the incision should extend approximately 8 to 10 cm distal to the tibial tubercle (**Figure 2**). Wide, full-thickness skin flaps should be lifted laterally, taking care to keep the musculature of the lower leg anterior compartment intact. The knee should be entered using the standard medial parapatellar arthrotomy. An extensive synovectomy should be performed as well. Attention should be focused on the medial aspect of the tibia at the level of the tibial tubercle.

The osteotomy fragment is planned and drawn out on the tibia around the tubercle using a surgical marker. The ideal location is 3 to 4 cm distal to the joint line, and the osteotomized fragment should be 4 cm wide, 6 to 8 cm long, and 2 to 4 cm deep (**Figure 3, A**). The proximal aspect of the osteotomized fragment should be configured to create a step cut on a slight angle (**Figure 3, B**). A microsagittal saw is used to perform the cuts sequentially: the proximal cut is made first, followed by the cut along the tibial crest in a medial-to-lateral direction (**Figure 4**). The cut should not extend completely across the tibia; the last few millimeters of bone and soft tissue should be left intact to serve as a hinge. The osteotomized fragment can then be lifted up carefully on the medial side (hinging on the soft tissues laterally) using a series of osteotomes, leaving a soft-tissue sleeve intact for ease of repair and reduction at the completion of the case and to maintain vascularity to the segment (**Figure 5**). At this point, the patella can be everted easily with the osteotomized fragment. The knee can be fully flexed, despite any preoperative limitations in ROM, and the surgeon can obtain easy access to the knee for component removal (including

Chapter 56: Revision Total Knee Arthroplasty via Tibial Tubercle Osteotomy

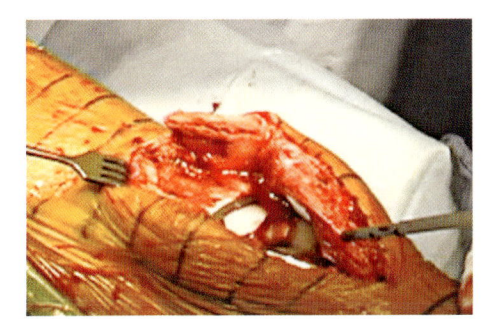

Figure 5 Intraoperative photograph shows the exposure obtained after the tibial tubercle osteotomy fragment is lifted laterally.

access to a tibial cement mantle if one exists), as in the case of a revised TKA with a long cemented stem.

When the final revision TKA prosthesis is in position, the osteotomy fragment is repaired. If fixation with wire is chosen, it is helpful to cut three or four pieces of wire beforehand. Each piece should be about 18 inches long. A hole is drilled from the medial aspect of the intact tibia, approximately 10 mm posterior and parallel to the osteotomy, using a 2.7-mm drill bit. The wire is then threaded through the hole. This should be repeated for a total of three wires, to ensure sufficient strength of the repair (**Figure 6, A**). Additional wires, may be used if desired, but they should be spaced an adequate distance apart. The fragment is then anatomically reduced back into its bony bed (**Figure 6, B and C**). This is usually done with the knee in full extension. It is most helpful to reduce the proximal segment back into the original step cut. The lateral limb of the wire is then easily bent over the TTO, and the wire is twisted and tightened down. The wire must be sufficiently tight and secure to ensure bony union of the TTO (**Figure 6, D**). A loose wire may not be strong enough to support healing of the TTO and may lead to pain or discomfort at the site. (On rare occasions, the wire may break or become prominent under the skin.) The wire ends are cut relatively short, tamped down using a bone tamp, and buried beneath soft tissue (**Figure 7**). The rest of the medial parapatellar arthrotomy may be closed in the standard fashion. Prior to closure, a medium Hemovac drain may be placed to help avoid an excessive hemarthrosis.

Complications
Complications that may arise after TTO include proximal migration of the osteotomized fragment, nonunion of the TTO, and prominent hardware. Two cases of tibia fracture after TTO have been reported.[5,6] Proximal migration of the fragment generally occurs when the step cut in the proximal aspect of the TTO is inadequate or not done. If this cut is not deep enough or is too thin, the fragment may fracture postoperatively, thus removing an essential buttress to counteract the cranially oriented pulling force of the quadriceps mechanism. Nonunion of the fragment is extremely rare because excellent vascularity usually exists through the proximal tibial metaphyseal bone. Finally, if the wire ends are not cut short enough or are not buried after being cut, they may become painful or prominent, necessitating removal after the TTO has healed.

Postoperative Care and Rehabilitation
In most cases, TTO should not affect the rehabilitation protocol after a difficult TKA or revision TKA. If the fixation of the TTO is adequate, patients may begin ROM exercises without limitation and bear weight as tolerated. If desired, a continuous passive motion machine may be implemented with a standard protocol to increase ROM. If the surgeon believes that fixation strength has been compromised, motion can simply be advanced more conservatively. A reasonable protocol in such situations might be to limit

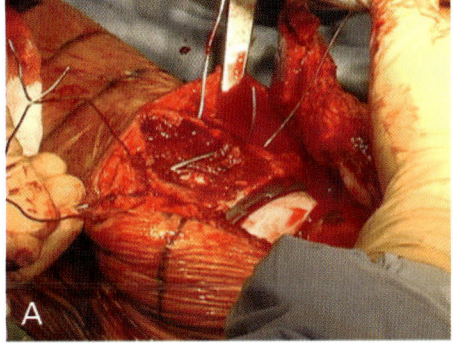

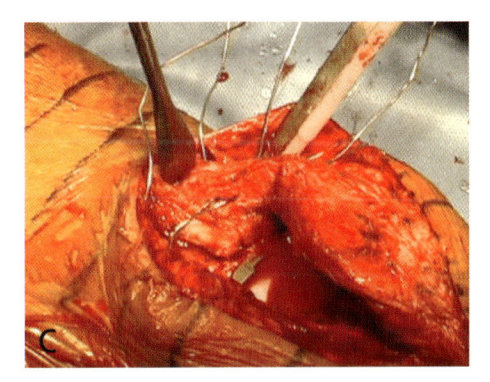

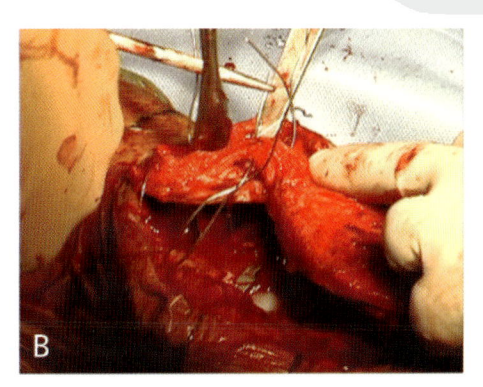

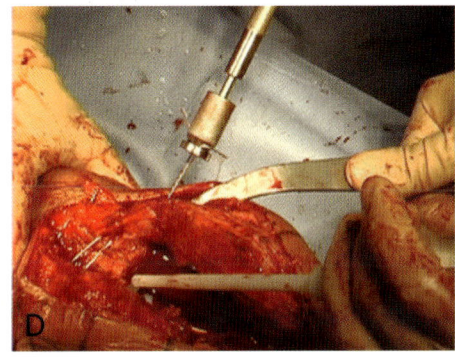

Figure 6 Intraoperative images demonstrate wire placement for tibial tubercle osteotomy repair. **A**, The wires are threaded through the drilled holes. **B**, The osteotomized fragment is being reduced back to the tibia. **C**, The arrangement of the wires is shown prior to the tightening and securing of the fragment. **D**, The fragment is secured using 18-gauge wire and a power wire tightener.

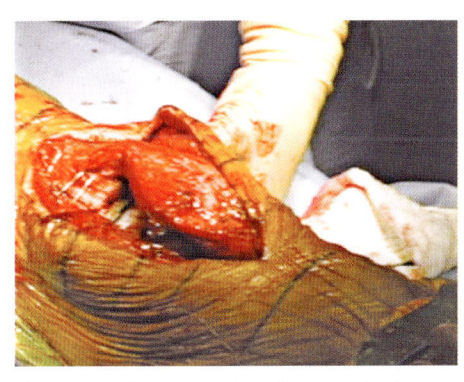

Figure 7 Intraoperative photograph shows the final tibial tubercle osteotomy repair, with the wire ends cut and buried beneath soft tissue.

ROM to 45° of flexion for the first 2 weeks, slowly advance to 90° by 4 weeks, and allow full ROM beyond 6 weeks.

Pearls
The two most important aspects of this approach are the keyed-in step cut in the proximal aspect of the TTO and the wire-tightening device used in the repair.

- The step cut should be thick enough to prevent proximal migration of the osteotomized fragment and should be angled so that the TTO keys in upon repair.
- The power attachment used to tighten the wires is extremely helpful. This

© 2013 American Academy of Orthopaedic Surgeons

makes securing the piece faster and stronger. Although the wires can be tightened by hand, a tightener provides more torque than can be achieved by hand and is significantly quicker.

References

1. Kurtz S, Ong K, Lau E, Mowat F, Halpern M: Projections of primary and revision hip and knee arthroplasty in the United States from 2005 to 2030. *J Bone Joint Surg Am* 2007;89(4):780-785.

2. Della Valle CJ, Berger RA, Rosenberg AG: Surgical exposures in revision total knee arthroplasty. *Clin Orthop Relat Res* 2006;446:59-68.

3. Whiteside LA: Exposure in difficult total knee arthroplasty using tibial tubercle osteotomy. *Clin Orthop Relat Res* 1995;321:32-35.

4. Caldwell PE, Bohlen BA, Owen JR, et al: Dynamic confirmation of fixation techniques of the tibial tubercle osteotomy. *Clin Orthop Relat Res* 2004;424:173-179.

5. Arredondo J, Worland RL, Jessup DE: Nonunion after a tibial shaft fracture complicating tibial tubercule osteotomy. *J Arthroplasty* 1998;13(8):958-960.

6. Ritter MA, Carr K, Keating EM, Faris PM, Meding JB: Tibial shaft fracture following tibial tubercle osteotomy. *J Arthroplasty* 1996;11(1):117-119.

Trauma

Section Editors
Lawrence X. Webb, MD
Eben A. Carroll, MD

57 General Principles of Surgical Débridement 369
Lawrence X. Webb, MD; Henry J. Dolch, DO

58 Fasciotomy for Compartment Syndrome of the Leg 371
Lawrence X. Webb, MD; Alireza Behboudi, DO

59 Open Reduction and Internal Fixation of Forearm Fractures......... 375
Thomas F. Varecka, MD

60 Open Reduction and Internal Fixation of Posterior Wall
Acetabular Fractures 385
Lawrence X. Webb, MD

61 Open Reduction and Internal Fixation of Femoral Neck Fractures 393
Lawrence X. Webb, MD; John C.P. Floyd, MD

62 Intertrochanteric Fracture Fixation Using a Sliding Hip Screw or
Cephalomedullary Nail...................................... 401
Alexandra K. Schwartz, MD; Christopher L. Sherman, DO, MS

63 Intramedullary Nailing of Diaphyseal Femur Fractures 407
Anna N. Miller, MD

64 Surgical Fixation of Fractures of the Distal Femur.................. 413
James F. Kellam, BSc, MD, FRCSC, FACS, FRCSI

65 Open Reduction and Internal Fixation of Tibial Plateau Fractures 421
James A. Goulet, MD; Mark E. Hake, MD

66 Tibial Diaphyseal Intramedullary Nailing 429
Clifford B. Jones, MD, FACS

67	**Open Reduction and Internal Fixation of the Tibial Plafond** 437
	Stephen K. Benirschke, MD; Patricia Kramer, PhD

68	**Surgical Treatment of Ankle Fractures** 443
	Eben A. Carroll, MD; Jason J. Halvorson, MD

69	**Surgical Management of Fractures of the Talus** 451
	John M. Tabit, DO; Lawrence X. Webb, MD

70	**Open Reduction and Internal Fixation of Calcaneal Fractures** 459
	Michael P. Clare, MD

71	**Open Reduction and Internal Fixation of Fracture-Dislocations of the Tarsometatarsal Joint** 467
	Terrence M. Philbin, DO; Gregory C. Berlet, MD

72	**Open Reduction and Internal Fixation of Proximal Fifth Metatarsal Fractures** 473
	Mark E. Easley, MD

Chapter 57
General Principles of Surgical Débridement

Lawrence X. Webb, MD   Henry J. Dolch, DO

Introduction
A wound characterized by tissue that is contaminated and/or devitalized is best managed with surgical débridement; that is, removal of contaminants as well as the devitalized tissue.[1] The goal of this process is to alter the wound environment so that healing can occur readily and free of infection. The surgeon must carefully assess the nature of the wound. If surgical extensions are needed to better evaluate and débride the wound, then they should be incorporated.

Video 57.1 Surgical Débridement. Lawrence X. Webb, MD; Henry J. Dolch, DO (6 min)

Procedure
Video Case
The video supplement shows a leg wound with an open knee joint at its base with degloved components of significance along with substantial gross contamination. The contaminants include mud and grass, which are ground into the tissue. This type of contamination and devitalization presents challenges to the surgeon, and transforming a wound like this to effect uneventful, infection-free healing with stable coverage and good preservation of knee function is a task that demands carefully staged and appropriately timed surgical interventions.

Surgical Technique
Grossly devitalized and highly contaminated tissues are removed with a knife and forceps. Subsequent techniques that are commonly used include high-pressure pulsatile lavage (HPPL) and low-pressure pulsatile lavage (LPPL). Recent studies show good effectiveness and minimal tissue damage and impairment of bone healing when LPPL is used.[2-7] We have found that a tangential excision tool is useful for removing contaminants in a wound like this.[8] This type of device works on the Bernoulli principle: a high-pressure saline stream across the working end of the tool creates a vacuum. The working end is dragged across the surface of the wound, allowing the vacuum it generates to pull the surface layer up into the high-pressure stream, which in turn tangentially excises the wound surface. In the process, the adsorbed mud and grass on the surface is pulled off with the tangential layer. This greatly facilitates the excision of these contaminants. Because of the violation of the joint space, the knee joint shown in the video was thoroughly irrigated with 3 L of saline solution.

Once the initial débridement is accomplished, we prefer to use a negative-pressure dressing with the pressure setting at –75 mm Hg. This helps to collect the edema (by wafting the interstitium and providing "microdrainage"), keep the soft tissue stable and the dessication-prone tissues moist, and avoid the need for often-painful dressing changes on the hospital ward or in the intensive care unit.[9-12] The patient is returned to the operating room at 48 to 72 hours for a "second look" at the wound. At that time, areas of necrosis not evident initially will have demarcated and are excised back to fully viable tissue. In the patient shown in the video case, the bulk of these demarcated tissues is part of the skin and subcutaneous tissue that was initially degloved. A low-pressure pulsed saline lavage is used at this time. A negative-pressure dressing is again applied, and it is changed at 48-hour intervals until the wound acquires some early granulations.

A split-thickness skin graft is then applied to these areas. Options for coverage of the exposed patellar tendon and adjoining fascia include local muscle flaps such as the medial head of the gastrocnemius. We elected instead to use an Integra bilayer (Integra LifeSciences) over this tissue, bolstered with a negative-pressure dressing. When the matrix portion of the bilayer had incorporated at day 5, a split-thickness skin graft was used over that area and again bolstered with a negative-pressure dressing with the pressure setting at –75 mm Hg. The graft incorporated over the next 7 days. These techniques derive from recent insights into accelerated incorporation of artificial dermis.[13-16] When the negative-pressure sponge was exchanged, the knee was gently manipulated, and a range of motion of 0° to 90° was readily achieved.

Postoperative Care and Rehabilitation
The patient used a continuous passive motion device for 2 hours three times daily to maintain knee motion. The newly grafted tissue was dressed in sterile saline–soaked gauze for protection, with dressing changes every day until epithelialization was complete. By week 6, the patient was mobilizing independently with a range of knee motion of 0° to 85° and had a stable soft-tissue cover (**Figure 1**).

Principles of Débridement
This case illustrates some of the important principles of débridement. The first involves thoroughly evaluating the wound. The patient shown in the video was initially prepared and draped by surgeons who assumed that the wound extent was slightly beyond the apparent wound. When they realized that the knee joint was violated, they requested an intraoperative consultation with us. The other wound component not originally appreciated by the first surgeons was the significant degloving, both proximal to (above the point of where the draping ended) and distal to the wound on the leg. The nature of the ground-in contaminants (soil organisms), the need for early coverage of exposed dessication-prone tissue, and the high-energy nature of the

---

Dr. Webb or an immediate family member is a member of a speakers' bureau or has made paid presentations on behalf of the Musculoskeletal Transplant Foundation; serves as a paid consultant to or is an employee of Zimmer; has received nonincome support (such as equipment or services), commercially derived honoraria, or other non–research-related funding (such as paid travel) from Synthes, Smith & Nephew, Stryker, Kinetic Concepts, and Doctors Group; and serves as a board member, owner, officer, or committee member of the Orthopaedic Trauma Association and the Southeastern Fracture Consortium Foundation. Neither Dr. Dolch nor any immediate family member has received anything of value from or has stock or stock options held in a commercial company or institution related directly or indirectly to the subject of this chapter.

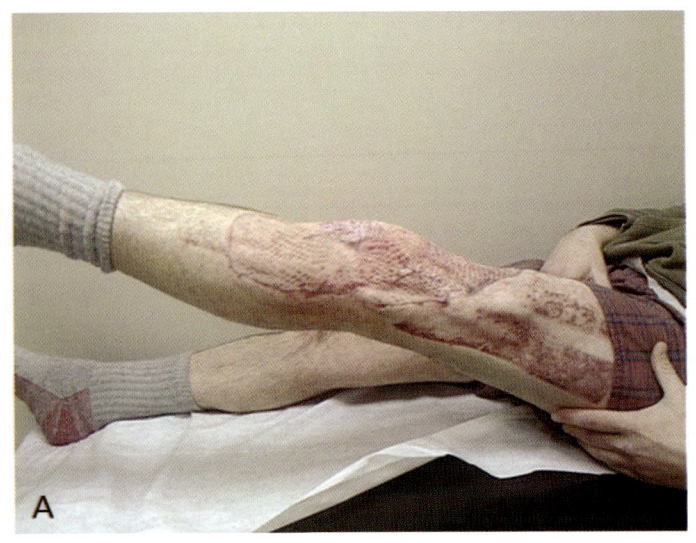

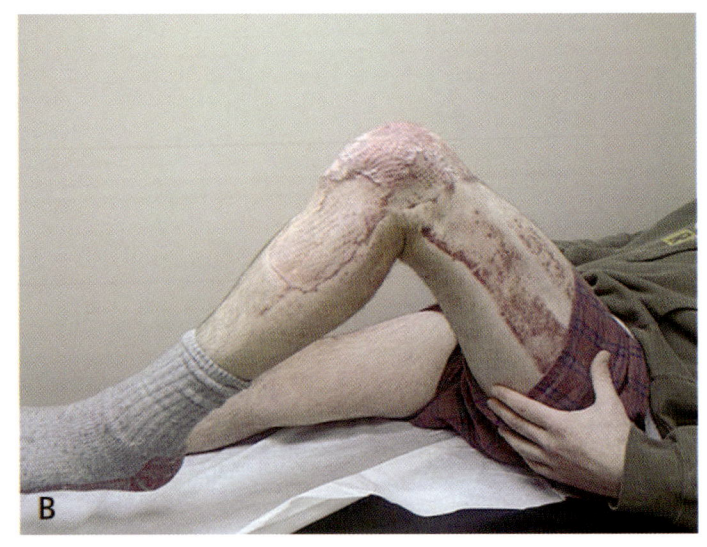

Figure 1 Clinical photographs of the patient shown in the video and discussed in the text at 12 weeks following the injury. The patient exhibits a range of motion of 0° (**A**) to 85° (**B**).

wound made secondary necrosis likely; therefore, the "second look" procedure was necessary.

The techniques discussed here encompass the following wound management principles for high-energy contaminated wounds: (1) thorough and timely débridement; (2) a second look at the wound at 48 hours to detect any demarcated tissue, with débridement of the implicated tissue; (3) arrangement for early wound coverage; and (4) early reestablishment of normal musculoskeletal function. This is exemplified in this case by the need for restoration of knee joint function. In the case of an open fracture wound, restoration of the structural integrity of the bone is needed.

References

1. Steed DL: Debridement. *Am J Surg* 2004;187(5A):71S-74S.
2. Dirschl DR, Duff GP, Dahners LE, Edin M, Rahn BA, Miclau T: High pressure pulsatile lavage irrigation of intraarticular fractures: Effects on fracture healing. *J Orthop Trauma* 1998;12(7):460-463.
3. Wheeler CB, Rodeheaver GT, Thacker JG, Edgerton MT, Edilich RF: Side-effects of high pressure irrigation. *Surg Gynecol Obstet* 1976;143(5):775-778.
4. Brown LL, Shelton HT, Bornside GH, Cohn I Jr: Evaluation of wound irrigation by pulsatile jet and conventional methods. *Ann Surg* 1978;187(2):170-173.
5. Bhandari M, Adili A, Lachowski RJ: High pressure pulsatile lavage of contaminated human tibiae: An in vitro study. *J Orthop Trauma* 1998;12(7):479-484.
6. Saxe A, Goldstein E, Dixon S, Ostrup R: Pulsatile lavage in the management of postoperative wound infections. *Am Surg* 1980;46(7):391-397.
7. Bhandari M, Schemitsch EH, Adili A, Lachowski RJ, Shaughnessy SG: High and low pressure pulsatile lavage of contaminated tibial fractures: An in vitro study of bacterial adherence and bone damage. *J Orthop Trauma* 1999;13(8):526-533.
8. Webb LX: New techniques in wound management: Vacuum-assisted wound closure. *J Am Acad Orthop Surg* 2002;10(5):303-311.
9. Tejwani N, Harvey E, Wolinsky P, Webb, LX: Initial management and wound coverage. *Inst Course Lect* 2011;60:15-25.
10. Morykwas MJ, Argenta LC, Shelton-Brown EI, McGuirt W: Vacuum-assisted closure: A new method for wound control and treatment. Animal studies and basic foundation. *Ann Plast Surg* 1997;38(6):553-562.
11. Argenta LC, Morykwas MJ: Vacuum-assisted closure: A new method for wound control and treatment. Clinical experience. *Ann Plast Surg* 1997;38(6):563-577.
12. Molnar JA, DeFranzo AJ, Hadaegh A, Morykwas MJ, Shen P, Argenta LC: Acceleration of Integra incorporation in complex tissue defects with subatmospheric pressure. *Plast Reconstr Surg* 2004;113(5):1339-1346.
13. Murray RC, Gordin EA, Saigal K, Leventhal D, Krein H, Heffelfinger RN: Reconstruction of the radial forearm free flap donor site using Integra artificial dermis. *Microsurgery* 2011;31(2):104-108.
14. Saxena V, Hwang CW, Huang S, Eichbaum Q, Ingber D, Orgill DP: Vacuum-assisted closure: Microdeformations of wounds and cell proliferation. *Plast Reconstr Surg* 2004;114(5):1086-1098.
15. Leffler M, Horch RE, Dragu A, Bach AD: The use of the artificial dermis (Integra) in combination with vacuum assisted closure for reconstruction of an extensive burn scar: A case report. *J Plast Reconstr Aesthet Surg* 2010;63(1):e32-e35.
16. Barnett TM, Shilt JS: Use of vacuum-assisted closure and a dermal regeneration template as an alternative to flap reconstruction in pediatric grade IIIB open lower-extremity injuries. *Am J Orthop (Belle Mead NJ)* 2009;38(6):301-305.

Chapter 58
Fasciotomy for Compartment Syndrome of the Leg

Lawrence X. Webb, MD   Alireza Behboudi, DO

Introduction

Compartment syndrome is caused by an elevation of pressure within the confines of an osseofascial compartment sufficient to compromise the microvascular blood flow of its contained tissue. If uncorrected, this leads to necrosis of the tissue within a few hours. The syndrome may arise in a host of clinical situations, with the most common being trauma.

Elevated pressure may be triggered by bleeding within the compartment and the accompanying tissue damage associated with the trauma.[1,2] A vicious circle of tissue trauma and inflammatory response, with release of inflammatory mediators that effect leaky capillaries and an outpouring of intravascular fluid to the tissue space (edema), contributes to the pathophysiology.[3,4] This outpouring of fluid occurs within the limited (and poorly yielding) osseofascial compartment space and causes an elevation of the tissue pressure within that space. With progression, this results in heightened capillary afterload at the microcirculatory level, with diminished capillary flow and compromised exchange of O^2 and CO^2 in the tissues. This process is a positive biofeedback loop, resulting in tissue ischemia and necrosis with lysis of cells and spillage of their contents into the interstitium. This causes an elevation of solute load within the space and an increased osmotic pressure. The determining factors for compartment syndrome are the tissue pressure within the compartment and its relationship to the diastolic blood pressure, with the critical threshold of a compartment pressure within 30 mm Hg of the diastolic blood pressure.[5-8] The relative protection afforded by hypertension (and the relative liability of hypotension) are easily understood by their positive and negative effects, respectively, on the microcirculatory flow in this setting.

This chapter describes compartment syndrome in the leg, but compartment syndrome can occur in other areas as well, including the thigh, the gluteal compartment, and the compartments of the foot, forearm, brachium and deltoid compartment. The pathophysiologic basis for each is the same as that described for the leg, and the remedy is the same: to decompress the compartment in a timely fashion so as to alleviate the embarrassment to the microcirculation of ischemic tissues.

Patient Selection

The first clinical symptom of compartment syndrome is pain. The earliest finding on physical examination is pain on passive stretch of the muscle in the affected compartment. Thus, if the anterior compartment of the leg is affected, pulling the toes into a plantarflexed position will elicit significant tenderness. If the deep posterior compartment is affected, dorsiflexion of the toes will elicit significant tenderness. Typically, the affected compartments have a tight (as opposed to soft and pliable) feel, and tenderness is elicited in the assessment (provided the process has not progressed to the point of blocking the nerves and anaesthetizing the leg). Over time, the pain increases and is less likely to be alleviated by narcotics. Numbness, paresthesias, diminished motor function, and ultimately pulselessness can ensue. Not uncommonly, at least some myonecrosis will have occurred if the syndrome progresses to the point of loss of sensation, with diminished motor function, and diminished pulse.[9] Alleviation of this situation is imperative and should proceed on an emergent basis with fasciotomy of all affected osseofascial compartments.

The accompanying video shows the technique for a two-incision fasciotomy.

Video 58.1 Technique for Two-Incision Leg Fasciotomy. Lawrence X. Webb, MD; John C.P. Floyd, MD (4 min)

Procedure
Surgical Technique

Our method of performing the release of all four osseofascial compartments uses a two-incision technique (**Figure 1**). Compartment pressures may be measured by several techniques, including that originally described by Whitesides et al.[10] Most commonly, a commercially available handheld pressure measurement device is used.

We release the anterior and lateral compartments through an anterolateral incision (**Figure 2, A**). The intermuscular septum is localized at the proximal part of the wound by means of a short, transverse incision (**Figure 2, B**). A small axial incision is made on the fascia anterior to the intermuscular septum; the incision should be long enough to admit the tip of curved Mayo scissors. The fasciotomy is then performed, both cephalad and caudally (**Figure 2, C**). This releases the anterior compartment. The underlying muscle is assessed for its color, consistency, contractility, and capillary refill. Similarly, the process is repeated for the fascia on the other side of the intermuscular septum to release the lateral compartment and assess the viability of its muscle (**Figure 2, D**).

For the release of the superficial and deep posterior compartments, an axially directed anteromedial incision is made approximately 2 cm medial to the posteromedial border of the tibia (**Figure 3, A**). The fascia is released directly under the incision for a short distance sufficient to admit the tip of curved Mayo scissors, which is directed cephalad and caudally to decompress the superficial posterior

---

Dr. Webb or an immediate family member is a member of a speakers' bureau or has made paid presentations on behalf of the Musculoskeletal Transplant Foundation; serves as a paid consultant to or is an employee of Zimmer; has received nonincome support (such as equipment or services), commercially derived honoraria, or other non–research-related funding (such as paid travel) from Synthes, Smith & Nephew, Stryker, Kinetic Concepts, and Doctors Group; and serves as a board member, owner, officer, or committee member of the Orthopaedic Trauma Association and the Southeastern Fracture Consortium Foundation. Neither Dr. Behboudi nor any immediate family member has received anything of value from or has stock or stock options held in a commercial company or institution related directly or indirectly to the subject of this chapter.

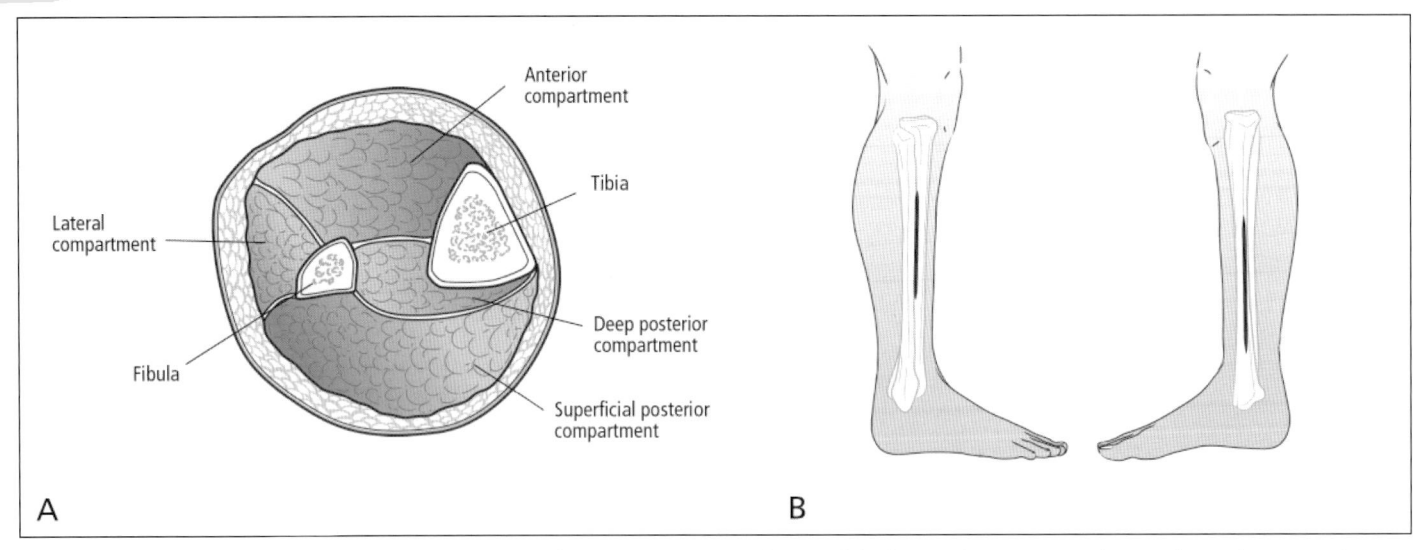

Section 5: Trauma

Figure 1 Illustrations depict a two-incision fasciotomy for compartment syndrome of the leg. **A,** Cross-sectional view shows the anatomic muscle compartments of the leg. **B,** Location of incisions on the lateral and medial aspects of the leg.

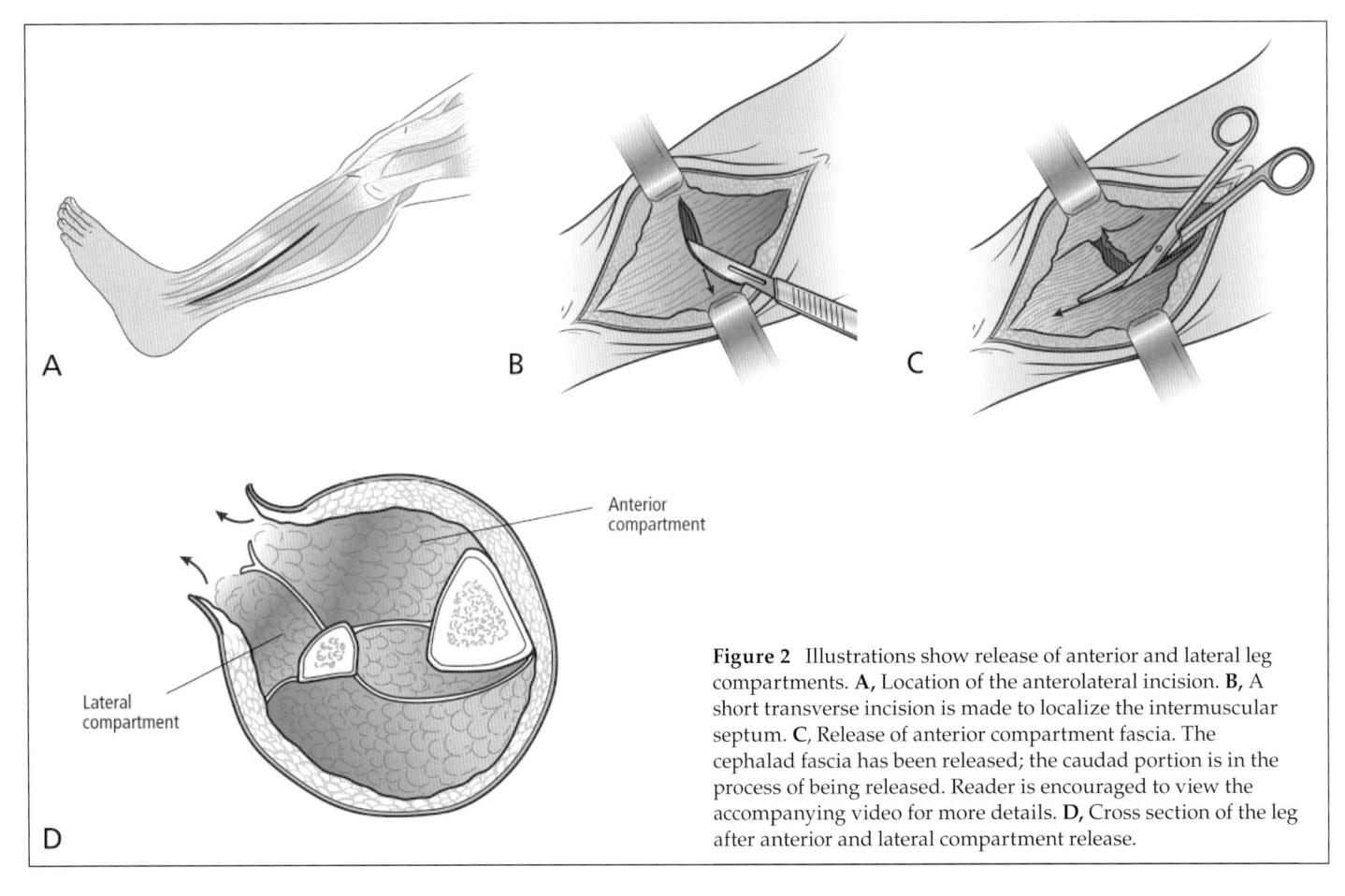

Figure 2 Illustrations show release of anterior and lateral leg compartments. **A,** Location of the anterolateral incision. **B,** A short transverse incision is made to localize the intermuscular septum. **C,** Release of anterior compartment fascia. The cephalad fascia has been released; the caudad portion is in the process of being released. Reader is encouraged to view the accompanying video for more details. **D,** Cross section of the leg after anterior and lateral compartment release.

compartment (**Figure 3, B**). The compartment musculature is then easily assessed. A second small, axially directed incision is made just off the posteromedial border of the tibia and is carried cephalad and caudad (**Figure 3, C**). When this is done correctly, the surgeon should be able to readily palpate the posteromedial portion of the bone and, following the release (**Figure 3, D**), assess the viability of the muscles of the compartment.

Once the fasciotomies have been performed, it is important to assess whether any extensions to the skin incisions are needed for the caudad and cephalad portions of the compartments. In severe cases, the skin itself in the proximal and distal aspects of the leg may be a continued tether and cause heightened underlying compartment pressure.

Complications

Scarring of the skin of the leg is the rule rather than the exception. Scarring is inherent in delayed wound closure and in the coverage provided by skin grafting.

A potential complication is injury to the superficial peroneal nerve. This nerve traverses the crural fascia at a variable point on the anterolateral aspect of the leg and supplies sensation to the anterolateral portion of the distal leg, the ankle, and the dorsum of the foot and toes, except for the web space between the great and second toe.

Postoperative Care and Rehabilitation

The wound can be dressed with moistened sterile gauze; however, we gener-

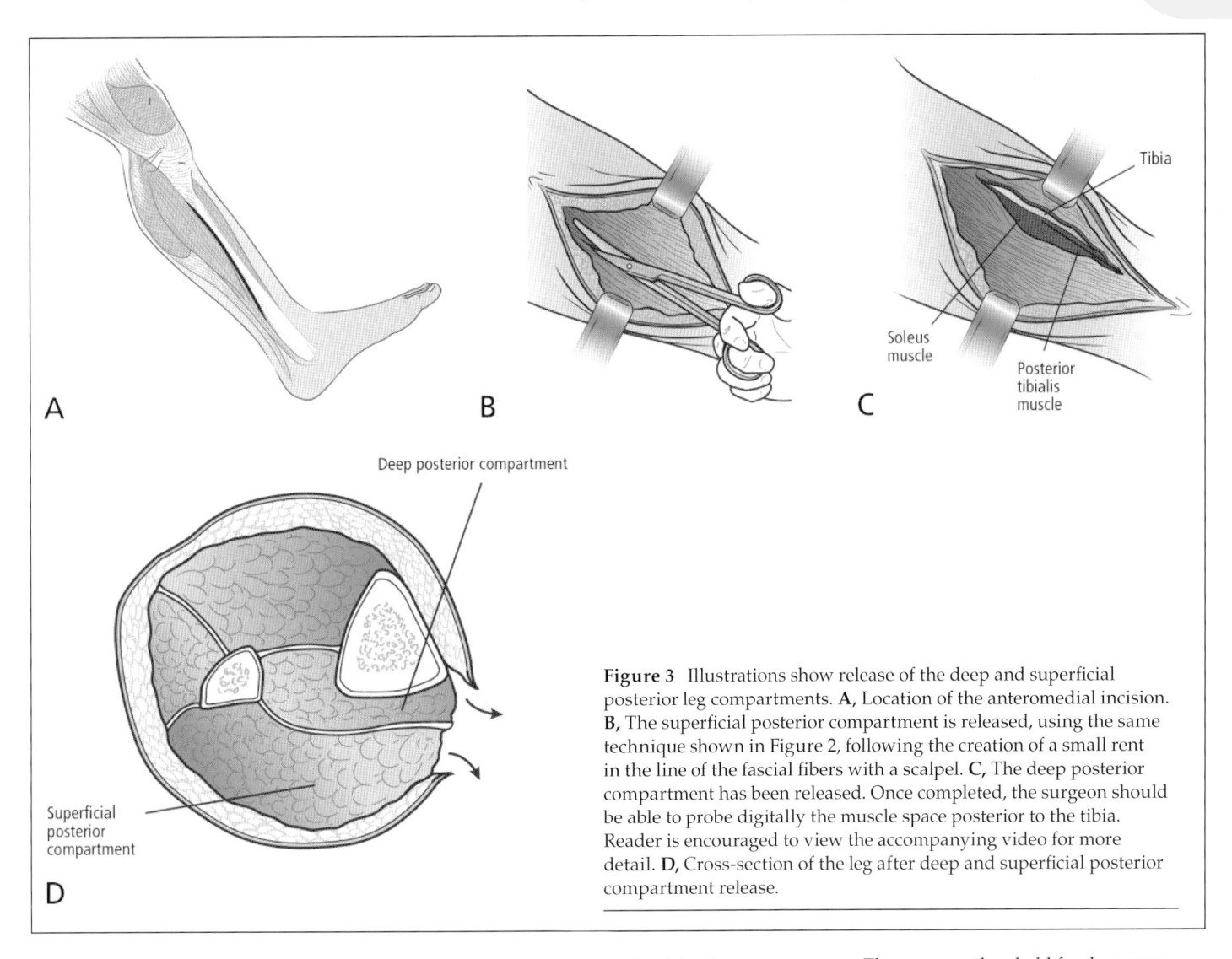

Figure 3 Illustrations show release of the deep and superficial posterior leg compartments. **A,** Location of the anteromedial incision. **B,** The superficial posterior compartment is released, using the same technique shown in Figure 2, following the creation of a small rent in the line of the fascial fibers with a scalpel. **C,** The deep posterior compartment has been released. Once completed, the surgeon should be able to probe digitally the muscle space posterior to the tibia. Reader is encouraged to view the accompanying video for more detail. **D,** Cross-section of the leg after deep and superficial posterior compartment release.

ally use a negative-pressure dressing (–50 mm Hg). The patient is returned to the operating room for staged revisiting of the wounds at 48 to 96 hours. At that time, further wound débridement, delayed primary wound closure, and/or split-thickness skin grafting as well as reapplication of a topical negative-pressure dressing are performed, depending on the condition of the wound.

Pearls

- A high index of suspicion for compartment syndrome is appropriate when a patient presents with severe unremitting limb pain and swelling.
- The sine qua non for the diagnosis of compartment syndrome is pain that is heightened on passive stretch of the muscles within the affected myofascial compartment.
- In patients with limited ability to appreciate pain (eg, a comatose patient or a patient with a traumatized neuropathic leg), measurement of compartment pressures may aid the diagnosis. Patients with tissue compartment pressures that rise to within 30 mm Hg of the diastolic blood pressure have a compartment syndrome.
- Once a diagnosis of compartment pressure is made, decompression of the affected compartment should proceed emergently.

References

1. Owen CA, Mubarak SJ, Hargens AR, Rutherford L, Garetto LP, Akeson WH: Intramuscular pressures with limb compression clarification of the pathogenesis of the drug-induced muscle-compartment syndrome. *N Engl J Med* 1979;300(21):1169-1172.
2. McQueen MM, Gaston P, Court-Brown CM: Acute compartment syndrome: Who is at risk? *J Bone Joint Surg Br* 2000;82(2):200-203.
3. Rorabeck CH, Macnab I: The pathophysiology of the anterior tibial compartmental syndrome. *Clin Orthop Relat Res* 1975;113:52-57.
4. Matsen FA III, Winquist RA, Krugmire RB Jr: Diagnosis and management of compartmental syndromes. *J Bone Joint Surg Am* 1980;62(2):286-291.
5. McQueen MM, Court-Brown CM: Compartment monitoring in tibial fractures: The pressure threshold for decompression. *J Bone Joint Surg Br* 1996;78(1):99-104.
6. Guyton AC, Hall JE: The microcirculation and the lymphatic system: Capillary fluid exchange, interstitial fluid, and lymph flow, in *Textbook of Medical Physiology*, ed 9. Philadelphia, PA, WB Saunders, 1996, pp 183-197.
7. Tornetta P III, Templeman D: Compartment syndrome associated with tibial fracture. *Instr Course Lect* 1997;46:303-308.
8. Meyer RS, White KK, Smith JM, Groppo ER, Mubarak SJ, Hargens AR: Intramuscular and blood pressures in legs positioned in the hemilithotomy position: Clarification of risk factors for well-leg acute compartment syndrome. *J Bone Joint Surg Am* 2002;84(10):1829-1835.
9. Ritenour AE, Dorlac WC, Fang R, et al: Complications after fasciotomy revision and delayed compartment release in combat patients. *J Trauma* 2008;64(2, suppl):S153-S162.
10. Whitesides TE Jr, Haney TC, Harada H, Holmes HE, Morimoto K: A simple method for tissue pressure determination. *Arch Surg* 1975;110(11):1311-1313.

Chapter 59
Open Reduction and Internal Fixation of Forearm Fractures

Thomas F. Varecka, MD

Introduction

The forearm is a unique regional structure within the musculoskeletal system. Not only does it serve as a platform for the origins and insertions of various muscle groups that produce elbow and wrist flexion and extension, it also is associated with its own intrinsic motions—supination and pronation. Anatomically, the forearm serves as a gantry, helping the terminal functional unit, the hand, to be placed three dimensionally within a person's environment to interact with the surroundings, thus facilitating the use of tools, self-care and feeding, and independence. Injuries to the forearm have the potential to seriously impair these functions. Given the role of the radius and ulna as a platform for muscle function, restoring stable, pain-free continuity to these bones is essential. Because the forearm itself functions as a joint with its own motion, accurate anatomic restoration is mandatory.[1-5]

Patient Selection

As the dual roles of anatomic and articular function of the forearm became more appreciated, the need to achieve stable, rigid fixation of fractures of the forearm became widely accepted.[1,2] Consequently, treatment of these fractures almost always involves open reduction and internal fixation (ORIF), usually with plates and screws (Figure 1). Because fracture instability is frequently quite marked when both the radius and ulna are broken and because of the variety of deforming forces exerted by the various forearm muscles when the skeleton has been disrupted (Figure 2), an open reduction almost invariably is required to reestablish anatomic alignment.[6,7] Plating is accepted as the most reliable means of maintaining rigid alignment once the fractures have been reduced.[8,9]

In addition to reducing the fractures of the radius and ulna, the surgeon also

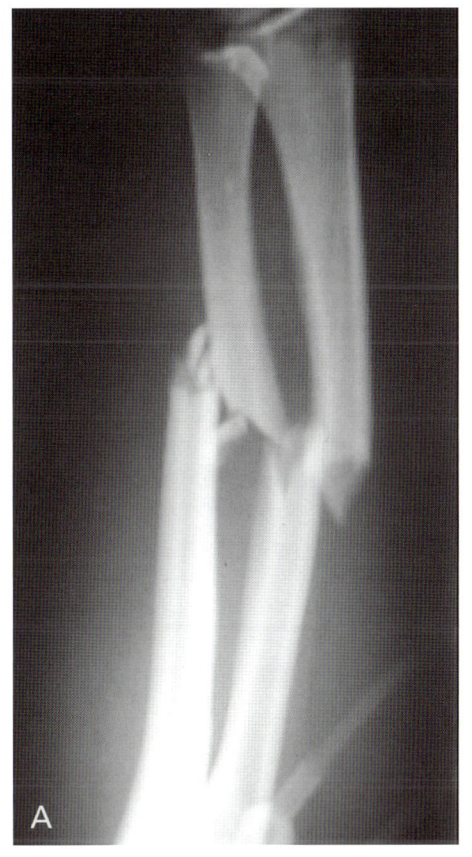

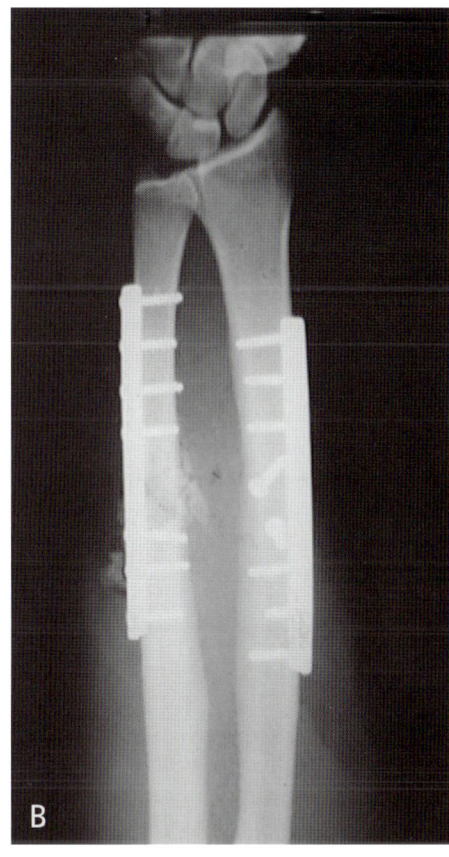

Figure 1 AP radiographs show a typical both-bone fracture of the forearm before (**A**) and after (**B**) open reduction and internal fixation.

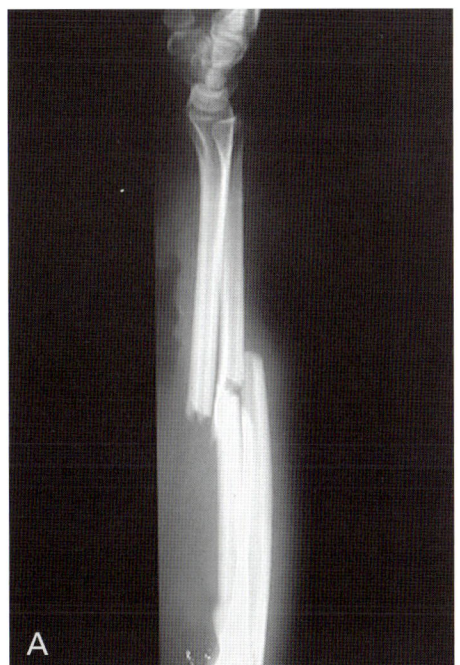

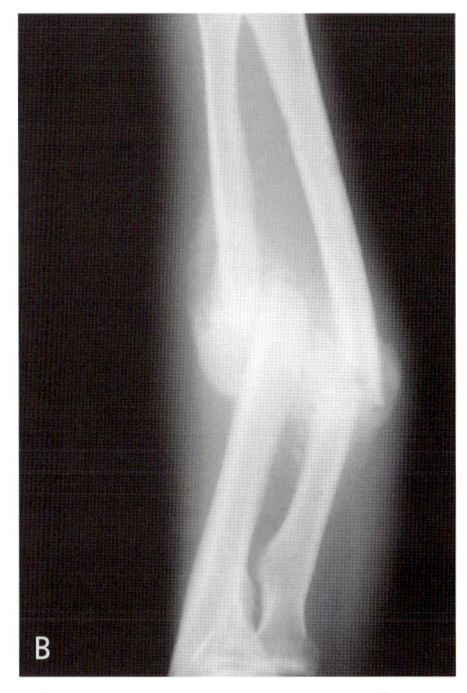

Figure 2 Radiographs show a both-bone forearm fracture. **A,** Lateral view shows the fracture before treatment, with malalignment and impending malunion. **B,** AP view shows the forearm following treatment with casting alone.

Dr. Varecka or an immediate family member is a member of a speakers' bureau or has made paid presentations on behalf of Stryker and Synthes and serves as an unpaid consultant to Stryker.

must pay attention to the proximal and distal radioulnar joints. Accurate and anatomic realignment of these articulations must be achieved if the forearm motions of supination and pronation are to be recovered. An accurate restoration of radial and ulnar diaphyseal anatomy usually will restore articular alignment by indirect means. Direct reduction of the proximal and distal radioulnar joints normally is not necessary, and accurate articular alignment generally can be assessed on intraoperative radiographs.

Few contraindications to ORIF of the forearm exist. In cases of severe skin compromise such as occurs with burns, or extensive and severe contamination such as occurs with fractures sustained in a farm setting, temporary stabilization of the fractures with an external fixator may be prudent. More simple open injuries with less extensive contamination are not in themselves contraindications to ORIF, even on an immediate basis.[2,10] Once the soft tissues or contamination has been addressed, however, proceeding with rigid internal fixation is indicated.

In addition to promoting recovery of forearm function, internal fixation has long been recommended as a means of allowing rapid recovery of the normal use and activity of the forearm, thus avoiding the development of so-called "fracture disease."[4] Fracture disease is the pathologic consequence of immobilizing normally mobile structures for long periods. It manifests as joint stiffness and pain, weakness from muscle deconditioning, hyperemia, skin atrophy, and allodynia. Although less common today than when forearm fractures were routinely treated for extended periods in long-arm casts, fracture disease still occurs. In its most egregious forms, fracture disease produces prolonged states of pain and disability and is termed complex regional pain syndrome.

Evaluation

The diagnosis of a forearm fracture usually is straightforward. A history of a fall on the outstretched arm or another form of indirect injury is quite common. More frequently, however, patients report having sustained a direct blow to the forearm by a rigid structure such as a baseball bat, a steering wheel, certain immovable objects (eg, trees or fences), or contact with the ground. Not uncommonly in urban environments, a gunshot injury is the cause. Pain, swelling, tenderness, and the inability to use the forearm are universal. When examining a patient with such a history, it is important to check for any associated openings in the skin, lacerations, or other evidence that the fracture may be open. Equally important and universally mandatory is the thorough evaluation and documentation of the patient's sensory, motor, and circulatory status. Also important is the recording of the circumstances of the injury, such as at the workplace or as a result of a motor vehicle collision or an altercation.

Preoperative Imaging

Standard radiographs should be obtained in the emergency department, with at least three separate projections—AP, lateral, and oblique—necessary to assess the fractures adequately for displacement, extent, comminution, presence of subcutaneous air (suggesting an open fracture), and presence of any foreign materials. These radiographs should routinely include the joints above and below (ie, the elbow and wrist) to exclude any involvement of these joints in the injury pattern. Rarely are special imaging techniques such as CT or MRI needed to establish the diagnosis of a both-bone forearm fracture.

Preoperative Planning

As with any challenging surgical exercise undertaken to fix a fracture, preoperative planning is highly recommended. A good preoperative plan should include an accurate drawing of the fracture(s) that details the position along the length of the bone, the degree of comminution and displacement, and the tentative location of any fixation devices. The position of all screws, including those to be placed outside the plates, should be indicated. Moreover, it is very helpful to generate a list of all equipment to be used in the order in which they will be used. All special devices should be noted, particularly when they may have to be procured from outside the hospital's routine equipment supply. The plan should include the need for imaging machines and the approximate points along the course of the procedure that will require intraoperative imaging. Another important element of the plan is dressing requirements, such as plaster bandages, the possible use of vacuum-assisted closure bandages, and other special needs. Preoperative plans allow all personnel involved to take part in the surgical activity more properly and efficiently. Finally, the preoperative plan should specify antibiotic coverage. Typically, a good broad-spectrum antibiotic, such as a cephalosporin, is chosen. In closed and uncomplicated fractures, the first dose should be administered in the preoperative holding area, and the antibiotic should be continued for about 24 hours postoperatively. In open fractures or grossly contaminated wounds, more aggressive antibiotic coverage may be necessary, and use of an aminoglycoside or a β-lactam–containing drug should be considered. In patients with true penicillin allergies with cephalosporin crossover, clindamycin is the usual recommended alternative.

Procedure

Patient Positioning/Room Setup

Forearm fractures ordinarily can be addressed with the patient in the supine position. A sturdy arm table extending from the regular operating room table is of great benefit in supporting the patient's arm during the procedure. The arm table allows the surgeon(s) and assistant(s) to be comfortably seated for the duration of the procedure. Prior to starting the surgery, it is useful to ensure that radiographic imaging devices can be moved easily into and out of the surgical field. Waiting to bring the C-arm or similar imaging device into optimum position until it is actually needed is inefficient and can lead to contamination of the surgical field (**Figure 3**).

ORIF of the forearm is best performed under tourniquet control. Checking that the tourniquet is accurately set and in proper working order before the start of surgery is strongly advised. Similarly, making sure that the internal fixation set is complete is recommended. Missing plates and/or inadequate numbers or varieties of screws should be determined before the start of surgery. A missing plate or an insufficient number of appropriate-length screws can compromise the quality and reliability of the surgical procedure, as well as the results.

Surgical Technique

The affected extremity is exsanguinated with an Esmarch wrap, and the tourniquet is inflated to approximately 100 to 125 mm Hg above systolic pressure. The particular incisions and surgical approaches used are usually determined by the fracture location and pattern. For most forearm fractures, an extensile approach, such as the volar approach of Henry[11] (**Figure 4**), is sufficient for the

Chapter 59: Open Reduction and Internal Fixation of Forearm Fractures

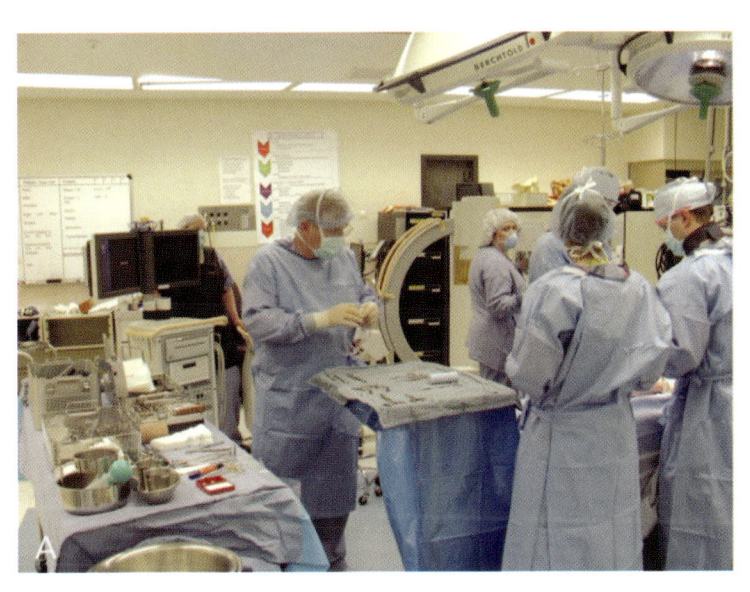

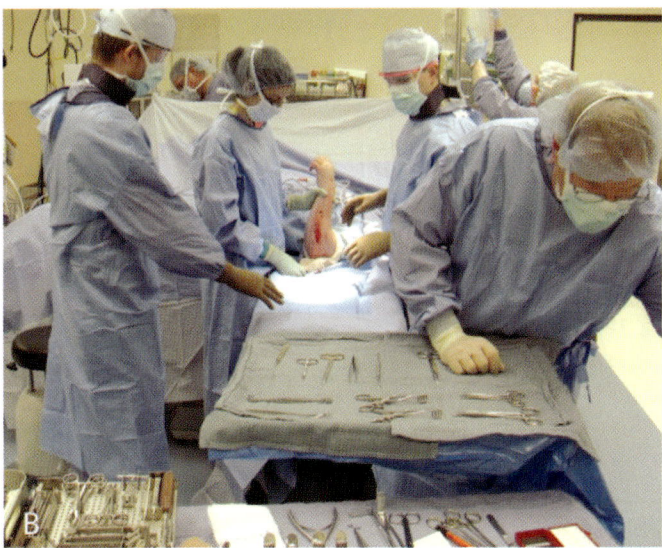

Figure 3 Photographs show the room setup and patient positioning for open reduction and internal fixation of a both-bone forearm fracture. **A,** The room setup, with C-arm, back table, and instruments prepared. **B,** The patient is positioned supine on the operating table with the injured arm supported on an arm table.

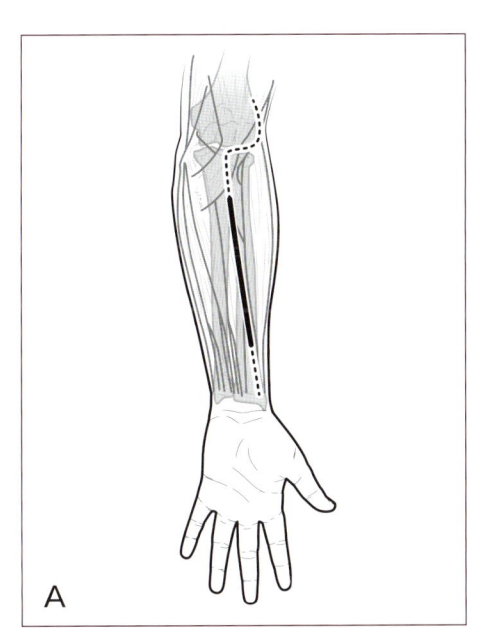

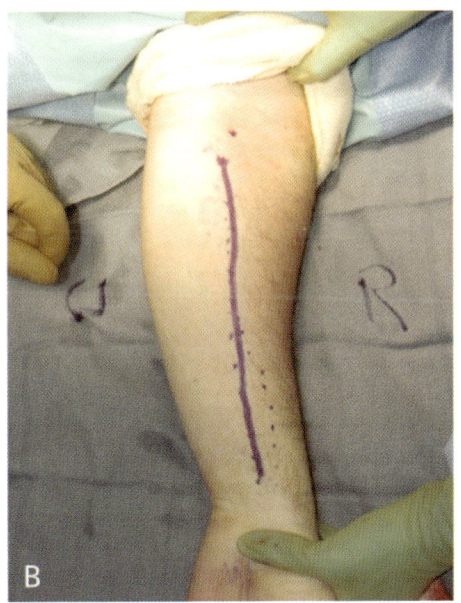

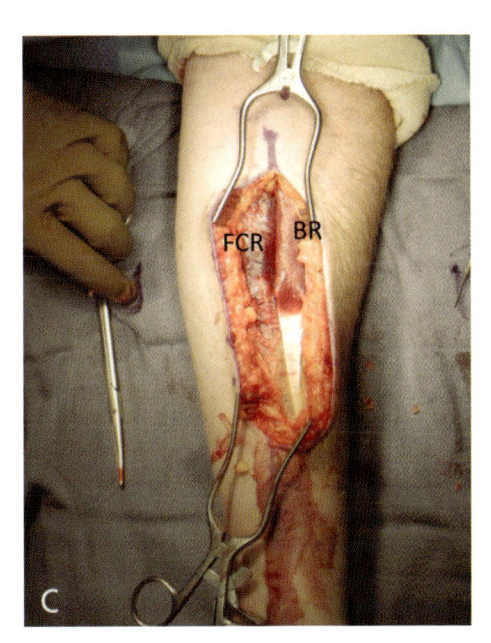

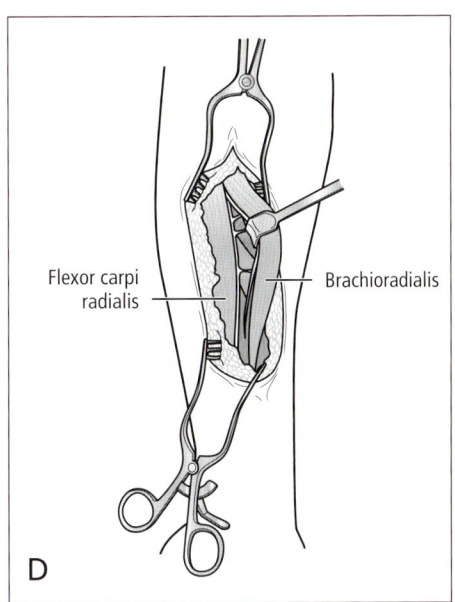

Figure 4 The volar approach of Henry. **A,** Illustration shows the incision. The incision used in panels **B** through **D** is represented by the solid portion of the line. **B,** Photograph shows the initial incision outlined on the skin. Intraoperative photograph (**C**) and illustration (**D**) show the initial exposure. A leash of vessels from the radial artery supplies the brachioradialis (BR) muscle. The vessels must be ligated to mobilize the brachioradialis muscle laterally. The superficial branch of the radial nerve is retracted with the brachioradialis muscle. FCR = flexor carpi radialis muscle.

© 2013 American Academy of Orthopaedic Surgeons

377

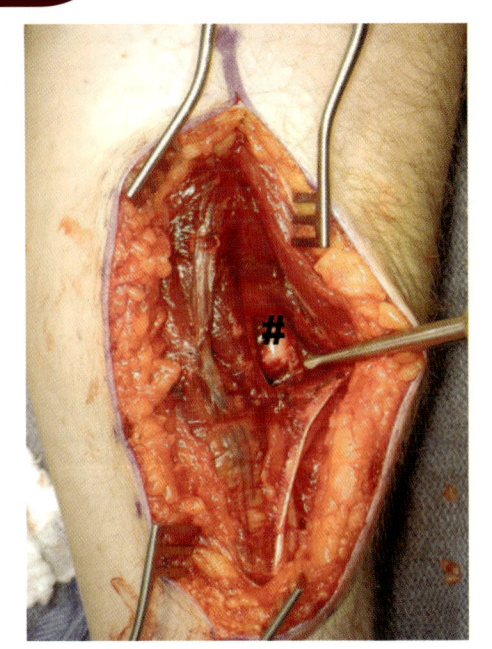

Figure 5 Intraoperative photograph shows proximal dissection for open reduction and internal fixation of a both-bone fracture. The brachioradialis and pronator teres muscles are retracted, exposing the fracture, which is denoted by the # sign.

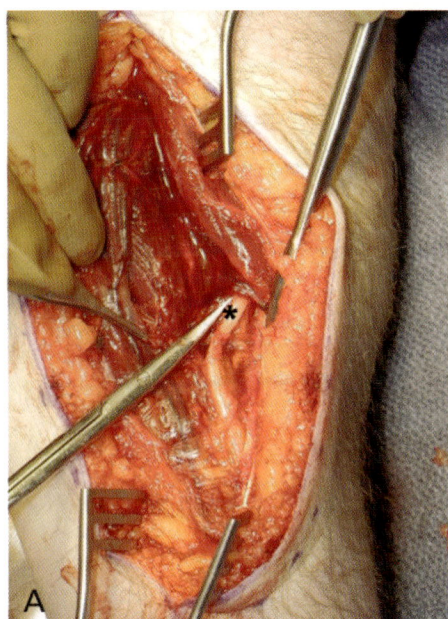

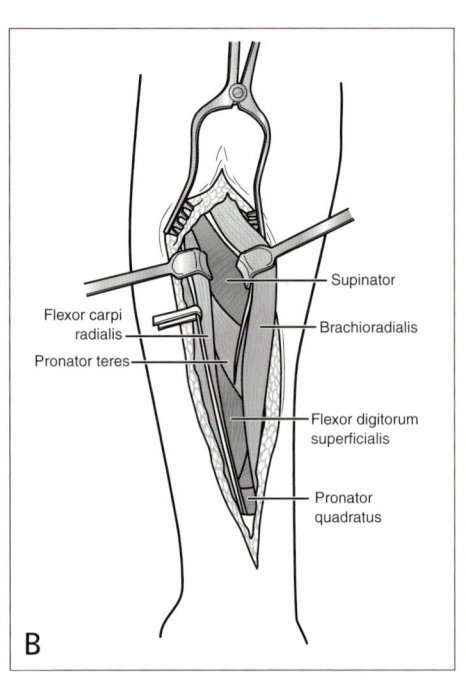

Figure 6 Dissection in the midforearm for open reduction and internal fixation of a both-bone fracture. **A,** Intraoperative photograph shows the brachioradialis muscle retracted. The superficial radial nerve is denoted by the asterisk. **B,** Deep to the brachioradialis and the flexor carpi radialis are the supinator muscles, the pronator teres, the flexor digitorum superficialis, and, most distally, the pronator quadratus.

radius; for the ulna, an ulnar midline approach usually is preferred.

In general, the bone with the more simple fracture pattern is addressed first. This fracture will be somewhat easier to reduce and fix and, once it is stabilized with a plate and screws, fixation of the second fracture can be a little less onerous. In fractures that are very unstable because of extensive associated soft-tissue disruption, however, fixing the ulna first can be a major challenge because of the need to hold the forearm in a suspended position as the plate and screws are being applied. This can make an already challenging task more trying and frustrating. Under these circumstances, fixing the radius first, even when it is the more severe fracture pattern, can simplify the surgical task.

Approach for Radial Fixation

The volar approach of Henry is an extensile incision that facilitates easy access to the fractured radius and permits the initial length of the incision to be increased if necessary to gain exposure of the entire length of the radius.[11] The initial incision is made anywhere along a line extending from the biceps tuberosity proximally to the prominence of the scaphoid tuberosity distally; the volar-ulnar border of the brachioradialis muscle is the most consistent landmark. The actual placement of the initial incision will be determined by the location of the fracture. Distally, the interval is generally between the brachioradialis muscle and the flexor carpi radialis (FCR) muscle (**Figure 4, C** and **D**). More proximally, the interval is between the brachioradialis muscle and the flexor digitorum superficialis muscle. Distally, as dissection is taken more deeply, the pronator quadratus muscle will be encountered, covering the broad, flat surface of the radius. More proximally, deeper dissection will reveal the pronator teres muscle (**Figure 5**) and the near-contiguous supinator muscle. In extreme circumstances, dissection can be carried even farther, between the brachioradialis muscle and the brachialis muscle, completely exposing the superficial radial nerve in the process.[11]

In the midforearm, the radial nerve will be encountered along the deep surface of the brachioradialis muscle (**Figure 6**). The nerve usually is found under the epimysium covering the muscle and should be specifically identified to avoid injury. More distally, the nerve gradually begins to emerge from under the brachioradialis muscle along its more volar margin. Similarly, several small perforating arterial branches from the radial artery that supply the brachioradialis usually are encountered at the junction of the middle and distal thirds of the radius. Careful recognition of these branches and preemptive cauterization or ligation when identified can save much valuable time and avoid potentially dangerous bleeding later.

Exposure of the fracture and surrounding bone should be done in a careful, measured manner and should be sharply performed (**Figure 7, A**). Only the surface of the bone to which the plate will be applied is exposed. Wide and indiscriminate periosteal elevation is discouraged because it can contribute to local bone ischemia, which adds further insult to an already damaged bone, possibly setting the stage for delayed union or nonunion and decreased resistance to infection. Indiscriminately scraping the bone with a dull periosteal elevator (or, worse, the tip of the suction device) is strongly discouraged.

Soft-tissue attachments to all bone fragments should be preserved. Stripping soft-tissue attachments from smaller fragments leads to devascularization and, ultimately, necrosis. If the anatomic reduction and internal fixation of intervening fragments necessitates removal of their soft-tissue attachments, then the surgeon may choose to bypass those fragments and include only the major proximal and distal fragments in the fixation construct. In this case, preserving the intervening fragments and their viability may provide an enhanced healing milieu.

Provisional Reduction of the Radial Fracture

Once the fracture has been exposed, provisional reduction can be performed

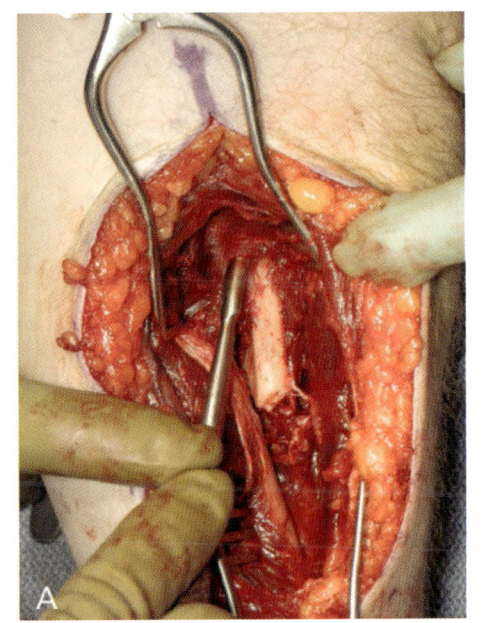

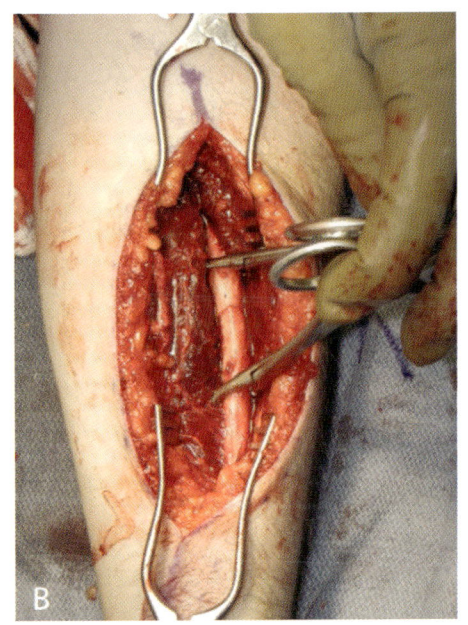

Figure 7 Intraoperative photographs demonstrate exposure and provisional reduction of the radial fracture in a both-bone fracture of the forearm. **A,** The fracture is exposed with a sharp periosteal elevator. **B,** Provisional reduction is achieved with bone clamps.

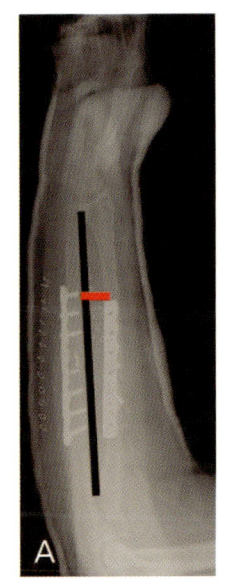

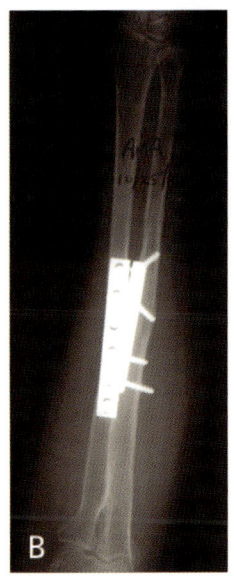

Figure 8 Radiographs obtained following open reduction and internal fixation of both-bone fractures demonstrate adequate restoration of the radial bow (**A**) and poor restoration of the radial bow (**B**).

(**Figure 7, B**). Cleaning the fracture ends of any debris, clotted blood, and organized hematoma will facilitate this effort. The provisional reduction can sometimes be maintained inherently in more stable fractures. Alternatively, using a temporary wire, bone clamps, or even the intended plate along with bone clamps can be considered. If the fracture pattern allows, insertion of interfragmentary screws frequently provides the surest form of provisional fixation. It is useful to check the adequacy of the reduction with intraoperative imaging before proceeding with definitive fixation. For the radius, the reduction can be deemed satisfactory only when the proper length and rotation and the appropriate radial bow have been reestablished. The radial bow is the normally occurring curvature of the radius in the coronal plane that allows it to rotate about the ulna as the forearm is supinated and pronated (**Figure 8, A**). Failure to reestablish the radial bow or reconstructing it inadequately or excessively can lead to malarticulation at the proximal or distal radioulnar joint or both, which can result in restriction in forearm rotation[9] (**Figure 8, B**).

Fixation of the Radial Fracture

Because of the multiplanar anatomy of the radius, some form of plate contouring is frequently necessary. Templating the shape of the radius in the vicinity of the intended fixation is useful when contouring of the plate is needed. Malleable aluminum templates are standard pieces of equipment in almost all commercially available fixation sets (**Figure 9**).

The appropriate plate should have been chosen as part of the preoperative plan. A thick, rigid plate designed for diaphyseal bone should be used. Evidence suggests that 3.5-mm plates are satisfactory.[12] Larger (4.5-mm) plates tend to produce excessive stress shielding and cortical atrophy in the region of the plate. In addition, the use of such excessively rigid plates can lead to fracture at the end of the plate because of stress concentration at the abrupt transition points between the portion of

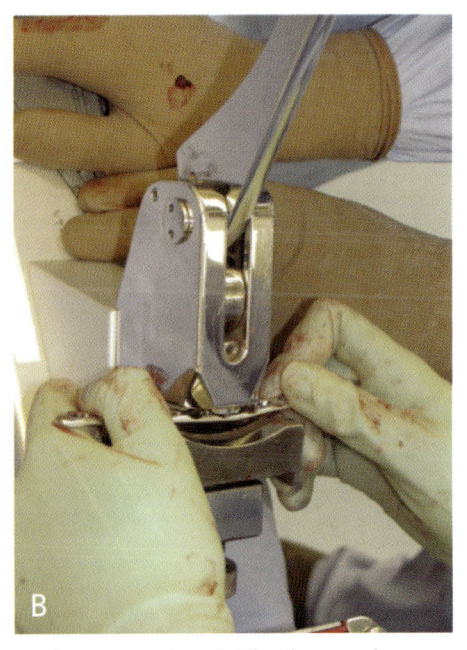

Figure 9 Intraoperative photographs demonstrate plate contouring. **A,** The shape and contour of the bone is determined with an aluminum template. **B,** Contouring of the plate.

the bone that has been fixed and the portions that are uncovered.[13,14] Thin plates, such as semitubular or one-third tubular plates, should be avoided because they are not strong enough to protect the bone or allow early range of motion.

The sequence of screw insertion is determined by the fracture pattern. If the fracture has a relatively short obliquity, applying the plate to the surface that allows for the creation of an acute angle between plate and bone surface is desirable. This allows the plate to function as a capturing buttress, as the screw pulls the plate to the bone surface, and allows the opposite fragment to be docked into this axillary construct, imparting significant stability. In more transverse patterns, the plate should be applied and fixed to the proximal fragment first because compression will be best achieved by applying it through the more mobile and controllable distal fragment (**Figure 10**). In the forearm, a minimum of three screws with bicortical purchase generally is required. Special plate applications, such as the bridging technique used for more comminuted fractures, may be adequately fixed with two pairs of screws—one set placed as close as possible to, but on the opposite side of, the fracture and the other set as far from the fracture as possible. With almost all plating techniques, however, deploying the screws over as great a distance along the bone as possible imparts optimal mechanical properties to the construct.

Standard plates are satisfactory for most diaphyseal forearm fractures. Locking plates may be desirable in unusual circumstances, such as fractures with bone loss and resulting severe instability; fractures extending into metadiaphyseal regions of the bone; or cases of pathologic bone, as is seen in neoplastic disease or severe osteomalacia caused by malnutrition or malabsorption.

In cases of severe bone loss, bone grafting may be needed. Evidence suggests that routine bone grafting is not indicated.[14-16] Although once thought to be necessary if significant comminution was present,[1] bone grafting is now reserved for situations in which disruption of the normal bone healing sequence is anticipated. In general, if any doubt exists about whether to bone graft, it probably is best to avoid doing so, because healing rates are approximately the same whether or not bone graft is used routinely.[14,15]

After fixation of the radius is completed, the wound can be packed with a moist sponge. Attention is then directed to the ulna.

Fixation of the Ulnar Fracture

Exposure of the ulnar fracture usually is completed along the ulnar midlateral border, entering the interval between the flexor carpi ulnaris muscle and the extensor carpi ulnaris muscle. This interval can be recognized readily in the more distal forearm and then developed more proximally if needed (**Figure 11, A**). Rarely, the approach may take a more volar route, between the flexor carpi ulnaris, with related ulnar neurovascular structures, and the flexor muscles and tendons in the ulnar bursa. Because of the potential for damage to the nerve and vessels, it is best to avoid this route unless absolutely necessary.

Fixation of the ulnar fracture (**Figure 11, B and C**) should follow the same principles as those outlined previously for the fixation of the radius. The determination of the appropriate plate and its application is similar.

Wound Closure

With completion of fixation, wound closure can commence. If a tourniquet has been used, it should be deflated before closure. Failure to identify sources of bleeding can lead to hematoma formation, wound drainage, infection, pain, return trips to the operating suite, and other undesirable consequences. The wounds should be closed in layers, avoiding severe, watertight closure of the deeper fascial tissues. Such extreme repairs can act as a restraint to swelling, leading to severe postoperative pain and even

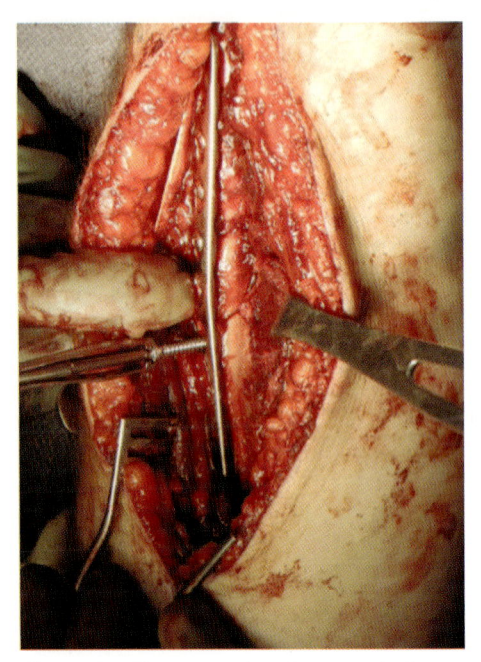

Figure 10 Intraoperative photograph shows the application of a plate to the radial fracture in a both-bone fracture. Note that the contour of the plate allows for reestablishment of radial bow.

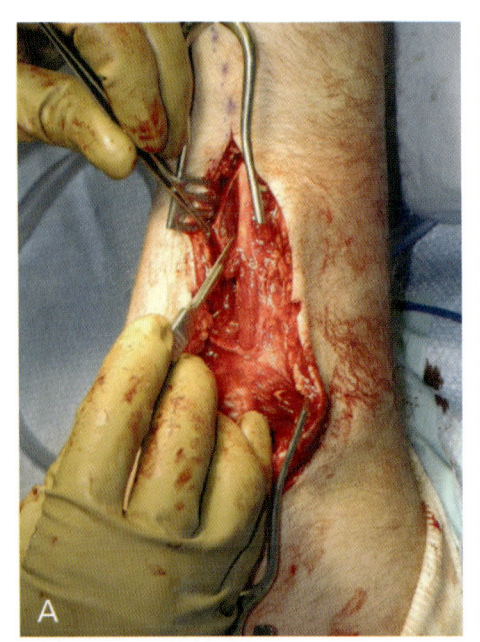

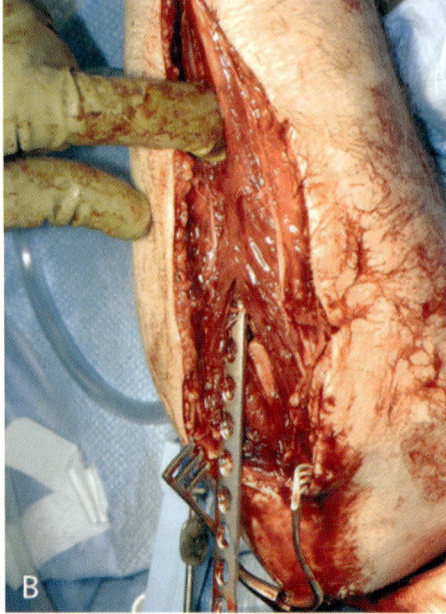

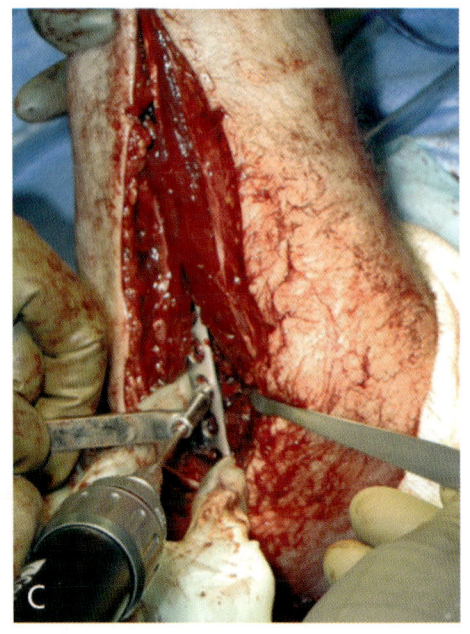

Figure 11 Intraoperative photographs demonstrate exposure and fixation of the ulnar fracture in a both-bone fracture. **A**, The ulna is exposed through a medial midaxial incision. **B**, The ulnar plate is inserted with limited submuscular technique. **C**, A screw hole is drilled for the ulnar plate. Note that the plate is partially covered because of the submuscular placement.

Chapter 59: Open Reduction and Internal Fixation of Forearm Fractures

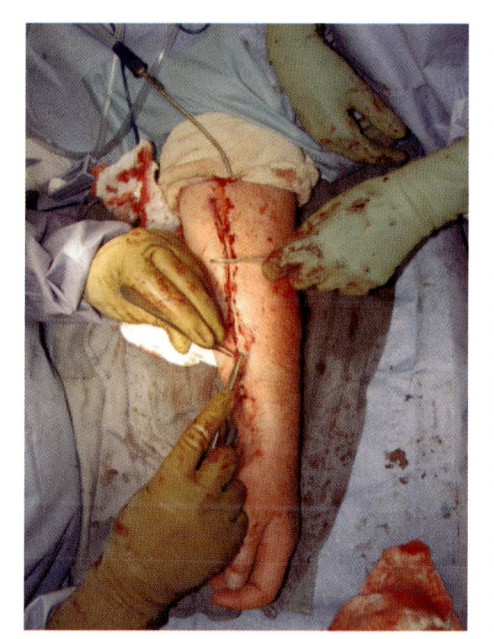

Figure 12 Intraoperative photograph shows wound closure following open reduction and internal fixation of a both-bone forearm fracture. The tourniquet was released before closure.

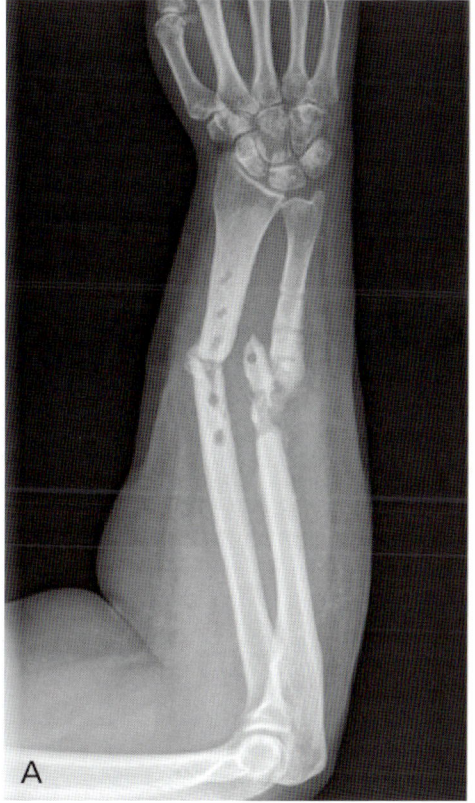

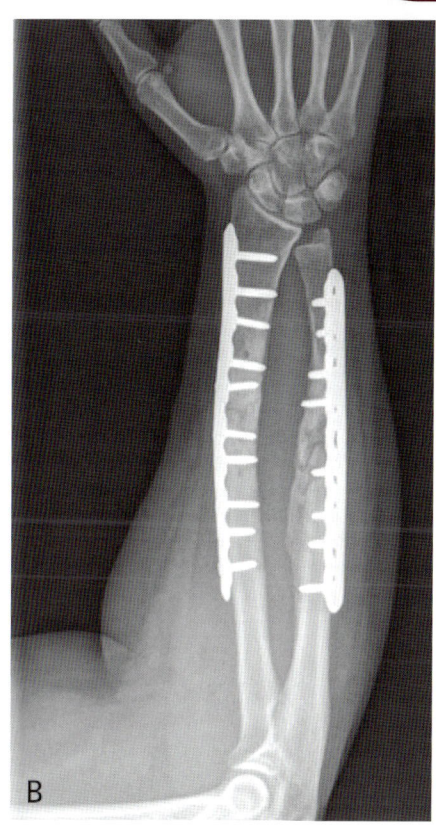

Figure 13 AP radiographs show a both-bone fracture following removal of plates and screws in the setting of an infection. The original injury was a highly contaminated open fracture that occurred on a farm. Once the fracture had been serially débrided (**A**) and subsequently reduced and stabilized, it went on to heal with complete resolution of the infection (**B**).

the development of compartment syndrome. More superficial subcutaneous tissue is closed with absorbable braided or monofilament suture. Skin closure is accomplished with nonabsorbable or absorbable sutures or skin staples, according to surgeon preference (**Figure 12**). When used appropriately, all methods give a satisfactory cosmetic result. Large, horizontal mattress sutures tend to leave unsightly "railroad track" scars and are best avoided.

Wound dressing also can be performed according to surgeon preference. Application of a nonadherent material under the gauze bandages usually is appreciated greatly by the patient at the time of dressing change. Whether to apply a plaster splint—and the nature of the splint—is determined by the fracture pattern, the security of the fracture fixation, and patient factors. In general, a plaster dressing should be as small as is deemed sufficient. In a child, a patient who lacks insight or understanding, or an uncooperative and noncompliant patient, a long-arm splint may be necessary. In a more compliant patient, a light short-arm splint or a bulky, soft compressive dressing is all that is needed. Dressings should be well padded, especially if plaster is used, but a complete, encircling plaster dressing should never be used because of the risk of pressure problems and compartment syndrome.

Complications

Perhaps the most universally feared complication is infection (**Figure 13**). Bone and soft-tissue destruction, nonhealing, chronic debilitation, and dysfunction are all potential end products of infection. The appropriate preparation of the patient preoperatively, meticulous surgical technique, and diligent postoperative vigilance are the cornerstones of minimizing complications of infection. The first sign of local sepsis, excessive wound drainage, or patient malaise—or other hints that infection may be developing—should signal that a return trip to the operating room is necessary. Relying on acute inflammatory markers, such as elevation in the erythrocyte sedimentation rate or C-reactive protein level, is inefficient and can delay the needed incision and drainage. When recognized early and addressed urgently, infection frequently can be controlled. In addition, it often is useful to engage the assistance of an infectious disease consultant for antibiotic management.

Nonunion is another infrequent but dreaded complication. Because the rigid fixation of forearm fractures usually is not accompanied by callus formation, nonunion or delayed union should be suspected whenever patients do not show the usual progression through the convalescence process. When pain persists longer than expected or the fracture remains tender and/or locally warm, a derangement in healing should be suspected. Ignoring such signs and delaying intervention until catastrophic hardware failure occurs is inefficient, costly, and lacking in compassion. The acute signs of fracture healing will resolve in most patients in 3 to 4 months. If this does not occur, the possibility of an unintended interruption in the healing process should be discussed frankly with the patient, and the patient should be prepared for the possible need for further surgery. Special imaging, such as CT, may be needed to confirm the presence of nonunion or delayed union (**Figure 14**).

Uncommon complications are encountered occasionally, the most devastating of which is the development of a radioulnar synostosis (**Figure 15**). Radioulnar synostosis is bone overgrowth that leads to a bridge forming between the radius and ulna; it is an absolute functional disaster. The synostosis deprives the forearm of its principal role of performing rotational motion. The hyperemia associated with a radioulnar synostosis often

© 2013 *American Academy of Orthopaedic Surgeons*

is uncomfortable, as is the resistance to the patient's persistent efforts to supinate and pronate the forearm. The preoperative recognition of a situation in which a synostosis is a possibility, such as highly comminuted both-bone fractures at the same level along the length of the radius and ulna with prominent hardware, can help the surgeon avoid this problem (Figure 16). The surgeon should meticulously avoid connecting the fracture sites intraoperatively. If bone grafting is needed, attention to detail when placing the grafts and avoidance of connecting the radial and ulnar fracture wounds is paramount. Routine prophylaxis for synostosis with postoperative irradiation or indomethacin is not recommended.

Most patients experience some loss of motion following a forearm fracture (Figure 17). Even the most meticulously performed surgery results in some scarring in excess of that incurred as a result of the injury.[3] Moreover, traumatic damage to the interosseous ligament and consequent soft-tissue fibrosis will lead to loss of motion, usually supination.[17] In addition, the elbow and wrist will lose some motion: in the elbow, a small amount of extension loss is seen; in the wrist, many patients lose some flexion. A frank discussion of these possibilities preoperatively or early in the postoperative period is advisable.

The routine removal of fixation hardware is no longer deemed a necessity. In the early experience with plate fixation of forearm fractures, such recommendations were common, but accumulated evidence now suggests that the retention of hardware usually is associated with fewer problems and complications than plate removal. It is suggested that plates and screws be removed only if they are themselves causing problems, are associated with the development of infection or nonunion, or are otherwise intolerably symptomatic.[8,12,13,18,19]

The most devastating complications frequently are those that are iatrogenic in nature. Intraoperative damage to nerve

Figure 14 Nonunion in a severe open fracture following crush injury to forearm. **A,** AP radiograph demonstrates the nonunion. **B,** Sagittal cut CT scan demonstrates radial nonunion 7 months later. **C,** Coronal cut CT scan demonstrates that ulnar nonunion also is present.

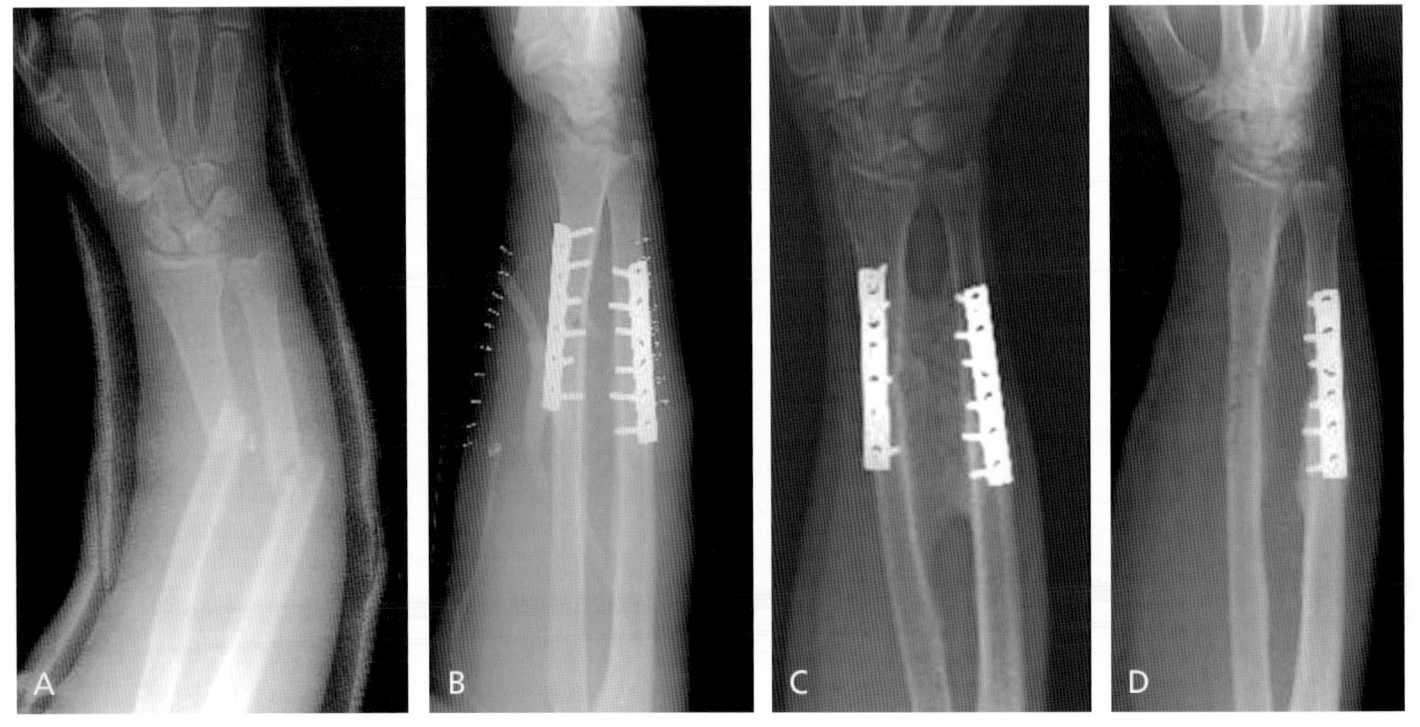

Figure 15 Radiographs demonstrate the development of a radioulnar synostosis. **A,** AP view demonstrates a routine both-bone forearm fracture. Note the fractures of the radius and ulna at the same level. **B,** Uncomplicated fixation is shown on the lateral view. **C,** The development of cross-union is seen. **D,** The fracture is shown after takedown of the cross-union. The patient never recovered full supination and pronation.

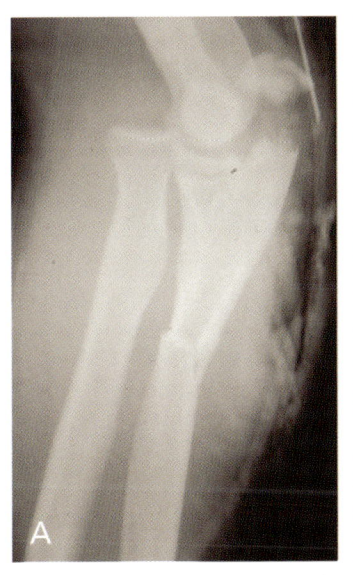

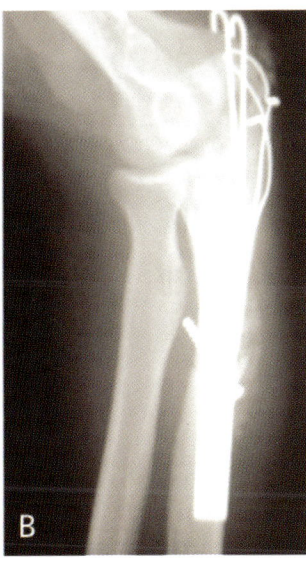

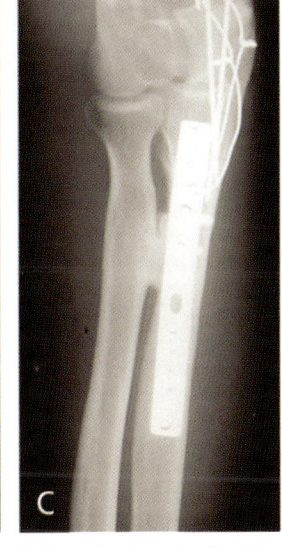

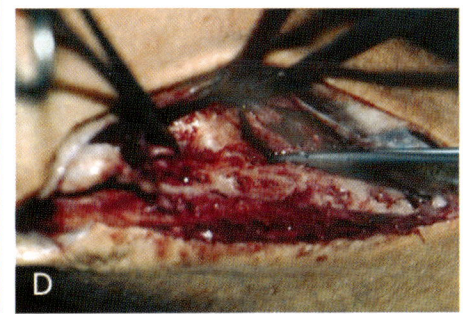

Figure 16 Highly comminuted both-bone fractures at the same level along the length of radius and ulna with prominent hardware. Lateral radiographs of the proximal forearm demonstrate transolecranon and ulnar shaft fractures before (**A**) and after (**B**) fixation. Note the excessively long oblique screw in panel B. **C**, Lateral view demonstrates a cross-union that developed secondary to the screw rubbing on the radial tuberosity. **D**, Intraoperative photograph depicts the cross-union at the time of surgical takedown.

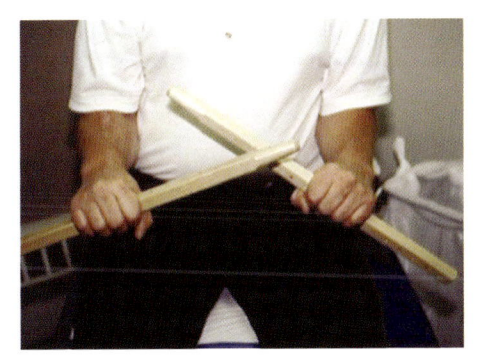

Figure 17 Clinical photograph shows a patient with loss of pronation following open reduction and internal fixation of a both-bone forearm fracture.

tissue is an avoidable complication and theoretically should never happen.[18] A review of the pertinent anatomy should be a routine part of the preoperative plan. A thorough preoperative neurologic examination with appropriate documentation is essential. If surgical problems do occur, an honest and timely discussion with the patient is mandatory.

Finally, and as discussed previously, fracture disease is a complication that can be readily avoided. Gentle handling of tissues, careful dissection around nerves, solid fixation, and early rehabilitation all can minimize this problem. If fracture disease does occur and the pathology progresses to complex regional pain syndrome, assistance from anesthesiology and pain management consultants who have an interest in this problem can be very helpful.

Postoperative Care and Rehabilitation

In the immediate postoperative phase, elevation and icing are very helpful in controlling swelling. In addition, gentle opening and closing of the fingers is extremely beneficial. The motion serves to pump edema fluid out of the fingers, hand, and forearm and encourages patients to begin taking responsibility for their rehabilitation. Patients usually are seen approximately 7 to 10 days postoperatively for wound evaluation and assessment. Most patients are comfortable enough at this time to begin gentle active and active-assisted range-of-motion exercises of the wrist, elbow, forearm, and shoulder. Frequently, in a compliant patient, a well-fitting elastic sleeve provides sufficient support. Occasionally, a prefabricated plastic forearm fracture brace is useful. Although such devices probably do not provide definitive protection, they are frequently welcomed by anxious or fearful patients as a means of providing some protection for the fracture.

Depending on the individual patient, formal physical therapy may or may not be initiated at this time. A formal physical therapy program supervised by a competent, caring therapist can be very helpful in reinforcing the need to move all parts of the affected upper extremity and allaying patient apprehension. Professional guidance through this part of the recovery ensures that the patient understands the exercise program, and intermittent measurement and recording of gains in motion provde the positive reinforcement that can help patients maintain motivation through a sometimes lengthy and arduous rehabilitation.

Strengthening exercises usually are deferred until most or all pain with range-of-motion activities has subsided, usually at about 6 weeks postoperatively. If pain is present, many patients will not do the strengthening exercises. It is sometimes necessary to emphasize to patients at this time that although the fracture has been "fixed," this is not synonymous with bone healing. The patient should understand the need to allow some bone healing to take place before initiating vigorous exercising. Athletes and other highly motivated patients frequently are most in need of such counseling.

Rigid fixation of fractures makes it difficult to assess fracture healing, so a somewhat more empirical approach frequently is required. Plating promotes primary bone healing; therefore, the formation of callus cannot be used as a sign of fracture consolidation. The presence or absence of the physical findings of a healing fracture should be sought on examination. As the fracture heals, no local warmth or tenderness should be present, and the patient should be free of pain with motion and gentle resistance and strengthening exercises. Only when these conditions are met should the patient be allowed to return to full and unrestricted activity. In adults, this normally occurs at 12 to 16 weeks.

© 2013 American Academy of Orthopaedic Surgeons

Pearls

- Displaced fractures of the radius and ulna disrupt the structure and function of the forearm. Unless the bony framework of the forearm is meticulously restored, the functional performance of the forearm will ultimately be compromised.
- Forearm fractures do best when rigid and stable fixation is performed in a timely fashion.
- The preoperative plan should include equipment needs, the surgical tactic, fixation options and plans, and an outline of postoperative management.
- The surgeon should avoid trying to fix both bones through a single incision.
- Postoperative rehabilitation should start early and be guided by a surgeon-therapist team.
- Some loss of motion usually follows a forearm fracture; however, the functional impairment usually is only slight.

References

1. Anderson LD, Sisk D, Tooms RE, Park WI III: Compression-plate fixation in acute diaphyseal fractures of the radius and ulna. *J Bone Joint Surg Am* 1975;57(3):287-297.
2. Dodge HS, Cady GW: Treatment of fractures of the radius and ulna with compression plates. *J Bone Joint Surg Am* 1972;54(6):1167-1176.
3. Droll KP, Perna P, Potter J, Harniman E, Schemitsch EH, McKee MD: Outcomes following plate fixation of fractures of both bones of the forearm in adults. *J Bone Joint Surg Am* 2007;89(12):2619-2624.
4. Grace TG, Eversmann WW Jr: Forearm fractures: Treatment by rigid fixation with early motion. *J Bone Joint Surg Am* 1980;62(3):433-438.
5. Schemitsch EH, Richards RR: The effect of malunion on functional outcome after plate fixation of fractures of both bones of the forearm in adults. *J Bone Joint Surg Am* 1992;74(7):1068-1078.
6. Evans EM: Fractures of the radius and ulna. *J Bone Joint Surg Br* 1951;33-B(4):548-561.
7. Knight RA, Purvis GD: Fractures of both bones of the forearm in adults. *J Bone Joint Surg Am* 1949;31A(4):755-764.
8. Langkamer VG, Ackroyd CE: Removal of forearm plates: A review of the complications. *J Bone Joint Surg Br* 1990;72(4):601-604.
9. Schemitsch EH, Jones D, Henley MB, Tencer AF: A comparison of malreduction after plate and intramedullary nail fixation of forearm fractures. *J Orthop Trauma* 1995;9(1):8-16.
10. Moed BR, Kellam JF, Foster RJ, Tile M, Hansen ST Jr: Immediate internal fixation of open fractures of the diaphysis of the forearm. *J Bone Joint Surg Am* 1986;68(7):1008-1017.
11. Henry AK: *Extensile Exposure*, ed 2. Edinburgh, Scotland, Churchill Livingstone, 1973.
12. Chapman MW, Gordon JE, Zissimos AG: Compression-plate fixation of acute fractures of the diaphyses of the radius and ulna. *J Bone Joint Surg Am* 1989;71(2):159-169.
13. Beaupre GS, Csongradi JJ: Refracture risk after plate removal in the forearm. *J Orthop Trauma* 1996;10(2):87-92.
14. Deluca PA, Lindsey RW, Ruwe PA: Refracture of bones of the forearm after the removal of compression plates. *J Bone Joint Surg Am* 1988;70(9):1372-1376.
15. Wei SY, Born CT, Abene A, Ong A, Hayda R, DeLong WG Jr: Diaphyseal forearm fractures treated with and without bone graft. *J Trauma* 1999;46(6):1045-1048.
16. Wright RR, Schmeling GJ, Schwab JP: The necessity of acute bone grafting in diaphyseal forearm fractures: A retrospective review. *J Orthop Trauma* 1997;11(4):288-294.
17. Pfaeffle HJ, Stabile KJ, Li ZM, Tomaino MM: Reconstruction of the interosseous ligament restores normal forearm compressive load transfer in cadavers. *J Hand Surg Am* 2005;30(2):319-325.
18. Hadden WA, Reschauer R, Seggl W: Results of AO plate fixation of forearm shaft fractures in adults. *Injury* 1983;15(1):44-52.
19. Labosky DA, Cermak MB, Waggy CA: Forearm fracture plates: to remove or not to remove. *J Hand Surg Am* 1990;15(2):294-301.

Chapter 60
Open Reduction and Internal Fixation of Posterior Wall Acetabular Fractures

Lawrence X. Webb, MD

Introduction
Classification
Fractures of the acetabulum are classified according to Letournel into two main groups: elementary fractures and associated fractures.[1] The classification is morphologic and is based on Judet oblique view radiographs.[2] Each group has five types (**Figure 1**). Posterior wall fractures are one of the elementary types; they also may occur as a component in two of the associated types—posterior column and posterior wall fractures, and transverse and posterior wall fractures. This chapter focuses on elementary posterior wall fractures. These are the most common of the ten types, accounting for approximately one fourth to one third of all acetabular fractures.[3,4]

Associated Injuries
Although posterior wall fractures are occasionally seen in isolation, these fractures are often the result of high-energy trauma, and associated injuries are not uncommon. Some of these are life threatening and should be identified and managed at the time of presentation, using ATLS (Advanced Trauma Life Support) protocols.[5]

The mechanism of injury is thought to be axial loading of the femur with the hip in the flexed position.[4] This occurs in motor vehicle accidents with frontal impact when the knee strikes the dashboard. The force is driven via the flexed hip against the posterior wall of the acetabulum, producing the fracture. The size of the fragment is thought to be determined by the degree of abduction or adduction at the time of impact.[4] With displacement of the fractured posterior wall, the femoral head is unconstrained, and it subluxates or dislocates posteriorly in 78% to 86% of

Video 60.1 Posterior Wall Fracture-Dislocation: Reduction and Traction Pin Placement. Lawrence X. Webb, MD; John M. Tabit, DO (4 min)

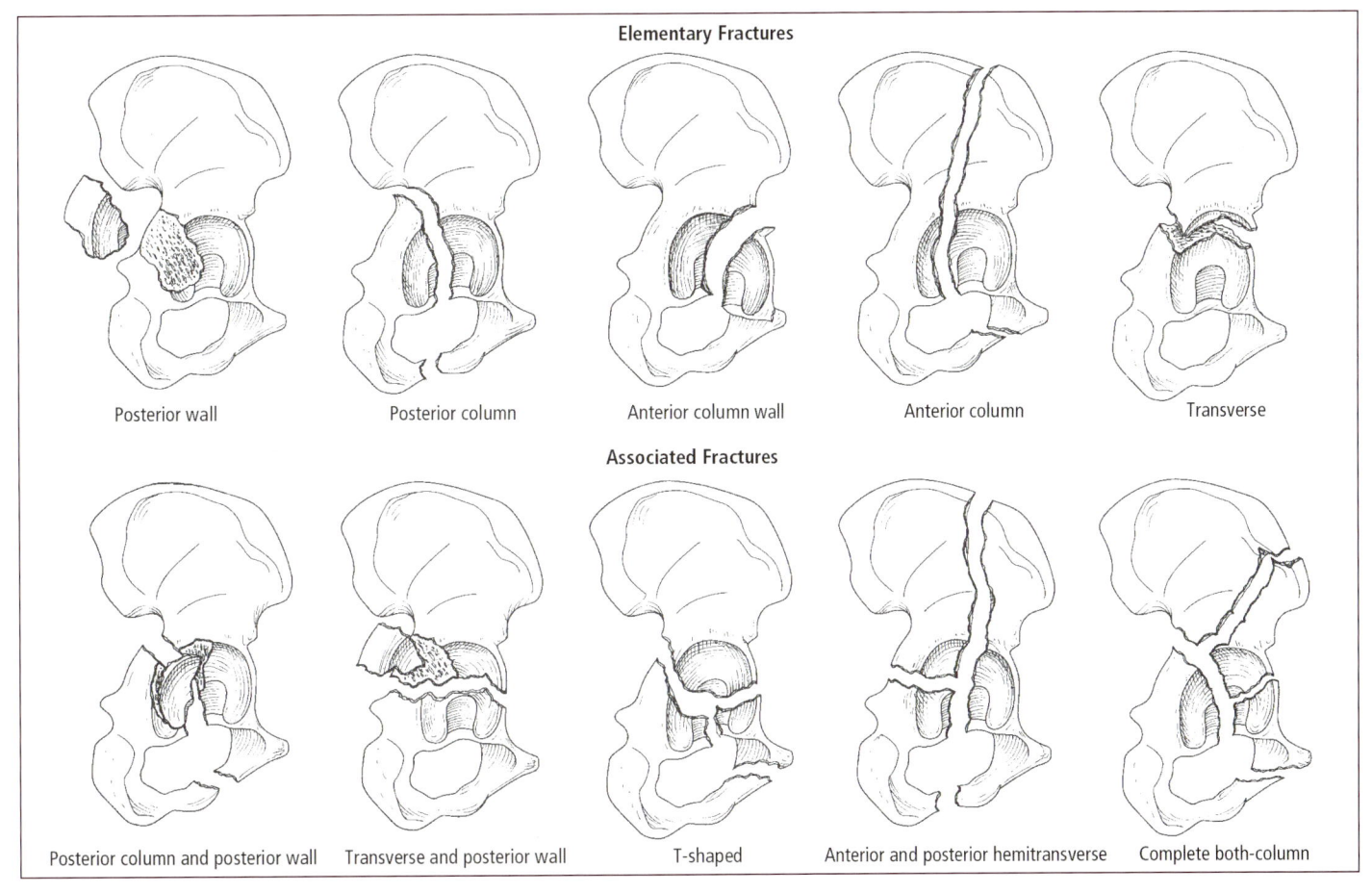

Figure 1 The Letournel classification of acetabular fractures.

Dr. Webb or an immediate family member is a member of a speakers' bureau or has made paid presentations on behalf of the Musculoskeletal Transplant Foundation; serves as a paid consultant to or is an employee of Zimmer; has received nonincome support (such as equipment or services), commercially derived honoraria, or other non–research-related funding (such as paid travel) from Synthes, Smith & Nephew, Stryker, Kinetic Concepts, and Doctors Group; and serves as a board member, owner, officer, or committee member of the Orthopaedic Trauma Association and the Southeastern Fracture Consortium Foundation.

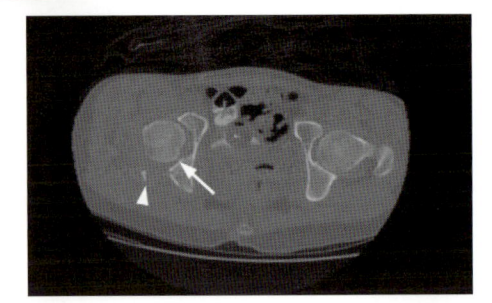

Figure 2 Axial CT scan of the pelvis clearly shows a marginal impaction fracture (arrow). The arrowhead indicates the edge of the posterior wall fragment.

the cases.[4,6] Also, as the femoral head displaces posteriorly, it may impact the edge of the fractured acetabular articular surface, resulting in a marginal impaction fracture. This accompanying fracture occurs in 27% to 46% of posterior wall fractures.[4,6] Other potential associated injuries include fracture of the femoral head, femoral neck, and femoral shaft as well as ligamentous injury to the knee.

Preoperative Imaging

In patients who present with multiple injuries, careful scrutiny of the initial pelvic radiograph will usually show the fracture. The fracture can be clearly seen and classified on Judet oblique views, particularly the obturator oblique view. CT helps in assessing the femoral head, the size and extent of segmentation or comminution of the posterior wall fragment(s), the size and location of intra-articular fragments, and associated marginal impaction fractures (**Figure 2**).

Procedure
Equipment/Implants

The following instruments are commonly used in the open reduction and internal fixation (ORIF) of posterior wall acetabular fractures:
- A self-retaining Charnley retractor
- Schanz pins (5.0-mm), hand chuck, small femoral distractor
- Sciatic nerve retractor, cobra retractor, Taylor retractor
- Adhesive plastic strips to temporarily hold retractors
- Standard and pituitary rongeurs (helpful in extracting joint fragments and debris)
- Cancellous bone allograft or bone graft substitute (to address marginal impaction)
- A ball-spike pusher
- 1.5- and 2.0-mm Kirschner wires (K-wires)
- Spring plates
- 3.5-mm reconstruction plates with corresponding aluminum templates and plate benders
- C-arm (preferably situated on the side of the table opposite the surgeon)

Early Management of Dislocation

Reduction of a hip dislocation in a timely fashion is important for pain relief as well as femoral head blood flow considerations. Protracted time (longer than 12 hours) with the hip dislocated is thought to have a deleterious effect on femoral head blood supply.[6-9] The reduction can be accomplished with conscious sedation in the emergency department or trauma bay or, if need be, with a general anesthetic with muscle relaxation in the operating room. Once the joint is reduced and this is verified on radiographs, the surgeon may choose to maintain the knee in extension with a splint (knee immobilizer).[10] For reductions that are unstable with large displaced fragments or those with intra-articular fragments, distal femoral skeletal pin traction should be used. In these instances, traction protects the head of the femur from the pressure of a fracture edge or an incarcerated intra-articular fragment that might otherwise focus localized heightened stress on the articular cartilage of the femoral head and corresponding acetabular surface.

Preoperative Planning and Patient Positioning

The nature of the posterior wall fragments, including their displacement, can be ascertained by study of the CT scan. This morphology can vary significantly.

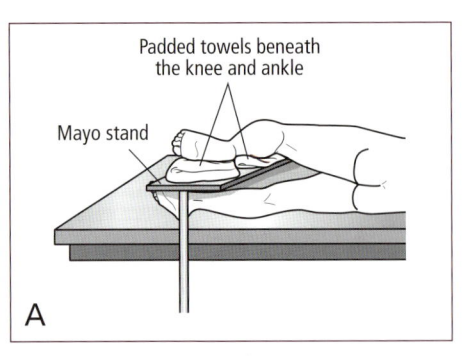

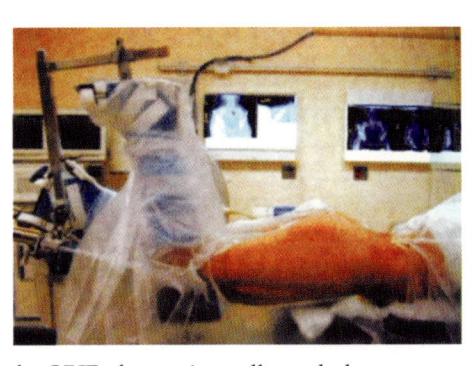

Figure 3 Illustrations show patient positioning for ORIF of posterior wall acetabular fractures. **A,** The lateral decubitus position. A Mayo stand, upon which the padded knee and leg rest, can be adjusted to effect hip adduction/abduction. Varying the height of a soft bump placed beneath the foot/ankle with the knee flexed is used to effect rotation. **B,** The prone position. Skeletal traction through a transfixing pin in the distal femur is used. The knee is maintained in the flexed position as shown. The unaffected leg is kept in extension. The patient's thighs and the peroneal post are appropriately padded. (Panel B reproduced with permission from Siegel J, Templeman DC: Open reduction and internal fixation of the posterior wall of the acetabulum, in Tornetta P III, Williams GR, Ramsey ML, Hunt TR III, Wiesel SW, eds: *Operative Techniques in Orthopaedic Trauma Surgery*. Philadelphia, PA, Lippincott Williams & Wilkins, 2011, p 315-325.)

The Kocher-Langenbeck approach is used. For this approach, the patient is placed in either the lateral decubitus position or the prone position. In either case, the knee is maintained in the flexed position to relax the sciatic nerve (**Figure 3**).

With the patient in the lateral decubitus position, neutral adduction/abduction can be facilitated by placing a padded Mayo stand beneath the flexed knee (**Figure 3, A**). Internal and external hip rotation can be achieved by raising or lowering the padded ankle and foot (while the knee is flexed and the skin is protected) using folded towels on a Mayo stand.

With the patient in the prone position, the use of a fracture table with maintenance of skeletal traction through a distal femoral transfixing pin is recommended, with the knee flexed to 80° using a fracture table boot over an appropriately padded foot and ankle (**Figure 3, B**). The radiopacity of gel rolls is a potential problem for C-arm imaging, so folded sheets should be used instead.[11] Care should be taken to appropriately pad the peroneal post on the fracture table to minimize the likelihood of a pudendal nerve palsy. The contralateral foot and ankle are padded well and placed in a fracture table boot with the knee extended. Both thighs are appropriately padded.

Surgical Technique
Exposure

As shown in the video, the incision calls for an obliquely directed limb in the line between the posterior superior iliac spine and the tip of the greater trochanter. The cephalad extent of the incision depends

Video 60.2 Fractures of the Pelvis and Acetabulum: Kocher-Langenbeck Approach. Emile Letournel, MD; Joel M. Matta, MD (20 min)

on the extent of posterior column exposure needed (as well as the patient's body morphotype). The incision is continued inferiorly at an angle of approximately 45°, proceeding axially over the lateral upper femur to the level of the gluteal crease, which corresponds to the level of insertion of the gluteus maximus tendon into the femur. The incision is deepened to the level of the fascia lata, which is incised in the line of the skin incision. This incision is continued cephalad, parallel to and between the in-line gluteus maximus fibers. The fibers are divided to the level just short of the neurovascular bundle, which thereby divides the fibers for the lower half of the muscle. At the inferior portion of the incision, a tenotomy of the femoral insertion of the gluteus maximus tendon is performed, approximately 1 cm from its insertion into the femur. This helps to allow the muscle to fall away from the posterior column and facilitates retraction and better visualization of the bony anatomy. The piriformis tendon and the obturator internus tendon and its associated gemelli muscles are identified, tagged with suture, and tenotomized approximately 1 cm from their insertion. The obturator internus tendon can be readily followed with the gloved finger to the lesser sciatic notch. The sciatic nerve can be identified on the side of the obturator internus away from the hip joint and traced from the upper border of the quadratus femoris to its point of issuance from the greater sciatic notch. The obturator internus tendon and the sciatic nerve behind it are retracted, enabling easy access to the lesser sciatic notch for placement of a retractor and visualization of the lower part of the posterior column. (I prefer to use a straight cobra retractor.) A sciatic nerve retractor is sometimes used in the greater notch at this point to facilitate the exposure of the cephalad aspect of the posterior column. Removal of a variable portion of gluteus minimus origin from the area cephaloposterior to the acetabulum helps to expose the upper portion of the posterior column and thwart the development of significant heterotopic bone postoperatively.[12] The lower part of the gluteus medius origin can then be elevated from the bone and retracted with a Taylor retractor. The posterior wall fragment(s) can be clearly visualized; tagging sutures are useful to enable direct visualization of the joint while hinging the fragment(s) on their capsular attachments. A Schanz pin can be placed in the trochanteric portion of the femur to facilitate traction on the femoral head and direct visualization of the joint space. Occasionally, this is better accomplished by means of a femoral distractor, which calls for placement of a second Schanz pin parallel to the first in the supra-acetabular position (**Figure 4**).

Figures 5 through **7** show cases that demonstrate various types of posterior wall fractures and the type of fixation used.

Intra-articular Fragments

Once distracted, the joint is carefully lavaged and all incarcerated chondro-osseous fragments are removed. Occasionally, an infolded posterior wall fragment critical to the anatomic reconstruction is delivered this way, as shown in **Figure 5, A**.

Marginal Impaction

If marginal impaction exists (**Figures 8** through **10**), it can be readily assessed. It should be addressed at this time, by hinged elevation with an osteotome, allowing the acetabular surface of the depressed fragment to congruently meet the reduced femoral head (**Figure 8, C** and **D**). The resulting void can be filled with either cancellous allograft or bone graft substitute. The posterior wall fragments are then meticulously fit back into their fracture bed anatomically, with care taken to maintain their capsular hinge, from which the blood supply is derived.

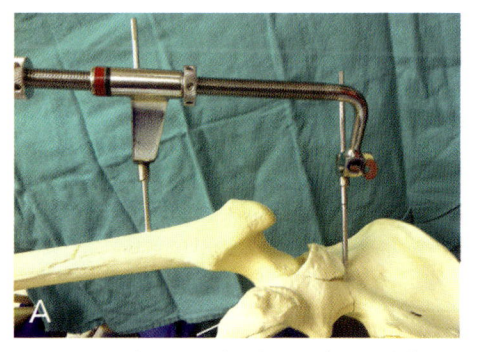

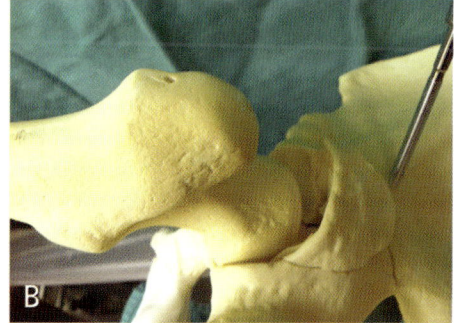

Figure 4 Photographs show a femoral distractor on a bone model of the hip. One pin is placed in the supra-acetabular ilium and one in the lateral proximal femur to effect traction (**A**) and enable direct visualization of the joint space (**B**).

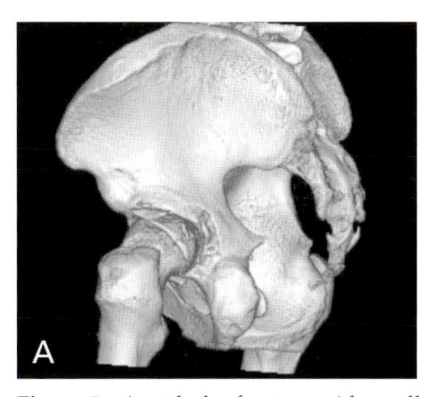

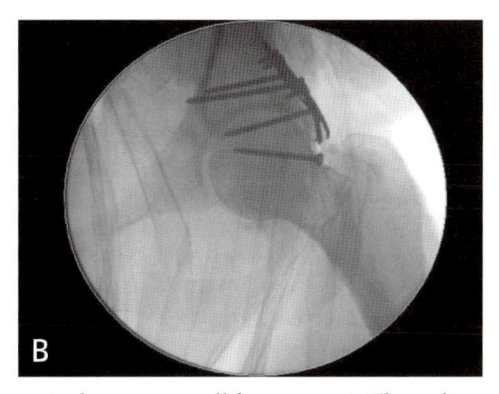

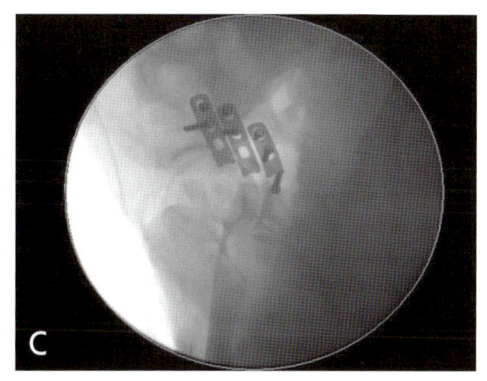

Figure 5 Acetabular fracture with small marginal posterior wall fragments. **A,** Three-dimensional CT reconstruction shows the fracture. During surgery, the joint space was cleared of infolded debris, and three of the marginal pieces were large enough to anatomically reduce using a dental pick and narrow Kirschner-wire provisional fixation. Fixation was provided by three spring (Zuelzer) plates, as shown on the obturator oblique (**B**) and iliac oblique (**C**) fluoroscopic views.

Section 5: Trauma

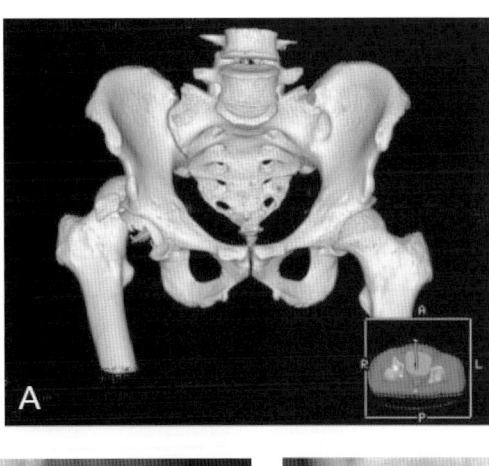

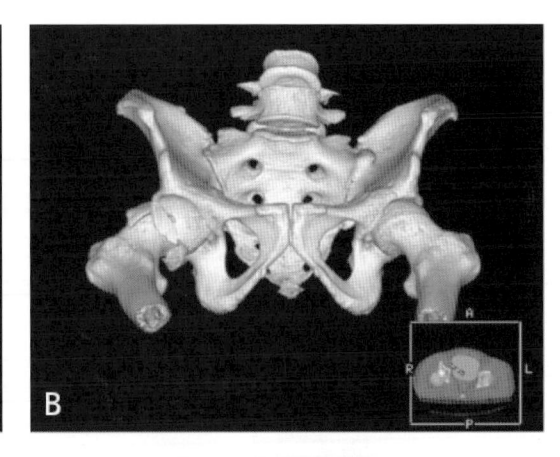

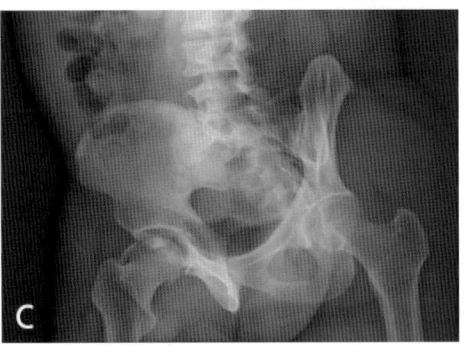

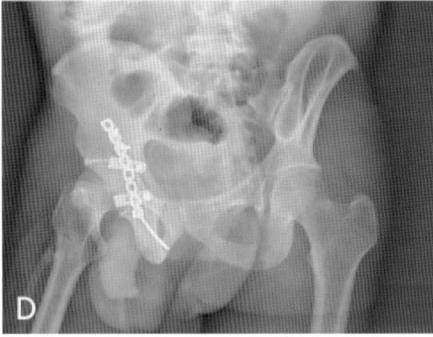

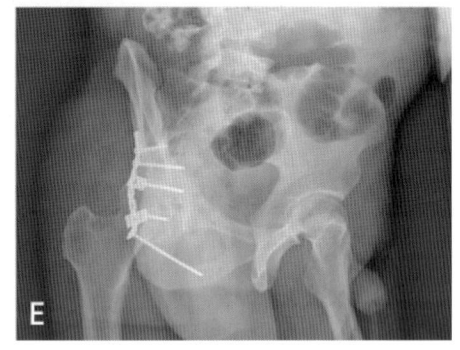

Figure 6 Posterior wall acetabular fracture in a multiply injured patient. **A** and **B**, Three-dimensional CT reconstructions obtained before reduction reveal a multifragmentary fracture. As seen on **B**, one of the fragments is nondisplaced but is situated in a position that makes it likely to fracture on reduction. This is exactly what occurred. **C**, Fluoroscopic image shows temporary femoral traction to distract the joint to take the stress off the articular cartilage of the femoral head as well as the acetabulum imposed by the incarcerated fragment. Iliac oblique (**D**) and obturator oblique (**E**) projections obtained after reduction show fixation with two spring (Zuelzer) plates and a spanning buttressing reconstruction plate.

Provisional Fixation

Provisional fixation of the reduced fragment/fractures is provided by the strategic placement of appropriately sized K-wire(s). These should be located in such a way as to avoid interference with definitive implant placement (**Figure 9, C**).

Implant Selection

Selection of an appropriate implant is dictated by the fracture pattern. Spring or Zuelzer[13] plates, either fashioned from one-third tubular plates[11] or available as implants, work well with small fragments near the edge of the acetabulum (**Figures 5 and 6**). Larger fragments may be amenable to interfragmentary screws and/or buttress plates (**Figure 7**). The fixation montage construct is dictated by the fracture pattern and the quality of the bone. A C-arm should be readily available during the case to check the reduction and implant placement in appropriate projections. The principles of anatomic reduction and secure fixation must be adhered to for a good outcome to be achieved in this major weight-bearing joint.

Wound Management

Once anatomic reduction and secure fixation have been obtained, the wound

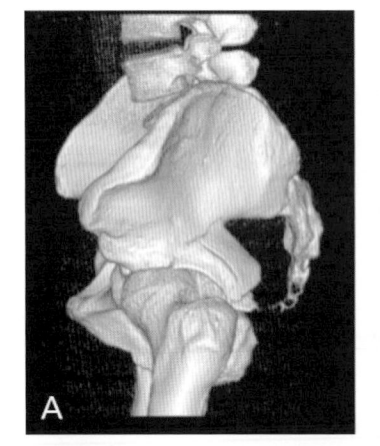

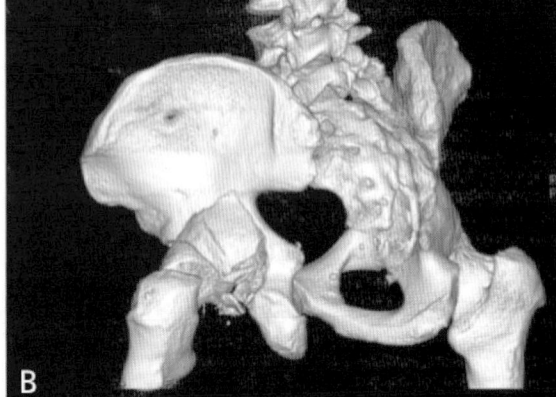

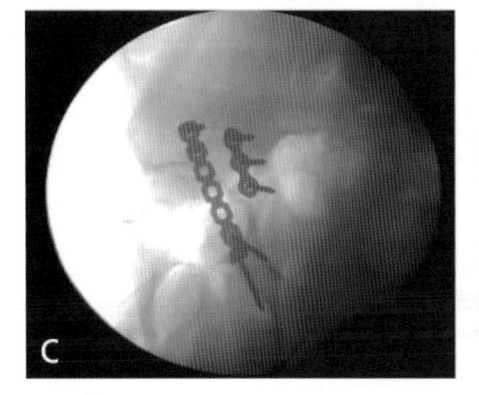

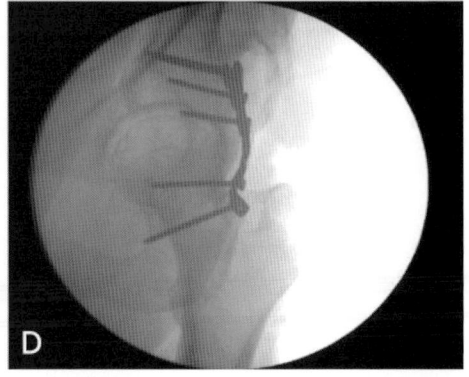

Figure 7 Posterior wall acetabular fracture with a large fragment and an incomplete secondary fracture line. Lateral (**A**) and iliac oblique (**B**) three-dimensional CT reconstructions show the fracture. The fragment was reduced and fixed with two buttressing reconstruction plates, as shown on iliac oblique (**C**) and obturator oblique (**D**) fluoroscopic images.

388   © 2013 American Academy of Orthopaedic Surgeons

Chapter 60: Open Reduction and Internal Fixation of Posterior Wall Acetabular Fractures

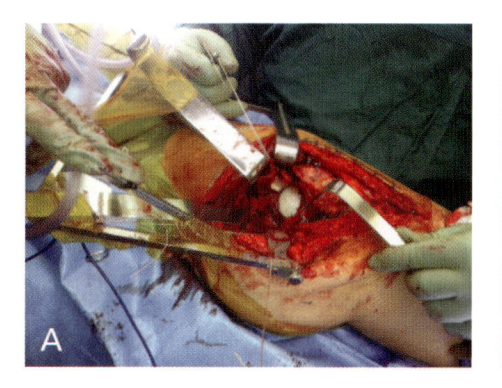

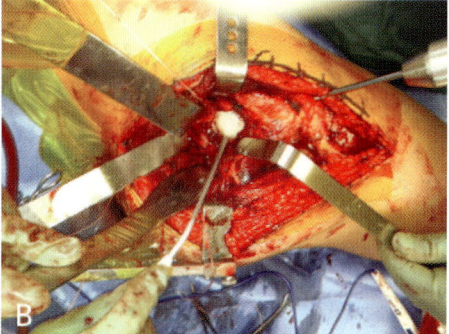

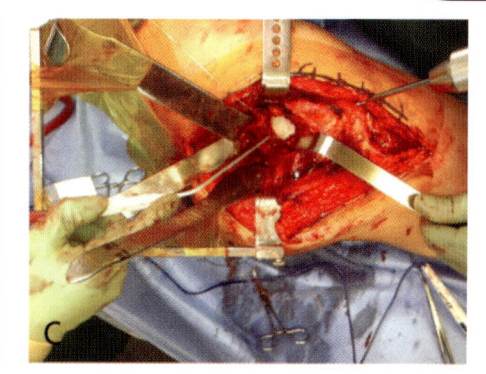

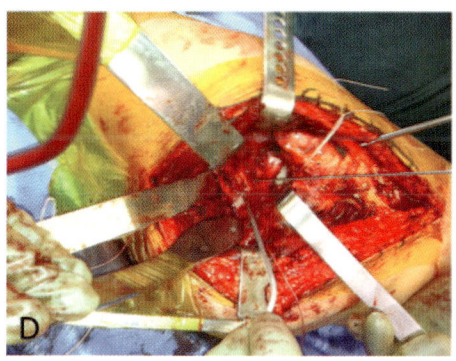

Figure 8 Intraoperative photographs show reduction and fixation of a posterior wall acetabular fracture with marginal impaction. **A,** The joint space is clearly visualized, with the major posterior wall fragment hinged on its intact capsule. **B,** Two small marginally impacted fragments are elevated from the fracture margin and positioned with their joint surfaces congruent with the femoral head. The more inferior fragment is seen here, supported by the terminal end of the small suction. **C,** The more cephalad fragment is seen here, supported by the terminal end of the small suction. **D,** Once the articular surface contact is concentrically restored and supported with allograft or synthetic bone, the main posterior wall fragments are reduced and provisionally fixed.

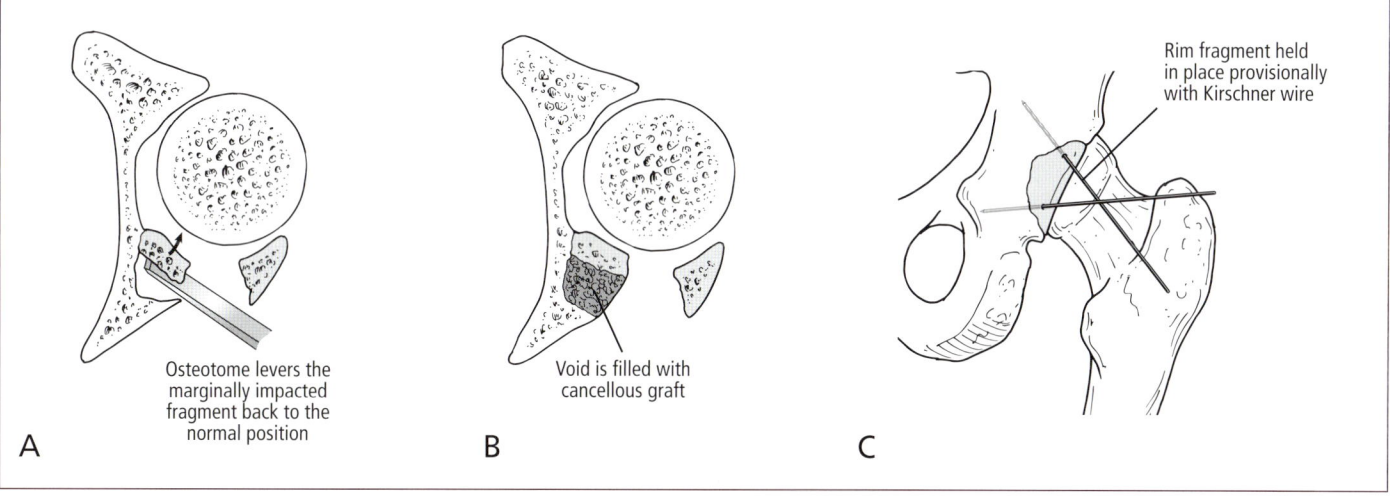

Figure 9 Illustrations show steps of reduction and provisional fixation of a posterior wall acetabular fracture with marginal impaction. **A,** Cross-sectional view illustrates the elevation of the marginal impacted fragment. **B,** Placement of bone graft. **C,** Provisional fixation with Kirschner wires of the overlying and now reduced posterior wall fragment.

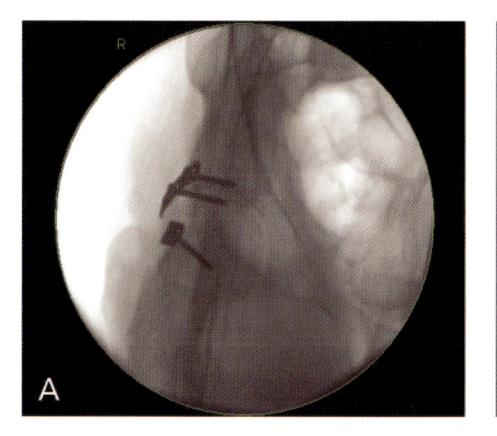

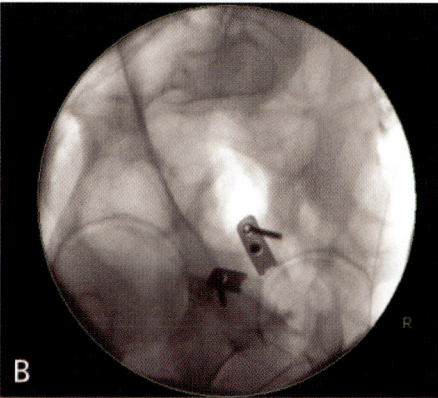

Figure 10 Obturator oblique (**A**) and iliac oblique (**B**) fluoroscopic views obtained intraoperatively are used to check the definitively fixed fragment and joint reduction.

is débrided and thoroughly lavaged. The sciatic nerve should be visualized and its integrity assessed. The piriformis and obturator internus tendon are reattached to their insertion points, and a layered closure is accomplished over a medium suction drain. I often use an incisional vacuum closure system as a dressing with xeroform as an intermediary between skin and sponge, with the pressure set at −50 mm Hg. This serves as a dynamic closed surgical dressing and is particularly helpful when the patient is obese, is returning to an intensive care unit, or has neighboring potentially draining wounds, a colostomy, or poorly controlled or uncontrolled bowel.[14-16] The vacuum closure system is placed in the sterile environment of the operating room and remains as a closed system until the wound has been dry for 24 to 36 hours, as judged by absence of fluid in the tube. When that occurs, the system is removed and replaced with a simple dressing.

Complications

Although the posterior wall fracture is considered an elementary fracture in Letournel's classification system, the surgical management of these injuries is often not so simple. Surgical complications can be significant and include infection (3%); venous thrombosis (7%); heterotopic ossification (37%); nerve injury, particularly the peroneal division of the sciatic nerve (10%); osteonecrosis of the femoral head (7%); and hip arthrosis (10% to 33%).[4,6,17,18]

The definitive surgical management of these fractures is best performed by a surgeon who is familiar with the surgical anatomy and skilled with the requisite reduction and fixation techniques. The early management of a posterior wall acetabular fracture by reduction of an associated dislocation and the institution of measures to maintain that reduction until the time of definitive surgery (including, if necessary, the use of skeletal traction) should be expeditiously performed by an orthopaedic surgeon on the hospital call panel.

In three small series of cases reported before 2002, posterior wall fractures were associated with an unsatisfactory outcome in approximately 30% of cases.[18-20] Tannast et al[21] recently reported on 2- to 20-year survivorship (measured by no need for total hip arthroplasty or an arthrodesis) of 107 surgically treated acetabular fractures with isolated posterior wall involvement. The survivorship for this group at 2 years was 88%, and at 20 years it was 76%. The median time to failure was 1.2 years.

Postoperative Care and Rehabilitation

Unless contraindicated, patients are usually started on an anticoagulant such as enoxaparin 40 mg subcutaneously daily. Thromboembolic stockings are applied. No consensus exists on the duration of antithrombotic pharmacologic prophylaxis, but I maintain it for 2 weeks postoperatively. I follow this with a combination of continued use of thromboembolic stockings and 81 mg aspirin daily until the patient has progressed to independent, aid-free, full–weight-bearing ambulation. A knee immobilizer is maintained for 3 weeks to safeguard hip flexion and thereby minimize loading of the posterior acetabulum.[10] Weight bearing is restricted to "weight of leg" for 12 weeks, at which time the patient is transitioned to full weight bearing.

Pearls

- Timely reduction of an associated posterior dislocation should occur with appropriate conscious sedation in the emergency department or with appropriate anesthesia and muscle relaxation in the operating room.
- Following reduction, Judet oblique views should be obtained and scrutinized. If there are loose fragments in the joint that widen the joint space in the weight-bearing areas, skeletal traction sufficient to distract the joint slightly is useful in alleviating the pressure on the articular cartilage. Traction should also be established in unstable reductions or when there is a question about stability.
- Regardless of whether the patient is in the prone or lateral position, the knee should be kept flexed (≥45°) during surgery to relax the sciatic nerve.
- The obturator internus and piriformis tendons should be tenotomized approximately 1 cm from their insertion and tagged to facilitate retraction and later repair.
- Tracing the acetabular portion of the retracted obturator internus with the surgeon's gloved finger leads to the lesser sciatic notch—often a good spot for seating a cobra-type retractor.
- One-sided adhesive plastic strips can be used to temporarily hold retractors.
- The acetabular rim portion of most posterior wall fracture fragments has a small extended portion of labrum; this is a good location to place a suture for traction on the fragment to enhance visualization of the distracted joint.
- Joint distraction is aided by appropriate muscle relaxation and placement of a 5-mm Schanz pin in the trochanteric portion of the femur. In certain cases, a second supra-acetabular Schanz pin can be placed for the purpose of using a femoral distractor.
- Marginal impaction is often best managed after clearing the joint of loose fragments and debris, reducing the head in the joint, and then levering the impacted fragment(s) to allow the corresponding articular surfaces to congruently "hug" each other while the void is back-filled with bone graft. I use cancellous bone allograft, but I have also used a quick-setting bone substitute, and I found both to be satisfactory. The final step in stabilization is to lock in this montage construct by perfectly reducing and appropriately fixing the rim fragment.
- The traumatized portion of the gluteus minimus should be resected to prevent heterotopic ossification.

References

1. Letournel E: Acetabulum fractures: Classification and management. *Clin Orthop Relat Res* 1980;151:81-106.
2. Judet R, Judet J, Letournel E: Fractures of the acetabulum: Classification and surgical approaches for open reduction. Preliminary report. *J Bone Joint Surg Am* 1964;46:1615-1646.
3. Laird A, Keating JF: Acetabular fractures: A 16-year prospective epidemiological study. *J Bone Joint Surg Br* 2005;87(7): 969-973.
4. Letournel E, Judet R: Posterior wall fractures, in *Fractures of the Acetabulum*, ed 2. Berlin, Germany, Springer Verlag, 1993, pp 67-85.
5. Committee on Trauma, American College of Surgeons: *ATLS Advanced Trauma Life Support for Doctors*, ed 8. Chicago, IL, American College of Surgeons, 2008.
6. Moed BR, WillsonCarr SE, Watson JT: Results of operative treatment of fractures of the posterior wall of the acetabulum. *J Bone Joint Surg Am* 2002;84(5):752-758.
7. Sahin V, Karakaş ES, Aksu S, Atlihan D, Turk CY, Halici M: Traumatic dislocation and fracture-dislocation of the hip: A long-term follow-up study. *J Trauma* 2003;54(3):520-529.
8. Brav EA: Traumatic dislocation of the hip: Army experience and results over a twelve year period. *J Bone Joint Surg Am* 1962;44:1115-1134.
9. Yang RS, Tsuang YH, Hang YS, Liu TK: Traumatic dislocation of the hip. *Clin Orthop Relat Res* 1991;265:218-227.
10. Alexander RD, Grimm L, Vrahas MS: The effect of knee immobilization on degree of hip flexion: A clinical correlation with posterior wall acetabular fractures. *Am J Orthop (Belle Mead NJ)* 1997;26(5):345-347.
11. Roberts ZV, Routt ML: Acetabular fractures, in Gardner MJ, Henley MB, eds: *Harborview Illustrated Tips and Tricks in Fracture Surgery*. Baltimore, MD, Lippincott Williams & Wilkins, 2011, pp 146-165.
12. Rath EM, Russell GV Jr, Washington WJ, Routt ML Jr: Gluteus minimus necrotic muscle debridement diminishes hetero-

topic ossification after acetabular fracture fixation. *Injury* 2002;33(9):751-756.
13. Zuelzer WA: An indirect method of fixation of small fractured fragments with the help of a hook-plate: A preliminary report. *Med Bull U S Army Eur Command Med Div* 1948;5(3):16-20.
14. Reddix RN Jr, Leng XI, Woodall J, Jackson B, Dedmond B, Webb LX: The effect of incisional negative pressure therapy on wound complications after acetabular fracture surgery. *J Surg Orthop Adv* 2010;19(2):91-97.
15. Reddix RN Jr, Tyler HK, Kulp B, Webb LX: Incisional vacuum-assisted wound closure in morbidly obese patients undergoing acetabular fracture surgery. *Am J Orthop (Belle Mead NJ)* 2009;38(9):446-449.
16. Stannard JP, Volgas DA, McGwin G III, et al: Incisional negative pressure wound therapy after high-risk lower extremity fractures. *J Orthop Trauma* 2012;26(1):37-42.
17. Pantazopoulos T, Nicolopoulos CS, Babis GC, Theodoropoulos T: Surgical treatment of acetabular posterior wall fractures. *Injury* 1993;24(5):319-323.
18. Saterbak AM, Marsh JL, Nepola JV, Brandser EA, Turbett T: Clinical failure after posterior wall acetabular fractures: The influence of initial fracture patterns. *J Orthop Trauma* 2000;14(4):230-237.
19. Aho AJ, Isberg UK, Katevuo VK: Acetabular posterior wall fracture: 38 cases followed for 5 years. *Acta Orthop Scand* 1986;57(2):101-105.
20. Chiu FY, Lo WH, Chen TH, Chen CM, Huang CK, Ma HL: Fractures of posterior wall of acetabulum. *Arch Orthop Trauma Surg* 1996;115(5):273-275.
21. Tannast M, Najibi S, Matta JM: Two to twenty-year survivorship of the hip in 810 patients with operatively treated acetabular fractures. *J Bone Joint Surg Am* 2012;94(17):1559-1567.

Video Reference

60.2 Letournel E, Matta JM: Video: *Fractures of the Pelvis and Acetabulum: Kocher-Langenbeck Approach.* Rosemont, IL, American Academy of Orthopaedic Surgeons, 1994.

Chapter 61
Open Reduction and Internal Fixation of Femoral Neck Fractures

Lawrence X. Webb, MD   John C.P. Floyd, MD

Introduction

Femoral neck fractures most frequently occur through low-energy mechanisms (typically falls) in older individuals. Osteoporosis, which is more common in women, is thought to be a major contributor to the high incidence of this fracture in the elderly. This fact and the greater longevity of women account for the 4 to 1 ratio of women to men in the occurrence of femoral neck fractures.[1]

Less commonly, femoral neck fractures occur in younger individuals through a high-energy mechanism. In this setting, accompanying injuries must be suspected, and early management using Advanced Trauma Life Support (ATLS) protocols is appropriate.[2]

Femoral neck fractures may be intracapsular or extracapsular. Extracapsular fractures (basicervical) behave biologically and mechanically like intertrochanteric fractures and usually can be managed with reduction and internal fixation using a fixed-angle device such as a sliding hip screw. This chapter focuses on the management of the intracapsular femoral neck fracture.

It is important to carefully assess the morphology of the fracture. To this end, the classification systems of Garden (**Figure 1**) and Pauwels (**Figure 2**) are relevant.[3,4] The alphanumeric AO/Orthopaedic Trauma Association classification system also is used. This system is quite detailed and is used primarily in the research and publication settings.[5]

Patient Selection

Femoral neck fractures generally are managed surgically because morbidity and mortality are significantly higher with nonsurgical management.[6] Surgical management with anatomic reduction (if the fracture is displaced) and secure fixation or arthroplasty is the best solution for pain control and patient mobilization. Nonsurgical management usually is reserved for patients who are medically extremely frail and in whom surgical intervention is contraindicated. Immobilization sets the stage for deep venous thrombosis, pulmonary emboli, and pneumonia. Pain associated with an unstable fracture presents the need for ongoing narcotic pain medication. Hip immobilization and prolonged patient recumbency make skin breakdown and hip flexion contractures more likely. In otherwise nonsurgical candidates with a nondisplaced or incomplete fracture, a local anesthetic and percutaneous screw fixation may be appropriate.[7] In nonsurgical candidates with displaced fractures, satisfactory relief of acute pain can be challenging. Consultation with a pain control service for regional anesthesia provided by way of an indwelling periarticular catheter may be useful, at least in the acute phase in select patients.[8,9]

Preoperative Imaging

The patient with a femoral neck fracture has pain in the affected hip area and tenderness with motion and axial loading. With a displaced fracture, the lower extremity is shortened and externally rotated. A radiograph obtained while gentle traction is maintained gives a better depiction of the fracture anatomy. This is especially important when the fracture is displaced. When an open reduction and internal fixation is planned and neck comminution or segmentation is present, a CT scan with three-dimensional reconstruction views is helpful. The fracture usually is seen clearly on radiographs. The exceptions are nondisplaced and incomplete fractures. When plain radiographs fail to reveal these fractures in patients with a consistent history and physical findings, MRI is indicated.[10]

Procedure

Instruments/Equipment/Implants

The equipment needed to successfully perform open reduction and internal fixation of femoral neck fractures includes the following: two Gelpi retractors;

Garden type I   Garden type II   Garden type III   Garden type IV

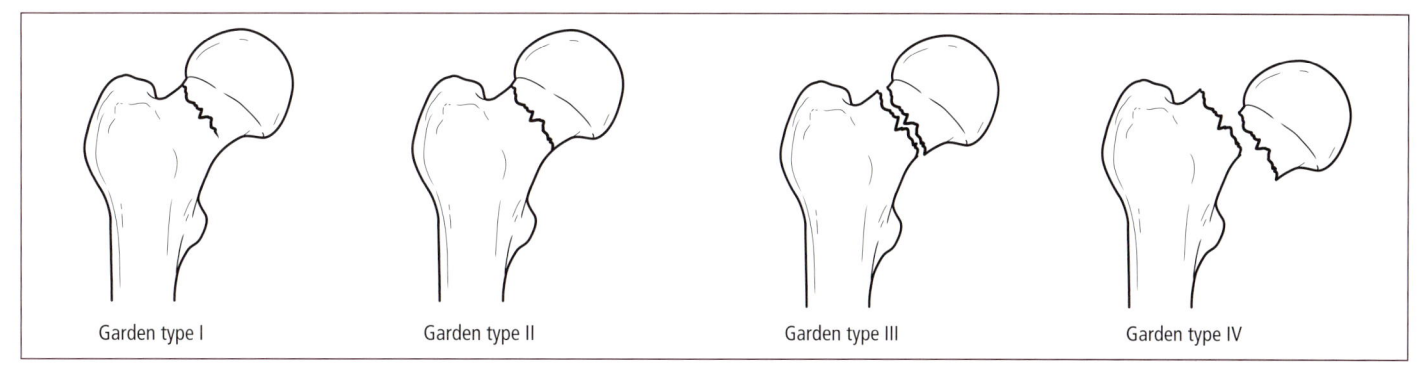

Figure 1 Illustration shows the Garden classification of femoral neck fractures. Garden I: incomplete (most often valgus-impacted). Garden II: complete, nondisplaced. Garden III: complete, incompletely displaced. Garden IV: complete, completely displaced.

Dr. Webb or an immediate family member is a member of a speakers' bureau or has made paid presentations on behalf of the Musculoskeletal Transplant Foundation; serves as a paid consultant to or is an employee of Zimmer; has received nonincome support (such as equipment or services), commercially derived honoraria, or other non–research-related funding (such as paid travel) from Synthes, Smith & Nephew, Stryker, Kinetic Concepts, and Doctors Group; and serves as a board member, owner, officer, or committee member of the Orthopaedic Trauma Association and the Southeastern Fracture Consortium Foundation. Dr. Floyd or an immediate family member is a member of a speakers' bureau or has made paid presentations on behalf of Smith & Nephew; serves as a paid consultant to or is an employee of Synthes; serves as an unpaid consultant to Bongiovi Medical and Health Technology; and has stock or stock options held in Bongiovi Medical and Health Technology.

Section 5: Trauma

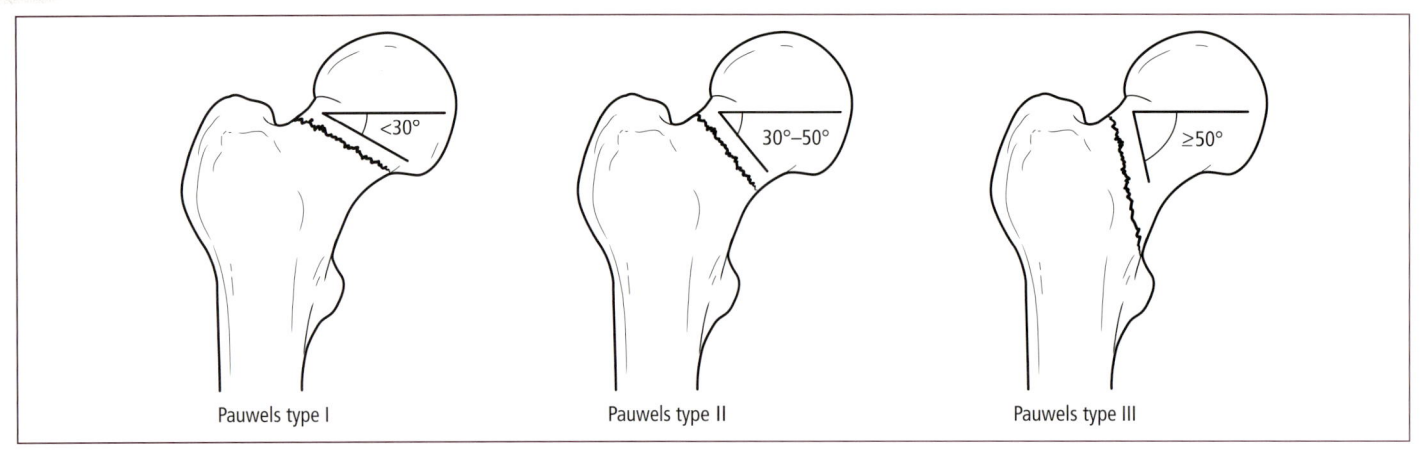

Figure 2 Illustration depicts the Pauwels classification of femoral neck fractures. Type I: The angle subtended by the horizontal and the line of the fracture on an AP radiograph is less than 30°. Type II: The angle subtended by the horizontal and the line of the fracture on an AP radiograph is between 30° and 50°. Type III: The angle subtended by the horizontal and the line of the fracture is greater than or equal to 50°.

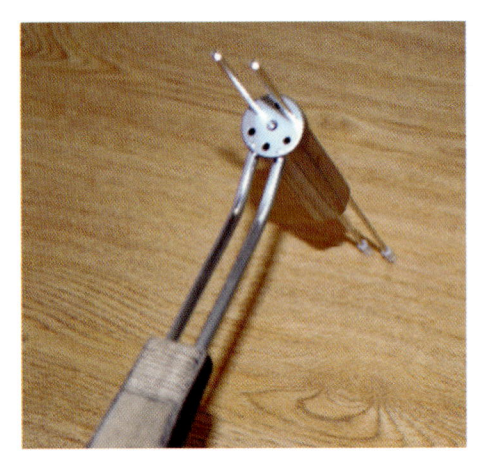

Figure 3 Photograph shows the parallel drill guide for 7.3-mm cannulated screws.

a C-arm; small, medium, and large pointed Weber tenaculum clamps; two Freer elevators; a dental pick; trocar-tipped terminally threaded Schantz pins (2.5 mm for the femoral head fragment and 5.0 mm for the distal trochanteric/femoral shaft fragment); and 2.0-mm Kirschner wires (K-wires). Required implants include 6.5- to 7.3-mm cannulated screws or, for Pauwels type III fractures, a 130° blade plate or its equivalent (eg, a spiral blade and side plate) and a bone graft if a need for grafting is anticipated. A mini-fragment set with 1.5- and 2.0-mm plates also should be in the room and available.

Surgical Technique

Internal fixation is appropriate for young patients (physiologic age <65 years) with an intracapsular femoral neck fracture. For patients with nondisplaced or minimally displaced fractures that are amenable to closed reduction, this is commonly accomplished on a fracture table. For patients with nondisplaced fractures (Garden types I and II) without the need for a reduction, this is commonly accomplished on a radiolucent table or a fracture table. Fixation can be provided by placement of parallel cannulated screws (**Figures 3** through **5**) or a sliding hip screw device, depending on the fracture pattern, bone quality, and surgeon preference. For patients with displaced fractures (Garden types III and IV), fixation is preceded by an open reduction that can be accomplished by a modified anterior (Smith Petersen) approach (**Figure 6**) or an anterolateral (Watson-Jones) approach[11,12] (**Figure 7**).

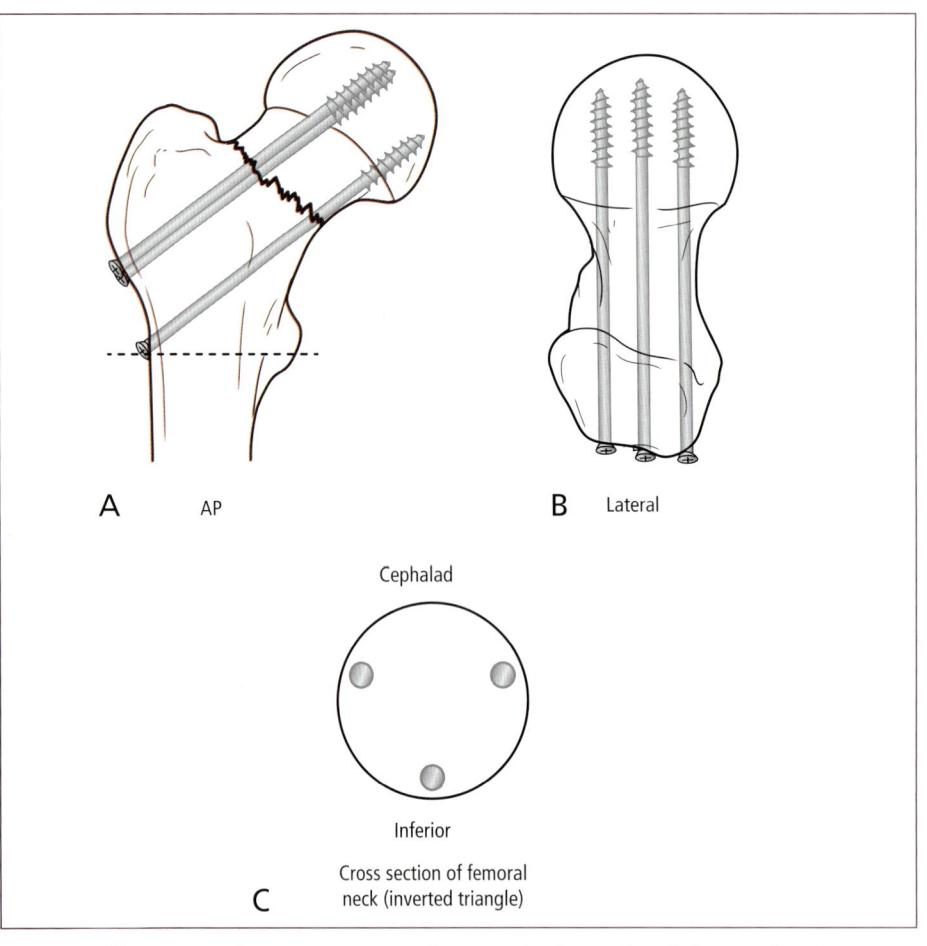

Figure 4 Illustrations show correct screw placement for femoral neck fracture fixation using three screws, which usually is sufficient. The pattern of screw placement is important. **A**, The first screw is directed tangential to and contiguous with the calcar at the level of the fracture on the AP view. Starting screws below the level of the lesser trochanter (dashed line) should be avoided to minimize the likelihood of an iatrogenic subtrochanteric fracture. **B**, On the lateral view, the first screw is seen bisecting the head and neck. **C**, The spread between the screws should be maximized, as shown on the cross-sectional view of the neck.

394 © 2013 American Academy of Orthopaedic Surgeons

Chapter 61: Open Reduction and Internal Fixation of Femoral Neck Fractures

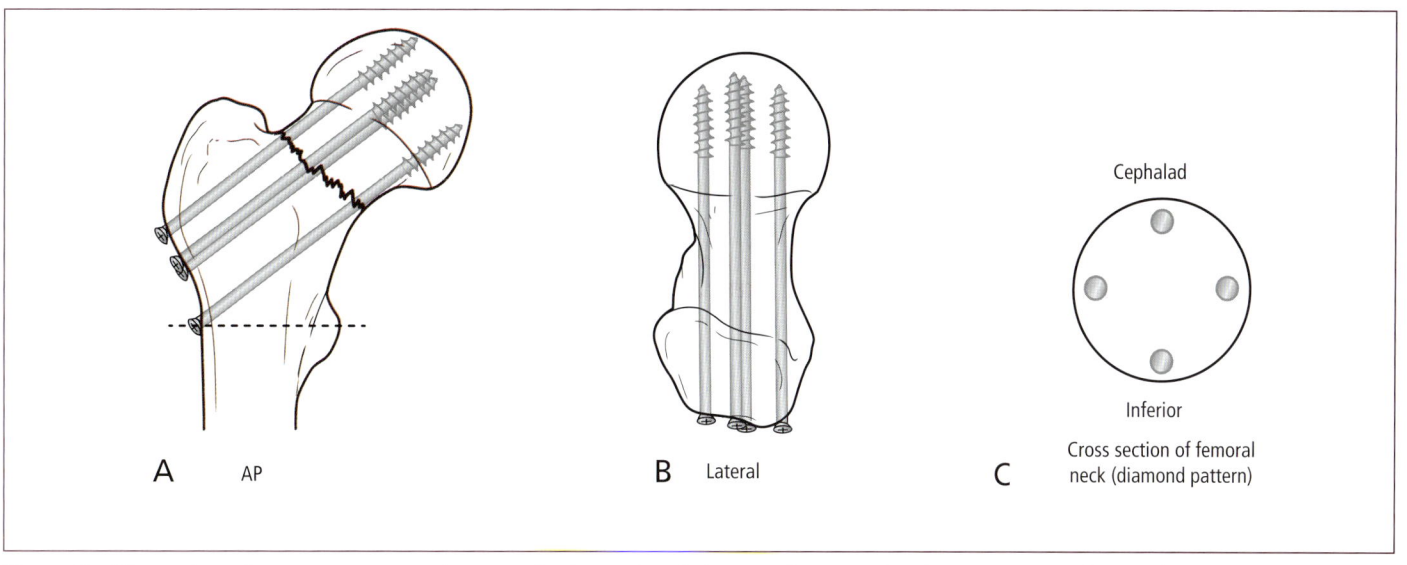

Figure 5 Illustrations show correct screw placement for femoral neck fracture fixation using four screws in a diamond pattern, which some authors recommend when posterior comminution is present. **A,** AP view shows all screws started above the level of the lesser trochanter (dashed line). **B,** Lateral view. **C,** Cross-sectional view of the femoral neck.

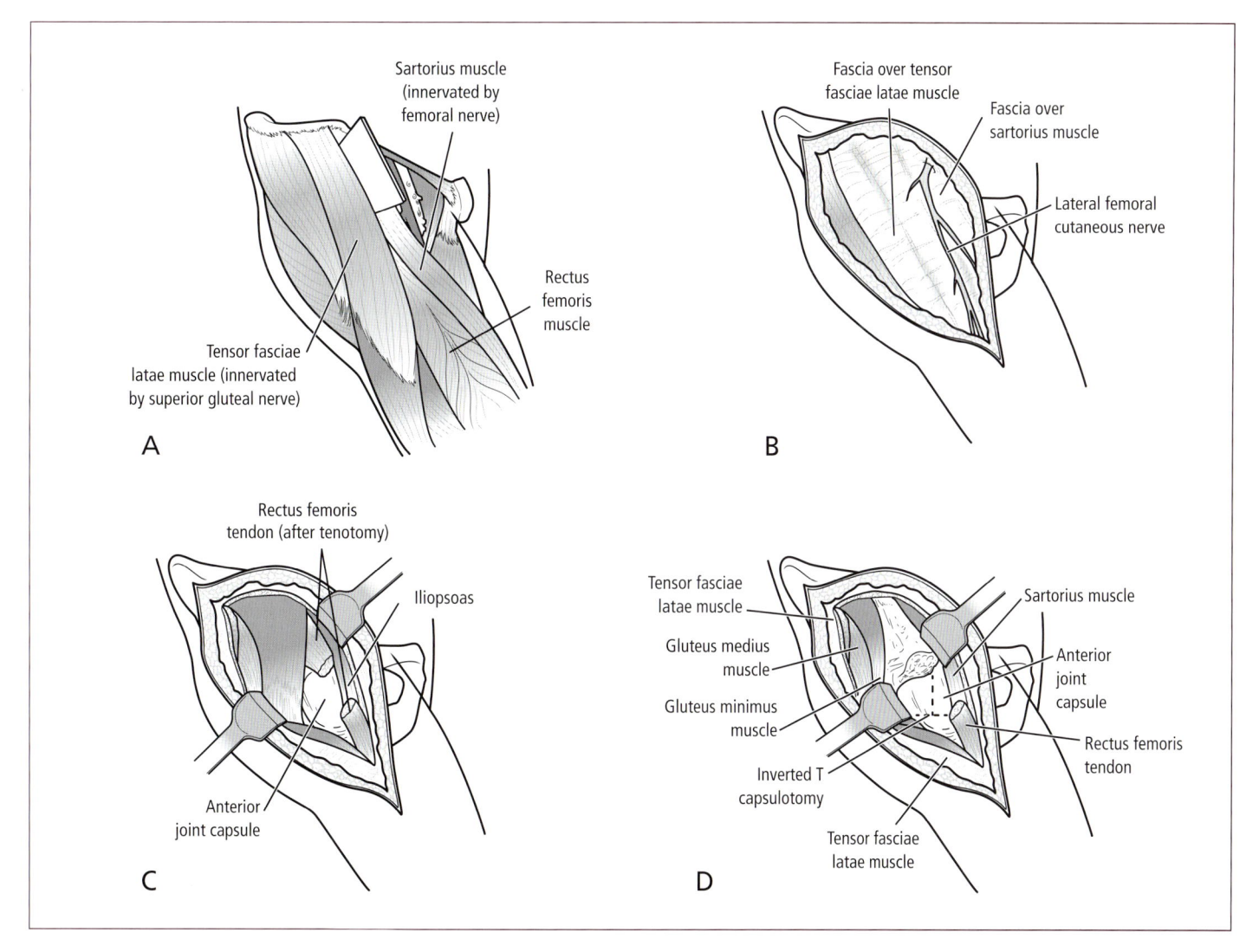

Figure 6 Illustrations demonstrate the modified Smith Petersen approach. **A,** The superficial plane of the approach. The rectus femoris muscle lies in the interval between the sartorius muscle, which is innervated by the femoral nerve, and the tensor fasciae latae muscle, which is innervated by the superior gluteal nerve. **B,** The surgeon must avoid injuring the lateral femoral cutaneous nerve, which pierces the fascia in the line between these muscles. **C,** The rectus femoris can be traced proximally to its tendinous attachment to the anterior inferior iliac spine. A tenotomy should be performed, with enough tendon retained on the anterior inferior iliac spine to allow a good repair at closure. **D,** The tenotomized rectus can be tagged and retracted inferiorly, exposing the underlying pericapsular tissue. An inverted T capsulotomy, with suture tagging and retraction of the capsular leaves, will enable a clear view of the fracture.

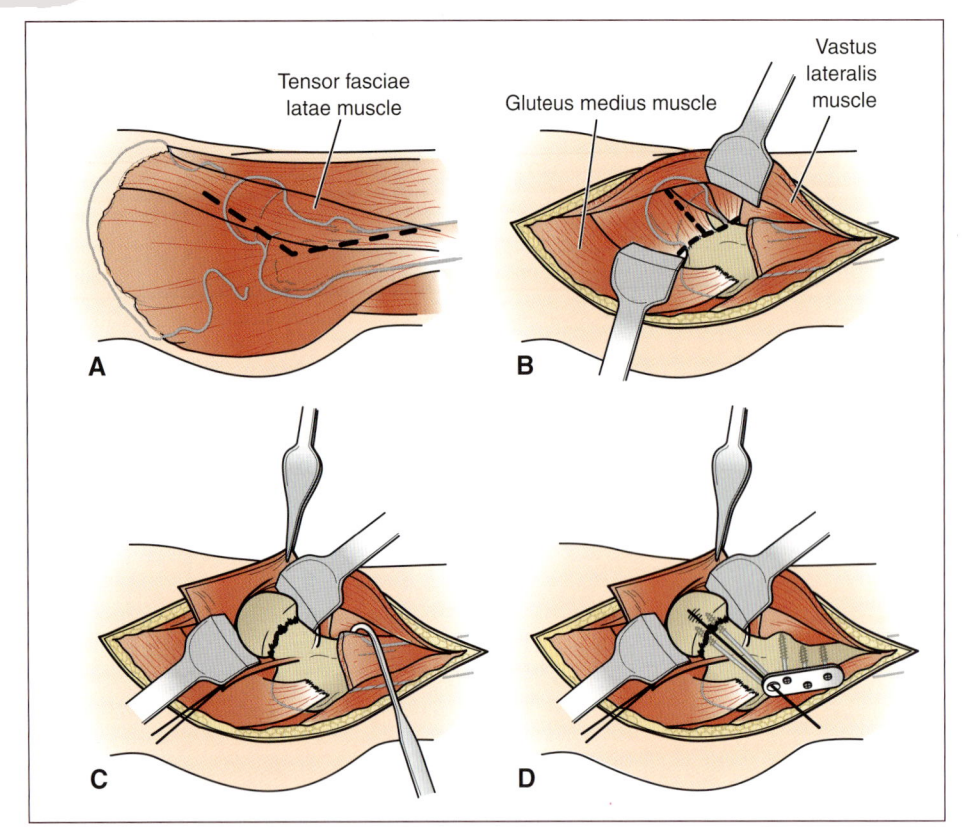

Figure 7 Illustrations demonstrate the anterolateral approach of Watson-Jones. **A,** The skin incision extends from the standard lateral incision over the proximal femoral shaft cephalad to the level of the tip of the greater trochanter and is angled toward the anterior superior iliac spine. The interval between the tensor fasciae latae and the gluteus medius is incised no more proximally than 5 cm cephaloanterior to the greater trochanter to avoid injury to the superior gluteal nerve. This enables exposure of the anterior hip capsule. **B,** An inverted T capsulotomy is performed. **C,** Suture tagging and retraction of the capsular leaves enables direct visualization of the fracture for reduction, and provisional fixation is facilitated. **D,** Definitive fixation can be accomplished through the inferior standard lateral portion of the approach.

Video 61.1 The Modified Smith Petersen Approach for Open Reduction and Internal Fixation of Femoral Neck Fractures. Lawrence X. Webb, MD; John C.P. Floyd, MD (5 min)

The modified Smith Petersen approach (**Figure 6**) can be used for the reduction and provisional fixation of the fractured femoral neck. In this approach, the patient is positioned supine on a radiolucent table with a folded sheet placed beneath the upper buttock on the affected side. This facilitates preparation and draping as well as obtaining a lateral C-arm view of the femoral neck and enables slight hip extension should it be needed in reduction. Following appropriate preparation and draping, the projected line between the anterior superior iliac spine and the lateral edge of the patella is incised caudally for approximately 15 cm, starting from 1 cm distal to the anterior superior iliac spine. The incision is deepened in the interval between the tensor fasciae latae muscle and the sartorius muscle, with care taken to avoid injury to the lateral femoral cutaneous nerve. The rectus femoris muscle lies at the base of the interval. The rectus femoris should be traced proximally to its tendon, which can be tagged with suture and tenotomized from its origin, leaving enough tendon attached to the anterior inferior iliac spine to afford an easy repair at closure. Once the muscle and its reflected head are elevated and retracted, the underlying hip capsule lies exposed and should be opened in an inverted T fashion. It may be helpful to guide the ideal placement of the incision in the capsule by pulling gentle traction through the femur and approximating the reduction. The capsular leaves are tagged with suture, and suitable Hohmann retractors are introduced to enable direct visualization of the fracture.

Once the fracture is visualized directly, the fragments can be manipulated carefully to effect an anatomic reduction under direct visualization. Helpful tools include a Freer elevator and a dental pick, along with saline irrigation to clear the fracture of infolded soft tissue and clotted blood. A stout K-wire or a 4-mm Schanz half pin can serve as a joystick for reducing the head fragment. The distal fragment can be managed with traction on the femoral shaft, appropriate rotation, and adduction/abduction (provided by an assistant). Adequate muscle relaxation provided by anesthesia is helpful here. Provisional fixation can be provided by placing a pointed tenaculum (Weber clamp) or a K-wire across the fracture. The use of a small plate with unicortical screws has been advocated by Molnar and Routt[11] to provide fixation in the setting of comminuted fracture patterns. Once a provisional fixation of the reduced fracture is completed and checked with a C-arm, definitive fixation follows. When the anterior approach is used for the reduction, a separate lateral incision or three small lateral incisions (if cannulated screws are placed percutaneously) are placed in the line of the projected axis of the reduced femoral neck for the definitive fixation. For Pauwels type I and II fractures, three or four parallel cannulated screws directed from the lateral proximal femur into the head will provide good fixation.[13-15] A C-arm and a parallel drill guide (**Figure 3**) are useful in helping to direct the guide pins for the cannulated screws in a manner that best ensures fracture stability (**Figures 4** and **5**).

An alternative to the anterior approach is the anterolateral approach of Watson-Jones, which uses the interval between the tensor fasciae latae muscle and the gluteus medius. The cephalad extent of the approach is limited to 5 cm cephaloanterior to the greater trochanter to avoid injury to the superior gluteal nerve (**Figure 7**). At the base of the interval between the two muscles, the pericapsular fat and underlying anterior hip capsule are exposed. The capsulotomy, followed by open reduction and provisional fixation, should proceed as described for the anterior approach. One advantage of the anterolateral approach is that fixation of the provisionally reduced fracture can be accomplished without the need for a second surgical wound.

For the highly vertical Pauwels type III fracture, parallel screws are not adequate to address the shear stresses imposed by the fracture[16] (**Figure 8**). Other fixation constructs, such as inclusion of nonparallel screws[17] or a 130° angle blade plate,[18]

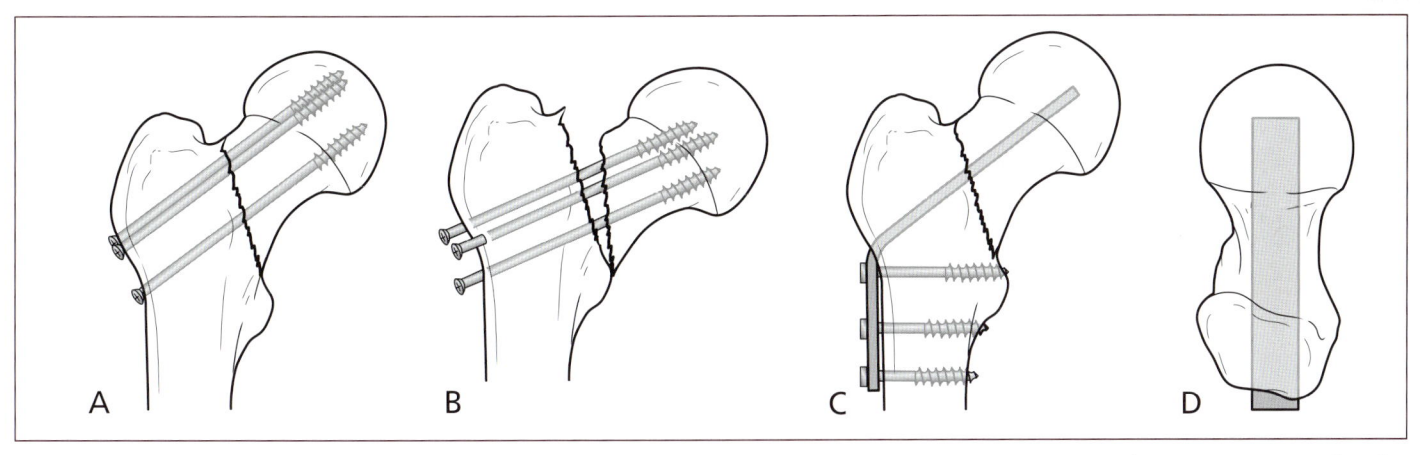

Figure 8 Illustrations demonstrate fixation of the highly vertical Pauwels type III fracture. **A,** A Pauwels type III fracture pattern is reduced and fixed with three parallel screws. **B,** Failure of screw fixation. Because of the poor ability of the fixation construct to negate the shear forces on this highly vertical fracture, it displaces, with offset in the neck and some backout of the screws. One proposed fixation of this fracture pattern that is more stable uses a 130° blade plate for fixation, shown in AP (**C**) and lateral (**D**) projections.

have been recommended for this pattern. In a multicenter study by Liporace et al[19] of 62 Pauwels type III fractures in 61 patients (37 treated with cannulated screw fixation and 25 stabilized with a fixed-angle device), good to excellent reduction was achieved in 59 (95%); however, the authors reported a 19% (7 of 37) nonunion rate for fractures treated with cannulated screw fixation and an 8% (2 of 25) nonunion rate for fractures stabilized with a fixed-angle device. The 11% difference in these rates is not statistically significant. No unanimity currently exists among experts regarding the ideal fixation for this challenging fracture pattern.

Postoperative Care and Rehabilitation

Once stabilized in an anatomic position, the patient can be mobilized with weight-of-leg ambulation, which should be enforced for 12 weeks. Return to weight bearing is contingent on fracture healing, which should be evident both radiographically and clinically, as evidenced by the patient being free from pain with axial stress.

Fracture Fixation in the Older Patient

No firm consensus exists on the management of femoral neck fractures in older (physiologic age >65 years) patients. In patients with incomplete fractures or with a complete fracture that is nondisplaced or valgus impacted, viable options include fixation in situ with parallel cannulated screws, as described previously for younger patients, or with a sliding hip screw device with a small side plate. A randomized prospective trial currently underway in centers in the United States and Canada is designed to address which of these fixation options is optimal (Mohit Bhandari, McMaster University, 2012).

In older patients with displaced fractures, arthroplasty is a good option, particularly when the higher reoperation rates associated with open reduction and internal fixation are considered.[20] The choices include cemented or uncemented hemiarthroplasty, cemented or uncemented bipolar hemiarthroplasty, and cemented or uncemented total hip arthroplasty (THA).

Little difference exists between unipolar hemiarthroplasty and bipolar hemiarthroplasty in the management of displaced femoral neck fractures.[21] THA is useful in patients with preexisting hip arthritis.[22] THA also should be considered for active community ambulators, in whom results of THA have been shown to be superior to cemented hemiarthroplasty, although with a potentially higher dislocation rate.[23] Given the liability of a higher dislocation rate for THA in this setting, an anterolateral surgical approach—such as a modified Hardinge[24] or an anterior approach as advocated by Matta et al[25]—as well as the use of larger diameter femoral heads should be considered.

Video 61.2 The Modified Hardinge Approach for Open Reduction and Internal Fixation of Femoral Neck Fractures. Lawrence X. Webb, MD; John C.P. Floyd, MD (8 min)

Complications

Osteonecrosis and nonunion correlate with initial fracture displacement. In a series of 30 femoral neck fractures in 28 patients managed with osteosynthesis with a minimum 2-year follow-up, Karaeminogullari et al[26] reported osteonecrosis and nonunion rates of 6% and 18%, respectively, in nondisplaced fractures. For displaced fractures, corresponding rates were 23% and 38%. The author found no correlation with time to fixation; rates of osteonecrosis and nonunion were 12.5% and 25%, respectively, in patients who underwent surgery before 12 hours and 14% and 27% in those who underwent surgery later. Nonunion is most often associated with varus neck positioning; a Pauwels valgus intertrochanteric osteotomy has been shown to effect healing in this setting[27-29] (**Figure 9**). Marti et al[27] reported that 6 patients in their series of 37 patients undergoing a detailed review who underwent osteotomy for nonunion had concomitant partial collapse of the femoral head. Only three of these patients required an arthroplasty, at a mean follow-up of 7.1 years.

Treatment options for osteonecrosis with femoral head collapse or precollapse include nonvascularized or vascularized strut grafts, osteotomies, and arthroplasty. The latter is usually the best option for the elderly patient.[30]

The increased incidence of dislocation of the hip following arthroplasty performed in the setting of femoral neck fracture and strategies for avoiding this complication were discussed previously. In addition to dislocation, complications include infection, thrombosis, heterotopic bone formation, loosening of components, wear, thigh pain, and periprosthetic fracture. Surgeons who perform hip arthroplasty should be familiar with the strategies for avoiding these complications as well as their early detection and management.

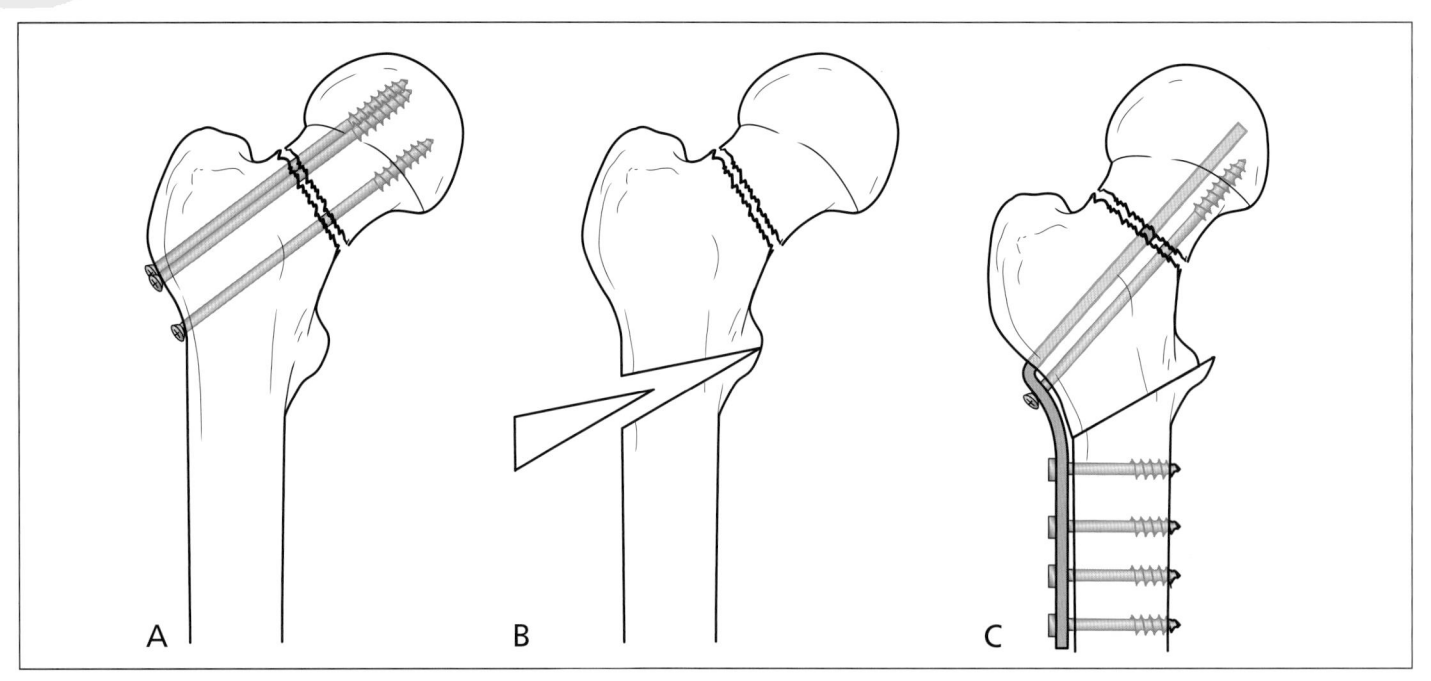

Figure 9 Illustrations demonstrate valgus intertrochanteric osteotomy for nonunion of a femoral neck fracture. The objective of the valgus intertrochanteric osteotomy is to enable the forces directed across the nonunited fracture to be predominantly compressive rather than shearing. **A,** Nonunion of the femoral neck fracture. **B,** The osteotomy. **C,** Lateral closure of the wedge and fixation with a 130° angled osteotomy blade plate.

Pearls

- For displaced fractures in younger patients with good bone in whom open reduction and internal fixation is appropriate, good traction views are necessary to determine the details of the fracture pattern and anticipated steps in reassembly of the bone. In cases of comminution or segmentation, a CT scan with three-dimensional reconstructed images is very helpful.
- Of the two recommended surgical approaches, we find the modified Smith Petersen approach affords better visualization, with ease of reduction and placement of clamps. The drawback is the need for placement of a second incision laterally for cannulated screws or a spiral blade and side plate device or its equivalent. The Watson-Jones incision can be carried inferiorly over the lateral thigh, and these implants can be applied through the lower extended limb of the incision. For a Pauwels type III fracture without comminution or segmentation, we prefer a Watson-Jones approach. For Pauwels type I and II fractures and all displaced femoral neck fractures with segmentation or comminution, a modified Smith Petersen approach and a second lateral incision are preferred.
- Some authors recommend a T capsulotomy, in which the horizontal limb is overlying but not detaching the labrum, or an inverted T capsulotomy. The latter is particularly helpful in visualizing and thereby ensuring the reduction of the inferiormost portion of a Pauwels type III fracture.
- Once the displaced fracture is exposed clearly, the 2.5-mm trocar-tipped, terminally threaded Schanz pin is seated in the femoral head fragment, and the 5.0-mm Schanz pin is seated in the femoral shaft fragment. An appropriate hand chuck is applied to each pin, and, with appropriate muscle relaxation, an anatomic reduction is effected and provisionally fixed, usually with K-wires and/or a Weber clamp. To facilitate this, Evans[31] reports an ingeniously devised Harborview modification of the Weber clamp, created by straightening the tines and applying them through drill holes.

References

1. Schürch MA, Rizzoli R, Mermillod B, Vasey H, Michel JP, Bonjour JP: A prospective study on socioeconomic aspects of fracture of the proximal femur. *J Bone Miner Res* 1996;11(12):1935-1942.
2. American College of Surgeons Committee on Trauma: *ATLS Advanced Trauma Life Support for Doctors,* ed 8. Chicago, IL, American College of Surgeons, 2008, pp 1-18.
3. Garden RS: Malreduction and avascular necrosis in subcapital fractures of the femur. *J Bone Joint Surg Br* 1971;53(2):183-197.
4. Bartoníček J: Pauwels' classification of femoral neck fractures: Correct interpretation of the original. *J Orthop Trauma* 2001;15(5):358-360.
5. Fracture and dislocation compendium: Orthopaedic Trauma Association Committee for Coding and Classification. *J Orthop Trauma* 1996;10(supp 1):v-ix, 1-154.
6. Hansen FF: Conservative vs surgical treatment of impacted subcapital fractures of the femoral neck. *Acta Orthop Scand Suppl* 1994;256:9.
7. Sher D, Biant LC: Subcapital fracture of the femoral neck in medically unwell patients: Technique for fixation using direct infiltration local anaesthetic rather than regional blockade. *Injury* 2007;38(10):1209-1213.
8. Kröll W, List WF: Pain treatment in the ICU: Intravenous, regional or both? *Eur J Anaesthesiol Suppl* 1997;15:49-52.
9. Shabat S, Stern A, Kollender Y, Nyska M: Continuous intra-articular patient-controlled analgesia in a cancer patient with a pathological hip fracture: A case report. *Acta Orthop Belg* 2001;67(3):304-306.
10. Speer KP, Spritzer CE, Harrelson JM, Nunley JA: Magnetic resonance imaging of the femoral head after acute intracap-

sular fracture of the femoral neck. *J Bone Joint Surg Am* 1990;72(1):98-103.

11. Molnar RB, Routt ML Jr: Open reduction of intracapsular hip fractures using a modified Smith-Petersen surgical exposure. *J Orthop Trauma* 2007;21(7):490-494.

12. Baumgaertner M, Higgins T: Femoral neck fractures, in Bucholz R, Heckman J, eds: *Fractures in Adults*, ed 5. Baltimore, MD, Lippincott, 2001, pp 1579-1634.

13. Swiontkowski MF, Harrington RM, Keller TS, Van Patten PK: Torsion and bending analysis of internal fixation techniques for femoral neck fractures: The role of implant design and bone density. *J Orthop Res* 1987;5(3):433-444.

14. Haidukewych GJ: Intracapsular hip fractures, in Stannard JP, Schmidt AH, Kregor PJ, eds: *Surgical Treatment of Orthopaedic Trauma*. New York, NY, Thieme, 2007, pp 539-566.

15. Kauffman JI, Simon JA, Kummer FJ, Pearlman CJ, Zuckerman JD, Koval KJ: Internal fixation of femoral neck fractures with posterior comminution: A biomechanical study. *J Orthop Trauma* 1999;13(3):155-159.

16. Haidukewych GJ, Rothwell WS, Jacofsky DJ, Torchia ME, Berry DJ: Operative treatment of femoral neck fractures in patients between the ages of fifteen and fifty years. *J Bone Joint Surg Am* 2004;86(8):1711-1716.

17. Parker MJ, Porter KM, Eastwood DM, Schembi Wismayer M, Bernard AA: Intracapsular fractures of the neck of femur: Parallel or crossed garden screws? *J Bone Joint Surg Br* 1991;73(5):826-827.

18. Broos PL, Vercruysse R, Fourneau I, Driesen R, Stappaerts KH: Unstable femoral neck fractures in young adults: Treatment with the AO 130-degree blade plate. *J Orthop Trauma* 1998;12(4):235-240.

19. Liporace F, Gaines R, Collinge C, Haidukewych GJ: Results of internal fixation of Pauwels type-3 vertical femoral neck fractures. *J Bone Joint Surg Am* 2008;90(8):1654-1659.

20. Lu-Yao GL, Keller RB, Littenberg B, Wennberg JE: Outcomes after displaced fractures of the femoral neck: A meta-analysis of one hundred and six published reports. *J Bone Joint Surg Am* 1994;76(1):15-25.

21. Ong BC, Maurer SG, Aharonoff GB, Zuckerman JD, Koval KJ: Unipolar versus bipolar hemiarthroplasty: Functional outcome after femoral neck fracture at a minimum of thirty-six months of follow-up. *J Orthop Trauma* 2002;16(5):317-322.

22. Lee BP, Berry DJ, Harmsen WS, Sim FH: Total hip arthroplasty for the treatment of an acute fracture of the femoral neck: Long-term results. *J Bone Joint Surg Am* 1998;80(1):70-75.

23. Keating JF, Grant A, Masson M, Scott NW, Forbes JF: Randomized comparison of reduction and fixation, bipolar hemiarthroplasty, and total hip arthroplasty: Treatment of displaced intracapsular hip fractures in healthy older patients. *J Bone Joint Surg Am* 2006;88(2):249-260.

24. Pai VS: A modified direct lateral approach in total hip arthroplasty. *J Orthop Surg (Hong Kong)* 2002;10(1):35-39.

25. Matta JM, Shahrdar C, Ferguson T: Single-incision anterior approach for total hip arthroplasty on an orthopaedic table. *Clin Orthop Relat Res* 2005;441:115-124.

26. Karaeminogullari O, Demirors H, Atabek M, Tuncay C, Tandogan R, Ozalay M: Avascular necrosis and nonunion after osteosynthesis of femoral neck fractures: Effect of fracture displacement and time to surgery. *Adv Ther* 2004;21(5):335-342.

27. Marti RK, Schüller HM, Raaymakers EL: Intertrochanteric osteotomy for nonunion of the femoral neck. *J Bone Joint Surg Br* 1989;71(5):782-787.

28. Ballmer FT, Ballmer PM, Baumgaertel F, Ganz R, Mast JW: Pauwels osteotomy for nonunions of the femoral neck. *Orthop Clin North Am* 1990;21(4):759-767.

29. Anglen JO: Intertrochanteric osteotomy for failed internal fixation of femoral neck fracture. *Clin Orthop Relat Res* 1997;341:175-182.

30. Franzén H, Nilsson LT, Strömqvist B, Johnsson R, Herrlin K: Secondary total hip replacement after fractures of the femoral neck. *J Bone Joint Surg Br* 1990;72(5):784-787.

31. Evans JM: Femoral neck fractures, in Gardner MJ, Henley MB, eds: *Harborview Illustrated Tips and Tricks in Fracture Surgery*. Philadelphia, PA, Lippincott Williams & Wilkins, 2011, pp 175-183.

Chapter 62
Intertrochanteric Fracture Fixation Using a Sliding Hip Screw or Cephalomedullary Nail

Alexandra K. Schwartz, MD   Christopher L. Sherman, DO, MS

Patient Selection
Approximately 340,000 patients sustain hip fractures in the United States each year. Intertrochanteric fractures are extracapsular hip fractures that occur primarily in elderly patients or patients with osteopenia or osteoporosis.

Indications
Surgical treatment is the standard of care for hip fractures. Nonsurgical treatment may be fraught with complications, including fracture displacement, pain, inability to transfer, decubitus ulcers, pulmonary complications, urinary tract infections, and deep venous thrombosis (DVT). Patients treated nonsurgically require active treatment with early mobilization and particular caution in avoiding the above-mentioned complications. A recent study analyzed a database of all hip fractures from Medicare claims in a 5-year period and found that approximately 6.2% of patients with hip fractures were treated nonsurgically.[1]

Contraindications
Surgery is contradicted primarily in the elderly, demented patient who was nonambulatory before the fracture and who has minimal pain. Rarely, a patient will be unable to undergo surgery because of severe medical comorbidities.

Preoperative Imaging
Good-quality plain radiographs are needed to assess the fracture pattern accurately and thereby make an accurate diagnosis. Failure to identify the fracture completely may lead to use of an inappropriate implant and, ultimately, failure of fixation. Preoperative images should include an AP view of the pelvis and AP and lateral views of the affected hip. A traction/internal rotation AP view of the hip (best obtained with gentle manual traction and 15° of internal rotation applied) is very helpful in delineating the fracture pattern (**Figure 1**).

The AP view of the pelvis is helpful because it demonstrates the native anatomy on the contralateral side, provided the contralateral hip has not sustained a fracture and is free of other pathology. A cross-table lateral is the preferred lateral view and is more comfortable for the patient than a frog-leg lateral. In approximately 2% to 10% of patients with a painful hip due to fracture after trauma, radiographic findings are negative. If the findings are negative but there is a high clinical suspicion for a fracture, further imaging is warranted. In the past, bone scans were commonly used. Bone scans may not show positive results until up to 72 hours postinjury, however, which can lead to a delay in diagnosis and treatment. In addition, a bone scan may not show the anatomic area of fracture, and therefore further imaging may still be required. CT is readily available and is often used. MRI is another alternative, although it is not always immediately available and is more expensive. Lubovsky et al[2] compared CT and MRI for the diagnosis of occult hip fractures. CT led to misdiagnosis in four of the six hips studied. MRI provided complete anatomic characterization of the fracture in the seven hips studied, eliminating the need for repeat or additional imaging. Patients who underwent CT scans and further imaging had a workup time of 56 hours, whereas those with MRI had a time to diagnosis of 32 hours.

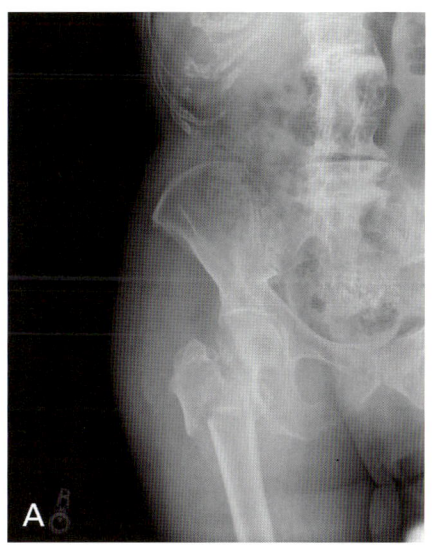

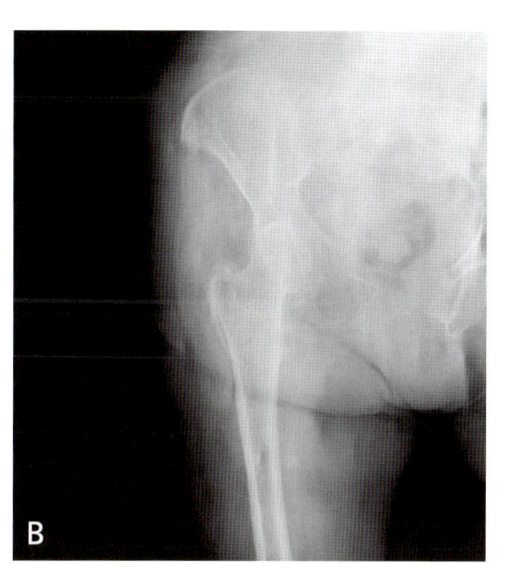

Figure 1 Radiographs demonstrate a comminuted proximal femur fracture. **A,** AP view of the hip. **B,** AP view obtained with the lower extremity in manual traction and internal rotation. The alignment of the hip with traction allows for better understanding of the fracture pattern and its behavior with closed reduction.

Procedure
Simple standard obliquity intertrochanteric fractures (on the Evans classification system) can be treated with either a sliding hip screw (SHS) or a cephalomedullary nail (CMN). Despite regional variations and surgeon preferences, the SHS is still the standard treatment because the CMN continues to have a higher rate of peri-implant fracture at the tip of the nail. No differences in blood loss, surgical time, or recovery have been reported.[3]

Reverse obliquity fractures, intertrochanteric fractures with lateral wall involvement, transverse intertrochanteric fractures, and fractures with subtrochanteric extension should not be treated with an SHS because of unacceptable rates of failure due to excessive collapse (**Figure 2**). Use of a CMN is indicated for these types of intertrochanteric fractures.[4]

Room Setup/Patient Positioning
After preoperative briefing, the patient is carefully positioned supine on the

---

Dr. Schwartz or an immediate family member is a member of a speakers' bureau or has made paid presentations on behalf of Synthes. Neither Dr. Sherman nor any immediate family member has received anything of value from or has stock or stock options held in a commercial company or institution related directly or indirectly to the subject of this chapter.

Section 5: Trauma

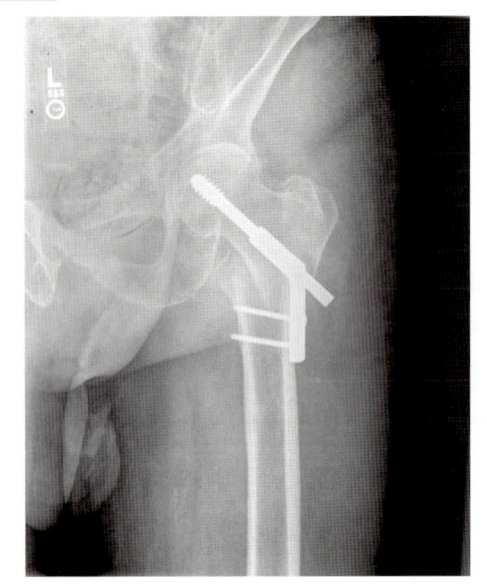

Figure 2 AP radiograph of the hip demonstrates an intertrochanteric fracture treated with a sliding hip screw. Excessive collapse has occurred because of a previously unrecognized lateral wall fracture.

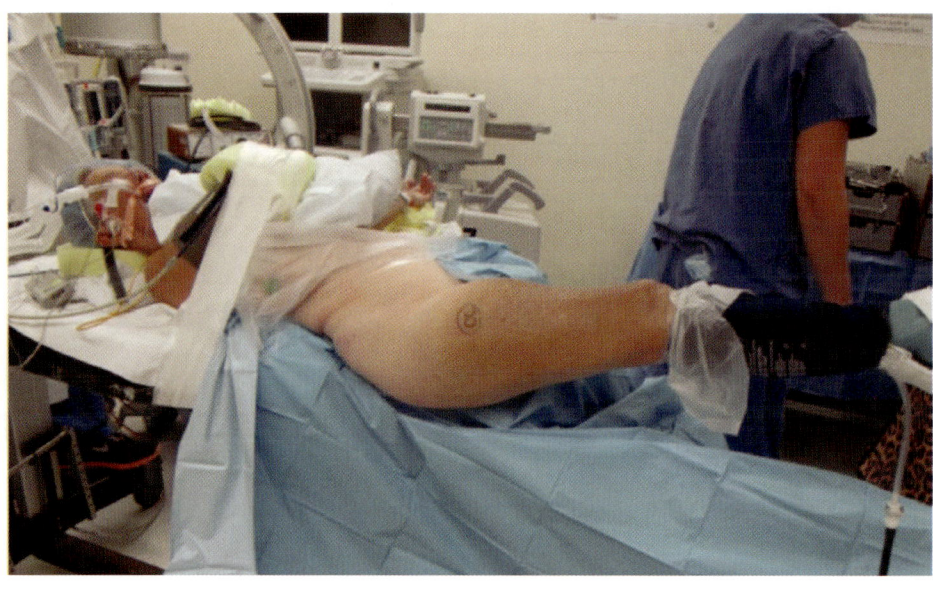

Figure 3 Photograph demonstrates typical setup and patient positioning on a fracture table for surgical fixation of an intertrochanteric fracture using an intramedullary nail. Note the proximal and posterior extent of draping required for intramedullary nail fixation and the intraoperative use of a compression device on bilateral lower extremities.

fracture table. The use of a fracture table is preferred for most intertrochanteric fractures, regardless of the implant chosen. The fracture table allows easy biplanar imaging without moving the fractured extremity, and it facilitates obtaining and maintaining an appropriate reduction. Obtaining fracture reduction before placement of either type of implant is critical. Boot traction rather than skeletal traction is usually adequate. Both feet and ankles are padded carefully to avoid pressure on bony prominences. Additional padding may be placed in the heel of the boot and over the dorsum of the feet. The legs are scissored with the surgical leg flexed and the contralateral leg extended. Care is taken to avoid hyperextension and excessive traction on the unaffected leg to avoid stretching of the femoral nerve. Placing the nonsurgical leg in a well-leg holder has been reported to cause compartment syndrome and is therefore not recommended.[5] A well-padded perineal post is placed. All bony prominences are carefully padded, the genitals are checked, and the patient is secured on the operating table. Lower extremity compressive devices are placed on both lower extremities. The arm on the surgical side is placed across the patient's chest with a pillow between the chest and arm. A foam pad is placed around the elbow to protect the olecranon. A towel is then placed over the adducted and internally rotated arm, and wide silk tape is used to secure the arm to the fracture table. This allows for improved imaging as well as appropriate access to the proximal femur for placement of a CMN (**Figure 3**).

Special Instruments/Equipment

Several reduction aids may be used. A laterally placed percutaneous ball-spike pusher allows correction of varus of the proximal fragment. A percutaneously placed Cobb elevator may be placed at the fracture site anteriorly to correct flexion deformity or posteriorly to correct extension deformity (**Figure 4**). Reduction clamps are also sometimes needed for more displaced fractures (**Figure 5**). It is critical to remember that the implant alone will not reduce the fracture.

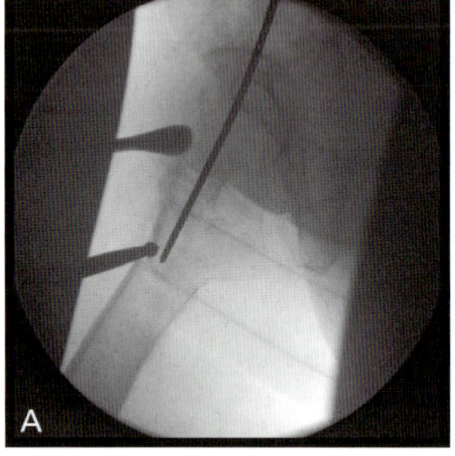

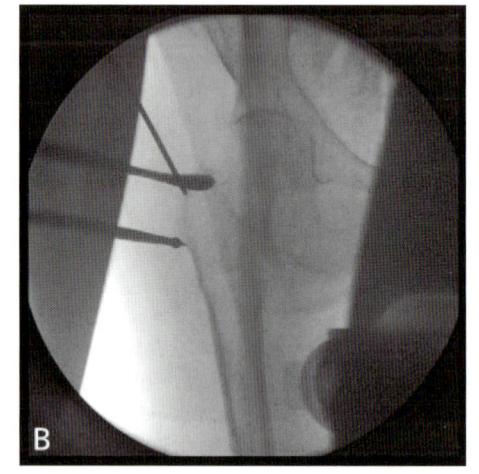

Figure 4 Intraoperative fluoroscopic views show reduction of an intertrochanteric fracture. **A**, Lateral view shows a Cobb elevator at the anterior neck to counteract flexion deformity of the proximal segment. A ball-spike pusher on the lateral cortex is also visualized. **B**, AP view shows a ball-spike pusher on the lateral cortex of the proximal segment, counteracting the abduction of the fragment.

Surgical Technique
Cephalomedullary Nail

Closed reduction is attempted under biplanar fluoroscopy. This is usually accomplished via internal rotation and traction. The tip of the greater trochanter should be at the level of the center of the femoral head to ensure that the hip is not malreduced in varus.[4] If reduction cannot be obtained, an open reduction will need to be performed.

Sterile preparation is performed using a preparatory solution about the hip, buttocks, and thigh. Care must be taken to prepare very proximally and posteriorly to gain access to the proximal femur for the correct starting point.

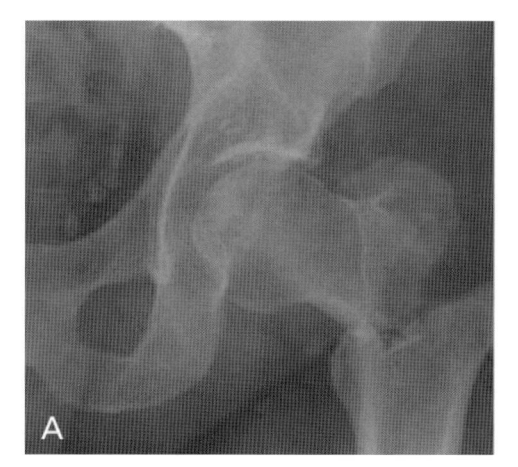

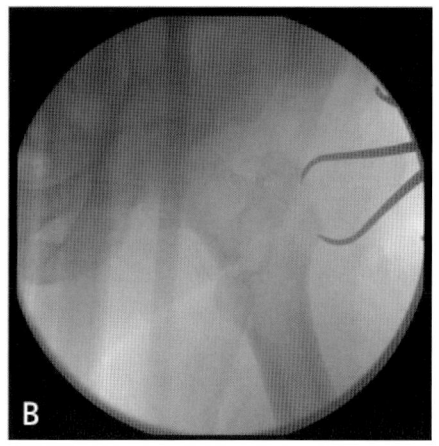

Figure 5 Images of a displaced intertrochanteric fracture. **A,** Preoperative AP radiograph shows the fracture, which was irreducible with traction alone. **B,** Intraoperative AP fluoroscopic view demonstrates open reduction of the fracture using a pointed reduction clamp.

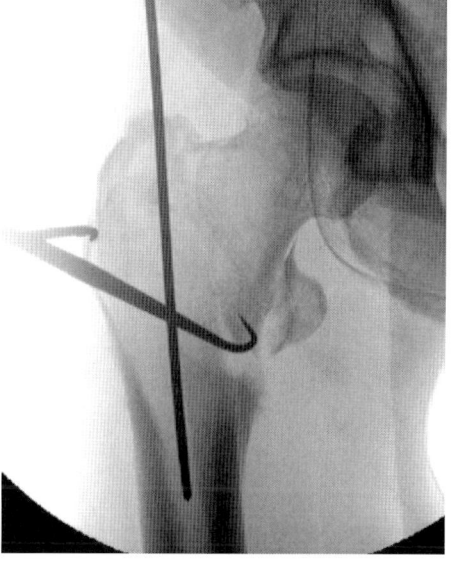

Figure 6 Intraoperative fluoroscopic AP view of the hip demonstrates the correct starting point for a cephalomedullary nail, just medial to the tip of the greater trochanter. This avoids accidental reaming out of the lateral cortex and minimizes the risk for varus malalignment.

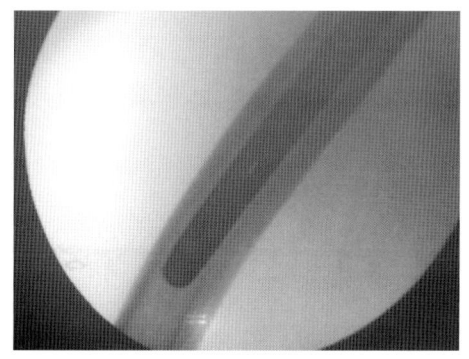

Figure 7 Intraoperative lateral fluoroscopic view of the femur demonstrates the potential risk of anterior cortex penetration when inserting a long cephalomedullary nail. Excessive manual force should be avoided when inserting these nails to avoid iatrogenic femur fracture during nail insertion.

The guide pin may be inserted percutaneously and the incision then based on the location of the pin. Alternatively, a 3.0-cm posterolateral proximal incision is extrapolated in line with the femur. Sharp dissection is performed through the subcutaneous tissue and fascia. The starting point is confirmed on AP and lateral fluorographic views. The starting point on the AP view should be just medial to the tip of the greater trochanter (**Figure 6**) and should be in line with the shaft of the femur on the lateral view. The guide pin is advanced into the proximal femoral metaphysis to the level of the lesser trochanter. An opening reamer is then advanced through the greater trochanter and through the femoral metaphysis to the level of the lesser trochanter. The opening reamer and guide pin are removed. If a long nail is to be placed, a ball-tipped guidewire is inserted into the intramedullary canal and advanced to the distal femoral physeal scar. The nail length is then measured. Incremental reaming of the diaphyseal canal can then ensue. The CMN selected is 1 to 1.5 mm smaller than the final reaming. If a short nail is chosen, reaming is not required.

The CMN is then inserted by hand. When inserting a long nail, the use of a mallet is avoided. The bow of the femur is greater in elderly patients, so using excessive force to insert the nail may cause perforation of the anterior cortex in osteopenic bone. Advancement of the nail is observed on fluoroscopic views of the distal femur to ensure that the nail does not impinge on or penetrate the anterior cortex (**Figure 7**). The final depth of seating of the nail is confirmed on an AP view of the hip. The final placement depends solely on the location of the lag screw, with the goal of placing it "center-center" and deep in the femoral head. The guide pin for the lag screw is then advanced. Once again, fluoroscopic evaluation in both the AP and lateral planes is performed, and the tip-apex distance (TAD) is calculated. The TAD is the sum of the distances between the center of the femoral head and the tip of the screw as measured on AP and lateral views of the hip. When the pin is in good position, the screw length is measured and subsequently inserted. Most systems use a set-screw, which is then tightened.

Distal interlocking screws may then be placed in axially and/or rotationally unstable fractures using freehand technique. Once acceptable alignment, rotation, and fracture position are confirmed, all wounds are copiously irrigated and closed.

Sliding Hip Screw

With the patient on a fracture table, closed reduction is attempted under fluoroscopic evaluation in both the AP and lateral planes. Patient positioning, surgical skin site preparation, and draping are similar to that used with the CMN technique described previously.

Fluoroscopy may be used to localize the appropriate site for surgical incision. Once the coordinates are obtained, a direct lateral approach to the proximal femur is performed with sharp dissection through the skin, subcutaneous tissue, and iliotibial band. The vastus lateralis musculature is preserved and reflected anteriorly off the iliotibial band, with subsequent exposure of the lateral proximal femur. The vastus lateralis and the iliotibial band are retracted with a Bennett-type retractor.

A guidewire is then advanced through the lateral aspect of the femur and into the femoral neck and head to the "center-center" position. Biplanar imaging assists with this step. The lag screw length is then measured over the guidewire. Reaming is performed to the appropriate depth. Once reaming is completed into the subchondral bone of the femoral head, the lag screw is placed. Final evaluation under fluoroscopy in both the AP and lateral planes is used to confirm proper screw placement. When the TAD is noted to be within all tolerances, the SHS plate with barrel is inserted. After accurate confirmation of the plate position on AP fluorography, two or more screws are placed. A single 6.5- or 7.3-mm cannulated screw may be added

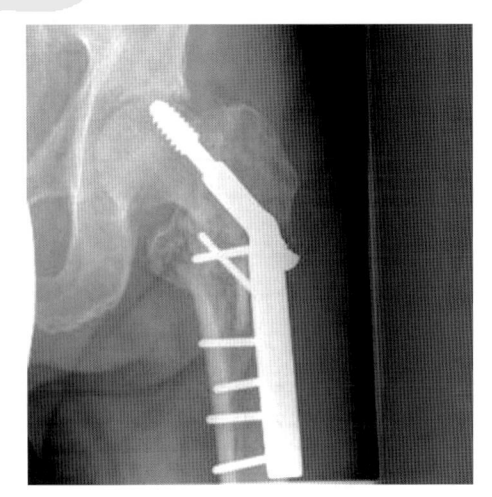

Figure 8 AP radiograph of the hip demonstrates failure of fixation and varus collapse following fixation of a transtrochanteric fracture treated with a sliding hip screw.

to provide rotational stability in basicervical fractures. The iliotibial band is closed securely, as are the subcutaneous tissue and skin.

Complications

Varus malunion is the most common biomechanical complication after surgical treatment of unstable intertrochanteric hip fractures, resulting in varus alignment, limb shortening, gluteal muscle imbalance, and abnormal gait (**Figure 8**). In addition, increased force is placed on the hip joint, which may lead to degenerative arthritis. Varus malunion is best avoided by obtaining an appropriate intraoperative reduction. A simple way to accomplish this is to ensure that the tip of the greater trochanter is in line with the center of the femoral head on the AP view. If the greater trochanter is proximal to the center of the femoral head, the alignment is varus. If the greater trochanter is distal to the center, the alignment is valgus.[4]

Another common and feared complication is displacement of the proximal segment leading to failure of fixation. Although this is often termed *screw cutout*, the screw does not actually cut through the bone. Rather, the fracture displaces and collapses, and the screw may ultimately protrude through the femoral head. The best way to prevent this is with proper placement of the lag screw. The optimal placement of the screw is deep and central within the femoral head. Baumgaertner et al[6] described the value of the TAD in predicting fixation failure in peritrochanteric fractures of the hip. A total TAD of less than 25 mm is associated with a significantly lower rate of screw cutout from the femoral head than is a total hip TAD that exceeds 25 mm.

A complication unique to CMNs, particularly the short CMN, is femoral fracture at the tip of the nail. Although the incidence of this complication has decreased with newer nail designs, it remains a concern. The 2010 Cochrane review[3] compared the SHS with various types of CMNs and found that CMNs were associated with an increased risk of femoral fracture intraoperatively and postoperatively. CMNs resulted in the need for reoperation in 1 of every 50 patients. Mortality and other long-term outcomes were similar between the implants. The review supports the use of the SHS for fixing the more common types of extracapsular hip fractures. Further research is needed to determine the outcomes of the newest generation of implants.

Postoperative Care and Rehabilitation

Patients should be mobilized immediately after surgery. Elderly patients are often unable to follow prescribed non–weight-bearing precautions because of upper extremity weakness, poor balance, and overall deconditioning. Therefore, the goal of surgical treatment is to obtain anatomic alignment and stable fixation to allow immediate postoperative weight bearing as tolerated. A study by Koval et al[7] showed that elderly patients who are allowed to bear weight as tolerated after surgical treatment of a hip fracture will voluntarily limit loading of the affected extremity. If there is concern about fracture stability and/or the implant, the patient will require wheelchair mobilization.

Without prophylaxis, the rate of DVT in patients with hip fractures is approximately 50% for all DVTs and 27% for proximal DVTs. This rate is reduced to 1.34% with current treatment modalities. The rate of fatal pulmonary embolism after hip fracture is 0.66% to 7.5%.[8] Protocols for DVT prophylaxis remain controversial. For patients undergoing routine hip fracture surgery, the Evidence-Based Clinical Practice Guidelines of the American College of Chest Physicians[9] (ACCP) include thromboprophylaxis using fondaparinux (grade 1A), low-molecular-weight heparin (LMWH) (grade 1B), adjusted-dose vitamin K antagonist (international normalized ratio [INR] target, 2.5; range, 2.0 to 3.0; grade 1B), or low-dose unfractionated heparin (grade 1B). The ACCP guidelines recommend against the use of aspirin alone. For patients in whom hip fracture surgery is likely to be delayed, the ACCP recommendation is thromboprophylaxis with LMWH or low-dose unfractionated heparin initiated during the time between hospital admission and surgery (grade 1C). For patients undergoing hip fracture surgery who have a high risk of bleeding, the recommendation is for the use of mechanical thromboprophylaxis (grade 1A). When the high bleeding risk decreases, pharmacologic thromboprophylaxis may be substituted for or added to the mechanical thromboprophylaxis (grade 1C).

The ACCP guidelines also give recommendations for the duration of prophylaxis.[9] For patients undergoing hip fracture surgery, thromboprophylaxis should be extended beyond 10 days and up to 35 days after surgery (grade 1A). The recommended options for extended thromboprophylaxis in hip fracture surgery include fondaparinux (grade 1A), LMWH (grade 1C), or a vitamin K antagonist (grade 1C). In general, pharmacologic thromboprophylaxis with fondaparinux or LMWH should be given to all patients with hip fractures unless contraindicated. The type and duration, however, are not clearly defined. The incidence of DVT is high in patients in whom fixation of the hip fracture is delayed; therefore, attention must be paid to preoperative prophylaxis.[8]

A recent systematic overview[10] of the evidence assessing best practices for elderly hip fracture patients noted the following conclusions regarding postoperative care: (1) antibiotic prophylaxis decreased wound infections and urinary tract infections; (2) suction wound drainage had no effect on infection rate, reoperation rate, or transfusion rate; (3) intermittent rather than indwelling urinary catheterization allowed earlier normal voiding patterns.

Pearls

- The appropriate implant must be chosen. An SHS is indicated for standard obliquity intertrochanteric fractures. A CMN is indicated for reverse obliquity fractures, transtrochanteric fractures, intertrochanteric fractures with subtrochanteric extension, and intertrochanteric fractures without an intact lateral wall.
- Caution and gentle technique are required when inserting a CMN because the anterior bow of the femur is often greater in elderly patients.

- The fracture must be reduced before placement of the implant. If the fracture is not reducible by closed means, percutaneous or open techniques should be used.
- The TAD is critical to success with both SHSs and CMNs, and it is one of the few factors under the surgeon's control. Using biplanar fluoroscopy, care should be taken to achieve a TAD of less than 25 mm.
- The starting point for a CMN is just medial to the tip of the greater trochanter.
- Adequate skin must be prepared and draped proximally and posteriorly for CMNs.

References

1. Neuman MD, Fleisher LA, Even-Shoshan O, Mi L, Silber JH: Nonoperative care for hip fracture in the elderly: The influence of race, income, and comorbidities. *Med Care* 2010;48(4):314-320.
2. Lubovsky O, Liebergall M, Mattan Y, Weil Y, Mosheiff R: Early diagnosis of occult hip fractures MRI versus CT scan. *Injury* 2005;36(6):788-792.
3. Parker MJ, Handoll HH: Gamma and other cephalocondylic intramedullary nails versus extramedullary implants for extracapsular hip fractures in adults. *Cochrane Database Syst Rev* 2010;(9):CD000093.
4. Haidukewych GJ: Intertrochanteric fractures: Ten tips to improve results. *J Bone Joint Surg Am* 2009;91(3):712-719.
5. Meyer RS, White KK, Smith JM, Groppo ER, Mubarak SJ, Hargens AR: Intramuscular and blood pressures in legs positioned in the hemilithotomy position: Clarification of risk factors for well-leg acute compartment syndrome. *J Bone Joint Surg Am* 2002;84(10):1829-1835.
6. Baumgaertner MR, Curtin SL, Lindskog DM, Keggi JM: The value of the tip-apex distance in predicting failure of fixation of peritrochanteric fractures of the hip. *J Bone Joint Surg Am* 1995;77(7):1058-1064.
7. Koval KJ, Sala DA, Kummer FJ, Zuckerman JD: Postoperative weight-bearing after a fracture of the femoral neck or an intertrochanteric fracture. *J Bone Joint Surg Am* 1998;80(3):352-356.
8. Marsland D, Mears SC, Kates SL: Venous thromboembolic prophylaxis for hip fractures. *Osteoporos Int* 2010; 21(suppl 4):S593-S604.
9. Geerts WH, Bergqvist D, Pineo GF, et al: Prevention of venous thromboembolism: American College of Chest Physicians Evidence-Based Clinical Practice Guidelines (8th Edition). *Chest* 2008; 133(6 Suppl):381S-453S.
10. Beaupre LA, Jones CA, Saunders LD, Johnston DW, Buckingham J, Majumdar SR: Best practices for elderly hip fracture patients: A systematic overview of the evidence. *J Gen Intern Med* 2005;20(11): 1019-1025.

Chapter 63
Intramedullary Nailing of Diaphyseal Femur Fractures

Anna N. Miller, MD

Patient Selection

Diaphyseal femur fractures (fractures of the femoral shaft) necessitate surgical fixation for several reasons. Surgical fixation allows patients with these injuries to mobilize more quickly after surgical fixation. Surgical treatment also decreases the risks of prolonged recumbency, including fat emboli syndrome, decubitus ulcers, and muscle atrophy.[1]

Indications

Intramedullary nailing is indicated for diaphyseal femur fractures in adult patients who can tolerate surgical intervention.[2]

Contraindications

Intramedullary nailing is contraindicated in patients who cannot tolerate surgical intervention. Relative contraindications include pediatric femur fractures (in some cases), highly contaminated open wounds (which may necessitate a staged procedure), and femoral fractures with proximal or distal involvement that may necessitate other fixation.[2] In addition, retrograde intramedullary nailing may be necessitated in extremely obese patients or considered in cases of bilateral femur fractures or ipsilateral femur and tibia fractures at the surgeon's discretion.

Preoperative Imaging

Adequate AP and lateral images of the entire femur, including the hip and knee joints, must be obtained before proceeding with surgical fixation. The surgeon should evaluate the femoral neck carefully for associated fractures.[3] In cases with comminution, it is advisable to get the same views of the uninjured femur if possible, to assess length and alignment for the fractured side.[4] In addition, if both legs are fractured, it is recommended that the simpler side be fixed first to assess length for the comminuted side. With comminution, rotation is also difficult to assess. A preoperative radiographic examination of the lesser trochanter on the uninjured side on an AP view obtained with the patella straight anterior is an excellent view to compare.[5] Femoral anteversion can be assessed by obtaining a direct lateral view of the knee with the proximal femur on the uninjured side to compare the version by the amount of C-arm rotation required to get a direct lateral view of each.[6,7]

Procedure

Room Setup/Patient Positioning

I recommend that this procedure be performed on a flat Jackson table. The use of a traction table increases the risks of complications due to traction and the perineal post.[8] The patient is positioned supine at the edge of the table such that the buttock/hip of the injured leg is hanging over the edge of the table (**Figure 1, A**). A bump is placed under the sacrum to elevate and provide complete access to the hip. I use a modified device built in the hospital's machine shop that provides intraoperative traction while keeping the leg free for manipulation (**Figure 1, B**). The patient's leg is elevated on a ramp to allow adequate lateral fluoroscopic imaging. The fluoroscopy unit is placed on the opposite side of the injured leg and rotated to approximately 10° above an horizontal to obtain image of the lateral femur.

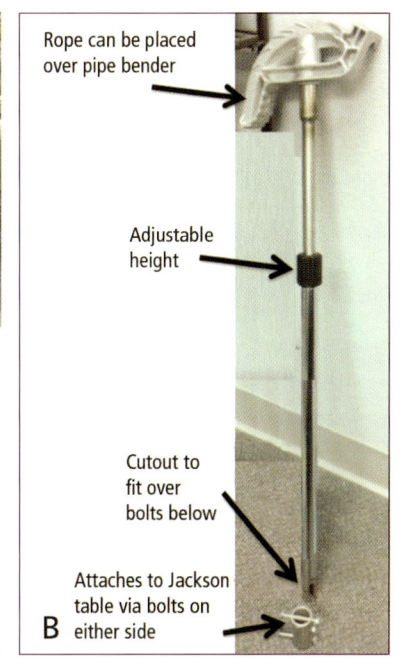

Special Instruments/Equipment/Implants

For this procedure, the following equipment should be available:

- Traction setup for the Jackson table
- Leg ramp and sacral bump
- Traction bow and sterile rope with 5/64-in Kirschner wire (K-wire) for traction
- Femoral nail and appropriate insertion equipment, reamers
- Reduction devices per surgeon's discretion (eg, ball-spike pusher and shoulder hook)

Surgical Technique

After the patient is positioned as described previously, the entire proximal femur is exposed; drapes should allow access up to the iliac crest and to the entire leg. A 5/64-in K-wire is placed in the distal femur. Care should be taken to place it very anterior to allow for intramedullary nail placement posterior to the wire (**Figure 2, A** and **B**). The tensioned traction bow is placed on the wire, a sterile rope is hung off the field on the pole at the end of the table, and approximately 10 lb of weights are hung from the rope. Traction is placed on the opposite side of the table from the fractured leg to allow for adduction.

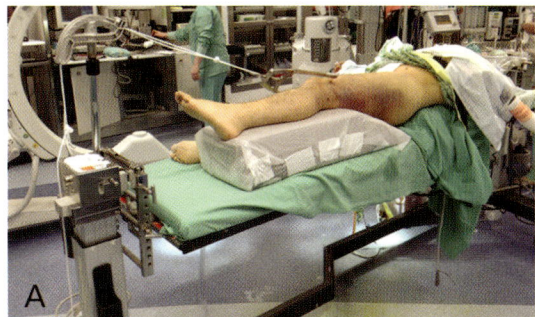

Figure 1 Photographs show patient positioning and room setup for intramedullary nailing of a femoral shaft fracture. **A**, The patient is supine on a Jackson table. His injured (left) hip has been moved laterally over the edge of the table, and the leg is elevated on a ramp (encased in plastic drapes). Traction is shown in place as an example. **B**, The traction setup that is attached to the Jackson table at the distal end on the opposite side of the injured leg to allow for adduction.

Dr. Miller or an immediate family member serves as a paid consultant to or is an employee of Synthes and has received nonincome support (such as equipment or services), commercially derived honoraria, or other non–research-related funding (such as paid travel) from Smith & Nephew.

Section 5: Trauma

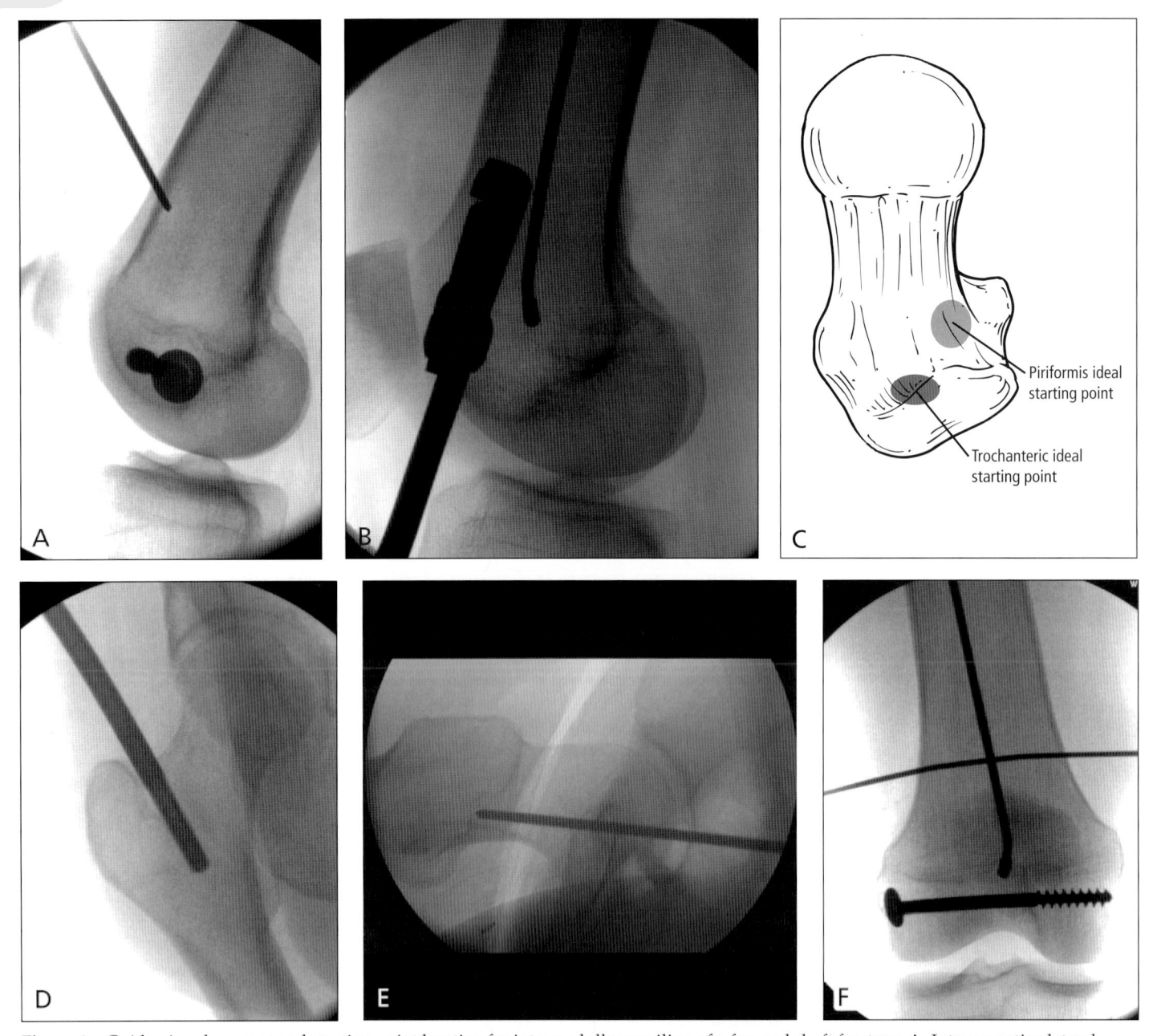

Figure 2 Guidewire placement and starting point location for intramedullary nailing of a femoral shaft fracture. **A,** Intraoperative lateral fluoroscopic image shows the anterior starting point for the 5/64-in Kirschner wire placement. **B,** Intraoperative lateral fluoroscopic image shows traction bow in front of the ball-tipped guidewire. Distal placement of the ball-tipped guidewire is also visible, with the wire well centered in the femur. **C,** Illustration of the axial view shows proper locations for piriformis and trochanteric entry sites. When a piriformis entry site is used, the nail should not be placed too far anteriorly because of the risk of iatrogenic fracture. When a trochanteric entry site is used, the nail should be placed medially on the trochanteric tip to avoid lateral wall blowout. **D,** Intraoperative AP fluoroscopic image of a right hip shows a dynamic hip screw reamer used to place the piriformis entry hole. **E,** Intraoperative lateral fluoroscopic image of a right hip shows proper placement of the piriformis starting point. **F,** Intraoperative AP fluoroscopic image of a right distal femur. Note the curved tip of the ball-tipped guidewire; the overall trajectory of the wire is toward the medial tibial spine.

The starting guidewire is percutaneously placed through the skin and to the appropriate starting point, either at the medial tip of the greater trochanter or the piriformis fossa, depending on the nail chosen by the surgeon. Care should be taken to access the appropriate starting point (**Figure 2, C**). A longitudinal incision is made around the wire in the skin and through subcutaneous tissue and fascia, taking care not to cut proximally into the region of the gluteal neurovascular bundle.

The opening reamer is placed over the guidewire as appropriate for the nail system to be used. A 9-mm dynamic hip screw (DHS) reamer can also be used as a starting reamer because this smaller diameter allows for more flexibility in directing the reamer (**Figure 2, D and E**). After the appropriate path is made, the ball-tipped guidewire is placed down the canal. If the DHS reamer was used as a starting reamer, it is important to use the same manufacturer's opening reamer subsequently to have an adequate opening for the proximal portion of the nail.

The ball-tipped guidewire should be very slightly bent at the tip to allow for directionality as it is placed down the canal (**Figure 2, F**). The femur itself should be aligned before placing the guidewire down; several methods can be used to facilitate this. First, the traction mentioned earlier will help achieve the desired length. The traction bow itself can also be manipulated to help achieve the desired alignment. A small hook as used in

408 © 2013 American Academy of Orthopaedic Surgeons

Chapter 63: Intramedullary Nailing of Diaphyseal Femur Fractures

open shoulder surgery and a ball spike (**Figure 3**) can be used to percutaneously pull and push on the fragments, respectively. After the guidewire is placed down the canal, this alignment should be maintained while reaming. The guidewire is placed as distally as possible in the distal femur and is located centrally on the lateral view, aiming slightly toward the medial tibial spine on the AP view (**Figures 2, B and D**).

After the ball-tipped guidewire is placed

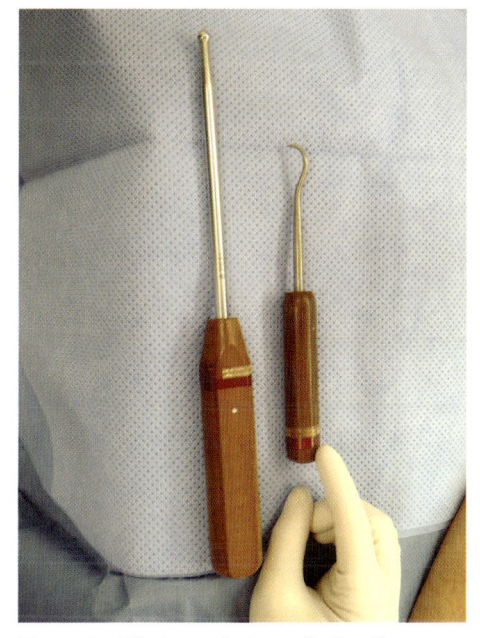

Figure 3 Photograph shows ball spike (left) and shoulder hook (right) used for percutaneous fracture manipulation.

and alignment is maintained, the measuring device should be used to estimate the length of the femur. It is important to confirm that the measuring device is all the way down to the starting point, either on the tip of the trochanter or into the piriformis fossa posterior to the femur. The longest nail possible should be used to avoid a metaphyseal end point for the nail, which can be a stress riser. Next, sequential reaming in 0.5-mm increments is recommended. The reaming should be performed to at least 1 mm over the size of the nail and until some chatter is heard in the femoral diaphysis.

The nail is checked proximally and distally to ensure it is then gently placed over the guidewire, taking care to ensure that length and rotation are maintained. If the guidewire has been bent and it is not certain that the bend will fit through the nail, the surgeon should consider replacing it with a straight wire before performing this step. The nail is checked proximally and distally to ensure it is well seated and of the appropriate length (**Figure 4, A**).

With a reconstruction-style or a cephalomedullary nail, the proximal screws should be placed first to confirm their location in the femoral head (**Figure 4, B**). In antegrade nails that do not have screws entering the femoral head, it is possible to place the distal screws first and backslap across the fracture if compression is needed. Traction should be removed at this time.

For proximal interlocking screws, the aiming arm for the nail is placed, and sleeves are used to estimate the sites of screw entry. Separate incisions can be made for each individual screw, or one incision can be made for both screws, taking care to incise the skin and fascia longitudinally. The trochar and sleeve are then placed down to bone, and the drill is placed through the aiming sleeve. The sleeve must remain secured to the bone during this process to avoid aiming errors. On lateral fluoroscopic imaging, the proximal screws for a cephalomedullary device should be in the exact center of the femoral head, and care should be taken not to penetrate through the articular surface of the femoral head. Depending on the system, screw length is measured from a calibrated drill bit or depth gauge, and screws are then placed through the aiming sleeves by hand.

After a final confirmation of length and rotation, distal interlocking screws are placed using the "perfect circle" technique. To obtain a perfect circle, I prefer to position the leg exactly perpendicular to the fluoroscopic imaging unit because having an assistant hold the leg tends to result in motion and error. Again, the skin is incised longitudinally for one or both incisions, and the incision is also taken down through the fascia. The drill is placed using fluoroscopic guidance, and then the hole is drilled exactly in line with the C-arm. If the surgeon starts to drill

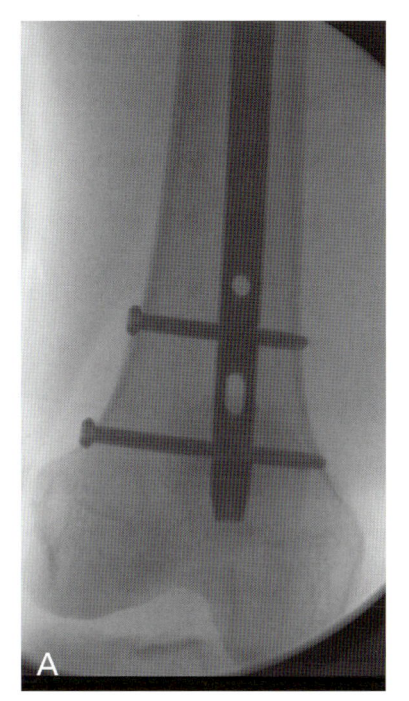

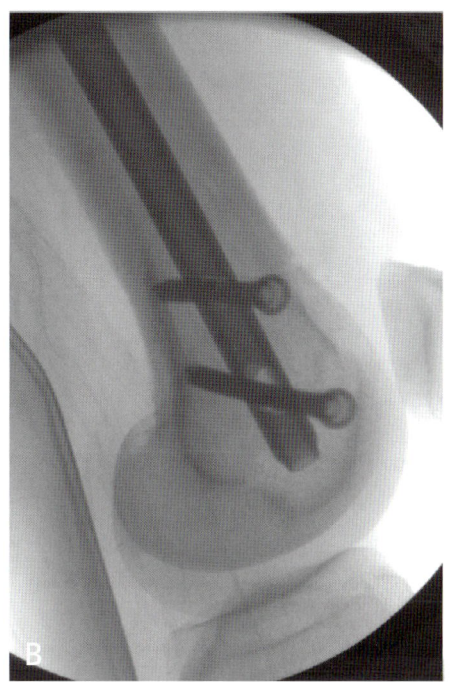

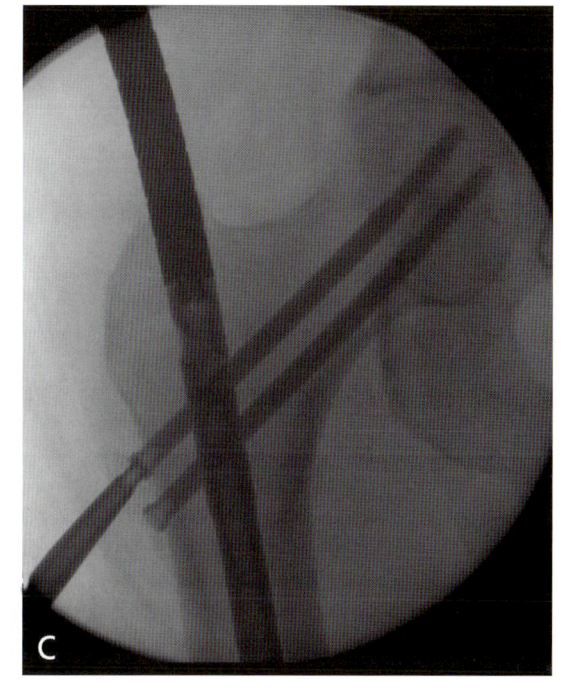

Figure 4 Intraoperative fluoroscopic images demonstrate correct placement of intramedullary nails. AP (**A**) and lateral (**B**) images show excellent distal placement of well-seated, long intramedullary nails. **C**, Intraoperative AP fluoroscopic image of a right hip shows well-placed proximal screws in the femoral head in a reconstruction-style nail.

© 2013 American Academy of Orthopaedic Surgeons

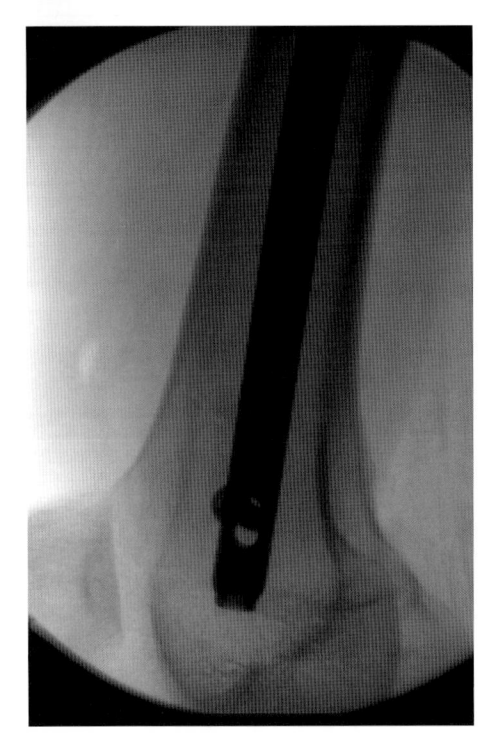

Figure 5 Intraoperative lateral fluoroscopic image of a distal femur after intramedullary nailing of a femoral shaft fracture shows that the distal interlocking screws are completely through the nail.

and finds that the drill gets entangled in soft tissue, it is advisable to recheck the fluoroscopic imaging before proceeding because soft tissue often moves the drill bit from the preferred starting point and can result in the drill bit missing the nail.

If no obstacles are encountered, the surgeon should continue to drill through the far cortex and then place the depth gauge, both for measurement purposes and to check fluoroscopically that the drill hole is through the nail. This saves the step of uncoupling the drill bit to check if the drill bit is through the nail, and then replacing the power on the drill bit to remove it before measuring. If the surgeon encounters resistance while drilling, then he or she should uncouple the drill and assess the drill bit trajectory fluoroscopically. The trajectory can then be manually corrected as necessary, assisted by a light mallet tap to place the drill bit through the far hole in the nail. Drilling can then proceed through the far cortex as described previously.

After measurement with a depth gauge, distal interlocking screws are placed by hand. It is essential that these screws not be overly long because this can result in irritation postoperatively. In addition, the surgeon should remember that the distal femur is trapezoidal in shape, so screws that appear appropriately sized on the AP view may actually be too long if visualized obliquely. Lateral images should be taken directly perpendicular to each screw to confirm that the screw is through the nail (**Figure 5**).

After the final placement of all hardware, final imaging should be performed for yet another assessment of length and rotation. Full-length radiographs can also be used to assess length and alignment. In addition, an internal rotation view of the femoral neck should be checked to reconfirm that there is no femoral neck fracture.

Wounds should then be copiously irrigated with saline. The deep fascia is closed with 0 Vicryl (Ethicon) figure-of-8 sutures, and the skin is reapproximated with 3-0 nylon mattress sutures. The wounds should be cleaned and dried a final time and a sterile dressing should be applied.

Complications

Infection rates reported in published series are low (less than 4%). Infections diagnosed within the first 3 months after surgery are usually treated with serial débridement and intravenous antibiotics. More chronic infections may necessitate hardware removal or exchange nailing as well as intravenous antibiotics.[9]

Malunion is most common in proximal or distal fractures, with a reported incidence of up to 30% in some series.[9] Rotational malunion is quite common and should not be underestimated if the patient reports symptoms of malalignment in the early postoperative period. Limb-length discrepancy can also be a problem with comminution, as described previously. CT evaluation is recommended for both of these problems. At the end of any procedure, the surgeon should evaluate the bilateral limbs for comparison of overall length, alignment, and rotation, including taking the hips through simultaneous internal and external rotation for comparison because malrotation is a commonly missed intraoperative complication.[9]

Nonunion is uncommon in femoral fractures. Treatment may start with dynamization whenever possible, but exchange nailing or even open bone grafting and fixation may be required, depending on the type of nonunion. In the absence of technical error, a metabolic workup should be performed in patients with nonunion.[9]

Femoral neck fracture may occur iatrogenically or during nail placement, and it may be missed pre- or postoperatively.[3] It is of utmost importance to evaluate the femoral neck for fracture before and at the end of the case. For best assessment of the neck for fracture, the surgeon should obtain a fluoroscopic image of the femoral neck in full internal rotation. It is also recommended that the hip be taken through a range of motion under live fluoroscopy to evaluate for any fractures.

Postoperative Care and Rehabilitation

Most patients are able to start weight bearing as tolerated immediately, usually with crutches or a walker for assistance. In cases of comminution with no intact cortical contact or with subtrochanteric fractures, patients should start with toe-touch weight bearing only. Patients should also start working on hip range of motion and abductor strengthening immediately because nail placement does cause some damage to the abductors and resultant weakness.

Pearls

- In cases with fracture comminution, it is advisable to obtain the same radiographic views of the uninjured femur if possible, to assess length and alignment for the fractured side.
- The patient is positioned on a flat Jackson table with a bump under the sacrum and the hip lateralized.
- Intraoperative traction and elevation on a radiolucent ramp help with reduction and imaging.
- For traction, a 5/64-in K-wire is placed in the distal femur, taking care to place it very anterior to allow for intramedullary nail placement posterior to the wire.
- A 9-mm DHS reamer can be used as a starting reamer because its smaller diameter allows for more flexibility in directing the reamer.
- The ball-tipped guidewire should be very slightly bent at the tip to allow for directionality as it is placed down the canal.
- The guidewire is placed as distally as possible in the distal femur, centrally located on the lateral view and aiming slightly toward the medial tibial spine on the AP view.
- If a reconstruction-style or cephalomedullary nail is used, the proximal screws should be placed first to confirm their location in the femoral head.
- To obtain perfect circles, the leg should be positioned exactly perpen-

dicular to the fluoroscopic imaging unit if possible because having an assistant hold the leg tends to result in motion and error.
- The surgeon should remember that the distal femur is trapezoidal in shape, so distal interlocking screws that appear appropriately sized on the AP view may actually be too long if visualized obliquely.
- At the conclusion of the case, an internal rotation view of the femoral neck should always be checked to reconfirm that there is no femoral neck fracture.

References

1. Bone LB, Johnson KD, Weigelt J, Scheinberg R: Early versus delayed stabilization of femoral fractures: A prospective randomized study. *J Bone Joint Surg Am* 1989;71(3):336-340.
2. de Boer P: Diaphyseal fractures: Principles, in Ruedi TP, Buckley RE, Moran CG, eds: *AO Principles of Fracture Management*, ed 2. Stuttgart, Germany, Thieme, 2007, pp 467-468.
3. Tornetta P III, Kain MS, Creevy WR: Diagnosis of femoral neck fractures in patients with a femoral shaft fracture: Improvement with a standard protocol. *J Bone Joint Surg Am* 2007;89(1):39-43.
4. Lindsey JD, Krieg JC: Femoral malrotation following intramedullary nail fixation. *J Am Acad Orthop Surg* 2011;19(1):17-26.
5. Deshmukh RG, Lou KK, Neo CB, Yew KS, Rozman I, George J: A technique to obtain correct rotational alignment during closed locked intramedullary nailing of the femur. *Injury* 1998;29(3):207-210.
6. Bråten M, Tveit K, Junk S, Aamodt A, Anda S, Terjesen T: The role of fluoroscopy in avoiding rotational deformity of treated femoral shaft fractures: An anatomical and clinical study. *Injury* 2000;31(5):311-315.
7. Tornetta P III, Ritz G, Kantor A: Femoral torsion after interlocked nailing of unstable femoral fractures. *J Trauma* 1995;38(2):213-219.
8. Flierl MA, Stahel PF, Hak DJ, Morgan SJ, Smith WR: Traction table-related complications in orthopaedic surgery. *J Am Acad Orthop Surg* 2010;18(11):668-675.
9. Ricci WM, Gallagher B, Haidukewych GJ: Intramedullary nailing of femoral shaft fractures: Current concepts. *J Am Acad Orthop Surg* 2009;17(5):296-305.

Chapter 64
Surgical Fixation of Fractures of the Distal Femur

James F. Kellam, BSc, MD, FRCSC, FACS, FRCSI

Introduction
Fractures of the distal femoral metaphysis still represent a significant challenge to the fracture surgeon.[1,2] The successful management of these fractures—either extra- or intra-articular—demands anatomic axial alignment with a precise reduction of the articular surface of this major lower extremity joint. The distal femur is defined by a square, the sides of which are the same length as the widest part of the distal femoral epiphysis in a child or the metaphysis in an adult (**Figure 1**). Any fracture that has its center inside this box is considered a distal femoral end–segment fracture. The intra-articular fractures may involve a part of the joint (partial articular fractures) in which one component of the joint is separated from the remainder of the joint that is still attached to the shaft or a complete articular fractures in which no part of the fractured articular segment remains attached to the metaphysis and/or diaphysis of the femur.

There are three major factors that make treatment of this fracture difficult:

- The high-energy distal femoral fracture by nature has significant soft-tissue stripping, and approximately 50% of the intra-articular fractures are open. In addition, the distal end of the femur is covered more by tendinous structure than by muscle bellies, thus leading to a poor environment for bone healing because of the lack of extraosseous vascularity so common in the more proximal femur.[1,2]
- The high-energy fracture patterns result in significant joint surface and metaphyseal fragmentation. This makes reduction difficult. It may also be impossible to reconstruct the articular surface, thus dooming the patient to early posttraumatic arthritis. This fragmentation in the metaphysis also contributes to the increased rate of delayed union and nonunion in these fractures.
- With the increasing incidence of osteoporosis, fractures of the distal femur are becoming more common. Advancing age is associated with the development of osteoarthritis requiring total knee arthroplasty and potentially an increased number of periprosthetic fractures. These fractures are associated with their own set of problems, which make management of this injury difficult.[3-7]

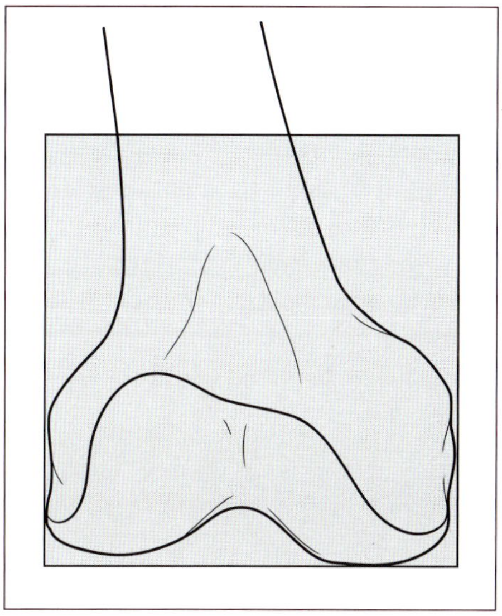

Patient Selection
Indications
The indication for surgery for distal femoral fractures is any displaced intra-articular fracture in an individual who is physiologically healthy, active, and ambulatory with or without aids. Displaced extra-articular fractures are indicated for surgical intervention in the majority of cases because the appropriate alignment of the distal femur is imperative to ensure long-term knee function.

Contraindications
Contraindications for surgical fixation include a completely nondisplaced fracture of the joint or metaphysis in a healthy individual who could mobilize with cast immobilization. This is extremely uncommon but will rarely result in knee stiffness. The other contraindications would be in individuals who are unfit for surgery and those who are nonambulators or significantly incapacitated such that they do not require their extremities for mobility. In the elderly patient with a multifragmented articular fracture in whom prolonged non–weight bearing will be difficult, consideration for total knee replacement may be advisable.

Preoperative Imaging
The first radiographs obtained for diagnostic purposes of distal femoral fractures are AP and lateral projections of the knee and the femoral shaft. It is imperative that good AP and lateral views centered on the knee be obtained. If the fracture is significantly displaced, these radiographs may be best performed after gentle traction and realignment has been performed. This will make the interpretation of the radiographs much easier. It is imperative to identify whether the fracture lines enter the joint, especially on the lateral projection, where coronal plane fractures of the medial or lateral condyle (Hoffa fracture) must be ruled out.[8] In high-energy open fractures, a significant number have occult or minimally displaced coronal-plane fractures.

Following reduction and immobilization with either a knee immobilizer or, more appropriately, tibial tubercle traction, a CT scan is indicated only if the surgeon's interpretation of the plain radiographs is uncertain as to articular involvement. Axial cuts and their associated coronal and sagittal reformations are excellent to determine the various intra-articular fracture pattern extensions. Three-dimensional CT reconstructions have not been used routinely in this fracture and are probably of little value.

Procedure
Timing
Surgical timing for this fracture should be as soon possible given the constraints of a healthy resuscitated patient, an adequate understanding of the injury, appropriate surgical conditions, and skilled

Figure 1 The distal end segment is defined by a square, the sides of which are the same length as the widest part of the distal femoral epiphysis in a child or the metaphysis in an adult.

Dr. Kellam or an immediate family member serves as a board member, owner, officer, or committee member of the Canadian Orthopaedic Association, the Orthopaedic Trauma Association, and the AO Foundation.

staff. These fractures are complex and require excellent preoperative planning and experienced surgical acumen. In a situation in which these conditions may not be met, consideration for joint-bridging external fixation is helpful as a method of stabilizing the patient's soft tissues, aligning the fracture, providing comfort, and awaiting the appropriate surgical team. For open fractures, the degree of soft-tissue disruption and contamination will determine the place of internal fixation. If in doubt, it is best to use a joint-spanning external fixator and allow the soft tissues to "declare" their intent (**Figure 2**).

Room Setup/Patient Positioning

A radiolucent table should be used for the operation. It is best if the whole table top is radiolucent, but if not, the surgeon can check to make sure that adequate radiographs of the complete femur in both the AP and lateral planes can be obtained. This is essential to ensure axial alignment. The use of fluoroscopy is important, and the fluoroscope is usually placed opposite the injured leg. The surgical team and scrub technicians are on the same side as the surgeon. The patient is placed on the operating table in the supine position, and the use of a sterile triangle or bump placed proximal to the fracture to allow flexion of the knee (**Figure 3, A**) is mandatory (flexion of up to 60° is very helpful). Another option is to place the patient's injured knee at the table break so that following draping, the lower end of the operating table is flexed to allow the knee to flex to whatever degree is required (**Figure 3, B**). This also allows some reverse Trendelenburg positioning to help with the exposure and surgical access. This will reduce the pull of the gastrocnemius and abductor magnus, preventing genu recurvatum and shortening. If a roll is placed under the buttock, care must be taken to avoid a malreduction, as this will internally ro-

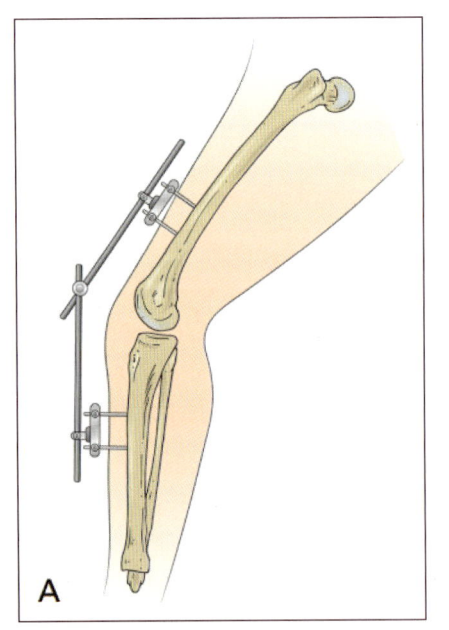

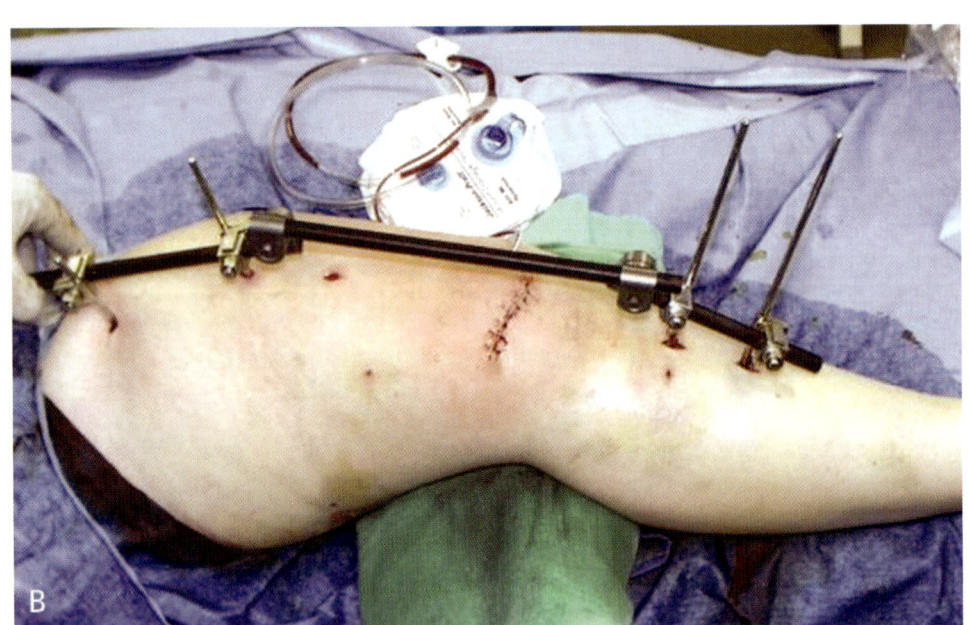

Figure 2 **A,** The joint-spanning external fixator. **B,** It is imperative that the Schanz screws are place outside of the proposed area for the surgical incisions for the fixation. (Courtesy of AO Archives and *AO Principles of Operative Management of Fractures*.)

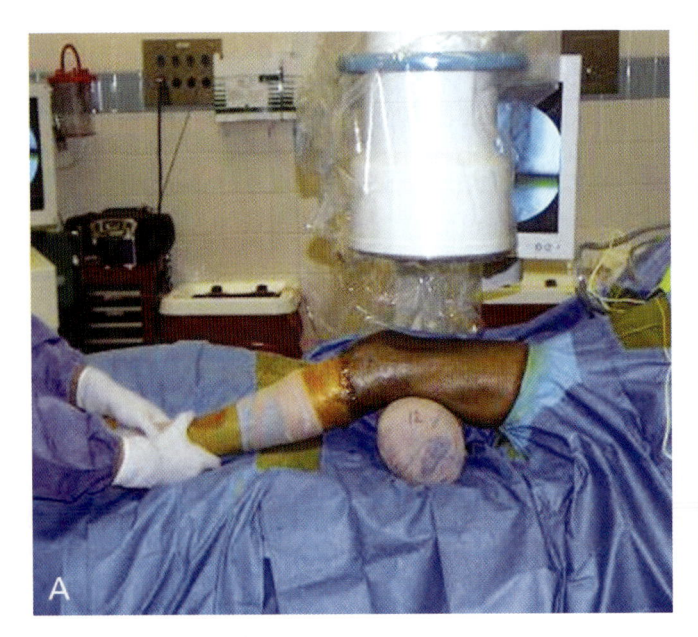

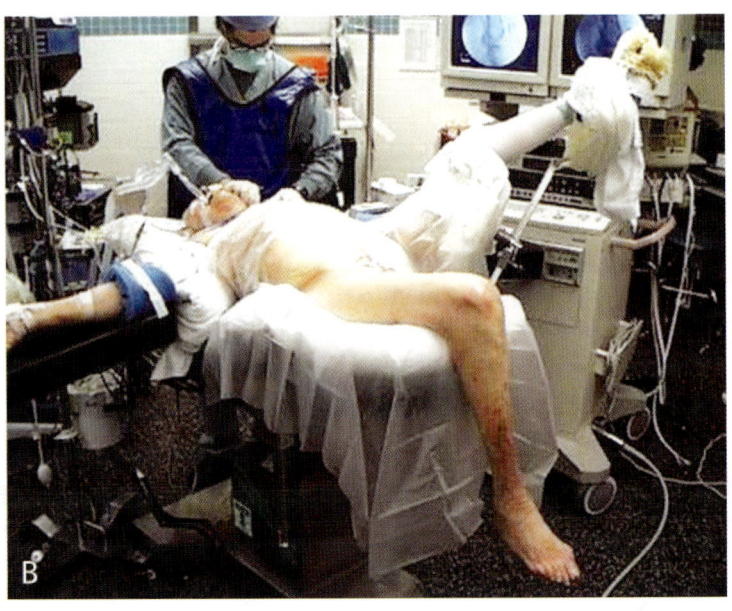

Figure 3 **A,** Patient position on radiolucent table with C-arm from the side opposite the fractured limb. Note the roll under the thigh providing a force for indirect reduction along with manual traction. (Courtesy of Steve Sims, MD, Charlotte, NC.) **B,** The patient is positioned on a regular operating table with the end flexed so as to allow access to the knee. (Courtesy of Eric Johnson, MD, Los Angeles, CA.)

Chapter 64: Surgical Fixation of Fractures of the Distal Femur

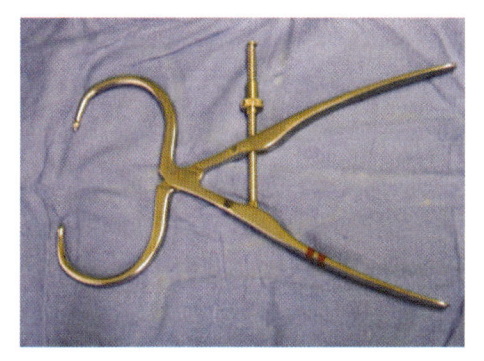

Figure 4 Wide-throated periarticular clamp.

tate the leg, resulting in a rotational malposition.

Special Instruments/Equipment/Implants

The first important aspect of this surgical procedure is the ability to obtain a reduction. If this is an intra-articular fracture, then the joint reduction must be anatomic. In order for this to be done, it is useful for the surgeon to have available multiple periarticular clamps of various throat sizes. These clamps should be pointed to get a good bite on the bone and minimize the soft-tissue disruption. For osteoporotic bone, the use of foot plates that can be attached to the ends of the reduction clamps will prevent the clamp from penetrating the weak metaphyseal cortical bone. A wide-throated clamp is usually used because of the width of the distal femoral metaphysis (**Figure 4**). The use of Kirschner wires (K-wires) as joysticks to manipulate fragments is also extremely helpful.

Implant choice begins with either cancellous or cortical screws of multiple sizes (2.7- to 6.5-mm screws). These are necessary for the stabilization of small and large intra-articular fragments. Presently, there is an increasing trend toward the use of 3.5-/4.0-mm screws for intra-articular stabilization. These screws provide more options for distal plate screw placement and may provide very good fixation due to their high pitch.

Currently, the most common plate is some form of a locking femoral condylar plate. The distal metaphyseal screw configuration is all round holes allowing locked screw insertion so as to enhance the angular stability of the metaphyseal component of the construct. The shaft holes of these plates may have round locking holes or combination holes that can allow both locking and regular cortical screws so axial compression may be obtained if needed (**Figure 5, A** and **B**). Another advantage of the combination hole is the ability to modify fixation and to angle screws to be able to better affect stabilization. Other implants for this region are retrograde femoral nails or fixed-angle devices such as the 95° blade plate or the dynamic condylar screw plate (**Figure 5, C** through **E**). The 95° devices are extremely appealing because with proper insertion, they allow reconstitution of the anatomic axis of the knee joint.[9-12]

A 3.5- or 4.5-mm T- or L-plate or a standard straight plate may be used as a buttress plate for a partial articular medial or lateral condylar fracture.

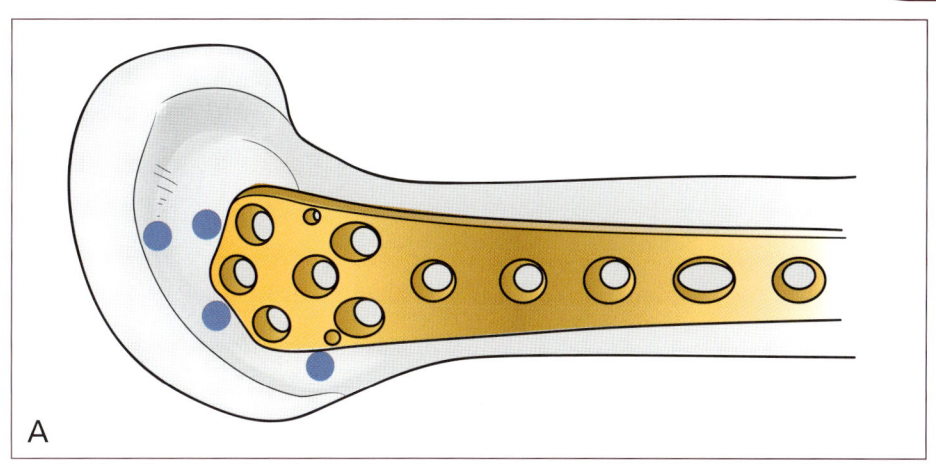

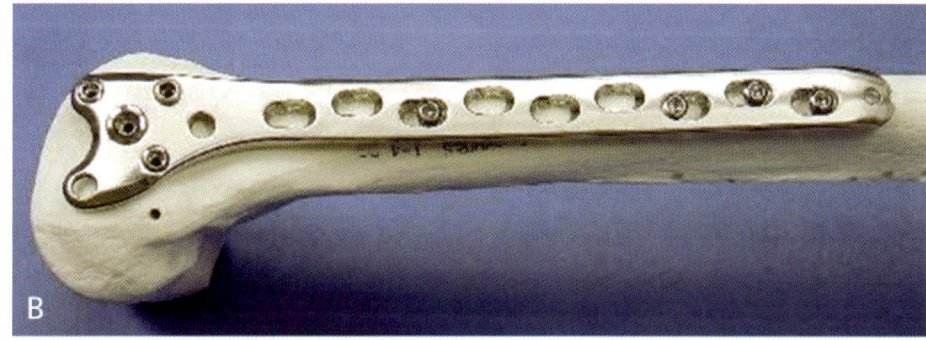

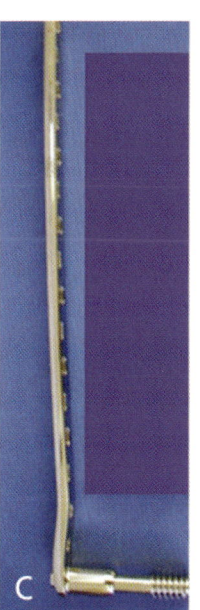

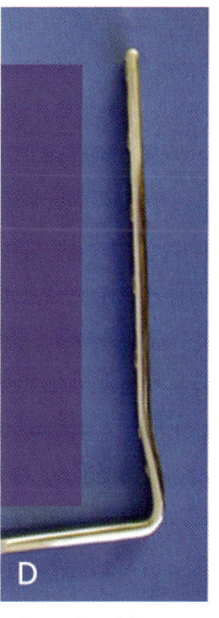

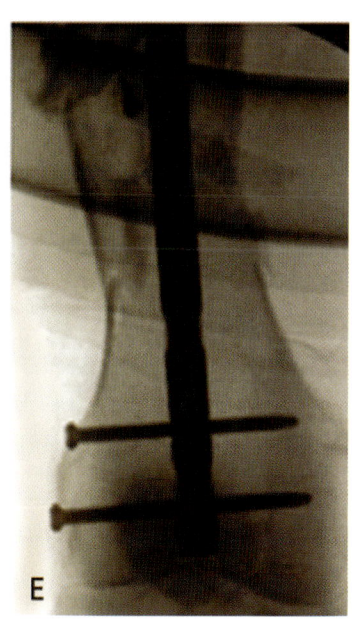

Figure 5 **A,** A round hole locking distal femoral plate. **B,** A distal femoral locking plate with a combination hole allowing the insertion of locking and nonlocking screws as well as axial compression and variable screw angulation when using nonlocking screws. Other implants for stabilization of distal femoral fractures: dynamic condylar screw (**C**), 95° blade plate (**D**), retrograde intramedullary nail (**E**).

Surgical Technique

The most important part of the surgical technique is the preoperative plan, which is based on the plain radiographs and the CT scan. A key aspect of the preoperative plan is to first look at the intra-articular fracture and identify the various frag-

© 2013 American Academy of Orthopaedic Surgeons

ments that will need to be reduced. A plan to establish the order of reduction is important. Usually, there is a main articular fracture fragment on which the other fragments can be built. This fracture will depend on the location of the intra-articular split into the joint, which commonly will enter the intercondylar notch. Screw placement must ensure that the screw heads are out of the footprint of the plate. Also, with coronal split fractures it is important to remember that these screws will be running anterior to posterior and must be placed to avoid the screws or blade from the plate. Consequently, time to plan the methods of reduction and screw placement is important.

Following this, determination of the plate length is required. In a simple metaphyseal fracture pattern, an anatomic reduction and interfragmentary compression of the fracture is necessary. A neutralization plate providing at least four cortices above the fracture will be required, along with tensioning of the plate. In multifragmentary metaphyseal-diaphyseal extension fractures, the plate will be much longer. It is recommended that the length of the plate be at least two to three times the length of the fragmented section of the fracture. Screw fill would be 50% of the holes in the shaft component of the plate. Stability at the fracture site is determined by the placement of the screws nearest to the fracture site. This can be adjusted by increasing the length of the plate and by moving screws away from the fracture site on the proximal end. Distal fixation is usually dictated by the fracture fragment, and the surgeon must apply as many screws as possible in the distal fragment for stability.

In older patients with osteoporotic bone, serious consideration should be given to using a plate long enough to span the femur up to the greater trochanter. In this circumstance, the surgeon must appreciate that the greater trochanter has a flare and the upper end of the plate will need to be contoured to accommodate this. The use of the screws through the plate up into the femoral neck will also provide a splint for the femoral neck in a patient with osteoporosis.

Approaches

Two approaches are best used for fixation. Because most fracture fixations are performed percutaneously, it is imperative to know whether or not an intra-

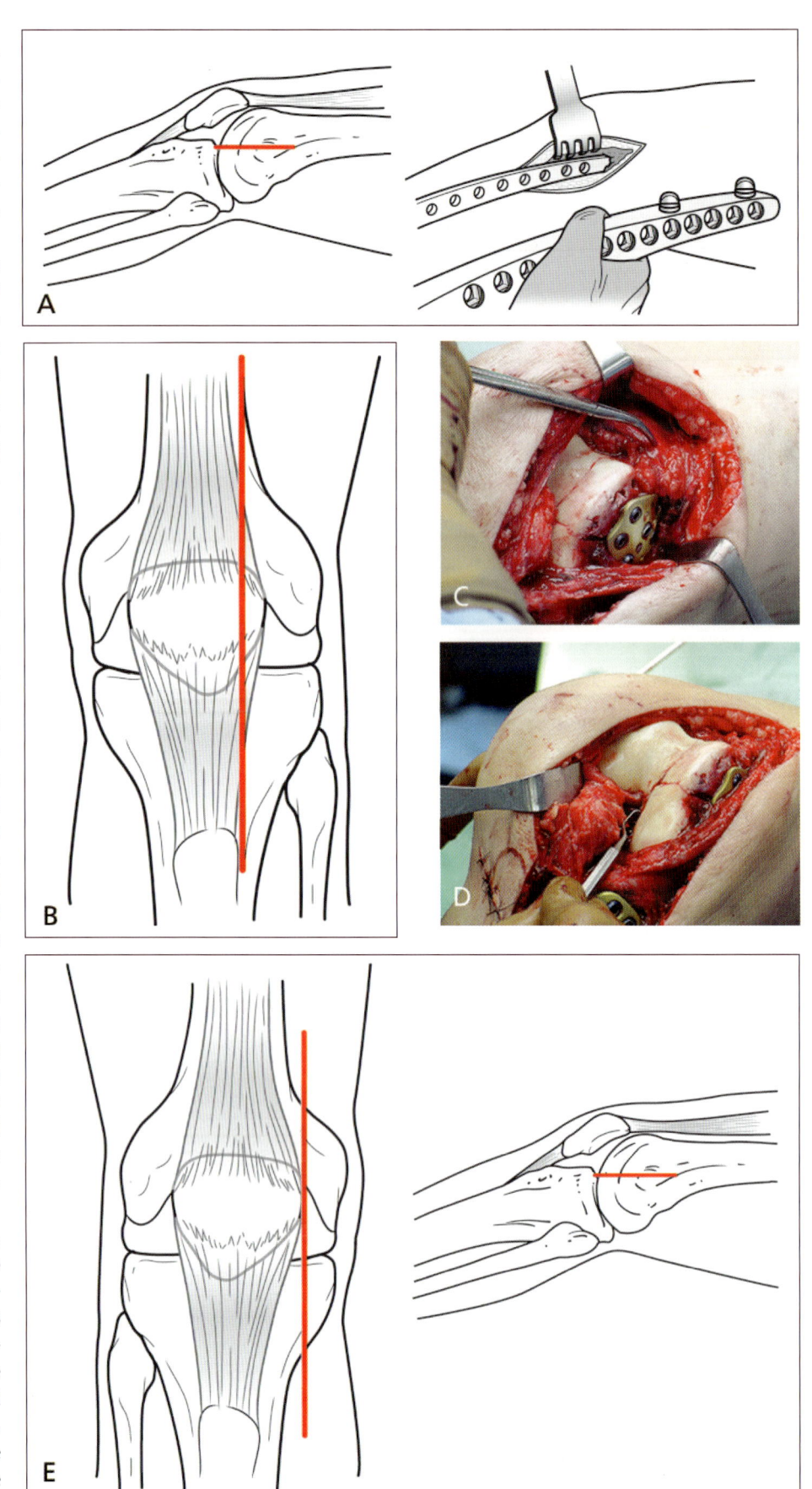

Figure 6 Approaches for fixation of distal femoral fractures. **A,** Illustrations show the lateral approach to the distal femur for plate insertion only. **B** through **D,** The anterolateral approach to the distal femur for open reduction and internal fixation of the joint surface and plate insertion. **B** shows the incision; **C** shows joint visualization; **D** shows the patella subluxated to improve visualization. **E,** Illustrations show the two-incision technique using a medial parapatellar incision *(left)* for joint access along with the lateral incision *(right)* for plate insertion. (Panels **C** and **D** courtesy of Steve Sims, MD, Charlotte, NC.)

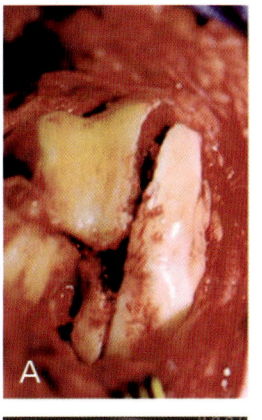

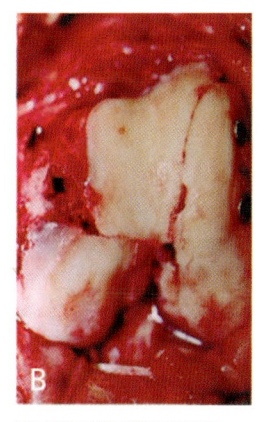

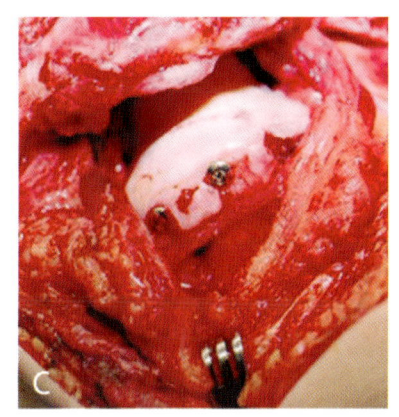

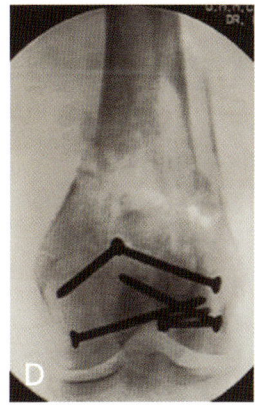

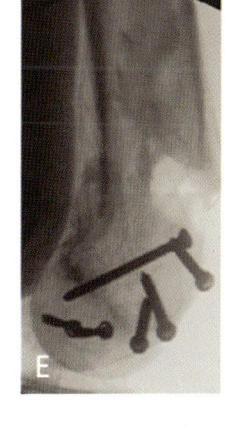

Figure 7 Steps in reduction and fixation of an intra-articular fracture of the distal femur. Intraoperative photographs show the unreduced fracture (**A**), the reduction (**B**), and screw placement (**C**). AP (**D**) and lateral (**E**) fluoroscopic views show the completed fixation.

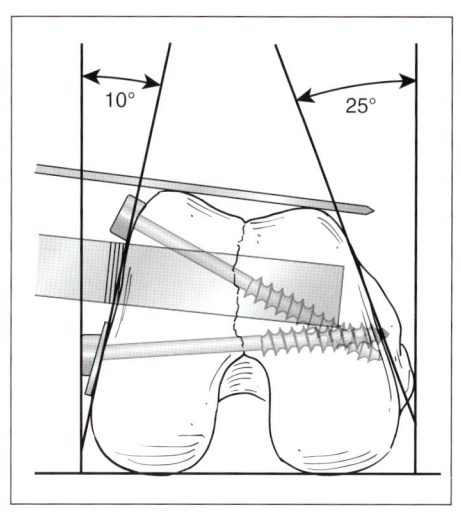

Figure 8 Illustration of the distal end of the femur in cross section shows correct placement of screws and plate for fixation of an intra-articular fracture.

articular reduction must be obtained. If no intra-articular reduction is needed, then a small incision centered over the middle of the distal lateral femoral condyle is made. This approach is through the skin and subcutaneous tissue and then through the iliotibial tract down onto the distal femur. Dissection of the synovium from the distal femur is performed, avoiding detachment of the lateral collateral ligament. Once the lateral face of the femur has been exposed, a long periosteal elevator (Cobb) or specifically designed plate-passing instrument is passed up the lateral aspect of the femur to develop a tunnel so that the plate may be inserted in a submuscular fashion. Where the upper end of the plate will lie, a small 4- to 6-cm incision (using a muscle-splitting technique to ensure that the plate is centered on the bone) may be helpful (**Figure 6, A**). There is a tendency for the tunnel to be created posteriorly, so fluoroscopically monitoring the tunneler's course in the lateral aspect is helpful.

If an intra-articular reduction is required, then an anterolateral (Henry's approach) or lateral parapatellar approach to the distal femur is performed. The lateral parapatellar approach is through a skin incision about 1 cm lateral to the patella that extends from 4 to 5 cm superior to the patella down to the tibial tubercle (**Figure 6, B**). The retinaculum of the lateral aspect of the knee is identified, as is the insertion of the vastus lateralis onto the rectus and patella. Sharp dissection is then performed to detach the vastus lateralis from the rectus and patella and then carried down through the joint capsule along the lateral edge of the patellar tendon. Care must be taken to avoid injuring the lateral meniscus. With this type of approach, medial subluxation or dislocation of the patella can occur. Once this has happened, there is excellent visualization of the distal femur (**Figure 6, C** and **D**). This approach is excellent for fractures through the middle to the lateral aspect of the intercondylar notch. However, at times it is difficult to reach the medial condyle if the fracture exits into the medial condyle or there is a medial coronal fracture. In this situation, a medial parapatellar incision is better to allow articular reduction and fixation, and the lateral approach as described for extra-articular fractures is used for inserting the plate (**Figure 6, E**).

Reduction Techniques

The intra-articular component is reduced (**Figure 7**) by repositioning the various fragments using joysticks and pointed clamps in the different fragments to help rotate and stabilize them. These fragments usually flex back due to the gastronemius pull; the joysticks will allow the articular fragment to be extended and reduced to its adjacent condyle. The surgeon can understand this displacement from the CT scan and direct visualization.

Once the articular surface is reduced, K-wires are placed across the fracture lines and the fracture fragments are stabilized using interfragmental compression by a variety of different screws, depending on the size and location of the fracture. It must be remembered that the distal femur is a trapezoid, with the medial side angled at 25° off the parallel. Consequently, on AP projections, the posterior aspect of the cortical margin of the medial condyle is seen; this makes screws appear to be in bone, but they could be long. It is imperative that a depth gauge be used and that the surgeon understand that in the anterior two thirds of the femoral condyle, the length of screws and plates must be very carefully obtained. Rotation of the distal femur to get an en face view of the medial cortex can be helpful (**Figure 8**).

Once the articular block has been reconstituted, the fracture is an extra-articular fracture. At this point, plate application is undertaken. The most important aspect at this point is to reconstitute the normal anatomic and mechanical axes of the distal femur. It must be remembered that all the plates that are designed for distal femoral fixation have a fixed angle of 90° or 95°. With proper insertion of these plates so that the plate's fixed blade or articular block segment screw is parallel to the joint surface, at right angles to the face of the lateral condyle and in the anterior half of the distal femoral condyle, the plate will line up down the shaft and appropriate axial alignment of the distal femur will occur. Hence, the proper application of the plate to the distal articular block becomes imperative. The important

Section 5: Trauma

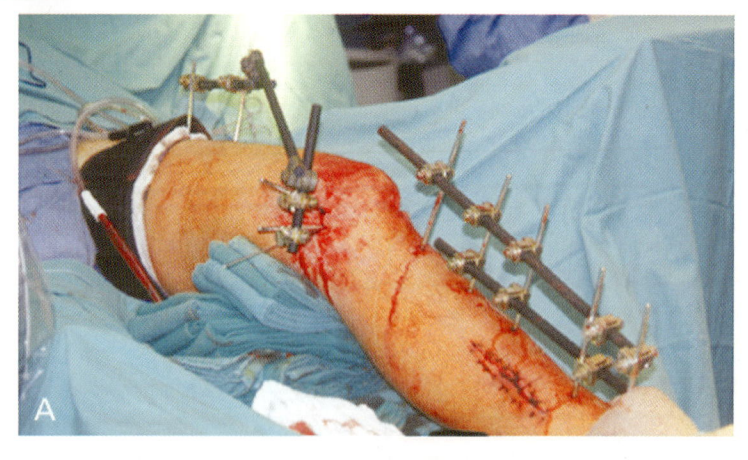

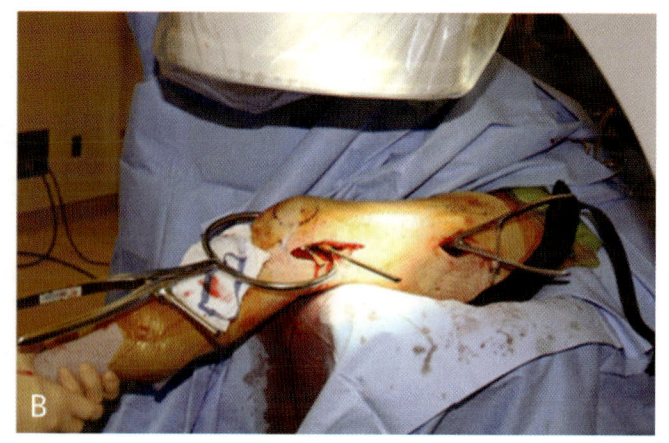

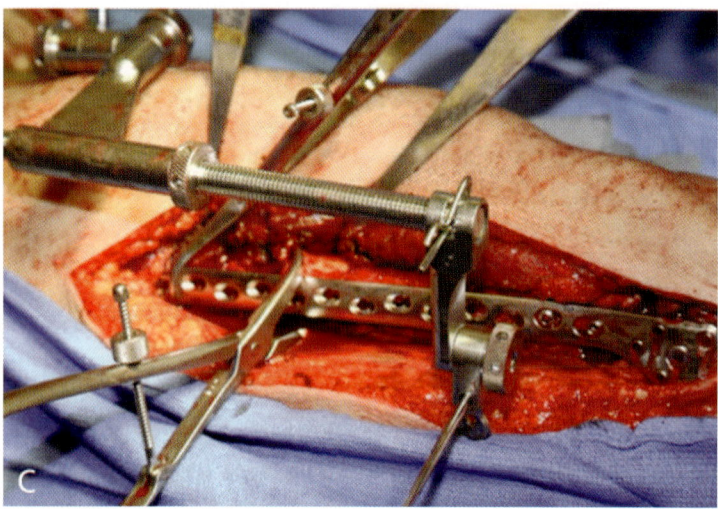

Figure 9 The techniques of obtaining axial alignment of the distal segment to the shaft: **A,** external fixator; **B,** manual traction; and **C,** femoral distractor.

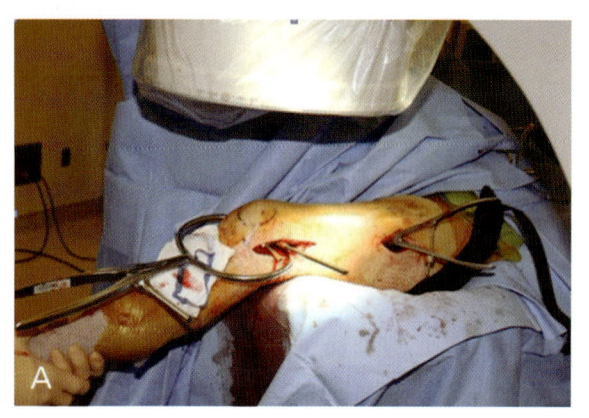

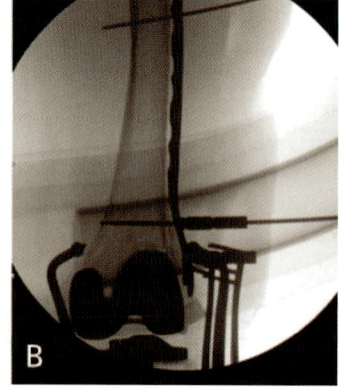

Figure 10 Clinical photograph (**A**) and radiograph (**B**) of plate inserted and stabilized with clamps. (Courtesy of Eric Johnson, MD, Los Angeles, CA.)

perils to remember are that whatever the initial locking device or fixed angle is, it must be parallel to the joint surface in the AP plane, and on the lateral plane the plate must sit flush to the lateral condylar face in its upper half. Should this not occur, the plate will tend to lie externally rotated on the distal block; thus, when attached to the femur, it will cause internal rotation of the distal fragment.

The next important aspect is the maintenance of length and rotation. Length must be obtained by traction. This may be manual, through an assistant, or with some form of distractor placed in the proximal femur in the AP plane and usually placed on the medial side into the extra-articular block. By distracting the distal fragment, reduction of length and, in fact, alignment can be obtained and rotation corrected (**Figure 9**). Another option is to place one distractor pin through a distal plate hole after the plate has been applied distally and a shaft pin proximal to the end of the plate on the lateral surface of the femur. It is extremely important to ensure that correct rotation is obtained when the plate is applied. This may mean placing a provisional screw, checking rotation, and then realigning the femur again.

Plate Insertion

The plates may be inserted percutaneously or through an open technique, according to the surgeon's preference. The open technique is accomplished through a lateral approach to the femur, with anterior displacement of the vastus lateralis. Care must be taken not to violate the medial aspect of the femur or the fracture site. Only the lateral cortex is exposed to allow placement of the plate.

In the percutaneous method, the plate is inserted through a small incision—through the anterolateral or small lateral incision and/or a second proximal incision. Most plates now have jigs that may be attached to allow percutaneous placement of the proximal screws as well as the distal screws. The plate is first passed up along the bone's lateral cortex in a submuscular tunnel. At this time, the surgeon should make sure that the track for the plate has been set by a periosteal elevator or specific plate guide so that it is not too anterior or posterior. This is important because it will be difficult to rotate the plate later on due to soft-tissue entrapment of the plate. When the plate is passed, it should be placed on the bone and the bone should be felt as the plate is passed up the shaft, to avoid malposition.

Chapter 64: Surgical Fixation of Fractures of the Distal Femur

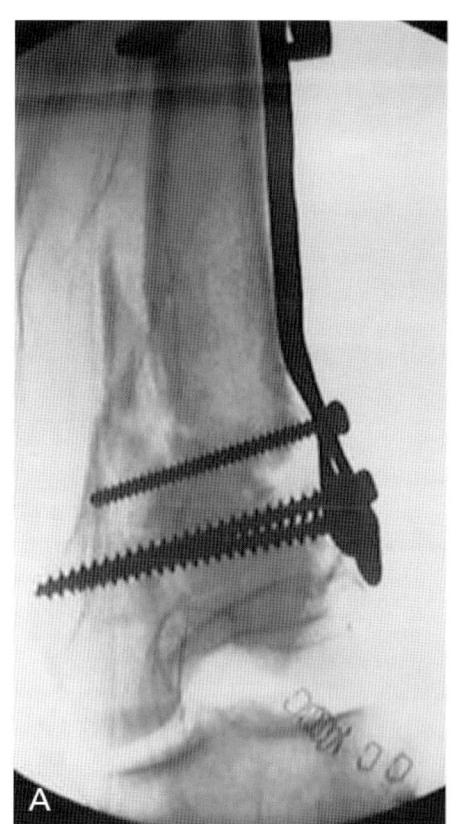

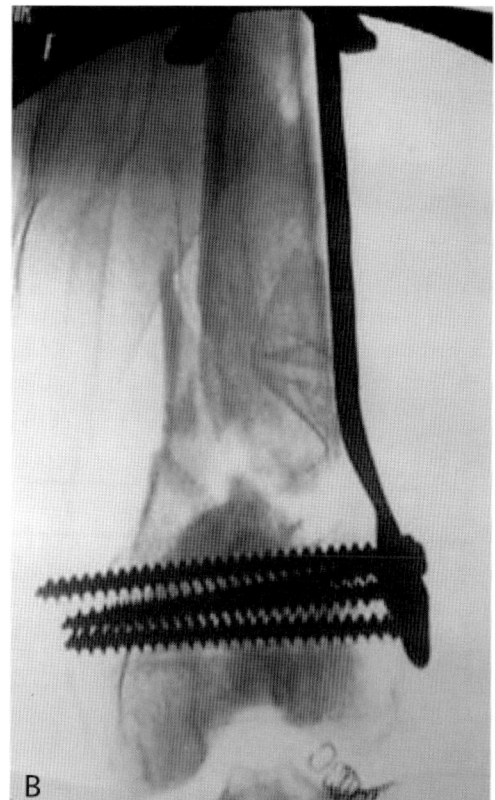

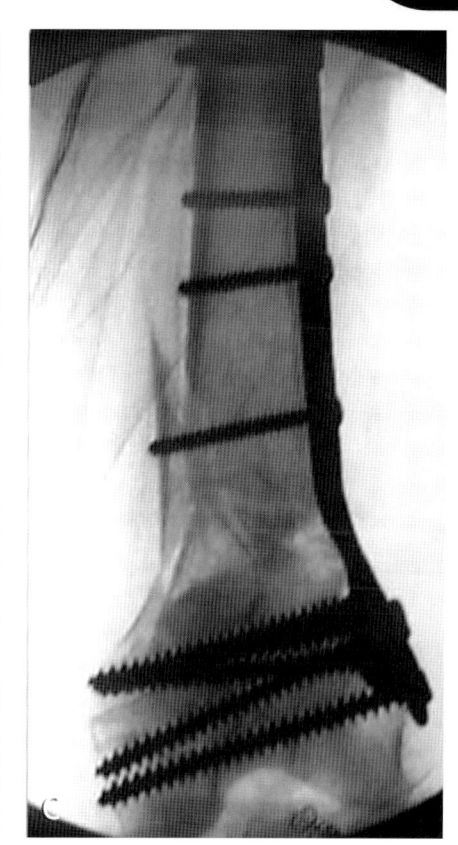

Figure 11 The importance of length in reestablishing axial alignment. **A,** Very short; **B,** short; and **C,** correct. (Radiographs courtesy of Eric Johnson, MD, Los Angeles, CA.)

This must be checked with the C-arm in both the AP and lateral planes. In the AP view, as long as the plate appears to be running along the lateral cortex and does not appear inside the cortex, it is safe to say it is on the lateral cortex. Once the plate has been passed proximally, it is affixed distally with a guidewire parallel to the joint surface.

Now, with the use of traction, the extra-articular component is reduced. At this time, it is important that the plate is provisionally fixed proximally with a 3.2-mm K-wire inserted into the most proximal plate hole, ensuring that the plate is centered on the lateral cortex (**Figure 10**). This can be done by visualizing the plate through a small muscle-splitting incision over the proximal end of the plate or percutaneously with a 3.2-mm K-wire or drill, ensuring that the wire or drill penetrates two distinct cortices and that the C-arm image confirms the plate is on the lateral cortex of the femur. The reduction is now checked to make sure that length and rotation are correct and the plate lies along the lateral cortex throughout its complete length (**Figure 11**). The reduction is verified using the C-arm and the technique of placing a radiodense line (cautery cord) from the center of the femoral head through the center of the ankle. If the line passes through the center of the knee, the correct mechanical axis has been achieved. There is a tendency for the distal part of the fracture to sag posteriorly, so the use of a bump or triangle to reduce this displacement may be necessary. Adjusting the flexion and extension of the knee may also help with the alignment (**Figure 12**).

Once the reduction is satisfactory and has been provisionally stabilized with at least two guide pins, four to six distal locking screws are placed, followed by the proximal plate screws either through the jig or freehand with C-arm

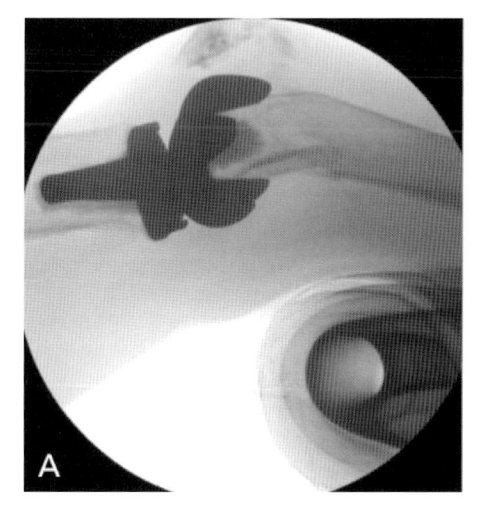

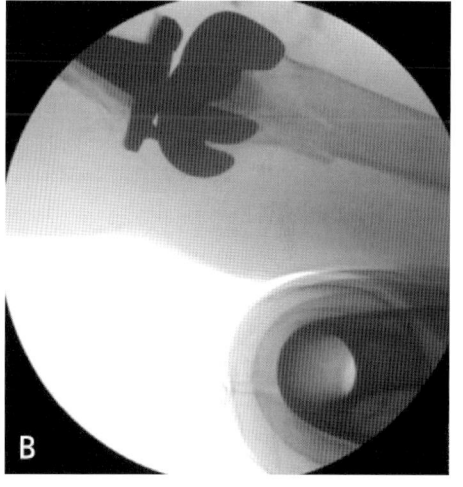

Figure 12 The importance of knee position in the reduction of the fracture. **A,** Knee in flexion, fracture apex anterior; **B,** knee extended, fracture reduced. (Courtesy of Eric Johnson, MD, Los Angeles, CA.)

assistance. There are a variety of different techniques to accomplish this; again, the implant chosen and the jigs that are used are a matter of surgeon preference. These may be nonlocking or locking, depending on the plate and the quality of the bone. If the plate is used as a reduction tool, then several nonlocking screws will be required proximally to draw the bone to the plate before any locking screws are placed, to avoid fixing the fracture in a malposition.

What must be remembered is that all nonlocking screws must be placed be-

© 2013 American Academy of Orthopaedic Surgeons

fore locking screws are placed. However, if the plate is being used as an internal fixator, the reduction will be obtained before plate application, and the plate fixed to the bone with locked screws to maintain the previously obtained reduction. It is not necessary that the plate sit on the bone in this situation, as it is acting as a fixator. The other use of locking screws is if the surgeon feels that the cortical bone is osteoporotic. In this situation, it is best to use predrilled bicortical locked screws because these enhance the fixation strength of the construct.[10,11] Generally, the distal metaphyseal block fixation consists of all locking screws, to maximize the angular stability of the distal fixation.

Complications

Complications usually occur with the inability to obtain length, alignment, or rotation. This must be checked immediately upon application of the plate to ensure that it is correct, and, if it is not, the reduction must be corrected. Placement of the plate too far posterior will tend to lead to varus misalignment and malrotation. Placement of the percutaneous screws must be bicortical. Should the plate be too anterior or posterior, these screws may be unicortical and cut out, leading to early fixation failure. This can be prevented by making sure on the lateral view that the guide holes of the insertion jig and the plate holes are perfectly aligned on the lateral cortex by getting perfect circles in the plate screw holes and ensuring that there is cortex above and below the plate on the C-arm image. This may also be checked by palpation through a small stab incision or open incision.

With higher-energy fractures, particularly open high-energy fractures, there is a high incidence of delayed union and nonunion. Consideration may be given in these circumstances to acute or early bone-grafting procedures. With the fixed-angle devices and locked plating, it is rarely necessary to use a medial plate.

Joint arthrofibrosis is uncommon unless the knee is immobilized and not allowed early active motion.

Postoperative Care and Rehabilitation

Postoperatively, the patients may be immobilized in a knee immobilizer for comfort for several days. They should be encouraged at this time to do static isometric quadriceps exercises and straight-leg raising. When the patient is comfortable, at 3 to 5 days, it is reasonable to remove the knee immobilizer and start active-assisted range of motion of the knee. The patient should be mobilized with a walker or crutches and can be weight-of-leg or touch-down weight bearing. Full weight bearing should not be instituted until healing is seen, between 3 and 4 months. The most important aspect of this stage is recovery of the range of motion. Also critical is that as the patient becomes more comfortable, strengthening of the thigh musculature is worked on as well. The use of continuous passive motion is another technique that can be used. This should be applied in the recovery room with the patient somewhat sedated and allowed to move between 0° to 45°. This can be increased rapidly, so that 90° of flexion should be obtained within 3 to 5 days. Thromboembolic prophylaxis is used while in the hospital and is a matter of surgeon choice, depending on patient mobility at the time of discharge.[13,14]

Pearls

- The distal intra-articular femoral fracture demands anatomic axial alignment with a precise reduction of the articular surface.
- Potential problems facing surgeons are high-energy injury, joint damage, and osteoporotic bone.
- It is imperative to identify whether the fracture lines enter the joint, especially on the lateral projection, where coronal plane fractures of the either the medial or lateral condyle (Hoffa fracture) must be ruled out with CT.
- These fractures are complex and require excellent preoperative planning and experienced surgical acumen.
- The surgical approach is determined by the need to reduce the articular surface.
- After articular reduction, the most important aspect is to reconstitute the normal anatomic and mechanical axes of the distal femur.
- During fracture stabilization, it is important not to violate the medial aspect of the femur or fracture site.

References

1. Gwathmey FW Jr, Jones-Quaidoo SM, Kahler D, Hurwitz S, Cui Q: Distal femoral fractures: Current concepts. *J Am Acad Orthop Surg* 2010;18(10):597-607.
2. Jahangir AA, Cross WW, Schmidt AH: Current management of distal femoral fractures. *Curr Orthop Pract* 2010;21(2):193-197.
3. Kolb W, Guhlmann H, Windisch C, Marx F, Koller H, Kolb K: Fixation of periprosthetic femur fractures above total knee arthroplasty with the less invasive stabilization system: A midterm follow-up study. *J Trauma* 2010;69(3):670-676.
4. Johnstone A, Carnegie C, Christie E, McCullough A: The challenges associated with treating distal femoral fractures with locking plates in the elderly: Differing patterns of failure with different locking plates. *J Bone Joint Surg Br* 2010;92(suppl 4):550.
5. Wähnert D, Hoffmeier KL, von Oldenburg G, Fröber R, Hofmann GO, Mückley T: Internal fixation of type-C distal femoral fractures in osteoporotic bone. *J Bone Joint Surg Am* 2010;92(6):1442-1452.
6. Platzer P, Schuster R, Aldrian S, et al: Management and outcome of periprosthetic fractures after total knee arthroplasty. *J Trauma* 2010;68(6):1464-1470.
7. Horwitz DS, Kubiak EN: Surgical treatment of osteoporotic fractures about the knee. *J Bone Joint Surg Am* 2009;91(12):2970-2982.
8. Nork SE, Segina DN, Aflatoon K, et al: The association between supracondylar-intercondylar distal femoral fractures and coronal plane fractures. *J Bone Joint Surg Am* 2005;87(3):564-569.
9. Kao FC, Tu YK, Su JY, Hsu KY, Wu CH, Chou MC: Treatment of distal femoral fracture by minimally invasive percutaneous plate osteosynthesis: Comparison between the dynamic condylar screw and the less invasive stabilization system. *J Trauma* 2009;67(4):719-726.
10. Schütz M, Müller M, Regazzoni P, et al: Use of the less invasive stabilization system (LISS) in patients with distal femoral (AO33) fractures: A prospective multicenter study. *Arch Orthop Trauma Surg* 2005;125(2):102-108.
11. Kregor PJ, Stannard JA, Zlowodzki M, Cole PA: Treatment of distal femur fractures using the less invasive stabilization system: Surgical experience and early clinical results in 103 fractures. *J Orthop Trauma* 2004;18(8):509-520.
12. Zlowodzki M, Williamson S, Cole PA, Zardiackas LD, Kregor PJ: Biomechanical evaluation of the less invasive stabilization system, angled blade plate, and retrograde intramedullary nail for the internal fixation of distal femur fractures. *J Orthop Trauma* 2004;18(8):494-502.
13. Rademakers MV, Kerkhoffs GM, Sierevelt IN, Raaymakers EL, Marti RK: Intra-articular fractures of the distal femur: A long-term follow-up study of surgically treated patients. *J Orthop Trauma* 2004;18(4):213-219.
14. Vincent A, Sharr J, Cockfield A, Bates P: LLSS fixation of distal femoral fractures. *J Bone Joint Surg Br* 2009;91:341.

Chapter 65
Open Reduction and Internal Fixation of Tibial Plateau Fractures

James A. Goulet, MD   Mark E. Hake, MD

Introduction
Fractures of the tibial plateau are challenging injuries. These fractures involve the joint surface and metaphysis of the proximal tibia and occur as a result of both high-energy and low-energy mechanisms. The severity of injury to the bone and surrounding soft tissue should be considered when deciding on the optimal course of treatment. Goals include anatomic reduction of the articular surface, restoration of the mechanical axis, stable fixation that allows early range of motion (ROM), preservation of the surrounding soft tissues, and avoidance of infection. Ligamentous repair or reconstruction also may be required to obtain a good outcome.

Patient Selection
Careful examination of the injured extremity is mandatory. Vascular injury, compartment syndrome, and open injuries should be noted and treated emergently. Knee stability and the condition of the soft-tissue envelope are vital in determining the imaging needed and timing involved in treatment.

Indications
Absolute indications for open treatment include fractures that are open or associated with compartment syndrome or vascular injury. Relative indications include fractures that cause joint instability or malalignment, medial condylar fractures, lateral plateau fractures with displacement greater than 3 mm, and condylar widening greater than 5 mm.[1,2] Fractures in the patient with multiple traumatic injuries also are more likely to be treated surgically to facilitate mobility. In general, fractures with less than 3 mm of displacement at the joint surface and with normal alignment and a stable knee in extension can be considered for closed treatment.

Contraindications
With all fractures, the patient's medical comorbidities and baseline activity level must be considered. Open treatment should be delayed until the surrounding soft tissues have been given adequate time to heal. Appropriate delay has been clearly shown to reduce the rate of wound breakdown and infection.[3,4] Temporary early external fixation should be applied in cases of gross instability or severe soft-tissue injury until definitive fixation can be performed. The goals of treatment have evolved to prioritize maintaining the viability of the soft tissues and preserving vascularity surrounding the fracture. Using indirect reduction techniques to restore limb alignment while obtaining anatomic reduction of the articular surface has been shown to lead to favorable outcomes.

Alternative Treatments
Some debate exists regarding the optimal treatment of bicondylar fractures. Given historically poor outcomes due to high rates of infection, alternative techniques have been explored. Small-wire external ring fixators have been shown to be a potential alternative to traditional open reduction and internal fixation (ORIF). A recent Level I study that compared this method with ORIF showed comparable outcomes with fewer complications than with ORIF.[5] The advent of locked plating led to the idea that bicondylar fractures could be stabilized by a single, laterally placed locked construct. Although several studies support this idea, a recent biomechanical study showed that dual plating allows less subsidence of the medial plateau than does a single, laterally based locked plate.[6] Bicortical screw placement used with a locking construct provides a stiffer construct with a higher maximum load compared with unicortical placement.[7]

Closed reduction and percutaneous fixation is an option for minimally displaced lateral split fractures with minimal joint surface comminution. Injury or incarceration of the lateral meniscus should be ruled out preoperatively with MRI. The reduction is obtained with a varus force or a laterally based femoral distractor. The reduction is maintained with large reduction forceps while two to three screws are placed to provide compression across the fracture. A small antiglide plate may be used in the setting of metaphyseal comminution or in patients with poor bone quality.

Arthroscopically assisted reduction and internal fixation may be beneficial for certain types of tibial plateau fractures with an intact or restorable cortical envelope. Although high-quality studies comparing outcomes of this technique with ORIF are lacking, cited benefits include minimal soft-tissue dissection, better visualization of reduction compared with open techniques, and the ability to diagnose and repair intra-articular soft-tissue injuries.[8] Shorter hospital stays and faster rehabilitation times also have been reported.[9]

Classification
The fracture pattern and severity of the soft-tissue injury will guide the decision about the optimal approach to use for reduction and stabilization. The two main classification systems used today describe the fracture pattern but do not take into account ligamentous injury or damage to the soft-tissue envelope, nor are they predictive of outcomes. The system described by Schatzker et al[10] divides fractures into six types. In general, types I, II, and III are low-energy injuries that involve the lateral plateau, and types IV, V, and VI involve a higher energy mechanism and medial condyle or bicondylar injury. The AO/OTA system classifies these fractures into extra-articular, partial articular, and complete articular, with further subdivisions based on the severity of the fracture.

Preoperative Imaging
Plain radiographs of the injured knee, including AP and lateral views, are

---

Dr. Goulet or an immediate family member has received royalties from Zimmer; is a member of a speakers' bureau or has made paid presentations on behalf of Smith & Nephew; has stock or stock options held in Pioneer Surgical Technology; and serves as a board member, owner, officer, or committee member of the American Orthopaedic Association, the Orthopaedic Trauma Association, and the Michigan Orthopaedic Society. Neither Dr. Hake nor any immediate family member has received anything of value from or has stock or stock options held in a commercial company or institution related directly or indirectly to the subject of this chapter.

obtained, along with internal and external rotation oblique views. An AP view with the beam directed 10° caudal shows displacement at the articular surface most clearly. CT with sagittal and coronal reconstructions has been shown to affect the surgical plan in many cases because articular depression can be difficult to evaluate on plain radiographs[11] (**Figure 1**). Obtaining preoperative MRI to evaluate for soft-tissue injury has become more common. Meniscal and ligamentous injuries have been shown to be common even in low-energy injuries. In a recent series of closed fractures evaluated arthroscopically, soft-tissue injuries were found in 70 of 98 cases (71%).[12] Meniscal injuries occurred with all fracture types, whereas anterior cruciate ligament tears were more common in Schatzker type IV and VI fractures. MRI is helpful to evaluate the need for ligamentous repair or reconstruction before hardware is placed.

Video 65.1 Open Reduction and Internal Fixation of Tibial Plateau Fractures. Mark E. Hake, MD; James A. Goulet, MD (21 min)

Procedure
Approaches

Many options have been described for treating low-energy and high-energy tibial plateau fractures. The anterolateral approach can be used for the most common types of these fractures. The anterolateral approach is used for ORIF of lateral plateau fractures (Schatzker types I, II, and III) as well as for fixation of the lateral plateau when using a dual-incision technique to repair bicondylar fractures. The Lobenhoffer posteromedial approach is used when fixation of the medial plateau is required. A posteromedial fragment has been shown to be present in approximately one third of AO/OTA C-type bicondylar tibial plateau fractures.[13] The Lobenhoffer approach, when used in combination with the anterolateral approach, leaves a wide skin bridge and provides sufficient soft-tissue coverage of the hardware, so later removal is rarely required.

Approaches that are required only rarely include the direct posterior approach, which is used for treating posterior shear–type injuries that are not accessible from the anterolateral or Lobenhoffer approaches.[14] We recommend against using a direct anterior approach with tibial tubercle osteotomy because it is associated with a high rate of nonunion.

Room Setup/Patient Positioning

Most patients treated with a single-incision or dual-incision technique can be placed supine on a radiolucent table. A high thigh tourniquet is placed. A radiolucent triangle is placed under the injured knee to facilitate access to the lateral plateau and aid in obtaining high-quality AP and lateral fluoroscopic images during the procedure. The C-arm is brought in from the contralateral side of the table. When using the Lobenhoffer approach, we prefer to place the patient prone, although a supine position also has been described.[15]

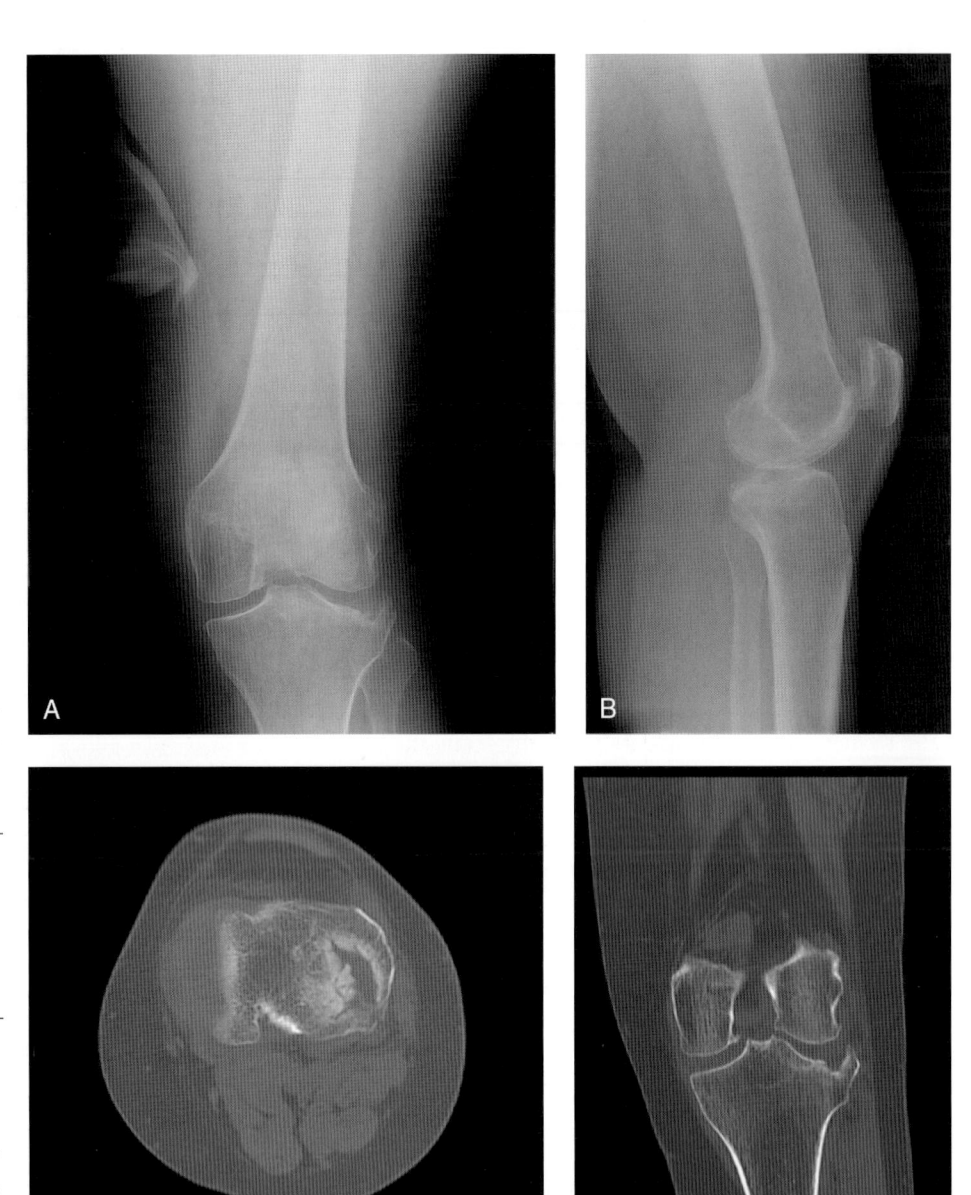

Figure 1 Schatzker type III tibial plateau fracture. AP (**A**) and lateral (**B**) radiographs. Axial (**C**) and coronal (**D**) CT cuts demonstrate a severe articular depression with no associated split in the cortex.

Special Instruments/Equipment/Implants

Several specialized instruments can be helpful when performing ORIF of tibial plateau fractures. A femoral distractor can prove useful for direct visualization of the joint surface, which is helpful when confirming adequate reduction. The distractor can be applied after a submeniscal arthrotomy is performed to confirm reduction of the fractured fragments. In many cases, the distractor provides axial traction to aid in reduction. If a femoral distractor is not available, a standard external fixator can be used in the same fashion to distract across the joint.

When an isolated depression of the joint surface is present, a cortical window is required to elevate the articular cartilage. This window can be created with a 2-mm drill and an osteotome. We have found that using a cannulated reamer from a hip compression screw set is useful for this purpose. The guidewire can be directed from the metaphysis directly at the depressed segment for accurate placement of the window. A curved bone tamp is used to reduce the displaced fragments. To fill the remaining defect, bone graft or a bone graft substitute is required to support the reduction. Autologous iliac crest bone graft was long considered the gold standard for this purpose, although it is associated with significant donor-site pain.[16,17] Alternatives such as allograft bone and calcium phosphate cement have largely supplanted autologous bone graft. Recent reports have shown that repairs with calcium phosphate cement have less subsidence and higher fatigue strength than autologous bone graft.[18] We typically use crushed cancellous allograft for this purpose because of its availability and ease of use.

Surgical Technique
Anterolateral Approach

The anterolateral approach is used for ORIF of the lateral plateau in Schatzker type I, II, and III fractures, which represent most tibial plateau fractures. It also is used in combination with a posteromedial approach when using a dual-incision technique to treat bicondylar fractures. Surgical treatment should be delayed until swelling has reduced and the soft-tissue envelope has been allowed time to heal.

The standard setup described previously is used. The incision is centered on the Gerdy tubercle in a lazy S fashion (**Figure 2**); a hockey stick–shaped incision also is commonly used. The incision is made midaxially at the joint line and sweeps anterior to run 1 to 2 cm lateral to the tibial crest. Proximally, the iliotibial band is cut in line with its fibers. The fascia over the anterior compartment is incised, and the tibialis anterior is elevated off the metaphysis gently using a Cobb elevator. A small cuff of fascia is left attached to the tibia to facilitate closure. It is helpful to use a Z-shaped retractor to put tension on the tibialis anterior while performing this step. At this point, the distal joint line can be palpated or found using a needle. A submeniscal arthrotomy is performed, taking great care not to injure the meniscus. The arthrotomy should involve only the anterior aspect of the joint, and care must be taken not to involve the lateral collateral ligament, which runs posterior to the lateral epicondyle of the femur to insert on the fibular head. A small portion of the coronary ligament should be left attached to the plateau to aid in later meniscal repair. Placement of a full-thickness stitch through the peripheral portion of the meniscus will aid in retraction and improve visualization of the joint surface (**Figure 3, A** and **B**).

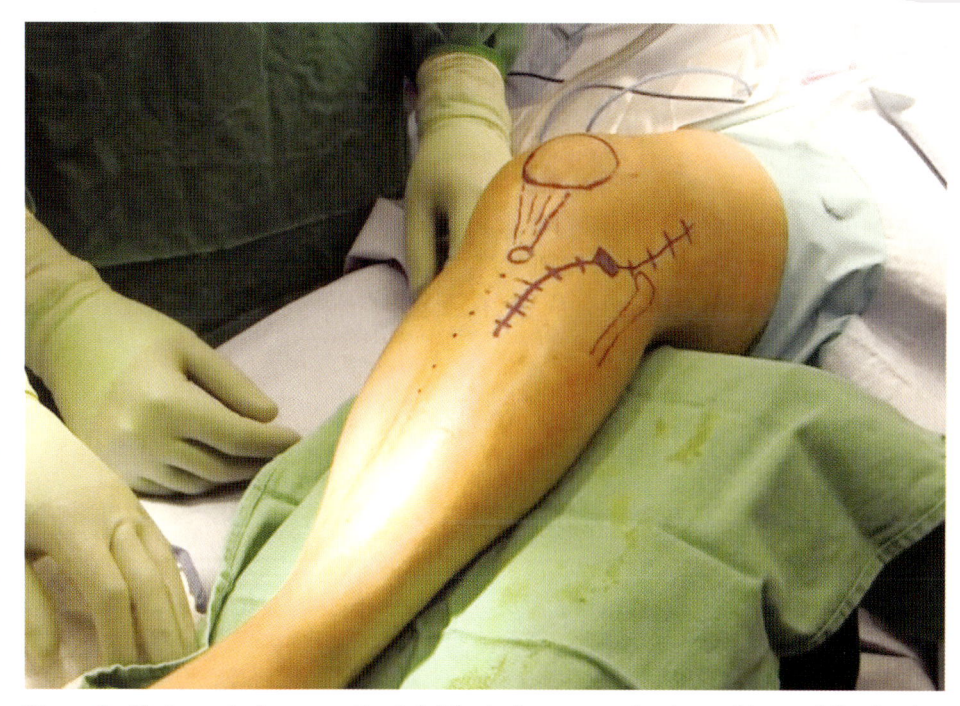

Figure 2 Photograph shows a patient's left leg before open reduction and internal fixation for a tibial plateau fracture. The leg is draped and the anterolateral incision is indicated, centered over the Gerdy tubercle. The patella, patellar tendon, tibial tubercle, and fibular head are drawn. A radiolucent triangle has been placed under the knee to aid in accessing the fracture and relaxing the collateral ligaments.

A femoral distractor can be applied, which provides an even greater view of the joint surface (**Figure 3, C**). Two Schanz pins are placed on either side of the joint. The proximal Schanz pin is placed in the lateral femoral metaphysis, parallel to the joint line. A second pin is placed in the lateral tibial shaft. This pin should be placed distal to the end of the plate that will be placed later. The distractor is then assembled posterior to the knee so that it does not interfere with visualization or imaging. It can be lengthened to provide up to 1 cm of additional distraction at the joint for improved visualization.

The next step depends on the type of fracture being treated. If only a simple lateral split exists, the fracture can be reduced and hardware placed. We typically use a precontoured plate for lateral plateau fixation because it is low profile and allows a row of rafting screws to be placed under the joint surface for support. Another advantage of this periarticular plate is the row of small holes for suture at the proximal end that facilitates closure of the submeniscal arthrotomy. Most patients will do well with a nonlocking plate. A locking construct may benefit patients with osteoporotic bone, although definite indications remain unclear. When using locked plates, one or two nonlocking screws should be placed first to provide interfragmentary compression.

When the fracture involves compression of the joint surface and a lateral split, the split portion of the fracture can be opened like a book to gain access to the compressed fragments. These fragments are then reduced to the joint surface. This should be performed from below the fragments and not through the defect in the articular surface. The depressed portion can be made to sit slightly proud to the intact joint. The void created is filled with bone graft or bone graft substitute. The split is closed and reduced, and the periarticular plate is placed. It is crucial in this step to place the row of rafting screws in the subchondral bone to support the repaired joint surface. Screws can be placed outside the plate if this will provide better support. If the proximal suture holes will be used to close the arthrotomy, suture should be placed through these holes before fixation of the plate (**Figure 3, D**).

Section 5: Trauma

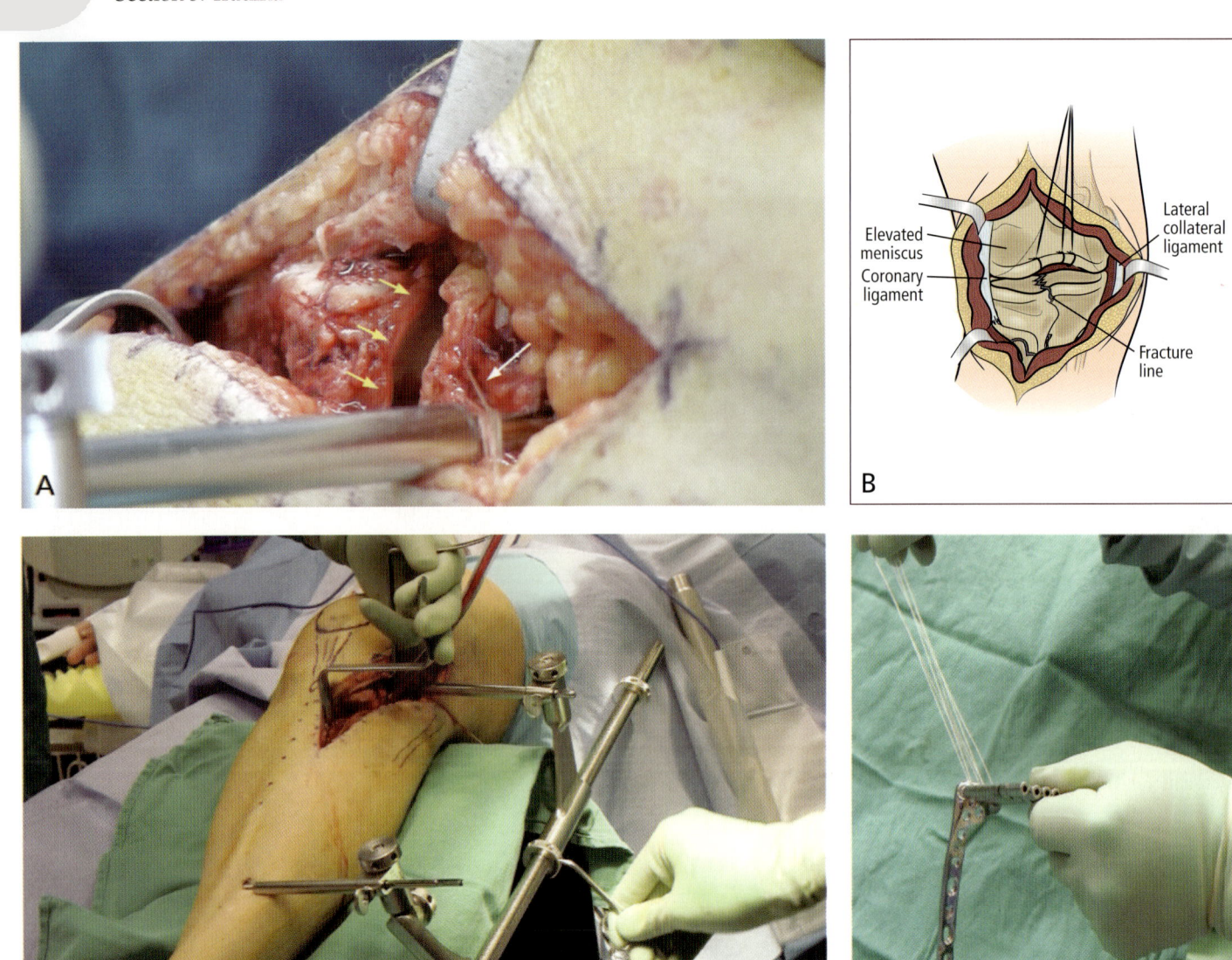

Figure 3 Open reduction and internal fixation (ORIF) of a lateral tibial plateau fracture via the anterolateral approach. **A,** Intraoperative photograph shows exposure for the ORIF. A submeniscal arthrotomy is made to allow direct evaluation of the joint surface. Care must be taken to not injure the lateral meniscus or lateral collateral ligament. The yellow arrows show a small cuff of the coronary ligament that is left on the tibia for closure. The white arrow highlights stay sutures that are placed for retraction of the meniscus. A headlamp may be required to visualize the joint surface. **B,** Illustration shows the submeniscal arthrotomy and fracture line running through the joint. **C,** Intraoperative photograph shows a femoral distractor in place on the lateral side of the patient's left knee. The main portion of the distractor remains posterior to the leg so that it does not interfere with access to or imaging of the fracture site. **D,** Photograph of a periarticular locking plate with sutures placed in the proximal small holes before application. These sutures will be used to close the submeniscal arthrotomy.

A cortical window can also be used to reduce areas of joint depression in Schatzker type III fractures. This technique is also used when a split is nondisplaced or when hinging it open would require extensive dissection of intact bone and periosteum. Traditionally, the window was made by drilling 2-mm holes in a diamond pattern and using an osteotome to break through the cortex. We prefer to use a cannulated reamer for this purpose (**Figure 4**). A guide pin is directed from the anterolateral metaphysis at the depressed joint surface. Fluoroscopy is used to confirm the location. A reamer is then used to ream up to the depressed fragments. Care should be taken to not damage pieces of the joint surface that have been depressed deep into the subchondral bone. A curved bone tamp is directed up to reduce the joint surface, and the remaining void is filled with allograft bone or cement (**Figure 5**). When using either technique, the surgeon should choose a plate that bypasses the window to stabilize this area (**Figure 6**).

Closure is performed in layers, beginning with the arthrotomy. The fascia is closed with interrupted braided, absorbable suture. We typically place a drain under the fascia. To ensure that the drain can be removed easily, the distal 2 cm of the drain is initially left extending from the distal portion of the fascial incision. Once the fascia is closed completely, the drain is pulled so that the distal end lies under the fascia. The skin is closed with a layer of deep dermal suture, followed by 2-0 nylon.

Lobenhoffer Approach

Schatzker type IV fractures with primarily posteromedial fragments (**Figure 7**) can be difficult to reduce and stabilize from a lateral or medial approach. The Lobenhoffer approach, first described in 2003, is used to access the medial plateau and is ideal for treating these fractures.

The patient is placed prone and the limb is exsanguinated. The incision runs along the border of the medial head of the gastrocnemius, extending from the joint line proximally for 6 to 8 cm (**Figure 8, A**). Once the fascia of the medial

Chapter 65: Open Reduction and Internal Fixation of Tibial Plateau Fractures

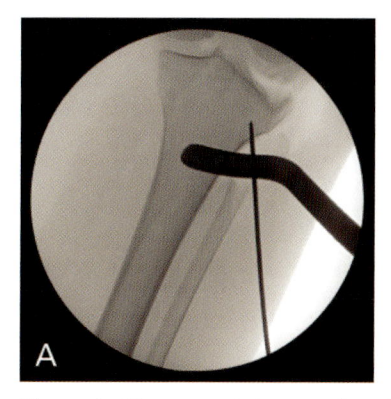

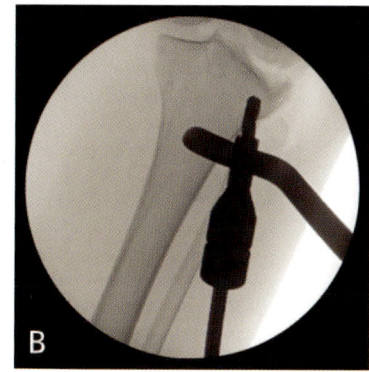

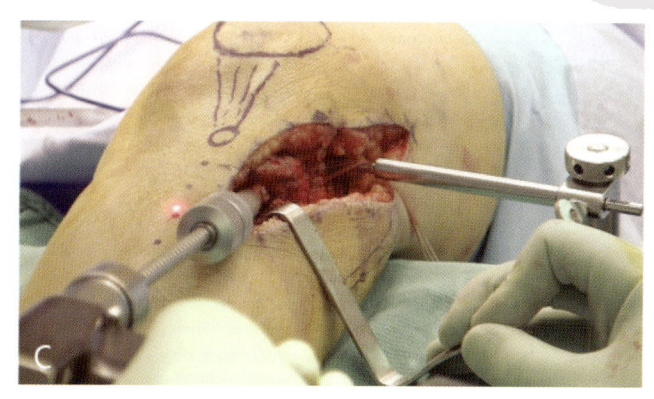

Figure 4 Fluoroscopic images show the creation of a cortical window for reduction of the joint surface. **A**, A guide pin is directed at the depressed fragments of the articular surface. **B**, A reamer is used to create a cortical window. **C**, Intraoperative photograph shows the cannulated reamer being directed toward the depression.

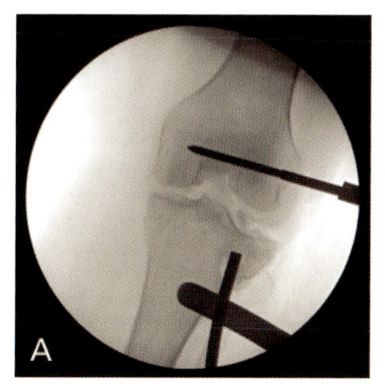

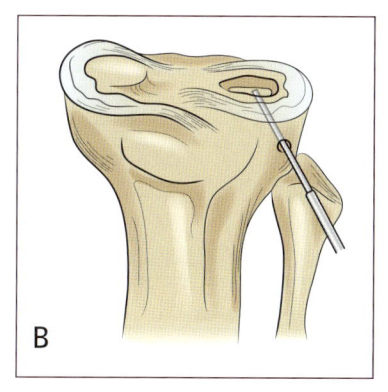

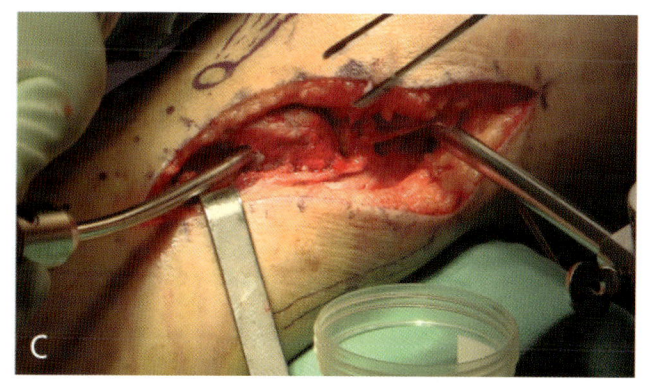

Figure 5 Reduction of area of fracture depression in a Schatzker type III tibial plateau fracture. AP fluoroscopic image (**A**) and illustration (**B**) depict a bone tamp being used to elevate the depressed fragments of the articular surface. **C**, Intraoperative photograph shows allograft cancellous bone being placed through the window to fill the void left in the metaphysis.

head of the gastrocnemius is incised, the pes anserinus tendons should be seen in the proximal portion of the wound. These tendons can be retracted anteriorly or, alternatively, released and later repaired at the end of the procedure. Blunt dissection between the medial gastrocnemius and the pes anserinus is taken down to the popliteus, which is released gently from the fragment in a subperiosteal fashion to reveal the fracture (**Figure 8, B** and **C**). A submeniscal arthrotomy is rarely needed with this approach because an anatomic reduction can be obtained using only visualization of the distal fracture line. Reduction of the fracture is aided by extension of the knee, axial traction, and an anteriorly directed force on the fracture fragment. A T-plate placed in an antiglide fashion will stabilize the fracture (**Figure 9**). The gastrocnemius, fascia, and skin can then be closed in layers.

Complications and Results

Complications are uncommon following surgical fixation of low-energy injuries, so recent studies focus on complex bicondylar fractures. In the past, the most common major complication associated with these injuries was deep infection. The in-

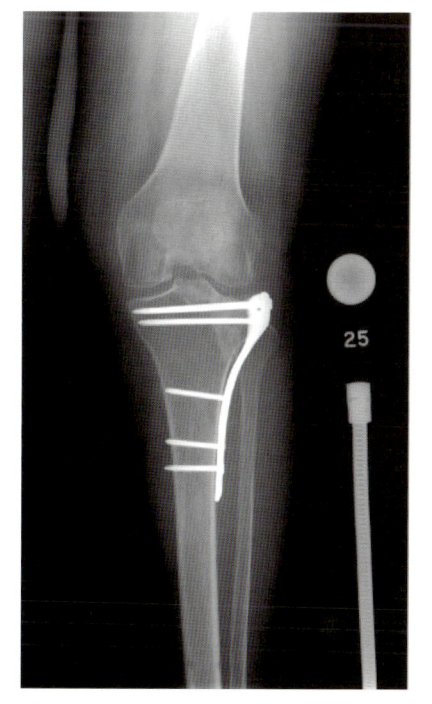

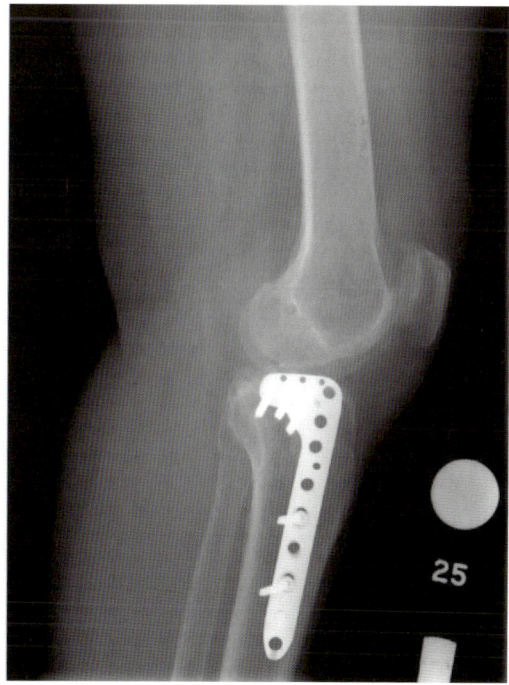

Figure 6 Postoperative AP (**A**) and lateral (**B**) radiographs demonstrate open reduction and internal fixation of a Schatzker type III tibial plateau fracture. A periarticular locking plate with a row of rafting screws is used to support the articular reduction. Note that the distal aspect of the plate bypasses the cortical window.

cidence of deep infection was reported to be as high as 80% when early definitive fixation and extensive soft-tissue dissec-

tion were performed.[19] With a better understanding of the injury, time allowed for recovery of the soft-tissue envelope,

© 2013 American Academy of Orthopaedic Surgeons

Section 5: Trauma

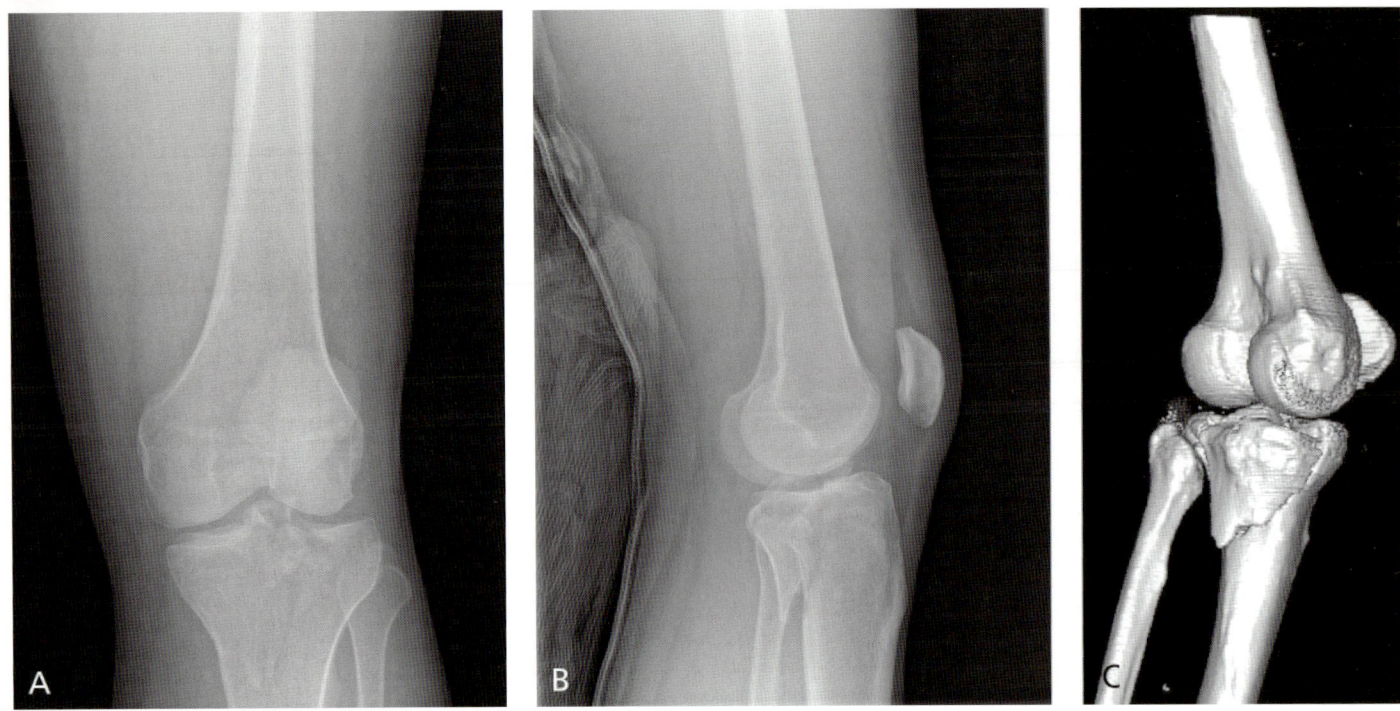

Figure 7 Schatzker type IV tibial plateau fracture. AP (**A**) and lateral (**B**) radiographs. **C**, Three-dimensional CT reconstruction demonstrates a large posteromedial fragment. The apex exits posterolaterally; therefore, a posterior plate will best buttress this fracture.

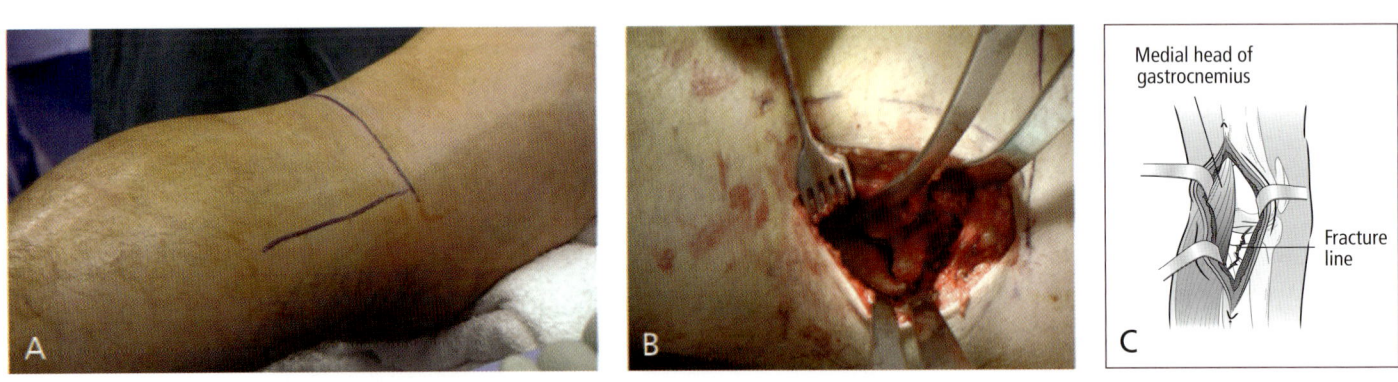

Figure 8 The Lobenhoffer approach for open reduction and internal fixation of a tibial plateau fracture. **A**, Photograph depicts the incision (solid longitudinal line) drawn on the patient's left leg. The patient is prone, and the head is to the right. The incision extends distally over the swollen calf from the joint line. It is 6 to 8 cm in length and runs along the border of the medial head of the gastrocnemius. **B**, Intraoperative photograph shows a posteromedial fragment visualized through the Lobenhoffer approach. The patient's head is to the right, and the foot is to the left. The upper retractors are on the posterior border of the tibia and are retracting the medial head of the gastrocnemius. **C**, Illustration shows the fracture with the anatomy and posteromedial fragment visualized through the Lobenhoffer approach.

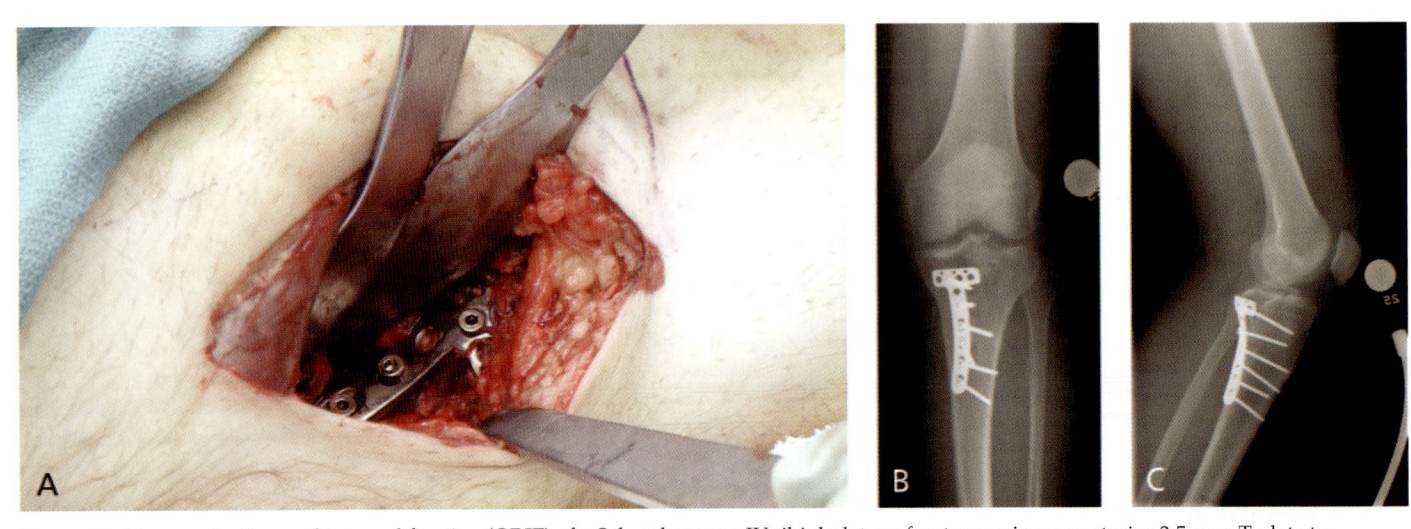

Figure 9 Open reduction and internal fixation (ORIF) of a Schatzker type IV tibial plateau fracture using a posterior 3.5-mm T-plate to buttress the posteromedial fragment. **A**, Intraoperative photograph shows the T-plate. Four screws are placed distal to the fracture, and two screws are placed across the fracture line in a lag fashion. Postoperative AP (**B**) and lateral (**C**) radiographs show the completed fixation.

and less invasive fixation methods, the incidence of wound complications has decreased significantly. Using a dual-incision technique with an average time to definitive treatment of 9.2 days, Barei et al[20] reported a deep infection rate of 8.4%. Infection rates generally are higher when compartment releases are performed. Union rates are approximately 95% regardless of the fixation method used. Malunion can occur with subsidence at the joint surface or with the loss of anatomic alignment at the fracture site, especially in the sagittal plane.[21] The rate of deep venous thrombosis has been reported to be 20% in high-energy fractures.[20]

Recent outcomes data have been encouraging. Rademakers et al[22] reported on 202 consecutive tibial plateau fractures, of which 69% were unicondylar and 31% bicondylar. At 1 year, the nonunion rate was 5% and the mean knee ROM was 130°. Just over half (54%) of the patients had a long-term follow-up at a mean of 14 years. Patients in this group with unicondylar fractures had statistically better results. Secondary arthritis developed in 31% of the patients, but this was well tolerated. Barei et al[4] used a dual-incision technique to treat 83 bicondylar tibial plateau fractures. Of these patients, 51% completed a Musculoskeletal Function Assessment (MFA) questionnaire, with a mean follow-up of 59 months. Patient age and the presence of multiple injuries were associated with a worse MFA score. A satisfactory articular reduction (<2 mm) was associated with a better MFA score. A standardized protocol with temporary spanning external fixation and delayed definitive treatment was used by Egol et al[3] to treat 57 high-energy tibial plateau fractures, 16 of which were open. The mean follow-up was 15.7 months. Definitive treatment took place at a mean of 15 days after the injury. The deep infection rate was 5%, and the nonunion rate was 4%. The mean knee ROM was 1° to 106°.

Postoperative Care and Rehabilitation

Patients are placed in a long-leg splint for comfort postoperatively. On postoperative day 1, the splint is removed and a hinged knee brace is placed. The brace is unlocked to encourage early ROM. Drains typically are removed on postoperative day 1 or 2. Patients remain toe-touch weight bearing for a total of 12 weeks. Early gentle ROM is encouraged under the supervision of a physical therapist. At 6 weeks, the knee brace is removed. The loss of muscle mass surrounding the knee can limit progress in these patients. We typically progress with low-stress strengthening exercises. Aquatic therapy and low-resistance stationary bike use are initiated after suture removal to help strengthen the injured extremity without putting excessive stress across the fracture site. When the Lobenhoffer approach is used, regaining full extension should be a main focus of rehabilitation.

Pearls

- The severity of injury to the bone and surrounding soft tissue should be considered when deciding on the optimal course of treatment.
- Relative indications include fractures that cause joint instability, most bicondylar and medial condylar fractures, lateral plateau fractures with displacement greater than 3 mm, and condylar widening greater than 5 mm.
- Temporary early external fixation should be applied in cases of gross instability or severe soft-tissue injury until definitive fixation can be performed.
- Evaluating for ligamentous injury in Schatzker type IV fractures with MRI before internal hardware is placed can guide surgical treatment.
- A femoral distractor can aid in reduction as well as visualization of the articular surface.
- A cannulated reamer can be used to make a cortical window in the tibial metaphysis to allow reduction of the depressed fragments with a bone tamp.

References

1. Honkonen SE: Indications for surgical treatment of tibial condyle fractures. *Clin Orthop Relat Res* 1994;302:199-205.
2. Brown TD, Anderson DD, Nepola JV, Singerman RJ, Pedersen DR, Brand RA: Contact stress aberrations following imprecise reduction of simple tibial plateau fractures. *J Orthop Res* 1988;6(6):851-862.
3. Egol KA, Tejwani NC, Capla EL, Wolinsky PL, Koval KJ: Staged management of high-energy proximal tibia fractures (OTA types 41): The results of a prospective, standardized protocol. *J Orthop Trauma* 2005;19(7):448-456.
4. Barei DP, Nork SE, Mills WJ, Coles CP, Henley MB, Benirschke SK: Functional outcomes of severe bicondylar tibial plateau fractures treated with dual incisions and medial and lateral plates. *J Bone Joint Surg Am* 2006;88(8):1713-1721.
5. Canadian Orthopaedic Trauma Society: Open reduction and internal fixation compared with circular fixator application for bicondylar tibial plateau fractures: Results of a multicenter, prospective, randomized clinical trial. *J Bone Joint Surg Am* 2006;88(12):2613-2623.
6. Higgins TF, Klatt J, Bachus KN: Biomechanical analysis of bicondylar tibial plateau fixation: How does lateral locking plate fixation compare to dual plate fixation? *J Orthop Trauma* 2007;21(5):301-306.
7. Dougherty PJ, Kim DG, Meisterling S, Wybo C, Yeni Y: Biomechanical comparison of bicortical versus unicortical screw placement of proximal tibia locking plates: A cadaveric model. *J Orthop Trauma* 2008;22(6):399-403.
8. Buchko GM, Johnson DH: Arthroscopy assisted operative management of tibial plateau fractures. *Clin Orthop Relat Res* 1996;332:29-36.
9. Cassard X, Beaufils P, Blin JL, Hardy P: Osteosynthesis under arthroscopic control of separated tibial plateau fractures: 26 case reports [French]. *Rev Chir Orthop Reparatrice Appar Mot* 1999;85(3):257-266.
10. Schatzker J, McBroom R, Bruce D: The tibial plateau fracture: The Toronto experience 1968-1975. *Clin Orthop Relat Res* 1979;138:94-104.
11. Chan PS, Klimkiewicz JJ, Luchetti WT, et al: Impact of CT scan on treatment plan and fracture classification of tibial plateau fractures. *J Orthop Trauma* 1997;11(7):484-489.
12. Abdel-Hamid MZ, Chang CH, Chan YS, et al: Arthroscopic evaluation of soft tissue injuries in tibial plateau fractures: Retrospective analysis of 98 cases. *Arthroscopy* 2006;22(6):669-675.
13. Barei DP, O'Mara TJ, Taitsman LA, Dunbar RP, Nork SE: Frequency and fracture morphology of the posteromedial fragment in bicondylar tibial plateau fracture patterns. *J Orthop Trauma* 2008;22(3):176-182.
14. Bhattacharyya T, McCarty LP III, Harris MB, et al: The posterior shearing tibial plateau fracture: Treatment and results via a posterior approach. *J Orthop Trauma* 2005;19(5):305-310.
15. Fakler JK, Ryzewicz M, Hartshorn C, Morgan SJ, Stahel PF, Smith WR: Optimizing the management of Moore type I postero-medial split fracture dislocations of the tibial head: Description of the Lobenhoffer approach. *J Orthop Trauma* 2007;21(5):330-336.
16. Segal D, Franchi AV, Campanile J: Iliac autograft for reconstruction of severely

depressed fracture of a lateral tibial plateau: Brief note. *J Bone Joint Surg Am* 1985;67(8):1270-1272.

17. Goulet JA, Senunas LE, DeSilva GL, Greenfield ML: Autogenous iliac crest bone graft: Complications and functional assessment. *Clin Orthop Relat Res* 1997;339:76-81.

18. McDonald E, Chu T, Tufaga M, et al: Tibial plateau fracture repairs augmented with calcium phosphate cement have higher in situ fatigue strength than those with autograft. *J Orthop Trauma* 2011;25(2):90-95.

19. Mallik AR, Covall DJ, Whitelaw GP: Internal versus external fixation of bicondylar tibial plateau fractures. *Orthop Rev* 1992;21(12):1433-1436.

20. Barei DP, Nork SE, Mills WJ, Henley MB, Benirschke SK: Complications associated with internal fixation of high-energy bicondylar tibial plateau fractures utilizing a two-incision technique. *J Orthop Trauma* 2004;18(10):649-657.

21. Streubel PN, Glasgow D, Wong A, Barei DP, Ricci WM, Gardner MJ: Sagittal plane deformity in bicondylar tibial plateau fractures. *J Orthop Trauma* 2011;25(9):560-565.

22. Rademakers MV, Kerkhoffs GM, Sierevelt IN, Raaymakers EL, Marti RK: Operative treatment of 109 tibial plateau fractures: Five- to 27-year follow-up results. *J Orthop Trauma* 2007;21(1):5-10.

Chapter 66
Tibial Diaphyseal Intramedullary Nailing

Clifford B. Jones, MD, FACS

Patient Selection
Indications
Most tibial diaphyseal fractures can be treated with an intramedullary nail. Nailing has been shown to be more beneficial than casting, with earlier return to function and maintenance of alignment.[1]

Contraindications
Contraindications to tibial intramedullary nailing that hinder nail insertion include preexisting osseous deformity and knee ligament repair (because of screws). Relative contraindications include total knee arthroplasty and morbid obesity, which hinders knee flexion. In open fractures with gross contamination, which require repeat excisional débridements, intramedullary nailing should potentially be delayed until débridements are completed.

Preoperative Imaging
Preoperative imaging requires AP and lateral radiographs to determine fracture pattern, comminution, and bone loss. The images should include the knee and ankle joints to diagnosis intra-articular extension. When radiographs are inconclusive for intra-articular extension or the pattern is unclear, CT scans can be beneficial. If bone loss is present, images of the contralateral tibia may predict symmetric tibial length.

Procedure
Room Setup/Patient Positioning
The patient is positioned supine on a radiolucent operating table (diving board or pelvic table). A radiolucent small bump (rolled towel or blanket, but not a beanbag, which is not radiolucent) is placed under the ipsilateral buttock to neutralize the normal lower extremity external rotation. The ipsilateral arm is placed out to the side or across the body. With extended surgical time and an obese patient, a bump under the buttock can increase the risk of shoulder hyperextension and/or brachial plexopathy. Placing a pad under the elbow and flexing the elbow can relieve this tension.

The surgeon should try to avoid tourniquet application or use. With an open fracture, venous injury, and exposed cancellous surfaces, however, limited or transient application of a sterile tourniquet can reduce blood loss.

The patient is prepared and draped to the midportion of the ipsilateral thigh. If warranted, the ipsilateral toes can be covered with an antimicrobial impervious drape to avoid additional contamination.

Fluoroscopy
The monitor should be at the end of the bed or angled 20° to 30° to enhance visualization. The fluoroscopy imaging arm and base should be placed at a 90° angle to the ipsilateral injured limb and table to facilitate consistency and mobilization. The fluoroscopy imaging base should be placed on the contralateral side of the table.

For AP imaging, the C-arm should be nearly parallel to the tibial diaphysis (**Figure 1**). With extreme knee flexion, the ipsilateral buttocks will overlap and obscure perpendicular views. True AP knee imaging is achieved when the proximal tibia overlays approximately 50% of the fibula. True lateral knee imaging occurs when the femoral condyles and tibial plateau are collinear. Increased knee flexion and tibial length (tall stature) hinder lateral imaging because the arc of the C-arm can impinge on the table and will be unable to elevate enough to image the knee.

Two nonpenetrating towel clamps are used to attach the large drape to the operating table and another two are used to stabilize the ends of the drape during lateral imaging. For AP imaging, the drape is folded in half and attached to the side of the operating table, with the clamps used to initially stabilize the ends of the drape.

Leg Positioning
The injured leg is positioned in a flexed position over a radiolucent triangle. The size of the triangle should allow for knee flexion of 100° to 120°. The foot should be suspended (**Figure 2, A**) and not rest on

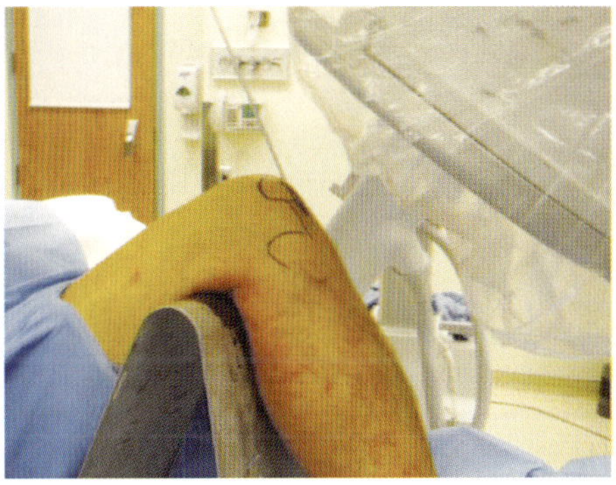

Figure 1 Fluoroscopic imaging for intramedullary nailing of the tibia. For AP imaging, the C-arm is positioned parallel to the tibial diaphysis.

the table (**Figure 2, B**).

The foot can be stabilized with towels, and smaller triangles can be used as bumps to correct for coronal and sagittal plane deformities. A cushion should be placed under the knee and calf of the contralateral leg. Also, if required, the uninjured limb should be secured to the table prior to preparation and draping to prevent it from falling off the table during the procedure. The drape over the uninjured limb and fluoroscopy C-arm can obscure the fallen limb and delay repositioning. Obese limbs are more problematic and may require a right angle to be placed under the table and alongside the limb.

Special Instruments/Equipment/Implants Required
- Complete intramedullary nail set of choice
- Complete reamer set of choice
- Ball-tipped guide rod
- Radiolucent table
- Large, medium, and small radiolucent triangles for limb positioning (**Figure 3**)
- Multiple small and large retractors
- Multiple large and small Weber bone reduction clamps (**Figure 4**)
- Dental picks
- Large universal distractor (in room, unopened)
- Multiple Schanz pins (2.5 and 5.0 mm)
- Small-fragment plate and screw set (in room, unopened) for provisional stabilization of open fractures and/or blocking screws

---

Dr. Jones or an immediate family member serves as a board member, owner, officer, or committee member of the American Orthopaedic Association, the Mid-America Orthopaedic Association, the Orthopaedic Trauma Association, and the Michigan Orthopaedic Society.

Section 5: Trauma

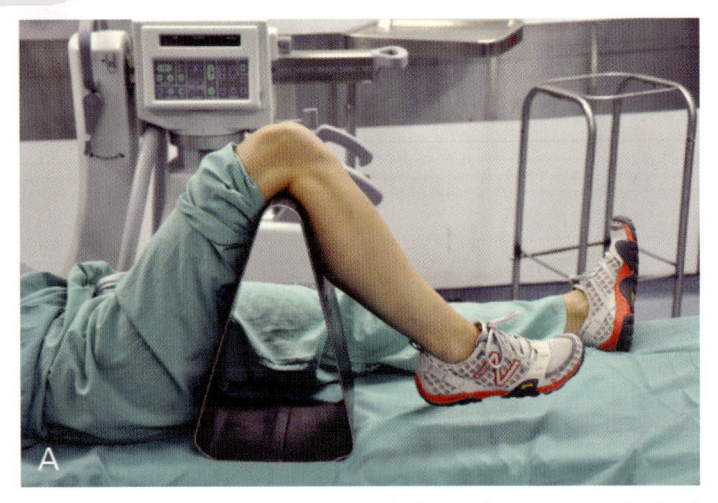

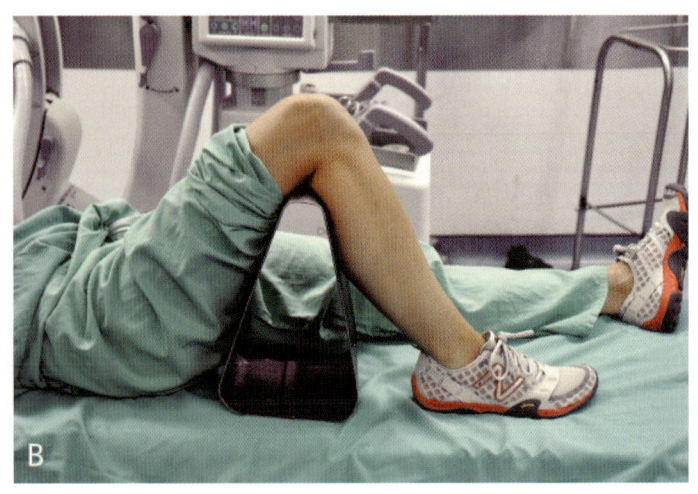

Figure 2 The foot should be suspended over the appropriately sized radiolucent triangle, not impinging or lying on the table. Photographs show correct (**A**) and incorrect (**B**) positioning. (Courtesy of Eben Carroll, MD, Winston-Salem, NC.)

- Additional large drapes for coverage of fluoroscopy machine during lateral visualization and coverage of the end of the table when the knee is flexed

Surgical Technique

Approach and Start Site

With the knee in flexion, the start site can be determined by fluoroscopic analysis.[1] The correct start site is based on surgeon experience and published cadaveric studies. In general, the best anatomic start site is along the medial aspect of the lateral tibial spine on the AP view (**Figure 5, A**) and on the apex of the anterior tibial slope on the lateral view[2,3] (**Figure 5, B**). To determine this start site, the guide pin is placed on the skin (**Figure 6**) and the position is confirmed with fluoroscopy. The pin site is marked on the skin.

Medial Parapatellar Approach

A 3- to 4-cm incision is made along the medial border of the patellar tendon. The paratenon is reflected, and the patellar fat pad is separated from the posterior aspect of the patella. The surgeon should exercise caution to avoid entrapment of the medial meniscus and coronary ligament. This approach was historically the approach of choice, but as anatomic studies provided a better understanding of the knee, this approach became rarely utilized.

Lateral Parapatellar Approach

This approach is useful for proximal third fractures, to facilitate nail placement along the lateral tibial cortex. A 3- to 4-cm incision is made along the lateral border of the patellar tendon. The paratenon is reflected, and the patellar fat pad is separated from the posterior aspect of the patella. The surgeon should take care to

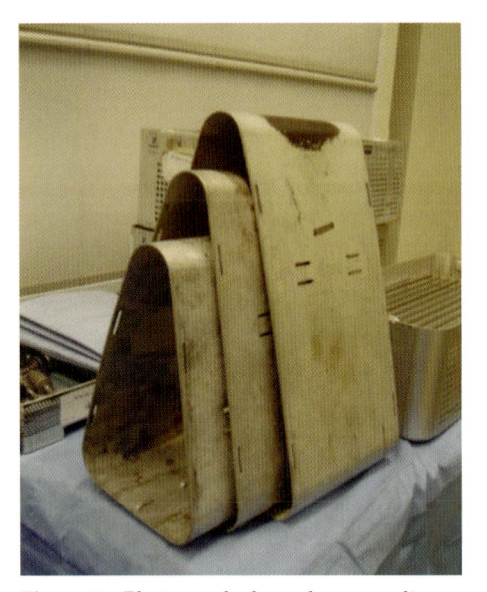

Figure 3 Photograph shows large, medium, and small triangles used to facilitate knee flexion and limb positioning.

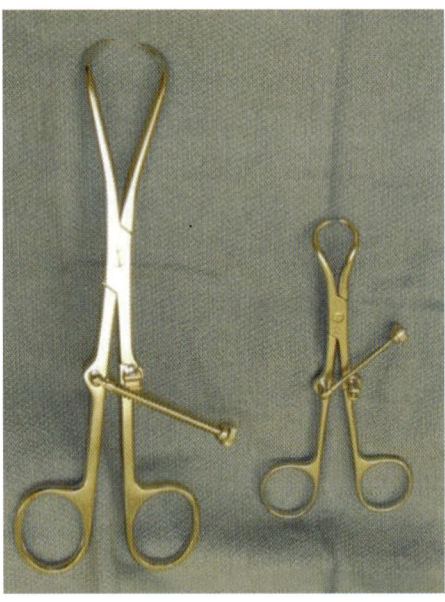

Figure 4 Photograph shows large and small "spin-down" Weber reduction clamps used to facilitate percutaneous fracture reduction.

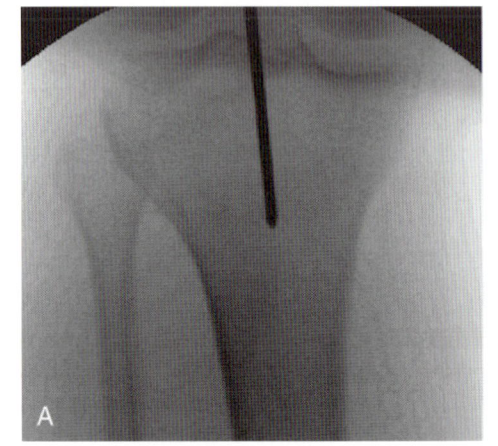

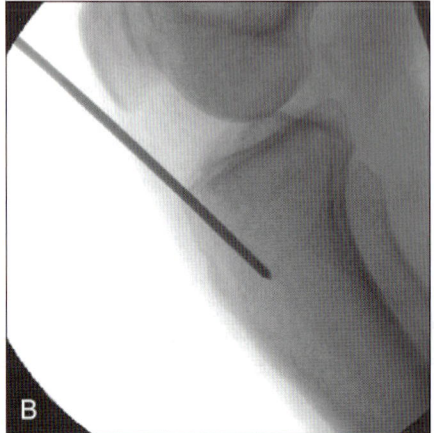

Figure 5 Fluorographic images show the start site for an intramedullary nail. **A**, AP image demonstrates alignment of the nail with the tibial diaphysis, with a start site just medial to the lateral tibial spine. **B**, Lateral image shows a starts site at the apex of the tibial metaphysis and collinear with the tibial diaphysis.

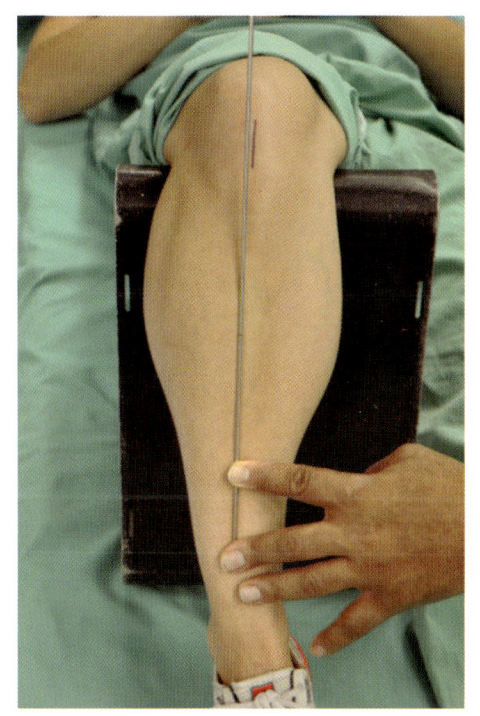

Figure 6 Photograph shows a guide pin placed on the skin to determine the start site for the intramedullary nail. The proximal tibial start site should line up with the tibial diaphysis. This determines the approach in relation to the patellar tendon. The position is then confirmed with fluoroscopy. (Courtesy of Eben Carroll, MD, Winston-Salem, NC.)

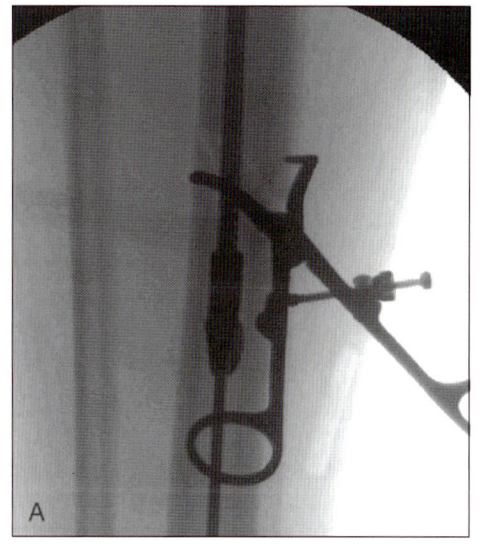

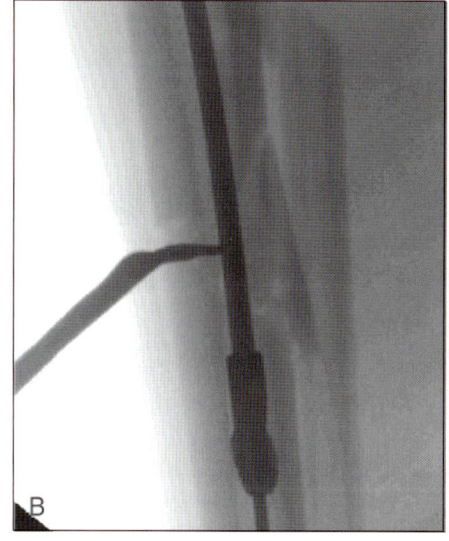

Figure 7 AP (**A**) and lateral (**B**) fluoroscopic images demonstrate a percutaneous clamp reducing the fracture and facilitating concentric reaming.

avoid entrapment of the lateral meniscus and coronary ligament.

Patellar Tendon–Splitting Approach
A 3- to 4-cm incision is made on the middle portion of the patellar tendon. The paratenon is split, and the patellar fat pad is separated from the posterior aspect of the patellar tendon. The surgeon must take care to avoid entrapment of the coronary ligament.

Percutaneous Patellar Tendon–Splitting Approach
A 2-cm incision is made over the distal third of the patella. The patellar tendon is split in a proximal-to-distal direction, starting at the inferior pole of the patella. The guide pin is placed along the posterior aspect of the patella. This is my preferred site and approach. It avoids cephalad compression/contusion of the skin from the guide pin, reamers, and nail with insertion.

Suprapatellar Approach
With the knee in a 20° to 30° flexion arc, a 2- to 3-cm incision is made over the rectus. The rectus is split in line with the fibers, and the dilating and instrument cannula is inserted.[4-7]

Medial Parapatellar Approach With Eversion of the Patella
This approach is used in knees with limited flexion from periarticular scarring, patella baja, and/or knee contracture. Without appropriate knee flexion, traditional approaches are impossible. An 8- to 10-cm incision is made over the medial half of the patella and patellar tendon with the knee in extension or slight flexion. An incision is made through the medial retinaculum. With a large enough retinacular incision, the patella is everted laterally. The knee is then flexed to the desired angle to facilitate pin insertion.

Fracture Reduction
The fracture must be reduced before guide pin insertion, reaming, and nail insertion to ensure optimal alignment, rotation, and length. The fracture reduction can be performed in many ways.

Transverse Fractures
To reduce a transverse fracture, the knee is flexed over the triangle and gentle traction is applied through the foot or ankle. With appropriate fracture distraction, the fracture is realigned and translated. All fracture edges must be keyed in for enhanced stability. Gentle compression is applied through the foot with bumps or manually to avoid gapping, translation, and/or rotation. Once the fracture is reduced, the guide pin is placed across the fracture site.

Oblique or Spiral Fractures
To reduce an oblique or spiral fracture with or without butterfly components, the fracture geometry is confirmed with preoperative radiographs. The extent of the fracture edges is determined with fluoroscopy and the skin is marked. Then 5- to 10-mm incisions are made on the medial/lateral and/or anterior/posterior aspects of the tibia.

The skin is spread with a hemostat. A spin-down Weber clamp is inserted through the skin, stopping once bone is reached. The clamp position is confirmed with fluoroscopy. With simultaneous traction and realignment, the clamp is compressed to reduce the fracture (**Figure 7**).

Once compression is achieved, fracture reduction is improved with gentle traction and rotation of the limb to facilitate cortical reapposition. The surgeon must be careful of underdiagnosed fracture extension or butterfly components. If compression is too firm, fracture extension and/or comminution may result. Once the fracture is reduced, the guide pin is placed across the fracture site.

Comminuted Fractures
Reduction of comminuted fractures requires extensive preplanning. If the fibular fracture is simple, it is reduced with a clamp, plate, or intramedullary device. If the fibula and tibia are both comminuted, radiographs of the contralateral tibia should be obtained for templating of length.

Segmental Fractures
With segmental fractures, both fractures are reduced under compression with the methods described above. Alternatively, open plate fixation can be used to ensure reduction and compression and decrease distraction at one or both of the fractures.

Section 5: Trauma

Open Fractures
Open fractures require the usual methods of excisional débridement and soft-tissue management. An open wound facilitates fracture reduction and clamp positioning. If needed, plate application under compression will ensure fracture reduction and facilitate nail insertion. The plate can be applied medially, laterally, or posteromedially. Screw length can be unicortical for medial or lateral plating. Screw length can be unicortical or bicortical for posteromedial plating. Plate application can be temporary—until nail insertion—or permanent if so desired. I avoid permanent plating along the medial tibial border under the thin and/or compromised skin.

Associated Proximal or Distal Articular Fractures
Any articular or periarticular fractures should be reduced initially and before nailing the diaphyseal fracture. Reduction of the metaphyseal/articular fracture can be performed open or percutaneously with Weber clamps. Maintaining clamp application and/or inserting strategically applied screws/plates can maintain the metaphyseal/articular fracture reduction.

Associated Ankle and/or Syndesmotic Fractures
Although rare, associated ankle and/or syndesmotic injuries are sometimes present and may be missed. The associated ankle and/or syndesmotic injury can be reduced, stabilized, and fixated before or after tibial diaphyseal treatment. In my opinion, performing tibial diaphyseal reduction first is preferable because it facilitates syndesmotic treatment by achieving overall length, alignment, and rotation of the limb. The ankle and/or syndesmotic hardware should be placed in strategic positions to avoid impedance of nail insertion.

Delayed or Severely Shortened Fractures
Either closed or open methods can be used to reduce severely shortened fractures or fractures for which treatment has been delayed.

Closed methods include traction applied from over a triangle as described previously. Other closed methods involve the use of an articulated distraction device attached via 5.0-mm Schanz pins or external fixation to achieve traction and, therefore, length.[8,9] Schanz pin positioning is parallel to the tibial plateau and plafond on the AP view and posterior to the axis of nail insertion on the lateral view.

Ball-Tipped Guide Rod
An opening to the intramedullary canal is created with a rigid cannulated reamer over a terminally threaded guide pin. Reaming should stop once the reamer has entered the diaphysis and has passed through the metaphyseal bone (**Figure 8**). The ball-tipped guide rod is then inserted through the medullary opening. The ball-tipped guide pin is used so that reaming does not extend past the tip of the guide rod and potentially into the ankle joint through fracture extension or osteoporotic bone and to extract broken cannulated instruments during the procedure.

The appropriate ball-tip size is determined with respect to the nail system and individual nail sizes. Smaller nails may demand smaller diameter ball-tipped guide rods and tips to achieve the appropriate inner diameter. Larger nails with corresponding larger inner diameters may allow standard ball-tipped guide pins to pass through the center without changing to a smooth-tipped guide pin through a radiolucent hollow exchange tube. The ball-tipped guide pin is inserted through this osseous opening.

The ball-tipped guide pin can be modified from a straight tip to a bent tip (**Figure 9**), which facilitates fracture reduction and strategic guide pin position. The bend can be accomplished with many different instruments, but it is best accomplished with a sharp bend over a small distance.

Reaming
The surgeon should not ream until the fracture is reduced. Errant reaming or reaming with the fracture unreduced prohibits optimal nail insertion and maintenance of fracture reduction. Proximally, the reamer is pushed gently through the soft tissues without reaming to avoid additional soft-tissue injury and/or soft-tissue entrapment. The reamer is then gently pushed into the canal through the start site to avoid eccentric anterior cortical reaming.[10]

The surgeon starts reaming using a small-diameter reamer with high rotational speed and slow advancement. Although controversial, reaming can be performed for both closed and open fractures. The reamer diameter is advanced in 1.0- or 0.5-mm increments. If the reamer does not advance without effort, the surgeon should reduce the reamer diameter and try again. Because cortical thickness, cortical density, and intramedullary diameter vary, the stopping point for medullary reaming varies based on surgeon experience, fracture characteristics, and soft-tissue injury.

To avoid reamer entrapment or cortical impaction, the surgeon should never stop the reamer rotation but should vary the rotation and/or advancement speed. The surgeon must be wary of cortical fragments at the fracture site or within the canal. Fracture fragments that are pulled into the canal or are in the canal can become trapped between the intact cortical wall and the reamer head. This usually occurs upon removal of the reamer head from distal to proximal within the distal segment. If fragments are becoming entrapped, placing the reamer in reverse can dislodge the intramedullary fragments. Attempting to pull out the reamer forcefully can extend the fracture line, comminute the fracture, or deform the reamer head.

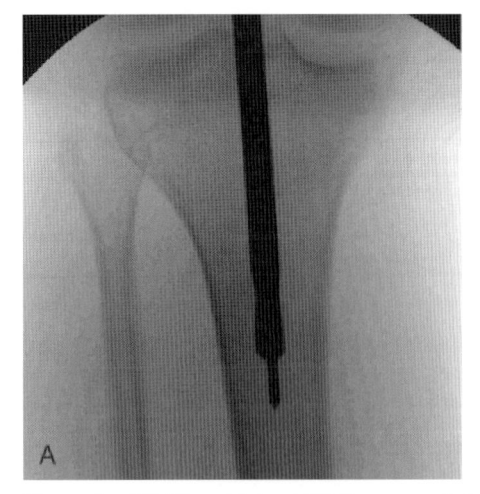

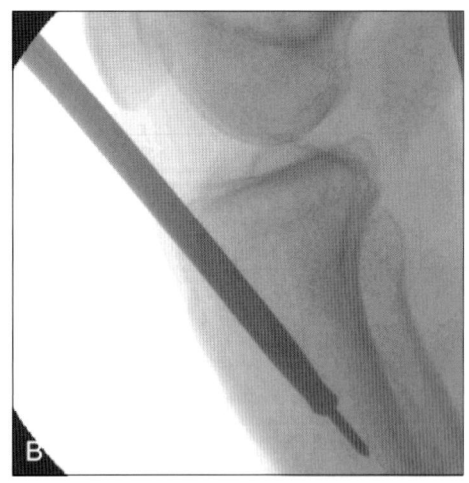

Figure 8 AP (**A**) and lateral (**B**) fluoroscopic images demonstrate a cannulated reamer system stopping at the metaphyseal-diaphyseal junction.

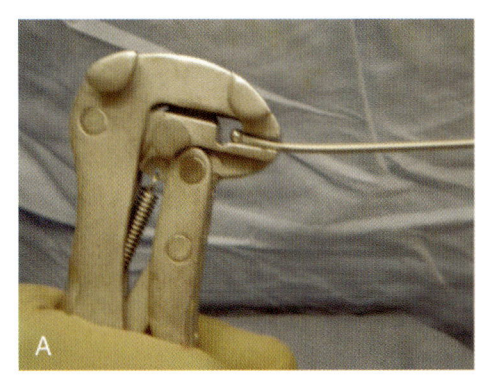

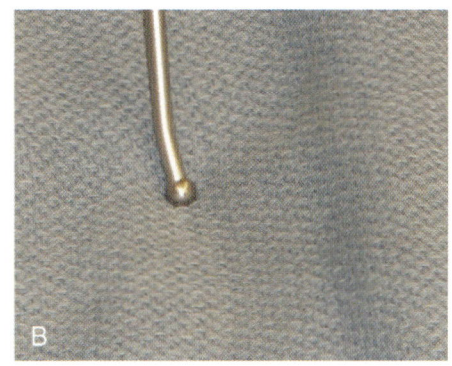

Figure 9 Photographs show modification of a ball-tipped guide rod from a straight tip (**A**) to a bent tip (**B**).

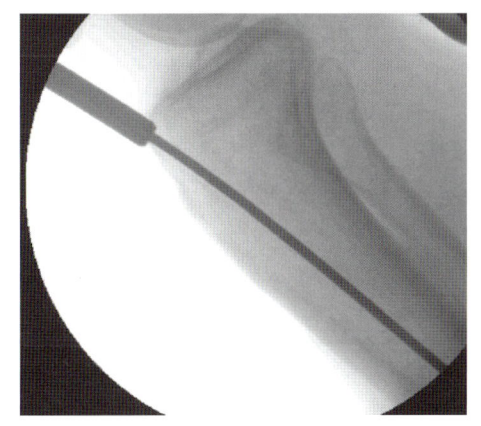

Figure 10 Nail length can be determined using a subtraction method of measurement, as demonstrated on this lateral fluoroscopic view.

Nail Insertion

Intramedullary nail diameter is based on surgeon experience, fracture characteristics, and the final stopping point of the reamer. In general, the nail diameter should be 0.5 to 1.0 mm larger than the final reamer diameter.

Nail length can be determined by comparing the length of the contralateral leg on preoperative images; by direct methods using external rulers that employ 10% to 15% image magnification; or by subtraction methods using rulers placed over the exposed end of the guide rod (**Figure 10**). Nail length is based on measuring technique and surgeon experience.

Nails should not be left prominent proximally. The nail must be inserted with the proper nail rotation. In general, the nail rotation and/or proximal guide direction is perpendicular to the anterior tibial crest. When attempting anterior-to-posterior distal screw insertion, the surgeon may insert the nail using slight internal rotation to enhance anterior-to-posterior screw insertion without tibialis anterior neurovascular bundle injury.

Compression of Fracture Distraction

In general, nails should be inserted down to the distal physeal scar. If attempting to insert nails distal to the distal physeal scar, the surgeon must ream across the physis. In young, dense bone, the nail will not pass the scar and will only distract the fracture. In older, osteoporotic bone, reaming or nail insertion without fluoroscopic imaging is dangerous. The reamer or nail may pass the distal physeal scar without a perceptible change when subchondral bone is entered, invading the joint through the plafond articular surface.

Once the nail is in the distal physeal scar bone, the fracture site should be checked on AP and lateral fluoroscopic images. If the fracture is distracted (**Figure 11, A**), it will require impaction (**Figure 11, B**). Backslapping the nail, applying longitudinal compression, and repeating nail insertion may facilitate fracture site compression. If the fracture will not compress with manual methods, the nail must be backslapped while engaged to the distal segment.

The drills are placed in both of the distal interlock sites. Alternatively, a Steinmann pin can be placed through the distal interlock sites. Placing small drill bits partially through the contralateral cortex or vigorous backslapping can deform the drill bits and interfere with their removal.

Backslapping should not be done with the final interlocking screws in position. This may inadvertently prestress the screws and potentiate early screw breakage. Once backslapped, the fracture site is rechecked in the AP and lateral planes to make sure inadvertent fracture site comminution or intussusception has not occurred.

Proximal Interlocking

Proximal interlocking screws are inserted through the nail guide drill sleeves. One, two, or three screws are placed proximally, depending on fracture configuration, nail configuration, and surgeon preference. If drilling from medial to lateral, the surgeon determines the drill sleeve to be flush with the medial proximal tibial cortical bone to avoid anterior nail drilling secondary to the medial cortical slope. When placing obliquely directed screws, the drill trajectory is determined before drilling all the way to the contralateral cortex. If the nail is not fully seated and/or the nail angulation is acute, the trajectory of the screw may pass through the tibial plateau articular surface (medial more common than lateral).[11] Also, rollover AP views should be obtained to avoid errant deep "past pointing" drilling, which can endanger the saphenous nerve medially and the peroneal nerve laterally.[12]

The screw length is confirmed with rollover and rollback AP views. Proper nail depth is confirmed before inserting screws and definitely before removing the proximal nail guide.

If the surgeon is having difficulty drilling and/or inserting the screws, guide rod removal is confirmed from inside the nail. If drilled with the guide rod in position initially, the nail or screw position will need to be changed to avoid creating an eccentric hole in the cortical bone, which would contribute to screw loosening.

Distal Interlocking

The distal interlocking screw is inserted using a freehand technique. Expensive radiolucent drill extenders can be used, but the freehand technique is not difficult or problematic. The "perfect circles" technique is the most efficient and most commonly used fluoroscopic technique. For this technique, the leg (and corresponding nail) is kept in a stable position distally. The fluoroscopic imaging unit is translated and rotated until a perfect circle is created by the distal interlock hole. Any angulation creating an elongated or imperfect appearance of the hole (**Figure 12, A**) can create an errant drill hole or screw impingement within the nail. Once the "perfect circle" is created (**Figure 12, B**), a radiopaque marker (eg, hemostat, drill bit, scalpel tip) is placed outside the skin to mark the incision site.

A vertical incision is made through the skin dermis only, and the soft tissue is carefully spread below the incision to avoid saphenous nerve or vein injury. The drill bit is inserted, either attached to

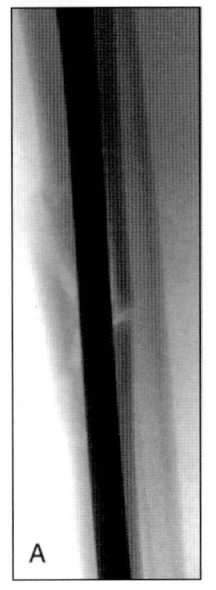

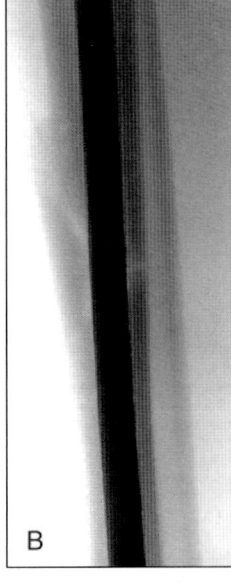

Figure 11 Fluoroscopic images of a tibial fracture fixed with an intramedullary nail. **A,** Distraction is seen along the posterior cortical bone. **B,** The fracture has been compressed.

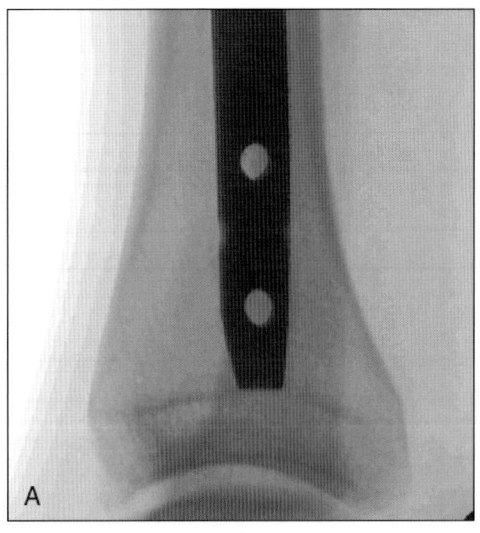

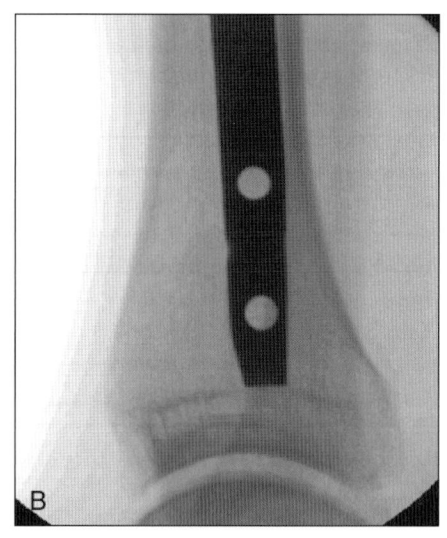

Figure 12 Fluoroscopic images demonstrate the "perfect circles" techniques for accurate placement of the distal interlocking screw. **A,** Lateral view demonstrates eccentric, or "imperfect," circles. **B,** Lateral view demonstrates correct ("perfect") circles.

the drill or held with a needle driver. The drill bit should be within the central portion of the radiolucent hole or circle from end to end. Again, if the drill bit is started or advanced off center, errant drilling or eccentric screw insertion will result. Once the drill bit is within the central portion of the nail, a confirmatory fluoroscopic image is obtained to ensure central drill placement.

The surgeon drills across the contralateral tibial cortex. Once the cortex has been crossed, lateral imaging is again used to confirm the position of the drill bit as being central. The surgeon must avoid drilling into the fibula except in special circumstances, such as osteoporotic bone, extremely distal fractures, and/or compromised skin that would preclude fibular fixation.

Poller Blocking Screws

In general, Poller blocking screws narrow the medullary osseous corridors.[13-15] The screws are used for errant start sites proximally, errant reaming tunnels distally, or with osteoporotic bone to narrow the medullary canal width. These screws are usually positioned along the concavity of the deformity and along the lateral aspect of the proximal segment in the anterior-posterior plane to force the nail medially and the proximal segment out of valgus. Poller blocking screws are usually inserted along the posterior aspect of the proximal fragment in the medial-lateral plane to force the nail anteriorly and out of apex anterior angulation.

The blocking screws, drill bits, Steinmann pins, or guide pins can be placed temporarily, until the nail and the interlock screws are inserted, or the blocking screws can be permanent. The screws should be 3.5-mm diameter or larger to avoid deformation and/or intramedullary breakage.

When reaming with blocking devices in place, the reamer is pushed across the site with the rotation turned off to avoid premature reamer wear and intramedullary metallic debris. When attempting to enhance nail stability in osteoporotic bone, blocking screws can be inserted in both the AP and lateral planes to diminish distal nail toggle.

The surgeon should keep in mind that the drill diameter is narrower than the screw diameter. When drilling next to the nail path, the surgeon must compensate for final screw insertion dimensions and position.

Interlocking Screw Enhancement

Interlocking screw enhancement can be achieved by taking advantage of new nail/screw technology or screw/plate interface geometry. Specifically engineered nails have been developed that allow for proximal nail cap insertion to entrap the most proximal interlock screw. In addition, specific interlocking hole geometry uses a tab or ridge in which specific screws engage upon insertion. This creates a "locking" interlocking screw. Screw/plate interface geometry can be used to enhance interlocking screw fixation as follows: screw insertion through a plate positioned extramedullary and the nail inserted intramedullary can achieve "locked" screw engineering. With a two-hole one-third tubular plate, the distance between the two screw holes is slightly larger than the distance between most nail holes distally. Therefore, when screws are inserted simultaneously and gradually, they tend to diverge medially within the plate and converge centrally within the nail. This forces the screw threads against the edges of the plate medially and the nail centrally, achieving a stable distal segment construct.

Nail Guide Removal

Only when nail position, interlocking screw insertion, and nail reduction are confirmed fluoroscopically can the proximal nail guide be removed. Also, confirmation should be obtained fluoroscopically that no proximal tibial plateau or distal tibial plafond fracture extension or surgeon-induced fractures are present. If the nail guide is inadvertently removed too early, the guide rod is reinserted within the proximal nail. The nail guide is placed over the guide rod and rotated into the correct position within the nail proximally. This is confirmed with fluoroscopy.

Incision Closure

In patients with skin compromise and high-energy injuries, I prefer closure of the incisions with 3.0-mm nylon sutures. I prefer Allgöwer-Donati sutures over vertical mattress or simple interrupted techniques.[16] Full-length elastic skin closure strips applied without tension across the incisions can enhance skin reapproximation and diminish skin tension during healing.

Intraoperative Splinting

After the sterile bandages have been applied, a splint is applied before the patient awakens, to reduce pain and equinus ankle deformities (**Figure 13**). The knee is bent to approximately 90° to relax the gastrocnemius muscle, and the ankle is positioned in neutral (90°) to maintain soft-tissue tension. To avoid equinus foot deformity and pressure to the posterior calcaneal area, the splint should be fully dry before the leg is placed onto the table or manual support is relaxed. Splint application is maintained for 2 to 14 days to reduce soft-tissue contracture.

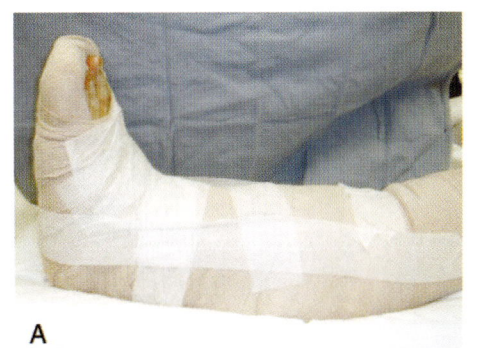

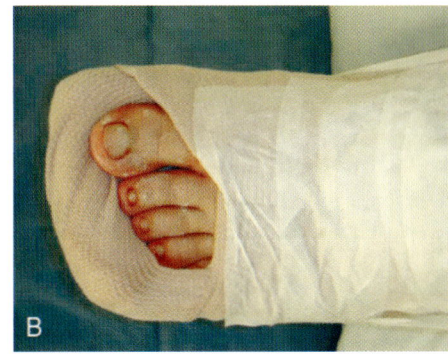

Figure 13 Photographs show splint applied following intramedullary nailing of a tibial diaphysis fracture. **A**, The appropriately applied short leg splint with sugar tong and extension to tip of toes is seen from the side. **B**, Dorsal view of the foot shows the splint protecting and supporting the toes.

Complications

The most common complication after intramedullary nailing for tibial fracture, occurring up to two thirds of the time, is knee pain.[2-11] The etiology is multifactorial, with no specific cause such as nail prominence, insertion site, or patellar tendon approach (medial, lateral, or split). The pain usually resolves with time, but rehabilitation focused on improving the resultant thigh weakness should not be delayed.[12] The second most common complication is nonunion. Nonunion, with a reported incidence of 1% to 50%, is more common in open fractures and with vascular injury, bone loss, infection, distraction, and relatively small nail insertion.[13-15] Infection is associated with open fractures. Other complications are malrotation, malalignment, leg length discrepancy, leg pain, and prominent hardware.

Postoperative Care and Rehabilitation

Splint removal is performed at 2 to 14 days. Range of motion is initiated with home exercises or formal physical therapy upon splint removal. Some authors advocate a short leg cast or splint application for up to 6 weeks to maintain a plantigrade foot, facilitate treatment of other ipsilateral injuries, and discourage noncompliant behavior.

Application of a brace with a removable splint, a foot-ankle orthosis, or a pneumatic boot can help protect the foot when the patient is convalescing, deconditioned, and beginning weight bearing. Weight bearing is begun based on patient compliance, fracture configuration, fracture stability, and surgeon preference. For simple transverse middiaphyseal fractures treated with proximal and distal interlocking screws, earlier weight bearing may be desirable. For complex metadiaphyseal and/or comminuted fractures, weight bearing until callus formation or after delayed bone grafting may be desirable.

Patients have varied outcomes once the tibial diaphyseal fracture is healed.[17]

Pearls

- A perfect tibial nailing depends on an accurate start site, fracture reduction, and central reaming; nondistracting nail insertion; and efficient interlocking.
- Only in middiaphyseal fractures with good canal fit of the nail within the cortices can indirect reduction of the fracture be accomplished.
- Treatment of tibial diaphyseal fractures early (within 3 to 5 days from injury) facilitates closed methods of alignment, translation, and rotational reduction.
- If unable to reduce the fracture with a single reduction method within 3 to 5 minutes, the surgeon should try another reduction method or revert to a minimally open soft-tissue protective method. The surgeon should not continue closed methods of reduction that compromise skin or future approaches.

References

1. Bone LB, Sucato D, Stegemann PM, Rohrbacher BJ: Displaced isolated fractures of the tibial shaft treated with either a cast or intramedullary nailing: An outcome analysis of matched pairs of patients. *J Bone Joint Surg Am* 1997;79(9):1336-1341.
2. Bhattacharyya T, Seng K, Nassif NA, Freedman I: Knee pain after tibial nailing: The role of nail prominence. *Clin Orthop Relat Res* 2006;449:303-307.
3. Cartwright-Terry M, Snow M, Nalwad H: The severity and prediction of anterior knee pain post tibial nail insertion. *J Orthop Trauma* 2007;21(6):381-385.
4. Darabos N, Bajs ID, Rutić Z, Darabos A, Poljak D, Dobsa J: Nail position has an influence on anterior knee pain after tibial intramedullary nailing. *Coll Antropol* 2011;35(3):873-877.
5. Katsoulis E, Court-Brown C, Giannoudis PV: Incidence and aetiology of anterior knee pain after intramedullary nailing of the femur and tibia. *J Bone Joint Surg Br* 2006;88(5):576-580.
6. Keating JF: Invited commentary: Anterior knee pain after intramedullary nailing of the tibia. Biomechanical effects of the nail entry zone and anterior cortical bone loss. *J Orthop Trauma* 2013;27(1):41-42.
7. Toivanen JA, Väistö O, Kannus P, Latvala K, Honkonen SE, Järvinen MJ: Anterior knee pain after intramedullary nailing of fractures of the tibial shaft: A prospective, randomized study comparing two different nail-insertion techniques. *J Bone Joint Surg Am* 2002;84-A(4):580-585.
8. Väistö O, Toivanen J, Kannus P, Järvinen M: Anterior knee pain after intramedullary nailing of fractures of the tibial shaft: An eight-year follow-up of a prospective, randomized study comparing two different nail-insertion techniques. *J Trauma* 2008;64(6):1511-1516.
9. Chen CY, Lin KC: Anterior knee pain. *J Orthop Trauma* 2013;27(1):e24.
10. Song SY, Chang HG, Byun JC, Kim TY: Anterior knee pain after tibial intramedullary nailing using a medial paratendinous approach. *J Orthop Trauma* 2012;26(3):172-177.
11. Ryan SP, Tornetta P III, Dielwart C, Kaye-Krall E: Knee pain correlates with union after tibial nailing. *J Orthop Trauma* 2011;25(12):731-735.
12. Väistö O, Toivanen J, Kannus P, Järvinen M: Anterior knee pain and thigh muscle strength after intramedullary nailing of a tibial shaft fracture: An 8-year follow-up of 28 consecutive cases. *J Orthop Trauma*

2007;21(3):165-171.

13. Yang JS, Otero J, McAndrew CM, Ricci WM, Gardner MJ: Can tibial nonunion be predicted at 3 months after intramedullary nailing? *J Orthop Trauma* 2013.

14. Court-Brown CM, McQueen MM: High success rate with exchange nailing to treat tibial shaft aseptic nonunion. *J Orthop Trauma* 1999;13(4):274.

15. Simunovic N, Walter S, Devereaux PJ, et al; SPRINT Investigators: Outcomes assessment in the SPRINT multicenter tibial fracture trial: Adjudication committee size has trivial effect on trial results. *J Clin Epidemiol* 2011;64(9):1023-1033.

16. Sagi HC, Papp S, Dipasquale T: The effect of suture pattern and tension on cutaneous blood flow as assessed by laser Doppler flowmetry in a pig model. *J Orthop Trauma* 2008;22(3):171-175.

17. Lefaivre KA, Guy P, Chan H, Blachut PA: Long-term follow-up of tibial shaft fractures treated with intramedullary nailing. *J Orthop Trauma* 2008;22(8):525-529.

Chapter 67
Open Reduction and Internal Fixation of the Tibial Plafond

Stephen K. Benirschke, MD   Patricia Kramer, PhD

Patient Selection
Indications
Patients who present with articular surface as well as gross metadiaphyseal malalignment of the tibial plafond are candidates for open reduction and internal fixation. Plafond injuries are characterized by an axial load applied to the tibia by the talus. Intrinsic articular surface impaction depends on the position of the foot at the time of impact and can occur across the entire joint surface. The medial edge of the plafond is injured preferentially when the foot is internally rotated/supinated, whereas the lateral edge is injured when the foot is externally rotated/pronated. Fibular involvement is common, and a Volkmann fragment with or without ligamentous avulsion is possible.

Contraindications
The most important concern related to surgical treatment in this patient group is evidence of noncompliance, especially with physician-directed changes in risk-prone psychosocial habits. Among these habits are nicotine (via smoking or chewing) and intravenous drug addictions, which can create serious postoperative complications with wound healing. Other potential issues include vascular status, venous insufficiency, and systemic disease, but these situations should be evaluated on a case-by-case basis, because with careful management these patients can be treated surgically. Neither extensive articular comminution nor open wounds should in and of themselves be contraindications to surgical repair.

Preoperative Imaging
A standard series of radiographs should be taken of the injured limb, including lateral and mortise views of the ankle, to determine the extent of injuries. When a tibial plafond fracture is diagnosed, imaging should be obtained throughout

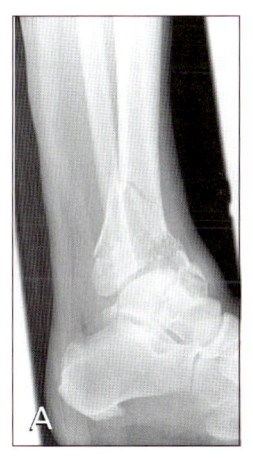

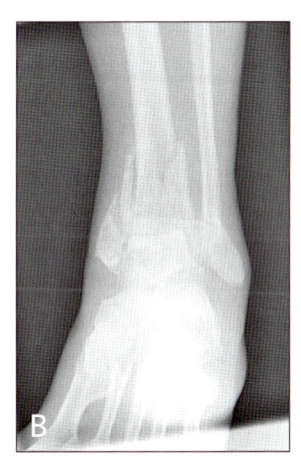

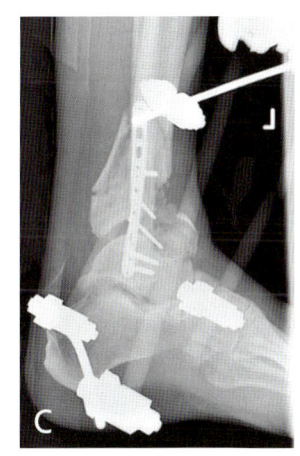

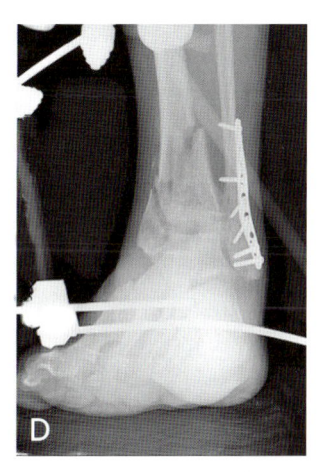

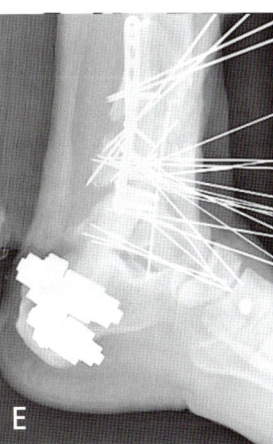

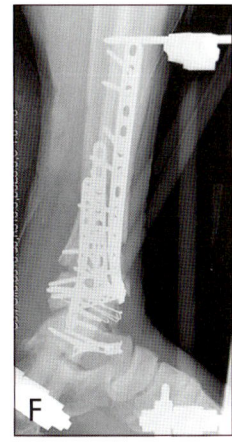

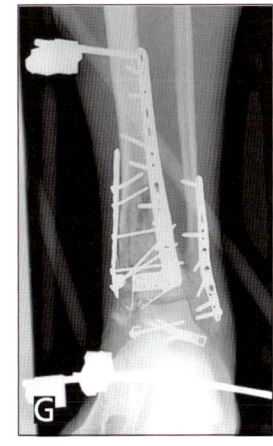

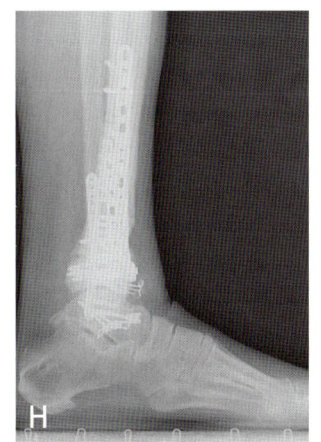

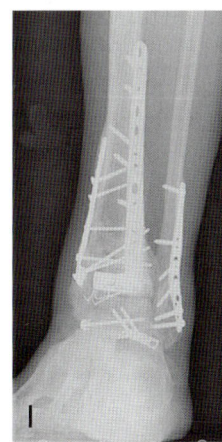

Figure 1 Radiographic series show initial injury, treatment, and outcome of a tibial plafond injury in patient A. **A**, Lateral radiograph of injured ankle and foot. **B**, Mortise radiograph of ankle and injured foot. **C**, Lateral radiograph after distraction and fixation of fibula. **D**, Mortise radiograph after distraction and fixation of fibula. Note that the Volkmann fragment no longer overlaps the tibial shaft. **E**, Intraoperative (definitive surgery) lateral radiograph demonstrating provisional fixation via Kirschner wires (a "K-wire jail"). **F**, Lateral postoperative radiograph. **G**, Mortise postoperative radiograph. Note that this patient required a medial buttress plate and that the frame was maintained in place for soft-tissue management. Lateral (**H**) and mortise (**I**) radiographs at 1.5-year follow-up.

Dr. Benirschke or an immediate family member serves as an unpaid consultant to Synthes and Zimmer. Neither Dr. Kramer nor any immediate family member has received anything of value from or has stock or stock options held in a commercial company or institution related directly or indirectly to the subject of this chapter.

Section 5: Trauma

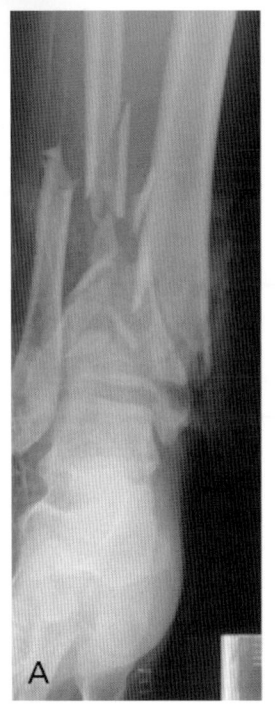

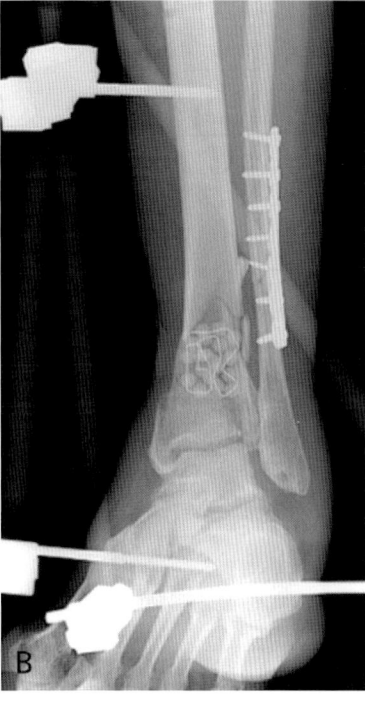

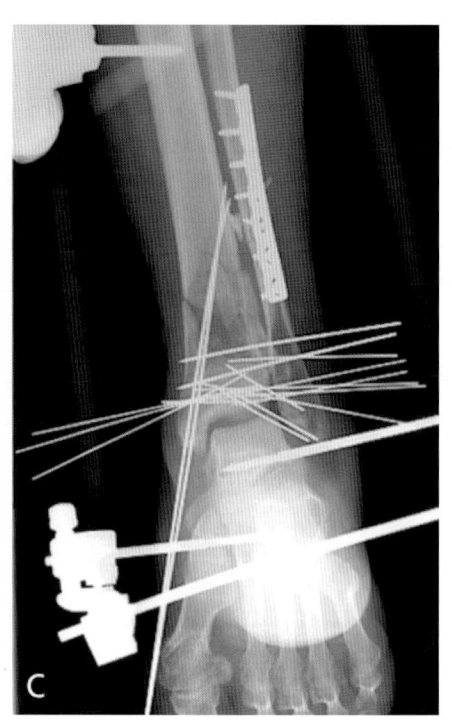

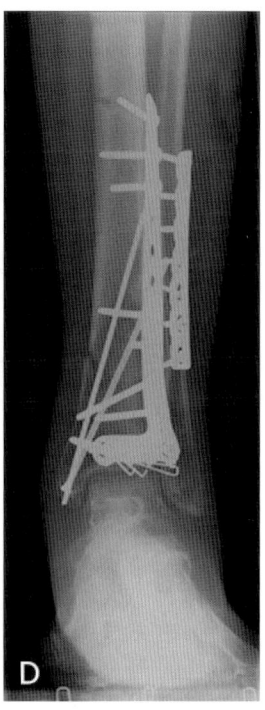

Figure 2 Mortise radiographic series shows the tibial plafond injury in patient B. **A**, Tibial plafond injury. **B**, An external fixator was applied and internal fixation of the fibula was performed. Antibiotic-impregnated beads were placed through the medial open wound into the osseous defect; they act as a void filler. The medial open wound was closed during this surgery. **C**, Provisional fixation with Kirschner wires. **D**, Definitive fixation including a medial strut screw.

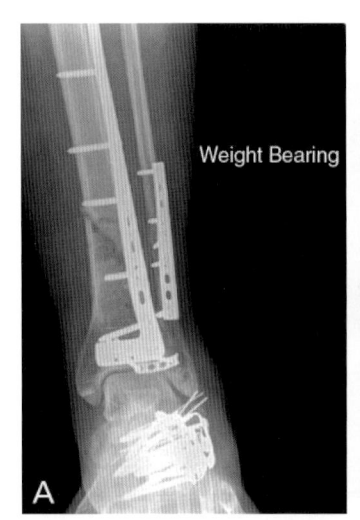

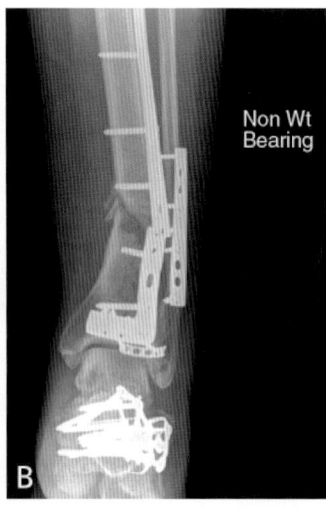

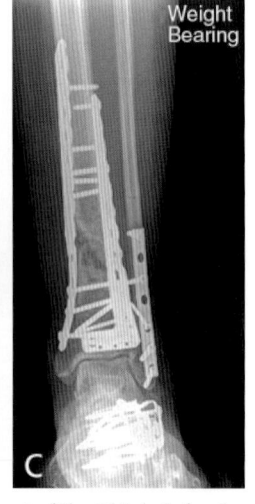

Figure 3 Postoperative mortise radiographic series shows the treatment of the tibial plafond injury in patient C. **A**, Two and a half months after definitive fixation. **B**, After 1 month of weight bearing. Note the broken implant. **C**, Five months after revision surgery. Note the medial buttress plate and replaced anterolateral plate.

the course of treatment. In this chapter, we describe three cases of tibial plafond fractures. The lateral and mortise radiographs of the first patient (A) are shown in **Figure 1**. These radiographs demonstrate the standard progression through treatment. The mortise radiographs of patient B are shown in **Figure 2**. This patient had a medial open wound; the injury required medial buttressing with screws. The radiographs of patient C are shown in **Figure 3**. Definitive fixation hardware failed in this patient and revision surgery was required.

Procedure

Room Setup/Patient Positioning

A similar surgical setup is used for both the index and definitive surgeries described here. The patient is placed supine on a pressure-relieving mattress on a radiolucent operating table without metal rails. A flank wedge is used under the ipsilateral hip to allow both external and internal rotation positioning of the ankle with a straight knee. For the index surgery, a more internally rotated position is used; for the definitive surgery, the leg should be able to rotate both internally and externally. The hip flank wedge creates a pressure point on the contralateral greater trochanter, which necessitates the use of the pressure-relieving mattress. A ramp pad is used under the ipsilateral limb to elevate the foot and ankle above the level of the contralateral foot. This positioning allows unimpeded access to the ankle by the surgical team and allows intraoperative radiographs to be taken without patient repositioning.

Surgical Technique

Two surgical interventions are generally necessary for management of a tibial plafond injury. The goal of the index surgery is to provide gross reduction of the ankle through distraction, which allows the talus to obtain a central position under the tibia, via application of the external fixation. Once this gross reduction has occurred, CT scans are taken, and planning for the definitive reduction and fixation can proceed. The definitive surgery occurs 10 to 21 days after injury.

Index Surgery

The index surgery is usually performed within hours of presentation, whether the patient is seeking initial treatment of the injury or has been referred from elsewhere. Early external fixation allows for earlier definitive treatment and better surgical outcome, but the Schanz pins must be placed carefully, avoiding neural

Chapter 67: Open Reduction and Internal Fixation of the Tibial Plafond

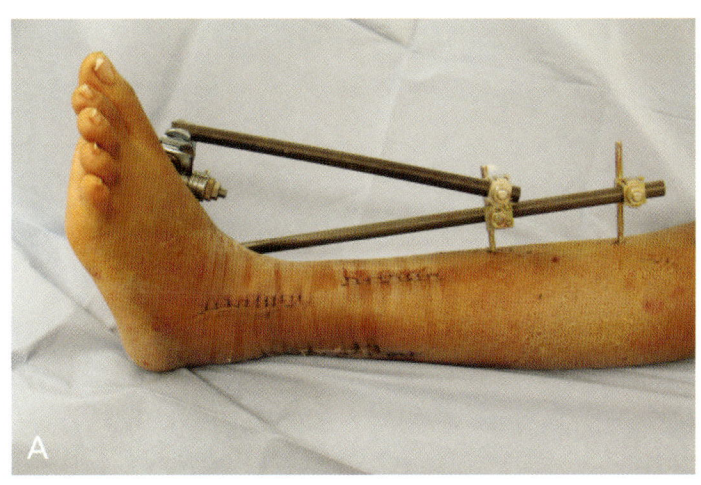

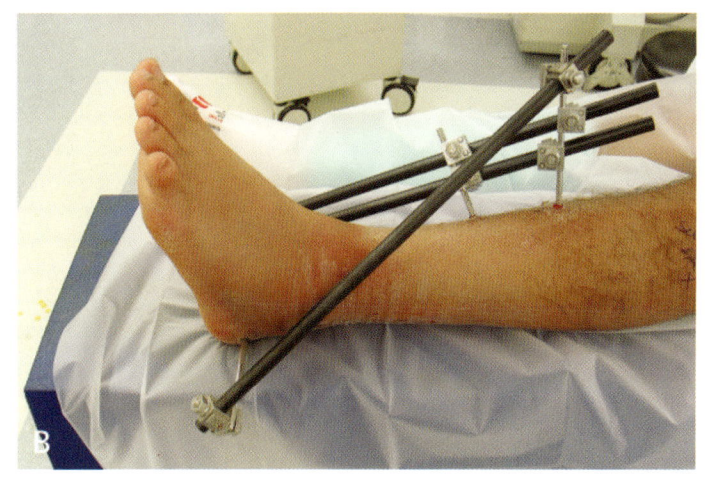

Figure 4 Photographs show an external fixation device. **A,** Unicolumnar frame, shown after definitive surgery. The two tibial pins are placed outside the affected area and as far apart as possible. Note the incisional wounds associated with the fibular fixation and the anterolateral approach. **B,** A typical bicolumnar frame. When a bicolumnar external fixation device is needed, the standard arrangement includes two bars to tie the two tibial pins to the medial calcaneus and midfoot (cuneiforms). This arrangement includes the components used in a unicolumnar medial application (shown in **A**), but the calcaneal pin exits the lateral side and a third bar ties it to the proximal tibial pin (as is shown in **B**). In the arrangement shown, the midfoot pin (through the cuneiforms) was not needed to provide adequate stability.

and vascular structures. Open fractures have external fixation applied at the time of initial irrigation and débridement.

Any fibular injury present is addressed first, using standard techniques. The key to the restoration of fibular anatomy is achieving correct fibular length, orientation, and rotation with the application of appropriate implants.[1] To restore normal ankle mechanics, most displaced fibular fractures require reduction, but fibular reduction is especially critical when these fractures are associated with tibial plafond injuries because the posterior (Volkmann) fragment is connected to the fibula via the posterior tibiofibular ligament. Unless this ligament is avulsed, reduction of the fibula will grossly reduce the Volkmann fragment, facilitating treatment of the tibial plafond. Consequently, fibular reduction is a critical step in the treatment of these fractures, and a less than anatomic fibular reduction is detrimental to the patient's outcome. Nonanatomic reductions must be revised, and the initial incision damages the soft-tissue envelope, making the revision more difficult. Although external fixation should be applied as soon as possible to minimize soft-tissue trauma, fibular fixation can wait until personnel with adequate training and equipment are available, which may require transfer from the referral center.

After the fibular fracture has been treated, an external fixation frame is attached. No tourniquet is used. The most basic frame is one applied along the medial column (**Figure 4, A**), but lateral injuries may require the addition of an additional bar, which makes a bicolumnar frame (**Figure 4, B**). The medial column frame is attached to the tibia, calcaneus, and cuneiforms. Four pins are placed to support the bar(s) through small incisions that follow the line of distraction. All pins are located outside of the anticipated location of the surgical incisions for definitive fracture treatment.

The calcaneal pin is inserted first. For medial column frames, the calcaneal pin is terminally threaded; for bicolumnar frames, the pin is centrally threaded (no threads on the ends). No predrilling is required. The pin is inserted from the medial surface of the calcaneus and, for bicolumnar frames, protrudes through the lateral surface of the foot. The calcaneal pin is placed in the posterior portion of the calcaneal tuberosity, posterior to a line that connects the superior and posterior edges. Placement of the calcaneal pin through this region will avoid the sural nerve and calcaneal branch of the tibial nerve.

The second pin is then inserted into the tibia; this is located at the proximal middle third junction of the tibia through its anteromedial surface, avoiding the saphenous nerve and vein. The proximal tibial pin is a 5-mm Schanz half pin (designed for bicortical applications). Predrilling is required for both tibial pins.

The third pin is inserted via a percutaneous stab wound through the medial surface of the medial cuneiform. This pin goes through the medial and intermediate cuneiforms and into the lateral cuneiform, but it does not transgress the base of the second metatarsal. No predrilling is required.

The final pin is the distal tibial pin, which is similar to the proximal tibial pin. Its location is determined by the tibial fracture. The pin should be located as distally as possible while remaining outside of the fracture area and forthcoming internal fixation.

Both tibial pins require predrilling because the cortices of the tibia are hard, but the pins in the foot do not need predrilling because the metadiaphyseal bone is softer. A small vertical incision is created in line with the limb perfusion. Both tibial pins and the soft tissues are carefully probed until the bone is exposed. Transverse incisions should never be used.

A triple-sleeve drilling attachment, which limits the amount of soft-tissue disruption, is inserted through the incision. A triple-fluted, sharp drill is used to underdrill a 3.2-mm pilot hole through the tibia. Underdrilling is preferable, especially in osteopenic bone, because it allows for good purchase of the screw threads in the cortical bone. Copious irrigation is maintained throughout the drilling process. It is critical to avoid thermal necrosis of the bone, and irrigation and the use of a sharp drill is the only way to avoid overheating the bone.[2,3] The fixator should be preassembled to facilitate its placement.

Although this attention to detail may seem overzealous, it comes from years of experience treating complications associated with less than accurate pin placement. Among the most serious of these potential complications are pin-tract infection, early loosening of the fixator, and

© 2013 American Academy of Orthopaedic Surgeons

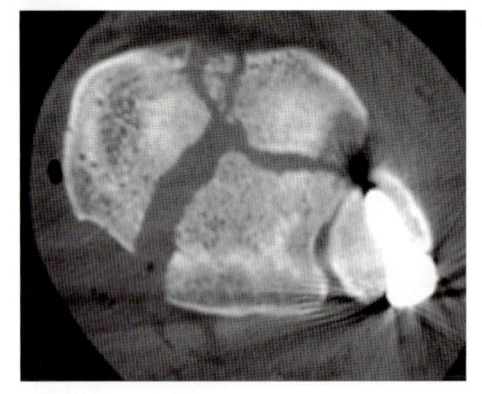

Figure 5 CT scan shows the three main fragments in a tibial plafond injury: the posterior or Volkmann fragment that is attached to the fibula via the tibiofibular ligament; the medial fragment, which in this case includes the malleolus; and the anterolateral or Chaput fragment.

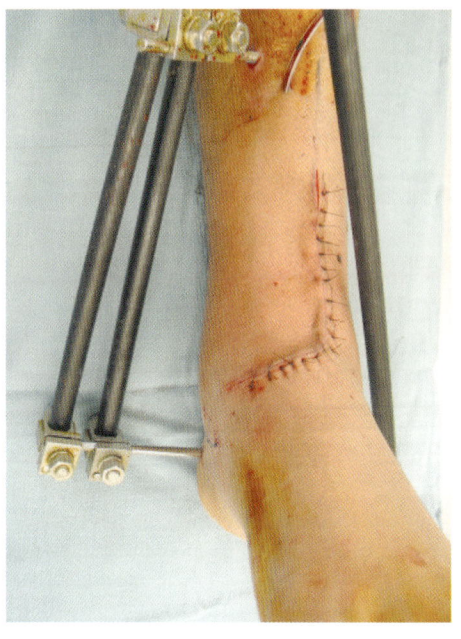

Figure 6 Photograph shows the closure of anteromedial approach. The surgical incision curves gently across the joint from lateral to medial and is closed with Algöwer sutures. Note that part of the bicolumnar external fixation frame is still in place and the drain exits superiorly.

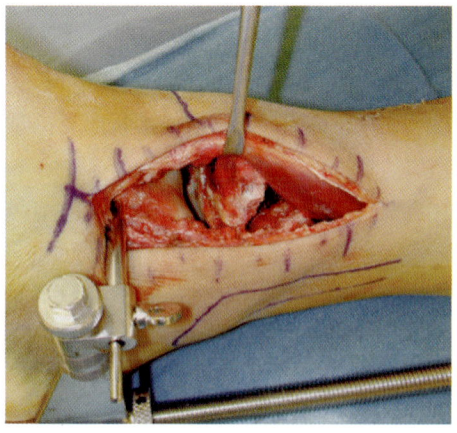

Figure 7 Intraoperative photograph shows the anterolateral approach with a Schanz pin in the talar neck. This allows the anterior joint to be distracted.

failure of fixation, all of which jeopardize the definitive surgery.

Slight distraction of the ankle joint is provided by the external fixator. Approximately 5 mm of space between the talar dome and the subchondral line of the fibula is sufficient. Distraction allows nonimpacted fragments to move, whereas impacted ones remain in place, allowing for detailed preoperative planning. The talus should be centrally located and its location checked with mortise and lateral radiographic views (**Figure 1, C** and **D**; **Figure 2, B**). The ankle should be in a neutral position, producing a plantigrade foot, but care should be taken to not overstretch the tibial and superficial peroneal nerves because overstretching can cause a dysesthetic foot. Preoperative physical examination should guide the surgeon to determine the appropriate ankle position.

After the external fixator is in place, the incisions used for pin placement are checked for signs that the skin is under pressure. These signs include ischemia of the skin and a lack of mobility of the skin adjacent to the pin. If the skin appears to be under pressure, the incision should be extended.

After the injury is grossly reduced, the pins are shortened so that the entire foot and ankle can be placed in a sterile short-leg splint. All external fixation pins are covered by the splint and the foot is held in a neutral position. A CT scan is completed at this time to discern which fragments are impacted and which responded to ligamentotaxis (**Figure 5**). The patient is instructed to avoid weight bearing and maintain continuous elevation of the foot at or slightly above cardiac level. Definitive fixation cannot occur until the swelling in the foot and ankle has resolved.

The splint is taken down approximately 10 days after external fixation is applied to ascertain the condition of the soft tissues. If the swelling has resolved, definitive fixation is scheduled. If the foot remains swollen, the short-leg splint is reapplied. At this time, compliance can be assessed using three criteria. The first is whether or not the patient has maintained strict elevation of the foot. Patients with substantial swelling at 10 days prompt the suspicion that elevation was not maintained. The condition of the splint can also be observed. Breaks, scuffing, or evidence of weight bearing should be pointed out and the consequences of early weight bearing discussed with the patient. Finally, attempts to change deleterious psychosocial habits should be discussed. Patients who have failed to attempt to quit smoking, for example, or who are untruthful in their responses may be contraindicated for surgical interventions due to potential wound-healing issues. Testing for nicotine usage (via a urine test for nicotine byproducts) is a tool that can be employed.

Duplex examination is done when the splint is removed. Patients with a deep venous thrombosis below the popliteal hiatus are treated with perioperative prophylactic anticoagulation, followed by full anticoagulation 48 hours after definitive tibial fixation. Deep venous thrombosis within 7 cm of the popliteal hiatus and above is treated with a prophylactic removable vena cava filter. After definitive surgery, the filter is removed and the patient is placed on therapeutic anticoagulation.

Definitive Surgery

Definitive stabilization occurs when the swelling has resolved and the soft tissues have "calmed down," which usually takes 10 to 21 days after external fixation. The surgical approach is determined by the injury characteristics and fracture patterns that are identified on the distracted joint based on CT images and the presumed mechanism of injury. Several approaches are possible.

The anteromedial approach is the classic approach to tibial plafond injuries (**Figure 6**). It allows for any medial impaction of the plafond to be addressed, visualization of the entire plafond, and control of the bone fragments. The surgical incision begins 1 cm lateral to the anterior crest, at the height where the anticipated proximal edge of plate will go (which is known from the surgical planning). The incision extends distally and curves gently, aiming for 1 cm distal to the tip of the medial malleolus. The anterior compartment is retracted laterally, including the tibialis anterior with its intact sheath. With this approach, the joint is visible but the lateral plafond is more difficult to visualize and lateral impaction, if present, is more difficult to reduce.

An alternative to the anteromedial approach is the anterolateral approach (**Figure 7**), which is appropriate for injuries with substantial lateral disruption. The surgical incision is lateral to the anterior crest of the tibia, in line with the space between the fourth and fifth metatarsals and lateral to the extensor mass. The anterior compartment is retracted laterally. The extensor retinaculum should be released along the lateral edge, because the tissue is more robust there. Another, more proximal incision is used to place the proximal screws through the plate. The anterolateral approach allows for optimal access to the anterolateral and posterolateral aspect of the plafond, but any medial impaction is more difficult to access and manipulation of medial gutter impaction is more difficult than with the anteromedial approach.

Finally, some situations make direct surgical access to the posterior injury seem attractive. For instance, the posteromedial or posterolateral approaches have been used for highly comminuted posterior injuries that require sequential reassembly to reestablish the posterior architecture of the ankle. Posterior approaches are rarely necessary and, if used, can lead to additional surgical complications and limit future salvage operations. It should be noted that adequate reduction of the fibula brings any posterior fragment into gross reduction, unless the tibiofibular ligament is avulsed. Consequently, surgical planning should use images obtained after fibular fixation, as discussed previously.

After the joint is accessed, a Schanz pin is inserted through the incision into the talar neck. This pin is used to rotate and distract the talus plantarly so that the anterior edge is open and the posterior surface can be visualized (**Figure 7**). This Schanz pin is used intraoperatively to improve access to the joint and is removed immediately before the incision is closed. Preliminary reductions are held in place with Kirschner wires (K-wires). A "K-wire jail" may be necessary to hold all the fragments in position before definitive fixation is applied and K-wires are ideally placed so that they can be maintained until definitive fixation has been placed (**Figure 1, E** and **Figure 2, C**).

Sequence of Reduction

1. Any Volkmann fragment is semi-reduced when fibular anatomy is addressed, unless the tibiofibular ligament is avulsed.

2. In the definitive surgery, the first step is to reduce any impaction within the Volkmann fragment. This step is critical because inadequately addressed impaction does not provide the correct "read" for reduction of the remaining articular fragments. When the posterior plafond is left impacted, the other plafond fragments tend to create an articular surface that is rotated, causing the anterior edge of the "roof" to be superior to its anatomic position. If the posterior plafond impaction is not addressed, the talar dome is not captured anteriorly and normal motion can cause the talus and foot to shift anteriorly relative to the leg. This can lead to pain, arthrosis, and the need for salvage surgeries such as ankle arthrodesis or arthroplasty.

3. The Volkmann fragment provides the anchor for the posteromedial fragment. The posteromedial fragment can also include the medial malleolar portion. If not, then the malleolar fragment is anchored to the posterior medial fragment.

4. Any central comminution is bought down to align with the Volkmann + posteromedial + medial malleolar portion. The goal is a smooth articular surface.

5. The last piece to be assembled is the tubercle of Chaput, which provides the anterior containment of the talus. If this fragment can be aligned with the anteromedial and posterolateral surfaces, then the reduction has been successfully accomplished. This process may be thought of as the Chaput fragment "closing the door" of the reduction.

In summary, the reduction proceeds from posterolateral to posteromedial to anteromedial to central to anterolateral. Implants are tailored to support the particular osseous injury (**Figure 1, F** and **G**). Substantial comminution or multiple fragments require stiffer implants like anteromedial and/or lateral buttress plates. K-wires provide provisional stabilization. Screws that are not integrated into an implant are rarely used. An exception to this is when the medial side needs stability but not buttressing, in which case strut screws are used (**Figure 2, D**).

Implants
Implants (plates) are slid up onto the tibia and their screws are inserted under direct visualization. With an anteromedial incision and an anteromedial plate, visualization should be through the initial incision, but with the anterolateral approach, a second incision is necessary to access the upper portion of the anterolateral plate. After making the second incision, the muscle bellies of the anterior compartment should not be skewered with screws; they should be retracted. Occasionally, with the anterolateral approach, a medial buttress plate is required. In this case, a small incision is made anteromedially near the distal-most tibia and the plate is slid proximally along the tibial surface. Screws for this plate are inserted percutaneously, because the medial tibial surface is covered by only a thin cutaneous layer (ie, there are no muscles to damage).

The frame usually comes off after the wound is closed, but if additional support is required, it can be left on for an additional 3 to 6 weeks, when the soft tissues have recovered (**Figure 4, A**).

Closure
The ankle joint capsule is closed with 2.0 Vicryl suture (Ethicon) in a figure-of-8 pattern. With the anteromedial approach, the periosteal layer of the tibia is also closed with figure-of-8 sutures. With the anterolateral approach, the ankle capsule, extensor retinaculum, and other tissues should be sutured. The skin is closed with Allgöwer sutures (**Figure 6**).

A 1/8-in Hemovac drain is placed under the anterior compartment, exiting anteriorly, and is left in place for 48 hours. Less than 10 mL of fluid per shift is expected by that time.

The leg is placed in a short-leg splint in 5° to 10° of dorsiflexion. Continuous indwelling peripheral nerve catheters provide pain control for the first 48 hours.

After the drain is removed, the patient is discharged to home. No oral antibiotics are supplied for use at home. The patient is instructed to continuously elevate the foot and maintain strict non–weight bearing. At 1 to 2 weeks after the definitive surgery, the splint is taken down and the patient initiates active range of motion of the ankle and subtalar joints and passive range of motion of the toes. A resting splint in 5° to 10° of dorsiflexion is applied.

Complications
Early complications include the possibility of deep venous thrombosis, delayed cutaneous healing, and deep infection.

Duplex examinations, described previously, are routinely done before the definitive surgery, and appropriate treatment is undertaken based on the location of the thrombosis. Delayed cutaneous healing of the apex of the skin flap is possible; this is usually associated with the anteromedial approach. Delayed wound healing can be associated with cellulitis. Meticulous soft-tissue care is required to optimize wound healing. The anterolateral approach is rarely associated with delayed wound-healing issues, which is one reason to use it whenever possible. Deep infections are also possible but can usually be avoided with meticulous care of the soft tissues.

Late complications include delayed union or nonunion of the metadiaphyseal junction, avascular collapse of the articular surface, and posttraumatic ankle arthrosis. The metadiaphyseal junction of the tibia can be difficult to heal, especially if sufficient buttressing did not occur in the definitive surgery. It can manifest with or without malalignment. If the junction appears slow to heal, additional buttressing can be provided to the junction. In the best case, the delayed union is noted before the primary implant has failed, but if the primary implant fails, it should be replaced at the same time that new buttressing is placed (**Figure 3, A** through **C**). Avascular collapse of the tibia usually occurs in the central region of the plafond, with the talus pushing through the avascular articular surface. When the initial injury is substantially comminuted or the fracture appears slow to heal, weight bearing should be delayed until radiographic evidence of healing is apparent. It is better to delay weight bearing than initiate collapse. Posttraumatic arthrosis of the ankle joint is also a possible sequela of plafond injuries. Meticulous reconstruction of the joint anatomy is the best way to avoid future problems because salvage options are limited.

Finally, nerve complications secondary to the initial injury are also possible and present long-term issues for the patient. It is imperative that disruption of the normal sensation in the foot caused by the initial injury be diagnosed before surgery. Careful soft-tissue dissection should limit any nerve complications from the surgery.

Postoperative Care and Rehabilitation

At 6-week follow-up, radiographs are taken to establish healing, and a support stocking is given to the patient. Although the patient remains non–weight bearing, more aggressive range of motion is allowed.

At 3 months, the patient is allowed to use a protective sock in a normal shoe with an insert and to initiate progressive weight bearing. Resumption of weight bearing is dependent on radiographic evidence of bone healing. It is better to delay weight bearing than to initiate it too soon.

At 6 months, the patient begins advanced gait training to increase muscular strength and balance. We typically follow patients at least 1 year and request a 2-year follow-up. At 1 year, most patients can still benefit from reinforcement of the skills learned in rehabilitation, even though most osseous healing is complete (**Figure 1, H** and **I**).

Pearls

- External fixation to obtain gross length, alignment, and rotation of the limb should occur as soon as possible to protect the soft-tissue envelope.
- Exacting attention to detail in external fixator pin placement is necessary to prevent complications, such as vascular or neural injury or bone necrosis.
- Fibular length, alignment, and rotation must be restored to anatomic configuration; surgical fibular reduction should occur when appropriate personnel and adequate equipment are available.
- Planning for the definitive surgery should be done using CT images obtained after fibular reduction and external fixator placement.
- Definitive surgery addresses anatomic reduction of the morphology of the plafond and metadiaphysis and should ensure that the metaphysis-shaft construct is stable enough to control the fracture fragments in the face of potential delayed bone healing.
- Impaction, particularly of the Volkmann fragment, must be addressed in order to create an anatomic joint surface.

References

1. Benirschke SK, Kramer PA: Malleolar fractures, in DiGiovanni C, Greigsburg J, eds: *Core Knowledge in Orthopaedics: Foot and Ankle.* New York, NY, Elsevier, 2007, pp 1-14.
2. Augustin G, Davila S, Mihoci K, Udiljak T, Vedrina DS, Antabak A: Thermal osteonecrosis and bone drilling parameters revisited. *Arch Orthop Trauma Surg* 2008;128(1):71-77.
3. Singh J, Davenport JH, Pegg DJ: A national survey of instrument sharpening guidelines. *Surgeon* 2010;8(3):136-139.

Chapter 68
Surgical Treatment of Ankle Fractures

Eben A. Carroll, MD *Jason J. Halvorson, MD*

Patient Selection

The ankle is the most frequently injured weight-bearing joint in the body, making ankle injuries commonplace to most orthopaedic surgeons.[1] Injury is usually the result of indirect rotational forces but also less commonly occurs after a direct blow. These forces result not only in bony fracture but also variable degrees of ligamentous and soft-tissue injury. Because ankle stability depends on both bony and ligamentous integrity, injury to both types of structures must be recognized and treated appropriately.

Fractures may be classified based on the anatomic site of injury or the mechanism of injury. The most common of the latter type is the Lauge-Hansen[2] classification system. This system predicts the position of the foot and the direction of the primary deforming force based on the displacement pattern, level, and morphology of the fibula fracture. The most common anatomic classification system is the Danis-Weber[3] system. This system uses the level of the lateral malleolar fracture in relation to the articular surface to classify these injuries.

As is true of many classification systems, neither of these systems perfectly predicts the need for surgical intervention. Each injury needs to be individualized and treatment decisions based on bone and ligamentous stability or lack thereof. Common to many of these injuries is some degree of dislocation or subluxation of the talus within the ankle mortise. It has long been established that even minimal mortise malalignment results in altered contact pressures and the risk of subsequent arthritis.[4] Imperative to successful management of these injuries is a stable, anatomically reduced ankle mortise. Stability is imparted by restoring the integrity of the bony injury and associated ligamentous injury.

Critical to decision making is the condition of the soft tissues. Marked swelling, the presence of fracture blisters, or other skin changes should delay surgery until the soft-tissue milieu resolves. Many ankle fractures can wait up to 3 weeks before undergoing definitive management without the need for significant change to surgical technique or any deleterious effect on outcome.[5] These considerations are of particular importance in the elderly and in those with diabetes.

All patients with suspected ankle injuries should get AP, mortise, and lateral radiographs. There are three important radiographic measurements with which all surgeons treating ankle fractures should be familiar: medial clear space (MCS), tibiofibular overlap, and tibiofibular clear space (**Figure 1**). In general, lateral shift of the talus 2 mm or greater (as measured by the MCS) or fracture displacement greater than 2 mm has been an indication for surgical intervention. The importance of dynamic stress views has recently been highlighted.[6] These views may demonstrate dynamic talar shift that may go unappreciated on static nonstress views (**Figure 2**). Similarly, injury

Figure 1 Illustration depicts the parameters commonly measured when assessing ankle stability. The medial clear space (MCS) should be 4 mm or less on the AP and mortise views. The tibiofibular overlap (TFO) should be 6 mm or more on the AP view and 1 mm or more on the mortise view. The tibiofibular clear space (TFCS) should be 6 mm or less on both AP and mortise views.

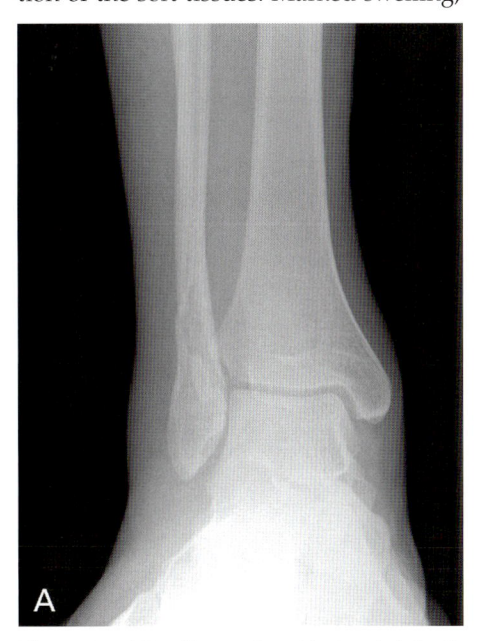

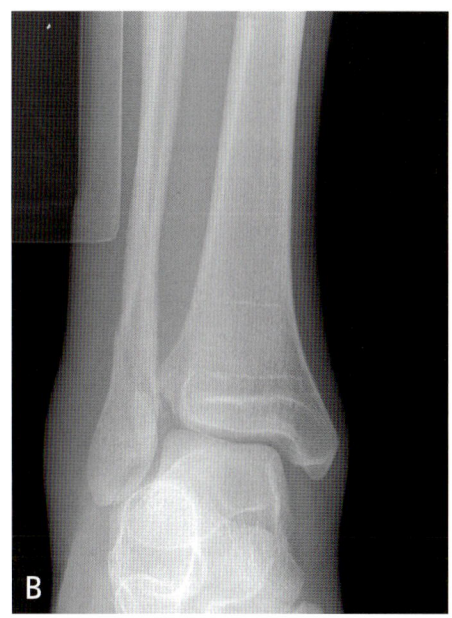

Figure 2 AP radiographs of isolated right distal fibula fracture. **A,** The medial clear space (MCS) appears normal on a static view. **B,** Note the increased MCS, suggestive of widening with gravity stress.

Dr. Carroll or an immediate family member has received research or institutional support from Synthes and Smith & Nephew and has received nonincome support (such as equipment or services), commercially derived honoraria, or other non–research-related funding (such as paid travel) from Synthes and Smith & Nephew. Neither Dr. Halvorson nor any immediate family member has received anything of value from or has stock or stock options held in a commercial company or institution related directly or indirectly to the subject of this chapter.

Section 5: Trauma

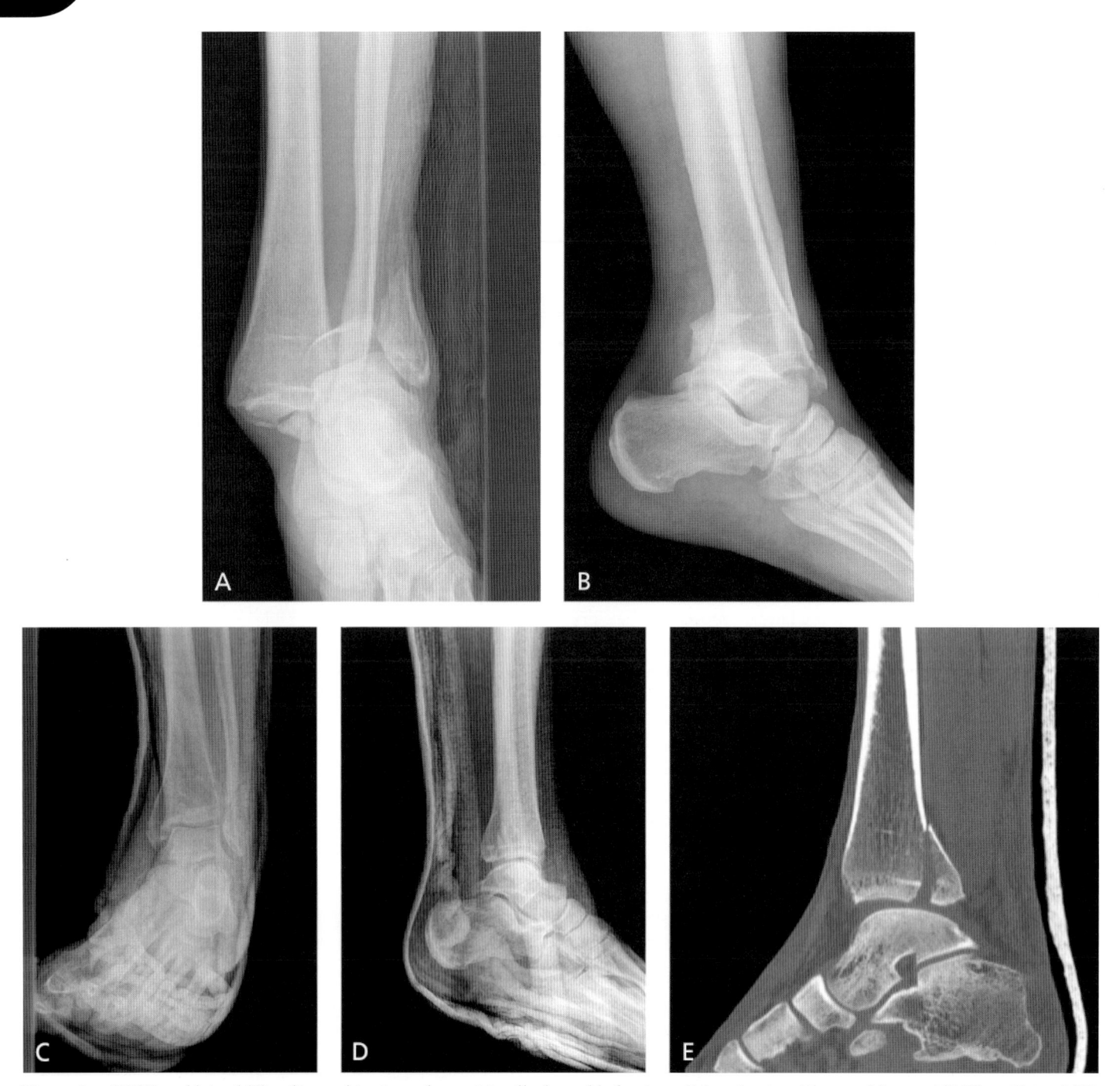

Figure 3 AP (**A**) and lateral (**B**) radiographic views show a trimalleolar ankle fracture-dislocation in a 76-year-old man. AP (**C**) and lateral (**D**) postreduction radiographs and sagittal reconstruction (**E**) of the posterior malleolar component. Note the now-reduced ankle mortise (**C**) and restoration of the tibiotalar relationship in the lateral plane (**D**). **E,** The size and displacement of the posterior malleolar fracture fragment are evident.

to the syndesmosis may be obvious with widening of the distal tibiofibular joint or appreciated only on dynamic stress examination.[7]

Monomalleolar fractures most commonly involve either the medial or lateral malleolus. Although long-term studies are lacking, most nondisplaced or minimally displaced (less than 2 mm) medial or lateral malleolar fractures are treated nonsurgically.[5] Monomalleolar injuries displaced more than 2 mm should undergo surgical intervention.[1] There is little role for nonsurgical management of bimalleolar and trimalleolar ankle fractures, fracture-dislocations, syndesmotic injuries, and open fractures; all of these injuries require surgical management in the absence of absolute contraindications to surgery.[1] Historic indications for the fixation of posterior malleolar fragments include those fractures that comprise greater than 25% of the tibial plafond and remain displaced greater than 2 mm after fibular fixation.[1] Recent literature, however, suggests that these indications may be expanding and that posterior malleolar fixation may improve fibular reduction and help restore the integrity of the syndesmosis by restoring the ligamentous connection between the fibula and the tibia via intact posteroinferior tibiofibular ligaments.[8,9]

Preoperative Imaging

The case described here is a 76-year-old man who sustained an ankle injury as a result of a motorcycle accident. He presented to the emergency department with a closed trimalleolar ankle fracture-dislocation (**Figure 3, A and B**). He underwent closed reduction under conscious sedation in the emergency department (**Figure 3 C through E**). He was subsequently discharged from the hospital

Chapter 68: Surgical Treatment of Ankle Fractures

and was brought back for formal surgical management 4 days after the injury when outpatient examination revealed resolution of swelling and a soft-tissue milieu appropriate for surgical intervention.

Video 68.1 Trimalleolar Ankle Fracture Fixation. Eben Carroll, MD; Jason Halvorson, MD (14 min)

Procedure

Room Setup/Patient Positioning

The room setup is depicted in **Figure 4**. The operating surgeon and the instrument table are on the same side as the ankle injury. Intraoperative C-arm imaging, which is required, is set up on the side opposite the surgical extremity. This setup allows the surgeon to work and gain concomitant imaging with little obstruction or frustration.

The position of the patient depends on the nature of the ankle injury. For most isolated monomalleolar fractures and bimalleolar injuries, the patient is positioned supine. A nonsterile bump is often placed under the affected hip, and a nonsterile tourniquet is applied. If there is a trimalleolar injury in which the posterior malleolar fracture needs to be addressed, we prefer the setup shown in **Figure 5, A**. In the patient depicted in **Figure 3**, there was a posterior malleolar fragment that needed to be addressed surgically. The patient was placed in a lateral position on a beanbag. This allows for a posterolateral approach to the fibula and posterior malleolus. The patient is then rolled into a supine position for fixation of the medial malleolar fracture (**Figure 5, B**).

Instruments/Equipment/Implants

A radiolucent table is used to maximize the ease of intraoperative imaging. Small-fragment plates and screws are usually sufficient to address most ankle fracture fixation dilemmas. On occasion, a wider variety of plates can be beneficial. In the case described here, 2.4- and 2.7-mm implants were used. Fracture-reducing clamps, dental picks, and tissue elevators also help to achieve the goals of surgery.

Surgical Technique

Our preference is to address the posterior malleolus and the fibula first, so the patient is initially placed in a lateral position. After preparation and draping, the injured extremity is exsanguinated with

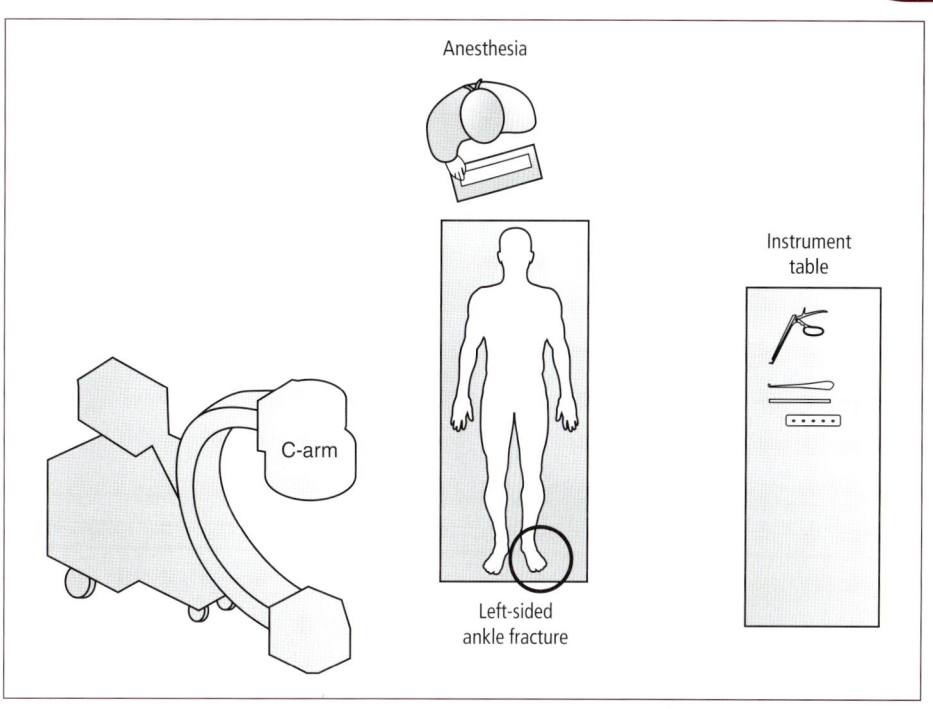

Figure 4 Illustration shows an example of the room setup for a patient with a left-sided ankle fracture. The scrub and the instrument table are set up on the same side as the injury, and the C-arm is set up on the side opposite the injury.

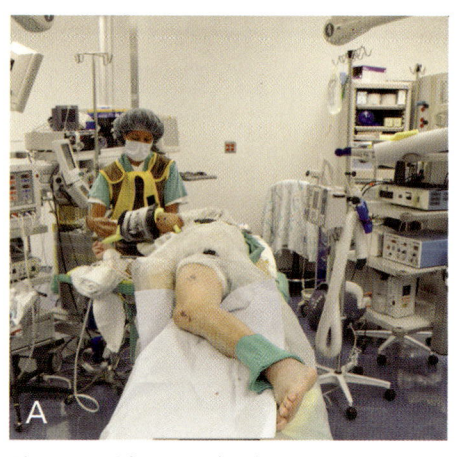

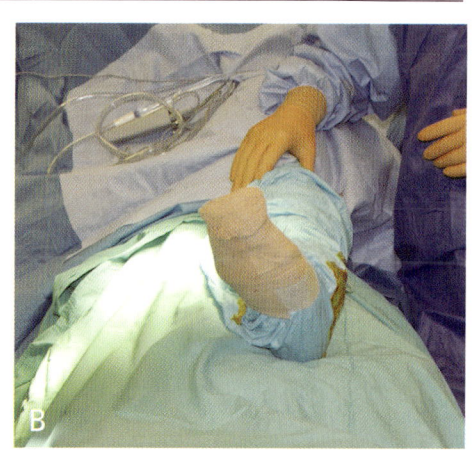

Figure 5 Photographs show patient positioning for surgical treatment of an ankle fracture. **A,** The patient is placed on a beanbag in the lateral decubitus position with the injured extremity up. **B,** After the fibula and/or posterior malleolar fractures are addressed, the beanbag is deflated and the patient is rolled into a supine position to allow access to the medial malleolus without the need for a separate preparation and draping.

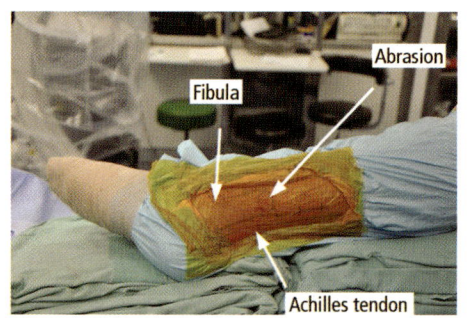

Figure 6 Photograph shows a left ankle with the patient in a right lateral decubitus position. Distal is to the left. Incision is made midway between the Achilles complex and the posterior border of the fibula. In this patient, the incision was created slightly more posterior, secondary to an abrasion in the path of the preferred incision.

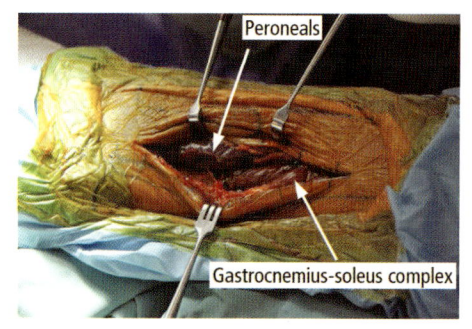

Figure 7 Intraoperative photograph shows a left ankle with the patient in a right lateral decubitus position. The superficial interval is between the peroneal musculature anteriorly and the gastrocnemius-soleus complex posteriorly.

© 2013 American Academy of Orthopaedic Surgeons

445

Section 5: Trauma

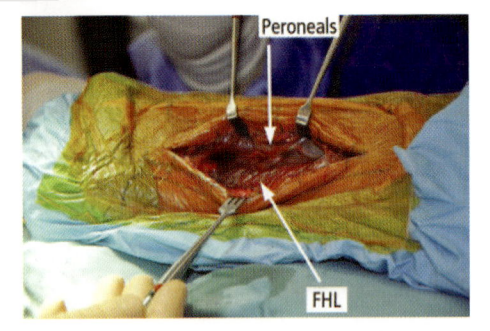

Figure 8 Intraoperative photograph shows the flexor hallucis longus (FHL) arising from the posterior surface of the fibula.

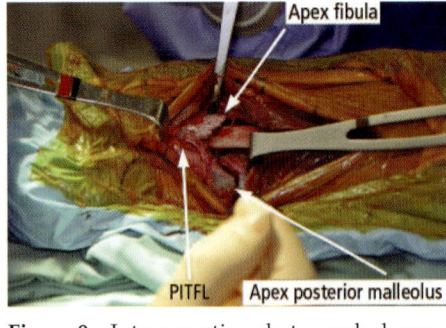

Figure 9 Intraoperative photograph shows the apexes of the fibular and posterior malleolar fractures. Note the intact posterior inferior tibiofibular ligament (PITFL).

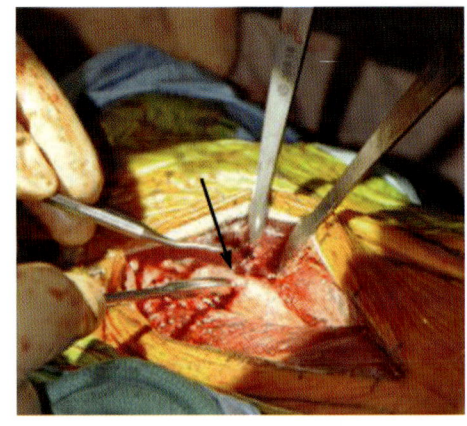

Figure 10 The fracture apex (arrow; in this figure, the fibula) is reduced with the help of a combination of clamps, ball-spike pushers, dental picks, and Kirschner wires.

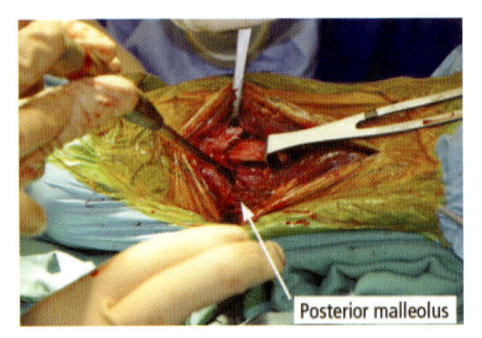

Figure 11 Intraoperative photograph shows the apex of the posterior malleolar fracture held provisionally and reduced with a Kirschner wire.

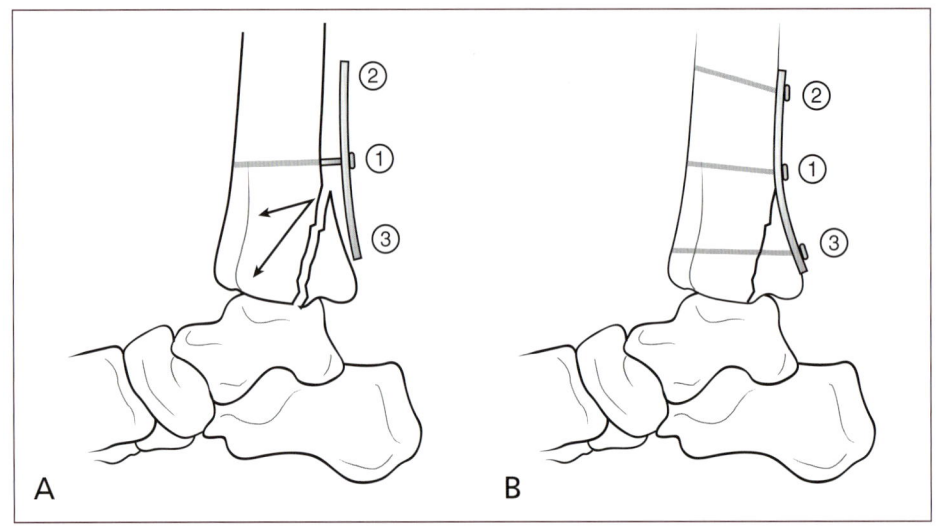

Figure 12 Illustration demonstrates reduction and neutralization of a posterior malleolar fracture using an antiglide plating technique. **A,** Screw 1 is inserted first, just proximal to the apex of the fracture line. With tightening of this screw, fracture reduction can be achieved with the distal anterior force vector applied via the plate. **B,** Screw 2 is then placed. Finally, any residual articular gapping is addressed with a lag screw in position 3. In a true antiglide construct, screw 3 may not always be necessary if no articular gapping is present.

an Esmarch bandage and the tourniquet is inflated to 250 mm Hg. The incision is made midway between the Achilles complex and the posterior border of the fibula (**Figure 6**). The surgical dissection uses the internervous plane between the gastrocnemius-soleus complex and the flexor hallucis longus muscle, innervated by the tibial nerve, and the peroneus brevis and longus, innervated by the superficial peroneal nerve.

Dissection is taken down to the deep fascia of the leg, with care taken to avoid damage to the short saphenous vein. Care must also be taken to protect the sural nerve, which is a safe distance from the surgical field proximally but may cross the incision at its more distal extension. The deep fascia of the leg is incised; the superficial interval lies between the peroneus longus and brevis anteriorly and the gastrocnemius-soleus complex posteriorly (**Figure 7**). The former muscles are retracted anterior and lateral, and the latter are retracted posterior and medial. Arising from the posterior surface of the fibula is the flexor hallucis longus (**Figure 8**). This muscle is detached from its origin on the posterior fibula and is retracted posterior and medial. Dissection is taken across the interosseous membrane until the posterior tibia is encountered. Care must be taken to not disrupt the posterior syndesmotic ligaments.

The apexes of the fibular and posterior malleolar fractures can be easily identified, delineated, and cleaned of obstructing soft-tissue debris via this interval (**Figure 9**). It has been shown that reduction of the fibula indirectly reduces the posterior malleolar fragment.[10] Similarly, reduction of the posterior malleolar fragment will usually help with reduction and restoration of length to the fibula. The posterior malleolar fragment often fails in tension, resulting in little comminution. This affords the surgeon an easy opportunity to help gauge rotation and length of the fibula, via an intact posterior syndesmosis, if the fibular fracture is not a simple pattern.

In the current case, the posterior malleolar fracture was reduced and fixed first, followed by the fibular component. Regardless of which fracture is addressed first, the process is the same. The fracture line is cleaned of obstructing soft-tissue debris. The fracture is reduced and held provisionally using a combination of clamps, ball-spike pushers, dental picks, and Kirschner wires (K-wires) as aids (**Figure 10**). Often, dorsiflexion of the foot can also be helpful to regain length. The fracture is held provisionally with a clamp or K-wire (**Figure 11**). The fracture is then neutralized with an antiglide plate and compressed with a lag screw as shown in **Figure 12**. In the current patient, we felt there was a small amount of residual diastasis at the level of the joint, so an additional lag screw was placed outside the posterior antiglide plate. With true antiglide plating, this may not always be necessary. This process was

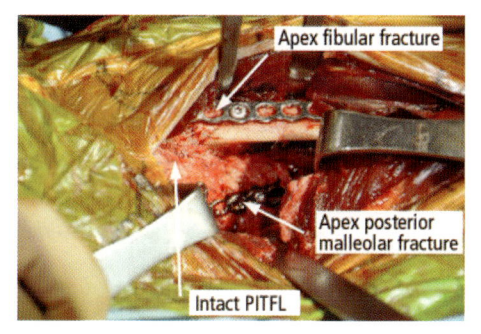

Chapter 68: Surgical Treatment of Ankle Fractures

Figure 13 Intraoperative photograph shows the posterior malleolar and fibular fractures reduced and neutralized with antiglide plates. Note the intact posterior inferior tibiofibular ligament (PITFL).

then repeated for the fibula (**Figure 13**). In the case described here, 2.7-mm plates were used, but one-third tubular small-fragment plates are standard for the ankle. The lateral side was copiously irrigated, and attention was turned toward the medial malleolus fracture.

If there is no posterior malleolar fracture requiring repair, the patient can be placed in a supine position and a direct lateral approach to the fibula can be made. The fibula is usually in a subcutaneous position, and the superficial peroneal nerve needs to protected, particularly for more proximal fibular fractures. From this approach, the fibula can be plated posteriorly, as described previously, although this is more difficult than via a posterolateral approach. Commonly, a one-third tubular small-fragment plate can be placed directly lateral to neutralize a reduced and lagged fibular fracture (**Figure 14**). This plate position may not be as strong a construct as the antiglide montage, and the lateral plate may be more prominent.[5]

As previously mentioned, after the posterolateral approach is complete, the beanbag is deflated, allowing the patient to return to a semisupine position. With gentle external rotation of the hip, an ideal position for addressing the medial malleolar fracture is achieved (**Figure 5, B**). The surgeon has several options for an incision to address the medial malleolar fracture fragment (**Figure 15**). In the case described here, a straight longitudinal incision centered over the medial malleolar fragment was made. The long saphenous vein must be identified and protected. The fracture line is cleaned of obstructing soft-tissue debris.

Quite often, portions of the deltoid ligament or the periosteum may be interposed between the medial malleolus and the tibia, and the surgeon needs to be sure to retrieve this soft tissue. Two

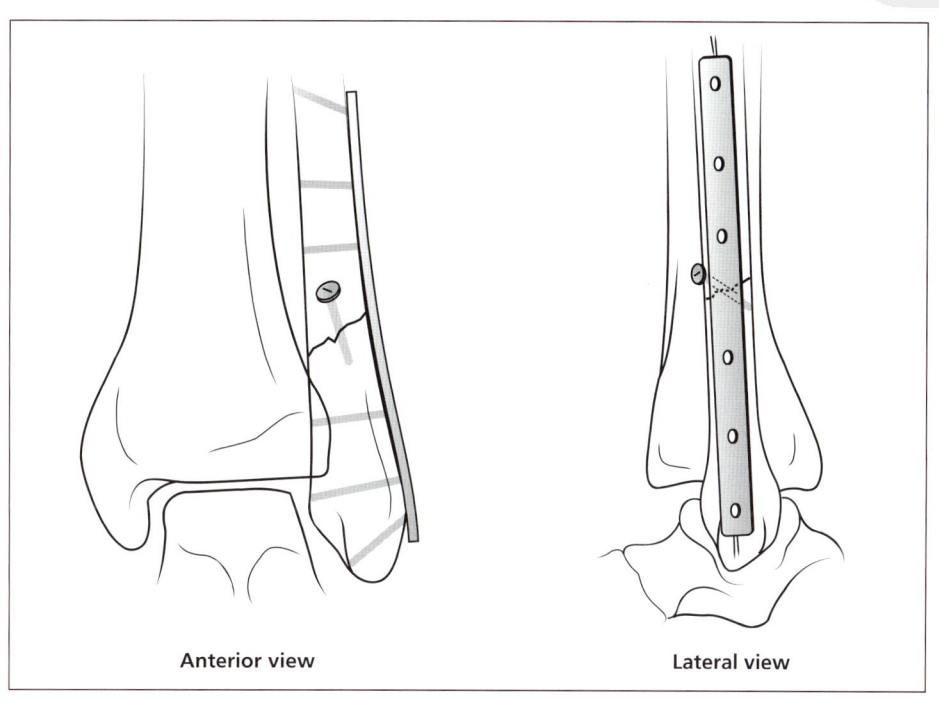

Figure 14 Illustration shows a commonly used fixation montage for laterally based fibular fixation. A one third tubular small-fragment plate can be placed directly lateral to neutralize a reduced and lagged fibular fracture. Too much obliquity of the distal screws must be avoided because this increases the risk of problems caused by hardware prominence.

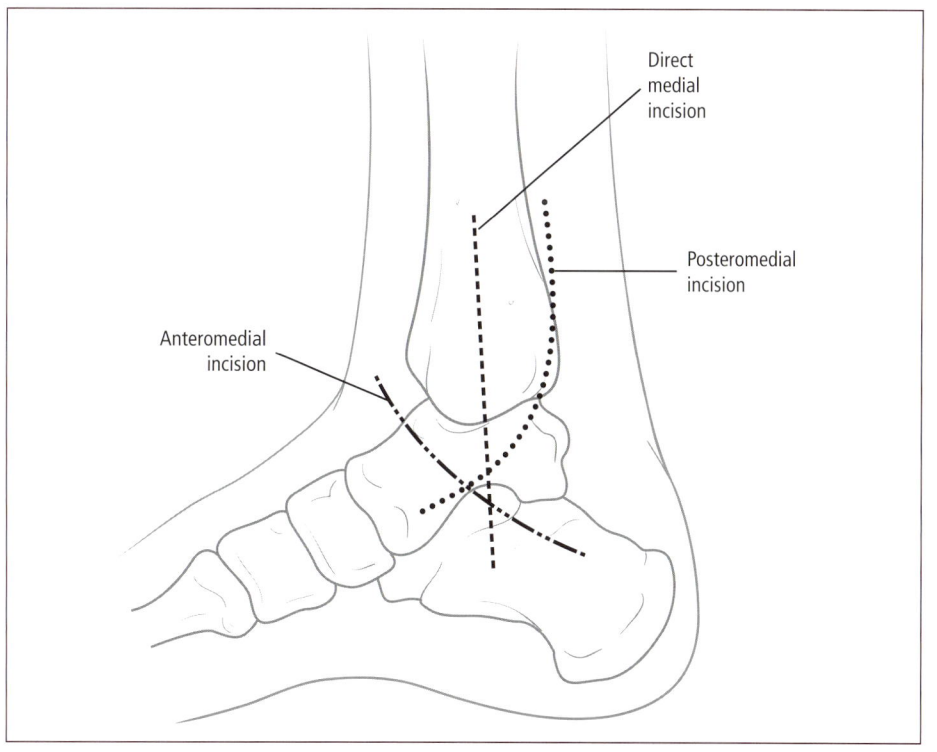

Figure 15 Illustration depicts options for incisions to address a medial malleolar fracture fragment.

K-wires are inserted into the medial malleolar fragment if it is of sufficient size. These two wires act as a joystick to reduce the fracture; they also have the advantage of being in prime position to act as provisional stabilization once the reduction is achieved. The medial reduction can be quite tricky, and we suggest that the reduction be gauged by direct visualization in two different areas, usually at the extra-articular medial fracture line and the anteromedial apex of the articular surface. This minimizes the chance for malrotation or malreduction. The intraoperative C-arm alone should not be relied upon to gauge reduction.

© 2013 American Academy of Orthopaedic Surgeons

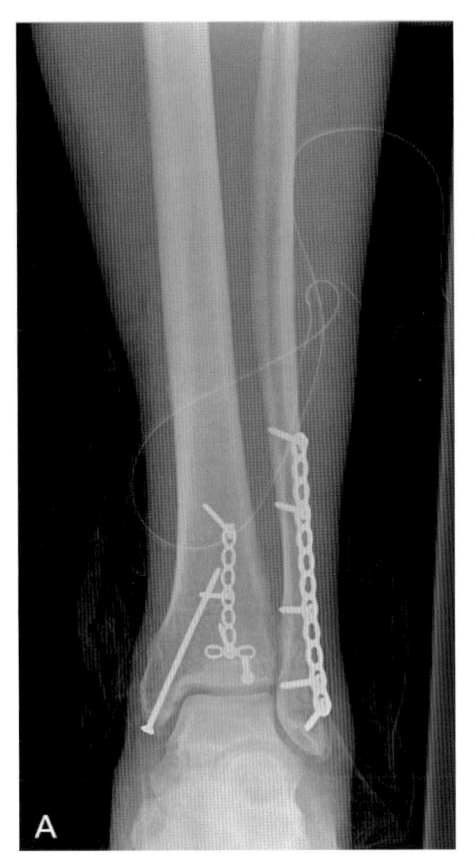

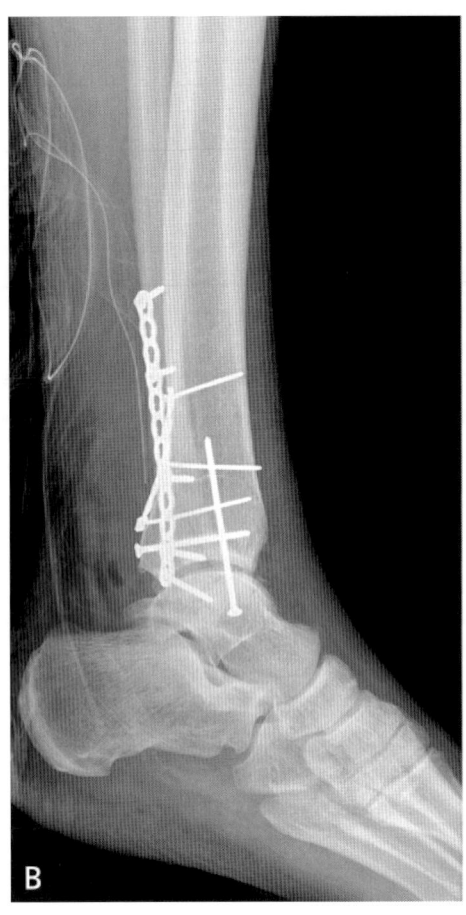

Figure 16 Final postoperative radiographs demonstrate re-establishment of mortise congruity and appropriate fixation of medial and lateral malleoli on the AP view (**A**) and the reduced and neutralized posterior malleolar fracture fragment on the lateral view (**B**).

Definitive fixation of the medial malleolar fragment is often performed with partially threaded 3.5- or 4.0-mm cannulated screws. Other options include noncannulated 2.7-, 3.5-, or 4.0-mm screws. Compression of the medial malleolar fragment should be achieved with partially threaded screws, fully threaded screws inserted with lag screw technique, or external compression with a clamp followed by set screw insertion. Often, unicortical screws are used, but there has been recent evidence that bicortical medial malleolar fixation may be advantageous.[11] Care should be taken to match the screw size to the size of the medial malleolar fragment to avoid iatrogenic comminution. In the case described here, the medial malleolar fragment was quite small, and a single 2.7-mm screw was used. Ideally, two points of fixation should be achieved in the medial malleolar fragment to control possible rotational displacement. The final fixation construct is shown in **Figure 16**.

Intraoperative fluoroscopic images and plain radiographs should be taken and scrutinized before closure. In particular the surgeon must ensure that syndesmotic stability has been restored. Historically, it was thought that only Danis-Weber type C injuries resulted in syndesmotic instability, but more recent work has demonstrated that syndesmotic injury can occur regardless of the level of the fibular fracture.[7] In the current case, after fracture fixation was complete, an intraoperative stress view was performed to ensure competency of the syndesmotic ligaments.

Once all static and dynamic radiographs have been inspected, the wounds are closed in a layered fashion over suction drains after copious irrigation. Nonabsorbable interrupted skin sutures should be used and staples avoided. Sterile dressings are applied and, before awakening, the patient is placed in a well-padded splint with the foot in neutral inversion/eversion and neutral dorsiflexion/plantar flexion.

Complications

The most commonly seen complications in the care of ankle fractures involve wound problems and infection. This occurs in 4% to 5% of cases,[5] which underscores the importance of careful and meticulous soft-tissue handling. Simple peri-incisional redness and superficial tissue necrosis may be observed or treated with antibiotics. More significant wound breakdown or exposed hardware may require consultation with a plastic surgeon. Frank wound infection or superficial infections that do not quickly resolve should undergo surgical débridement and culture-directed antibiotic therapy.

Malunion has dire consequences on contact pressures in the ankle.[4,12] Treating surgeons should make every effort at the initial surgical intervention to ensure anatomic reduction because correction of malunion becomes more difficult after the initial surgery. Nonunion is uncommon around the ankle but most commonly occurs with displaced medial malleolar fractures. As previously discussed, it is not uncommon for soft tissue to invaginate within the fracture cleft, which may predispose to nonunion. The surgeon must be careful to retrieve any such intervening soft tissue during medial malleolar fracture reduction.

It is not uncommon, given the subcutaneous position of the fibula and medial malleolus at the level of the ankle, for hardware in these areas to be symptomatic. Although there is little literature to guide recommendations, hardware removal is usually delayed until a year after surgery but often results in symptomatic improvement for patients. Technical factors such as posterolateral fibular plating, decreasing the obliquity of screws placed in a laterally based fibular plate, and smaller medial malleolar screws may decrease the incidence of symptomatic hardware.

Postoperative Care and Rehabilitation

There is little good evidence in the literature to guide postoperative treatment in terms of time to weight bearing and duration of immobilization. Some evidence exists that early range of motion may be of benefit.[13] Routinely, the patient is maintained in a splint for the initial 2-week postoperative period. After suture removal, if the soft-tissue milieu appears amenable, patients are placed in a fracture boot and allowed to remove the brace and begin gentle range-of-motion exercises. Weight bearing is delayed for a period of 6 to 8 weeks. If diabetes is a complicating comorbidity, then cast immobilization is continued for 8 weeks and weight bearing is delayed until 12 weeks after surgical intervention.

Pearls

- The condition of the soft tissue is of critical importance. Definitive surgical intervention should be delayed until the soft-tissue milieu is amenable to surgery.
- The manner in which the soft tissue is handled has direct implications for postoperative complications such as wound slough and infection.
- Dynamic radiographs (stress views) are required before assuming that a monomalleolar fibular fracture is stable and the deltoid ligament is intact.
- The ankle joint is unforgiving of malreduction; anatomic reduction should be achieved at the initial surgical setting.
- Posterolateral fibular plating, decreasing the obliquity of distal screws in a laterally based fibular plate, and proper size and location of medial malleolar screws may decrease the incidence of symptomatic hardware.
- A well-padded cast with the foot in neutral inversion/eversion and a neutral dorsiflexion/plantar flexion position is placed immediately postoperatively and is maintained until the soft tissue looks amenable to allow for range of motion.
- Weight bearing is progressed cautiously in diabetic patients.

References

1. Michelson JD: Ankle fractures resulting from rotational injuries. *J Am Acad Orthop Surg* 2003;11(6):403-412.
2. Lauge N: Fractures of the ankle: Analytic historic survey as the basis of new experimental, roentgenologic and clinical investigations. *Arch Surg* 1948;56(3):259-317.
3. Weber BG: Die Verletzungen des Oberen Sprunggelenkes, in *Aktuelle Probleme in der Chirurgie*, ed 3. Bern, Switzerland, Verlag Hans Huber, 1977.
4. Ramsey PL, Hamilton W: Changes in tibiotalar area of contact caused by lateral talar shift. *J Bone Joint Surg Am* 1976;58(3):356-357.
5. Collinge CA, Heier K: Ankle fractures and dislocations, in Stannard JP, Schmidt AH, Kregor PJ, eds: *Surgical Treatment of Orthopaedic Trauma*. New York, NY, Thieme Medical Publishers, 2007, pp 792-814.
6. Michelson JD, Varner KE, Checcone M: Diagnosing deltoid injury in ankle fractures: The gravity stress view. *Clin Orthop Relat Res* 2001;387:178-182.
7. Stark E, Tornetta P III, Creevy WR: Syndesmotic instability in Weber B ankle fractures: A clinical evaluation. *J Orthop Trauma* 2007;21(9):643-646.
8. Gardner MJ, Brodsky A, Briggs SM, Nielson JH, Lorich DG: Fixation of posterior malleolar fractures provides greater syndesmotic stability. *Clin Orthop Relat Res* 2006;447:165-171.
9. Miller AN, Carroll EA, Parker RJ, Helfet DL, Lorich DG: Posterior malleolar stabilization of syndesmotic injuries is equivalent to screw fixation. *Clin Orthop Relat Res* 2010;468(4):1129-1135.
10. Harper MC, Hardin G: Posterior malleolar fractures of the ankle associated with external rotation-abduction injuries: Results with and without internal fixation. *J Bone Joint Surg Am* 1988;70(9):1348-1356.
11. Ricci WM, Tornetta P, Borrelli J Jr: Lag screw fixation of medial malleolar fractures: A biomechanical, radiographic, and clinical comparison of unicortical partially threaded lag screws and bicortical fully threaded lag screws. *J Orthop Trauma* 2012;26(10):602-606.
12. Vrahas M, Fu F, Veenis B: Intraarticular contact stresses with simulated ankle malunions. *J Orthop Trauma* 1994;8(2):159-166.
13. Egol KA, Dolan R, Koval KJ: Functional outcome of surgery for fractures of the ankle: A prospective, randomised comparison of management in a cast or a functional brace. *J Bone Joint Surg Br* 2000;82(2):246-249.

Chapter 69
Surgical Management of Fractures of the Talus

John M. Tabit, DO   Lawrence X. Webb, MD

Introduction

Anatomy

The talus consists of the head, neck, body, lateral process, and posterior process. The posterior process is divided into a medial tubercle and a lateral tubercle by the groove corresponding to the flexor hallucis longus (FHL) tendon. The talus and its constituent parts are illustrated in **Figure 1**. Sixty percent of the talus is covered by hyaline cartilage, and this feature is pivotal to its role as a major contributor to the motion of the midfoot, hindfoot, and ankle. There are no muscle or tendon attachments directly to the bone (**Figure 2**). The talus receives its blood supply from all three major arteries that supply the foot and ankle, including the peroneal, anterior tibial, and posterior tibial arteries.[1,2] Locally, the bone receives its blood supply from the arteries that derive from these three: the artery of the tarsal canal, the deltoid artery, and the artery of the sinus tarsi (**Figure 3**). Recent studies have shown that the talus has a rich and redundant intraosseous blood supply.[3] This may help to explain why osteonecrosis is seldom associated with nondisplaced fractures of the talar neck. It also may explain the enhanced potential for vascular recovery in displaced fractures following open reduction and internal fixation (ORIF).[3-5]

Mechanism of Injury

Talar neck fractures occur most commonly as a result of hyperdorsiflexion of the foot. The low bone density and small cross-sectional area of the talar neck make it susceptible to fracture at the "giving way point," as the stressed talus strikes the much denser anterior tibia. Based on laboratory studies and clinical data, it has been estimated that up to 26% of talar neck fractures have concomitant medial malleolar fractures, with hindfoot supination playing a significant role in the

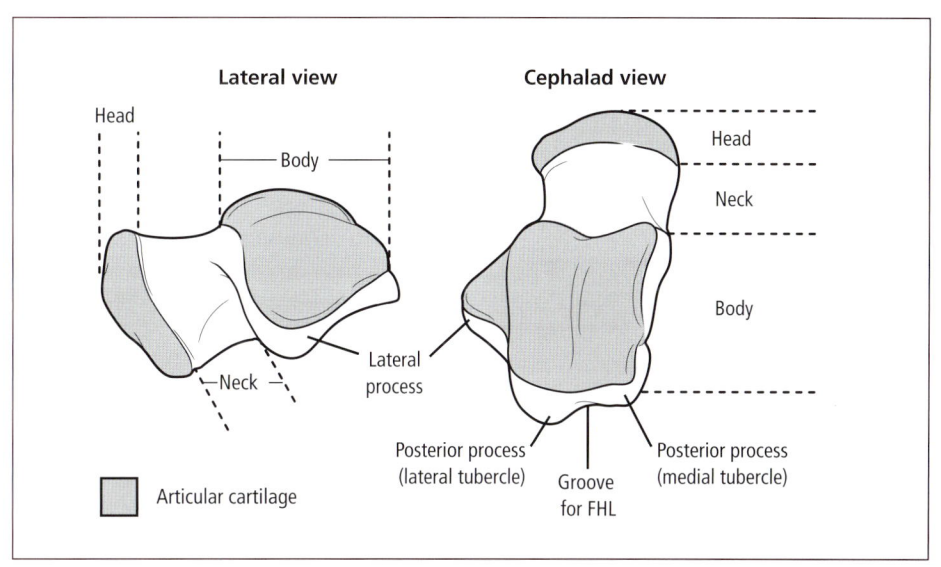

Figure 1 Illustration depicts two views of the talus. FHL = flexor hallucis longus.

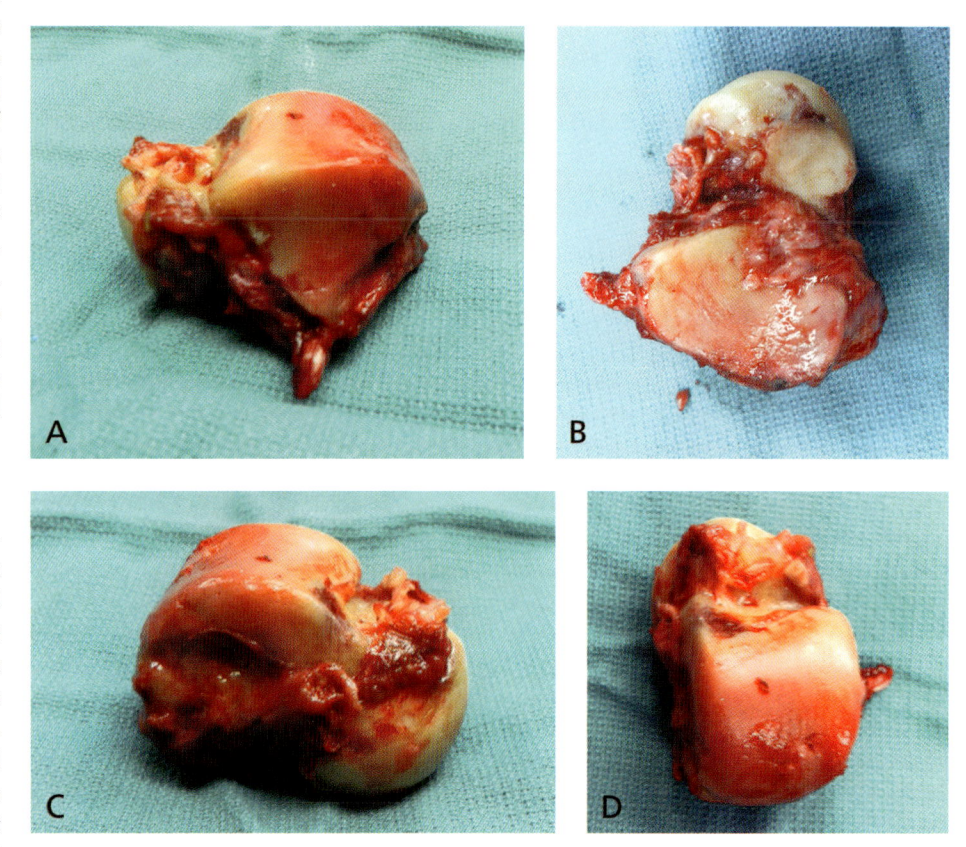

Figure 2 Photographs show the lateral (**A**), inferior (**B**), medial (**C**), and cephalad (**D**) aspects of a fresh talus specimen from a right ankle.

Dr. Webb or an immediate family member is a member of a speakers' bureau or has made paid presentations on behalf of the Musculoskeletal Transplant Foundation; serves as a paid consultant to or is an employee of Zimmer; has received nonincome support (such as equipment or services), commercially derived honoraria, or other non–research-related funding (such as paid travel) from Synthes, Smith & Nephew, Stryker, Kinetic Concepts, and Doctors Group; and serves as a board member, owner, officer, or committee member of the Orthopaedic Trauma Association and the Southeastern Fracture Consortium Foundation. Neither Dr. Tabit nor any immediate family member has received anything of value from or has stock or stock optins held in a commercial company or institution related directly or indirectly to the subject of this chapter.

© 2013 American Academy of Orthopaedic Surgeons

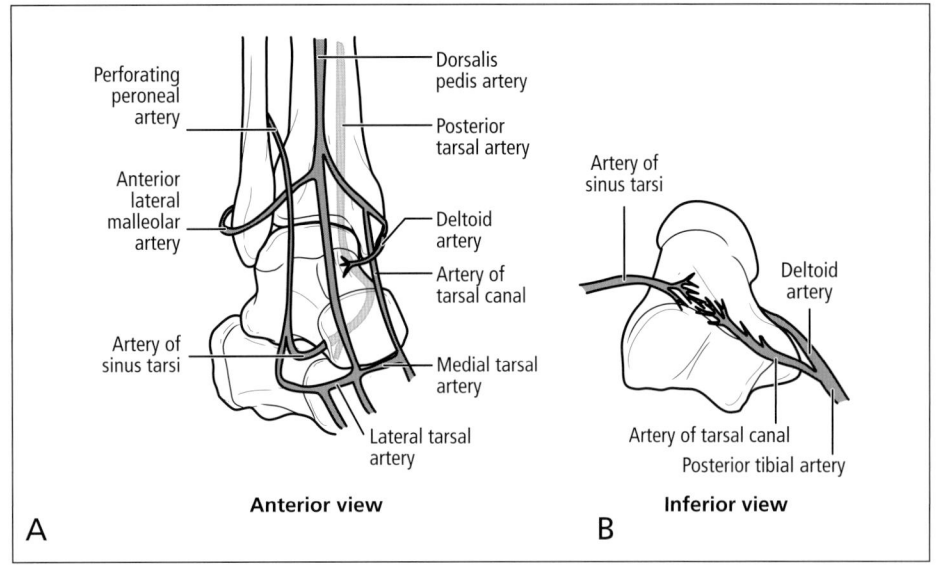

Figure 3 Illustrations show anterior (**A**) and inferior (**B**) views of the talus with its blood supply. The blood supply is derived from an anastamotic ring with contributions from the posterior tibial artery by way of its deltoid artery branch and the artery of the tarsal canal. The dorsalis pedis artery and the perforating peroneal artery also contribute, by way of their branches, to the artery of the sinus tarsi and the lateral tarsal artery, respectively. (Adapted from Fortin P, Balazsy J: Talus fractures: Evaluation and treatment. *J Am Acad Orthop Surg* 2001;9[6]: pp114-127.)

mechanism of injury.[6,7] These fractures are often high-energy injuries, resulting in significant comminution and displacement and having a high incidence of associated fractures (64%) and disruptions of the soft-tissue envelope (21% are open injuries).[6]

Classification

The most widely used classification system for talar neck fractures is the one described by Hawkins in 1970.[6] The Hawkins classification defines type I fractures as nondisplaced, type II fractures as displaced with subluxation or dislocation of the subtalar joint and an intact tibiotalar joint, and type III fractures as displaced with subluxation or dislocation of both the subtalar and tibiotalar joints. The rates of osteonecrosis of the talar body correlate with this classification, and the risk of vascular disruption increases with the extent of displacement. Osteonecrosis rates have been reported to be 0% to 13%, 20% to 50%, and 83% to 100% for Hawkins types I, II, and III fractures, respectively.[6,8] Improved techniques for open reduction and internal fixation of the talus have resulted in an overall diminution in the osteonecrosis rates for Hawkins type II and III fractures.[5,9,10] Canale and Kelly[8] later added a type IV talar neck fracture, characterized as a Hawkins type III injury with an accompanying dislocation of the talonavicular joint.

The Hawkins classification system is confined to fracture-dislocations of the neck of the talus alone; the AO/Orthopaedic Trauma Association (AO/OTA) classification is more encyclopedic. Although the AO/OTA system is used infrequently in common clinical orthopaedic parlance, it is of great value in research.[11]

Patient Selection
Indications

Truly nondisplaced fractures, as assessed on radiographs and CT scans as described below, can be managed nonsurgically in a short leg splint with conversion to a cast once the swelling has subsided. Non–weight bearing should be enforced for 8 to 12 weeks, with subsequent protected graduated weight bearing. Radiographic views obtained at office follow-up visits with the foot out of the cast should include an ankle mortise view, a lateral view, and a Canale view. At 8 weeks, the mortise radiographic view should be inspected for the presence of a Hawkins sign, which is a subchondral lucency of the talar body that indicates bone resorption and vascularity. A good prognostic Hawkins sign is seen in 95% of nondisplaced talar neck fractures. Tezval et al[12] studied the prognostic reliability of the Hawkins sign for avascular necrosis in patients with displaced fractures and demonstrated a sensitivity of 100% and a specificity of 58%.

Most talar fractures are displaced and require surgical management. Patients generally present with edema and ecchymosis of the ankle or foot. Gross deformity may be present in higher grade fracture-dislocations (**Figure 4**). In the acute setting, closed reduction of dislocations of the peritalar joints should be attempted, especially if the soft-tissue envelope is compromised by the displacement. Immobilization can be accomplished with a posterior splint or a bridging external fixator. Definitive management of the fracture with open reduction and internal fixation should proceed if closed reduction of the dislocation is unsuccessful. If closed reduction is satisfactory, an open reduction and internal fixation of the fracture should follow as soon as possible but is not emergent. In the recent past, controversy existed regarding the timing of reduction and fixation of talar fractures. A delay in reduction was thought to be related to a higher incidence of osteonecrosis. Several recent retrospective reviews, however, support the concept that the timing of reduction and fixation do not influence the incidence of osteonecrosis and posttraumatic arthritis.[4,13,14]

Contraindications

Contraindications to a surgical repair include preexisting active or indolent bone infection involving the talus, severe neuropathic foot, and uncorrectable vascular impairment with a high likelihood of impaired wound healing. In such situations, a tibiocalcaneal fusion or an amputation and early fitting with a prosthesis is indicated.

Isolated nondisplaced lateral or posterior process fractures also may be managed nonsurgically. Displaced fractures should be reduced and stably fixed.

Isolated osteochondral fractures may accompany ankle sprains. If they are sizable with involvement of the subchondral bone, they may be amenable to reduction and stabilization with countersunk minifragment screws or headless screws. When the fragments are small and displaced in the joint, they may need to be excised. If unrecognized, these intraarticular fragments may cause persisting ankle pain and mechanical symptoms if the fracture is treated as a simple sprain.

Preoperative Imaging

Routine ankle and foot radiographs, including mortise, lateral ankle, and Canale views, should be obtained, as well as CT scans (**Figure 5**). The lateral view shows the neck and highlights talona-

Chapter 69: Surgical Management of Fractures of the Talus

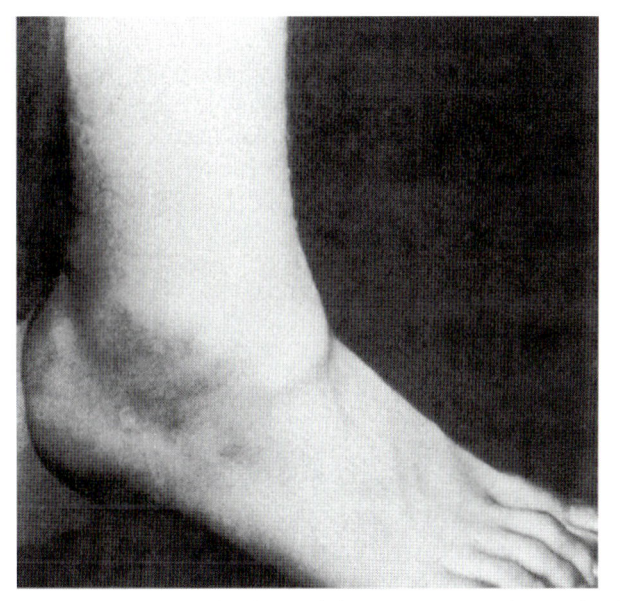

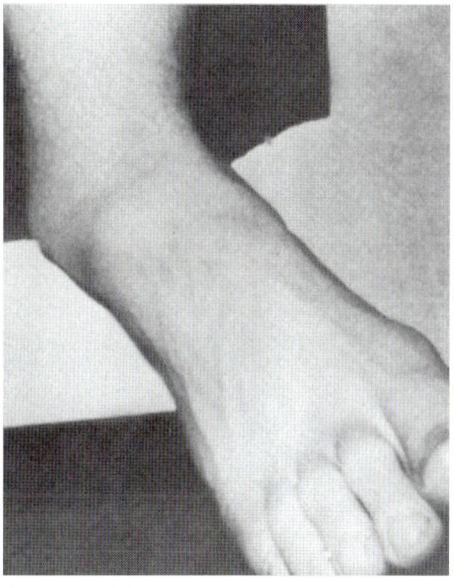

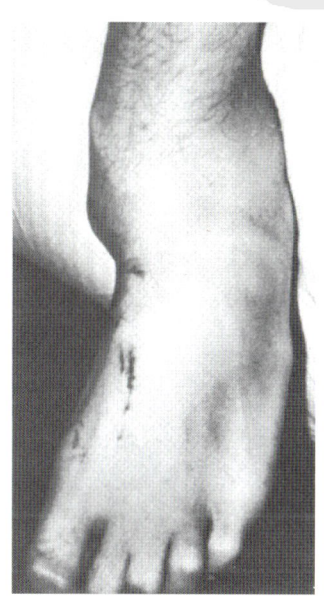

Figure 4 Photographs depict deformity associated with the dislocation of the subtalar joint. In this medial subtalar dislocation, the head of the talus is palpable on the dorsum of the foot (**A**), and the heel is displaced medially (**B**). **C,** In this lateral subtalar dislocation, the head of the talus is prominent medially, while the rest of the foot is dislocated laterally. (Reproduced with permission from Buckingham WW Jr, LeFlore I: Subtalar dislocation of the foot. *J Trauma* 1973;13(9):753-765.)

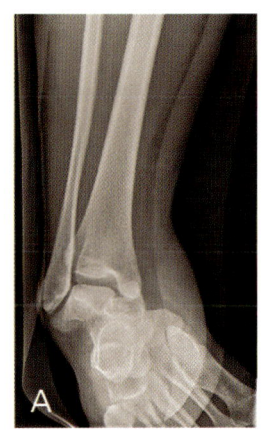

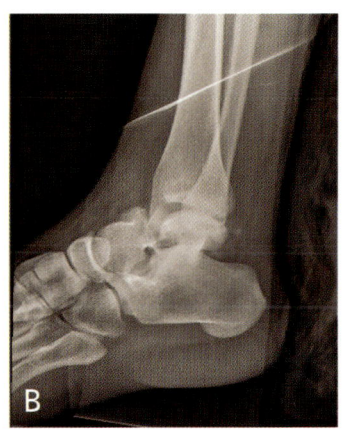

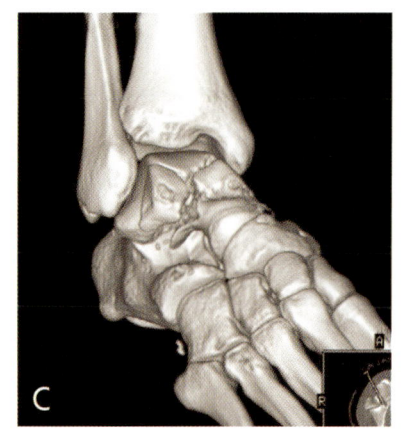

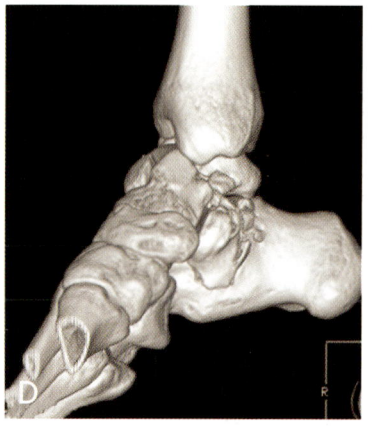

Figure 5 Fracture of the talus in a 20-year-old woman. Mortise (**A**) and lateral (**B**) views of the ankle. **C,** Three-dimensional CT reconstruction image reveals a combination neck and body fracture. **D,** An associated minimally displaced fracture of the sustentaculum is seen on this three-dimensional CT reconstruction image.

Video 69.1 Talar Neck Fracture and Lateral Process Open Reduction and Internal Fixation. John M. Tabit, DO; Lawrence X. Webb, MD (5 min)

vicular, tibiotalar, and talocalcaneal joint incongruities. The AP view of the foot and the mortise ankle view show talonavicular and tibiotalar joint incongruities, respectively. The Canale view shows the neck in profile. It is obtained with the foot in maximal plantar flexion and internally rotated 15°. The beam is angled 75° from the horizontal plane.[8] CT, including high-quality three-dimensional images, is essential for preoperative planning. It is very helpful in characterizing the extent of comminution and displacement and in understanding the subtleties of the fracture as well as the presence and characteristics of neighboring associated fractures.

Procedure
Patient Positioning
For talar head, neck, and most body fractures, the patient can be positioned supine with the feet at the end of a radiolucent cantilever type table. A soft bump is placed under the affected extremity at the buttock. If desired, a tourniquet is placed on the proximal thigh, and the C-arm is brought in from the opposite side of the table. For an isolated lateral process fracture, the patient can be placed in the lateral decubitus position with the affected side up. For posterior process fractures, the patient should be positioned prone on a radiolucent cantilever type table.

Instruments/Equipment/Implants
Common items needed for an open reduction of a talar fracture include small and medium Gelpi retractors and lamina spreaders, a headlamp, a wire driver/drill, an assortment of 1.0-, 1.25-, 1.6-, and 2.0-mm Kirschner wires (K-wires) and small trocar-tipped terminally threaded Schanz pins, small pointed tenaculum (Weber) clamps, two dental picks, and a femoral distractor. An unopened external fixator set should be available in the operating room. If a medial malleolar osteotomy is planned, an oscillating saw, small osteotome, and partially threaded 4.0-mm screws (usually 35-mm long) will also be needed. Minifragment and small-fragment sets containing multiple sizes (1.5-, 2.0-, 2.4-, 2.7-, and 3.5-mm) of plates and screws, with lengths up to 60 mm, should be available. If marginal im-

© 2013 *American Academy of Orthopaedic Surgeons*

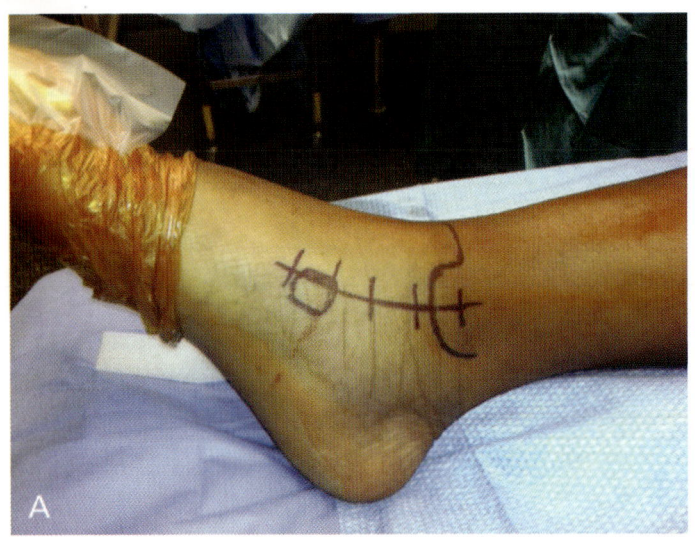

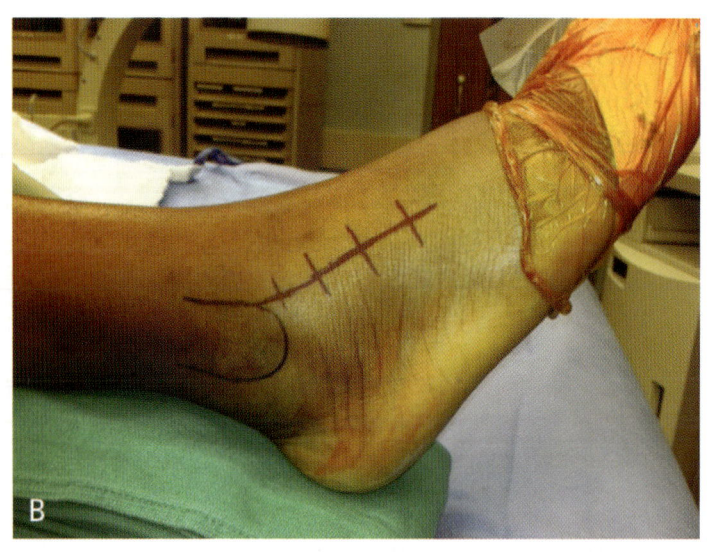

Figure 6 Photographs show the medial and lateral incisions for surgical repair of the talus. **A,** The medial incision begins at the medial malleolus and extends to the navicular tuberosity. **B,** The lateral incision begins at the anterior border of the lateral malleolus and is in line with the fourth ray.

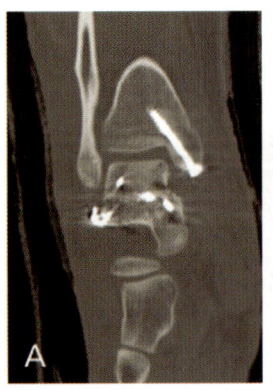

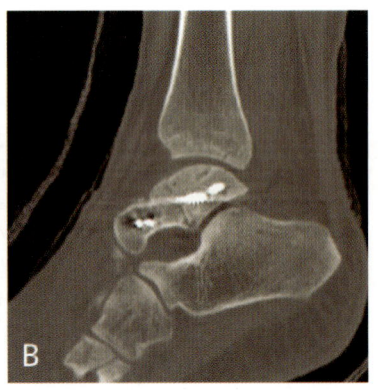

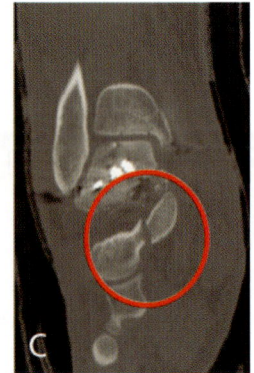

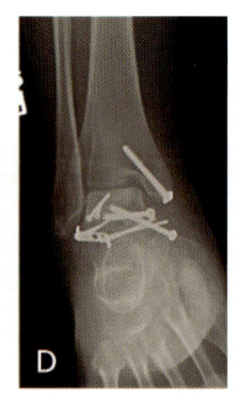

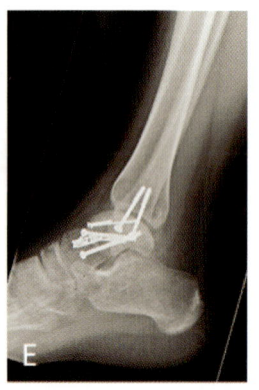

Figure 7 Management of the combination neck and body talar fracture in the patient shown in Figure 5. Postoperative coronal (**A**) and sagittal (**B**) CT scans show good reduction of the talus following a medial malleolar osteotomy. **C,** Coronal CT scan shows satisfactory position of the associated fracture of the sustentaculum. AP (**D**) and lateral (**E**) views at 5 months, at which time the patient had no swelling or pain. She had resumed weight bearing, reacclimatized to shoe wear, and ambulated independently without a limp.

paction or an impression fracture of the talar articular surface is a component of the injury, cancellous allograft and/or a juvenile cartilage tissue graft may be needed.

Surgical Technique
Fractures of the Talar Neck and Body

For talar neck and most body fractures, the bone most often is approached by simultaneous medial and lateral incisions because the adequacy of reduction is difficult to assess through a single incision. The medial incision is started at the medial malleolus and extends to the navicular tuberosity (**Figure 6, A**). Care is taken to establish full-thickness flaps and to preserve the deltoid ligament. The ankle joint capsule is incised, exposing the dorsomedial talar neck and the anterior part of the medial talar body. Excessive dissection over the dorsum of the talus should be avoided to preserve the blood supply. In fractures that involve the talar body or have posterior body fragments, a medial malleolar osteotomy can facilitate exposure.

The lateral incision begins at the anterior border of the inferior part of the lateral malleolus and continues in line with the fourth ray of the foot (**Figure 6, B**). Care is taken to preserve the superficial peroneal nerve, which is frequently encountered in the proximal part of the incision. Dissection continues sharply through the extensor retinaculum, developing full-thickness flaps. The interval between the extensor digitorum longus tendon and the extensor brevis musculature is used. The fat pad of the sinus tarsi is excised to visualize the lateral talar neck, lateral process, lateral talar head, and lateral talar dome. The subtalar joint and lateral process also may be accessed through the lateral incision taken slightly farther proximally, facilitating the reduction and fixation of small displaced fragments or the removal of fracture debris. **Figure 7** shows the treatment of a combination neck and body fracture with an associated minimally displaced fracture of the sustentaculum.

Isolated Displaced Lateral Process Fractures

For isolated displaced lateral process fractures, a small (1- to 2-in) incision directed parallel to the posterior facet of the subtalar joint, just distal to the fibula, is appropriate. As discussed previously, in this situation, the patient can be positioned laterally with the affected side up.

Displaced Posterior Fractures of the Talar Body or Displaced Medial Tubercle Posterior Process Fractures

Displaced posterior fractures of the talar body or displaced medial tubercle posterior process fractures may require a posteromedial approach (**Figure 8, A**). For this approach, the patient is placed in the prone position and a longitudinal incision is made parallel to and approximately one fingerbreadth medial to the Achilles tendon. A two-pin distractor with one pin in the tuberosity of the calcaneus and one in the tibia is useful here (**Figure 8, B**). Care is taken to protect the neurovascular bundle medially. We isolate the bundle with vessel loops. The FHL is then elevated and retracted. A strategically located K-wire is helpful in retraction for exposure. Next, the joint capsule is incised sharply, exposing the posterior talus. With ankle dorsiflexion and posterior distraction aided by the distractor (or single-pin external fixator), a large portion of the talar dome can be visualized.

Displaced Fractures of the Lateral Tubercle of the Posterior Process

For displaced fractures of the lateral tubercle of the posterior process, the patient is positioned prone and the skin incision is made parallel to and approximately 1 cm lateral to the Achilles tendon (**Figure 9, A**). The dissection is medial to the sural nerve, in the interval between the peroneal tendons and the FHL. As with the medial tubercle, visualization can be enhanced by using a headlight, a K-wire to retract the FHL tendon, and a two-pin distractor or external fixator with one pin in the fibula and one in the tuberosity of the os calcis (**Figure 9, B**). Once reduced, posterior process fractures can be fixed with a minifragment plate and/or screws.

Percutaneous Fixation

When soft tissues preclude a formal open reduction and internal fixation and the fracture can be accurately reduced by closed or semi-open methods, low-profile fixation accomplished through neighboring healthy tissues is a potential strategy (**Figure 10**).

Complications

Complications include infection,[17] osteonecrosis, posttraumatic arthritis, and malunion. The incidence of radiographic osteonecrosis ranges from 11% to 100% for displaced neck fractures,[6,8-10,18] and the incidence of posttraumatic arthritis ranges from 45% to 70%.[19-21] Sanders et al[5] reported malunion in 36% of the patients in a series of 102 patients with 104 displaced talar neck fractures, with the most common malpositions being varus and hyperextension.

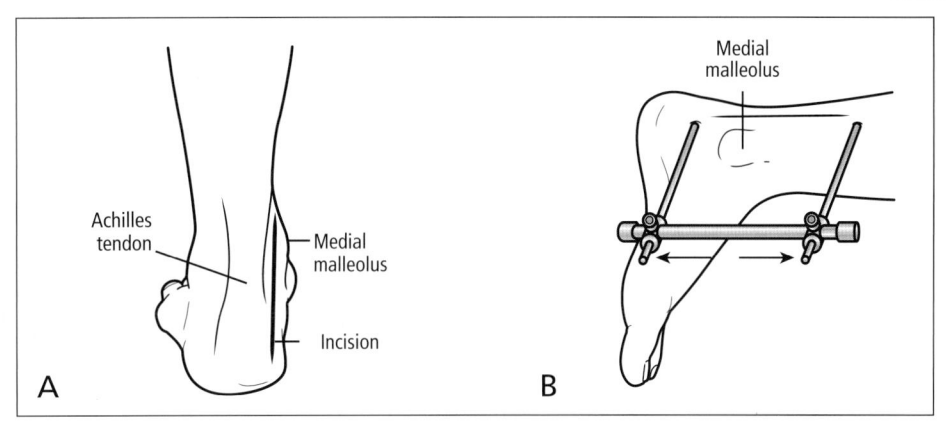

Figure 8 Illustrations depict the incision (**A**) and two-pin distraction external fixator (**B**) for the posteromedial approach.

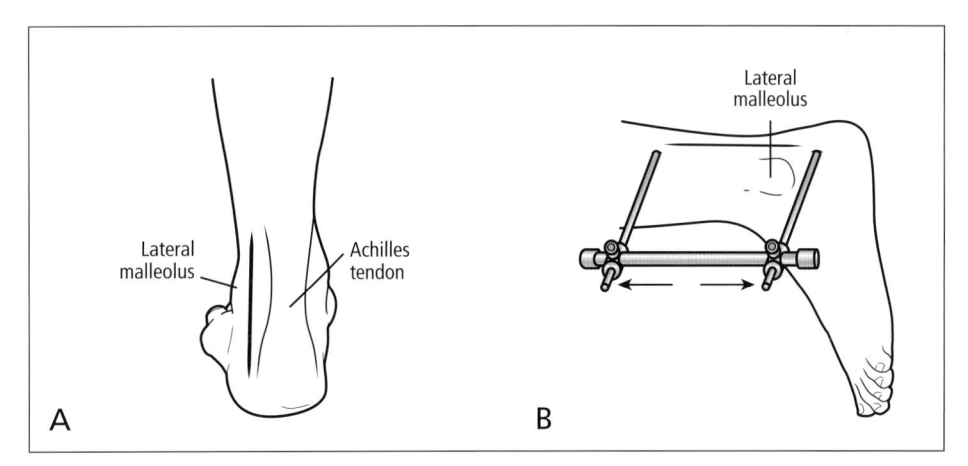

Figure 9 Illustrations depict the incision (**A**) and two-pin distraction external fixator (**B**) for a displaced lateral tubercle posterior process fracture.

Postoperative Care and Rehabilitation

After fixation, a standard closure is performed over a medium suction drain. At our institution, an incisional negative-pressure wound therapy system is applied over a nonadherent dressing with continuous suction at -50 mm Hg. This is a dynamic surgical dressing that can be applied in the sterile environment of the operating room and left in place on the hospital ward until the wound is dry. A recent prospective trial comprised of surgically managed calcaneal, tibial plafond, and tibial plateau fractures randomized between negative-pressure wound therapy and standard dressings showed a significantly lower infection rate in the former group.[22] A short leg posterior splint is applied and converted to a short leg cast when swelling has subsided. The patient should remain non–weight bearing on the affected leg for 12 weeks. If the fracture is stable and the patient is reliable, protection can be provided at 6 weeks by a removable controlled ankle motion (CAM) boot, with time out of the boot daily for range-of-motion exercises of the ankle and foot. The patient should not bear weight for the full 12 weeks.

Pearls

- The surgeon must be mindful of the high incidence of fractures associated with displaced talar neck fractures. CT scans and mortise, lateral ankle, and Canale view radiographs should be scrutinized for such associated fractures.
- The surgeon should develop a careful preoperative plan and be mindful of the blood supply and soft tissues.
- Displaced neck fractures should be approached, reduced, and stably fixed from both the medial and lateral incisions simultaneously, not sequentially.
- For lateral fixation, a contoured minifragment plate can be used in the axilla of the talar neck.
- The surgeon must be mindful of the close relationship of the posterior tibial tendon to the posterior aspect of the medial malleolus when performing a medial malleolar osteotomy.
- A negative-pressure wound therapy system is useful in protecting the

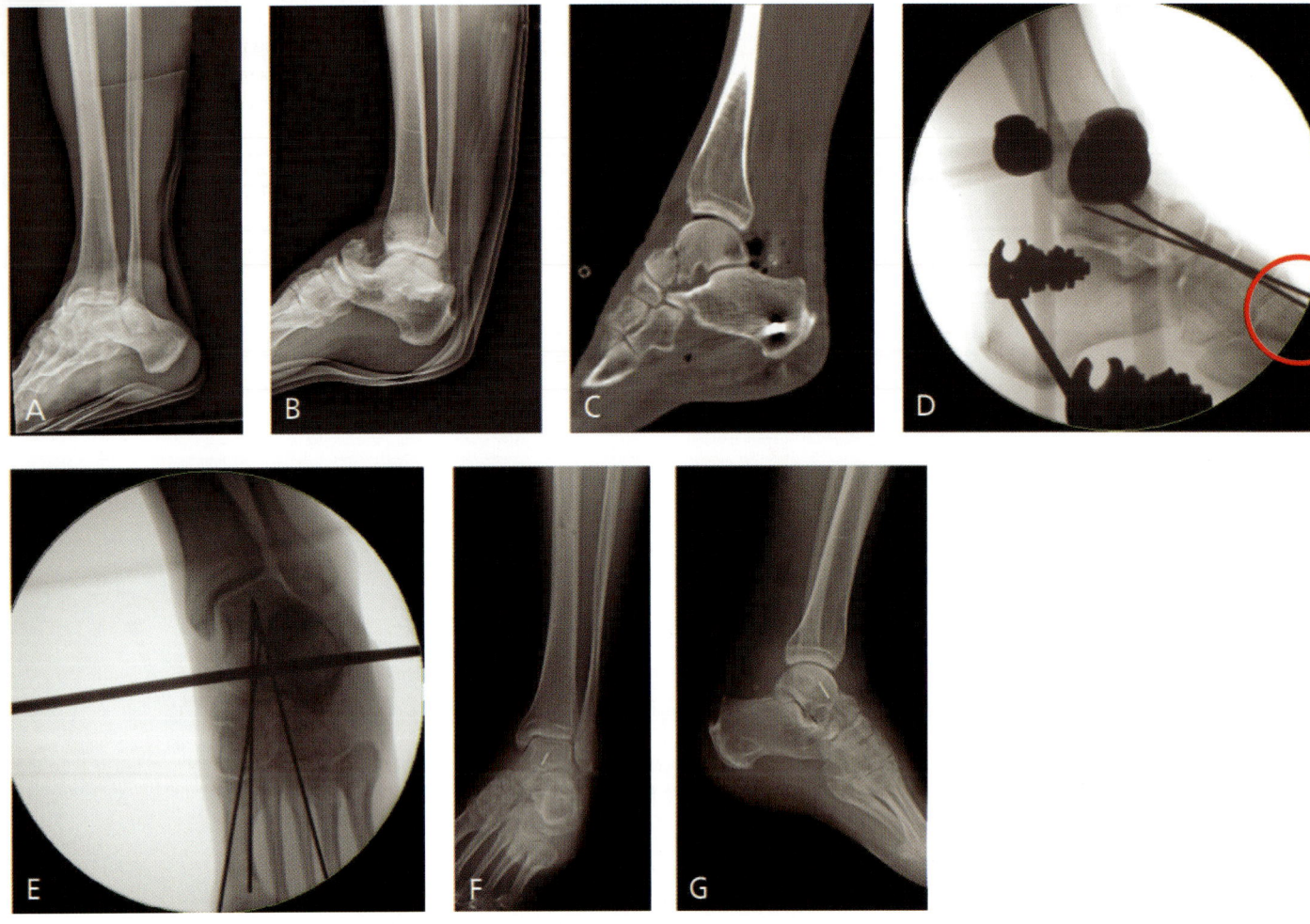

Figure 10 Open fracture of the talar neck with significant soft-tissue compromise over the fracture managed with bridging external fixation and percutaneous pin fixation. **A** and **B** are orthogonal radiographs of the patient's severely displaced ankle and foot. The talar neck fracture was open and the wound was débrided. The reduction was stabilized with a bridging external fixation frame and percutaneously applied Schanz pins. **C,** Sagittal CT scan obtained after application of the bridging frame shows excellent position of the neck fracture. Lateral (**D**) and AP/Canale (**E**) fluoroscopic views obtained at "second-look" surgery at 48 hours postoperatively. At this time the wound was cleaned and the fracture was stabilized by means of three small Schanz pins directed from the normal-appearing area of skin and soft tissue distally on the dorsum (circle in panel D). Postoperative AP (**F**) and lateral (**G**) views of the ankle obtained at 6 months. At this time the patient was fully ambulatory and had no pain, swelling, or limp. A terminal portion of one of the pins had broken off and can be seen in the talar body.

surgical wound and may aid in the resolution of edema that invariably accompanies this injury.

References

1. Fortin PT, Balazsy JE: Talus fractures: Evaluation and treatment. *J Am Acad Orthop Surg* 2001;9(2):114-127.
2. Mulfinger GL, Trueta J: The blood supply of the talus. *J Bone Joint Surg Br* 1970;52(1):160-167.
3. Miller AN, Prasarn ML, Dyke JP, Helfet DL, Lorich DG: Quantitative assessment of the vascularity of the talus with gadolinium-enhanced magnetic resonance imaging. *J Bone Joint Surg Am* 2011;93(12):1116-1121.
4. Vallier HA, Nork SE, Barei DP, Benirschke SK, Sangeorzan BJ: Talar neck fractures: Results and outcomes. *J Bone Joint Surg Am* 2004;86-A(8):1616-1624.
5. Sanders DW, Busam M, Hattwick E, Edwards JR, McAndrew MP, Johnson KD: Functional outcomes following displaced talar neck fractures. *J Orthop Trauma* 2004;18(5):265-270.
6. Hawkins LG: Fractures of the neck of the talus. *J Bone Joint Surg Am* 1970;52(5):991-1002.
7. Peterson L, Romanus B, Dahlberg E: Fracture of the collum tali—an experimental study. *J Biomech* 1976;9(4):277-279.
8. Canale ST, Kelly FB Jr: Fractures of the neck of the talus: Long-term evaluation of seventy-one cases. *J Bone Joint Surg Am* 1978;60(2):143-156.
9. Elgafy H, Ebraheim NA, Tile M, Stephen D, Kase J: Fractures of the talus: Experience of two level 1 trauma centers. *Foot Ankle Int* 2000;21(12):1023-1029.
10. Peterson L, Goldie IF, Irstam L: Fracture of the neck of the talus: A clinical study. *Acta Orthop Scand* 1977;48(6):696-706.
11. Marsh JL, Slongo TF, Agel J, et al: Fracture and dislocation classification compendium - 2007: Orthopaedic Trauma Association classification, database and outcomes committee. *J Orthop Trauma* 2007;21(10, Suppl)S1-S133.
12. Tezval M, Dumont C, Stürmer KM: Prognostic reliability of the Hawkins sign in fractures of the talus. *J Orthop Trauma* 2007;21(8):538-543.
13. Mayo KA: Fractures of the talus: Principles of management and techniques of treatment. *Tech Orthop* 1987;2:42-54.
14. Lindvall E, Haidukewych G, DiPasquale T, Herscovici D Jr, Sanders R: Open reduction and stable fixation of isolated, displaced talar neck and body fractures. *J Bone Joint Surg Am* 2004;86-A(10):2229-2234.

15. Bojanic I, Bergovec M, Smoljanovic T: Combined anterior and posterior arthroscopic portals for loose body removal and synovectomy for synovial chondromatosis. *Foot Ankle Int* 2009;30(11):1120-1123.

16. Jerosch J: Arthroscopic ankle surgery: Indications, methods, results, complications [German]. *Orthopade* 1999;28(6):538-549.

17. Marsh JL, Saltzman CL, Iverson M, Shapiro DS: Major open injuries of the talus. *J Orthop Trauma* 1995;9(5):371-376.

18. Metzger MJ, Levin JS, Clancy JT: Talar neck fractures and rates of avascular necrosis. *J Foot Ankle Surg* 1999;38(2):154-162.

19. Canale ST: Fractures of the neck of the talus. *Orthopedics* 1990;13(10):1105-1115.

20. Schulze W, Richter J, Russe O, Ingelfinger P, Muhr G: Surgical treatment of talus fractures: A retrospective study of 80 cases followed for 1-15 years. *Acta Orthop Scand* 2002;73(3):344-351.

21. Szyszkowitz R, Reschauer R, Seggl W: Eighty-five talus fractures treated by ORIF with five to eight years of follow-up study of 69 patients. *Clin Orthop Relat Res* 1985;199:97-107.

22. Stannard JP, Volgas DA, McGwin G III, et al: Incisional negative pressure wound therapy after high-risk lower extremity fractures. *J Orthop Trauma* 2012;26(1):37-42.

Chapter 70
Open Reduction and Internal Fixation of Calcaneal Fractures

Michael P. Clare, MD

Patient Selection
Indications
Fractures of the calcaneus generally occur in the setting of high-energy trauma, resulting in complex, three-dimensionally oriented fracture patterns. The exact pattern of fracture lines and the extent of comminution are influenced by the position of the foot at impact, the extent of force involved, and the overall bone quality of the patient. Surgical management is generally indicated for displaced intra-articular fractures involving the posterior facet. The primary goal of surgery is anatomic restoration of alignment and return of function without pain. Although a variety of surgical approaches have been described, the extensile lateral approach is currently generally preferred for displaced intra-articular fractures because it consistently allows reduction of the calcaneal body; restoration of calcaneal height, width, and overall morphology, in addition to the posterior facet articular surface where possible; and a late in situ arthrodesis as a means of salvage in the event of posttraumatic arthritis.[1]

Contraindications
Nonsurgical management is best reserved for intra-articular fractures that are truly nondisplaced (Sanders type I) on CT.[2] Other specific indications for nonsurgical management include fractures in patients with severe peripheral vascular disease or type I diabetes mellitus, fractures in patients with medical comorbidities prohibiting surgery, and fractures in elderly patients who are minimal (household) ambulators.[3] Chronologic age itself is not necessarily a contraindication to surgical treatment because many older patients are healthy and active well into their seventies.[4] Nonsurgical management also may be necessary in certain instances in which injury severity precludes early surgical intervention, including fractures associated with severe blistering or massive prolonged edema, fractures with large open wounds, and patients with life-threatening injuries. In these instances, the injury may be managed later as a calcaneal malunion.[5]

Preoperative Imaging
Plain Radiography
Plain radiographic evaluation includes a lateral view of the hindfoot, an AP view of the foot, a Harris axial view of the heel, and a mortise view of the ankle. These views should reveal almost any fracture, dislocation, or subluxation in the hindfoot.

Typically, a fracture of the calcaneus is most easily identified on the lateral view of the hindfoot (**Figure 1**). With an intra-articular fracture, loss of height in the posterior facet is seen. The articular surface is impacted within the body of the calcaneus and is usually rotated anteriorly up to 90° relative to the remaining subtalar joint. A decreased tuber angle of Böhler and an increased crucial angle of Gissane are seen in fracture patterns in which the entire posterior facet is separated from the sustentaculum and depressed; if only the lateral portion of the posterior facet is involved, the split in the articular surface manifests as a double density sign, in which case the tuber angle of Böhler and the crucial angle of Gissane may remain normal.[3] The lateral view also allows delineation as to whether the fracture is a joint depression or a tongue-type fracture.[6]

The AP view of the foot will usually reveal the extension of fracture lines into the calcaneocuboid joint and also may demonstrate anterolateral fragments and expansion of the lateral calcaneal wall. This view otherwise offers only limited information and can thus be omitted in most cases. The Harris axial view of the heel shows a loss of calcaneal height as well as increased width and (typically) varus angulation of the tuberosity fragment. The Harris view also provides visualization of the articular surface. This view is unfortunately difficult to obtain with acute fractures because of pain. A mortise view of the ankle will usually demonstrate involvement of the posterior facet.

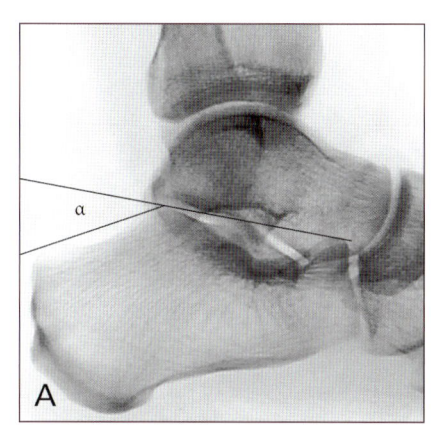

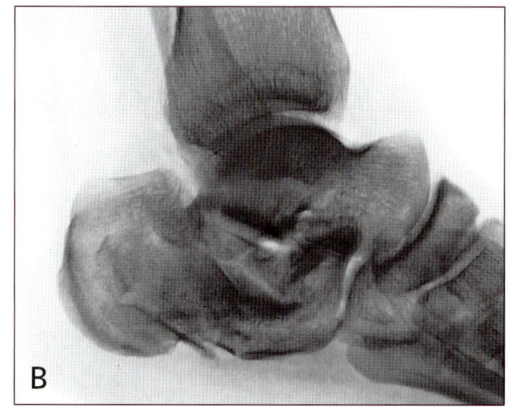

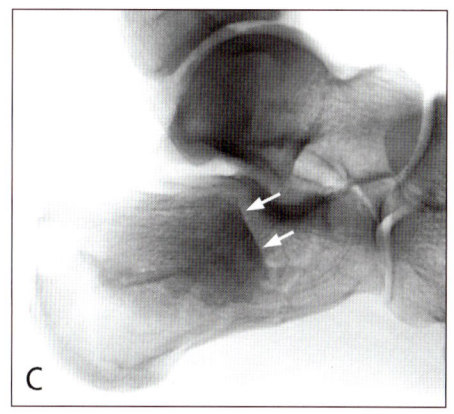

Figure 1 Lateral hindfoot radiographs demonstrate radiographic signs used to assess for a calcaneal fracture. **A,** A normal tuber angle of Böhler (angle α) is seen in this uninjured foot. **B,** View of a foot with a calcaneal fracture demonstrates a decreased angle of Böhler. Note also the marked loss of calcaneal height with relative horizontalization of the talus. **C,** View of a foot with a calcaneal fracture. Impaction of the superolateral fragment manifests as double-density sign (arrows).

Dr. Clare or an immediate family member serves as a paid consultant to or is an employee of BESPA Medical.

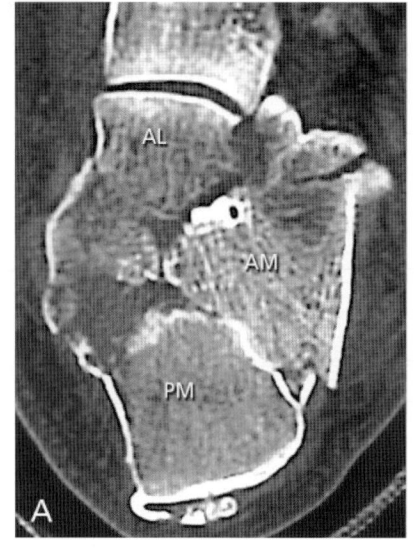

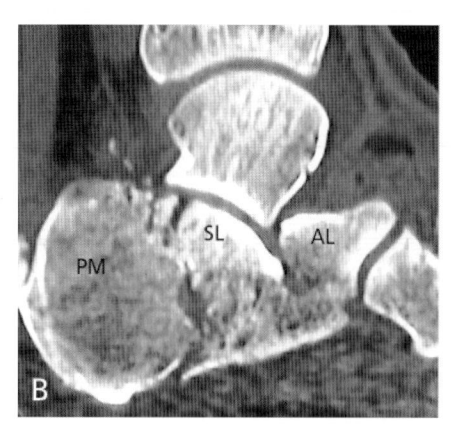

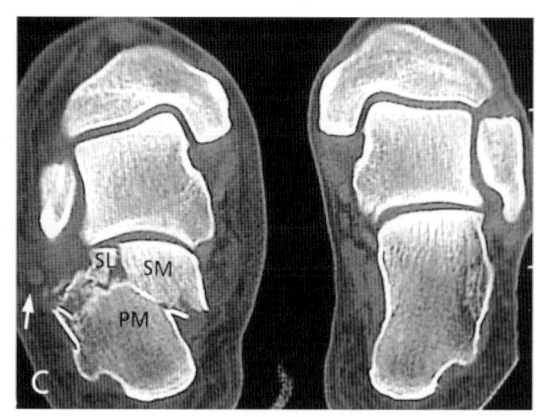

Figure 2 Axial (**A**), sagittal (**B**), and semicoronal (**C**) CT images delineate typical calcaneal fracture fragments. In the semicoronal image of the injured side (left image of C), note the potential impingement of the expanded lateral wall against the peroneal tendons (arrow). AL = anterolateral; AM = anterior main; PM = posterior main; SL = superolateral; SM = superomedial.

Computed Tomography

CT is indicated if the plain radiographs reveal an intra-articular extension of the calcaneal fracture. Images are obtained at 2- to 3-mm intervals in the axial, sagittal, and 30° semicoronal planes.

The axial or transverse cuts will reveal extension of fracture lines into the anterior process and the calcaneocuboid joint, as well as the sustentaculum tali and the anteroinferior margin of the posterior facet (**Figure 2, A**). The sagittal reconstruction views will demonstrate displacement of the tuberosity fragment; the extent of involvement of the anterior process region, including superior displacement of the anterolateral fragment; the anterior rotational displacement of the superolateral posterior facet fragment; and delineation of the fracture as a joint depression or tongue-type pattern[6] (**Figure 2, B**). The 30° semicoronal images will show displacement of articular fragments in the posterior facet, the sustentaculum tali, the extent of widening and shortening of the calcaneal body, expansion of the lateral calcaneal wall, varus angulation of the tuberosity, and the position of the flexor hallucis longus and peroneal tendons (**Figure 2, C**).

Pathoanatomy

In a displaced intra-articular calcaneal fracture, the loss of height through the calcaneus results in a shortened and widened heel, classically with varus malalignment of the tuberosity. This loss of height is reflected in a decreased tuber angle of Böhler, such that the normal declination of the talus is diminished and the talus becomes relatively more horizontal, which leads to secondary loss of ankle dorsiflexion (**Figure 1, B**). As the superolateral fragment of the posterior facet is impacted plantarward, the thin lateral wall explodes laterally just posterior to the crucial angle of Gissane. This lateral wall expansion may trap the peroneal tendons against the lateral malleolus and also affect subtalar motion; in some cases, a violent contracture of the peroneal tendons may avulse the tendon sheath from the fibula, resulting in an avulsion fracture of the lateral malleolus and dislocation of the peroneal tendons. The anterior process typically displaces superiorly, which directly limits subtalar joint motion by impinging against the lateral process of the talus.

Clarification of fragment terminology is necessary to understand the pathoanatomy of displaced intra-articular calcaneal fractures (**Figure 2**). The anterolateral fragment encompasses the lateral wall of the anterior process, is typically pyramidal in shape, and may include a portion of the calcaneocuboid articular surface. The anterior main fragment is the large fragment anterior to the primary fracture line, which usually includes the anterior portion of the sustentaculum and the anterior process. The superomedial fragment, also known as the sustentacular, or constant, fragment, is the fragment of variable size found posterior to the primary fracture line; this fragment almost always remains attached to the talus through the deltoid ligament complex and is therefore stable. The superolateral fragment, also referred to as the semilunar (comet) fragment, is the lateral portion of the posterior facet that is sheared from the remaining posterior facet in joint depression fractures. The tongue fragment refers to the superolateral fragment that remains attached to a portion of the posterior tuberosity, including the Achilles tendon insertion, and is found in tongue-type fractures. The posterior main fragment represents the posterior tuberosity.

Fracture-Dislocation Patterns

Fracture-dislocation patterns, which occur when the superolateral fragment remains contiguous with the lateral wall and the posterior tuberosity, are relatively rare.[7] The resulting large posterolateral fragment dislocates laterally and is forcefully driven into the talofibular joint, often producing a fracture of the lateral malleolus, dislocation of the peroneal tendons, and disruption of the lateral ligamentous complex of the ankle. The hindfoot inverts through the ankle joint as the limb recoils; this is seen on plain radiographs as increased lateral talar tilt. The fracture pattern, which is confirmed on CT evaluation (**Figure 3**), is most commonly a simple two-part split fracture, such that as the dislocation is reduced, the articular fragments typically align anatomically. As with most dislocations, the sooner it is reduced, the easier the reduction tends to be; with delayed treatment, a formal open reduction will usually be required.[8]

Procedure

Resolution of Soft-Tissue Swelling

Surgery is ideally performed within the first 3 weeks after injury, before early consolidation of the fracture. Once con-

Chapter 70: Open Reduction and Internal Fixation of Calcaneal Fractures

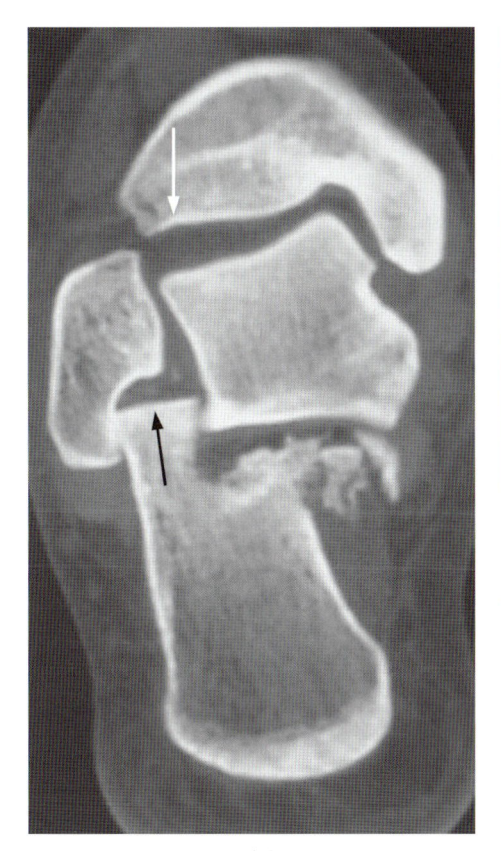

Figure 3 Semicoronal CT image demonstrates a variant calcaneal fracture-dislocation pattern. Note the posterolateral fragment wedged within the talofibular joint (black arrow) and the varus tilt of the talus within the ankle mortise (white arrow).

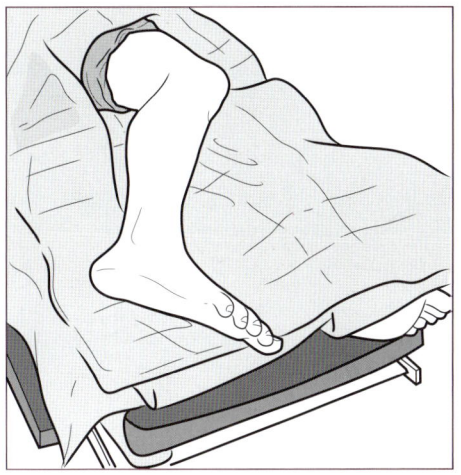

Figure 4 Illustration shows intraoperative positioning for the extensile lateral approach for open reduction and internal fixation of a calcaneal fracture. Note the scissor positioning of the surgical and nonsurgical limbs and the operating platform, which facilitate intraoperative fluoroscopy.

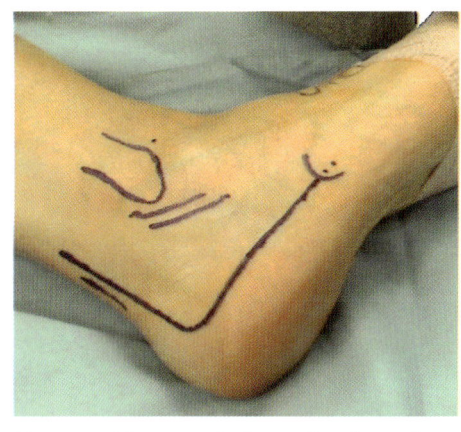

Figure 5 Photograph shows the planned extensile lateral incision for open reduction and internal fixation of a calcaneal fracture. The vertical limb, which runs immediately lateral to the Achilles tendon and thus posterior to the sural nerve and the lateral calcaneal artery, preserves vascular supply to the flap.

solidation ensues, the fragments become increasingly difficult to separate to obtain an adequate reduction, and the articular cartilage may delaminate from the underlying subchondral bone. Surgery must be delayed, however, until the associated soft-tissue swelling has adequately dissipated, which may require up to 3 weeks. Splint immobilization and limb elevation are performed initially, and the patient is later converted to a compression stocking and a fracture boot. Full resolution of soft-tissue edema is demonstrated by the wrinkle test; a positive result indicates that surgical intervention may be safely undertaken.[3]

Room Setup/Patient Positioning
For isolated injuries, the patient is placed in the lateral decubitus position on a beanbag. The lower extremities are positioned in a scissor configuration: the surgical limb is flexed at the knee and angled toward the distal, posterior corner of the operating table, and the nonsurgical limb is extended at the knee and lies away from the eventual surgical field. Protective padding is placed beneath the contralateral limb for protection of the peroneal nerve, and an operating "platform" is created with blankets and foam padding to elevate the surgical limb (**Figure 4**). Alternatively, the prone position may be used in the event of bilateral injuries.

Special Instruments/Equipment/Implants
As with almost any periarticular fracture in the foot and ankle, instruments that are invaluable in assisting with calcaneal fracture reduction include dental picks, Freer elevators, sharp and blunt periosteal elevators, Schanz pins, and a laminar spreader. Several low-profile, anatomic plates specific to the calcaneus are also available, with both locking and nonlocking screw holes as fixation options. Although locking plates have not been shown to be superior to nonlocking plates in the treatment of displaced intra-articular calcaneal fractures, locking plates may be beneficial in maintaining calcaneal height, particularly with joint depression–type fracture patterns, or in patients with marginal bone quality.

Improving Efficiency
Because of the complex three-dimensional nature of fracture patterns in the calcaneus, preoperative planning and a meticulous review of the injury radiographs and CT scans are essential in anticipating the nature of the fracture pattern and the technical maneuvers needed to achieve fracture reduction. The procedure should be completed within 120 to 130 minutes of tourniquet time to minimize potential wound complications. Tourniquet time must therefore be adequately budgeted: the surgical approach should be completed within 20 minutes; fracture reduction, within 60 minutes; definitive stabilization, within 20 to 30 minutes; and wound closure, within 20 minutes.[3]

Video 70.1 Extensile Lateral Approach for Joint Depression–Type Calcaneal Fractures. Michael P. Clare, MD (6 min)

Surgical Technique
The extensile lateral approach for joint depression–type fractures is described here.

Incision/Approach
Soft-tissue complications following the surgical management of calcaneal fractures remain a major source of morbidity with these injuries. Thus, careful attention to detail with respect to placement of the incision and gentle handling of the soft tissues are of paramount importance. The incision begins approximately 2 cm proximal to the tip of the lateral malleolus, immediately lateral to the Achilles tendon and thus posterior to the sural nerve and the lateral calcaneal artery, and the vertical limb extends toward the plantar foot. The horizontal limb continues at the junction of the skin of the lateral foot and the heel pad and extends to the base of the fifth metatarsal, with a gentle curve connecting the two limbs of the incision (**Figure 5**). Dissection is specifically taken "straight to bone" at the level of the calcaneal tuberosity proximally, avoiding any

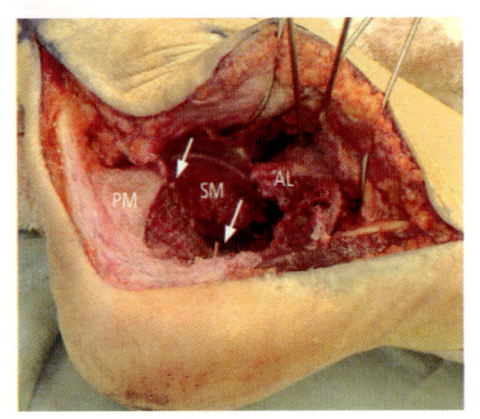

Figure 6 Intraoperative view following excision of the lateral wall fragment and superolateral fragment during open reduction and internal fixation of a calcaneal fracture. Mobilization is through the primary fracture line (white arrows). AL = anterolateral; SM = superomedial; PM = posterior main.

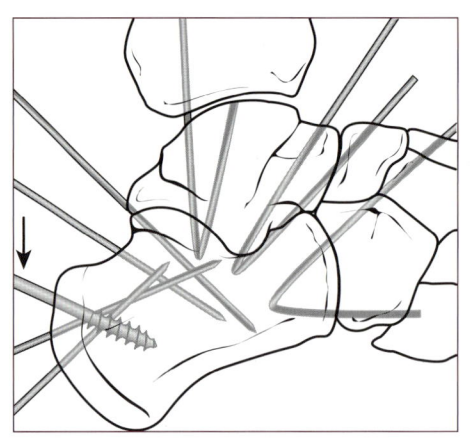

Figure 7 Illustration shows the Essex-Lopresti reduction technique for an intra-articular split-tongue pattern. Note the placement of the Schanz pin within the tongue fragment (arrow) to neutralize the pull of the Achilles tendon.

beveling of the skin, and continues to the midpoint of the horizontal limb.

A full-thickness, subperiosteal flap is then raised, starting at the apex. The use of retractors is specifically avoided until a sizable subperiosteal flap is developed, which prevents separation of the skin from the underlying subcutaneous tissue. The calcaneofibular ligament is sharply released from the lateral calcaneal wall, and the adjacent peroneal tendons are released from the peroneal tubercle through the cartilaginous "pulley." A periosteal elevator is then used to gently mobilize the tendons along the distal portion of the incision, thereby exposing the anterolateral calcaneus. Thus, the peroneal tendons, the sural nerve, and the lateral calcaneal artery are contained entirely within the flap, and devascularization of the lateral skin is minimized.

Deep dissection continues to the sinus tarsi and the anterior process region anteriorly and to the superiormost portion of the calcaneal tuberosity posteriorly for "window" visualization of the posterior facet. Using a "no touch" technique, three 1.6-mm Kirschner wires (K-wires) are placed for retraction of the subperiosteal flap: One into the fibula as the peroneal tendons are slightly subluxated anterior to the lateral malleolus, a second wire in the talar neck, and a third wire in the cuboid as the peroneal tendons are levered away from the anterolateral calcaneus with a periosteal elevator.

Mobilization of the Fragments
The expanded lateral wall fragment is gently mobilized, débrided of residual hematoma, and preserved in saline on the back table, as is the adjacent, impacted superolateral articular fragment of the posterior facet. The articular surface of the fragment is assessed for chondral damage. Removal of the articular fragment thus affords exposure of the medial sustentacular (constant) fragment, the tuberosity fragment, and the obliquely oriented primary fracture line medially (**Figure 6**). A blunt periosteal elevator is introduced into the primary fracture line and levered plantarward, thereby disimpacting the posterior main fragment from the superomedial fragment and restoring calcaneal height and length along the medial calcaneal wall. A 4.5-mm Schanz pin is placed in the posteroinferior corner of the calcaneal tuberosity for further manipulation.[9]

Reduction of the Articular Surface
The superolateral fragment (Sanders type II fracture) is brought back into the wound, and two parallel 1.6-mm K-wires are placed to facilitate reduction; in the event of two separate fragments (Sanders type III fracture), the central articular fragment is first reduced to the superomedial fragment and stabilized with 1.5-mm bioresorbable poly-L-lactide pins. The protruding ends of the bioresorbable pins are removed flush with the bony surface with a handheld electrocautery unit. The superolateral (lateralmost articular) fragment is then reduced and provisionally stabilized with 1.6-mm K-wires to the central and superomedial fragments. The articular fragment(s) must be precisely reduced such that (superior-inferior) height, (anterior-posterior) rotation, and coronal plane (varus-valgus) alignment are correct.

Split Tongue–Type Variant Patterns
With intra-articular (split) tongue-type patterns (Sanders type IIA or IIB and type III), the pull of the Achilles tendon on the tongue fragment may preclude reduction of the lateral articular surface in proper sagittal plane rotation. In this instance, the Essex-Lopresti reduction technique is performed on the tongue fragment with a 4.5-mm Schanz pin placed percutaneously into the tongue fragment, which neutralizes the deforming forces of the Achilles tendon and allows anatomic reduction of the articular surface in the sagittal plane[10] (**Figure 7**).

Reduction of the Anterior Process
The anterior process fragments are next pulled inferiorly and provisionally secured with 1.6-mm K-wires. Fracture lines through the anterior process often vary, in that there may be three separate fragments and, as the anterolateral fragment is reduced, the central fragment may remain displaced superiorly. A lamina spreader may then be used to facilitate reduction of the central fragment. A transverse fracture line may be present through the crucial angle of Gissane, in essence rotating the superomedial fragment beneath the anterior main fragment. In this case, before reduction of the superolateral articular fragment, the superomedial fragment must be derotated, reduced, and provisionally stabilized to the anterior main fragment to prevent malrotation of the entire posterior facet articular surface.

The articular reduction is verified through window visualization: the superolateral and superomedial fragments should align both anteriorly and posteriorly. Full visualization of the articular surface posteriorly may be facilitated with a small retractor placed at the posterior margin of the joint surface. Failure to visualize the posterior facet from both sides of the window may lead to malreduction of the fragment(s) in the sagittal plane. At this point, the posterior edge of the anterolateral fragment should "key" into the anteroinferior edge of the superolateral fragment, indicating restoration of the crucial angle of Gissane. The lateral wall and the body of the calcaneus should align with simple valgus manipulation of the Schanz pin, and the previously excised lateral wall fragment should anatomically reduce, confirming at least that the lateral column is anatomically restored.

The reduction is then confirmed by intraoperative fluoroscopy, including

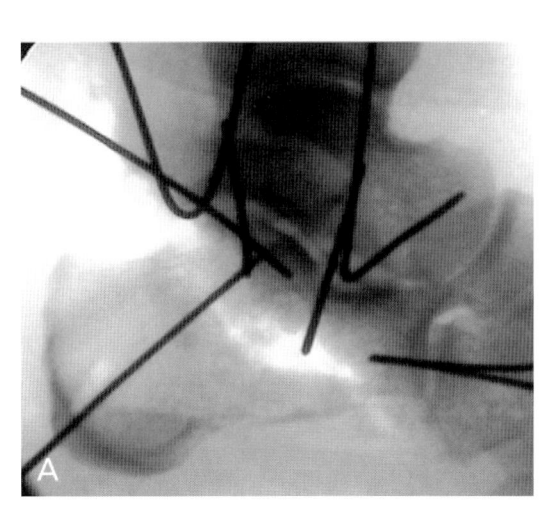

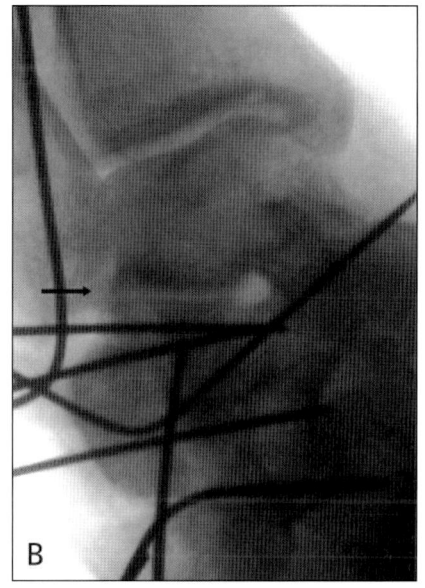

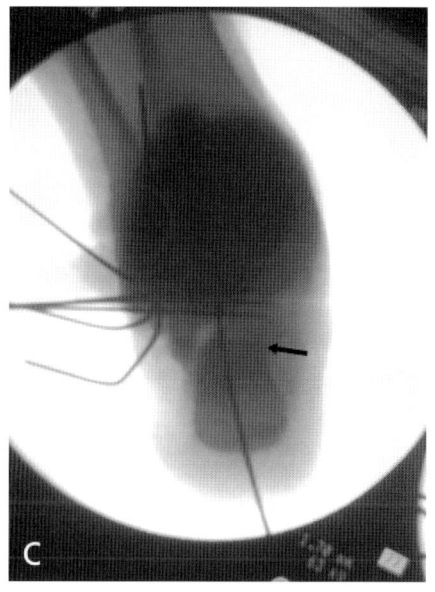

Figure 8 Intraoperative lateral (**A**), Broden (**B**), and axial (**C**) fluoroscopic images of a joint depression–type calcaneal fracture pattern demonstrate provisional reduction. Arrows indicate the anatomic alignment of the posterior facet articular surface (**B**) and restoration of calcaneal length (**C**).

lateral, Broden, and axial views. The lateral view should be a true lateral view of the talus at the ankle joint to accurately assess the calcaneus (**Figure 8, A**). Next, the limb is externally rotated 45° while the fluoroscope is kept in the same position. The beam is then canted 10° toward the foot of the bed to obtain a Broden view, which reveals the posterior facet. The entire facet is visualized under live fluoroscopy through dorsiflexion and plantar flexion of the foot (**Figure 8, B**). Finally, the limb is externally rotated 90°, and the foot is maximally dorsiflexed through the midfoot. The beam is further angled 30° toward the foot of the bed, demonstrating a clear axial view of the calcaneus (**Figure 8, C**).

Definitive Fixation

The posterior facet is then secured with 2.7-mm or 3.5-mm cortical lag screws placed just beneath the articular surface and angling toward the sustentaculum. An anatomic calcaneal plate is then selected and secured with 3.5-mm cortical screws, starting with the distalmost screw holes overlying the anterior process. The oblique orientation of the calcaneocuboid articulation is accommodated by aiming slightly posteriorly. Screw placement on power will bring the plate to bone, thus restoring calcaneal width. Next, the calcaneal tuberosity is secured to the plate while a simultaneous lateral-to-medial force is maintained on the plate and a valgus-directed force is maintained on the tuberosity. The main components of the calcaneus (anterior process, posterior tuberosity, and articular surface) are further secured to the plate such that two screws traverse each component. With split tongue–type variant patterns, an additional screw may be placed from the superior edge of the tuberosity perpendicular to the tongue fracture line for orthogonal fixation. One or two additional locking screws may be placed beneath the posterior facet articular block for rafter effect, particularly for joint depression–type patterns. Final lateral, Broden, and axial fluoroscopic images are obtained, confirming the final reduction and placement of implants (**Figure 9**).

Assessing the Peroneal Tendons

With removal of the K-wires, the peroneal tendons should reduce into the peroneal groove along the posterior edge of the lateral malleolus. The peroneal tendons are assessed for stability by advancing a Freer elevator within the peroneal tendon sheath to the level of the lateral malleolus and levering forward (**Figure 10**). If the superior peroneal retinaculum (SPR) and the tendon sheath remain intact, a firm end point will be encountered; if the retinaculum and the tendon sheath are detached, the elevator will easily slide anterior to the fibula, in which case an SPR repair is required.[11] The extensile lateral flap is then closed to reestablish tension on the peroneal tendon sheath. The SPR repair may be completed with the tourniquet deflated if insufficient time remains.

Acute SPR Repair

A small (<3-cm) incision is made along the posterolateral edge of the lateral malleolus, which should provide sufficient skin bridge to the vertical limb of the extensile lateral incision. The peroneal sheath is incised, and the false pouch is identified. Two suture anchors are placed along the posterolateral rim of the lateral malleolus, and the nonabsorbable sutures are passed in horizontal mattress fashion into the detached retinaculum. By advancing the sutures anteriorly, the SPR is tensioned toward the posterolateral rim, thereby eliminating the false pouch. With the peroneal tendons held reduced in the peroneal groove, the sutures are then tied down, which reestablishes a checkrein on the peroneal tendons. Tendon stability is confirmed by taking the involved limb through a range of motion passively. The tendon sheath is closed with interrupted, figure-of-8 No. 2-0 nonabsorbable sutures.

Wound Closure

The full-thickness flap is closed over a deep drain with deep No. 0 absorbable sutures placed in interrupted fashion starting at the proximal and distal ends and progressing toward the apex of the incision. The sutures are hand-tied sequentially in similar fashion to eliminate tension at the apex of the incision. The skin layer is closed with 3-0 monofilament suture using the modified Allgöwer-Donati technique. The tourniquet is deflated and sterile dressings are

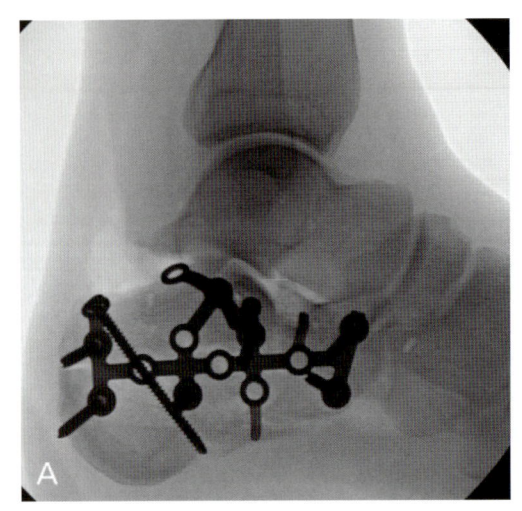

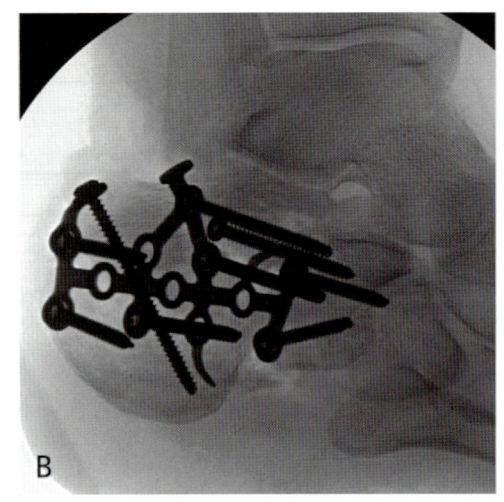

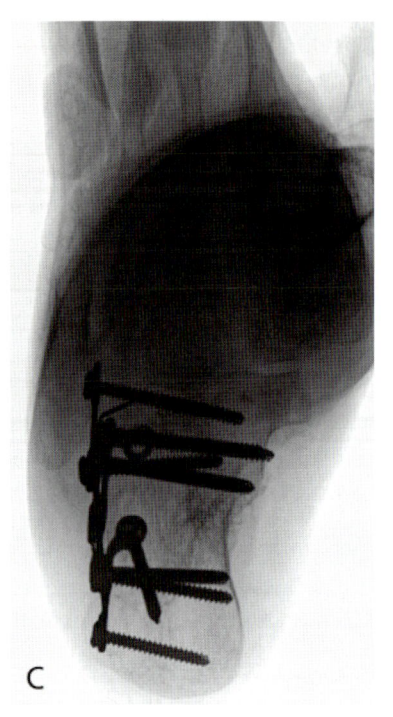

Figure 9 Intraoperative lateral (**A**), Broden (**B**), and axial (**C**) fluoroscopic images demonstrating definitive fixation and final reduction of a split tongue–type calcaneal fracture pattern.

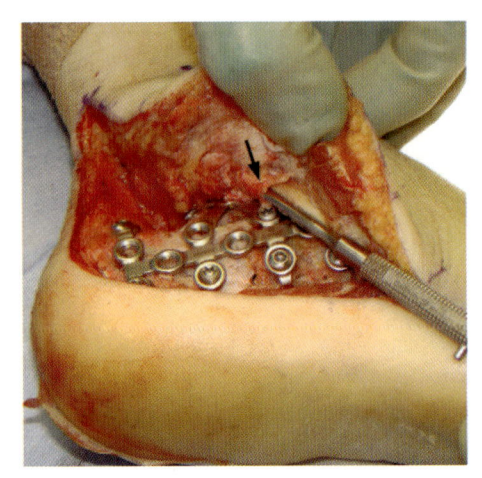

Figure 10 Intraoperative photograph shows assessment of the superior peroneal retinaculum in a foot with a calcaneal fracture. Note the Freer elevator within the peroneal tendon sheath (arrow).

placed, followed by a bulky Jones dressing and a Weber splint.

Complications
Delayed Wound Healing/Wound Dehiscence

The most common complication following surgical treatment of a calcaneal fracture is wound dehiscence, which occurs in up to 25% of cases.[2,3,9,12] Despite relatively easy approximation at the time of surgical closure, the wound may later separate, typically at the apex of the incision, even up to 4 weeks following surgery. Most wounds ultimately heal; deep infection and osteomyelitis develop in only 1% to 4% of closed fractures.[2,3,9,12]

If a wound dehiscence occurs, all range-of-motion exercise is discontinued to prevent further wound separation. The wound is managed with serial whirlpool treatments, damp-to-dry dressing changes, and oral antibiotics. Alternatively, cast immobilization may be instituted with window access for dressing changes. Once the wound seals, range-of-motion exercises are reinstituted. Negative-pressure wound therapy may be used for recalcitrant wounds. A recent randomized prospective study in which negative-pressure wound therapy was used as an "incisional VAC" at the time of wound closure reported a lower relative risk of wound infection by a factor of 1.9.[13]

Posttraumatic Subtalar Arthritis

A principal goal of internal fixation is anatomic restoration of the posterior facet articular surface. Posttraumatic arthritis may still develop, however, as a result of cartilage damage at the time of injury.[3] In this instance, because calcaneal height and morphology have already been restored, implant removal and an in situ subtalar arthrodesis may be performed.[1]

Postoperative Care and Rehabilitation

Following splint immobilization, a compression stocking and a fracture boot are used at 2 weeks postoperatively, and early ankle and subtalar range-of-motion exercises are begun. The sutures are removed once the incision is fully sealed and dry, typically at 4 to 5 weeks; however, weight bearing is not initiated until 10 to 12 weeks postoperatively. The patient is gradually transitioned to regular shoe wear as weight bearing is advanced. Formal physical therapy is not typically necessary, provided the patient makes sufficient progress in regaining ankle and hindfoot motion before the progression of weight bearing. Balance, proprioception, and eversion strengthening are emphasized before activity progression.

Pearls

- The surgeon must thoroughly understand the pathoanatomy of a calcaneal fracture to properly treat the injury. I believe the learning curve is approximately 100 fractures before reproducible results are consistently achieved.
- Soft-tissue management is arguably as important as the treatment of the bony injury; attention to detail with placement of the incision and gentle, meticulous soft-tissue handling is of paramount importance.
- Restoration of calcaneal morphology (calcaneal height, length, width, and the crucial angle of Gissane) is arguably as important as the reduction of the posterior facet articular surface.
- Definitive fixation typically consists of nonlocking screws placed through an anatomic calcaneal plate in box configuration and cortical lag screws

stabilizing the posterior facet articular fragments. In joint depression patterns, one or two locking screws are placed beneath the articular block for a rafter effect to maintain height.
- Prior to flap closure, the integrity of the superior peroneal retinaculum must be assessed. The farther lateral the fracture line in the posterior facet extends, the greater the likelihood of peroneal tendon dislocation.
- Gentle ankle range-of-motion exercises are begun at 2 weeks postoperatively; subtalar motion exercises are delayed until 4 to 5 weeks postoperatively, at which time the incision should be sealed and dry. Proprioceptive exercises and eversion strengthening are emphasized thereafter.

References

1. Radnay CS, Clare MP, Sanders RW: Subtalar fusion after displaced intra-articular calcaneal fractures: Does initial operative treatment matter? *J Bone Joint Surg Am* 2009;91(3):541-546.
2. Sanders R, Fortin P, DiPasquale T, Walling A: Operative treatment in 120 displaced intraarticular calcaneal fractures: Results using a prognostic computed tomography scan classification. *Clin Orthop Relat Res* 1993;290:87-95.
3. Sanders R: Displaced intra-articular fractures of the calcaneus. *J Bone Joint Surg Am* 2000;82(2):225-250.
4. Herscovici D Jr, Widmaier J, Scaduto JM, Sanders RW, Walling A: Operative treatment of calcaneal fractures in elderly patients. *J Bone Joint Surg Am* 2005;87(6):1260-1264.
5. Clare MP, Lee WE III, Sanders RW: Intermediate to long-term results of a treatment protocol for calcaneal fracture malunions. *J Bone Joint Surg Am* 2005;87(5):963-973.
6. Essex-Lopresti P: The mechanism, reduction technique, and results in fractures of the os calcis. *Br J Surg* 1952;39(157):395-419.
7. Eastwood DM, Maxwell-Armstrong CA, Atkins RM: Fracture of the lateral malleolus with talar tilt: Primarily a calcaneal fracture not an ankle injury. *Injury* 1993;24(2):109-112.
8. Sanders RW, Clare MP: Calcaneus fractures, in Bucholz RW, Heckman JD, Court-Brown CM, Koval KJ, Tornetta P III, Wirth MA, eds: *Rockwood and Green's Fractures in Adults,* ed 7. Philadelphia, PA, Lippincott Williams & Wilkins, 2010, pp 2064-2109.
9. Harvey EJ, Grujic L, Early JS, Benirschke SK, Sangeorzan BJ: Morbidity associated with ORIF of intra-articular calcaneus fractures using a lateral approach. *Foot Ankle Int* 2001;22(11):868-873.
10. Tornetta P III: The Essex-Lopresti reduction for calcaneal fractures revisited. *J Orthop Trauma* 1998;12(7):469-473.
11. Clare MP: Acute and chronic peroneal tendon dislocations. *Tech Foot Ankle Surg* 2009;8:112-118.
12. Benirschke SK, Kramer PA: Wound healing complications in closed and open calcaneal fractures. *J Orthop Trauma* 2004;18(1):1-6.
13. Stannard JP, Volgas DA, McGwin G III, et al: Incisional negative pressure wound therapy after high-risk lower extremity fractures. *J Orthop Trauma* 2012;26(1):37-42.

Chapter 71
Open Reduction and Internal Fixation of Fracture-Dislocations of the Tarsometatarsal Joint

Terrence M. Philbin, DO Gregory C. Berlet, MD

Patient Selection
Fracture-dislocations of the midfoot will forever be linked to the Napoleonic-era surgeon Jacques Lisfranc, who described midfoot amputation as a treatment of the injury we now refer to as a Lisfranc. Injuries to the tarsometatarsal (TMT) joint occur in less than 1% of all fractures, with a frequency of 1 in 55,000 persons.[1] The clinical results of missed or inappropriately treated TMT fracture-dislocations are poor. Chronic joint instability can lead to persistent pain, deformity, and midfoot arthritis.[2]

The indications for open reduction and internal fixation (ORIF) of the TMT joint are injuries with displacement and instability.[3] Midfoot arthritis has been reported as a frequent result of significant TMT joint injury and instability. The contraindications to ORIF of the TMT joint include active infection and vascular insufficiency. A delayed ORIF should be considered when there is massive edema to the midfoot. Approximate reduction and provisional fixation can be used in the form of external fixation or percutaneous pinning to reduce any tenting of the skin from the fracture and to allow soft tissue to recover prior to definitive fixation (**Figure 1**).

Video 71.1 Open Reduction and Internal Fixation of an Unstable Midfoot Injury. Terrence M. Philbin, DO; Gregory C. Berlet, MD (1 min)

Preoperative Imaging
The most common mechanism of injury to the midfoot is an axial load to a hyper plantar-flexed foot. A recent study reviewing front-end motor vehicle accidents with airbag deployment revealed that 38% of the injuries involved the foot and ankle.[4] Up to 20% of TMT joint injuries are missed or misdiagnosed, potentially leading to long-term sequelae.[5] A plantar ecchymosis sign can be pathognomonic for a high-grade midfoot injury (**Figure 2**).

Preoperative imaging should always start with AP, lateral, and oblique radiographs, weight bearing if possible. On the AP view, the first and second TMT joints are assessed for fracture and diastasis. The oblique view is best to assess the alignment of the lateral column. Non–weight-bearing radiographs have a 50% rate of misdiagnosis of unstable midfoot injuries[6] (**Figure 3**). A fleck sign (small bone avulsion) can be a clue that an unstable injury is present (**Figure 4**). If radiographic results are not diagnostic, several options are available for diagnostic imaging. Stress radiographs under anesthesia are very useful to delineate any diastasis or displacement at the TMT joints. CT is helpful in diagnosing associated fractures and quantifying the extent of joint injury (**Figure 5**). MRI is most

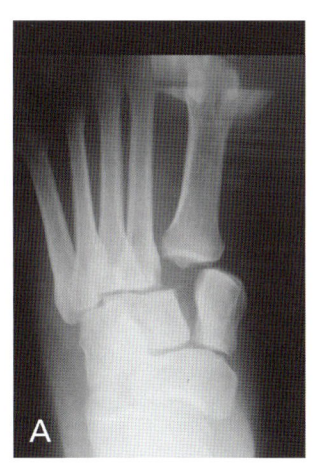

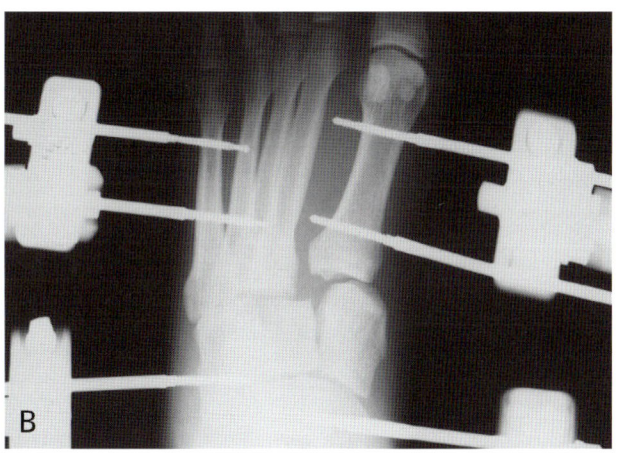

Figure 1 AP radiographs show tarsometatarsal joint injury before (**A**) and after (**B**) provisional external fixation.

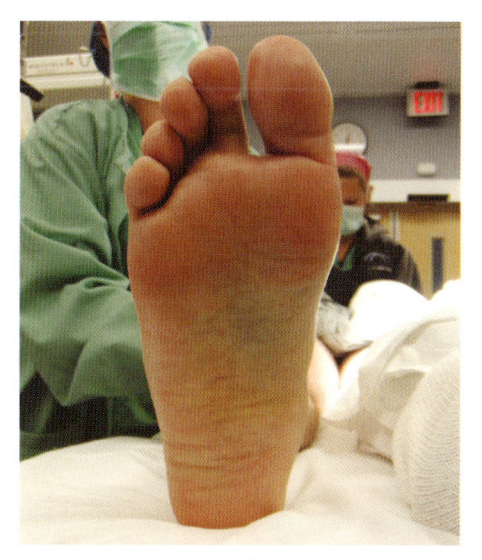

Figure 2 Photograph shows the plantar ecchymosis sign.

Dr. Philbin or an immediate family member has received royalties from Orthohelix, Biomet, and Stryker; is a member of a speakers' bureau or has made paid presentations on behalf of DJ Orthopaedics, Pfizer, Biomet, Footmax, Orthohelix, and Stryker; serves as a paid consultant to or is an employee of Biomet, Orthohelix, Pfizer, DJ Orthopaedics, Lifenet, Amniox, and Stryker; has stock or stock options held in Orthohelix; has received research or institutional support from Biomet, DJ Orthopaedics, Pfizer, Biomimetic, and Artilon; and serves as a board member, owner, officer, or committee member of the Arthritis Foundation, the American Orthopaedic Foot & Ankle Society, the American Academy of Orthopaedic Surgeons, the American Osteopathic Academy of Orthopedics, and the ADA. Dr. Berlet or an immediate family member has received royalties from Bledsoe Brace and Wright Medical Technology; is a member of a speakers' bureau or has made paid presentations on behalf of Wright Medical Technology; serves as a paid consultant to or is an employee of Medtronic, Wright Medical Technology, Biomet, Stryker, and DJ Orthopaedics; has stock or stock options held in Bledsoe Technologies and Wright Medical Technology; has received research or institutional support from DJ Orthopaedics, Zimmer, and BioMimetic Therapeutics; and serves as a board member, owner, officer, or committee member of the American Academy of Orthopaedic Surgeons and the American Orthopaedic Foot & Ankle Society.

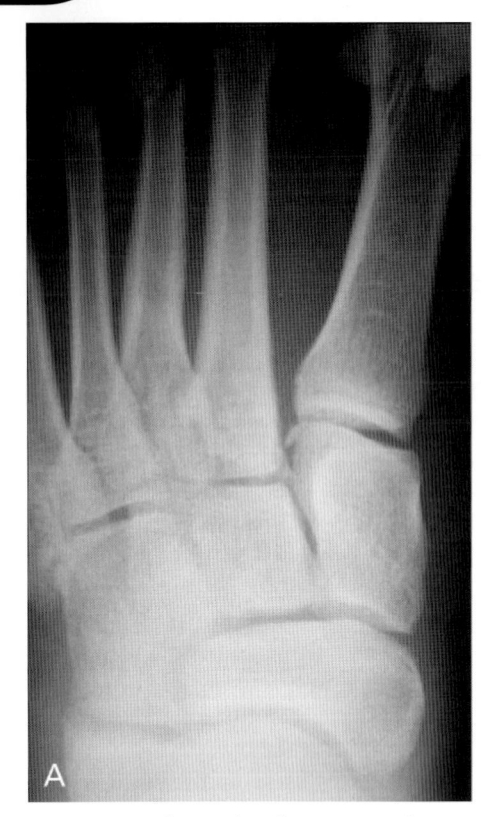

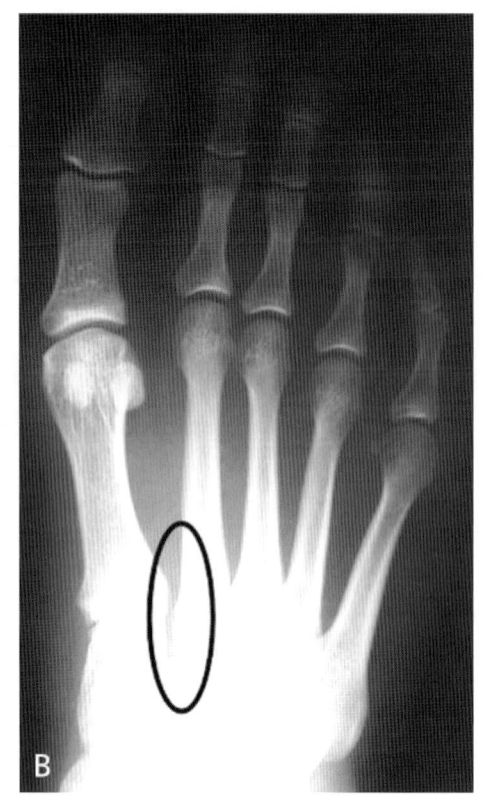

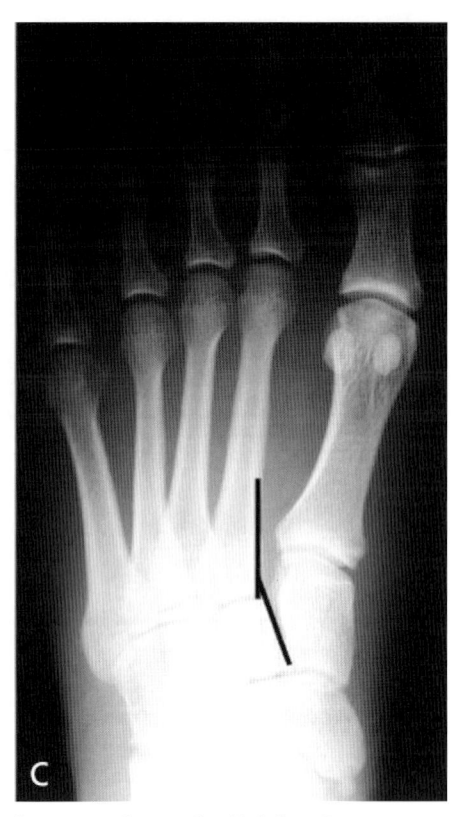

Figure 3 Radiographs of a patient with an unstable midfoot injury of the left foot. **A,** Non–weight-bearing radiograph of left foot. Injury is not apparent. **B,** Oval indicates contralateral (normal) foot. **C,** Weight-bearing radiograph of the left foot demonstrates diastasis (lines).

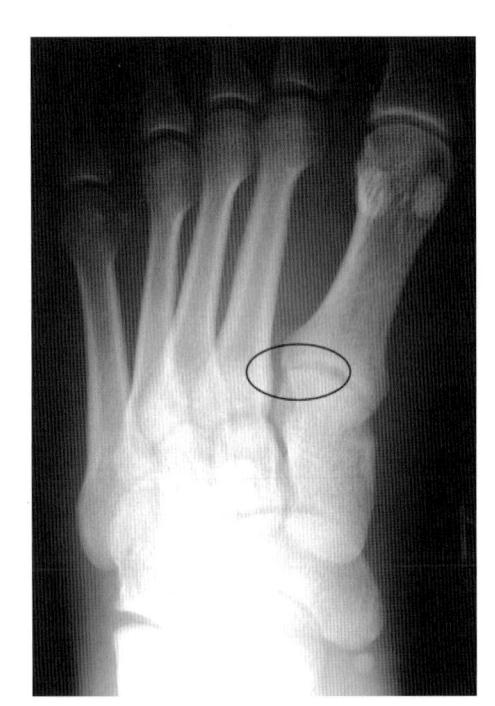

Figure 4 AP radiograph of the left foot shows the fleck sign.

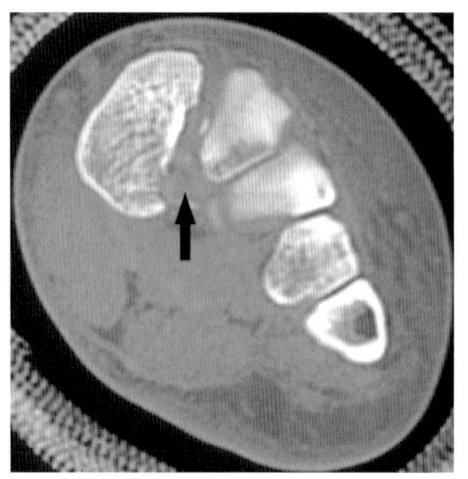

Figure 5 CT scan shows diastasis in the midfoot with a comminuted fracture.

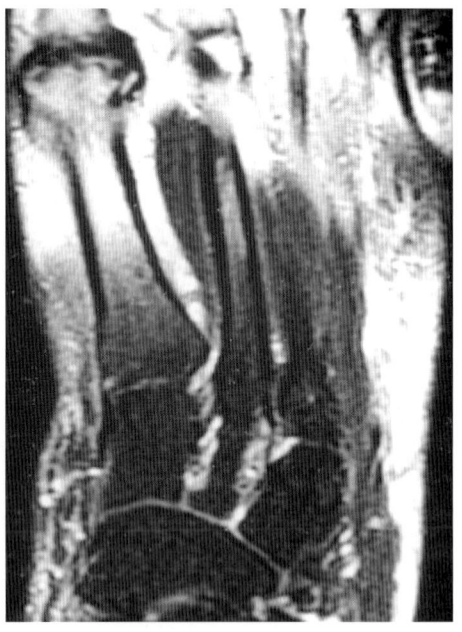

Figure 6 T2-weighted MRI shows intact Lisfranc ligaments.

useful in identifying the soft-tissue component of the injury, a Lisfranc ligament tear (**Figure 6**).[7]

Fracture-dislocations of the TMT joint have no universal classification system. The current classification systems focus on the mechanism of injury and/or the patterns of displacement. The Myerson classification is a modification of the original descriptions from Quenu and Kuss in 1909, modified by Hardcastle et al in 1982 (**Figure 7**).[5,8]

Procedure
Room Setup/Patient Positioning
The patient is placed in the supine position with a bump under the ipsilateral hip. The fluoroscopy unit should be placed on the side of the surgical foot and opposite the surgical table. In a semielective setting, some surgeons prefer a preoperative ankle or popliteal block as an augment to general anesthesia for postoperative pain control.

Special Instruments/Equipment/Implants
The following equipment should be available for this procedure: a standard small-fragment set with cannulated or solid screws based on the surgeon's preference, Kirschner wires (K-wires) and pointed reduction forceps large enough to reduce the medial cuneiform to the lateral second TMT base, a dental pick, an

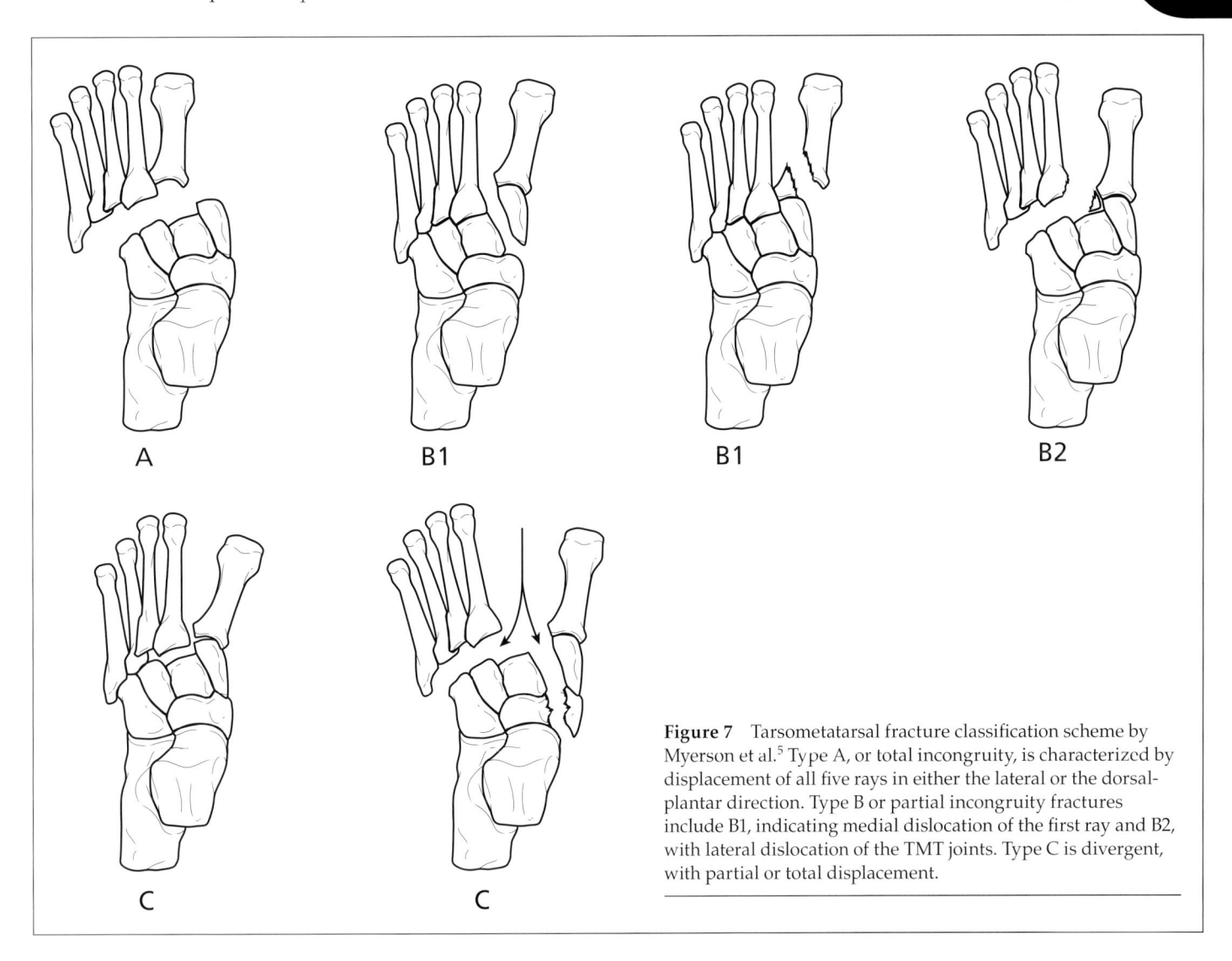

Figure 7 Tarsometatarsal fracture classification scheme by Myerson et al.[5] Type A, or total incongruity, is characterized by displacement of all five rays in either the lateral or the dorsal-plantar direction. Type B or partial incongruity fractures include B1, indicating medial dislocation of the first ray and B2, with lateral dislocation of the TMT joints. Type C is divergent, with partial or total displacement.

anterior cruciate ligament aiming guide, long drill bits, and a burr or countersink.

Surgical Technique

Prior to making an incision, it is helpful to obtain stress views of the midfoot to determine which joints are unstable. Two different incisions can be used based on the extent of injury. The dorsomedial incision allows good visualization to the first and second TMT joint, the cuneiforms, the medial third TMT joint, and the joints proximal in the medial column if necessary. Occasionally, a dorsolateral incision will be needed to expose the lateral column of the foot. It is paramount to preserve a good soft-tissue bridge between the dorsomedial and dorsolateral incisions to prevent wound complications. Care should be taken to not disrupt the dorsal pedis artery because it provides the main blood supply to the dorsal flap.

The dorsomedial incision is placed directly over the first TMT joint (**Figure 8**). The longitudinal incision is deepened between the extensor hallucis longus and the extensor hallucis brevis tendons. The dorsal pedis artery and nerve are deep to the extensor hallucis brevis muscle–tendon junction and must be protected. The capsule and the periosteum over the first TMT, second TMT, and intercuneiform joints (if necessary) should be sharply dissected, giving the surgeon exposure to ensure precise reduction to the injured joints. Care should be taken to avoid the communicating branch of the dorsal pedis as it dives plantarly between the first and second TMT joints. Typically, this incision will allow visualization up to the medial third TMT base.

The dorsolateral incision is placed over the fourth TMT joint (**Figure 9**). As the incision is deepened, the extensor digitorum brevis and the extensor digitorum communis tendons are retracted. This incision allows exposure of the lateral third TMT, the fourth TMT, and the fifth TMT joints.

The joints are ready for anatomic reduction once all the fracture debris has been removed, allowing for proper alignment. Precise anatomic reduction has been shown to achieve good results and prevent arthritis. Reduction should be performed in a systematic manner from proximal medial to distal lateral. The intercuneiform joint should be provisionally fixed first if there is evidence of fracture with instability (**Figure 10**). Reduction forceps are then used to realign the intermediate cuneiform and the base of the second TMT joint. The first TMT joint is then provisionally fixed (**Figure 11**). At this point in the surgery, it is important to verify clinically as well as with fluoroscopy that there is precise anatomic reduction. Further provisional fixation should be placed if there is a lateral column injury.

The first screw will be put in transversely from medial to lateral across the cuneiforms. The first TMT screw is directed from distal to proximal across the joint. Countersinking of the screw or a pocket hole should be used to prevent breaking of the dorsal cortex and screw prominence.[9] The "home-run" screw is placed from the medial cuneiform to the base of the second TMT joint (**Figure 12**). An anterior cruciate ligament–type aim-

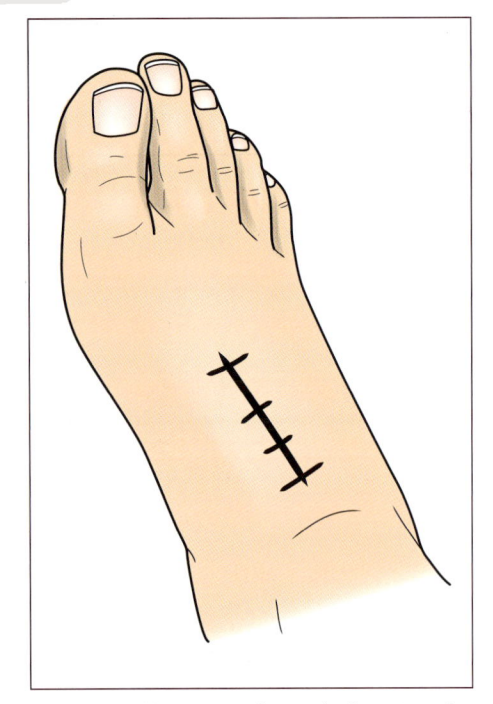

Figure 8 Illustration shows the location of the dorsomedial incision.

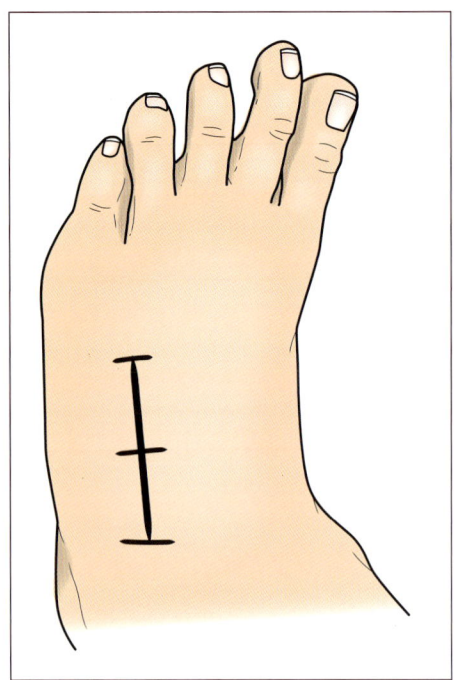

Figure 9 Illustration shows the location of the dorsolateral incision.

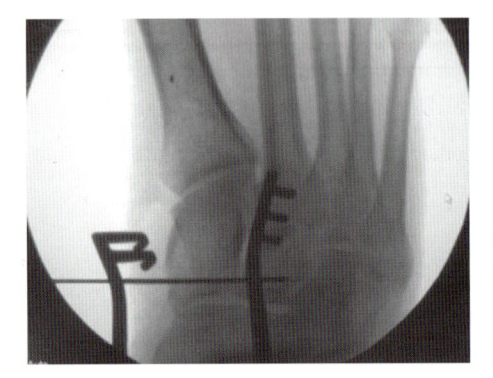

Figure 10 Fluoroscopic image shows provisional fixation in the intercuneiform joint.

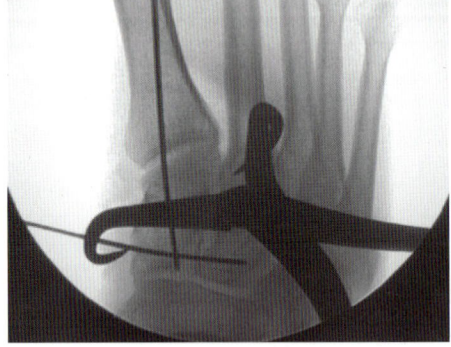

Figure 11 Fluoroscopic image shows reduction of the medial cuneiform to the base of the second TMT joint and provisional fixation in the first TMT joint.

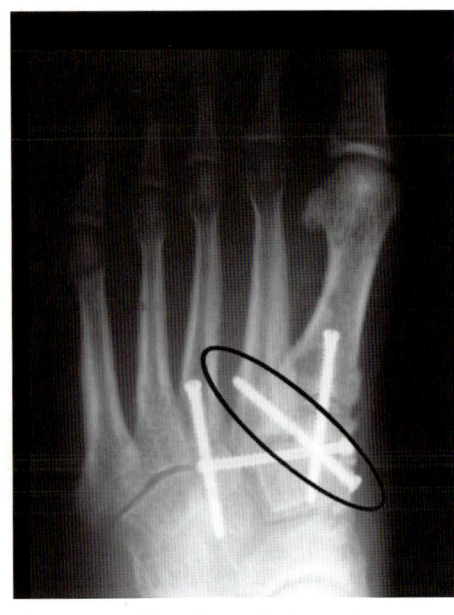

Figure 12 AP radiograph shows placement of the "home-run" screw (oval).

ing guide may be useful in obtaining the direction of the screw. For lateral column injuries, screw fixation should be considered for the third TMT joint from distal to proximal into the middle or lateral cuneiform. K-wire fixation is advised for the fourth and fifth TMT joint.

Closure of the capsule and periosteum should be attempted if the soft tissue is viable following injury. The external skin should be closed with a no-touch technique to help prevent skin compromise. The patient is then placed into a well-padded dressing, cotton roll, and a posterior splint.

Complications

Patients who sustain high-energy TMT fracture-dislocations are at risk for postoperative wound complications and infection. The best way to prevent wound problems after surgery is to make good decisions before surgery. The timing of the definitive ORIF incision is paramount. Any significantly displaced fracture should be reduced and provisionally fixed until the soft tissue is ready.

Midfoot arthritis is still a concern even after ORIF of the TMT joints. Precise anatomic reduction following fracture-dislocation of the midfoot has been shown to minimize the need for fusion.[10] Midfoot posttraumatic arthritis can be treated with nonsteroidal anti-inflammatory drugs, cortisone injections, full-length carbon fiber inserts, a rocker-bottom shoe, and a midfoot fusion.[1]

Postoperative Care and Rehabilitation

The patient is kept non–weight bearing for 6 weeks. At 3 weeks postoperatively, sutures are removed, the patient is placed into a CAM (controlled ankle motion) walker boot, and therapy is initiated to begin range-of-motion exercises on the forefoot and the ankle. At 6 weeks, K-wires are removed (if necessary) and weight bearing is started in the boot. After 9 weeks, patients are allowed to start weaning out of the boot into custom inserts with carbon fiber in good supportive shoewear and progressed in physical therapy. Hardware is generally removed from joints of high stress, like the first TMT joint, after 4 months.

Pearls

- Prior to making any incisions, stress radiographs should be obtained to determine which joints are unstable and affected.
- Preoperative planning is key to making appropriate incisions so that the surgeon can access the joints properly.
- Open versus percutaneous reduction is recommended so the surgeon can obtain direct visualization of the joint reduction.
- Bridge plating over the joints should be considered as an alternative to screw fixation through the joint.

References

1. Patel A, Rao S, Nawoczenski D, Flemister AS, DiGiovanni B, Baumhauer JF: Midfoot arthritis. *J Am Acad Orthop Surg* 2010;18(7):417-425.
2. Philbin T, Rosenberg G, Sferra JJ: Complications of missed or untreated Lisfranc injuries. *Foot Ankle Clin* 2003;8(1):61-71.
3. Ly TV, Coetzee JC: Treatment of primar-

ily ligamentous Lisfranc joint injuries: Primary arthrodesis compared with open reduction and internal fixation. A prospective, randomized study. *J Bone Joint Surg Am* 2006;88(3):514-520.

4. Chong M, Sochor M, Ipaktchi K, Brede C, Poster C, Wang S: The interaction of occupant factors on the lower extremity fractures in frontal collision of motor vehicle crashes based on a level I trauma center. *J Trauma* 2007;62(3):720-729.

5. Myerson MS, Fisher RT, Burgess AR, Kenzora JE: Fracture dislocations of the tarsometatarsal joints: End results correlated with pathology and treatment. *Foot Ankle* 1986;6(5):225-242.

6. Nunley JA, Vertullo CJ: Classification, investigation, and management of midfoot sprains: Lisfranc injuries in the athlete. *Am J Sports Med* 2002;30(6):871-878.

7. Raikin SM, Elias I, Dheer S, Besser MP, Morrison WB, Zoga AC: Prediction of midfoot instability in the subtle Lisfranc injury: Comparison of magnetic resonance imaging with intraoperative findings. *J Bone Joint Surg Am* 2009;91(4):892-899.

8. Hardcastle PH, Reschauer R, Kutscha-Lissberg E, Schoffmann W: Injuries to the tarsometatarsal joint: Incidence, classification and treatment. *J Bone Joint Surg Br* 1982;64(3):349-356.

9. Sands A: Open reduction and internal fixation of Lisfranc/tarsometatarsal injuries, in Pfeffer GB, Easley ME, Frey C, Hintermann B, Sands AK, eds: *Operative Techniques: Foot and Ankle Surgery*. Philadelphia, PA, Saunders Elsevier, 2010, pp 246-256.

10. Rammelt S, Schneiders W, Schikore H, Holch M, Heineck J, Zwipp H: Primary open reduction and fixation compared with delayed corrective arthrodesis in the treatment of tarsometatarsal (Lisfranc) fracture dislocation. *J Bone Joint Surg Br* 2008;90(11):1499-1506.

Chapter 72
Open Reduction and Internal Fixation of Proximal Fifth Metatarsal Fractures

Mark E. Easley, MD

Patient Selection
Indications
Open reduction and internal fixation (ORIF) is indicated for patients with proximal fifth metatarsal fractures in zone II (Jones fractures) or zone III (stress fractures), particularly for delayed union of a fracture treated nonsurgically and for an acute fracture in an athlete[1-5] (**Figure 1**).

Contraindications
Contraindications to ORIF include skin compromise or active infection on the surgical foot, particularly the lateral midfoot; vascular insufficiency; an immunocompromised patient (on immunosuppressive medications that may lead to delayed healing); neuropathy; and a patient with varus heel and a tendency for lateral foot overload.[6] In the last situation, ORIF should not be performed in isolation but should be considered with concomitant correction of hindfoot malalignment, either with surgical realignment or with orthoses.

Specific correction of hindfoot alignment depends on the etiology of hindfoot varus, including the following in isolation or in combination: calcaneal malunion, distal tibial malunion, peroneal tendon insufficiency, chronic lateral ankle instability, forefoot-driven hindfoot varus (rigidly plantar flexed first ray), and cavus foot with or without neuromuscular imbalance. With a hindfoot that can easily be positioned in physiologic valgus, an orthosis may suffice.

Preoperative Imaging
Plain radiographs, including AP, oblique, and lateral views of the proximal fifth metatarsal fracture, are sufficient (**Figure 2**). CT or MRI is rarely, if ever, indicated.

Procedure
Room Setup/Patient Positioning
The patient is positioned supine, with a bolster under the ipsilateral hip, to provide improved access to the lateral foot (**Figure 3, A**). The surgical foot should be on edge of the operating table, directly where the surgeon is positioned.

There should be ample clearance for the fluoroscopy unit to be placed immediately adjacent to the operating table and surgical foot. The fluoroscopy unit must have a sterile cover so that it can serve as an extension of the table for portions of the procedure (**Figure 3, B**).

A tourniquet may be used to avoid bleeding that may obscure structures at risk at the surgical site. A calf or ankle tourniquet is typically adequate. A calf tourniquet is placed distal to the fibular head to avoid untoward pressure on the common peroneal nerve.

Special Instruments/Equipment/Implants
The following equipment should be on hand for this procedure:
- Fluoroscopy unit
- Cannulated drill system
- Graduated taps
- Solid screws (generally stronger than cannulated screws, and my preference)[7-10]
- Dedicated instrument and implant sets. These are commercially available and obviate the need to collect equipment from multiple sets.

Surgical Technique
Approach
The surgical approach is similar to intramedullary fixation of a long bone. A lon-

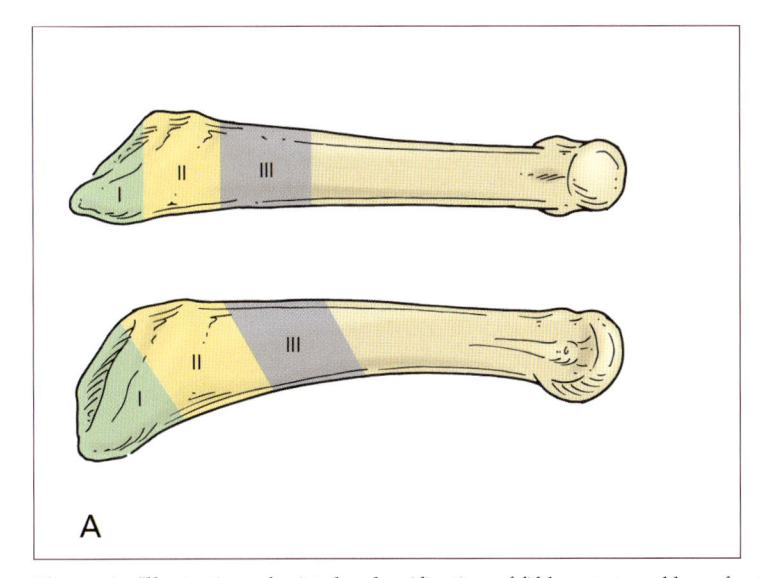

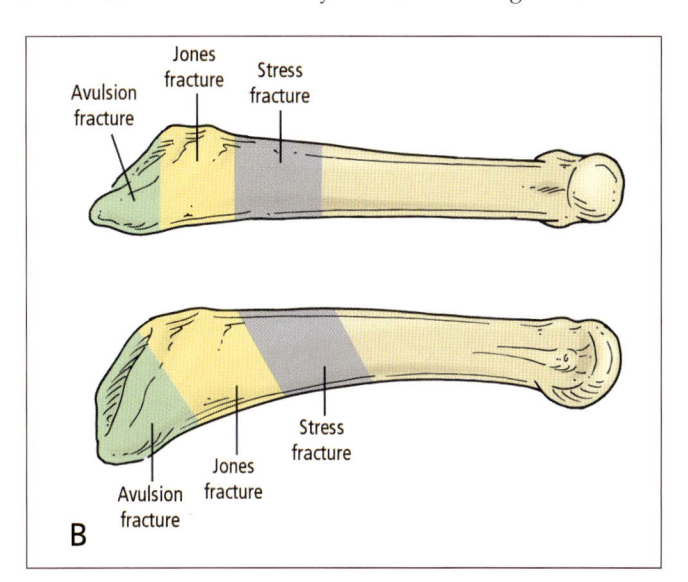

Figure 1 Illustrations depict the classification of fifth metatarsal base fractures. **A,** Zones of the base of the fifth metatarsal. **B,** Designation of fracture types in the proximal fifth metatarsal.

Dr. Easley or an immediate family member is a member of a speakers' bureau or has made paid presentations on behalf of Small Bone Innovations and Datatrace, DT MedSurg; serves as a paid consultant to or is an employee of Exactech, Small Bone Innovations, Integra LifeSciences, and Tornier; has received research or institutional support from Biomimetic; and serves as a board member, owner, officer, or committee member of the American Orthopaedic Foot & Ankle Society.

Section 5: Trauma

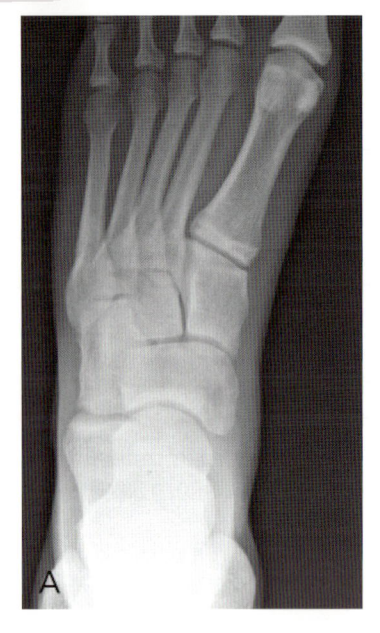

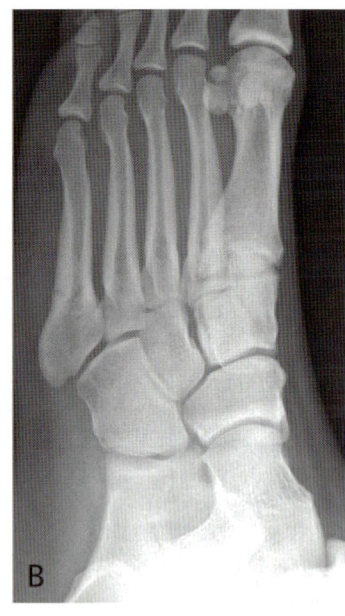

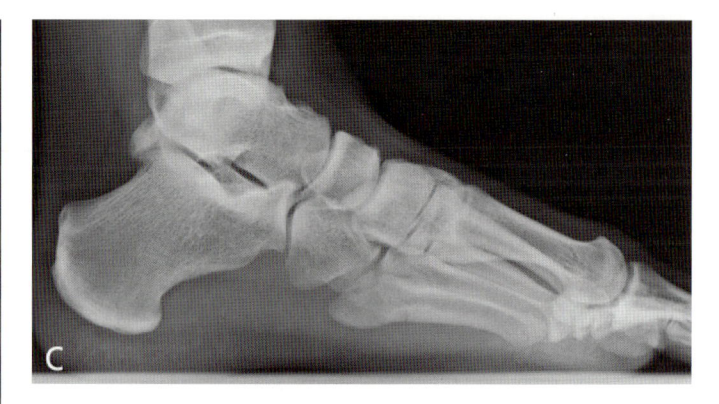

Figure 2 Non–weight-bearing AP (**A**), oblique (**B**), and lateral (**C**) radiographs of the foot of a 22-year-old college athlete with a zone II base of the fifth metatarsal fracture (Jones fracture). Note that the subtle fracture, most readily seen on the oblique view, extends into the articulation between the fourth and fifth metatarsal bases, thus designating this fracture as a zone II injury.

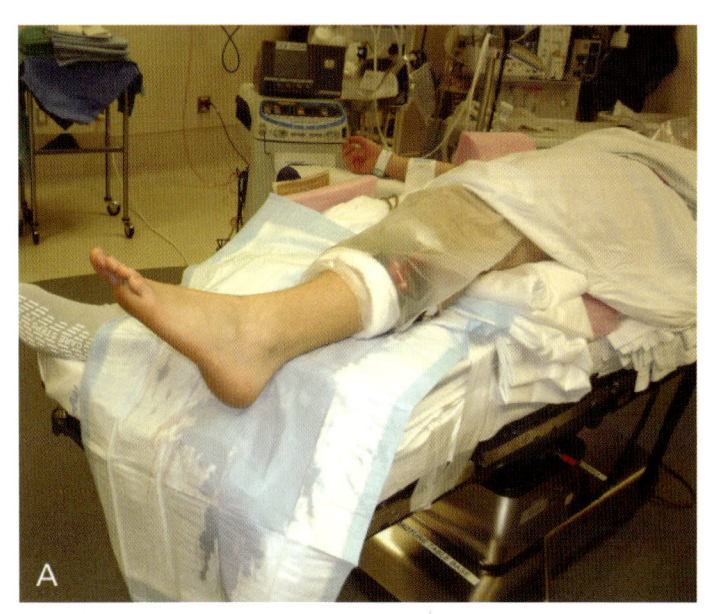

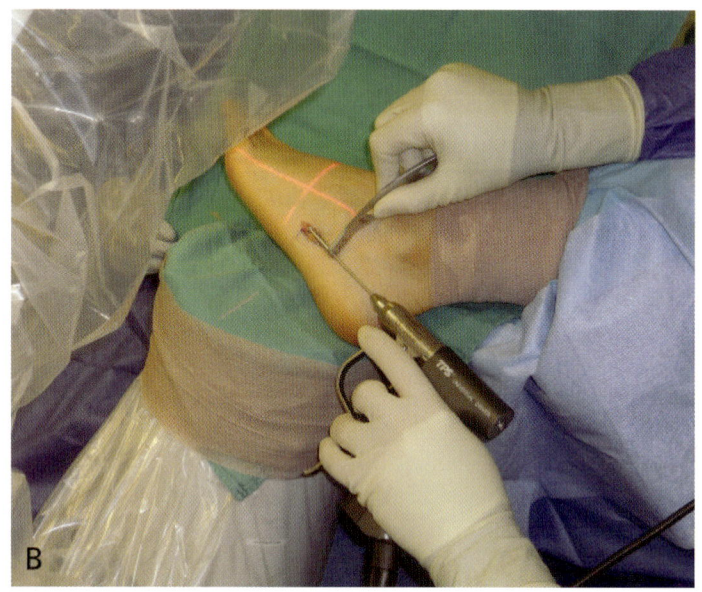

Figure 3 Intraoperative photographs show patient positioning for open reduction and internal fixation of a proximal fifth metatarsal fracture. **A**, The patient is positioned on the edge of the operating table with support under the ipsilateral hip and lower leg. This position allows satisfactory access to the base of the fifth metatarsal. **B**, The fluoroscopy unit may easily be positioned adjacent to the table so that it can serve as a lateral extension to the operating table, to support the surgical foot during the fluoroscopic portions of the procedure.

gitudinal incision is made on the lateral foot, approximately 1 cm proximal to the base of the fifth metatarsal (**Figure 4**). The goal is to achieve the "high and inside" starting position for the guide pin and screw on the fifth metatarsal base (**Figure 5**). This position facilitates directing the screw in line with the metatarsal shaft. High and inside implies superior and medial on the proximal end of the metatarsal to optimally direct the screw along the longitudinal axis of the fifth metatarsal.[2] If the starting point is too plantar or too lateral, the screw cannot be directed properly.

The structures at risk are shown in **Figure 6**. The sural nerve courses directly at the incision site for this procedure.[11] The peroneus brevis inserts on the dorsal base of the fifth metatarsal, and the peroneus longus courses lateral to and then plantar to the cuboid, immediately proximal to the fifth metatarsal base. The sural nerve and peroneus brevis are typically retracted dorsally, while the peroneus longus is typically retracted plantarward.

With the structures at risk protected, the high and inside position should be easily accessible with the cannulated drill's guide pin. A drill guide should be used with the guide pin, drill, and tap to further protect the structures at risk injury.

Guide Pin Positioning and Drilling

The guide pin for the cannulated drill must be directed into the center of the intramedullary canal of the fifth metatarsal, and its position must be confirmed in three planes (AP, oblique, and lateral). Two of three views may suggest an ideal position for the guide pin while the third does not; thus, it is necessary to confirm proper guide pin position in all three planes.[2]

Once the optimal starting point for the guide pin (high and inside; **Figure 5**) is confirmed fluoroscopically in one plane (typically, the oblique plane, as this places the metatarsal in profile and is the easi-

474 © 2013 American Academy of Orthopaedic Surgeons

Chapter 72: Open Reduction and Internal Fixation of Proximal Fifth Metatarsal Fractures

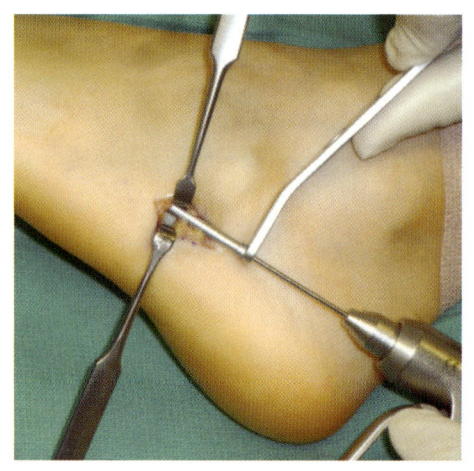

Figure 4 Intraoperative photograph shows surgical approach for open reduction and internal fixation of a proximal fifth metatarsal fracture. An incision is made approximately 1 to 2 cm proximal to the fifth metatarsal base, in line with the fifth metatarsal shaft. The assistant retracts the peroneus brevis tendon and sural nerve dorsally and the peroneus longus tendon plantarward, while the surgeon uses a protective sleeve for guide pin, drill, and tap.

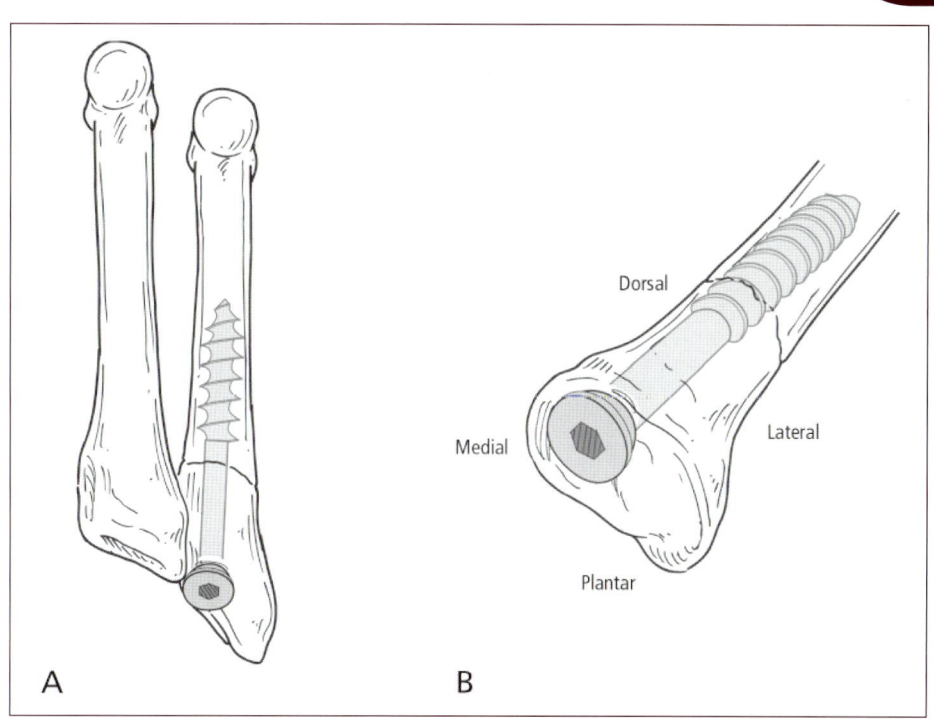

Figure 5 Illustrations demonstrate the "high and inside" starting position for the guide pin and screw for open reduction and internal fixation of a proximal fifth metatarsal fracture. A medial and superior starting position aligns the trajectory of the screw with the metatarsal shaft. **A,** Longitudinal aspect. **B,** End-on view of the proximal fifth metatarsal base.

est position in which to interpret the pin's position on fluoroscopy), it is essential to confirm its proper position in the other two planes (**Figure 7, A** through **C**).

The ideal starting point should be determined before advancing the guide pin because it is difficult to make subtle adjustments with a guide pin once a hole has been created close to the ideal starting position. (If a hole has been improperly placed 1 to 2 mm from the ideal starting point, the pin will tend to fall back into the improperly placed hole.) Once the optimal starting point is confirmed in all three planes, the guide pin may be partially advanced and its position confirmed in all three planes. After the ideal trajectory is confirmed, the guide pin may be advanced farther, across the fracture or nonunion site (**Figure 7, D** through **F**).

The fifth metatarsal is a curved bone, and intramedullary fixation is performed with a straight screw. The guide pin, drill, tap, and screw only need to be advanced beyond the fracture/nonunion site to accommodate all of the desired screw's thread length, which typically only involves the proximal 50% of the metatarsal. If the final screw is advanced far beyond the fracture site, it may impinge on the distal medial cortex of the curved fifth metatarsal, thereby creating a lateral cortical gap at the fracture site and potentially promoting nonunion. If there is a concern that the guide pin will dislodge with use of the cannulated drill or the tap, then the guide pin may be advanced farther down the fifth metatarsal, but there is no need to drill or tap that far.

With the guide pin properly positioned

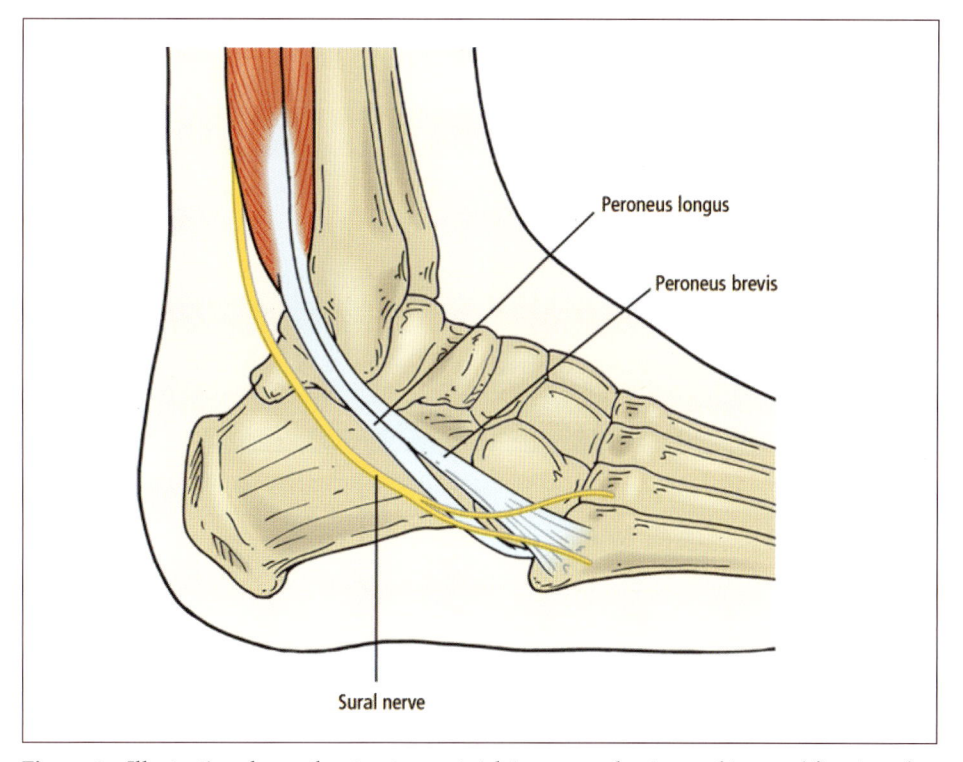

Figure 6 Illustration shows the structures at risk in open reduction and internal fixation of a proximal fifth metatarsal fracture. Typically, the peroneus brevis tendon and sural nerve are retracted dorsally and the peroneus longus tendon is retracted plantarward.

in all three planes and the structures at risk protected, the cannulated drill (used with a drill sleeve to further protect the structures at risk) is used to overdrill the guide pin, just beyond the fracture site (**Figure 8**).

© 2013 American Academy of Orthopaedic Surgeons

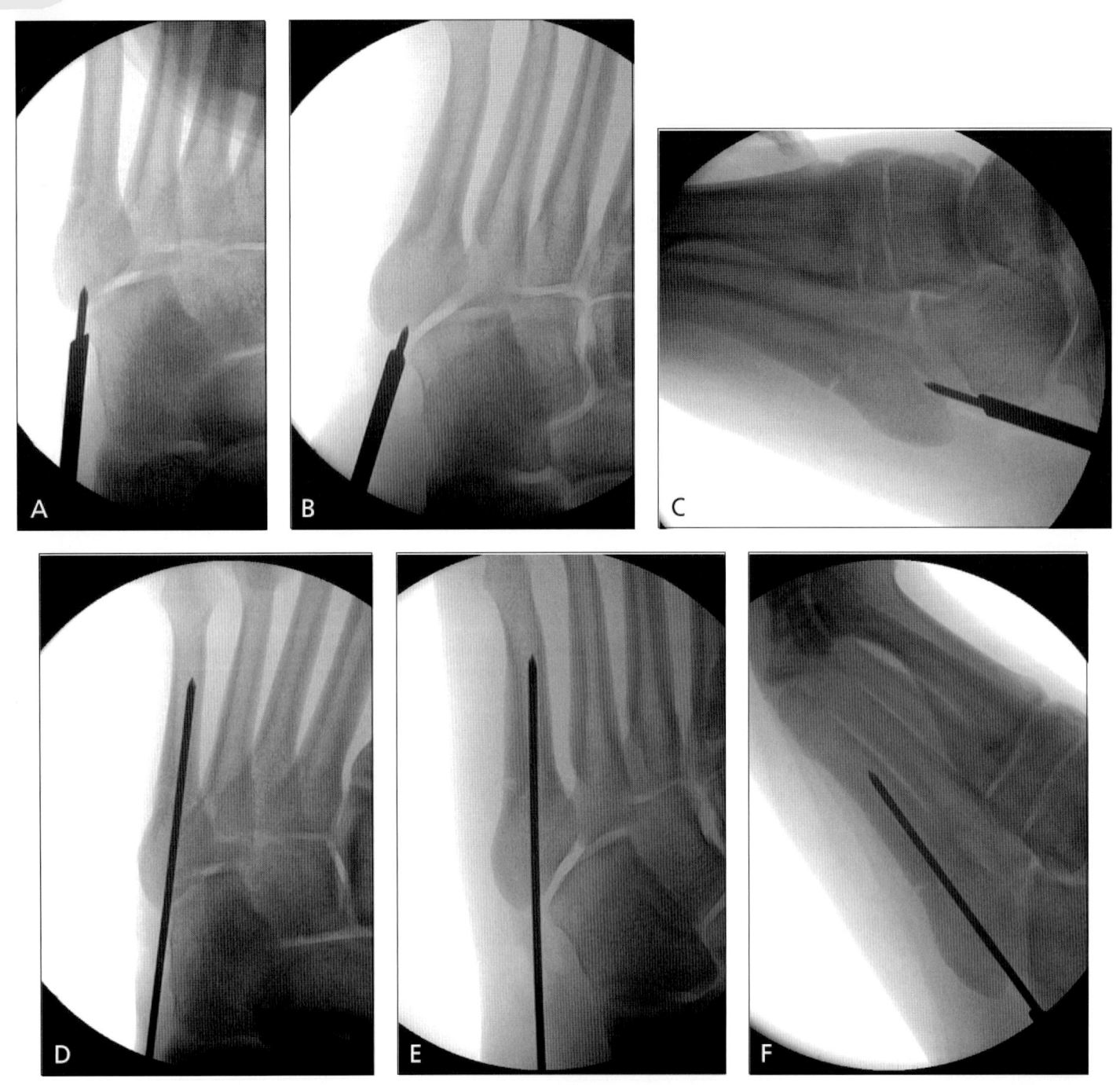

Figure 7 Fluoroscopic images show guide pin positioning for open reduction and internal fixation of a proximal fifth metatarsal fracture. AP (**A**), oblique (**B**), and lateral (**C**) views show the starting point for the guide pin/screw. AP (**D**), oblique (**E**), and lateral (**F**) views show the guide pin advanced past the fracture. Note that the guide pin is not advanced the entire length of the metatarsal.

In the setting of nonunion, the guide pin may be extracted, and a small-diameter drill may be introduced to drill the sclerotic bone at the nonunion site to promote fracture healing. The guide pin will need to be replaced and its optimal position again confirmed fluoroscopically.

Use of the Tap

The tap is introduced over the guide pin. The tap serves two purposes: it prepares the canal for the screw and gauges the size of screw that will afford the best purchase in the distal fragment.[2]

Because the structures at risk must be protected, it is prudent to use a protective sleeve over the tap (**Figure 9, A**). The tap size that engages the distal fragment to the point of torquing it with each turn typically represents the optimal screw size. Because there is no need to advance the screw to the distal fifth metatarsal and it needs to be advanced only far enough for all threads to cross the fracture or nonunion site, a relatively large screw diameter typically can be used, even in average-size individuals (**Figure 9, B**). Because screw diameter is dictated by the tap's diameter, a set of graduated taps is preferred to make this determination.

While advancing the screw with one hand, the surgeon holds the distal aspect of the metatarsal with the other hand to gauge and resist torque that is created as the tap is advanced into the distal fragment. The optimal screw diameter is determined by the tap that creates a firm torque on the distal fragment with each turn of the screw.

The tap and guide pin are removed from the canal, but the guide pin should be left

Chapter 72: Open Reduction and Internal Fixation of Proximal Fifth Metatarsal Fractures

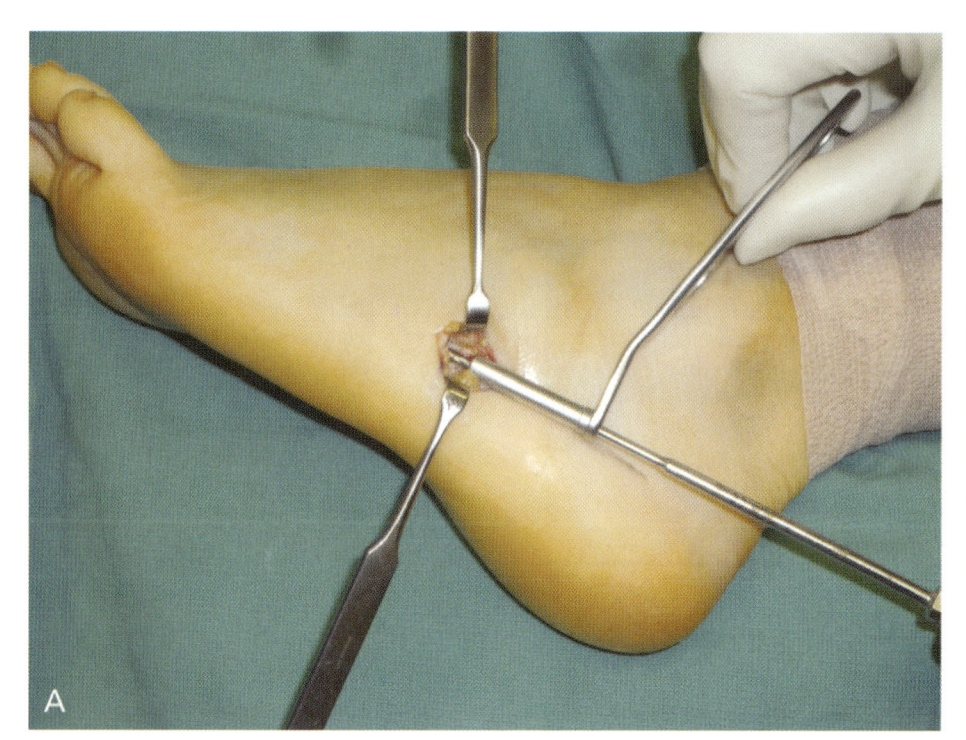

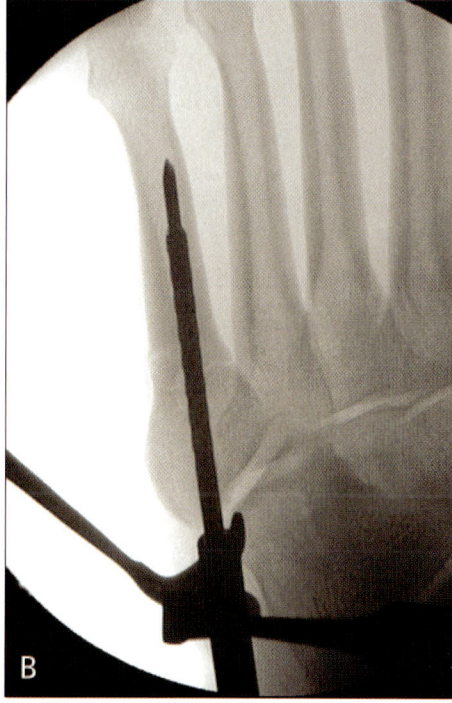

Figure 8 Drilling for open reduction and internal fixation of a proximal fifth metatarsal fracture. **A,** Intraoperative photograph shows a protective drill sleeve used to protect structures at risk, in addition to retraction of the peroneal tendons and sural nerve. **B,** Fluoroscopic image. Note that drilling is necessary only to the level that will allow the threads of the partially threaded screw to cross the fracture site.

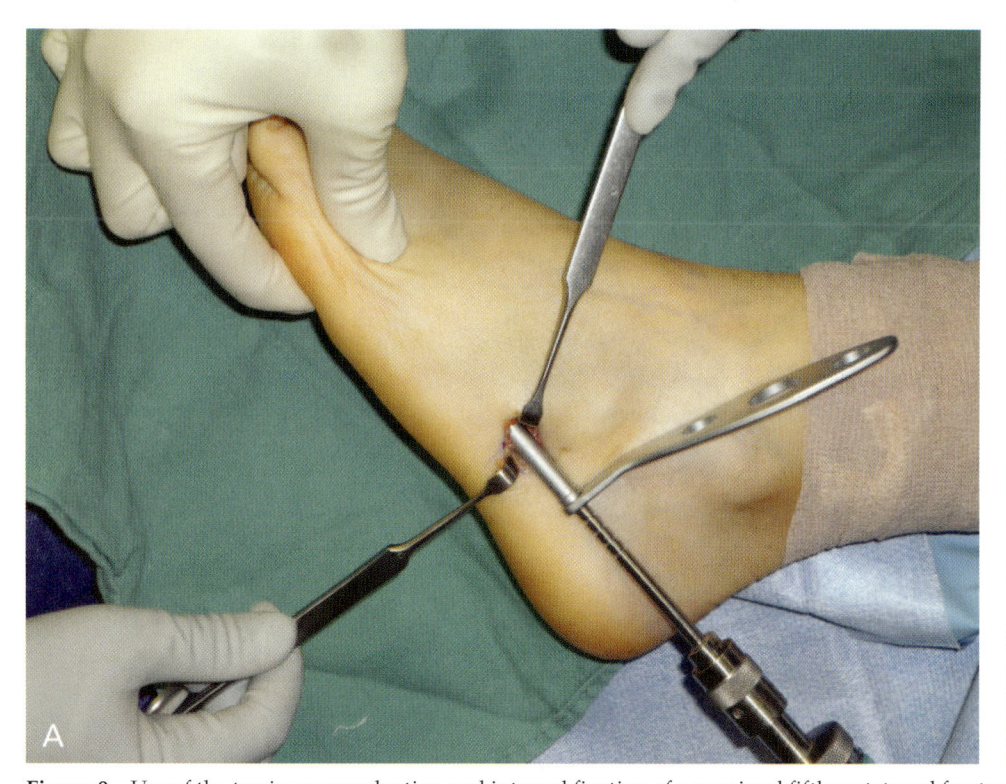

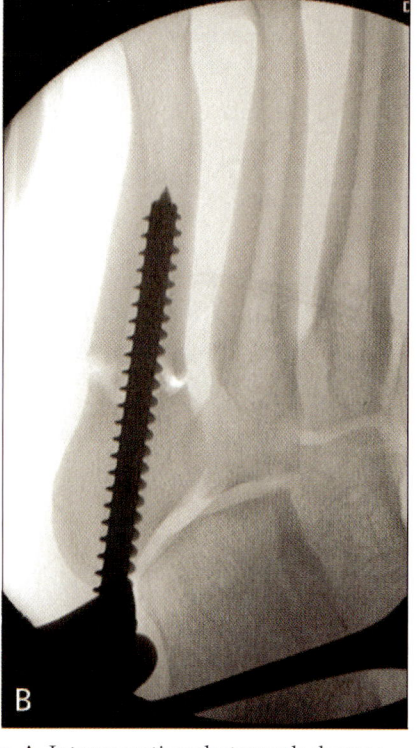

Figure 9 Use of the tap in open reduction and internal fixation of a proximal fifth metatarsal fracture. **A,** Intraoperative photograph shows a protective sleeve being used. Note that the distal fragment is being held as the tap is advanced. This allows the surgeon to gauge the optimal screw size as progressively larger taps are used until the proper tap engages the inner cortex. **B,** Fluoroscopic image shows the tap engaged to the point that it started to distract the fracture. Note that the tap is advanced only far enough to allow the threads of the partially threaded screw to cross the fracture.

in place if it is to be used to measure for the optimal screw length. Determining screw length is described in the next section.

Screws
Screw Diameter
The optimal screw diameter is determined by the diameter of the tap that best engages the distal fragment. Although biomechanical data exist that suggest improved fracture fixation with larger screw diameter,[7-10] the clinical evidence to support using larger screw diameters is weak.[12]

© 2013 American Academy of Orthopaedic Surgeons

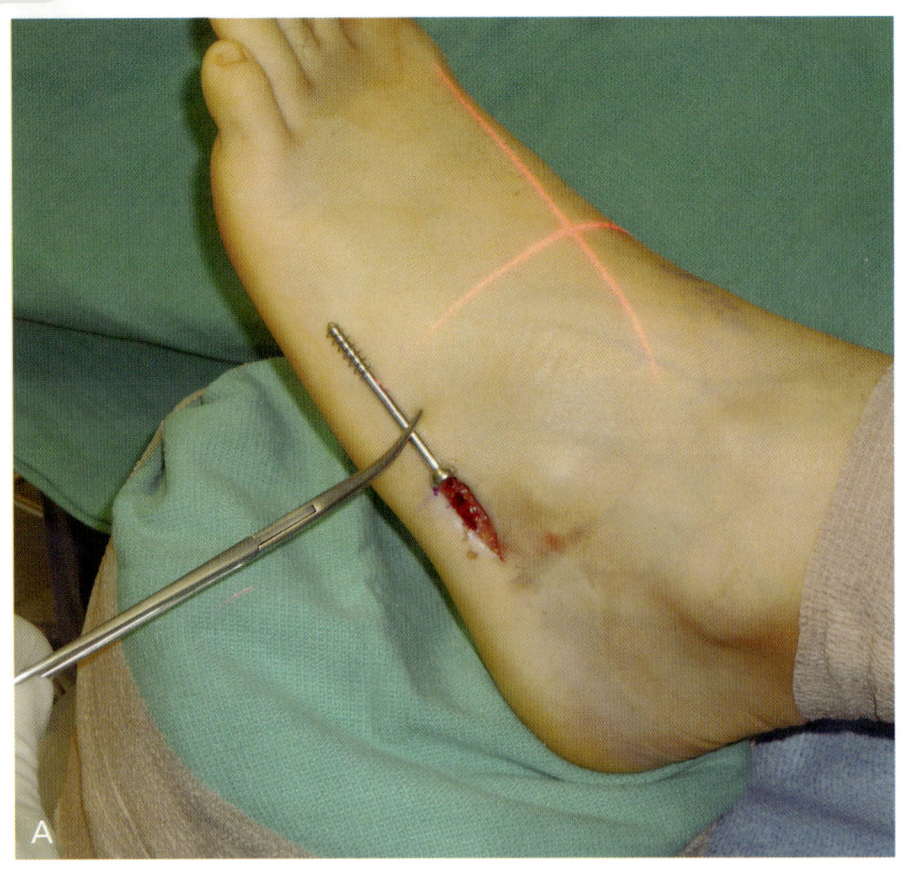

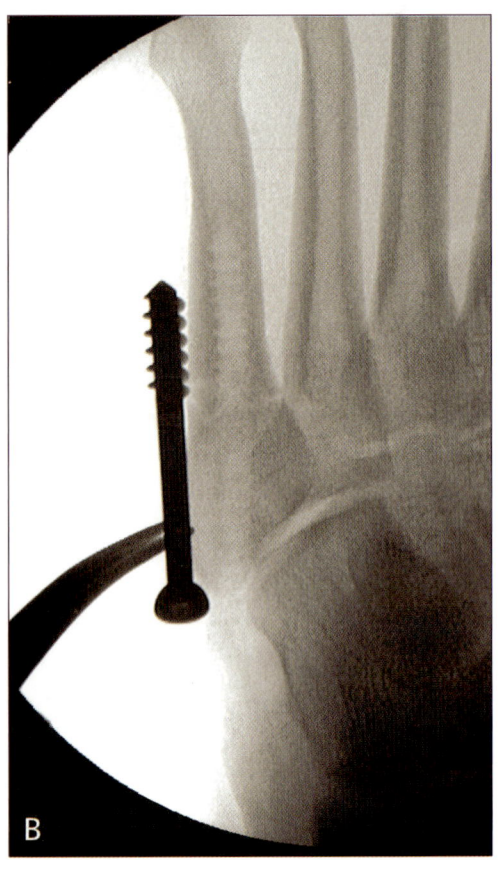

Figure 10 Determining screw length for open reduction and internal fixation of a proximal fifth metatarsal fracture. Intraoperative photograph (**A**) and fluoroscopic image (**B**) show the surgeon holding the screw adjacent to the metatarsal for a fluoroscopic image. Although the surgeon must account for magnification error, this technique provides some guidance as to the length of screw needed for the threads to cross the fracture. A screw that is too long will tend to contact the medical cortex distally and potentially gap the lateral aspect of the fracture.

Screw Length

The optimal screw length is the length that most effectively allows all threads to cross the fracture site. The screw must not be so long that it contacts the distal medial cortex in the distal fragment, or it may promote gapping of the lateral cortex at the fracture site and potentially lead to nonunion.[1,2]

Screw length may be determined by the following three methods (if there is any question, more than one method should be used to confirm proper screw length): (1) using a cannulated depth gauge with the guide pin in optimal position (ie, the tip of the guide pin in the desired position for the tip of the screw); (2) using two guide pins and measuring the difference, with the intramedullary guide pin in the optimal position and the second placed to the level of the base of the fifth metatarsal (the position of both guide pins must be confirmed fluoroscopically); and (3) holding the screw immediately adjacent to the fifth metatarsal base to determine if the threads will cross the fracture site (must account for a slight magnification effect) (**Figure 10**).

Screw Insertion

With the ideal screw diameter and length determined, the screw is advanced into the prepared canal while protecting the structures at risk (**Figure 11, A**). As the screw engages the distal fragment, the surgeon must (1) resist the torque that is created by the screw in the distal fragment so that the screw fully advances in the metatarsal, and (2) apply an axial force on the distal fragment as the screw is advanced to again ensure that the screw fully advances, with all threads crossing the fracture site. All three planes are checked to confirm that the screw is fully seated and that the fracture site is reduced and compressed as much as possible (**Figure 11, B** through **D**).

Video

This technique in the video demonstrates an ORIF of a fifth metatarsal stress fracture with delayed union/nonunion. This patient was treated after the fracture failed to progress to union despite 6 months of appropriate nonsurgical management at an outside institution.

Video 72.1 Open Reduction and Internal Fixation of Proximal 5th Metatarsal Fracture. Mark E. Easley, MD (9 min)

Complications

Complications of ORIF of these fractures include infection, sural neuralgia,[11] injury to the peroneus brevis or longus tendons, delayed union or nonunion (**Figure 12**), prominent hardware (screw head), refracture (sometimes with broken screw), and distal fracture at the tip of the screw (peri-implant fracture).

Postoperative Care and Rehabilitation

The patient undergoes protected weight bearing in a splint, controlled ankle motion (CAM) walker, or cast for 4 to 5 weeks. Gradual progression of weight bearing in a CAM walker is instituted between 5 and 8 weeks. With radiographic evidence of healing, weight bearing may be advanced in a regular shoe.[1,4,5]

The patient should be restricted from athletic activity until the fracture site is

Chapter 72: Open Reduction and Internal Fixation of Proximal Fifth Metatarsal Fractures

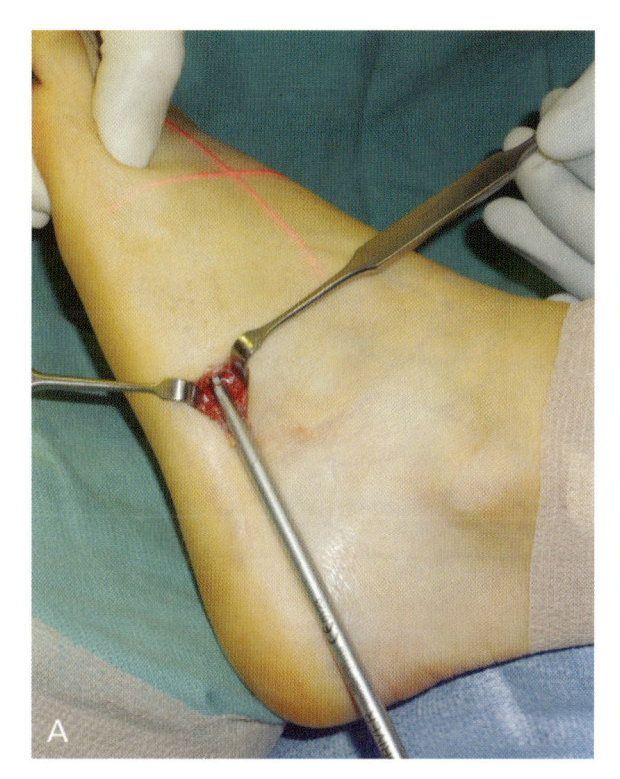

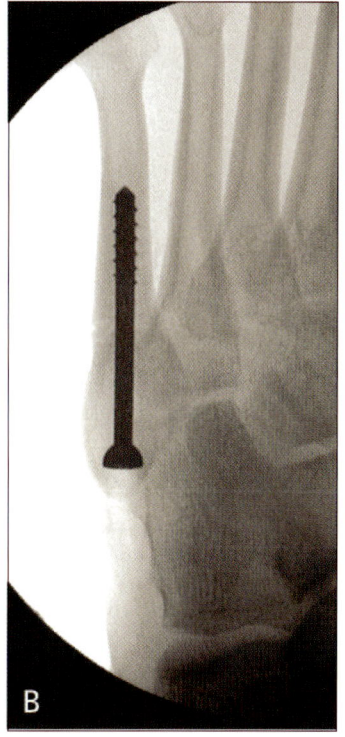

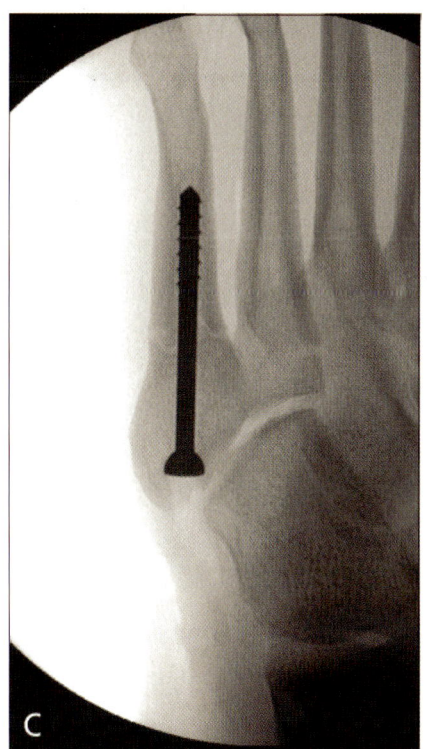

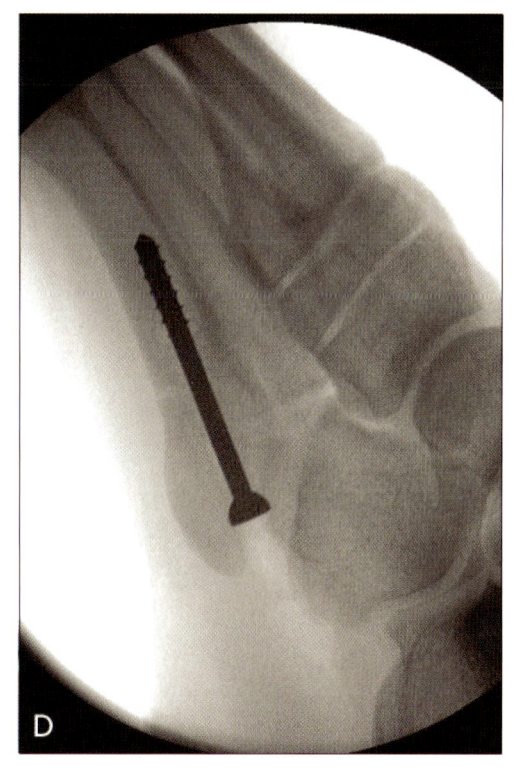

Figure 11 Screw insertion in open reduction and internal fixation of a proximal fifth metatarsal fracture. **A,** Intraoperative photograph shows the surgeon holding the distal fragment with one hand while placing the screw with the other. This technique allows for axial compression and assessment of how well the screw engages the inner cortex of the distal fragment. Intraoperative AP (**B**), oblique (**C**), and lateral (**D**) fluoroscopic images confirm that the screw is in proper position, the fracture is reduced, and there are no associated stress fractures.

nontender and radiographs suggest progression toward full healing (usually by 10 to 12 weeks; Figure 13).

If there is evidence of delayed union, weight bearing should be restricted, a CAM walker boot should be continued, and an external bone stimulator may be considered. If the radiographic interpretation of suspected delayed union is difficult, CT may be considered to assess fracture healing. When there is no radiographic evidence for progression toward healing, reoperation needs to be considered with bone grafting, external bone stimulation, revision ORIF screw removal, and exchange to a larger screw, much like treatment of nonunion in a long-bone fracture.

Pearls

- The structures at risk (sural nerve, peroneal tendons) must be protected.
- The base of the fifth metatarsal is subject to a watershed area of poor vascularity; zone II and some zone III fractures are notorious for delayed healing. (Preoperative patient education is essential because even a perfect surgery may lead to delayed union.)
- Because delay in healing of base of fifth metatarsal fractures is relatively common, I prefer to use the largest solid screw as possible to stabilize the fracture.
- The screw should not extend into the distal aspect of the metatarsal. A longer screw will potentially abut against the distal medial cortex, thereby creating a gap at the lateral cortex fracture site and leading to delay in healing or even nonunion.

© 2013 American Academy of Orthopaedic Surgeons

Section 5: Trauma

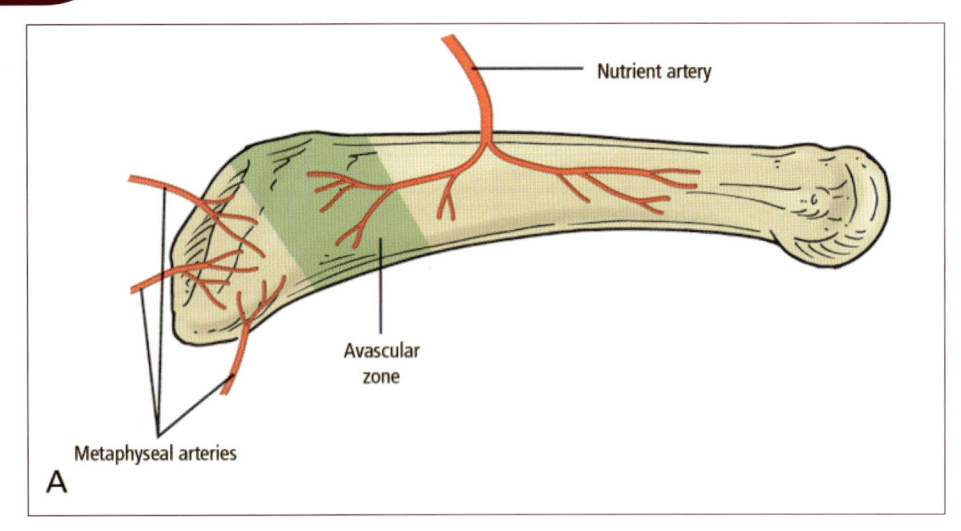

Figure 12 **A,** Illustration shows vascularity of the fifth metatarsal. Zone II (the green area) is the location for the Jones fracture, which is notorious for delayed union and even nonunion due to the watershed that leaves that segment of the fifth metatarsal with a marginal blood supply. **B,** Oblique radiograph obtained at 8-month follow-up after open reduction and internal fixation (ORIF) of acute fifth metatarsal fracture suggests nonunion rather than refracture. This athlete had apparent clinical and radiographic healing 4 months after ORIF of an acute fifth metatarsal base fracture but then experienced recurrent symptoms 8 months after surgery, despite 4 months of pain-free participation in sports after being released to play.

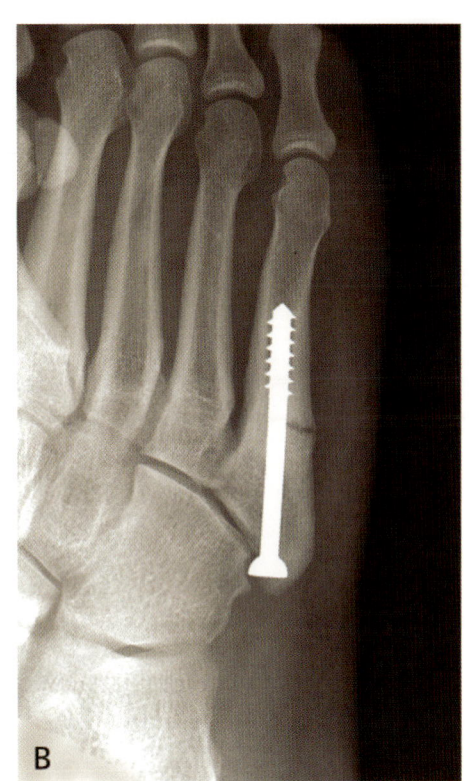

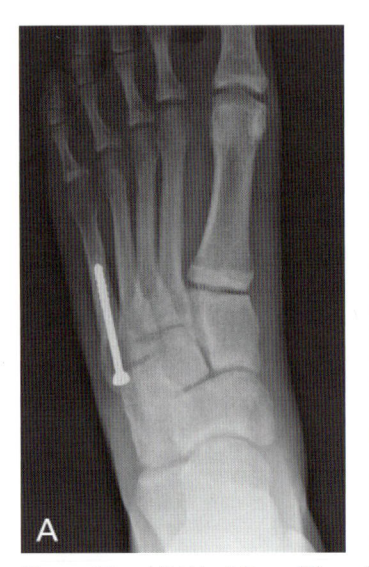

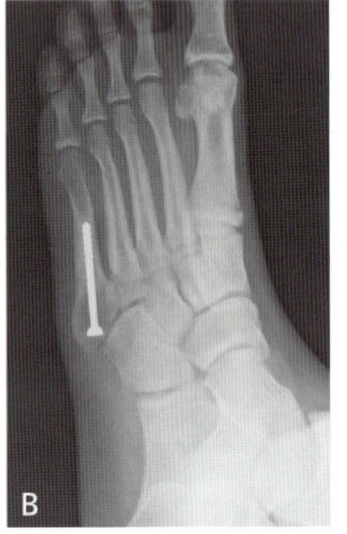

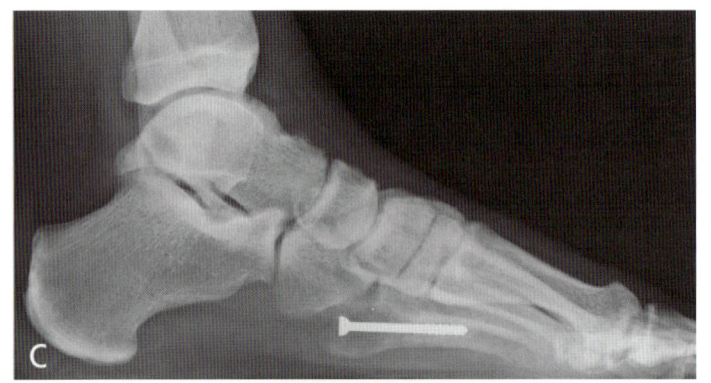

Figure 13 AP (**A**), oblique (**B**), and lateral (**C**) radiographs obtained at 3-month follow-up for the patient described as the case example in this chapter. The foot was nontender on clinical examination, and bridging trabeculation at the fracture site is suggested on all three radiographic views.

- This procedure involves a straight screw being inserted into a curved bone. It only needs to be inserted far enough for the threads to cross the fracture site, thereby allowing a relatively large screw diameter and promoting compression at the fracture.
- Ideal screw position depends on an ideal starting point. The screw should be inserted in the high and inside position on the proximal end of the fifth metatarsal (ie, superior and medial).
- The operated foot is placed on the operating table in such a way that is easy to position the fluoroscopy unit adjacent to the table, so that it can be easily used to confirm proper guide pin and screw position.

References

1. Nunley JA: Fractures of the base of the fifth metatarsal: The Jones fracture. *Orthop Clin North Am* 2001;32(1):171-180.
2. Easley ME, Nunley JA: Open reduction and internal fixation of proximal fifth metatarsal (Jones' or stress) fracture, in Pfeffer GB, Frey C, Hintermann B, Sands AK, eds: *Foot and Ankle Surgery*. Philadelphia, PA, Saunders-Elsevier, 2010, pp 277-286.
3. Chuckpaiwong B, Queen RM, Easley ME, Nunley JA: Distinguishing Jones and proximal diaphyseal fractures of the fifth metatarsal. *Clin Orthop Relat Res* 2008;466(8):1966-1970.
4. Porter DA, Duncan M, Meyer SJ: Fifth metatarsal Jones fracture fixation with a 4.5-mm cannulated stainless steel screw in the competitive and recreational athlete: A clinical and radiographic evaluation. *Am J Sports Med* 2005;33(5):726-733.
5. Portland G, Kelikian A, Kodros S: Acute surgical management of Jones' fractures. *Foot Ankle Int* 2003;24(11):829-833.
6. Raikin SM, Slenker N, Ratigan B: The association of a varus hindfoot and fracture

of the fifth metatarsal metaphyseal-diaphyseal junction: The Jones fracture. *Am J Sports Med* 2008;36(7):1367-1372.

7. Horst F, Gilbert BJ, Glisson RR, Nunley JA: Torque resistance after fixation of Jones fractures with intramedullary screws. *Foot Ankle Int* 2004;25(12):914-919.

8. Kelly IP, Glisson RR, Fink C, Easley ME, Nunley JA: Intramedullary screw fixation of Jones fractures. *Foot Ankle Int* 2001;22(7):585-589.

9. Sides SD, Fetter NL, Glisson R, Nunley JA: Bending stiffness and pull-out strength of tapered, variable pitch screws, and 6.5-mm cancellous screws in acute Jones fractures. *Foot Ankle Int* 2006;27(10):821-825.

10. Vertullo CJ, Glisson RR, Nunley JA: Torsional strains in the proximal fifth metatarsal: Implications for Jones and stress fracture management. *Foot Ankle Int* 2004;25(9):650-656.

11. Donley BG, McCollum MJ, Murphy GA, Richardson EG: Risk of sural nerve injury with intramedullary screw fixation of fifth metatarsal fractures: A cadaver study. *Foot Ankle Int* 1999;20(3):182-184.

12. Porter DA, Rund AM, Dobslaw R, Duncan M: Comparison of 4.5- and 5.5-mm cannulated stainless steel screws for fifth metatarsal Jones fracture fixation. *Foot Ankle Int* 2009;30(1):27-33.

Foot and Ankle

Section Editor
Michael Pinzur, MD

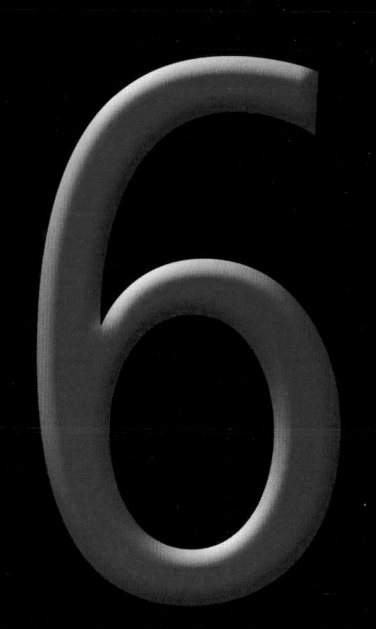

73 Ankle Arthroscopy: Diagnostics, Débridement, and
Removal of Loose Bodies 485
Carol Frey, MD

74 Arthroscopic Treatment of Osteochondral Lesions of the Talus 491
Steven M. Raikin, MD; Nicholas R. Slenker, MD

75 Augmented Lateral Ankle Ligament Reconstruction for
Persistent Ankle Instability 499
Nicholas A. Abidi, MD

76 Achilles Tendon Rupture Repair 505
Stanley C. Graves, MD; Jaycen Brown, BS

77 Tibiotalar Arthrodesis 509
Siddhant K. Mehta, MD; Nicholas A. Abidi, MD; Sheldon S. Lin, MD

78 Subtalar Arthrodesis 515
James B. Carr, MD

79 Arthrodesis of the Tarsometatarsal Joint 519
J. Chris Coetzee, MD, FRCSC; Pascal Rippstein, MD

80 Surgical Treatment of Navicular Stress Fractures 527
Bethany Gallagher, MD; Arthur K. Walling, MD

81 Arthrodesis of the Hallux Metatarsophalangeal Joint 531
Chirag S. Patel, MD; Loretta Chou, MD

82 Proximal and Distal First Metatarsal Osteotomies for
Hallux Valgus 535
Christopher B. Hirose, MD; Michael J. Coughlin, MD

83   **Chronic Exertional Compartment Syndrome and Release** **541**
Emily A. Wagstrom, MD; Annunziato Amendola, MD;
Brian R. Wolf, MD, MS

84   **Transtibial Amputation** **545**
COL James R. Ficke, MD; MAJ Daniel J. Stinner, MD

85   **Midfoot Amputations** **551**
Terrence M. Philbin, DO; Bryan Witt, DO

Chapter 73
Ankle Arthroscopy: Diagnostics, Débridement, and Removal of Loose Bodies

Carol Frey, MD

Patient Selection
Indications
The most common reasons for ankle arthroscopy are given in **Table 1**. One of the most common indications for ankle arthroscopy is anterior ankle impingement. Anterior impingement is generally caused by soft-tissue or bone obstruction. Anterior tibial spurs are a common source of anterior impingement. Anterior impingement and spurs are common in athletes, especially those who dorsiflex their ankles with force, such as runners, dancers, and football players. An incidence of 45% was reported in football players and 59% in dancers.[1] Physical examination will reveal anterior ankle pain, exacerbated by forced dorsiflexion of the ankle. The pain is usually localized along the anterior ridge of the tibia.

Although the cause of anterior spurs is unknown, they most likely result from repetitive minor injuries rather than one traumatic episode. They may be part of an early degenerative process in the ankle. Although anterior spurs are usually asymptomatic, surgery may be required when they are painful. The procedure is recommended for patients who have persistent anterior ankle pain and loss of dorsiflexion after nonsurgical treatment has failed. Anterior spurs on the tibia and talus can be removed with the arthroscope.

Anterolateral soft-tissue impingement, another cause of anterior ankle impingement, occurs mainly in three sites: the superior portion of the anterior inferior tibiofibular ligament (AITFL), the distal portion of the AITFL, and along the anterior talofibular ligament (ATFL) and the lateral gutter near the area of the lateral talar dome. Physical examination will again reveal anterior ankle pain, made worse by forced dorsiflexion of the ankle. The pain is usually present in the lateral gutter area of the ankle. Anterolateral impingement of the ankle should be considered in a patient with chronic anterolateral pain after an inversion injury, regardless of the stability of the ankle joint. Anterior soft-tissue impingement lesions may be removed with the arthroscope.[1-5]

Contraindications
Contraindications can include infection, severe peripheral neuropathy, complex regional pain syndrome, or significant psychiatric disorder.

Preoperative Imaging
Radiographs obtained in the early stages of anterior bone impingement may be negative. A lateral radiograph may reveal the spur. A forced dorsiflexion lateral radiograph may confirm anterior impingement. The talus may show secondary dorsal spur formation (**Figure 1**), and loose bodies may be seen.

MRI will often show cartilage thinning and soft-tissue reaction, in addition to an osteophyte. Although not indicated in all cases of anterior impingement of the ankle, MRI can be useful in cases where additional pathology in the ankle or subtalar joint must be evaluated. In the diagnosis of anterior soft-tissue impingement, MRI has been reported to be approximately 79% accurate and 84% sensitive.[4] As noted previously, anterolateral soft-tissue impingement occurs mainly in three sites: the superior portion of the AITFL; the distal portion of the AITFL, which may have a separate fascicle involved; and along the ATFL and the lateral gutter near the area of the lateral talar

Table 1 Conditions That Can Be Treated Arthroscopically

Diagnosis/Indications	Percentage of Cases That Can Be Treated Arthroscopically
Ankle arthritis	25
Loose body	90
Synovectomy	90
Acute infection	80
Lateral impingement	95–100
Osteochondral defects	95–100
Anterior osteophytes	80–90
Stabilization	25
Ankle arthrodesis	25
Foreign body	90–100

(Reproduced with permission from Frey C: Foot and ankle arthroscopy and endoscopy, in Myerson MS, ed: *Foot and Ankle Disorders*. Philadelphia, PA, WB Saunders, 2000, vol 2, p 1478.)

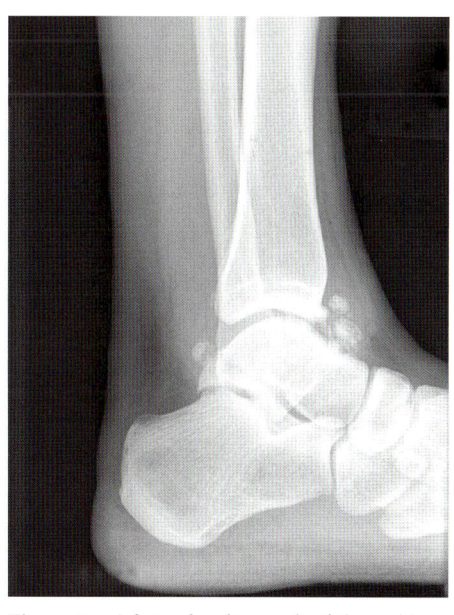

Figure 1 A lateral radiograph of the ankle reveals an anterior tibial spur.

Dr. Frey or an immediate family member is a member of a speakers' bureau or has made paid presentations on behalf of Össur; serves as an unpaid consultant to Össur; and serves as a board member, owner, officer, or committee member of the Arthroscopy Association of North America.

dome. All these areas can be visualized on MRI. Sagittal T1-weighted and STIR (short tau inversion recovery) images are particularly useful. Displacement of subcutaneous fat by fluid (effusion) or soft tissue can be seen using these sequences (Figure 2).

Ultrasonography has been found to be accurate in detecting synovial lesions in the anterior lateral gutter, demonstrating ligament injuries, and differentiating soft-tissue from bone impingement. Ultrasonography will not show osteochondral lesions or stress fracture. It may also overlook some loose bodies.[6]

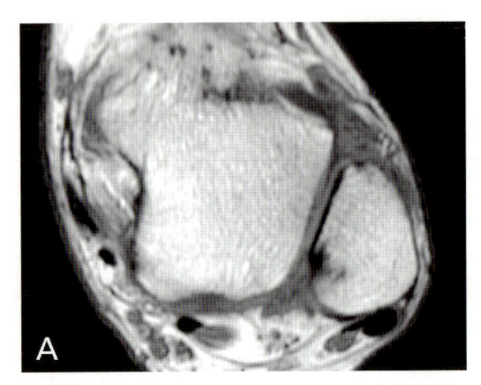

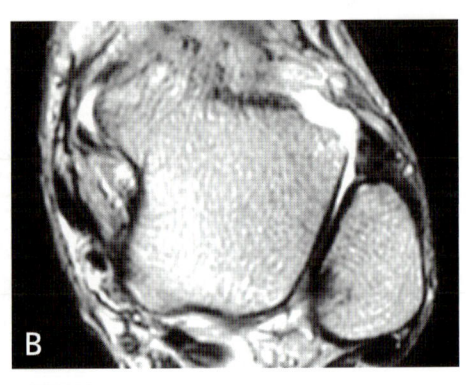

Figure 2 Axial T1-weighted (**A**) and fast spin-echo T2-weighted (**B**) MRIs of the ankle of a 39-year-old man with anterolateral ankle impingement. Thickening and scarring of the distal fascicle is evident in these images taken 3 months after an anterior inferior tibiofibular ligament injury.

Video 73.1 Subtalar Arthroscopy. Richard D. Ferkel, MD (9 min)

Procedure

Room Setup/Patient Positioning

Ankle arthroscopy is usually performed as an outpatient procedure. The use of spinal anesthesia is preferred, although general anesthesia can be administered. In carefully selected patients, ankle block anesthesia using 1% lidocaine is appropriate, but this is rarely used.

The patient is placed in the supine position on the operating room table with a well-padded tourniquet on the proximal thigh. The limb is prepared and draped with a standard lower limb extremity set, and a bolster is placed under the thigh to elevate the extremity off the table. A well-padded thigh holder can also be used. The limb is exsanguinated, and the tourniquet is inflated. The well-padded straps or stirrups of a noninvasive distraction device are then applied (Figure 3).

Noninvasive distraction is recommended for this procedure to allow for better access to the spur and to prevent cartilage damage. Care must be taken not to excessively distract the joint because this will pull the synovium and capsule tight up against the spur and make visualization and access difficult.

Special Instruments/Equipment

The following instruments and equipment should be on hand: a No. 11 scalpel; a straight mosquito clamp; a 20-mL syringe; an 18-gauge spinal needle; a lightweight camera with compatible light source; a video/TV monitor; a blunt trochar/cannula; a thigh holder/large sterile bump; a 2.9-mm arthroscope, with 30° and 70° angulations; small curets; a rasp; small grasping forceps, probes, and biters; a 2.9- to 3.5-mm arthroscopic full radius shaver; an acromionizer (burr); a radiofrequency wand; a high-flow infusion pump; and a noninvasive distractor.

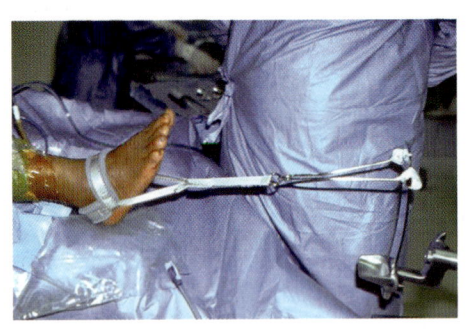

Figure 3 Photograph shows the standard setup and patient positioning for ankle arthroscopy.

Surgical Technique

The superficial anatomy is used to guide proper placement of the portals. A skin marker is used to outline the extra-articular anatomy, including the joint line, the greater saphenous vein, the superficial peroneal nerve and its branches, the saphenous nerve, and the dorsalis pedis artery.

The anterolateral portal is placed just lateral to the peroneus tertius, entering the joint between the fibula and the talus just distal to the joint line. The anteromedial portal is located at the level of the joint line just medial to the tibialis anterior tendon (Figure 4).

An 18-gauge needle is introduced into the joint medial to the tibialis anterior tendon, and 15 to 20 mL of normal saline is injected to distend the joint. The dorsiflexion motion of the foot indicates proper placement of the fluid into the joint. A No. 11 blade is used to make a small vertical skin incision, avoiding the surrounding tendons and neurovascular structures. A small, straight mosquito clamp is used to spread the subcutaneous tissue to the level of the joint capsule. The cannula of the 2.9-mm arthroscope with a blunt trochar is inserted, followed by the arthroscope. Saline solution inflow is connected to the arthroscope for continuous joint distention. An 18-gauge spinal needle is inserted under direct visualization to confirm placement of the anterolateral portal. An incision is made lateral to the peroneus tertius tendon. If the problem is known to be located posterior, a posterolateral portal is made under direct visualization by placing the arthroscope through the medial notch to view posteriorly. An 18-gauge spinal needle is then inserted lateral to the Achilles tendon at a 5° angle toward the medial malleolus. Special care must be taken to avoid the short saphenous vein, the sural nerve, and the peroneal tendons (Figure 5).

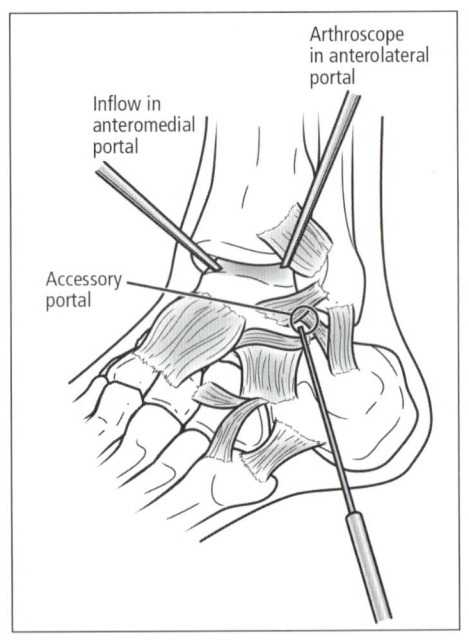

Figure 4 Illustration shows the anterolateral and anteromedial portals used for the treatment of anterior ankle impingement. Accessory portals may be helpful.

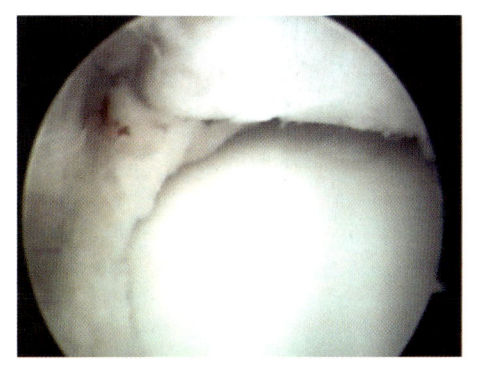

Figure 5 Arthroscopic view shows the placement of the posterolateral portal. Care is taken to avoid the sural nerve.

The anteromedial and anterolateral portals are used to visualize the anterior joint, including the medial, central, and lateral talus and the anterior tibial rim. By directing the arthroscope through the medial gutter, the surgeon can examine the medial talomalleolar space and the deltoid ligament. Directing the arthroscope toward the lateral gutter reveals the distal one third of the anterior tibiofibular ligament. At the distal aspect of the lateral gutter, the discrete thickening of the anterior lateral joint capsule that is made up of the fibers of the ATFL can be seen. The lateral dome of the talus is well seen. The calcaneofibular ligament cannot be seen because it is extra-articular.

Continuing on this path, through the lateral gutter (the lateral talomalleolar space), the ATFL and the posterior talofibular ligament are examined. If the foot is plantar flexed, the arthroscope can often pass over the talar dome into the posterior compartment, allowing visualization of the posterolateral and posteromedial aspects of the joint as well as the posterior capsule. The arthroscope can be rotated 180° to allow visualization of the plafond.

Placement of the arthroscope through the posterolateral portal allows further examination of the posteromedial and posterolateral gutters. The posterior tibiotalar joint is better visualized, as are the posteromedial and posterolateral articulations of the tibia, talus, and fibula.

With distraction, the anteromedial, anterolateral, and posterolateral portals can be used to obtain nearly complete access to all compartments of the ankle joint with relatively minimal risk of neuromuscular injury. The entire tibial plafond can be accessed by a combination of these portals. Furthermore, these portals allow débridement of all lesions in these areas.

Anterior impingement osteophytes occur between the anterior tibial edge and the proximal talar neck at the anterior capsular insertion sites. An anterior lateral placement of the arthroscope with an anteromedial placement of the curet allows access to the capsular insertion on the anterior talus. Because of the more anterior position of the medial malleolus, the combination of the anteromedial arthroscope and the anterolateral curet does not allow adequate access to the anterior capsular insertion into the talus. Using a 30° arthroscope, significant leverage would be required to visualize this area and would damage the arthroscope. A 70° arthroscope may help to visualize this area and is occasionally used (**Figure 6**).

Soft-tissue lesions and loose bodies can occur in any compartment of the ankle joint. Anterior compartment lesions can be approached through anterior portals. Anterolateral lesions can be accessed by means of these portals as well. Posterior compartment pathology as seen with hypertrophy of the posterior talofibular ligament and posterior impingement lesions should be approached with the addition of the posterolateral portal (**Figure 7**).

Dorsiflexion and plantar flexion may be necessary to visualize the impinging structures. Posterior portals are not necessary for the removal of anterior spurs on the talus and tibia. For the removal of anterior bone spurs, a 2.9-mm arthroscope, a high-flow system, and an arthroscopic pump are used. Excessive synovium is cleared away with a full-radius power shaver or a radiofrequency wand. The spur is visualized and removed with a 4.0-mm power burr. The acromionizer works well for removing the exostosis.

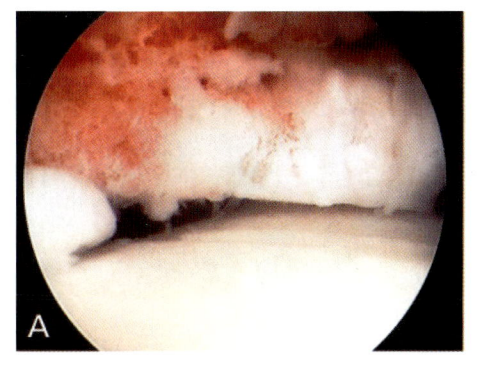

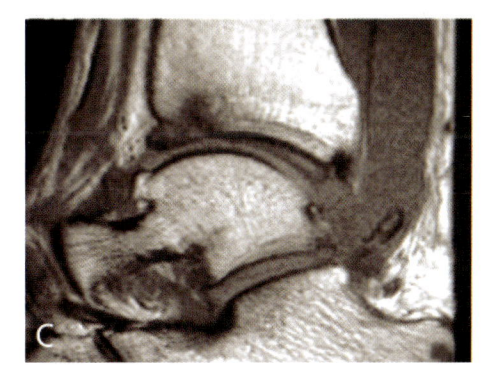

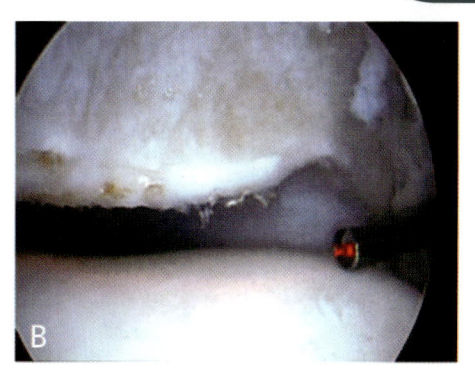

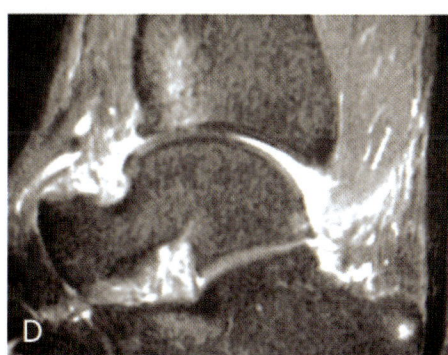

Figure 6 Arthroscopic views of a large anterior tibial spur before (**A**) and after (**B**) débridement with the acromionizer. Sagittal T1-weighted (**C**) and short tau inversion recovery (**D**) MRIs show anterior osteophytes of the distal tibia and talus, anterior tibiotalar joint capsular hypertrophy, and subchondral marrow edema within the anterior distal aspect of the tibia.

Once the spur is removed, the anterior surface is smoothed with a full-radius shaver or a curet. Care must be taken to inspect the joint for loose bodies. The origin and development of loose bodies should be kept in mind when reviewing the history and physical findings and while performing the arthroscopy. When symptomatic, loose bodies should be removed, and this is easily done arthroscopically. Depending on the size, number, and position of the loose bodies, a distraction technique is usually required.

After completion of the arthroscopic examination, all instruments are removed, and the remaining irrigation fluids are expressed from the joint. All wounds are closed with 4-0 nylon suture. The wounds are covered with sterile dressings, and a soft, bulky dressing is applied.

Complications

The reported complication rate associated with arthroscopy of the ankle joint is 0.7% to 9%.[1-12] Most of the complications were

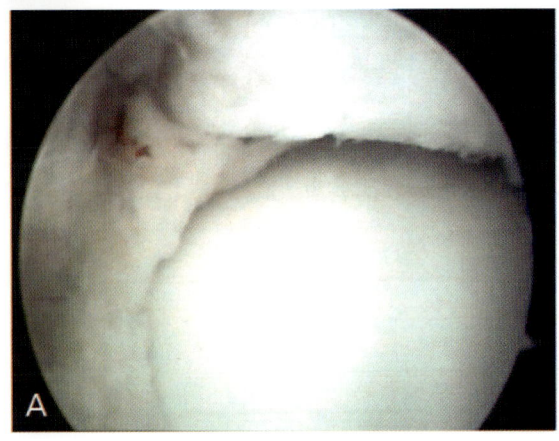

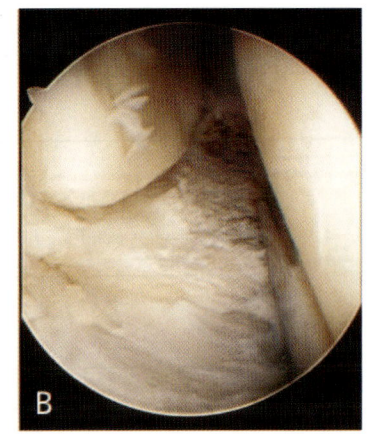

Figure 7 Arthroscopic views before (**A**) and after (**B**) treatment of a soft-tissue anterior impingement lesion of the ankle. The distal one third of the anterior tibiofibular ligament is intra-articular and can be débrided if it is hypertrophied, injured, or a source of impingement.

neuralgic conditions, which accounted for 49% of the complications. Injury to the superficial peroneal nerve was the most common nerve injury, followed by the sural nerve, saphenous nerve, and deep peroneal nerve. All the nerve injuries occurred through direct injury, by portal or distraction pin placement. Other possible complications include vascular injury, tendon injury, complex regional pain syndrome (rare), infection, deep venous thrombosis, sinus tract formation, skin necrosis, and cartilage damage.

Postoperative Care and Rehabilitation

The ankle is placed in a bulky dressing with or without a cryotherapy unit incorporated into the dressing. The patient is allowed to bear weight at 5 days, when the inflammation has decreased. Sutures are removed at 10 to 14 days. Physical therapy starts after the sutures are removed, with range-of-motion activities, modalities, and stretching of the Achilles tendon. This is followed by strengthening, proprioception, and closed-chain activities. Patients with anterior impingement, with and without fragmentation, will take approximately 6 weeks to recover postoperatively. Patients with arthritic changes in the ankle joint will take approximately 12 weeks to recover. Some soft-tissue swelling may be present for up to 6 months postoperatively.

Outcomes

Arthroscopic treatment of anterior ankle pain provides reliable improvement in function, decrease in pain, and improvement in clinical scores for most patients, including athletes.[3]

At long-term follow up, the results have been reported to be approximately 92% to 95% good to excellent in patients without joint space narrowing. In athletes, around 80% were able to return to sports at the same level of performance.[1,7] Some reports indicate that osteophytes usually recur to some extent, and most patients do not feel that range of dorsiflexion returns to normal.[8] Symptomatic relief, however, allows most to return to function. As expected, the results in nonarthritic joints are the best. Patients with anterolateral soft-tissue impingement after an ankle scope and débridement do better overall, when compared with those with anterior bone impingement.[5] Furthermore, outcomes have not been reported to be as good if there is some combination of associated joint pathology, such as chondral lesions, syndesmosis injury, or a new inversion injury of the ankle, after the arthroscopy.[11]

The evidence-based literature leads to a recommendation for ankle arthroscopy for the management of ankle impingement (grade B). The removal of loose bodies is supported by only poor-quality evidence (grade C).[5] This may be because most loose bodies are associated with other pathology, such as osteoarthritis. It has been suggested that increasing degrees of preexisting osteoarthritis correlate with poor outcomes.[12]

Some authors have noted the rate of infection in ankle arthroscopy to be higher than that in the knee.[5] It has been reported to be as high as 4% in one study.[5] If infection occurs, however, treatment is successful the majority of the time.

Pearls

- Noninvasive distraction is recommended for spur removal to allow for better access to the spur and to prevent cartilage damage. However, care must be taken not to excessively distract the joint because this will pull the synovium and the capsule tight up against the spur and make visualization and access difficult.
- Dorsiflexion or plantar flexion may be necessary to visualize the impinging structures.
- Excessive synovium is cleared away with a 3.5- to 4-mm full-radius power shaver. The spur is then removed with a 4-mm power burr. The acromionizer works well for removing the exostosis, or the 5- and 7-mm osteotomes can be used. Once the spur is removed, the bone surface is smoothed with a 4-mm full-radius shaver or a curet. Care must be taken to inspect the joint for loose bodies at the conclusion of the procedure. Posterior portals are not necessary for removing anterior spurs on the talus or the tibia.
- In general, loose body removal by arthroscopic methods is preferred over arthrotomy. In addition to other disadvantages, arthrotomy gives no more assurance of removal.
- Although the postoperative results may be similar for open versus arthroscopic removal of anterior spurs, the recovery is shorter for the arthroscopic group.[9]

References

1. Coull R, Raffiq T, James LE, Stephens MM: Open treatment of anterior impingement of the ankle. *J Bone Joint Surg Br* 2003;85(4):550-553.
2. Branca A, Di Palma L, Bucca C, Visconti CS, Di Mille M: Arthroscopic treatment of anterior ankle impingement. *Foot Ankle Int* 1997;18(7):418-423.
3. Baums MH, Kahl E, Schultz W, Klinger HM: Clinical outcome of the arthroscopic management of sports-related "anterior ankle pain": A prospective study. *Knee Surg Sports Traumatol Arthrosc* 2006;14(5):482-486.
4. Ferkel RD, Tyorkin M, Applegate GR, Heinen GT: MRI evaluation of anterolateral soft tissue impingement of the ankle. *Foot Ankle Int* 2010;31(8):655-661.
5. Glazebrook MA, Ganapathy V, Bridge MA, Stone JW, Allard JP: Evidence-based indications for ankle arthroscopy. *Arthroscopy* 2009;25(12):1478-1490.
6. McCarthy CL, Wilson DJ, Coltman TP: Anterolateral ankle impingement: Findings and diagnostic accuracy with ultrasound imaging. *Skeletal Radiol* 2008;37(3):209-216.
7. Murawski CD, Kennedy JG: Anteromedial impingement in the ankle joint:

Outcomes following arthroscopy. *Am J Sports Med* 2010;38(10):2017-2024.

8. Rasmussen S, Hjorth Jensen C: Arthroscopic treatment of impingement of the ankle reduces pain and enhances function. *Scand J Med Sci Sports* 2002;12(2):69-72.

9. Scranton PE Jr, McDermott JE: Anterior tibiotalar spurs: A comparison of open versus arthroscopic debridement. *Foot Ankle* 1992;13(3):125-129.

10. Tol JL, Verheyen CP, van Dijk CN: Arthroscopic treatment of anterior impingement in the ankle. *J Bone Joint Surg Br* 2001;83(1):9-13.

11. Urgüden M, Söyüncü Y, Ozdemir H, Sekban H, Akyildiz FF, Aydin AT: Arthroscopic treatment of anterolateral soft tissue impingement of the ankle: Evaluation of factors affecting outcome. *Arthroscopy* 2005;21(3):317-322.

12. van Dijk CN, Tol JL, Verheyen CC: A prospective study of prognostic factors concerning the outcome of arthroscopic surgery for anterior ankle impingement. *Am J Sports Med* 1997;25(6):737-745.

Video Reference

73.1 Ferkel RD: Subtalar Arthroscopy, in Tasto JP: Video: *Surgical Techniques in Orthopaedics: Principles in Arthroscopy.* Rosemont, IL, American Academy of Orthopaedic Surgeons, 2003.

Chapter 74
Arthroscopic Treatment of Osteochondral Lesions of the Talus

Steven M. Raikin, MD   Nicholas R. Slenker, MD

Introduction

Osteochondral lesions of the talus (OLTs) are a common source of ankle pain and instability. They are defined as a defect in the articular hyaline cartilage, predominantly within the weight-bearing area of the talar dome, and with involvement of the underlying bone. Although trauma is implicated in many cases, it does not account for the etiology of every lesion. The etiology of OLTs has been debated since 1888, when König first described "osteochondritis dissecans" of the knee, which he suggested was the result of spontaneous necrosis.[1] Talar involvement was then described in 1922 by Kappis,[2] who identified a strong association with prior trauma. The initial classification of talar lesions was described in 1959 by Berndt and Harty,[3] who proposed an anatomic rationale for the association of these "transchondral fractures of the talar dome" with intra-articular trauma. In their review that included 582 patients with OLTs, a history of ankle trauma was reported in 76% of patients.[3] However, the etiology of OLTs in patients without a history of trauma remains unknown. Repetitive microtrauma, vascular abnormalities resulting in osteonecrosis, and congenital factors have been speculated to play a role.

Historically, the majority of OLTs were described as occurring either posterior-medial or anterior-lateral, and there has been a stronger association between lateral lesions and a history of trauma. More recently, Elias et al[4] developed an anatomic grid that divides the talar dome into nine equal zones. They analyzed MRI examinations of 424 patients with OLTs using this grid and determined that 62% of the lesions were medial and 34% were lateral. More striking was that in the sagittal plane, most of the lesions (80%) were central. They also confirmed an earlier observation that medial lesions were wider and deeper than lateral le-

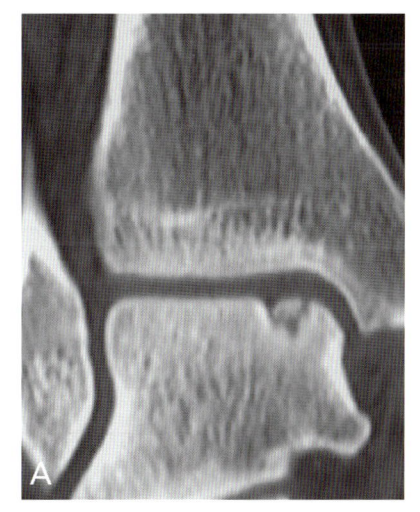

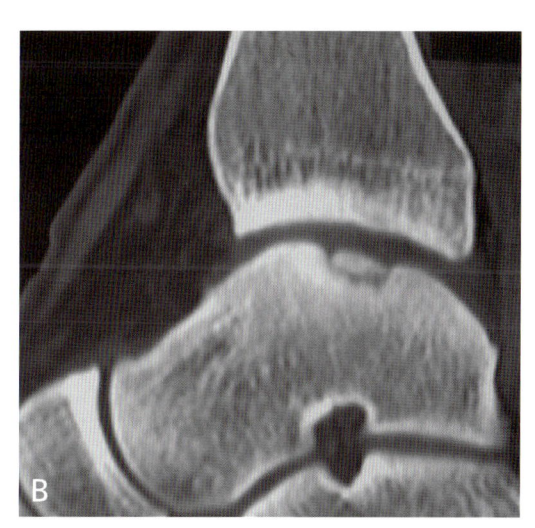

Figure 1 Coronal (**A**) and sagittal (**B**) CT scans demonstrate a stage III medial osteochondral lesion of the talus.

sions. This is consistent with the mechanism originally proposed by Berndt and Harty, in which lateral lesions are typically caused by shear between the talus and the fibula that causes shallow, displaced, "wafer-shaped" lesions on the lateral dome of the talus, whereas medial lesions result from torsion and impaction of the tibia on the talus, resulting in deeper, "cup-shaped" lesions.

Symptomatic OLTs typically present with pain, catching, instability, and/or swelling of the ankle. Lesions are commonly seen on radiographic studies but may be incidental findings. Although often nonspecific, a meticulous clinical evaluation is essential to differentiate among the many potential diagnoses, including ligamentous injury, fractures of the fibula, and fractures of the tibial plafond. The index of suspicion should be high in the setting of ankle pain without any recognized trauma or with persistent ankle pain after an acute injury has resolved.

Diagnostic Imaging

Diagnostic imaging should begin with AP, lateral, and mortise weight-bearing radiographs of the ankle. However, after an acute injury with a nondisplaced lesion, plain radiographs may be unrevealing. A chronic lesion with displacement, osteonecrosis, or cystic change may be clearly evident on plain radiographs. The limitations of radiographs include a low sensitivity, inability to assess the articular cartilage, and an inability to assess the extent of the lesion. MRI has proven to be very sensitive and specific in the diagnosis of OLTs and allows good visualization of the articular surface.[5] The benefits of MRI include an accurate assessment of the location and extent of the lesion and the presence of bone marrow edema, which is suggestive of an active lesion, and an evaluation of the vascular status of the fragment. However, excessive edema can sometimes obscure the bony extent of the lesion. Polyaxial CT scanning accurately delineates the bony defect (**Figure 1**). In clinical practice, MRI is typically obtained before CT to evaluate a patient with unexplained pain because MRI can detect a variety of pathologic conditions. Frequently, a CT scan is then obtained to characterize bony lesions more fully when the MRI findings are inconclusive.

Classification

The classification system introduced by Berndt and Harty in 1959 remains the most widely used method of describing an OLT.[3] It is based on the appearance of the lesion on plain radiographs and

---

Dr. Raikin or an immediate family member is a member of a speakers' bureau or has made paid presentations on behalf of DePuy and has received research or institutional support from Biomimetic. Neither Dr. Slenker nor any immediate family member has received anything of value from or has stock or stock options held in a commercial company or institution related directly or indirectly to the subject of this chapter.

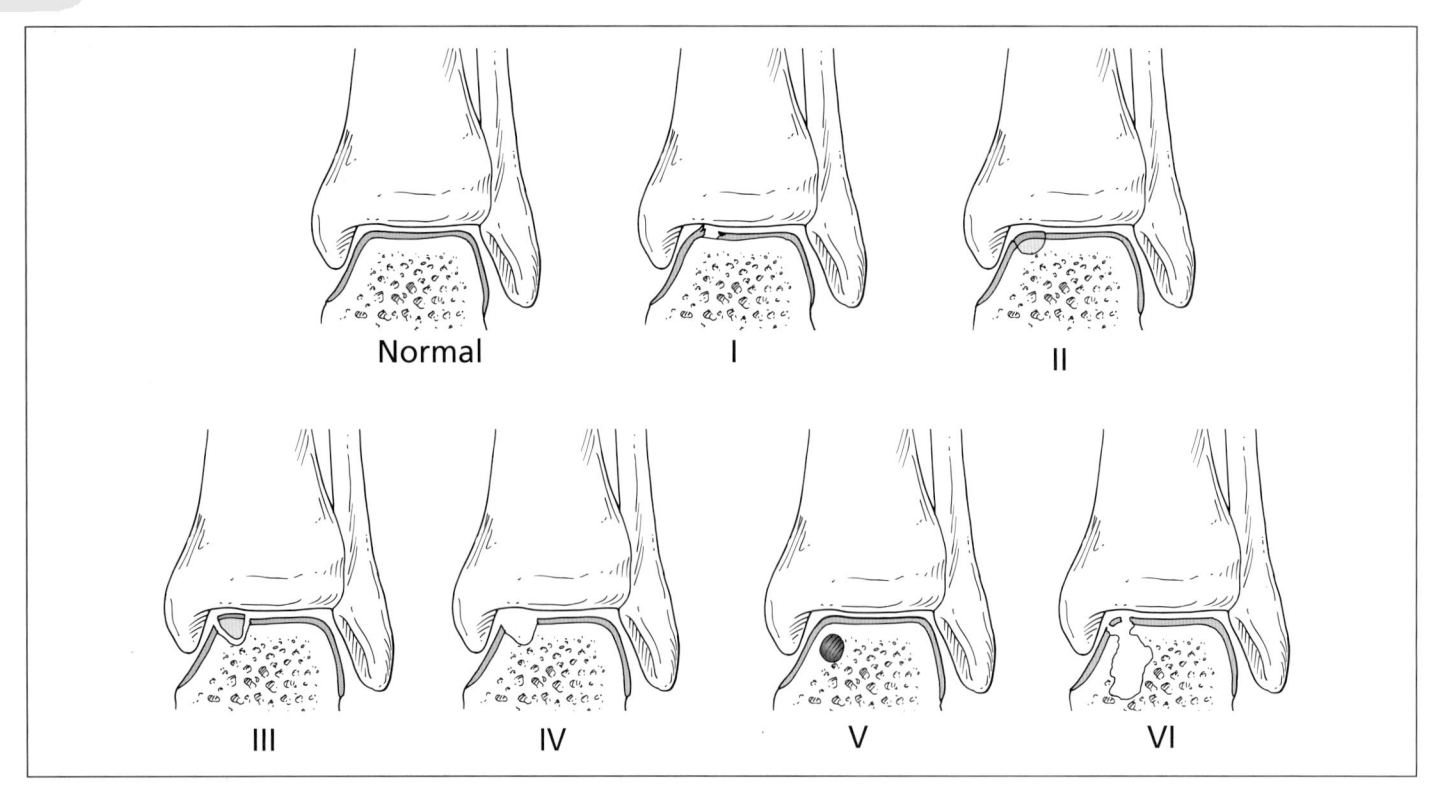

Figure 2 Illustrations show the senior author's (S.M.R.'s) grading system for osteochondral lesions of the talus (shown as medial lesions). See text for descriptions.

includes four stages. Since its introduction, several authors have revised the original classification to include findings on MRI, CT, and arthroscopy. In particular, a fifth and a sixth stage have been added to describe cystic changes and massive-volume lesions, respectively.[6,7] The senior author (S.M.R.) has proposed a grading system that is a combination of the various modality-specific systems described previously (**Figure 2**).

Stage I lesions involve an isolated cartilaginous flap, without subchondral bony compromise. Radiographs and CT scans are usually negative. MRI demonstrates edema in the underlying bone without evidence of fracture. Symptoms are commonly mechanical and include painful catching and giving way of the ankle.

Stage II lesions involve an incomplete or completely nondisplaced fracture of the underlying bone (Berndt and Harty stage I and II). This is often not visible on plain radiographs, but it is clearly discernible on MRI or CT scans. These lesions are stable and unlikely to displace, and they may respond best to nonsurgical treatment.

Stage III lesions are unstable and displaced. The fragment usually remains in its bed or crater, covered by dysmorphic cartilage, and can be balloted arthroscopically. These lesions are clearly visible on plain radiographs, MRI, or CT. Large acute fragments may maintain their vascularity and can potentially be reduced and fixed with a bioabsorbable pin, particularly in the acute traumatic setting. If the fragment is avascular, treatment is by arthroscopic resection, débridement, and microfracture of the lesion base.

Stage IV lesions involve a defect devoid of any remaining bony fragments. The fragments may be free floating within the joint as loose bodies or crushed and no longer present. The lesion base may still be covered by damaged cartilage or unstable fibrocartilage that, in symptomatic cases, should be arthroscopically débrided and the base microfractured.

Stage V lesions are subchondral cysts, often with an intact cartilaginous cap. These have been shown to do poorly with arthroscopic débridement and microfracture.[7] Treatment options include retrograde drilling and bone grafting of the lesion (arthroscopic confirmation of an intact and healthy cartilage cap is an essential part of the procedure) or osteochondral autologous transfer.

Stage VI lesions are very large and include either a large surface area of chondral damage and/or a large subchondral cyst communicating with the joint (ie, osteochondral cyst). These lesions are too large to treat arthroscopically or with an osteochondral autologous transfer procedure and require fresh osteochondral allograft transplantation.[8-10]

Treatment Options/Indications

A trial of nonsurgical management is advocated for all nondisplaced OLTs.[11] The main contraindication to nonsurgical management is acute injuries with displaced osteochondral fragments. In these cases, immediate surgical management is warranted to either resect or reduce and internally fixate the fragment. Generally, nonsurgical treatment involves an initial period of non–weight bearing with cast immobilization, followed by progressive weight bearing and mobilization to full ambulation by 12 to 16 weeks. Studies by Shearer et al[12] and Elias et al[5] demonstrated 54% and 45% success rates, respectively, for nonsurgical treatment of OLTs. Although good results may be obtained without surgery, some lesions remain symptomatic after a course of nonsurgical management. The indications for surgical intervention include symptomatic lesions refractory to nonsurgical care regardless of the stage. The presence of advanced grade III or IV lesions often necessitates surgical intervention as well.[13,14] A meta-analysis conducted by Tol et al[11] in 2000 showed only a 45% success rate in nonsurgical treatment of grade I, grade II, and medial grade III osteochondral defects of the talus. Furthermore, the results of excision and drilling were encouraging compared with nonsurgical treatment. They found excision, curettage, and drilling to have had good to excellent results in 88% of patients with grade III and higher lesions (16 studies, 165 patients). However, simple excision and curettage without drilling (9 studies, 111 patients) had a success rate of 78%, and excision alone (5 studies, 63 patients) had a success rate of 38%.

Multiple surgical treatment options exist, including débridement with or without bone marrow stimulation, autologous chondrocyte implantation, allograft transplantation, and osteochondral autograft transplantation or mosaicplasty. Despite advancements in some of these options, arthroscopic débridement combined with bone marrow stimulation remains one of the most effective treatments.[13,14] It is considered the treatment of choice for primary lesions not exceeding 15 mm in diameter.[11] Multiple arthroscopically assisted techniques for stimulating the release of marrow cells to heal an OLT have been described. These techniques include abrasion chondroplasty, curettage, antegrade and retrograde drilling, and débridement with microfracture. All of these techniques are designed to penetrate the subchondral bone and fill the débrided talar lesion with blood and cytokines that will mediate a healing response to form reparative fibrocartilage. This chapter will focus on arthroscopic débridement and microfracture of the talus.

Video 74.1 Arthroscopic Treatment of Osteochondral Lesions of the Talus. Steven M. Raikin, MD; Nicholas Slenker, MD (10 min)

Procedure

Setup/Patient Positioning

Arthroscopy of the ankle may be performed with general, regional, or local anesthesia. The position of the patient may also vary, depending on surgeon preference. We prefer supine placement of the patient, with the surgical limb held in a well-padded arthroscopic leg holder, with the end of the operating table maximally bent (beyond 90°), allowing the leg to hang free with the knee flexed. This permits distraction by gravity or by an assistant or traction device. Either a thigh or calf tourniquet is applied. The procedure may not need to be done under tourniquet if an arthroscopic pump is used. Alternatively, the patient can be positioned completely supine with the leg extended. A resistance bump is placed below the slightly flexed thigh, and an external noninvasive traction system is attached to the ankle via a sling, through which the joint is distracted. Finally, invasive distraction can be used with a tibial pin and a talar or calcaneal pin with a mechanical distractor device; however, noninvasive distraction techniques with skin traction are much more common. Typically, the decision to perform distraction is made at the time of surgery and depends on the laxity of the joint and the location of the pathologic tissue that is to be addressed. Using the gravity technique, if additional traction is required, this can easily be achieved by applying the distraction sling around the hindfoot attached to a looped gauze bandage. The amount of distraction force can then either be applied by the surgeon's control using his or her foot or with external weight. Regardless of technique, no more than 156 to 222 N of force should be exerted for more than 90 minutes. Excessive use of force for prolonged periods of time may cause bothersome paresthesias in the superficial peroneal nerve. Periodic release is recommended in long procedures.

Equipment

A 2.7-mm, 30° short arthroscope is preferred because of both the shorter lever arm and the ease of accessibility to the joint. A 70° scope should be available for difficult-to-visualize regions of the ankle. Small-joint arthroscopic instruments that should be available include a small hooked probe, a set of small-joint arthroscopic graspers, small thin-necked curets (usually 4-0 or 5-0 size), a small-joint motorized shaving system (we usually use a 2.5-mm or 3.2-mm full-radius shaver depending on joint size, laxity, and accessibility of the lesion), and a set of micropicks. If micropicks are not available, antegrade drilling of the lesion can be performed using a 0.062-in Kirschner wire (K-wire) and a drill. A microvector guide system is required to ensure accurate arthroscopic placement of the K-wire during drilling. An arthroscopic pump can be used, but extreme caution must be exercised to avoid complications.

Surgical Technique

An understanding of the surface and intra-articular anatomy is essential to the successful performance of ankle arthroscopy. The superficial anatomy serves as a guide to safe portal placement in the ankle. The neurovascular and tendinous structures are most at risk. It is important to mark the anatomic landmarks, including the joint line, the dorsalis pedis artery, the great saphenous vein, the anterior tibial tendon, and the peroneus tertius tendon. The superficial peroneal nerve and its branches must also be respected because of their proximity to the anterolateral portal. The superficial peroneal nerve divides into the intermediate and dorsal cutaneous branches approximately 6.5 cm proximal to the tip of the fibula.

The anteromedial, anterolateral, and posterolateral portals are the most commonly used because these are the safest areas for insertion away from neurovascular structures (**Figure 3**).

The anteromedial portal is made just medial to the anterior tibialis tendon, at or just proximal to the joint line. This is located approximately 5 mm proximal to the medial malleolus. This portal is made first because it is easy to establish and is in a region without any major neurovascular structures. The great saphenous vein and nerve are at risk when establishing this portal, lying 7 to 9 mm medial to the portal.

The anterolateral portal is made just lateral to the peroneus tertius tendon at the level of the joint line. The branches of the superficial peroneal nerve are most at risk. The intermediate branch of the superficial peroneal nerve lies approximately 6 mm lateral to the anterolateral portal.

An anterocentral portal has been described between the tendons of the extensor digitorum communis; however, use of this portal is discouraged because of the extremely close proximity of the dorsalis pedis artery and the deep peroneal nerve.

A posterolateral portal can be established just lateral to the Achilles tendon, approximately 1 cm proximal to the distal tip of the fibula. This portal can be made under direct visualization looking posteriorly from the anteromedial portal. The lesser saphenous vein and the sural nerve are at risk in establishing this portal. These two structures run parallel to each other along the posterolateral aspect of the ankle joint.

A posterocentral, or trans-Achilles, portal can be made through the middle of the Achilles tendon at the level of the joint line. This portal is not recommended because of both limited mobility and the associated morbidity to the tendon.

The posteromedial portal is generally contraindicated because of the proximity of the posterior tibial artery and nerve.

Section 6: Foot and Ankle

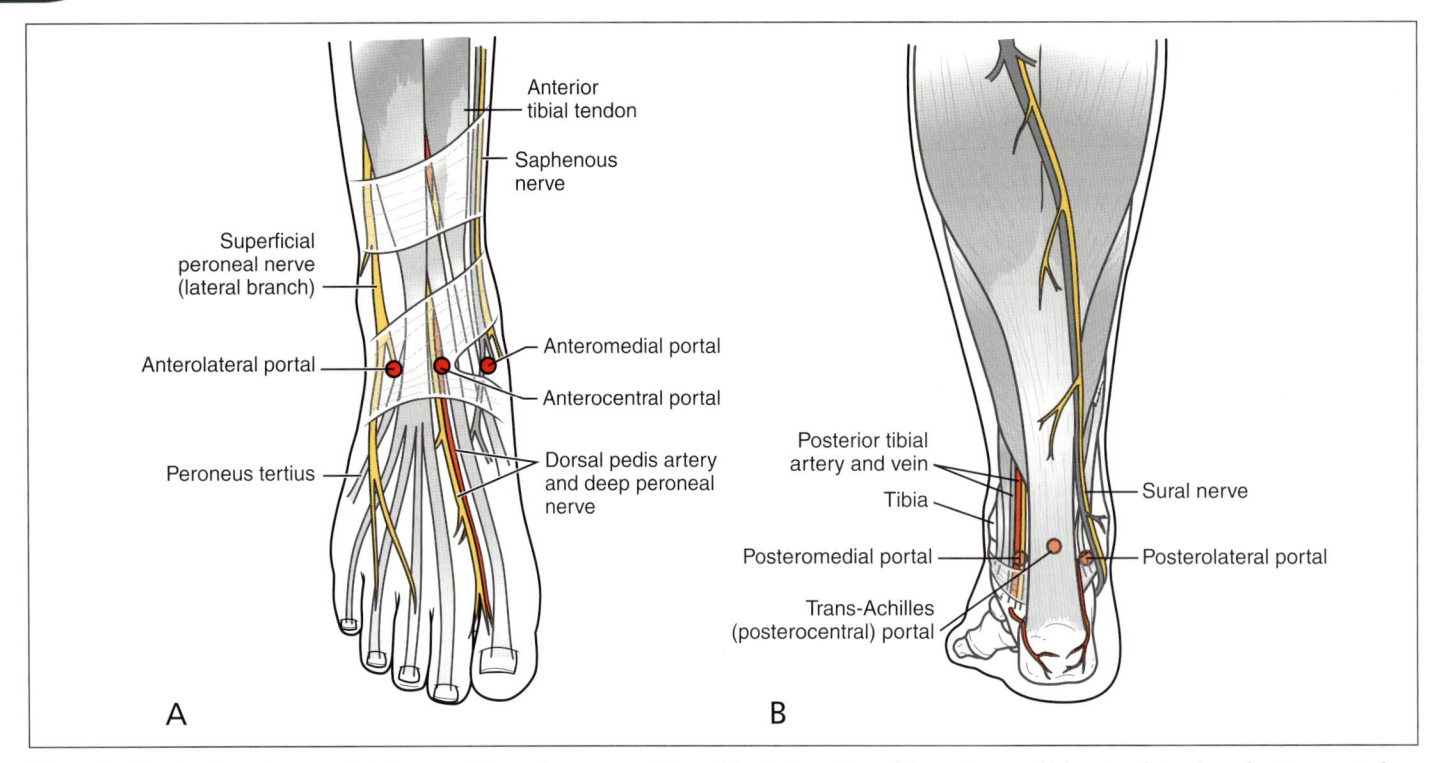

Figure 3 Illustrations show portal placement for arthroscopy of the ankle. **A,** Location of the anteromedial, anterolateral, and anterocentral portals. **B,** Location of the posteromedial, trans-Achilles, and posterolateral portals. (Adapted from Stetson WB, Ferkel RD: Ankle arthroscopy: I. Technique and complications. *J Am Acad Orthop Surg* 1996;4:17-23.)

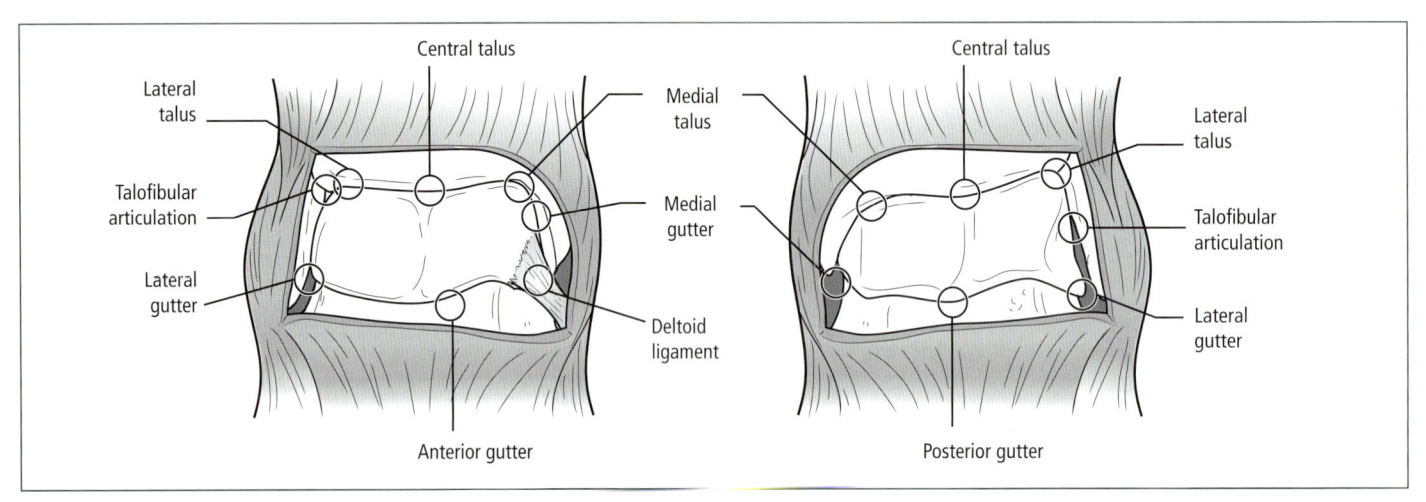

Figure 4 Illustration shows the eight-point anterior (left) and seven-point posterior (right) arthroscopic examination. (Adapted from Stetson WB, Ferkel RD: Ankle arthroscopy I: Technique and complications. *J Am Acad Orthop Surg* 1996;4:17-23.)

Before portal placement, the ankle joint should be distended with 20 to 30 mL of lactated Ringer solution injected medial to the anterior tibialis tendon with an 18- to 20-gauge needle. Epinephrine (1:200,000) can be added to the solution to limit bleeding during the procedure. This injection helps to establish the exact location of the anteromedial portal. To prevent injury to the neurovascular structures, the incisions for the portals should be made vertically and through skin only. Using a No. 11 blade, the skin is moved over the blade to keep the incision superficial. The deeper layers are spread bluntly with a hemostat down into the ankle capsule. The ankle joint is then penetrated with a blunt probe through the arthroscopic cannula. Probe insertion is best done under traction and joint distension to minimize damage to the articular cartilage. Additionally, the ankle should be plantar flexed, bringing the narrowest portion of the talus into the mortise, allowing additional room for atraumatic scope insertion. It is important to remember that the probe, although blunt, can still cause significant cartilage disruption. The blunt probe is then removed from the cannula. If the joint has been distended prior to insertion of the cannula, a backflow of lactated Ringer solution occurs when the probe is removed, confirming appropriate placement within the joint capsule. With the arthroscope introduced into the joint, the anterolateral portal can then be established under direct visualization with a 25-gauge needle. It is usually located just lateral to the peroneus tertius at the level of the ankle joint. This portal can sometimes be determined more easily by transilluminating the skin with the arthroscope to assist in the identification of the neurovascular structures and tendons.

A standardized diagnostic arthroscopic examination is always performed first. It is initially done through the anterome-

Chapter 74: Arthroscopic Treatment of Osteochondral Lesions of the Talus

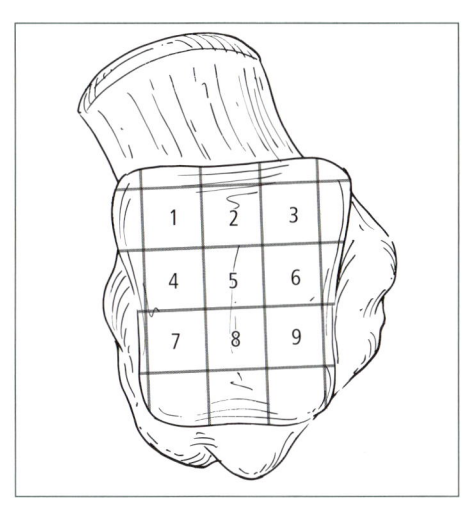

Figure 5 Illustration shows the nine-zone localization grid on the talar dome.

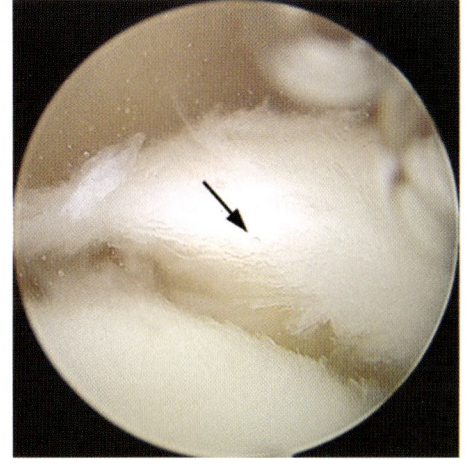

Figure 6 Arthroscopic view shows an unstable cartilaginous flap of a medial osteochondral lesion of the talus (arrow) as seen from the lateral portal.

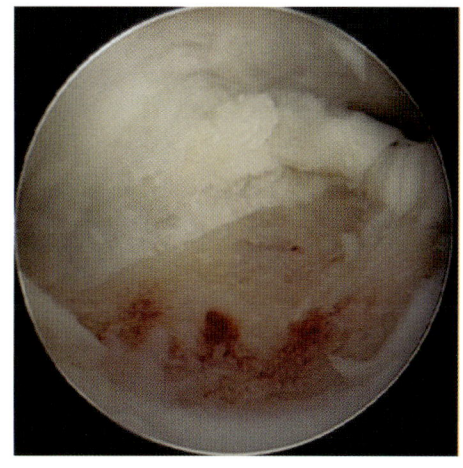

Figure 7 Arthroscopic view of the talus following débridement shows the lesion now has a stable base with a rounded cartilaginous rim.

dial portal and subsequently through the anterolateral and posterolateral portals. An "eight-point anterior" and "seven-point posterior" arthroscopic examination enables a thorough and systematic evaluation of all areas of the ankle (**Figure 4**). This guarantees that all areas of the ankle are carefully inspected and any intra-articular lesions can be identified in their corresponding zones.

The osteochondral lesion is usually best visualized from the opposite-side portal (ie, medial lesions through the lateral portal and lateral lesions through the medial portal) and worked on through the same-side portal, as demonstrated in the video. The surgeon should be familiar with the exact location of the lesion before surgery using the nine-zone localizing system described by Elias et al[3] (**Figure 5**). After the lesion is identified, the border of the lesion is established with a probe (**Figure 6**). Normal articular cartilage is firm and not easily penetrated with probing. Degenerative and unstable cartilage is friable and easily penetrated, lifted, and delaminated off the underlying lesion. A grade III lesion may have an apparently intact cartilaginous cap, but the unstable bony fragment can easily be ballotted under the cap, which is easily penetrated with the probe. The unstable cartilage flaps and fragments are débrided. This is accomplished by using a combination of the mini-probe, curets, and a motorized shaver. When the articular cartilage is soft on palpation or is fibrillated or degenerated, even though it may appear stable, excision is recommended. Excision of the subchondral fragment and curettage of the lesion's surface is done to remove debris, fibrous tissue, and devitalized cartilage. The bone at the

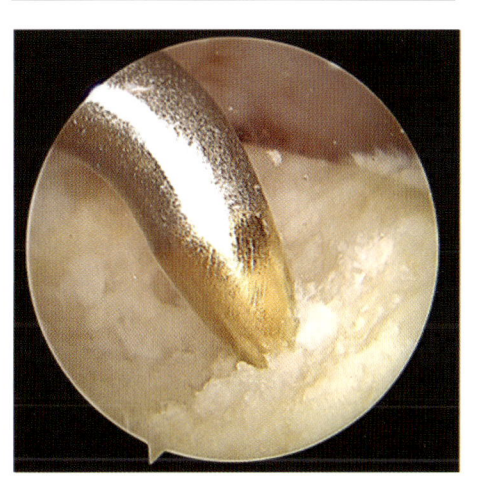

Figure 8 Arthroscopic view of the talus shows a 40° microfracture pick placed within the base of the lesion. The gold tip measures 3 mm and should be buried by impaction with a mallet.

base of the lesion may be soft and dysvascular (especially in cup-shaped medial lesions), and this needs to be removed down to a stable healthy bone base. Once a stable rim of intact cartilage and a stable bony base is attained (**Figure 7**), a marrow stimulation technique can be performed on the exposed lesion. Vascular access channels are created in the underlying subchondral bone using an awl, a drill, or an arthroscopic shaver. This allows marrow elements to migrate into the site of injury and produce fibrocartilage to cover the lesion.

Bone marrow stimulation by means of microfracture picks (**Figure 8**) has recently gained popularity. One of the advantages of this approach in the ankle is it avoids the unaffected cartilage of the tibial plafond side of the joint, which is frequently penetrated during antegrade drilling techniques. Sets of anatomically

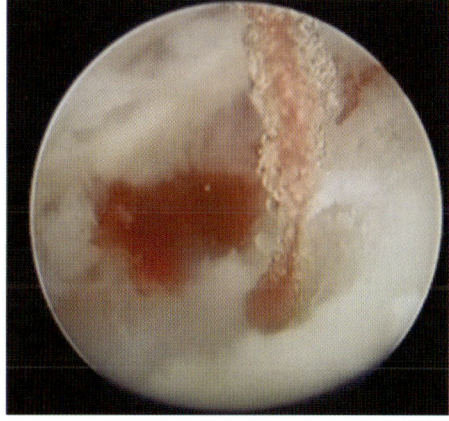

Figure 9 Arthroscopic view of the talus after tourniquet release and pick removal. Bleeding can be seen from two of the pick holes.

shaped picks or awls are commercially available for use in the ankle. A microfracture pick, typically angled at 40°, 60°, or 90°, is introduced through one of the portals. It is then malleted so as to pierce the subchondral plate in the base of the lesion to a depth of 3 mm (this is seen by the gold-colored tips of the picks, which should be buried during insertion). Multiple pick holes should be created at intervals of approximately 3 mm, the number depending on the size of the lesion. The tourniquet is subsequently released and the pump is turned off to confirm that healthy egress of marrow (seen as fat droplets) and bleeding from the underlying bone has been achieved (**Figure 9**).

Alternatively, antegrade drilling of an OLT is performed with a 0.062-in K-wire using a transmalleolar technique. An arthroscopic targeting guide, similar to that used during anterior cruciate ligament reconstruction, is used, placing the guide ball at the location within the

© 2013 American Academy of Orthopaedic Surgeons

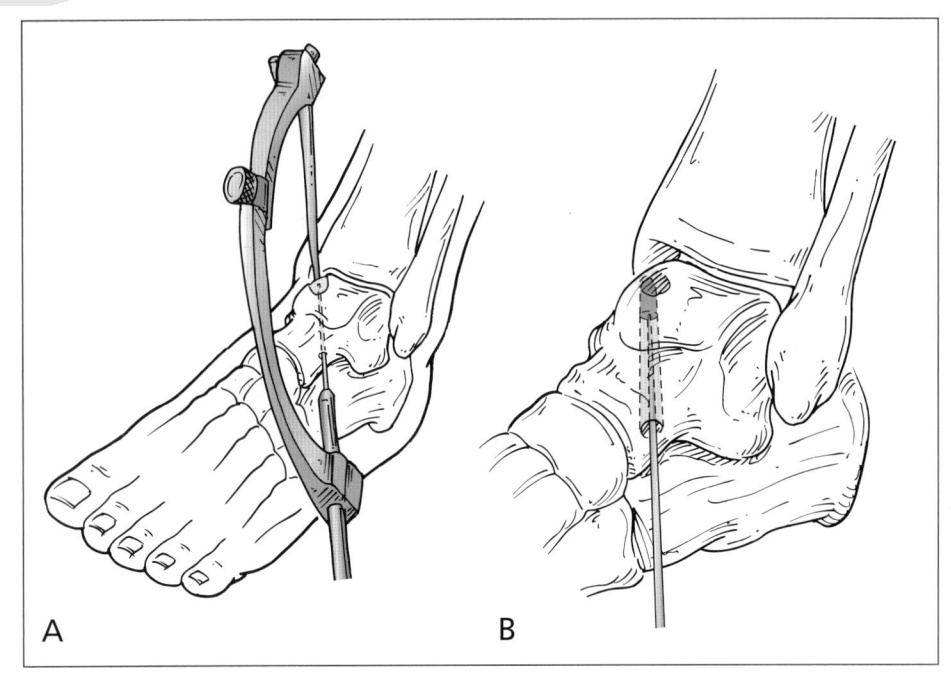

Figure 10 Illustrations show retrograde drilling with drill guide placement (**A**) and bone grafting (**B**).

lesion where the drill hole is planned. The K-wire is inserted from about 3 cm proximal to the tip of the malleolus and is directed into the lesion under arthroscopic visualization. The wire is drilled into the lesion and then withdrawn to the articular surface at the distal end of the tibia; drilling is then continued at a few other sites after slightly changing the angle of plantar flexion or dorsiflexion of the ankle joint. Drilling is continued until healthy bleeding from the bone marrow is confirmed. Next, the angle of insertion of the K-wire is changed, and the same procedure is repeated until the entire lesion has been addressed.

An important subset of OLTs possesses an intact dome of overlying cartilage coupled with an underlying bony defect or cyst (stage V lesion). Despite the intact cartilage, these lesions are frequently symptomatic. In an effort to preserve cartilage, retrograde drilling of this type of lesion was proposed by Taranow et al[14] in 1999 (**Figure 10**). This technique is achieved by placing a small-joint drill guide through the anteromedial portal and positioning it over the center of the OLT. The drill guide is positioned to allow guidewire insertion percutaneously into the lateral aspect of the sinus tarsi at the junction of the neck and body of the talus. The tip of the guidewire is then advanced to lie within the center of the OLT. It should not penetrate the subchondral plate of the talar dome. A 3.5- or 4.5-mm cannulated drill set is then used, depending on the size of the lesion. After the drill and guidewire are removed, the lesion is curetted through the drill hole. The resulting bone defect is then packed with autologous bone graft, typically harvested from the calcaneus. It is critical that great care is taken during this procedure to avoid penetrating the subchondral plate.

After completion of the arthroscopic procedure, all wounds are closed with a 4-0 nonabsorbable nylon suture, and a compressive dressing is applied. The patient is immediately placed into a fracture boot. A cold therapy system can be used for postoperative pain and swelling control.

Complications

Several complications have been described, including injury to neurovascular structures, instrument breakage, articular surface damage, neuroma formation, infection, and reflex sympathetic dystrophy. The superficial peroneal nerve is at highest risk, and injury to this nerve is associated with the anterolateral portal. In the largest series to date, Ferkel et al[15] found an overall complication rate of 9%. Neurologic complications were most common (49%), with injury to the superficial peroneal nerve happening most frequently (56%), followed by the sural nerve (22%) and the saphenous nerve (18%). Superficial wound infections occurred in six patients; the infections appeared to be related to close portal placement, the type of cannula used, and early mobilization. Deep wound infection developed in only two patients and was correlated with a lack of preoperative antibiotic therapy in both cases.

The thinness of the skin and the lack of subcutaneous tissues around the ankle joint make postoperative swelling common. This usually responds well to elevation, compression, and application of ice. Compartment syndrome has not been reported in association with ankle arthroscopy; however, patients should be monitored appropriately for excessive pain.

Postoperative Care

Patients remain non–weight bearing in the fracture boot for a period of 6 weeks. They are allowed to remove the boot for range-of-motion exercises as soon as they are comfortable. At 6 weeks postoperatively, patients are transitioned to full weight bearing in the fracture boot, while more aggressive physical therapy is initiated out of the boot. Subsequent gradual weaning from the boot is allowed over the next 6 weeks.

Pearls

- Portal placement is the most important part of the procedure. Poorly placed incisions will limit access to the joint and increase the risk of neurovascular or tendinous injury. All topical landmarks should be identified before joint distention because these areas may become distorted.
- Distending the joint with a large syringe and 25 to 30 mL of saline before portal placement will allow the joint to "inflate" and ease the entrance of the equipment.
- In certain instances, débridement of hypertrophic synovium or adhesed capsule may be necessary to adequately maneuver within the joint.
- Using distraction devices, either invasive or noninvasive, can enhance access to different areas of the ankle joint, although gravity alone is usually sufficient. Using additional traction systems can increase the complication rate associated with this procedure.
- When using the two-portal technique, the surgeon may need to exchange the camera between portals to evaluate the joint completely, both before and after addressing the OTL itself.
- For marrow stimulation techniques that rely on reparative cartilage healing, non–weight bearing with early range of motion in the postoperative period is vitally important to surgical success.

References

1. König F: Über freie Körper in den gelenken. *Deutsch Z Chir* 1888;27:90-109.
2. Kappis M: Weitere Beitrage zur traumatisch-mechanischen Entstehung der "spontanen" Knorpelablosungen. *Deutsch Z Chir* 1922;171:13-29.
3. Berndt AL, Harty M: Transchondral fractures (osteochondritis dissecans) of the talus. *J Bone Joint Surg Am* 1959;41-A: 988-1020.
4. Elias I, Zoga AC, Morrison WB, Besser MP, Schweitzer ME, Raikin SM: Osteochondral lesions of the talus: Localization and morphologic data from 424 patients using a novel anatomical grid scheme. *Foot Ankle Int* 2007;28(2):154-161.
5. Elias I, Jung JW, Raikin SM, Schweitzer MW, Carrino JA, Morrison WB: Osteochondral lesions of the talus: Change in MRI findings over time in talar lesions without operative intervention and implications for staging systems. *Foot Ankle Int* 2006;27(3):157-166.
6. Raikin SM: Stage VI: Massive osteochondral defects of the talus. *Foot Ankle Clin* 2004;9(4):737-744, vi.
7. Scranton PE Jr, McDermott JE: Treatment of type V osteochondral lesions of the talus with ipsilateral knee osteochondral autografts. *Foot Ankle Int* 2001;22(5):380-384.
8. Görtz S, De Young AJ, Bugbee WD: Fresh osteochondral allografting for osteochondral lesions of the talus. *Foot Ankle Int* 2010;31(4):283-290.
9. Hahn DB, Aanstoos ME, Wilkins RM: Osteochondral lesions of the talus treated with fresh talar allografts. *Foot Ankle Int* 2010;31(4):277-282.
10. Raikin SM: Fresh osteochondral allografts for large-volume cystic osteochondral defects of the talus. *J Bone Joint Surg Am* 2009;91(12):2818-2826.
11. Tol JL, Struijs PA, Bossuyt PM, Verhagen RA, van Dijk CN: Treatment strategies in osteochondral defects of the talar dome: A systematic review. *Foot Ankle Int* 2000;21(2):119-126.
12. Shearer C, Loomer R, Clement D: Nonoperatively managed stage 5 osteochondral talar lesions. *Foot Ankle Int* 2002;23(7):651-654.
13. Ferkel RD, Zanotti RM, Komenda GA, et al: Arthroscopic treatment of chronic osteochondral lesions of the talus: Long-term results. *Am J Sports Med* 2008;36(9):1750-1762.
14. Gobbi A, Francisco RA, Lubowitz JH, Allegra F, Canata G: Osteochondral lesions of the talus: Randomized controlled trial comparing chondroplasty, microfracture, and osteochondral autograft transplantation. *Arthroscopy* 2006;22(10):1085-1092.
15. Taranow WS, Bisignani GA, Towers JD, Conti SF: Retrograde drilling of osteochondral lesions of the medial talar dome. *Foot Ankle Int* 1999;20(8):474-480.
16. Ferkel RD, Heath DD, Guhl JF: Neurological complications of ankle arthroscopy. *Arthroscopy* 1996;12(2):200-208.

Chapter 75
Augmented Lateral Ankle Ligament Reconstruction for Persistent Ankle Instability

Nicholas A. Abidi, MD

Patient Selection
Indications
There are up to 27,000 ankle sprains in the United States every day.[1] If evaluated and treated shortly after the initial injury, the majority of sprains can be successfully treated nonsurgically. Patients with persistent ankle pain, locking, giving way, and swelling should be considered for further investigation into the etiology of the symptoms. Older patients with instability of the knee or ankle can fall unexpectedly and sustain wrist and hip fractures. Surgery should not be considered in patients with chronic lateral ankle ligament instability until a course of treatment with ankle bracing and physical therapy has failed. Many of these patients can develop osteochondral defects of the talus, impinging spurs, and tibiotalar joint osteoarthritis.[2] Surgical reconstruction of the ankle ligaments should be considered before the sequelae of chronic instability develop. Patients with thick, native, attenuated ligaments can be considered for traditional lateral ankle ligament reconstruction. Patients with underlying hyperlaxity, more than 10 years of instability, and nonexistent ligaments intraoperative inspection should undergo tendon augmentation or native lateral ankle ligament reconstruction.[3]

Contraindications
There are some contraindications to ankle ligament reconstruction. Patients with significant underlying arthritis should not undergo ankle ligament reconstruction expecting that it would be a definitive procedure. These patients are typically more suitable for arthrodesis or total ankle arthroplasty. Some arthroplasty patients may actually require lateral ankle ligament reconstruction before undergoing total ankle arthroplasty to stabilize the prosthesis. Older patients who cannot participate in rehabilitation are not optimal surgical candidates. In addition, patients with suspected acute posterior tibial tendon rupture would not do well postoperatively. Patients with poor blood supply and previous scar tissue formation laterally should undergo reconstruction along with plastic surgery advice. Neuropathic patients who are at risk of Charcot arthropathy are not acceptable candidates for lateral ankle ligament reconstruction.

We will describe lateral ankle ligament reconstruction with native ligaments,[4] peroneus longus tendon strip autograft, or hamstring autograft/allograft.[5]

Preoperative Imaging
Stress ankle radiographs have been used in the past as the diagnostic standard for demonstrating ankle instability. However, there are groups of patients who present with functional instability and have negative stress radiographs. Stress ankle radiographs are cumbersome and inaccurate. Commercially available instability devices do not appear to correlate well with clinical ankle instability. In addition, these studies are painful to patients. Studies have pointed out the inconsistencies among MRI, stress radiography, and intraoperative arthroscopic findings.[6]

Weight-bearing radiographs of the foot and ankle are necessary to determine articular space and alignment. Patients with varus tibiotalar joint degenerative changes may not be candidates for lateral ankle ligament stabilization alone (**Figure 1**). Younger patients with this deformity may be candidates for supramalleolar osteotomy. However, removing periarticular osteophytes can occasionally result in a plantigrade ankle that is amenable to lateral ankle stabilization. Patients with varus heel alignment on examination and plain radiographs may require lateralizing calcaneal osteotomy at the time of lateral ankle ligament stabilization. A lateral foot radiograph may determine that the patient has excessive plantar flexion of the first ray, which might lead to excessive varus moment on the hindfoot and ankle.[7] This may require dorsiflexion osteotomy of the first metatarsal shaft in addition to the lateral ankle ligament stabilization (**Figure 2**).

MRI of the ankle, preferably in at least a 1.5-T scanner with an extremity coil, provides images that can evaluate bony surfaces and portions of the anterior talofibular ligament (ATFL) and calcaneofibular ligament (CFL). Most experienced surgeons use MRI to look for unexpected problems in the tendons or joint that require planning and additional attention at the time of surgery. The diagnosis of instability is typically based on a history of instability and the clinical evaluation (**Figure 3**).

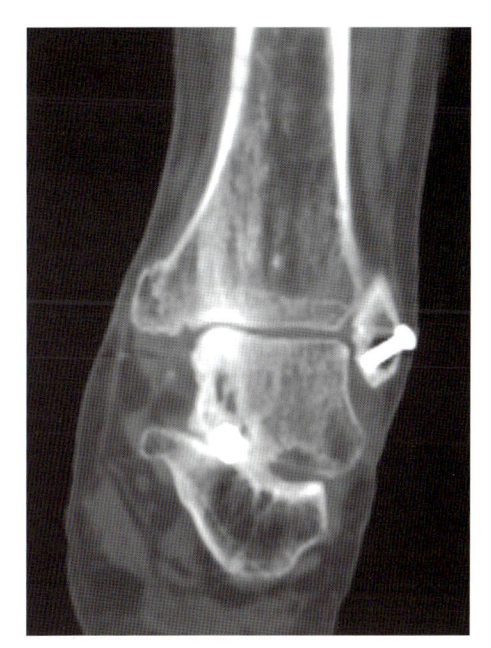

Figure 1 CT scan demonstrates medial tibial degenerative joint disease and supramalleolar varus deformity.

Video 75.1 Augmented Lateral Ankle Ligament Reconstruction. Nicholas A. Abidi, MD; Brian Martin, PA-C (25 min)

Procedure
Patient Positioning
Patient positioning must take into account procedures that are performed at the same time as lateral ankle ligament reconstruction. I typically perform

---
Dr. Abidi or an immediate family member has received royalties from Arthrex; is a member of a speakers' bureau or has made paid presentations on behalf of Acumed and Arthrex; serves as a paid consultant to or is an employee of Acumed, Arthrex, and Biomet; owns stock or stock options held in Global Orthopaedic Solutions; and serves as a board member, owner, officer, or committee member of the American Orthopaedic Foot & Ankle Society.

Section 6: Foot and Ankle

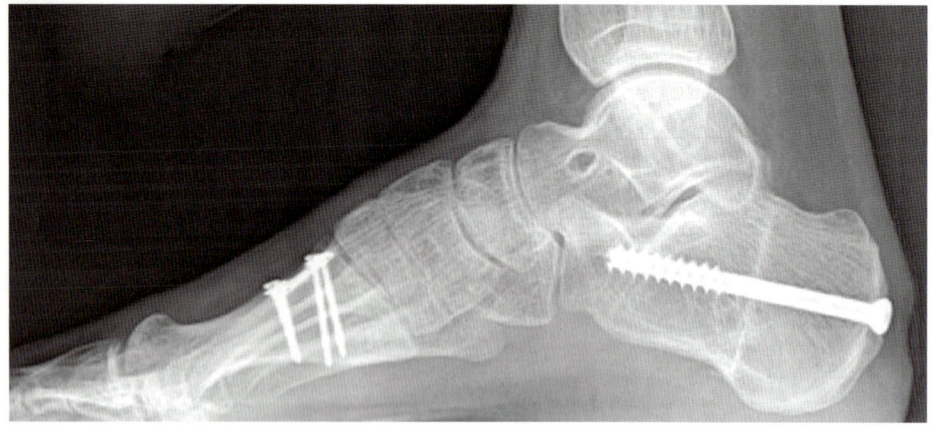

Figure 2 Postoperative lateral radiograph shows a first metatarsal dorsiflexion osteotomy combined with calcaneal osteotomy.

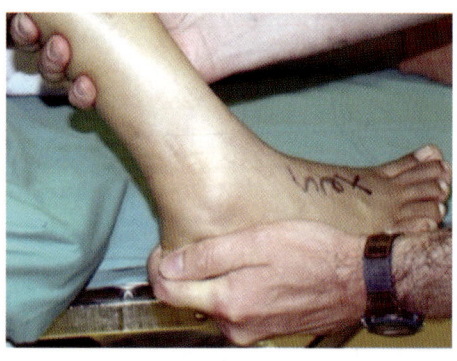

Figure 3 Photograph shows the anterior drawer test. The foot is slightly plantar flexed and internally rotated. The examiner's right hand stabilizes the tibia while the left hand exerts an anterior pull.

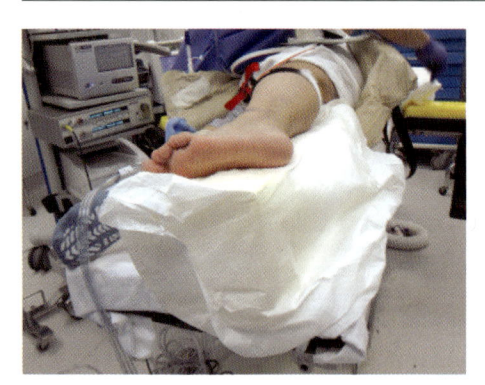

Figure 4 Photograph shows setup and patient positioning for lateral ankle ligament reconstruction. The surgical leg is elevated on a foam block. The peroneal nerve of the nonsurgical leg and all bony prominences are shielded from any pressure.

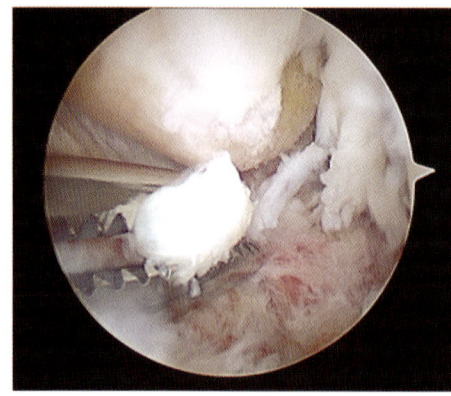

Figure 5 Arthroscopic view shows a loose body being removed from the tibiotalar joint.

simultaneous ankle arthroscopy and occasionally fluoroscopy. Patients are placed on a beanbag in a semilateral position. The patient's feet should be at the end of the operating table to facilitate dorsiflexion of the foot during ligament tensioning at the end of the ligament reconstruction. The range of motion of the hip joint and the leg should be checked to be sure that access will be appropriate for all the planned procedures before prepping and draping. It is important to be able to externally rotate the ankle and leg enough to have access to the medial and lateral ankle arthroscopic portals during the initial phase of the case (**Figure 4**).

Anesthesia

Patients undergo a popliteal block anesthetic that can be supplemented with a spinal or general anesthetic as necessary. The saphenous nerve should undergo a regional block to manage medial postoperative pain.

Surgical Technique

I routinely perform ankle arthroscopy to débride the distal portion of the anterior tibiofibular ligament, the impinging tibiotalar osteophytes, and loose bodies from the anterior tibiotalar joint (**Figure 5**). In addition, the talus is carefully inspected for osteochondral defects on the medial and lateral talar dome. This is done before the open lateral ankle ligament stabilization procedure but during the same surgical session. Open ankle ligament stabilization will not be described here because the indications and the technique of the arthroscopic procedure in the presence of ankle instability have been described by multiple authors.[2,8-11] The accompanying video outlines ankle arthroscopy in addition to the augmented Broström ligament reconstruction involving a split free peroneus longus tendon autograft.

An incision is made from 5 cm above the tip of the lateral malleolus, traveling over the mid-malleolus and coursing distally over the peroneal tendons toward the base of the fifth metatarsal. During the dissection, the sural nerve is avoided.

The peroneal tendons are inspected for tears inferior and superior to the superior peroneal retinaculum. The superior peroneal retinaculum is preserved. The inferior peroneal retinaculum is frequently released if it appears to create stenosis of the peroneal tendon sheath.

If it is determined that there is posterior impingement of the posterolateral process of the talus or os trigonum, an interval is created between the peroneal and Achilles tendons to expose the posterior aspect of the ankle joint. A posterior ankle arthrotomy is created. The posterior process of the talus or os trigonum is excised. The raw bone surface is covered with bone wax to prevent heterotopic ossification. The flexor hallucis longus tendon is inspected for impingement and damage.

Following the incision, the lateral ankle joint capsule around the distal fibula is sharply detached, along with the ATFL and the CFL (**Figure 6**). All loose and avulsed bone and cartilage fragments are excised. A distal fibular periosteal flap is created with proximal retraction of the flap. The superior peroneal retinaculum is maintained. Approximately 4 cm above the tip of the fibula, a small opening is made in the peroneal retinacular sheath proximal to the superior peroneal retinaculum. The peroneus longus tendon is identified between the distal fibula and the peroneus brevis tendon. One third of the tendon's diameter (4-5 mm) is harvested in the cephalad direction using a pigtailed tendon stripper (**Figure 7, A**). This tendon graft is approximately 15 cm in length.

The tissue between the peroneal tendons and the CFL is separated, visualizing the CFL ligament (**Figure 7, B**). Visualizing the caudal-most section of the calcaneal insertion of the CFL, the area is débrided. A guide pin for a cannulated drill bit is placed along the origin of the CFL. This is drilled with a 4.5-mm drill bit to a depth of 20 to 25 mm. An anterior cruciate ligament notch punch is used to create a keyhole along the cephalad portion

Chapter 75: Augmented Lateral Ankle Ligament Reconstruction for Persistent Ankle Instability

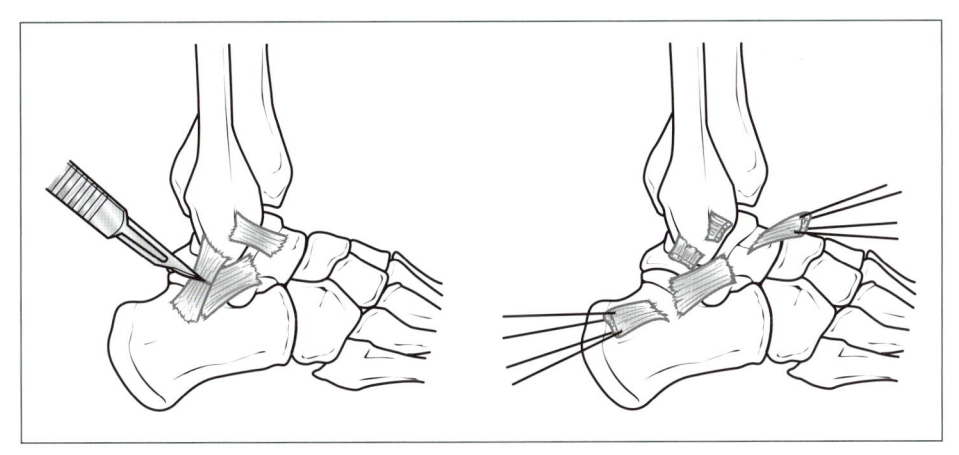

Figure 6 Illustrations show initial steps in lateral ankle ligament reconstruction. The lateral ankle joint capsule around the distal fibula is sharply detached, along with the ATFL and the CFL.

of the drill hole for the tendon to slide into alongside an interference anchor (**Figure 7, C**). The free peroneus longus tendon graft is whipstitched with 2-0 FiberWire (Arthrex) that allows anchoring to the calcaneus with the use of an interference anchor (PEEK [polyetheretherketone] 4.75 × 15 mm, Arthrex) (**Figure 7, D and E**). The free tendon is brought under the peroneal tendons toward the fibula. A guide pin for a cannulated drill bit is placed from the tip of the fibula at the CFL insertion point toward the origin of the ATFL. A tunnel is created in the distal fibula by drilling with a 4.0-mm drill bit from the distal tip of the fibula at the insertion of the CFL to slightly cephalad to

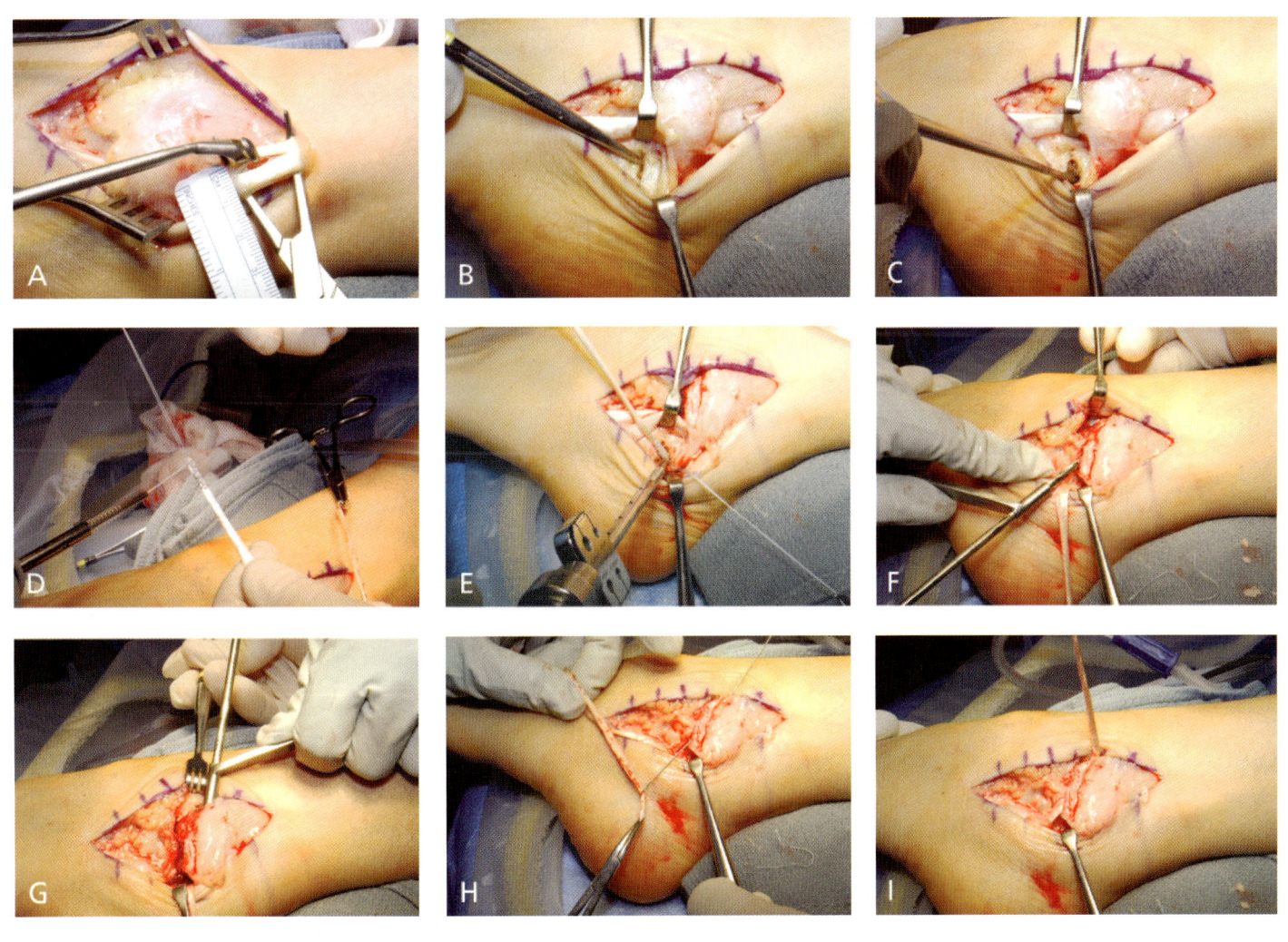

Figure 7 Intraoperative photographs demonstrate steps in lateral ankle ligament reconstruction. **A**, A pigtailed tendon stripper is used to harvest a 4-mm–thick section of the peroneus longus tendon above the superior peroneal retinaculum. **B**, The natural origin of the CFL is exposed. **C**, A drill hole is made at the origin of the native CFL. An anterior cruciate ligament notch puncher is used to create a cephalad notch in the drill hole. This notch will create a place to slide the peroneus longus tendon graft alongside the tenodesis interference anchor. **D**, The peroneus longus tendon graft is captured with a No. 2 nonabsorbable suture and the tenodesis interference anchor system. **E**, The first limb of the peroneus longus tendon autograft is placed into the drill hole at the origin of the CFL. The anchor is screwed into the tunnel, providing an interference fit against the whipstitched tendon. **F**, A 4.0-mm cannulated drill bit is drilled over a guide pin in the end of the fibula that travels from the CFL insertion to the ATFL origin. **G**, The two ends of the tunnel in the fibula are connected over a guide pin with a 4.0-mm cannulated drill bit. **H**, A nitinol wire tendon-passing tool is used to pass the peroneus longus tendon graft through the tunnel that was drilled in the fibula. **I**, The peroneus longus graft is passed through the tunnel from the insertion of the CFL to the origin of the ATFL. It is tensioned, and excursion of the tendon is confirmed by examining tensioning at the origin of the CFL.

© 2013 American Academy of Orthopaedic Surgeons

Section 6: Foot and Ankle

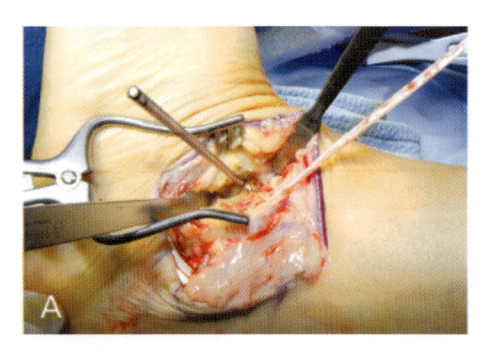

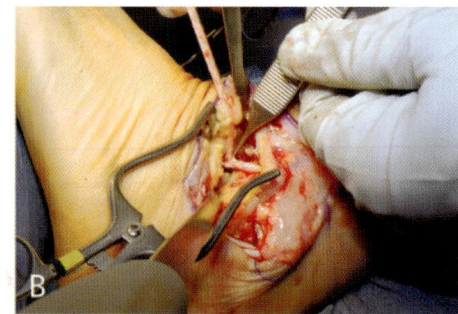

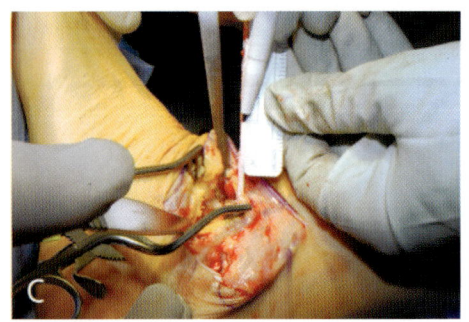

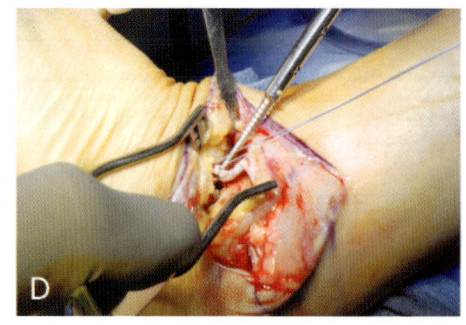

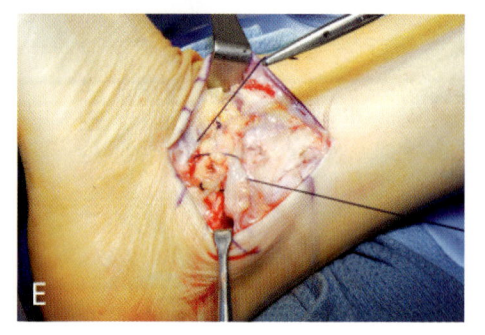

Figure 8 Intraoperative photographs demonstrate final steps in lateral ankle ligament reconstruction. **A,** A cannulated guide pin is drilled into the insertion point of the ATFL. This will be drilled with a cannulated 4.5-mm drill bit and notched with an anterior cruciate ligament notch puncher. **B,** The peroneus longus tendon autograft is tensioned with the foot held dorsiflexed and externally rotated, and the insertion point at the ATFL is approximated. **C,** The peroneus longus tendon autograft is whipstitched with a nonabsorbable suture 17 mm beyond where the edge of the ATFL insertion point was measured on the tendon. The excess tendon beyond this point is truncated. This 17 mm will represent 15 mm placed within the tunnel and 2 mm as it rounds the edge of the tunnel. **D,** With the foot and ankle dorsiflexed and externally rotated, the peroneus longus tendon autograft is captured with the No. 2 nonabsorbable suture along with the tenodesis anchor system. The tenodesis system is used to place the graft under tension prior to screwing the interference anchor into place. **E,** The Broström-Karlsson procedure is performed after the tendon transfer by imbricating the perosteal flap that was created at the end of the fibula. This repair can also be augmented with the Gould modification by also imbricating the inferior extensor retinaculum to the edge of the distal periosteal flap.

the origin of the ATFL (**Figure 7, F**). The tunnel is connected directly from the origin of the ATFL with a cannulated guide pin and a 4.0-mm drill bit (**Figure 7, G**). The free peroneus longus tendon graft is passed through the tunnel with the assistance of a nitinol wire (**Figure 7, H and I**). The tunnel can be lubricated with irrigation fluid to assist with the passage of the strip of peroneus longus tendon. It can also be enlarged with a curet.

A distal capsular interval is created over the insertion of the ATFL, perpendicular to the talar neck at the junction of the capsule and the inferior extensor retinaculum. Care is taken to avoid damaging the extensor tendons or neurovascular structures of the ankle along the lateral ankle capsule. Two mini Hohmann retractors are placed on both sides of the talar neck. This helps to centralize the footprint of the insertion of the tendon transfer at the ATFL insertion. A small Weitlaner retractor is used to separate the ankle capsule and the inferior extensor retinaculum.

A guide pin for a cannulated drill is placed into the distal insertion point of the ATFL, on the neck of the talus perpendicular to the talar neck, with care to leave enough margins for the drill bit (**Figure 8, A**). The talar neck is drilled with a 4.5-mm drill to a depth of 20 to 25 mm perpendicular to the neck of the talus. A notch punch is used to create a keyhole on the side of the hole that is closest to the fibula. The tendon is passed under the anterolateral capsule and out the capsular interval toward the talar head parallel with the talar neck. The tendon graft is tensioned by the assistant, while maximum foot dorsiflexion and eversion of the ankle is maintained. The tendon is marked at the proximal edge of the drill hole and again 17 mm distally (**Figure 8, B and C**). This approximates the length of the interference anchor and permits adequate tendon tensioning during implantation.

Once measured, the tendon is whipstitched with 2-0 FiberWire suture along the 17-mm excursion and secured into the hole in the talar neck with an interference Bio-Tenodesis anchor (Arthrex) (**Figure 8, D**). The end of the tendon is grasped with a No. 2 diameter FiberWire suture that is placed through the hollow handle of the anchor insertional tool. Care is taken to ensure that the distal end of the insertion handle does not bottom out with the tendon into the anchor hole in the talar neck.

This permits tensioning of the tendon before securing the anchor. The tendon is placed into the notch that was placed on the proximal side of the talar neck anchor hole to permit smooth tendon passage into the hole and prevent tendon disruption during screw placement.

The patient's foot is held in dorsiflexion and eversion by the assistant. Appropriate tendon tension is confirmed with forward pressure on the insertion handle before advancing the interference screw into the anchoring hole while holding the paddle on the handle in place. Strength and tension of the tendon transfer are confirmed with inversion and plantar flexion of the foot before removing the insertion handle.

The Broström/Karlsson capsular repair is performed with No. 1 Vicryl suture (Ethicon) in a horizontal mattress pants-over-vest fashion through the periosteal capsule close to the bone, the ATFL, the CFL, and the capsular tissue with a stout needle if possible. The Gould modification is also performed with figure-of-8 suture technique using No. 1 Vicryl suture (**Figure 8, E**). Care is taken to avoid incorporating the surrounding tendons or neurovascular structures into the repair.

Vicryl suture is used in this layer because this portion of the repair is designed to prevent soft-tissue impingement and support the tendon transfer, which is the primary support for the ankle ligament reconstruction. The Vicryl suture dissolves rapidly and no longer will provide structural support within 2 weeks of implantation.

Closure

The incision is closed with 2-0 or 3-0 polydioxanone (PDS) interrupted sutures (Ethicon) for incision alignment. A running layer of 3-0 or 4-0 PDS suture is used for the subcuticular closure. Staples and/or liquid skin adhesive can be used as a final layer. This type of closure allows early range of motion of the ankle at 2 weeks after surgery and provides an incision that is resistant to water and sweat. The patient's knee is flexed to 90° to permit maximum dorsiflexion of the ankle during splint placement. The patient is placed into a bulky Jones dressing of cast padding and a fiberglass 5-in × 30-in splint. All bony prominences are padded with gauze before splint placement. The outer layer of the splint consists of bias wrap as opposed to an elastic bandage.

Complications

Complications can stem from intraoperative variability in patient bone density as well as inability to harvest adequate peroneus longus tendon graft in length or diameter. When a patient's bone density is low, the calcaneal interference anchors can loosen. Care is taken during drilling and notch placement to avoid overenlargement of the pilot hole for the interference anchor. While using the pigtailed tendon stripper, care should be taken to make sure that it is sharp enough to harvest adequate length and width of peroneus longus tendon. The tendon graft should be between 4 and 4.5 mm in diameter, and the length should be enough to span the distance between the CFL insertion site, the fibular tunnel, and the insertion of the ATFL on the neck of the talus. Inadequate peroneus longus graft might necessitate the use of hamstring autograft or allograft.

Postoperative Care

Patients are instructed to ice and elevate the surgical limb for 10 to 14 days postoperatively. They are evaluated in the office and placed into a removable cast boot with a rocker-bottom sole for 2 more weeks. If there are no significant articular cartilage defects treated intraoperatively, patients are permitted to advance to full weight bearing at the first postoperative visit. Physical therapy, similar to an ankle sprain rehabilitation protocol, is initiated at this visit. Patients typically undergo 12 sessions of physical therapy after this surgical procedure. The number of physical therapy sessions varies by patient habitus and demand levels. Patients are placed into a figure-of-8 ASO (ankle stabilizing orthosis) lace-up brace at the fourth week postoperatively to encourage nonantalgic, plantigrade ambulation. This is tapered off as rapidly as possible depending on patient strength and compliance with physical therapy. Patients are tapered from the ASO lace-up brace into off-the-shelf orthoses to improve inversion during gait and loosen up the subtalar joint by the sixth week postoperatively. Patient calf diameters are monitored postoperatively for improvements in strength. Patients are permitted to start straight-line running as soon as they approach 85% motor strength. Patients can start cutting and pivoting activities by 12 weeks postoperatively in most cases.

Pearls

Exposure to the ligament attachment points on the calcaneus and the talar neck are key. Improper exposure in these areas set up improper biomechanics postoperatively.

Care should also be taken not to damage the superior peroneal retinaculum during peroneus longus tendon harvesting. If the diameter of the harvested tendon is much smaller than 4 mm but the tendon is long, it can be doubled up to provide more strength in a larger patient. In addition, tensioning the graft with the foot held in dorsiflexion and eversion is important, as the graft may stretch with time and should be tightest during surgery.

When notching the holes, care must be taken to not make the initial notch too large; it can always be made larger if necessary, but it cannot be made smaller. Caution should also be exercised to avoid plunging when making the tunnel notches. A small, narrow anterior cruciate ligament tunnel notcher should be used. The tendon size and bone density should be taken into account when making the notch. The talar neck tunnel should be directed plantarward, away from the talar neck, to avoid a talar neck fracture or cutout dorsally.

Informing patients about the possibility of numbness in the sural nerve distribution postoperatively due to scarring is very important. Starting early rehabilitation is key to avoiding excessive tightness and scarring after surgery. The surgeon must be careful to decompress the posterior aspect of the ankle when necessary, to improve postoperative range of motion and prevent posterior ankle impingement.

Conclusions

Lateral ankle ligament reconstruction is a reliable, reproducible surgical procedure. Many ankle sprains occur each day. The majority of these patients are treated successfully with physical therapy and bracing. For patients with chronic instability, underlying general laxity, or extensive ankle ligament damage, traditional lateral ankle ligament reconstruction as described by Broström may not be sufficient to provide long-term, reliable ankle stability. Traditional lateral ankle ligament reconstruction can be augmented reliably with peroneus tendon allograft or autograft with very little accompanying morbidity. In a 2-year prospective study (unpublished data, presented at Specialty Day, 2007 AAOS Annual Meeting), I noted high patient satisfaction, extremely low recurrent injury rate, and rapid recovery after augmented lateral ankle ligament reconstruction. Since switching to this technique, I have noted much more consistently reproducible, excellent results than previously experienced with traditional lateral ankle ligament reconstruction techniques.

References

1. Mizel MS, Hecht PJ, Marymont JV, Temple HT: Evaluation and treatment of chronic ankle pain. *Instr Course Lect* 2004;53:311-321.
2. Harrington KD: Degenerative arthritis of the ankle secondary to long-standing lateral ligament instability. *J Bone Joint Surg Am* 1979;61(3):354-361.
3. Colville MR: Surgical treatment of the unstable ankle. *J Am Acad Orthop Surg* 1998;6(6):368-377.
4. Broström L: Sprained ankles: VI. Surgical treatment of "chronic" ligament ruptures. *Acta Chir Scand* 1966;132(5):551-565.
5. Takao M, Oae K, Uchio Y, Ochi M, Yamamoto H: Anatomical reconstruction of the lateral ligaments of the ankle with a gracilis autograft: A new technique using an interference fit anchoring system. *Am J Sports Med* 2005;33(6):814-823.
6. Takao M, Innami K, Matsushita T, Uchio Y, Ochi M: Arthroscopic and magnetic resonance image appearance and

reconstruction of the anterior talofibular ligament in cases of apparent functional ankle instability. *Am J Sports Med* 2008;36(8):1542-1547.

7. Fortin PT, Guettler J, Manoli A II: Idiopathic cavovarus and lateral ankle instability: Recognition and treatment implications relating to ankle arthritis. *Foot Ankle Int* 2002;23(11):1031-1037.

8. Sugimoto K, Takakura Y, Okahashi K, Samoto N, Kawate K, Iwai M: Chondral injuries of the ankle with recurrent lateral instability: An arthroscopic study. *J Bone Joint Surg Am* 2009;91(1):99-106.

9. Ferran NA, Oliva F, Maffulli N: Ankle instability. *Sports Med Arthrosc* 2009;17(2):139-145.

10. Maffulli N, Ferran NA: Management of acute and chronic ankle instability. *J Am Acad Orthop Surg* 2008;16(10):608-615.

11. Hua Y, Chen S, Li Y, Chen J, Li H: Combination of modified Broström procedure with ankle arthroscopy for chronic ankle instability accompanied by intra-articular symptoms. *Arthroscopy* 2010;26(4):524-528.

Video Reference

75.1 Abidi NA, Martin B: *Augmented Lateral Ankle Ligament Reconstruction.* Rosemont, IL, American Academy of Orthopaedic Surgeons, 2009.

Chapter 76
Achilles Tendon Rupture Repair

Stanley C. Graves, MD   Jaycen Brown, BS

Introduction

Intrasubstance rupture of the Achilles tendon is commonly a sports-related injury of patients in their 40s or 50s. Patients commonly give this history: "I feel like someone shot me in the back of the leg." A palpable gap is present in the substance of the Achilles tendon. There is often weakness in voluntary plantar flexion and increased passive ankle dorsiflexion in comparison to the opposite side. The classic examination is the Thompson test. With the patient kneeling on a chair or a stool, the examiner squeezes the calf. If the tendon is ruptured, the foot will not actively plantar flex. Diagnosis is generally straightforward. The American Academy of Orthopaedic Surgeons' Clinical Practice Guidelines generally support surgical repair but advise caution in patients with diabetes, neuropathy, immunocompromised states, peripheral vascular disease, or local/systemic dermatologic disorders as well as in patients who are older than 65 years, use tobacco, have a sedentary lifestyle, or are obese.[1]

Until recently, consensus in the United States favored acute surgical repair, with the thought that surgery provides greater strength with a decreased risk for rerupture.[2-4] Surgery can be open, limited open, or percutaneous, with and without assistive devices.[5-15] A recent controversial paper suggested comparable outcomes with a structured nonsurgical protocol.[16] Augmentation with synthetic, biologic, or allogenic material has been reported in both animal models and limited case series.[17-19]

This chapter will discuss the open technique used by the authors. This technique appears both safe and reliable for surgeons who only occasionally encounter such patients. When exposed, the ruptured ends are classically described as looking like the ends of a mop. The ends are frayed, and the tearing occurs diffusely throughout a significant length of the proximal and distal parts of the tendon. The surgeon should beware if the tear appears "clean" because this situation is likely representative of attempted healing in a previously injured tendon. This tissue should be excised to achieve a solid repair at an appropriate tendon length and tension.

Procedure
Acute Achilles Tendon Rupture Repair
Surgical Technique

Patients have historically been positioned prone for ease of access. Alternatively, if the patient is not obese, and the ipsilateral leg will sufficiently externally rotate, a sandbag or "bump" can be placed under the contralateral hip to allow access for the posterior midline incision using figure-of-4 positioning. This avoids the risks associated with the prone position, which include the need for intubation, lung compression with ventilation-perfusion mismatches, and outflow obstruction of the lower extremity. A second benefit when the patient is positioned in this fashion is the ease of access to the flexor hallucis longus (FHL) tendon from the medial arch. After positioning is completed, access should be checked before making the incision.

An extensile form of incision should be considered to address wound breakdown or tendon rerupture, generally avoiding a curvilinear or transverse incision. A relatively midline incision allows distal extension if the FHL needs to be harvested to replace nonfunctional tendon or for augmentation of poor-quality tissue.

The poor-quality, stringy tissue on both the proximal and distal aspects of the rupture should be débrided. The ankle can be plantar flexed to take tension off the repair. The surgeon should remember that most cadaver models of Achilles tendon repair are based on mechanical testing of tendons that have been surgically transected instead of violently ruptured.[7,10,20] The method of repair is likely not as crucial as the method used in flexor tendon repair in the hand. A sound repair with a minimal amount of nonabsorbable suture material is probably best. I prefer the Krackow pattern, using a heavier suture material (No. 2 nonabsorbable suture) that will not easily tear out or fail (**Figure 1**). The peritenon is generally shredded and will add little to the repair. After the repair is completed, the ankle should be gently dorsiflexed to 90° to determine the stability of the repair. This will allow confidence during the postoperative rehabilitation period. Augmentation with cultured fibroblast material, synthetic mesh, or allograft is rarely necessary in primary repair performed within a few weeks of injury. The use of drains to prevent postoperative hematoma is generally recommended but is optional. Skin closure should be meticulous, minimizing surgical trauma from retraction during the surgery or tissue forceps during the repair. The authors favor carefully placed sutures as opposed to skin clips.[21] The ankle should be immobilized in slight (5° to 10°) equinus to optimize blood flow to the posterior skin and avoid pinching of the skin around the posterior incision. The authors prefer a large bulky dressing underneath the splint (**Figure 2**).

Postoperative Care

Recent investigations support an accelerated rehabilitation program following surgical repair of an acute Achilles tendon rupture.[8] Postoperatively, the ankle is immobilized in slight (5° to 10°) equinus. At the first postoperative visit (usually 5 to 10 days following surgery), if the repair is considered secure, active motion can be initiated. At this phase of the rehabilitation program, active motion is performed several times daily, with a resting splint used at all other times. Many authors will allow weight bearing with a removable fracture boot when the patient can actively dorsiflex the ankle to neutral (90°) and the wound is stable and closed—typically after 3 weeks. The fracture boot is then used as a dorsiflexion-block "splint" during this phase of the rehabilitation process. The fracture boot is removed at 8 weeks following surgery, when physical therapy can be initiated. If the surgeon feels that the repair is tenuous, a cast can be applied and changed at 3 weeks, when the sutures are removed.

Neither of the following authors nor any immediate family member has received anything of value from or has stock or stock options held in a commercial company or institution related directly or indirectly to the subject of this chapter: Dr. Graves and Mr. Brown.

Video 76.1 Chronic Achilles Tendon Repair. Stanley C. Graves, MD (8 min)

Chronic or Neglected Achilles Tendon Rupture

Although less studied, the treatment of undiagnosed Achilles tendon rupture employs similar principles to those employed in the treatment of acute injuries. These patients present late, either because they never sought treatment following the original injury or because the injury was missed. The diagnosis at this time is relatively straightforward. These patients will be able to actively plantar flex the ankle using either the toe flexors or the early scarring within the Achilles tendon sheath. Patients will generally have a palpable defect at the site of the tendon rupture. Passive dorsiflexion will generally be increased, and there will be relative weakness in active plantar flexion. Patients will generally be unable to perform a single-leg raise.

Surgical Planning

The goals of surgery are to replace the damaged retracted tissue with healthy viable tissue to restore appropriate strength and tension. The guiding available literature is based on small retrospective case series.[22-27] Most authors indicate that predictable acceptable results can be achieved, but all state that the ultimate outcome will not be as satisfying as that achieved with primary repair.[28]

Standard tendon reconstruction techniques include V-Y advancement, fascial turndown, autograft, and allograft. Repair with V-Y advancement is used for small gaps of 2 to 3 cm (**Figure 3**). Depending on the local anatomy, fascial turndown can generally be used for gaps of between 3 and 8 cm (**Figure 4**). Autograft or allograft may well be necessary when the gap is greater than 5 cm. Autograft can be harvested from the fascia lata/iliotibial band, the plantaris, the hamstring tendon, and the long flexor tendons to the foot. The most favored autograft tendon is the FHL.[23,24]

MRI is not absolutely necessary but can be beneficial to measure the gap and evaluate the tissue available for reconstruction.

Surgical Technique

Surgical positioning is generally supine rather than prone, as with acute repairs.

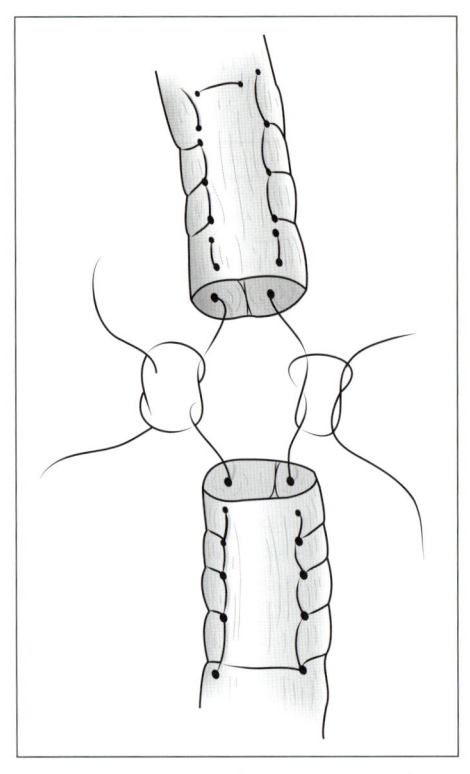

Figure 1 Illustration demonstrates tendon reapproximation with a Krackow suture pattern.

We favor using a sandbag or bump under the opposite hip and accessing the posterior leg with figure-of-4 positioning. A longitudinal midline incision is used.[29] This type of incision requires less undermining of the soft tissues and can be extended both proximally and distally as necessary. It can be extended proximally, to obtain healthy tissue for repair, and distally to secure the FHL transfer to bone. Once the posterior incision has been completed, the healthy tendon ends can be identified, removing the structurally poor intervening scar tissue.

Our preferred surgical technique employs the FHL tendon as autograft for reconstruction. Following débridement of the injured tendon, attention is directed to harvesting the FHL tendon. The proximal tendon is identified by opening the deep posterior compartment. Dissection should be started lateral to the neurovascular bundle. Care should be taken to avoid injury to the posterior tibial nerve.

To secure sufficient length for the reconstruction, a separate incision is made in the medial arch. The abductor muscle is reflected plantarly, and the intermuscular septum is divided to reveal the knot of Henry, where the FHL and flexor digitorum longus cross. (This dissection is easier with the patient in the supine position than the prone position.) After the

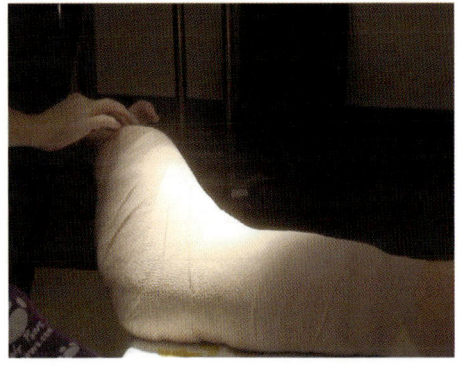

Figure 2 A Robert Jones dressing provides bulky compression with room for swelling.

two tendons are identified, the interconnections between the two tendons are released. The distal stump of the FHL tendon is then sewn to either the flexor digitorum longus or the flexor hallucis brevis tendon. The FHL tendon is then cut proximal to the tenodesis and retracted into the posterior incision. During the release of the interconnections between the two flexor tendons, care should be taken to avoid damage to the plantar nerves.

The FHL tendon can be dissected through the posterior incision and released from the medial ankle. However, to gain enough length for securing it in the calcaneus, some blind dissection is necessary, placing the tibial nerve at risk for blunt injury. With the foot held in slight equinus equal to the opposite ankle, the gap between the Achilles tendon ends is measured. A nonabsorbable suture is placed in the distal end of the FHL tendon. The gap will generally measure between 8 and 12 cm. Because the gap is usually very large, the incision must be extended proximally, taking care to avoid injury to the sural nerve, as it is more centrally located in this region than one might expect.

Although the distal end of the FHL tendon transfer can be attached to the remaining distal stump of the Achilles tendon, I prefer to place the tendon through a drill hole in the calcaneus. This construct provides an extremely stable repair for the reconstruction, allowing early motion and relatively early weight bearing. The hole is drilled parallel with the tibia. The tendon is passed through the hole and sewn back on itself.

A 2- to 3-cm rectangle is created in the proximal Achilles muscle stump. Tissue is cut from the muscle beneath it and then rotated inward on its hinge. By rotating the flap inward, the lump that is left at the hinge is smaller (**Figure 4**). Sutures are now placed in the distal stump as well as

Chapter 76: Achilles Tendon Rupture Repair

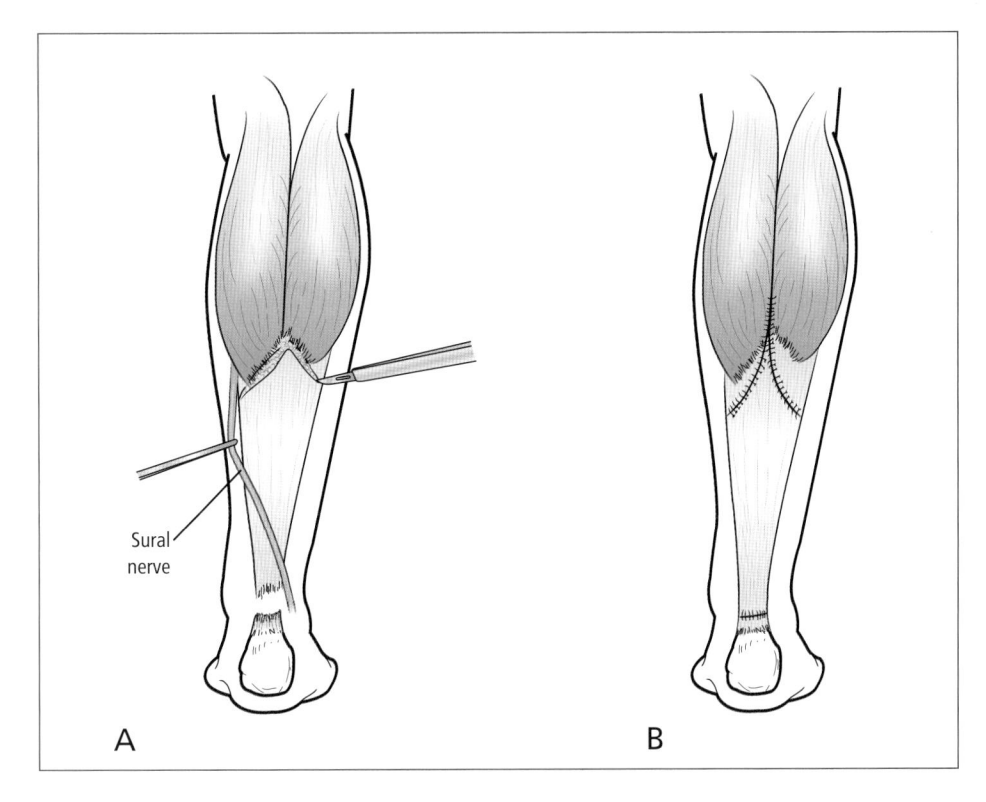

Figure 3 Illustrations show V-Y advancement. **A,** After careful dissection proximally to the Achilles aponeurosis, being attentive to the location of the sural nerve, two oblique fascial incisions should be made along the inferior border of the muscle. **B,** The Achilles tendon rupture can then be repaired because of the increased extensibility of the gastrocnemius-soleus complex. After the repair of the rupture has been completed, the fascial incisions can be sutured while the foot is held in dorsiflexion, so as to keep from getting a tight Achilles tendon postoperatively.

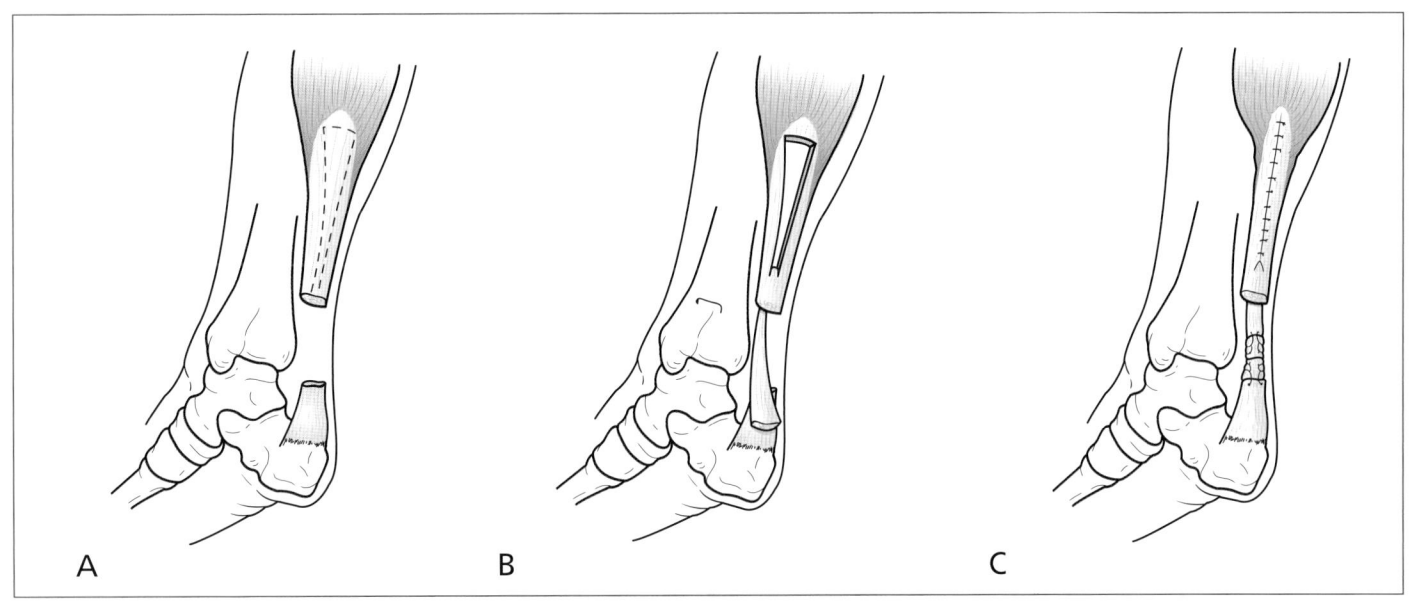

Figure 4 Illustrations demonstrate fascial turndown. **A,** The dashed outline shows an incision that will allow a repair that matches up the distal component of the tendon uniformly. **B,** The proximal portion of the tendon should be reflected anteriorly to minimize the palpable thickening where the two tendons are overlapping. **C,** With the foot held in a neutral position equal to the unaffected side, the rupture site can be repaired with the reflected proximal tendon. After this has been completed, the harvest site should be repaired to produce a stronger tendon overall.

the fascial turndown, preparing for the reconstruction.

After the FHL tendon transfer has been secured through the drill hole in the bone and the tension has been set, the distal stump and proximal turndown can be sewn to each other and secured to the FHL tendon distally and FHL muscle proximally. After the reconstruction is completed, the surgeon should stress the repair by bringing the ankle to neutral with no fear of rupturing the reconstruction.

Wound closure and immobilization are accomplished with the same decision process as used with acute repair.

Postoperative Care
Considerations for postoperative care are similar to those for acute tendon repair.

Complications
Due to the tenuous vascularity of this region, before modern plastic surgery soft-tissue transfer techniques and negative-pressure wound therapy were available, wound complications often led to transtibial amputation. Because of the limited vascularity of the tendon in acute repair or the graft in late reconstruction, aggressive management of early wound complications should be applied. Aggressive débridement and the use of negative-pressure wound therapy and modern plastic surgery will generally avoid wound complications.

Rerupture is unusual. This complication is addressed nonsurgically with an ankle-foot orthosis and surgically with the same methods as described in this chapter.

Pearls

- Positioning the patient supine allows easier harvesting of the FHL, if necessary, and is safer than prone positioning with regard to anesthesia.
- The linear incision along the midline of the leg allows for an easily extensible incision, complete visualization of the affected area, and healing, provided the skin is handled with care during the operation.
- To achieve a repair that is neither too loose nor too tight, the repair should be secured with the foot in the same position as the contralateral foot at rest.
- Keeping the insertion point of the FHL transfer close to the original insertion of the Achilles tendon will approximate the FHL muscle belly to the Achilles tendon repair and will increase blood supply to promote better healing of the repair.

References

1. Chiodo CP, Glazebrook M, Bluman EM, et al: Diagnosis and treatment of acute Achilles tendon rupture. *J Am Acad Orthop Surg* 2010;18(8):503-510.
2. Khan RJ, Carey Smith RL: Surgical interventions for treating acute Achilles tendon ruptures. *Cochrane Database Syst Rev* 2010;9(9):CD003674.
3. Neumayer F, Mouhsine E, Arlettaz Y, Gremion G, Wettstein M, Crevoisier X: A new conservative-dynamic treatment for the acute ruptured Achilles tendon. *Arch Orthop Trauma Surg* 2010;130(3):363-368.
4. Davies MS, Solan M: Minimal incision techniques for acute Achilles repair. *Foot Ankle Clin* 2009;14(4):685-697.
5. Aktas S, Kocaoglu B: Open versus minimal invasive repair with Achillon device. *Foot Ankle Int* 2009;30(5):391-397.
6. Maffulli N, Longo UG, Ronga M, Khanna A, Denaro V: Favorable outcome of percutaneous repair of Achilles tendon ruptures in the elderly. *Clin Orthop Relat Res* 2010;468(4):1039-1046.
7. Huffard B, O'Loughlin PF, Wright T, Deland J, Kennedy JG: Achilles tendon repair: Achillon system vs. Krackow suture. An anatomic in vitro biomechanical study. *Clin Biomech (Bristol, Avon)* 2008;23(9):1158-1164.
8. Suchak AA, Bostick GP, Beaupré LA, Durand DC, Jomha NM: The influence of early weight-bearing compared with non-weight-bearing after surgical repair of the Achilles tendon. *J Bone Joint Surg Am* 2008;90(9):1876-1883.
9. Fortis AP, Dimas A, Lamprakis AA: Repair of Achilles tendon rupture under endoscopic control. *Arthroscopy* 2008;24(6):683-688.
10. Lee SJ, Goldsmith S, Nicholas SJ, McHugh M, Kremenic I, Ben-Avi S: Optimizing Achilles tendon repair: Effect of epitendinous suture augmentation on the strength of Achilles tendon repairs. *Foot Ankle Int* 2008;29(4):427-432.
11. Jacob KM, Paterson R: Surgical repair followed by functional rehabilitation for acute and chronic Achilles tendon injuries: Excellent functional results, patient satisfaction and no reruptures. *ANZ J Surg* 2007;77(4):287-291.
12. Ozkaya U, Parmaksizoglu AS, Kabukcuoglu Y, Sokucu S, Basilgan S: Open minimally invasive Achilles tendon repair with early rehabilitation: Functional results of 25 consecutive patients. *Injury* 2009;40(6):669-672.
13. Lansdaal JR, Goslings JC, Reichart M, et al: The results of 163 Achilles tendon ruptures treated by a minimally invasive surgical technique and functional aftertreatment. *Injury* 2007;38(7):839-844.
14. Tang KL, Thermann H, Dai G, Chen GX, Guo L, Yang L: Arthroscopically assisted percutaneous repair of fresh closed Achilles tendon rupture by Kessler's suture. *Am J Sports Med* 2007;35(4):589-596.
15. Labib SA, Rolf R, Dacus R, Hutton WC: The "Giftbox" repair of the Achilles tendon: A modification of the Krackow technique. *Foot Ankle Int* 2009;30(5):410-414.
16. Tan G, Sabb B, Kadakia AR: Non-surgical management of Achilles ruptures. *Foot Ankle Clin* 2009;14(4):675-684.
17. Barber FA, McGarry JE, Herbert MA, Anderson RB: A biomechanical study of Achilles tendon repair augmentation using GraftJacket matrix. *Foot Ankle Int* 2008;29(3):329-333.
18. Hohendorff B, Siepen W, Spiering L, Staub L, Schmuck T, Boss A: Long-term results after operatively treated Achilles tendon rupture: Fibrin glue versus suture. *J Foot Ankle Surg* 2008;47(5):392-399.
19. Sánchez M, Anitua E, Azofra J, Andía I, Padilla S, Mujika I: Comparison of surgically repaired Achilles tendon tears using platelet-rich fibrin matrices. *Am J Sports Med* 2007;35(2):245-251.
20. Herbort M, Haber A, Zantop T, et al: Biomechanical comparison of the primary stability of suturing Achilles tendon rupture: A cadaver study of Bunnell and Kessler techniques under cyclic loading conditions. *Arch Orthop Trauma Surg* 2008;128(11):1273-1277.
21. Syed KA, Gandhi R, Davey JR, Mahomed NN: Risk of wound infection is greater after skin closure with staples than with sutures in orthopaedic surgery. *J Bone Joint Surg Am* 2010;92(16):2732.
22. Yasuda T, Kinoshita M, Okuda R: Reconstruction of chronic Achilles tendon rupture with the use of interposed tissue between the stumps. *Am J Sports Med* 2007;35(4):582-588.
23. Mann RA, Holmes GB Jr, Seale KS, Collins DN: Chronic rupture of the Achilles tendon: A new technique of repair. *J Bone Joint Surg Am* 1991;73(2):214-219.
24. Wapner KL, Pavlock GS, Hecht PJ, Naselli F, Walther R: Repair of chronic Achilles tendon rupture with flexor hallucis longus tendon transfer. *Foot Ankle* 1993;14(8):443-449.
25. Lee DK: Achilles tendon repair with acellular tissue graft augmentation in neglected ruptures. *J Foot Ankle Surg* 2007;46(6):451-455.
26. Maffulli N, Ajis A, Longo UG, Denaro V: Chronic rupture of tendo Achillis. *Foot Ankle Clin* 2007;12(4):583-596, vi.
27. El Shewy MT, El Barbary HM, Abdel-Ghani H: Repair of chronic rupture of the Achilles tendon using 2 intratendinous flaps from the proximal gastrocnemius-soleus complex. *Am J Sports Med* 2009;37(8):1570-1577.
28. Maffulli N, Ajis A: Management of chronic ruptures of the Achilles tendon. *J Bone Joint Surg Am* 2008;90(6):1348-1360.
29. Attinger CE, Evans KK, Bulan E, Blume P, Cooper P: Angiosomes of the foot and ankle and clinical implications for limb salvage: Reconstruction, incisions, and revascularization. *Plast Reconstr Surg* 2006;117(7, suppl):261S-293S.

Chapter 77
Tibiotalar Arthrodesis

Siddhant K. Mehta, MD   Nicholas A. Abidi, MD   Sheldon S. Lin, MD

Introduction
Ankle arthritis represents degenerative changes of the tibiotalar joint that often result in limited range of motion, severe pain, and difficulty in ambulation. Surgical management must be considered in patients with end-stage ankle arthritis refractory to nonsurgical treatment. Tibiotalar (ankle) arthrodesis has been the mainstay of treatment for over 50 years, providing predictable symptomatic relief in patients with severe, end-stage ankle arthritis. This chapter will discuss indications and contraindications, describe general principles and preoperative imaging, and detail the surgical technique for open ankle arthrodesis.

Patient Selection
Indications
Appropriate patient selection for ankle arthrodesis is of paramount importance to achieve favorable outcomes.[1] The most common indication for ankle arthrodesis is posttraumatic arthritis, which can occur secondary to ankle fractures, tibial plafond fractures, or, less commonly, chronic ankle instability. Other indications include rheumatoid arthritis, infection, primary osteoarthritis, or salvage of a failed total ankle arthroplasty. Relative indications for this procedure include deformity—varus, valgus, or equinus—that may cause pain or interfere with activities of daily living.

Contraindications
Contraindications to ankle arthrodesis include acute infection or chronic untreated osteomyelitis, as well as osteonecrosis of a significant portion of the talar body. Severe osteopenia is a relative contraindication, as it would hinder optimal screw purchase for a stable fixation. Peripheral neuropathy, such as in patients with diabetes mellitus, may also be a relative contraindication as a higher incidence of nonunion or postoperative infection has been observed.

Preoperative Imaging
Radiographic assessment is performed with conventional radiographs (weight-bearing ankle series) and advanced imaging modalities (MRI, CT, nuclear imaging). Routine radiographs should include weight-bearing AP, mortise, and lateral views of the ankle (**Figure 1**). A weight-bearing study is critical in providing a more accurate approximation of the presence and degree of cartilage thinning than a non–weight-bearing study.

Typical degenerative changes include joint space narrowing, osteophyte formation, subchondral bone cysts, and subchondral bone sclerosis. The presence of joint incongruency, malalignment, or dislocation should also be noted. Additionally, in inflammatory arthritis, joint subluxation, large erosions, and bone destruction may be observed. End-stage rheumatoid arthritis is noted by malalignment, displacement, and ankylosis of the joints of the foot and ankle. Furthermore, advanced imaging can allow evaluation of the subtalar joint for concomitant arthritis (CT scan), as well as provide useful preoperative information, such as evidence of osteonecrosis of the talus (MRI) or the presence of infection (nuclear medicine study).

General Principles
Rigid fixation, adequate compression, and a favorable biologic environment are known to be key components for osseous healing and a successful fusion construct across the tibiotalar articulation. A stable fixation can be achieved through an external fixator device or internal fixation, performed arthroscopically or through an open approach. Selection of the surgical technique should be based on the

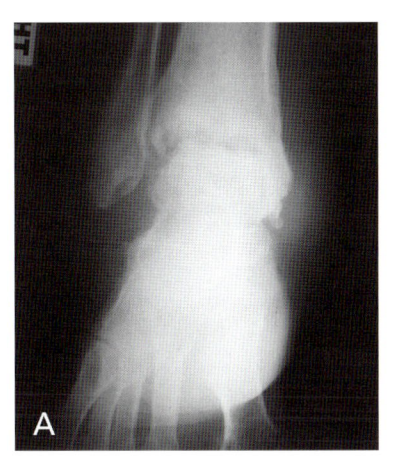

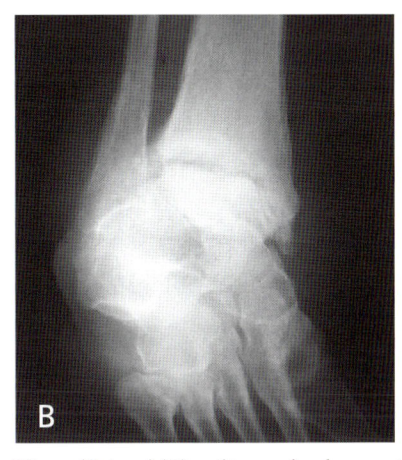

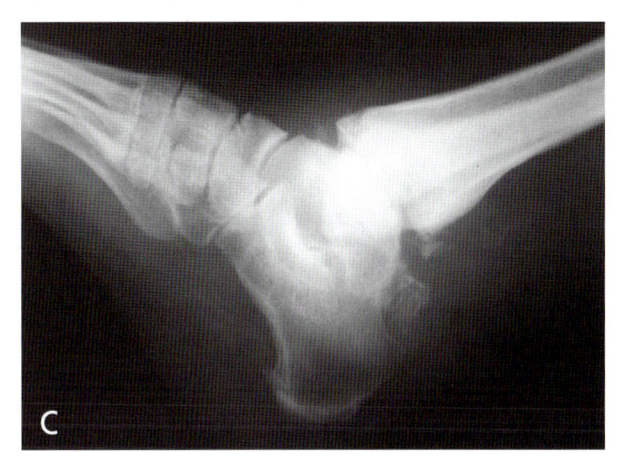

Figure 1 Preoperative AP (**A**), mortise (**B**), and lateral (**C**) radiographs demonstrate severe, end-stage tibiotalar arthritis.

Dr. Abidi or an immediate family member has received royalties from Arthrex; is a member of a speakers' bureau or has made paid presentations on behalf of Acumed and Arthrex; serves as a paid consultant to or is an employee of Acumed, Arthex, and Biomet; has stock or stock options held in Global Orthopaedic Solutions; and serves as a board member, owner, officer, or committee member of the American Orthopaedic Foot & Ankle Society. Dr. Lin or an immediate family member serves as a paid consultant to or is an employee of Biomimetic, Zimmer, and Tissuegene; has received research or institutional support from Biomimetic, EBI, and Tornier; and serves as a board member, owner, officer, or committee member of the American Orthopaedic Foot & Ankle Society. Neither Dr. Mehta nor any immediate family member has received anything of value from or has stock or stock options held in a commercial company or institution related directly or indirectly to the subject of this chapter.

Section 6: Foot & Ankle

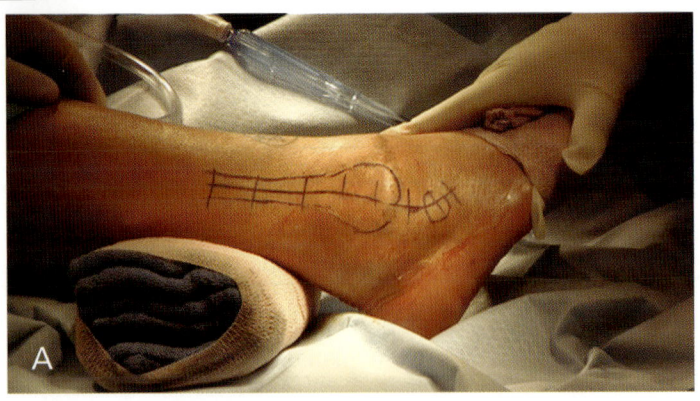

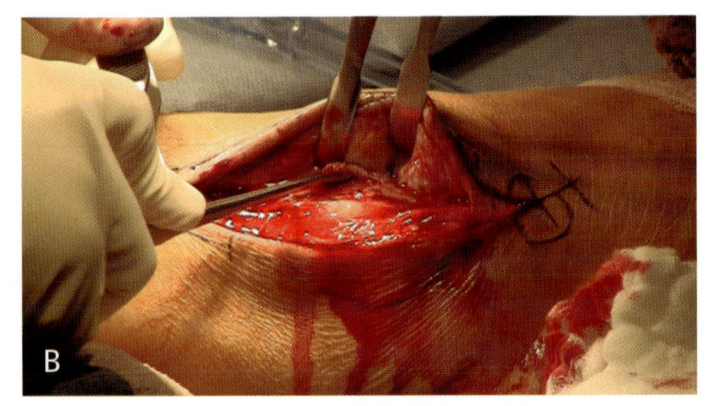

Figure 2 Intraoperative photographs show ankle arthrodesis. **A,** The lateral landmarks and planned incision are drawn on the skin. **B,** The periosteum is stripped from the anterior aspect and, minimally, from the posterior aspect to fully expose the distal fibula.

underlying disorder. As a general rule, external fixators are preferred for patients undergoing arthrodesis for a preexisting septic joint and for patients with severe osteopenia. Arthroscopic arthrodesis or the "mini-open" arthrodesis should be used only for patients with minimal deformity. Open arthrodesis is appropriate for patients with significant ankle deformity and foot and ankle malalignment.[1]

Regardless of the surgical technique chosen, the optimal postoperative position of the affected foot and ankle joint is the same. The foot should be externally rotated 20° to 30° relative to the tibia, with the ankle joint in neutral flexion (0°), 5° to 10° of external rotation, and slight valgus (5°).[2] This position provides the best extremity alignment and accommodation of hip and knee motion during ambulation. Fusion of the ankle in plantar flexion results in genu recurvatum when placing the foot flat on the floor. Subsequently, laxity of the medial collateral ligament of the knee develops, secondary to the externally rotated gait that patients adopt to avoid "rolling over" a plantar-flexed foot.[2]

Although internal compression arthrodesis with two or three cannulated screws is successful and continues to be a common procedure for the management of ankle arthritis, it may not be adequate for certain patient groups.[1] The arthrodesis technique must be modified for patients with compromised soft tissues, with nonunion after previous arthrodesis attempts, or with neuropathic ankle joints. Patients with symptomatic nonunion, osteonecrosis of the talus, or Charcot arthropathy frequently require substantial débridement of devitalized bone from the talus. Bone grafting, with or without the use of orthobiologics, can be used in these patients to regain some of the lost height, but often tibiotalocalcaneal arthrodesis is required to achieve a successful fusion. More rigid internal fixation is a part of almost all fusion techniques used in these difficult situations. Furthermore, supplemental plating at the medial, lateral, or anterior aspect of the tibiotalar joint has been shown to provide a secure fixation and thus it increases fusion rates and improves stability at the fusion site.[3-6]

Procedure

Patient Positioning

The patient is placed in a supine position at the immediate edge of the operating table. A sandbag is placed under the ipsilateral hip to internally rotate the leg and improve exposure of the lateral aspect of the foot and ankle. The limb is prepared and draped appropriately to ensure adequate exposure. The foot and ankle are exsanguinated with an Esmarch elastic wrap, and a tourniquet is inflated on the upper third of the thigh. The surgeon operates from the foot of the table.

Video 77.1 Tibiotalar Arthrodesis. Siddhant K. Mehta, MD; Nicholas A. Abidi, MD; Sheldon S. Lin, MD (6 min)

Special Instruments/Equipment/Implants

The following instruments and equipment should be on hand: microsagittal saw and/or osteotomes, curets/osteotomes, 7.3-mm cannulated screws, 4.0- or 4.5-mm cannulated screws, and plating systems (optional).

Surgical Technique

Numerous approaches and techniques exist to achieve a stable ankle arthrodesis.[7] This section will focus on open ankle arthrodesis using a two-incision transfibular exposure, and a transarticular cross-screw fixation technique supplemented with fibular-onlay strut grafting and anterior plating. The complete procedure can be seen in the video supplement.

Open ankle arthrodesis can be used for any patient but is particularly useful for patients with severe ankle joint deformity because it provides better visualization of the joint and improved access for bone resection, correction of deformity, and screw placement. It is performed through a two-incision transfibular exposure. The first incision is marked and made directly over the fibula, beginning approximately 10 cm proximal to the tip of the fibula and extending distally along the fibular shaft toward the base of the fourth metatarsal (**Figure 2, A**). This incision uses the internervous plane that lies between the peroneal muscles (superficial peroneal nerve) and extensors (deep peroneal nerve) as the dissection is being performed down to subcutaneous bone. After the distal 10 cm of the fibula has been exposed, the superior peroneal retinaculum is incised posteriorly and the peroneal tendons are mobilized while the sural and superficial peroneal nerves are protected. The exposure is performed carefully to maintain full-thickness flaps and to identify and protect tendons and neurovascular structures.

The periosteum is stripped from the fibula anteriorly and minimally posteriorly using an osteotome or curet (**Figure 2, B**). The deep incision is then extended across medially to expose the distal tibia and the tibiotalar articulation and distally to expose the posterior facet of the subtalar joint and the sinus tarsi area. The soft tissue from the distal end of the tibia and the talar neck to the medial malleolus is stripped with a periosteal elevator.

© 2013 American Academy of Orthopaedic Surgeons

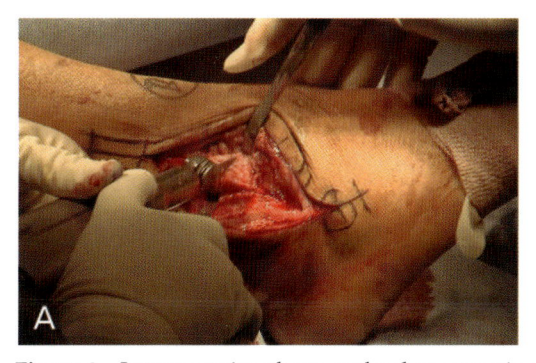

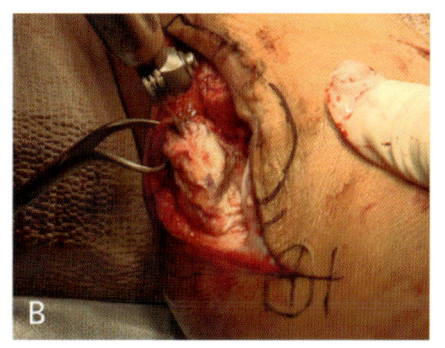

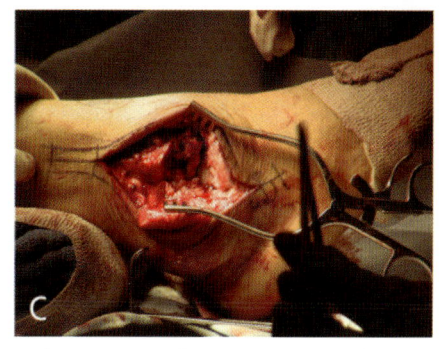

Figure 3 Intraoperative photographs show steps in ankle arthrodesis. **A,** A fibular osteotomy is created approximately 4 to 6 cm proximal to the tip of the lateral malleolus. **B,** The distal fibula is split in half in the sagittal plane. The medial fragment will later be morcellized to serve as autologous bone graft, and the lateral fragment will be lagged to the tibia and the talus to provide lateral stability. **C,** The distal fibula is turned down and away from the arthrodesis site to provide adequate exposure to the posteromedial tibia.

An oscillating saw is used to create a fibular osteotomy approximately 4 to 6 cm proximal to the tip of the lateral malleolus while the soft-tissue attachments at the posterolateral aspect and distal end of the fibula are preserved (**Figure 3, A**). The syndesmosis is then débrided of intervening cartilage, soft tissues, and cortical bone, after which exposure of the tibiotalar joint can be enhanced. A sagittal cut of the fibula is made to resect the medial fibular fragment to be morcellized and used for autologous bone grafting (**Figure 3, B**). The remaining fibula is then turned down and away from the arthrodesis site to provide adequate exposure to the posteromedial aspect of the tibia (**Figure 3, C**). The blood supply to this lateral fibular fragment is maintained because of the preserved ligamentous attachments this fragment is later used as a fibular-onlay strut graft to serve as a lateral buttress.

Sharp dissection is used through the lateral incision to elevate the scarred ankle capsule and strip soft-tissue attachments from the joint both anteriorly and posteriorly. Retractors are placed as needed to expose the ankle mortise and protect soft tissues while bone cuts are made. The tibiotalar joint is then manually denuded of cartilage and subchondral cortical bone with curets and/or osteotomes. Following joint preparation, tibiotalar fusion alignment should be inspected directly and via fluoroscopic image intensification. Additional correction can be achieved using osteotomes or, if needed, autologous bone block placement.

One option (which we prefer not to perform because of its potential to "burn the bone") is to create two flat surfaces. Using a broad osteotome or an oscillating saw, a cut perpendicular to the long axis of the tibia is made at the level of the apex of the dome of the articular surface, allowing removal of the tibial plafond. The cut should cross the ankle joint but stop just where the medial malleolus begins. The medial malleolus serves to provide an area of solid fixation for the lateral-to-medial screw and preserve the medial blood supply to the talus through the deltoid ligament.

Next, the foot is placed in proper alignment for arthrodesis. The talus is positioned so that the forefoot is in 5° to 10° of external rotation and the hindfoot is in 5° of valgus, with 0° of dorsiflexion and displacement so that the posterior margins of the talus and tibia are flush. A cut through the dome of the talus is then made parallel to the distal tibial cut, resecting approximately 3 to 5 mm of bone. The joint surfaces are brought together, and alignment is assessed. To correct for malalignment, further bony resection from the distal tibial end is performed.

The second incision is made after distal tibial and talar bony resection. Exposure of the medial malleolus is achieved through a longitudinal 6-cm anteromedial incision made along the anterior third of the medial malleolus, dissecting through subcutaneous tissue and fat while full-thickness flaps are maintained (**Figure 4**). The ankle capsule and periosteum are carefully removed. The remaining joint surfaces are inspected carefully for residual cartilage and sclerotic bone. All joint surfaces are drilled or cureted until bleeding bone is noted. The tibiotalar joint surfaces are apposed, and satisfactory alignment is obtained.

After the surface congruency and varus-valgus, dorsiflexion–plantar flexion, and rotational alignment have been checked, the joint position is secured with two guide pins for large (7.0- to 7.3-mm) cannulated, partially threaded cancellous screws to provide compression at the fusion site. The first guide pin is placed starting at the base of the talar neck, directed proximally in a posteromedial direction (**Figure 5, A**). The second guide pin is placed starting just above the posterior facet and anterior to the lateral process in a posteromedial direction, parallel to the first guide pin (**Figure 5, B**). Extreme caution must be taken to avoid violating the subtalar joint while placing the guide pins. Care must be taken to translate the foot posteriorly (foot relative to the tibia on lateral view) to reduce the lever arm and the forces across the ankle arthrodesis site. Fluoroscopic image intensification is used to confirm pin placement and bone apposition (**Figure 5, C**), after which the compression screws are placed and the guide pins are removed. This transfibular two-screw ankle fusion technique has been described by Mann et al[8] (**Figure 6**).

Another common technique incorporates multiple screws crossing at 90° angles. The first home-run cannulated screw is placed from the posterolateral tibia down the center of the talus (**Figure 7, A**). The second screw is placed from the anterolateral aspect of the talus and directed proximally into the medial cortex of the tibia (**Figure 7, B**). Alterna-

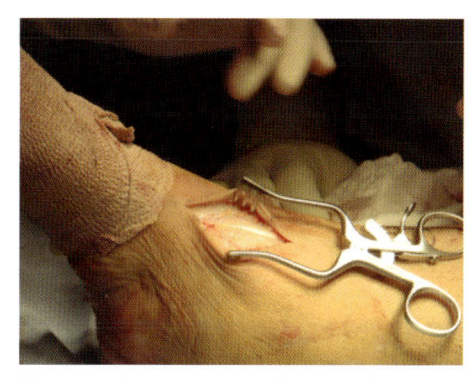

Figure 4 Intraoperative photograph shows exposure to the medial aspect of the tibiotalar articulation obtained through a 6-cm anteromedial incision made along the anterior third of the medial malleolus.

Section 6: Foot & Ankle

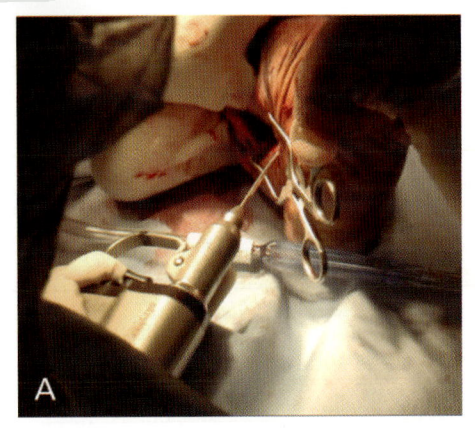

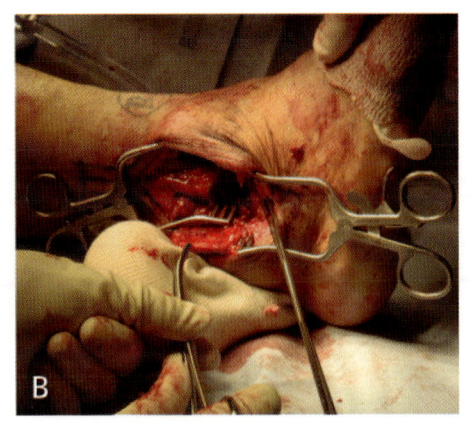

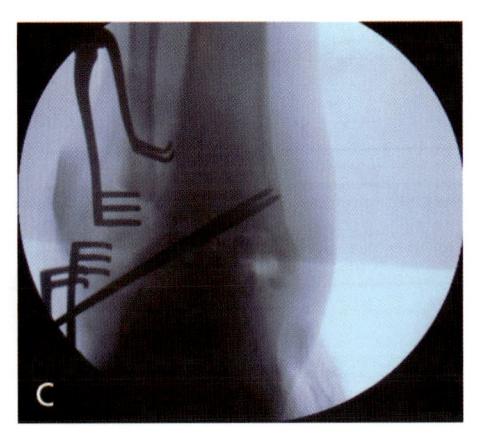

Figure 5 Placement of guide pins for fixation in ankle arthrodesis. Two parallel guide pins are placed across the arthrodesis site. **A,** Intraoperative photograph shows the first guide pin being placed, starting at the base of the talar neck and directed proximally in a posteromedial direction. **B,** Intraoperative photograph shows the second guide pin being placed, starting from just above the posterior facet and anterior to the lateral process. **C,** Fluoroscopic image shows both guide pins in place.

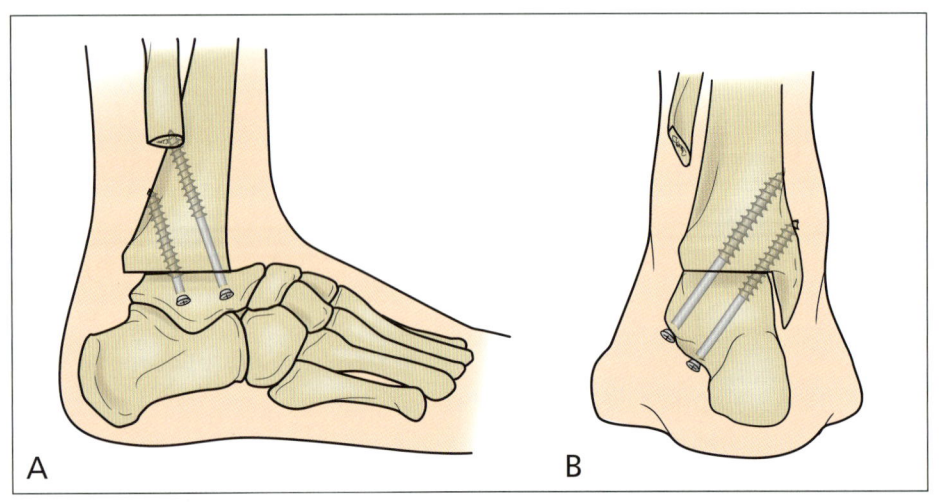

Figure 6 Illustrations of the lateral (A) and posterior (B) aspects of the foot show the placement of cancellous screws across the arthrodesis site as described by Mann et al.[8]

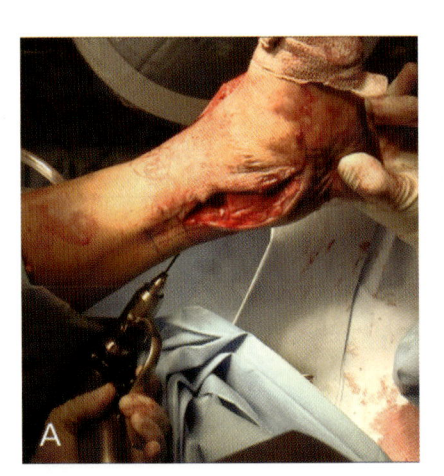

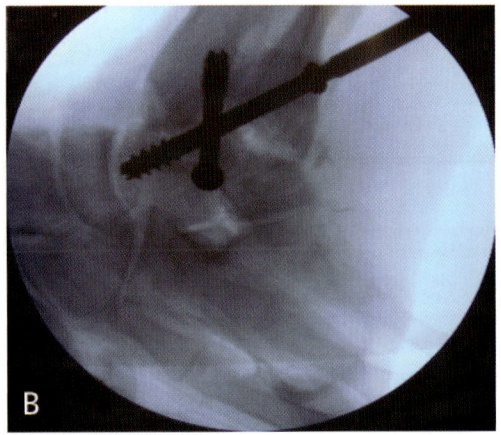

Figure 7 Cross-screw fixation technique for ankle arthrodesis. **A,** Intraoperative photograph shows the guide pin for the first cancellous screw being placed from the posterolateral tibia down the center of the talus. **B,** Fluoroscopic image shows the second screw in place, from the anterolateral aspect of the talus directed proximally into the medial cortex of the tibia.

tively, the first screw may be placed from the medial malleolus into the lateral aspect of the talus. The final compression screw is placed in the lateral aspect of the tibia and directed distally and medially into the talus.

After compression and stable screw fixation is achieved at the arthrodesis site, morcellized autologous bone graft obtained from the medial fibular fragment is packed at the arthrodesis site (Figure 8, A). The distal fibular-onlay strut graft is positioned across the lateral aspect of the tibiotalar arthrodesis in its original anatomic position and subsequently lagged to the tibia and the talus with two 4.0- or 4.5-mm screws (Figure 8, B and C). The fibular-onlay strut graft serves as a lateral buttress to provide additional lateral stability to the arthrodesis site and assist in preventing lateral drifting of the talus[9,10] (Figure 9).

One potential adjunct is the application of an anatomically contoured tibiotalar plate with fully threaded screws to supplement the arthrodesis construct[3] (Figure 10). An anterior plate is positioned through the anteromedial incision onto the anterior aspect of the tibiotalar articulation. With the arthrodesis maintained under axial compression, the anterior plate is secured to the tibia and talus with three or four 3.5-mm cortical screws inserted anterior to posterior through the holes in the plate. Care must be taken to avoid penetration of the subtalar joint at the time of screw placement. The alignment and length of the screws should be confirmed with fluoroscopy (Figure 11).

The wounds are closed with a two-layer technique, taking care to protect the adjacent nerves.

Outcomes/Complications

There are several predictable outcomes in patients undergoing tibiotalar arthrodesis. Ankle arthrodesis results in a 60% to 70% loss of sagittal motion, as well as decreased motion at the subtalar joint.[11] Conceptually, sacrificing ankle motion to relieve pain puts greater stress on the surrounding joints. Gait studies and cadaveric studies have shown that a tibiotalar fusion decreases walking speed by 16% and places increased stresses on the subtalar and midfoot joints as a result of the

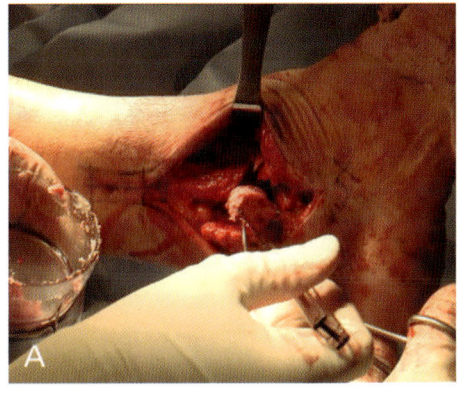

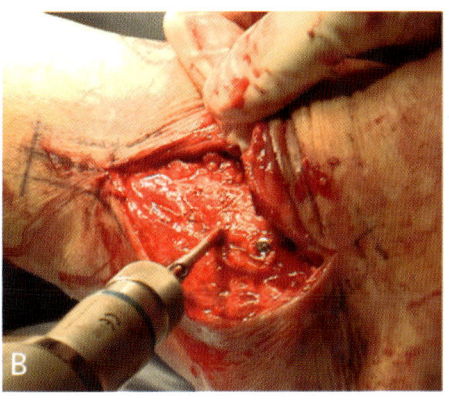

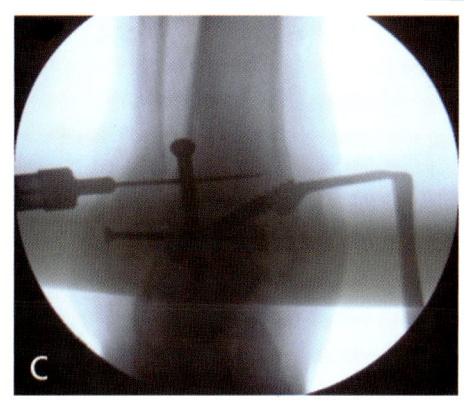

Chapter 77: Tibiotalar Arthrodesis

Figure 8 Grafting in ankle arthrodesis. **A,** Intraoperative photograph shows morcellized autologous bone graft obtained from the medial fibular fragment being packed at the arthrodesis site. The distal fibular-onlay strut graft is then positioned across the lateral aspect of the tibiotalar arthrodesis in its original anatomic position. It is subsequently lagged to the tibia and the talus with two 4.0- or 4.5-mm fully threaded cortical screws. Intraoperative photograph (**B**) and fluoroscopic image (**C**) show the distal lag screw in place and the proximal hole being drilled.

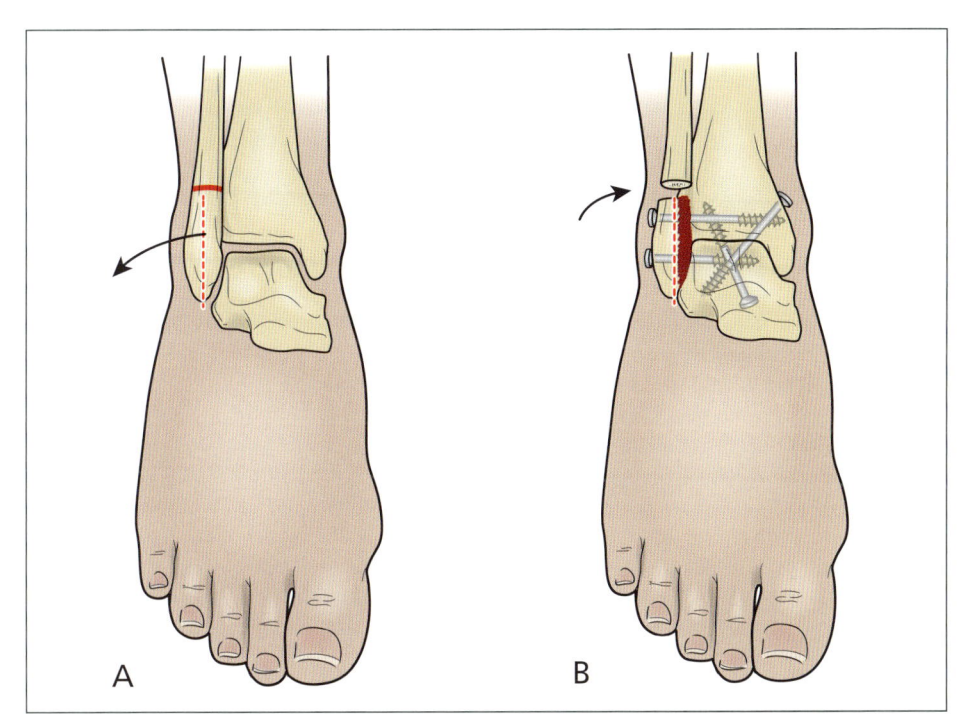

Figure 9 Illustrations show ankle arthrodesis. **A,** The fibular osteotomy is achieved while distal fibular soft-tissue attachments are maintained. **B,** After cross-screw fixation, the fibula is lagged to the tibia and the talus in its anatomic position, to serve as a lateral buttress.

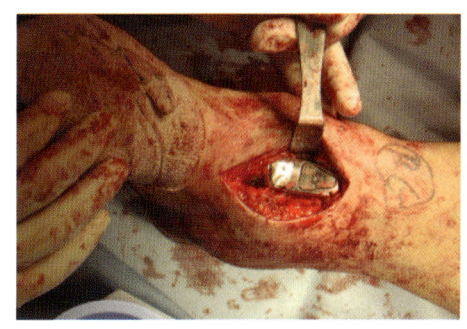

Figure 10 Intraoperative photograph shows the application of an anatomically contoured tibiotalar plate with fully threaded screws to supplement the arthrodesis construct.

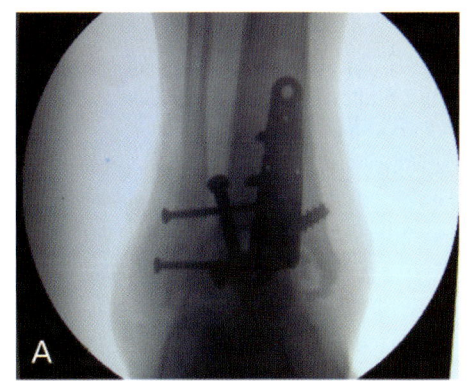

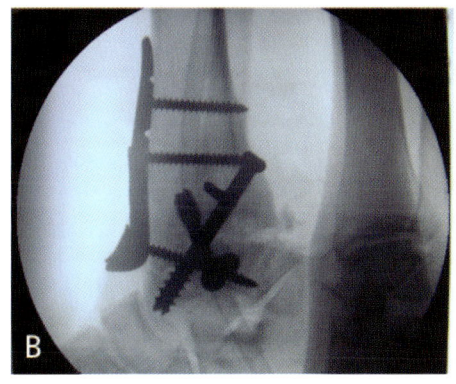

Figure 11 Final fluoroscopic AP (**A**) and lateral (**B**) views demonstrate a stable ankle arthrodesis with cross-screw fixation supplemented with a fibular-onlay strut graft and anterior tibiotalar plating.

transmission of gait forces to these surrounding joints. Over time, this can lead to progressive degeneration and arthritis with the possible need for further fusions of these joints.[12]

Additionally, ankle arthrodesis is a technically demanding orthopaedic procedure that may result in complications, including nonunion, infection, impaired wound healing, and neurovascular injury.[13] Nonunion at the fusion site can occur in up to 10% of cases. An increased rate of nonunion has been associated with several risk factors, including initial high-grade traumatic fracture, open injury, evidence of osteonecrosis of the talus, major medical comorbidities, neuropathy, local infection, and tobacco use.[14] Patient age, a history of undergoing a subtalar or triple arthrodesis, and the surgical arthrodesis technique selected are not associated risk factors for nonunion.

Careful patient selection with screening for identifiable risk factors can reduce the incidence of nonunion. Additionally, various strategies have been described to achieve a stable fixation, including using multiple compression screws and larger diameter screws to improve mechanical stability and compression. More recently, the utility of electrical bone stimulation and biologic adjuncts, such as platelet-rich plasma, recombinant bone morphogenetic proteins, and recombi-

© 2013 American Academy of Orthopaedic Surgeons

nant platelet-derived growth factor, have been described to enhance fusion rates in high-risk patients.[15]

Furthermore, careful surgical dissection and soft-tissue preservation are paramount to achieving favorable outcomes. Gentle handling of the soft-tissue attachments to the distal fibular segment and meticulous resection of articular cartilage with preservation of bone length are essential for minimizing associated postoperative complications such as infection, wound healing problems, and neurovascular injury.

Postoperative Care

After wound closure, the extremity is placed in a bulky cast padding and a plaster splint dressing, which is maintained for 2 weeks. A non–weight-bearing short leg cast is then applied, and weight bearing is not permitted until evidence of arthrodesis is observed on the follow-up radiographs, which usually occurs 8 to 12 weeks postoperatively.

Pearls

- For satisfactory short- and long-term results of tibiotalar arthrodesis, it is paramount that correct alignment is achieved and the ankle be positioned in neutral flexion, 5° to 10° of external rotation, and approximately 5° of valgus.
- The amount of rigid fixation used and the technique(s) employed to obtain a successful arthrodesis across the tibiotalar joint are ultimately predicated on host factors and bone quality. The techniques discussed in this chapter include both basic and supplemental methods for adequate fixation.
- Care must be taken to appropriately identify risk factors for impaired osseous healing—advanced age, systemic diseases (eg, diabetes mellitus), smoking, poor nutritional status, chronic use of corticosteroids, and immunosuppressive therapy (chemotherapy, radiotherapy). In these high-risk patients, bone grafting with or without the use of orthobiologics (eg, local growth factor augmentation with platelet-rich plasma, bone morphogenetic proteins, or recombinant human platelet-derived growth factor) or biophysical bone stimulation with low-intensity pulsed ultrasound, direct current, or pulsed electromagnetic fields may improve clinical outcomes after tibiotalar arthrodesis.

References

1. Abidi NA, Gruen GS, Conti SF: Ankle arthrodesis: Indications and techniques. *J Am Acad Orthop Surg* 2000;8(3):200-209.
2. Buck P, Morrey BF, Chao EY: The optimum position of arthrodesis of the ankle: A gait study of the knee and ankle. *J Bone Joint Surg Am* 1987;69(7):1052-1062.
3. Tarkin IS, Mormino MA, Clare MP, Haider H, Walling AK, Sanders RW: Anterior plate supplementation increases ankle arthrodesis construct rigidity. *Foot Ankle Int* 2007;28(2):219-223.
4. Mears DC, Gordon RG, Kann SE, Kann JN: Ankle arthrodesis with an anterior tension plate. *Clin Orthop Relat Res* 1991;268:70-77.
5. Scranton PE Jr, Fu FH, Brown TD: Ankle arthrodesis: A comparative clinical and biomechanical evaluation. *Clin Orthop Relat Res* 1980;151:234-243.
6. Scranton PE Jr: Use of internal compression in arthrodesis of the ankle. *J Bone Joint Surg Am* 1985;67(4):550-555.
7. Pickering R: Arthrodesis of the ankle, knee, and hip, in Canale S, ed: *Campbell's Operative Orthopaedics*, ed 11. Philadelphia, PA, Mosby, 2003, vol. 1, pp 155-198.
8. Mann RA, Van Manen JW, Wapner K, Martin J: Ankle fusion. *Clin Orthop Relat Res* 1991;268:49-55.
9. Horst F, Nunley JA II: Ankle arthrodesis. *J Surg Orthop Adv* 2004;13(2):81-90.
10. Thordarson DB, Markolf KL, Cracchiolo A III: Arthrodesis of the ankle with cancellous-bone screws and fibular strut graft: Biomechanical analysis. *J Bone Joint Surg Am* 1990;72(9):1359-1363.
11. Hintermann B, Nigg BM: Influence of arthrodeses on kinematics of the axially loaded ankle complex during dorsiflexion/plantarflexion. *Foot Ankle Int* 1995;16(10):633-636.
12. Coester LM, Saltzman CL, Leupold J, Pontarelli W: Long-term results following ankle arthrodesis for post-traumatic arthritis. *J Bone Joint Surg Am* 2001;83-A(2):219-228.
13. Raikin SM, Rampuri V: An approach to the failed ankle arthrodesis. *Foot Ankle Clin* 2008;13(3):401-416, viii.
14. Frey C, Halikus NM, Vu-Rose T, Ebramzadeh E: A review of ankle arthrodesis: Predisposing factors to nonunion. *Foot Ankle Int* 1994;15(11):581-584.
15. Mehta SK, Breitbart EA, Berberian WS, Liporace FA, Lin SS: Bone and wound healing in the diabetic patient. *Foot Ankle Clin* 2010;15(3):411-437.

Chapter 78
Subtalar Arthrodesis

James B. Carr, MD

Patient Selection
Indications
The primary indication for subtalar arthrodesis is painful arthritis.[1] Common causes of arthritis include osteoarthritis, posttraumatic arthritis, and arthritis from inflammatory diseases.[2] These etiologies may cause alterations in the normal foot alignment—an important consideration in preoperative planning. For example, a severe valgus alignment associated with posterior tibial tendon insufficiency must be corrected in addition to the goal of obtaining an arthrodesis. Surgical treatment is considered after nonsurgical treatment—such as cortisone injections, medications, inserts, and rocker-bottom shoes—has failed.

Contraindications
There are no absolute contraindications to subtalar arthrodesis, but certain situations make a satisfactory result less likely.[3] Charcot arthropathy places the limb at much higher risk of failure with either infection or nonunion. Smoking and prior hindfoot surgery also increase the chance of poor healing. Active infection should be controlled before the definitive arthrodesis and may require alternative techniques such as external fixation. It can be difficult to localize the source of posttraumatic pain, especially if chronic narcotics are being used. A local anesthetic injection is useful in such situations. The midfoot and forefoot should be carefully checked for alignment, stability, and arthritis. If present, these conditions may require a more extensive procedure than subtalar arthrodesis. Poor vascularity or skin condition can contraindicate surgery on the hindfoot.

Preoperative Imaging
The initial diagnostic workup should include AP, lateral, and axial views of the hindfoot. If the alignment of the hindfoot is abnormal, a long weight-bearing axial view including the distal tibia will delineate calcaneal-tibial alignment (**Figure 1**). Broden views may be used to focus on the subtalar joint but are most useful intraoperatively to judge implant placement.

The definitive imaging modality for defining the bony anatomy is CT. This will accurately define the presence/severity of arthritis, image adjacent joints, and provide useful information about the alignment of the hindfoot. In complex cases, a three-dimensional image can be obtained and provide a readily understandable method to visualize the anatomy of the situation. The surgeon can also plan the length and direction of implants if desired. The status of healing is also better determined with CT scanning.[4]

MRI is also useful in imaging the subtalar joint preoperatively. One example would be its use in cases of subtle subtalar symptoms that may not be apparent on routine imaging. Areas of bone marrow edema adjacent to the articular surfaces correlate with symptomatic regions of the joint. MRI is also the best tool for assessing vascularity of the talus in cases of osteonecrosis (eg, after talus fracture).

Procedure
Setup/Patient Positioning
The room setup includes tourniquet control, a "bump" under the ipsilateral hip, and a plan to access the point of the heel for an axially directed screw. Methods include the figure-of-4 position, flexion of the knee to place the point of the heel off the side of the bed, or positioning that leaves the point of the heel off the foot of the bed. A C-arm is brought in from the opposite side of the bed.

Implants
I prefer to use an axially directed large-fragment lag screw (6.5 mm). Larger screws can be used if the 6.5-mm screw strips its threads during placement. It is placed from the point of the heel through a stab incision be countersunk to avoid irritation from the screw head. A second screw is directed from the lateral talar process into the medial calcaneus. This provides an out-of-plane screw to the axial one and improves fixation. A 4.0-mm

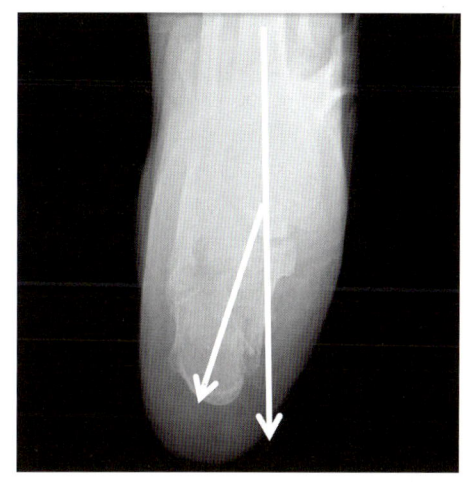

Figure 1 Long axial radiograph of the tibia, talus, and calcaneus demonstrates the weight-bearing line falling medial to the calcaneus. The calcaneus is in excessive valgus and thus would require correction if subtalar arthrodesis were performed.

cannulated screw is used. While excellent fusion rates have been reported with a single screw,[5] my anecdotal experience is that the second screw results in faster union with less pain (**Figure 2**).

Surgical Technique: In Situ Arthrodesis
Under tourniquet control, a 4- to 6-cm incision is made starting just distal to the tip of the fibula and overlying the anterior process of the calcaneus (**Figure 3**). The dissection may encounter the peroneal tendons but should leave them undisturbed in their sheath. The sural nerve should lie plantar to the incision. Dissection is carried sharply over the anterior process of the calcaneus. The tissues from the floor of the sinus tarsi are elevated. This will lead to the posterior facet of the subtalar joint. Exposure is improved if the talocalcaneal interosseous ligament is released. This allows for better separation of the joint surfaces for exposure. It also exposes the middle and anterior facets.

A small lamina spreader is introduced between the talus and calcaneus to distract the two surfaces. Occasionally, large osteophytes will have to be removed from the lateral process of the talus to improve exposure. At this point, a series of curets and osteotomes is used to denude the calcaneal and talar joint surfaces to bleeding subchondral bone. Care must

---

Dr. Carr is deceased. At the time this chapter was written, Dr. Carr or an immediate family member had received royalties from DePuy; was a member of a speakers' bureau or had made paid presentations on behalf of Stryker; and served as a paid consultant to or was an employee of Stryker and Biomet.

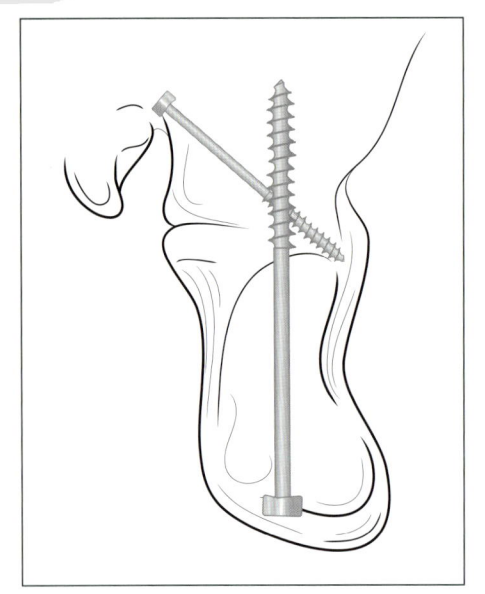

Figure 2 Illustration shows two screws used for subtalar arthrodesis. The larger screw is directed in an axial manner from the calcaneus into the talus. The second, smaller-diameter screw is directed from the lateral process of the talus into the medial wall of the calcaneus.

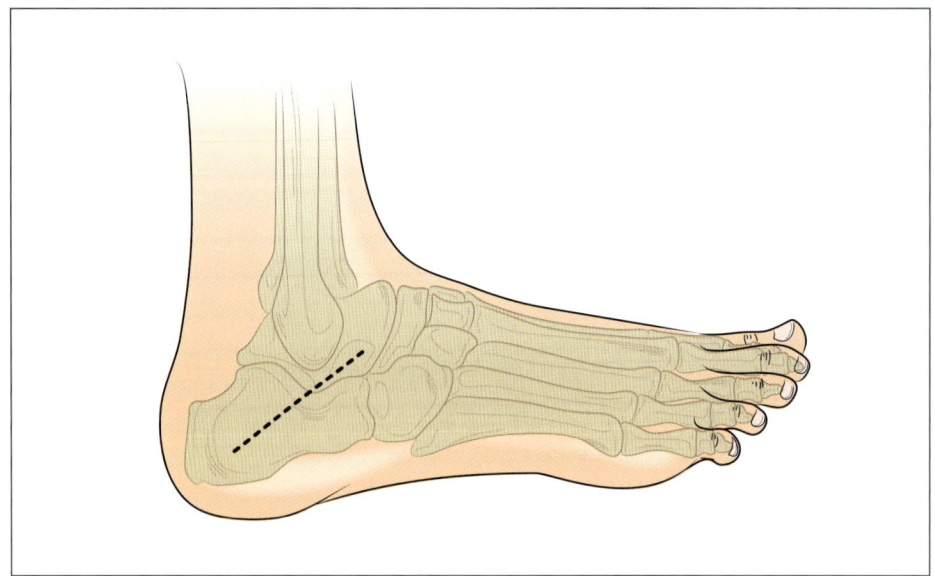

Figure 3 Illustration shows the sinus tarsi incision starts at the tip of the fibula and extends anteriorly along the anterior process of the calcaneus.

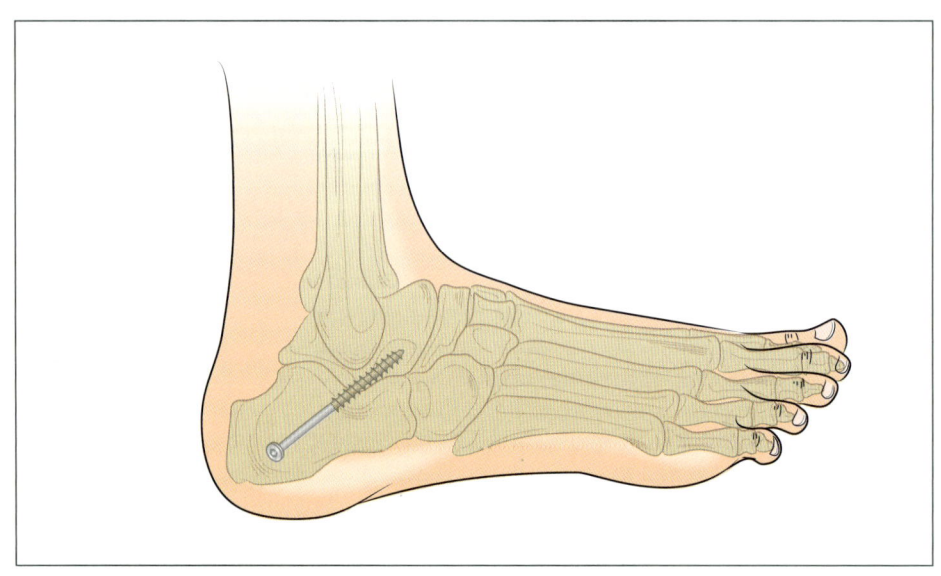

Figure 4 Illustration shows the axial screw is inserted from the tuberosity of the calcaneus, centrally into the talus.

be given to the deep, curvilinear shape of the posterior facet, which is difficult to thoroughly prepare. The anterior and middle facets should also be prepared to bleeding bone. Not only will this assist in healing, but it will also prevent the two facets from keeping the surfaces separated.

Once the bone surfaces are prepared, a 2.0-mm drill should be used to make multiple perforations. The subtalar joint is now compressed together to assess the bone contact. Any bone causing separation is resected. The ideal heel alignment is 7° of valgus. It can be assessed by radiographic means—views incorporating the tibia and calcaneus—and clinically. Min and Sanders[6] have also described assessment of the heel position on the mortise view of the ankle. Provisional fixation with a large wire is useful at this stage. Once the bone is adequately prepared and positioned, fixation is performed.

Fixation is performed with two screws (**Figure 2**). The first is a large-fragment screw directed from the tuberosity of the calcaneus into the body of the talus (**Figure 4**). The screw head should be countersunk to prevent symptomatic irritation, which may necessitate later removal. It may be cannulated according to surgeon preference. A 6.5- to 8.0-mm large-fragment screw with "short threads" (ie, 16 to 22 mm) should be chosen. The short thread length will avoid penetration of the ankle joint. It will also keep threads from crossing the arthrodesis site, aiding compression and bone healing. This screw position is assessed with the C-arm, using the lateral foot, AP ankle, and axial calcaneal views.

A second small-fragment lag screw is aimed from the lateral talar process into the medial wall of the calcaneus. The screw size can be either 4.0 mm or 3.5 mm. This screw head must also be countersunk well because it is inserted through the articular surface of the talus. Its insertion may require a separate anterior stab incision to obtain the proper insertion angle. Avoiding penetration of the medial calcaneal wall will prevent damage to the neurovascular and tendinous structures of the hindfoot. This screw depth is best judged on the axial view of the calcaneus. The purpose of the second screw is to augment fixation strength, as documented by Chuckpaiwong et al.[7] Additionally, because the axially directed large-fragment screw is placed in the rotational axis of the subtalar joint, the second screw will prevent this motion.

Bone graft is typically not used for an in situ arthrodesis. If desired, it may be harvested locally; for example, from the distal or proximal tibia. Bone graft substitutes are also an option, but they are not routinely used. The wound is closed in layered fashion. The patient is placed in either a posterior splint or a well-padded cast that will allow for postoperative swelling. Alternatively, the cast can be bivalved to accommodate swelling.

Deformity Correction

The most common reason for subtalar arthrodesis in a general practice is arthritis.

Chapter 78: Subtalar Arthrodesis

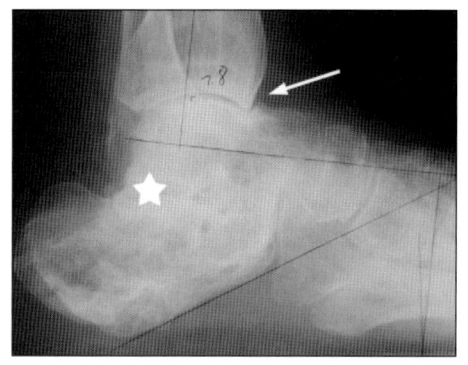

Figure 5 Lateral radiograph demonstrates a talus that is "horizontal" in relationship to the calcaneus. This produces tibiotalar neck impingement (arrow) with anterior ankle pain and restricts ankle dorsiflexion. It is most commonly seen after calcaneal fracture, but occasionally occurs in conditions like Charcot arthritis. The star indicates subtalar arthritis.

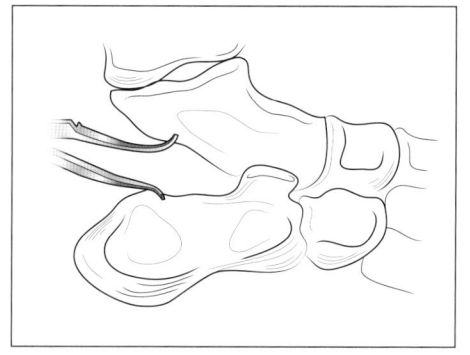

Figure 6 Illustration shows one method to correct a horizontal talus. The space between the calcaneus and talus is distracted with a lamina spreader. A tricortical bone graft is then placed in the resulting gap.

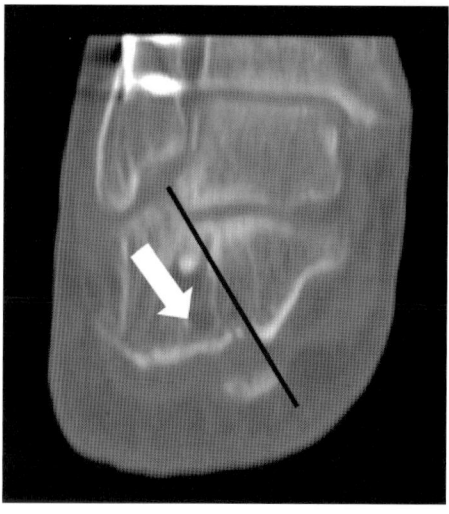

Figure 7 Axial CT scan of the calcaneus/talus demonstrates a Romash osteotomy. This re-creates the primary fracture line. The tuberosity of the calcaneus can then be shifted distally and medially to restore its anatomic alignment. The arrow denotes the direction of correction.

There may be a hindfoot deformity that needs to be addressed. A common deformity is valgus from end-stage posterior tibial tendon dysfunction (stage 4). In this instance, the valgus results from both lateral bone loss and rotation about the subtalar joint. In most cases, the deformity can be corrected with standard exposure and bone preparation. Attention must be paid to the middle and anterior facets. If they are not addressed, full correction of the valgus is difficult. If not prepared and contoured, they can serve as a medial strut that not only tilts the heel into more valgus but separates the posterior facet surfaces as well. Finally, in severe deformities without bone loss, release of the medial subtalar ligaments can free up the calcaneus to allow appropriate rotation and correction of malposition.

Maintaining the lateral talocalcaneal angle between 25° and 40° is possible in most cases. In extreme instances, such as a calcaneal malunion, a tricortical bone graft can be added to the subtalar joint if the lateral talocalcaneal angle is less than 25° after surface preparation (**Figures 5 and 6**).[8-10] This needs to be anticipated, as the graft is best applied through a posterolateral approach in the lateral decubitus position as described by Carr et al.[8] An alternative method for correction of calcaneal malunion is the Romash osteotomy (**Figure 7**). This osteotomy re-creates the original fracture line, allowing the tuberosity to be shifted back under the talus and thus regaining a more normal talocalcaneal relationship.

Varus alignment can almost always be corrected with standard bone preparation techniques. The use of screws with the shorter thread length tends to avoid both penetration of the ankle joint and allowing threads to cross the fusion site, hence decreasing the ability to apply compression and achieve rigid internal fixation. The position of this screw is assessed with fluoroscopy in the lateral foot, AP ankle, and axial views. Once again, all three facets must be prepared to properly free up the subtalar articulation. Release of the medial subtalar capsule is also useful and helps derotate the calcaneus. Failure to correct hindfoot varus will lock the transverse tarsal joint, resulting in a varus forefoot and excessive pressure through the lateral column of the foot.

Complications

The most common complication following subtalar arthrodesis is nonunion.[11] Coughlin et al[4] reported a nonunion rate of 35% at 6 months as demonstrated by CT scanning. Importantly, plain radiographs suggested union had occurred in 86%. Smoking, diabetes, and prior surgery are risk factors leading to higher nonunion rates. Nonunion may be treated with noninvasive bone stimulators, but many cases require reoperation. Bone grafting and refixation is advisable. Also, addition of the second screw as described above should be considered if a revision surgery is required.

Malunion is another complication of subtalar arthrodesis. Most commonly, this involves varus of the calcaneus. The patient notes "rolling in" of the ankle and walks with extra pressure on the lateral border of the foot. This situation is best evaluated with CT. If a varus deformity associated with a firm union is demonstrated on CT, the deformity can be corrected with a Dwyer laterally based closing wedge osteotomy. However, if there is significant malrotation of the entire hindfoot, the best method of correction involves osteotomy and recreation of the original subtalar joint. This will allow appropriate rotation of the calcaneus, in addition to corrective bone removal. Most commonly, this situation presents itself in the presence of a triple arthrodesis, in which case an additional transverse tarsal osteotomy is needed.

Postoperative Care and Rehabilitation

Postoperatively, the patient is kept non–weight bearing for the first 2 weeks, and strict elevation is encouraged. This will keep swelling down and assist pain control. At 2 weeks, the stitches are removed and a weight-bearing short leg cast is applied. Alternatively, a removable short leg orthosis ("walker boot") may be used. At 6 weeks, a radiograph is obtained and function is progressed based on the healing. Typically, a walking orthosis is recommended for 1 more month and then discontinued. Osseous union should be obtained by 3 months. If there are any questions regarding healing at this stage, a CT scan can be obtained.[4]

Outcomes

Reported union rates are 85 to 95%.[1-3] Subtalar arthrodesis should be considered a salvage procedure. Because subtalar motion is by definition obliterated, an important "shock absorbing" function of the foot is lost. This is the likely reason for the difficulty patients experience with activities such as walking on uneven surfaces. However, the pain relief for advanced arthritis can be gratifying, especially if deformity is also corrected. Most outcome studies show American Orthopaedic Foot & Ankle Society hindfoot scores in the upper 70s to middle 80s following subtalar arthrodesis.[11]

Pearls

- A preoperative CT scan is useful in determining the degree of subtalar arthritis and alignment. A three-dimensional reconstruction is useful for severe deformities and preoperative planning.
- The preoperative plan should determine if an in situ arthrodesis is appropriate. The goal should be the restoration of normal talocalcaneal relationships.
- Correction of deformity can be done with capsular release and bone shaping in most cases.
- Bone block distraction arthrodesis can correct loss of height in addition to calcaneal bone loss.
- Arthroscopic arthrodesis has been described using a prone position and two portals.[12,13]
- Countersinking of screws merits special attention, as they can cause symptoms if left prominent.
- The mortise view of the ankle will demonstrate heel valgus, in addition to confirming correct screw placement in the talus/calcaneus. Normal valgus will appear as the calcaneus aligned in slight lateral angulation in relation to the tibial axis.
- Release of the talocalcaneal ligament and medial capsule will allow distraction of the subtalar joint and improve access to the posterior portions of the joint.

References

1. Davies MB, Rosenfeld PF, Stavrou P, Saxby TS: A comprehensive review of subtalar arthrodesis. *Foot Ankle Int* 2007;28(3):295-297.
2. Easley ME, Trnka HJ, Schon LC, Myerson MS: Isolated subtalar arthrodesis. *J Bone Joint Surg Am* 2000;82(5):613-624.
3. Chahal J, Stephen DJ, Bulmer B, Daniels T, Kreder HJ: Factors associated with outcome after subtalar arthrodesis. *J Orthop Trauma* 2006;20(8):555-561.
4. Coughlin MJ, Grimes JS, Traughber PD, Jones CP: Comparison of radiographs and CT scans in the prospective evaluation of the fusion of hindfoot arthrodesis. *Foot Ankle Int* 2006;27(10):780-787.
5. DeCarbo WT, Berlet GC, Hyer CF, Smith WB: Single-screw fixation for subtalar joint fusion does not increase nonunion rate. *Foot Ankle Spec* 2010;3(4):164-166.
6. Min W, Sanders RW: The use of the mortise view of the ankle to determine hindfoot alignment: Technique tip. *Foot Ankle Int* 2010;31(9):823-827.
7. Chuckpaiwong B, Easley ME, Glisson RR: Screw placement in subtalar arthrodesis: A biomechanical study. *Foot Ankle Int* 2009;30(2):133-141.
8. Carr JB, Hansen ST, Benirschke SK: Subtalar distraction bone block fusion for late complications of os calcis fractures. *Foot Ankle* 1988;9(2):81-86.
9. Radnay CS, Clare MP, Sanders RW: Subtalar fusion after displaced intra-articular calcaneal fractures: Does initial operative treatment matter? Surgical technique. *J Bone Joint Surg Am* 2010;92(Suppl 1, Pt 1):32-43.
10. Deorio JK, Leaseburg JT, Shapiro SA: Subtalar distraction arthrodesis through a posterior approach. *Foot Ankle Int* 2008;29(12):1189-1194.
11. Diezi C, Favre P, Vienne P: Primary isolated subtalar arthrodesis: Outcome after 2 to 5 years followup. *Foot Ankle Int* 2008;29(12):1195-1202.
12. Amendola A, Lee KB, Saltzman CL, Suh JS: Technique and early experience with posterior arthroscopic subtalar arthrodesis. *Foot Ankle Int* 2007;28(3):298-302.
13. Glanzmann MC, Sanhueza-Hernandez R: Arthroscopic subtalar arthrodesis for symptomatic osteoarthritis of the hindfoot: A prospective study of 41 cases. *Foot Ankle Int* 2007;28(1):2-7.

Chapter 79
Arthrodesis of the Tarsometatarsal Joint

J. Chris Coetzee, MD, FRCSC   Pascal Rippstein, MD

Introduction
Anatomy
The unique anatomy of the tarsometatarsal (TMT) joint complex, also called the Lisfranc joint, contributes to the spectrum of injury patterns. The stability of the TMT joint complex is maintained by a combination of the wedge-shaped configuration of the metatarsal bases and their corresponding cuneiform articulations, as well as by ligamentous support (**Figure 1**).

The Lisfranc ligament is composed of three portions, running from the medial cuneiform to the base of the second metatarsal. The strongest part is the plantar portion of the ligament, which is the main stabilizing component of the first and second metatarsal interspace. There is very little motion at the second and third TMT joints, 10° to 20° at the fourth and fifth metatarsal-cuboid, and 5° to 10° at the first TMT joint.

The second TMT joint is recessed between the medial and lateral cuneiforms. The strong plantar ligaments "lock" the metatarsals to the midfoot.

A very important factor to remember is that Lisfranc joints have no inherent stability. The joints are flat on flat surfaces and rely on ligamentous stability to maintain reduction (compared with the inherent stability of a ball-and-socket joint).

Patient Selection
Indications
TMT arthrodesis, or fusion, can be indicated for a variety of problems, including acute fracture or instability, but most of these procedures are done for chronic deformity and pain.[1] Chronic deformity and pain can be secondary to prior Lisfranc injury; they also can be due to primary degenerative changes or Charcot neuroarthropathy.

Indications for primary fusions of TMT joints include (1) major ligamentous disruptions with multidirectional instability/dislocation of the Lisfranc joints, (2) comminuted intra-articular fractures at the base of the first or second metatarsal, and (3) crush injuries of the midfoot with intra-articular fracture-dislocation.[2,3]

Indications for secondary TMT fusions include (1) posttraumatic degenerative joint disease (DJD) after Lisfranc injuries, (2) idiopathic/primary TMT DJD, (3) rheumatoid arthritis, and (4) stable/chronic Charcot neuroarthropathy or other complications of diabetes.[4-6]

Figures 2, 3, and **4** show three different scenarios where a TMT fusion is indicated. Each creates a different challenge in treatment, but the surgical principles stay the same.

Contraindications
Contraindications for fusion of the TMT joints are (1) skeletal immaturity/open physes; (2) acute Charcot neuroarthropathy (relative); (3) simple, incomplete ligamentous injuries; and (4) active infection. Charcot neuroarthropathy can be approached with care; it should be dealt with acutely only if there is impending skin breakdown.

Procedure
Surgical Technique
The surgical approach for a TMT fusion is exactly the same as the approach commonly used for an open reduction and internal fixation of a Lisfranc injury. A calf or thigh tourniquet is used and inflated to 250 mm Hg. Depending on the number of TMT joints involved in the injury or arthritic process, one or two dorsal, longitudinal incisions are made.

The first incision is made between the first and second metatarsals (**Figure 5**). This will allow access to the first TMT joint and most of the second. Pathology involving only the medial two TMT joints can be corrected with this single incision. If there is any concern about the accuracy of the reduction, it is advisable to do a second, more lateral incision to facilitate exposure and visualization of the joint.[2]

If there is a reason to fuse the third TMT joint, a second lateral incision should always be made. We believe that it is advisable to be liberal with the use of a two-incision approach; adequate exposure of the lateral corner of the second metatarsal base and the lateral cuneiform through a single dorsomedial incision can be very hard to obtain.

It is extremely rare that the fourth and fifth TMT joints would need to be fused. The only time when it is reasonable is in severe deformities secondary to Charcot neuroarthropathy, where the lateral border of the foot needs to be elevated.

The second incision is centered over the fourth metatarsal; in reality it is much farther lateral than what is appreciated. The most common mistake is to make the incision too far medial. Incision placement may be aided by fluoroscopic guidance and the identification of the intended bony targets. The foot should be internally rotated to obtain an end-on view of the fourth metatarsal. If the radiograph is taken with the foot in a neutral position,

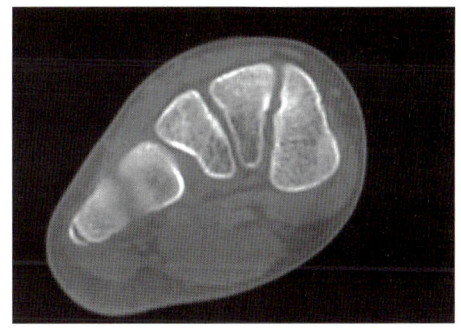

Figure 1 CT scan demonstrates the configuration of the Lisfranc complex, which mimics a "Roman arch," in which the stability is dependent upon the bony configuration and ligament stability. There is no inherent joint stability.

Dr. Coetzee or an immediate family member has received royalties from Arthrex, DePuy, and MMI; is a member of a speakers' bureau or has made paid presentations on behalf of Arthrex and Tornier; serves as a paid consultant to or is an employee of Arthrex, Tornier, Zimmer, and Allosource; owns stock or stock options in Tornier; has received research or institutional support from DePuy, Zimmer, and Allosource; and serves as a board member, owner, officer, or committee member of the American Orthopaedic Foot & Ankle Society and the American Academy of Orthopaedic Surgeons. Dr. Rippstein or an immediate family member has received royalties from DePuy; is a member of a speakers' bureau or has made paid presentations on behalf of DePuy; and serves as a paid consultant to or is an employee of DePuy.

Section 6: Foot and Ankle

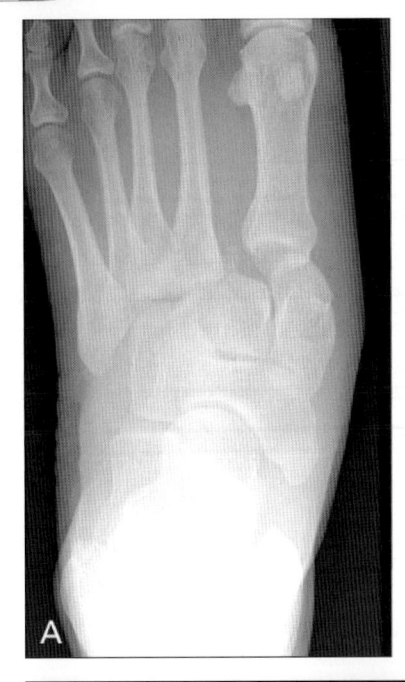

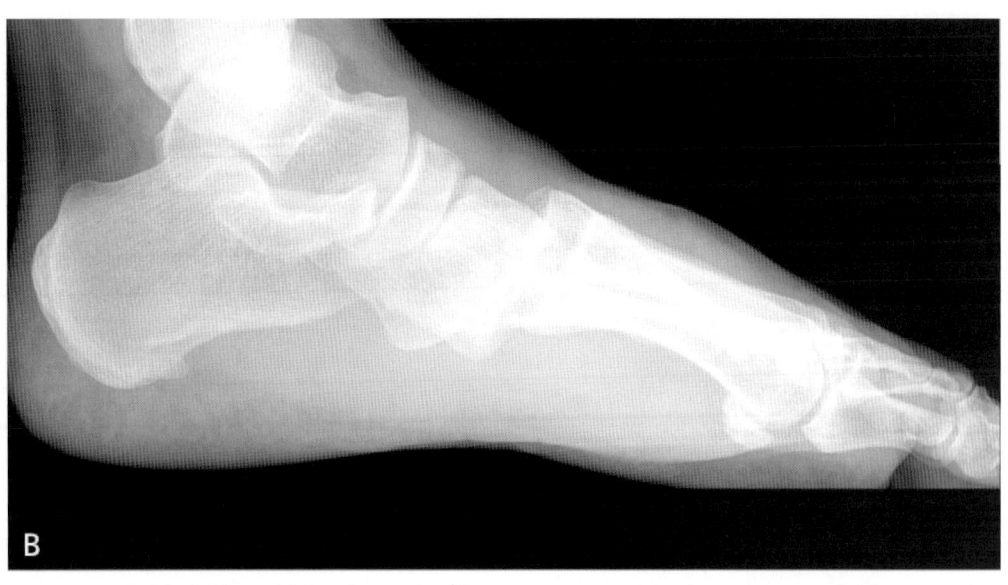

Figure 2 AP (**A**) and lateral (**B**) radiographs of an acute traumatic Lisfranc fracture-dislocation with signs of intra-articular fractures.

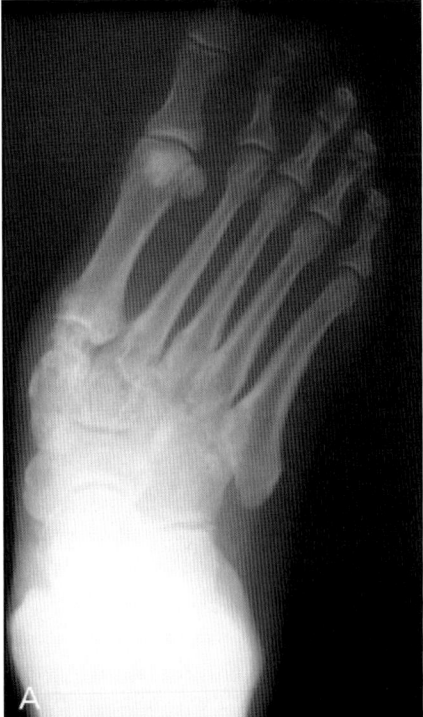

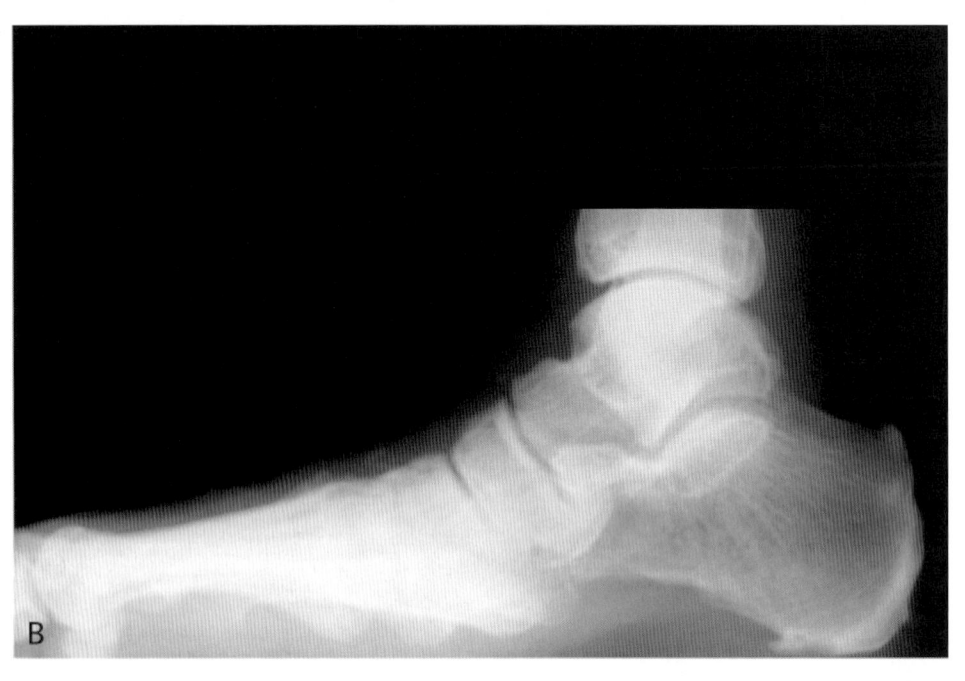

Figure 3 AP (**A**) and lateral (**B**) radiographs show severe deformity in the sagittal and coronal planes secondary to an untreated or poorly treated Lisfranc injury 15 years earlier.

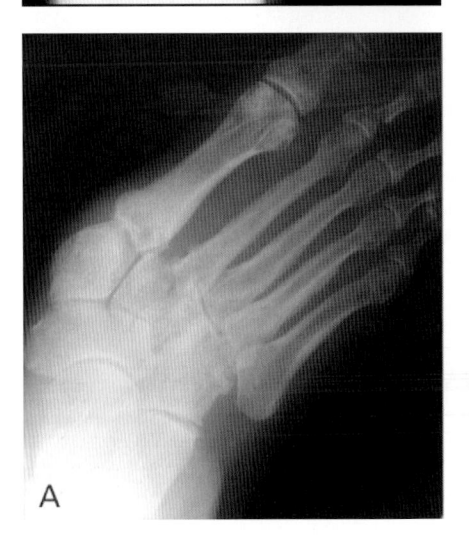

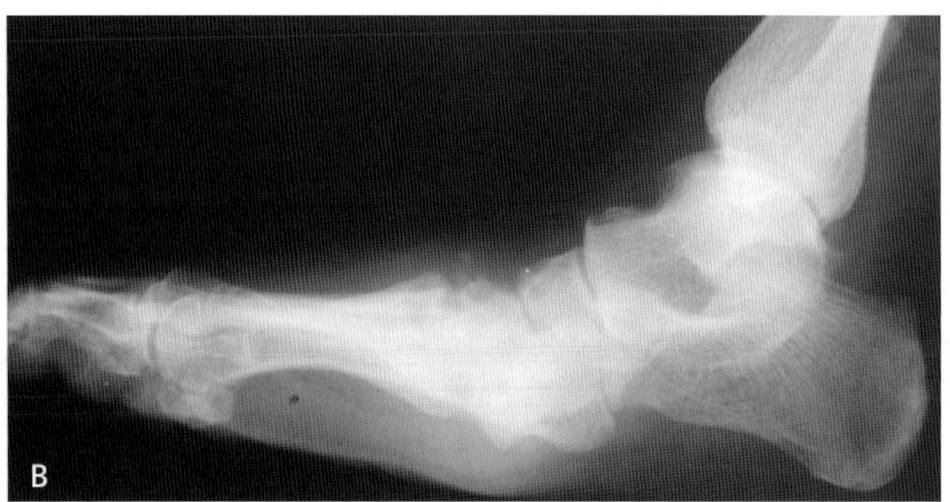

Figure 4 AP (**A**) and lateral (**B**) radiographs demonstrate severe deformity in all planes secondary to Charcot neuroarthropathy in patient with type 1 diabetes.

Chapter 79: Arthrodesis of the Tarsometatarsal Joint

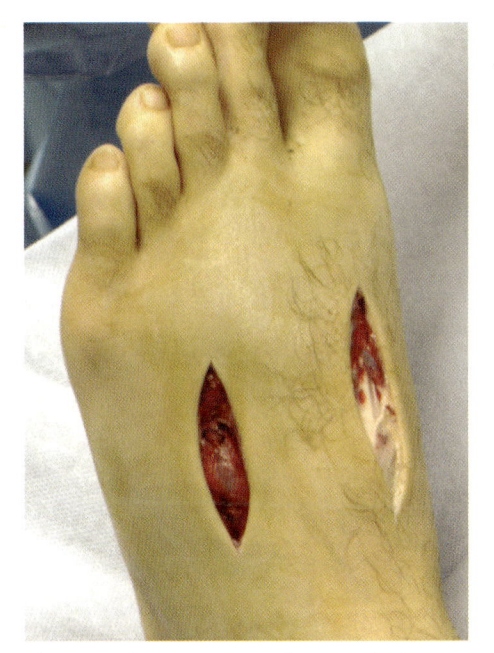

Figure 5 Intraoperative photograph shows the surgical approaches for a tarsometatarsal joint fusion in a left foot. The medial incision is between the first and second metatarsals, just lateral to the extensor hallucis tendon. The lateral incision is at least 4 cm farther lateral, overlying the fourth metatarsal.

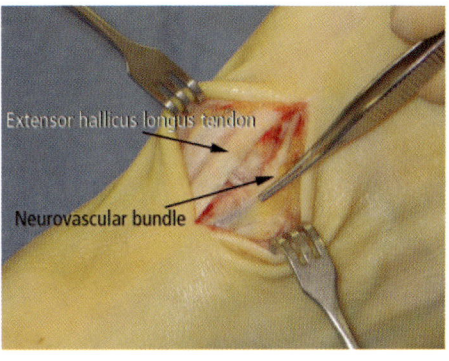

Figure 6 In this close-up intraoperative photograph of a left foot, the extensor hallucis longus tendon is medial. The dorsalis pedis artery and the deep peroneal nerve are lateral to the tendon and will be encountered during the exposure. A branch of the superficial peroneal nerve usually runs from lateral to medial across the distal portion of the exposure.

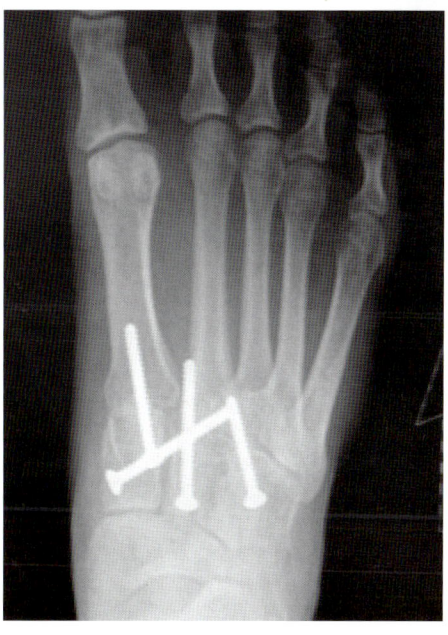

Figure 7 AP radiograph shows typical screw placement in reduction of a dislocation of the first through third TMT joints. The first ray is immobilized first, followed by the second and then the third.

there is too much overlap between the third, fourth, and fifth metatarsals to accurately determine the position of the fourth ray.

This incision endangers the lateral branches of the superficial peroneal nerve, and they should also be protected. The incision is usually just lateral to the extensor digitorum longus tendon, which is easily retracted to expose the underlying extensor digitorum brevis. The brevis muscle belly is divided longitudinally by sharp dissection. This allows visualization of the third, fourth, and lateral half of the second TMT joints.

The structures to protect with the medial incision include the superficial and deep peroneal nerves and the dorsalis pedis artery. A 6-cm incision is made just lateral to the extensor hallucis tendon. The distal end of the incision extends to about 3 cm distal to the first TMT joint level. The sensory branches of the superficial peroneal nerve are retracted laterally with the dorsalis pedis artery. At the distal end of the incision is a vein typically found crossing the field; this should be cauterized if it is in the way (**Figure 6**).

Due to the ligamentous disruption, the unstable segments are usually easily recognized in acute trauma. Most often the dorsal capsular and ligamentous structures will also be disrupted. The hematoma is evacuated from the joints to allow adequate exposure and visualization. Typically, even in ligamentous injuries, a small avulsion fracture is seen at the medial base of the second metatarsal where the Lisfranc ligament attaches.

It is important at this point to determine which joints are involved in the instability pattern. This is accomplished visually and under fluoroscopy. The hindfoot is stabilized while the forefoot is manipulated, first with an abduction and adduction force, followed by plantar flexion and dorsiflexion stress.

In the chronic situation with advanced DJD, there is often significant deformity of the TMT joints with lateral (adduction) deviation as well as dorsiflexion collapse of the metatarsals. An in situ fusion is very rarely indicated, and the goal should be to have an anatomic restoration in all planes.[1]

The TMT joints should therefore be adequately mobilized to allow reduction in all planes. This usually requires a fairly extensile soft-tissue release around the involved joints.

Fusion for primary indications is no more difficult than an open reduction and internal fixation. Care is taken to adequately débride the joints. Any small, free pieces of cartilage should be removed. The articular cartilage is then removed from the opposing surfaces of the joints. This is done with small rongeurs, curets, and small osteotomes. The goal is to remove only the cartilage and expose subchondral bone. It is not necessary or advisable to use a saw to prepare the surfaces. Saw cuts might shorten the metatarsal and the cuneiform, which is not of any benefit.

The first TMT joint is about 30 mm deep. A small lamina spreader is very helpful in allowing full visualization of the entire joint. In the absence of full exposure of the depth of the joint, there is a tendency to fuse the joint in dorsiflexion.

After complete removal of the cartilage, the surfaces are prepared for fusion by feathering the opposing surfaces with a small osteotome or small-diameter drill.

As a general rule, the first TMT joint is secured first. The reduction and alignment are confirmed visually and under fluoroscopy. A temporary Kirschner wire (K-wire) is inserted to stabilize the joint. This is followed by the use of a 3-mm, 4-mm, or 5-mm cortical screw, depending on the size of the patient, to internally fix the joint. We typically place the screw from the medial cuneiform into the first metatarsal, but it can also be done from the first metatarsal to the medial cuneiform. This allows for a stable medial column as a foundation to which the remaining metatarsals may be secured. The next step is to reduce the second metatarsal base into the keystone position. A clamp is used to pull the metatarsal base onto the lateral aspect of the first metatarsal and the adjacent medial cuneiform (**Figure 7**).

The most common mistake made here is to inadvertently elevate the second metatarsal in the process of screw placement. It is therefore imperative to visually—but also radiographically—check the align-

© 2013 American Academy of Orthopaedic Surgeons

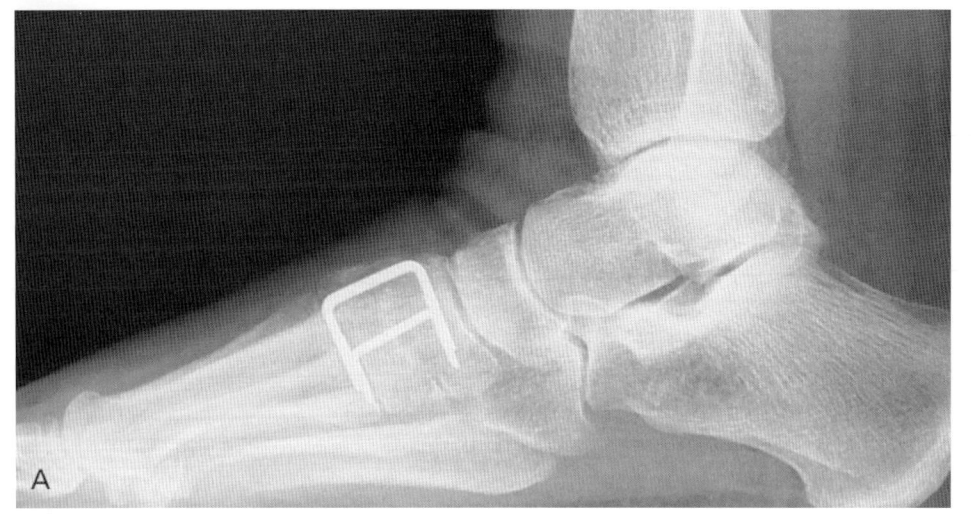

Figure 8 Lateral (**A**) and AP (**B**) radiographs show staple fixation of the second and third TMT joints. This is technically easier than screws.

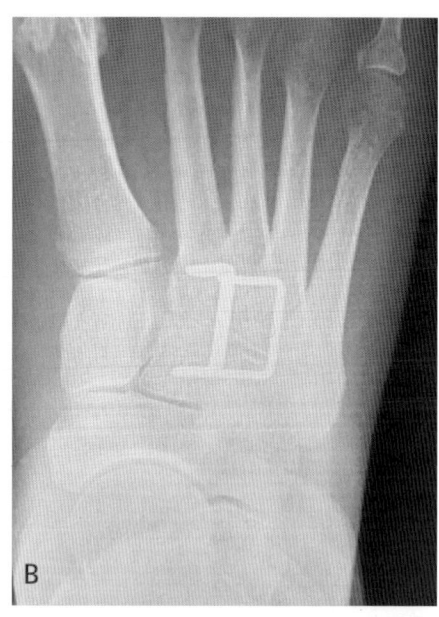

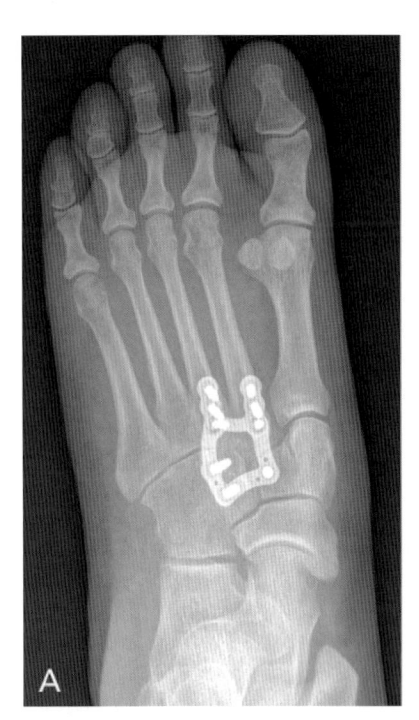

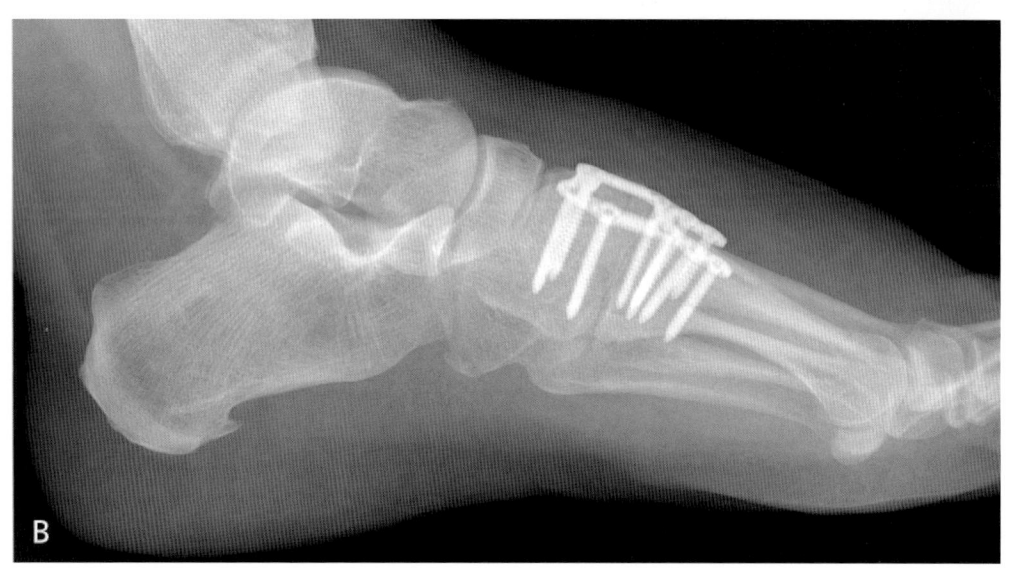

Figure 9 AP (**A**) and lateral (**B**) radiographs show plate fixation, which is a better option than screws or staples for significant communication of the metatarsal bases. With the plate construct, the surgeon can maintain length and alignment while immobilizing the joints.

ment of the metatarsal. The second screw is inserted from the medial cuneiform into the base of the second metatarsal.

If there is intercuneiform instability or DJD, the same incision is used, and the screw from the medial aspect of the medial cuneiform and the base of the second metatarsal is augmented with an intercuneiform screw.

The technique and method of further fixation is somewhat dependent on the individual situation and personal preference. There should be at least one more fixation point across the second and, if needed, the third TMT joints. This could be done with additional screws, staples, or plate fixation.

The technically simplest method for the second and third TMT joints is to use any of the commercially available compression staples (**Figure 8**). This is acceptable if the joints are well aligned and reduced. Especially for the third TMT joint, this is simpler than a screw. The acute angle required to insert the screw can make it difficult, especially in small patients.

If a fusion is done for an acute, comminuted intra-articular or proximal metatarsal fracture, a dorsal plate might be indicated to span and immobilize the fractured portion of the metatarsal as well (**Figure 9**). There are several plating systems available that are specifically designed for this purpose.

In the garden-variety primary fusion, bone graft is seldom needed. There are usually no voids to fill, and joint apposition is excellent.

These screw and/or staple constructs are usually sufficient for the indications for primary TMT fusions, but more often than not these constructs provide inadequate fixation in the secondary group, especially for a post-Charcot collapse. Whether the deformity is due to chronic posttraumatic DJD or Charcot, the loss of ligamentous integrity leads to deformity in the sagittal and coronal planes. There is a combination of metatarsus adductus and dorsiflexion of varying degrees. It could range from a subtle collapse on one end of the spectrum to a severe deformity resulting in a plantar or plantar-medial ulcer due to pressure on the medial cuneiform on the other end of the spectrum.

In long-standing cases, there are secondary bony changes that make the surgical correction much more complicated (**Figures 3** and **4**). These fusions are more challenging, as can be expected. It is imperative to completely mobilize all the joints with adequate soft-tissue dissection to allow reduction in all planes. With severe deformities, it is often advisable to add a plantar-medial incision (Figure 10). This will greatly aid in achieving reduction, removing the prominence and allowing for plate fixation on the tension side of the Lisfranc joints.[6]

With this incision, the insertion of the tibialis anterior attachment on the cuneiform and metatarsals will invariably be in the way. If it is not possible to work around the tendon, there should be a low threshold to detach it as far as needed to achieve reduction, with the understanding that it should be reattached at the end of the procedure.

We believe one should, at least initially, be very careful not to make saw cuts to achieve reduction. We prefer to do a complete soft-tissue release, remove whatever cartilage is left, remove osteophytes, and then reduce the TMT joints and do a temporary K-wire fixation.

At this point, the surgeon will be able to access the bone loss and actual apposition of the joints. Due to the extension/adduction collapse, the bone defects will be dorsal and lateral. If the defects are relatively small, they could be filled with autologous bone graft. If the defects are large and there is limited contact between the metatarsals and corresponding cuneiform, one could do very careful bone resections to allow for a larger contact area before grafting and fixation. It is best to start plantar medial and work across to the lateral side. The second and third joints are prepared through the dorsal incisions. Bone cuts should start small. It is deceptively easy to create larger defects than what one started with.

If there is excellent apposition of the joints, the fixation could be as described for primary fusions. In reality, however, most secondary fusions need more powerful fixation.

A plantar-medial plate can be a very secure and powerful way to reduce and align the medial column. A compression screw is first inserted across the first TMT joint, followed by the plantar plate. The dorsal and lateral joint defects are then grafted, followed by fixation. There are several excellent plate options available that could span the first, second, and third TMT joints, depending on the situation.

Figures 11 through 13 show the postoperative results of the surgical procedures done for the index cases shown in Figures 2 through 4. As illustrated in the figures, the more severe the deformity, the harder it is to make it look perfect on a radiograph.

Complications

The pitfalls for surgery around the TMT joints are similar, whether the surgeon does an open reduction and internal fixation or a primary or a secondary fusion.

Superficial sensory nerve injury could cause considerable morbidity to the patient if a neuroma forms in this area.

The dorsalis pedis and the deep peroneal nerve are in the interval between the extensor hallucis longus and brevis. The dorsalis pedis courses from dorsal to plantar in the foot between the first and second metatarsals about 1 cm distal to the first TMT joint. With the "home run screw" from the medial cuneiform to the base of the second metatarsal, this artery is at risk and could be damaged.

The third TMT joint is much farther lateral than appreciated. There should therefore be at least a 4-cm bridge between the two incisions, and it is preferable to confirm one's location under fluoroscopy before making the second incision.

Due to the angle required to insert screws, it is sometimes very hard to get a good compression screw into the third TMT joint. An alternative is to use a staple, which is usually easier to position and insert.

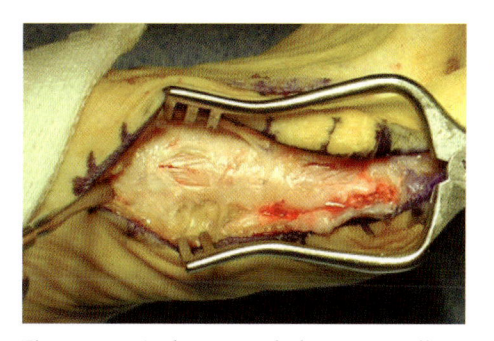

Figure 10 A plantar-medial incision will greatly aid in the ability to correct severe deformities in the TMT area. The Freer elevator in this intraoperative photograph shows the tibialis anterior tendon, which is encountered with this incision.

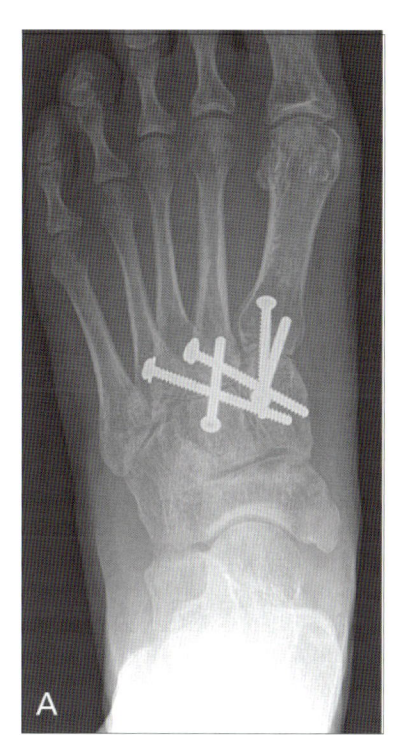

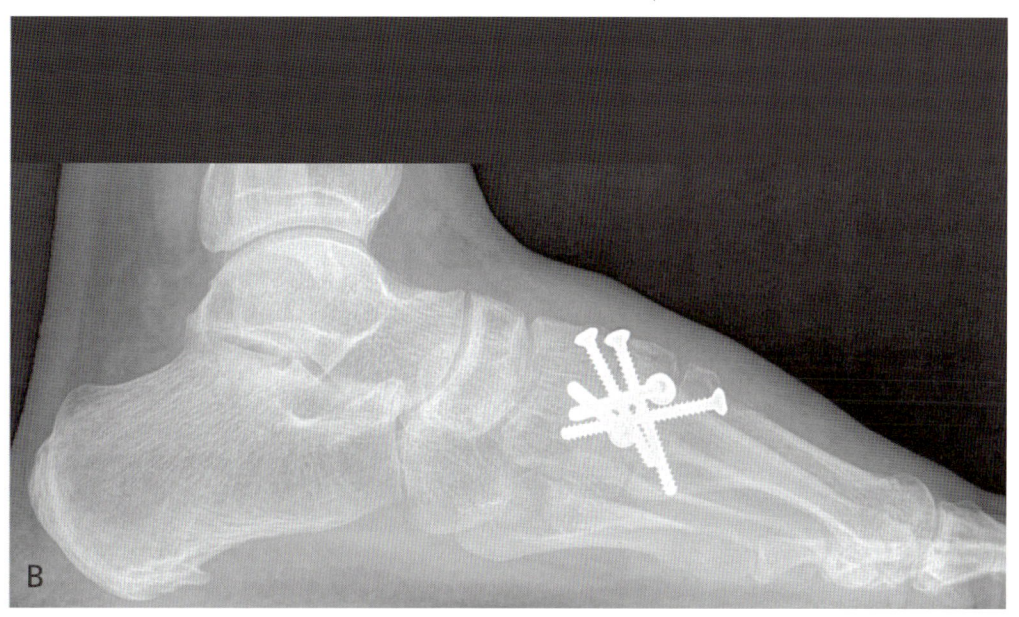

Figure 11 AP (**A**) and lateral (**B**) radiographs of the patient in Figure 2 after a fusion using screws. Reduction and alignment is fairly predictable if done early.

Section 6: Foot and Ankle

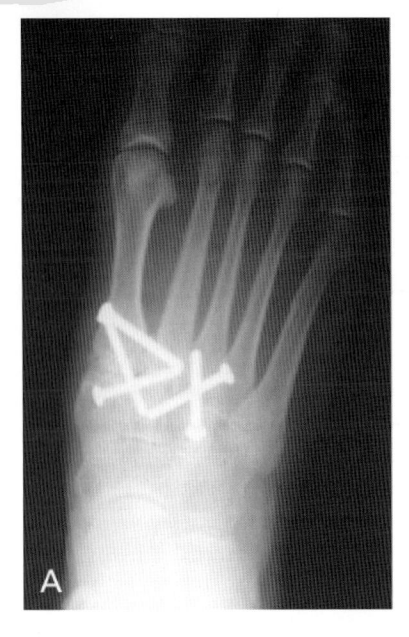

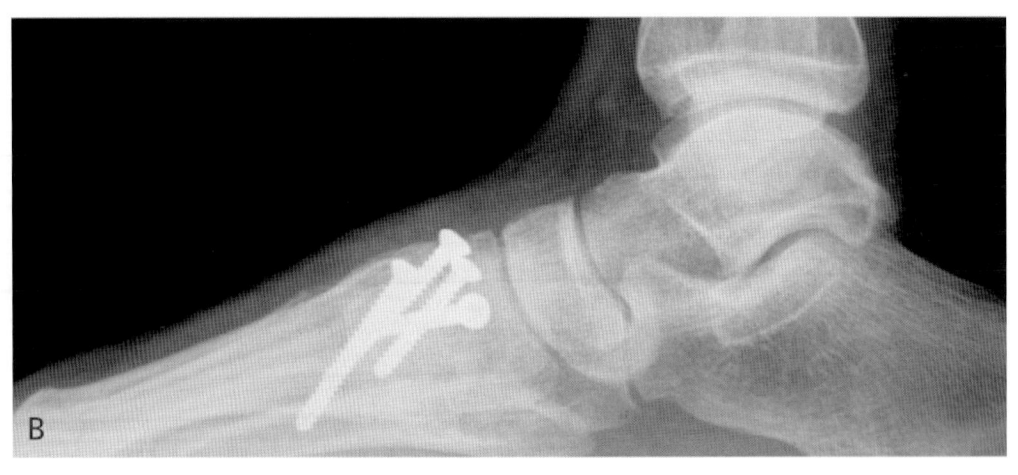

Figure 12 AP (**A**) and lateral (**B**) radiographs of the patient in Figure 3 after a fusion. The sagittal plane reduction is much improved but not perfect. Coronal alignment is perfect, with excellent restoration of the longitudinal arch of the foot.

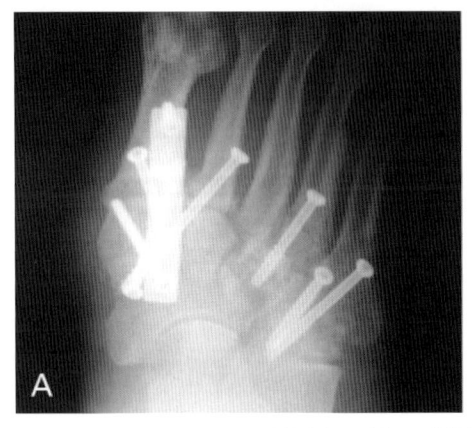

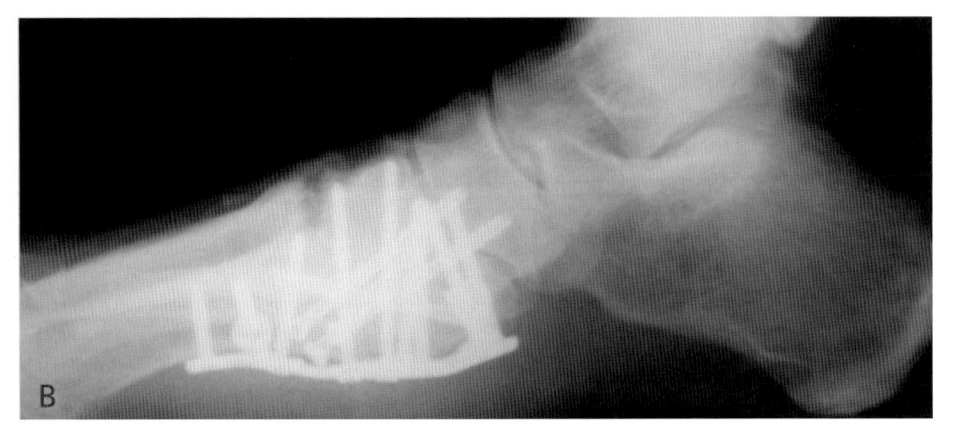

Figure 13 Postoperative AP (**A**) and lateral (**B**) radiographs of the patient in Figure 4 show satisfactory sagittal and coronal plane reduction using a combination of a plantar plate for the medial ray and screws for the lateral rays. A plantar plate can provide excellent strength and stability on the tension side of the joint in severe deformities. This is one of the few cases where a fusion of the lateral two rays is done to also restore the lateral border after severe collapse due to the Charcot process.

The first TMT joint is about 30 mm deep. Without adequate exposure and distraction, the surgeon might not be able to remove all of the cartilage from the plantar third of the joint, which would place the metatarsal in a dorsiflexed position if compressed for arthrodesis.

Postoperative Care and Rehabilitation

Due to the shear, instead of axial, forces on the TMT joints, postoperative care is important. As a general rule, the patient is immobilized in a cast splint after surgery. The patient should be non–weight bearing for the first 2 weeks with the aid of crutches or a knee scooter.

Sutures are removed at 2 weeks and the patient is placed in a pneumatic removable walker. From week 2 to week 6, the patient should still be essentially non–weight bearing but could be heel weight bearing in the shower. It is advisable to remove the walker boot several times a day to do active range of motion of the ankle. Most patients are comfortable enough that they do not have to sleep with the boot after 4 weeks.

At 6 weeks, radiographs are taken to evaluate the fusion. If it looks good, the patient can start to bear weight flat-footed in the walker boot and start physical therapy.

Initial therapy is geared toward reduction of swelling and active range of motion. Straight-line activities can be resumed if comfortable. Active single-leg heel raises should be avoided for the first 3 months after surgery, unless there is very clear evidence that the fusion is completely solid.

At 3 months, rehabilitation moves into a more restorative phase, and the patient is allowed to be without the boot and increase proprioception, endurance, and strength. Agility training can usually start by the fourth month, but it takes at least 6 months to return to full unrestricted activity and footwear.

Pearls
- The neurovascular structures must be protected.
- An adequate exposure and soft-tissue release are necessary to allow reduction.
- A deformity should not be fused in situ.
- Bone graft is used only as needed, especially if there are dorsal and lateral defects after reduction.
- Adequate fixation must be used because of the large forces over the TMT joints.

References
1. Sangeorzan BJ, Veith RG, Hansen ST Jr: Salvage of Lisfranc's tarsometatarsal joint by arthrodesis. *Foot Ankle* 1990;10(4): 193-200.
2. Coetzee JC, Ly TV: Treatment of primarily ligamentous Lisfranc joint injuries: Primary arthrodesis compared with open reduction and internal fixation.

Surgical technique. *J Bone Joint Surg Am* 2007;89(Suppl 2 Pt 1):122-127.

3. Henning JA, Jones CB, Sietsema DL, Bohay DR, Anderson JG: Open reduction internal fixation versus primary arthrodesis for Lisfranc injuries: A prospective randomized study. *Foot Ankle Int* 2009;30(10):913-922.

4. Rammelt S, Schneiders W, Schikore H, Holch M, Heineck J, Zwipp H: Primary open reduction and fixation compared with delayed corrective arthrodesis in the treatment of tarsometatarsal (Lisfranc) fracture dislocation. *J Bone Joint Surg Br* 2008;90(11):1499-1506.

5. Teng AL, Pinzur MS, Lomasney L, Mahoney L, Havey R: Functional outcome following anatomic restoration of tarsal-metatarsal fracture dislocation. *Foot Ankle Int* 2002;23(10):922-926.

6. Simon SR, Tejwani SG, Wilson DL, Santner TJ, Denniston NL: Arthrodesis as an early alternative to nonoperative management of Charcot arthropathy of the diabetic foot. *J Bone Joint Surg Am* 2000;82-A(7):939-950.

Chapter 80
Surgical Treatment of Navicular Stress Fractures

Bethany Gallagher, MD   Arthur K. Walling, MD

Patient Selection

Navicular stress fractures are most frequently seen in active patients who participate in demanding, high-impact/explosive athletics involving sprinting and jumping. These injuries require a high level of suspicion, as the presenting symptoms are nonspecific and have an insidious onset.[1,2] Patients present with a host of foot symptoms, from vague arch "cramping" to prolonged swelling and midfoot tenderness. The symptoms are quite difficult to localize and initially are troublesome only during the activity. Ultimately, they progress to more debilitating and consistent pain.[1]

Frequently, there is a delay in diagnosis and initiation of appropriate treatment, ranging from 4 to 7.2 months.[3] This delay is attributed to the nonspecific symptoms as well as initial misdiagnosis. The clinical findings and history can often be confused with posterior/anterior tibial tendinitis, midfoot sprain, and ankle sprains. Only when patients fail to improve is further imaging performed and the treatment redirected.

To guide treatment of a navicular stress fracture, a classification scheme was developed to identify displaced versus nondisplaced and complete versus incomplete fracture patterns. This is important in the discussion with the patient regarding options and potential surgical intervention. Nonsurgical management is frequently offered to patients with complete nondisplaced or partial fractures of the navicular. This involves a minimum of 6 to 8 weeks of dedicated time in a non–weight-bearing cast before advancing weight bearing. Multiple studies have consistently shown that immobilization with weight bearing leads to treatment failure, nonunion, and inability to return to preinjury activity.[1,3,4] However, in the compliant patient population, studies have reported successful outcomes with non–weight-bearing immobilization for a minimum of 6 weeks. Torg et al[3] showed 100% fracture union, and Khan et al[4] reported 86% return to sports at an average of 5.6 months. Navicular stress fractures successfully treated with this protocol were incomplete or nondisplaced patterns. Patients with displaced fractures, patients who cannot tolerate prolonged immobilization, or those in whom nonunion develops despite immobilization are offered surgical intervention.[3,5-7]

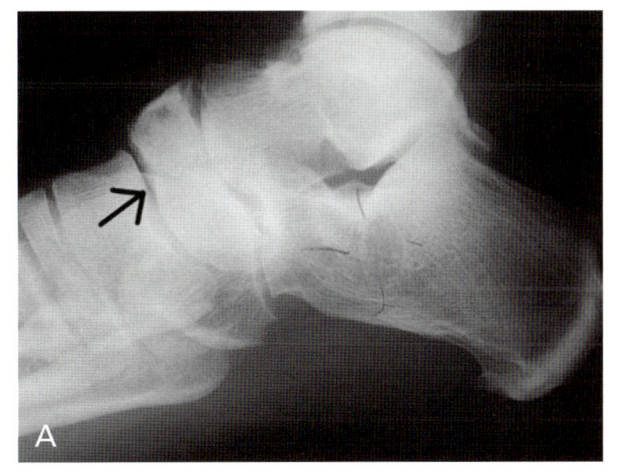

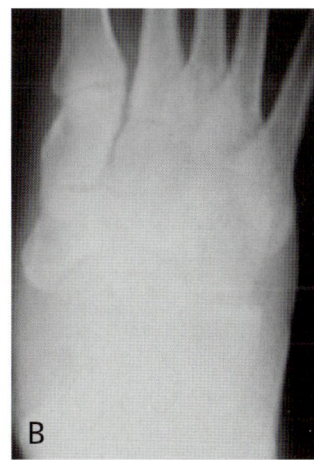

Figure 1 Lateral (**A**) and AP (**B**) weight-bearing radiographs of a foot with a displaced navicular stress fracture (arrow).

Preoperative Imaging

On initial evaluation, the patient undergoes a standard weight-bearing radiographic series of the foot, including AP, oblique, and lateral views. Often, these provide little information because a stress injury is difficult to visualize on radiographs. Several studies have confirmed the significantly low rate of detection on radiographs, ranging from 67% to 82%.[3,4] However, weight-bearing radiographs are low-cost initial screening instruments that can show displacement of a complete navicular stress fracture and cystic change or progressive arthritic change of the talonavicular joint, as well as overall foot alignment, which may be important in a discussion of reconstruction and may eliminate the need for further costly imaging modalities (**Figure 1**).

The next stage of imaging is often dependent on the initial radiographs. If the fracture is identified on radiographs or if they show navicular sclerosis suggestive of further pathology, the patient is sent for a CT scan to further delineate the fracture pattern, any associated arthritic change, and any degenerative cyst development[2] (**Figure 2**). When the initial radiographs are not diagnostic but the history and examination are consistent with a potential stress injury, a bone scan or an MRI can be used to identify bony uptake or edema and fracture lines, respectively (**Figures 3 and 4**).[1] Bone scans are 100% sensitive for injury, but positive findings are unfortunately nonspecific.[3,4] MRI reduces radiation exposure and shows additional soft-tissue detail but has limited capability to accurately identify all navicular stress fractures.[8] MRI may be most beneficial in the early stage of diagnosis to identify a stress reaction before fracture. Therefore, these patients still require a conclusive CT scan following a positive result. The most typical navicular stress fracture pattern on CT is an incomplete fracture in the central third of the bone extending from dorsal-medial to plantar-lateral.[1] The CT scan is the most critical imaging modality for fracture classification and surgical planning with navicular stress fractures.[9]

Procedure
Patient Positioning

The patient is placed in the supine position with a small bump under the

---

Dr. Walling or an immediate family member is a member of a speakers' bureau or has made paid presentations on behalf of SBI and Synthes and serves as a board member, owner, officer, or committee member of the American Academy of Orthopaedic Surgeons. Neither Dr. Gallagher nor any immediate family member has received anything of value from or owns stock in a commercial company or institution related directly or indirectly to the subject of this chapter.

Section 6: Foot and Ankle

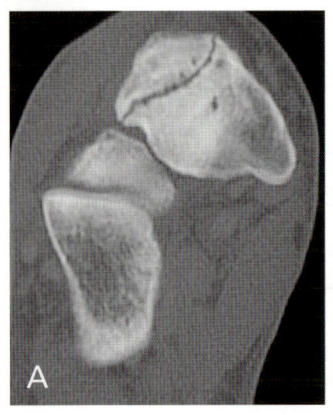

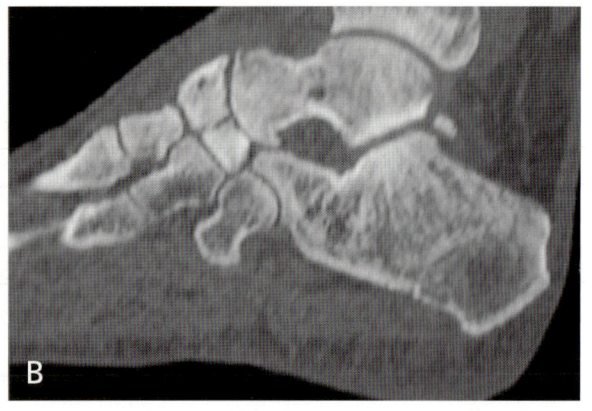

Figure 2 Axial (**A**) and sagittal (**B**) CT scan cuts show a complete navicular stress fracture pattern.

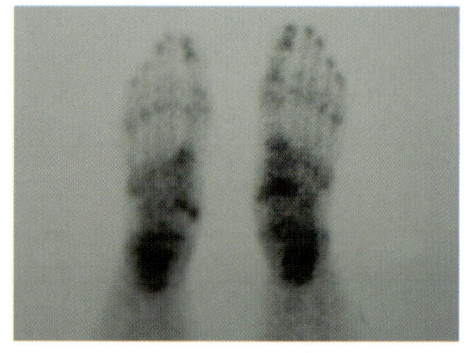

Figure 3 Positive bone scan for navicular stress fracture in the right foot.

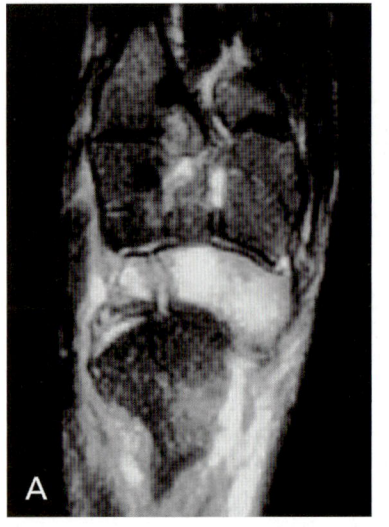

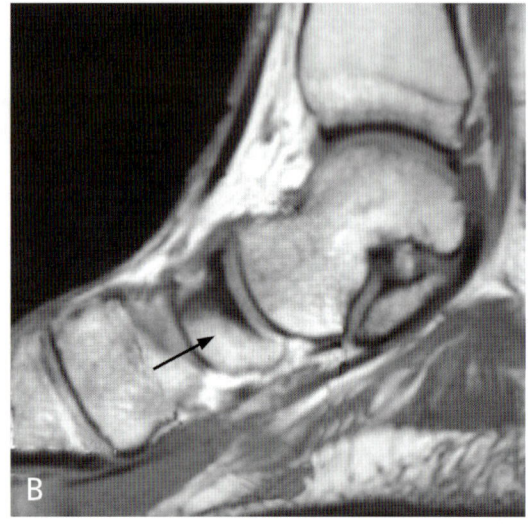

Figure 4 Axial (**A**) and sagittal (**B**) MRIs show a navicular stress fracture (arrow) with associated bone edema and fracture line.

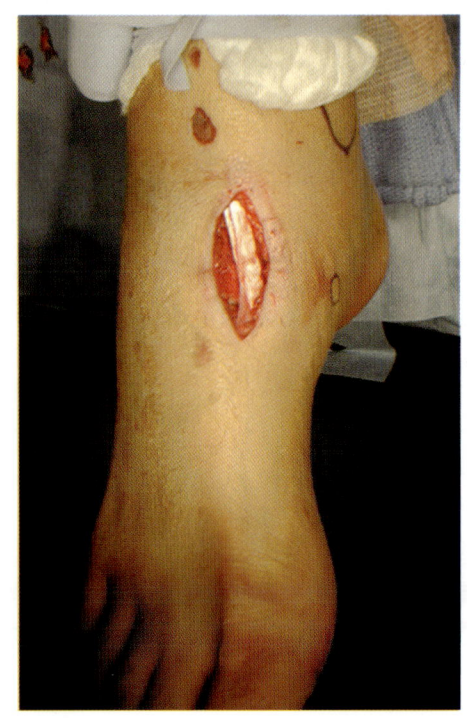

Figure 5 Intraoperative photograph shows the surgical approach to the navicular.

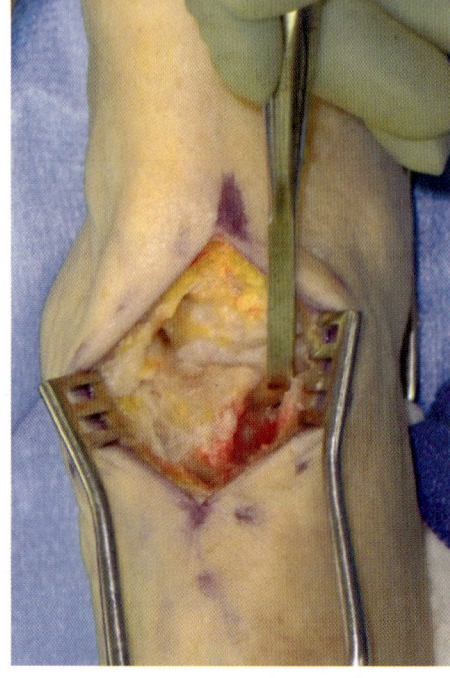

Figure 6 Intraoperative photograph shows exposure of the talonavicular joint and identification of the navicular fracture plane.

ipsilateral hip. A nonsterile tourniquet is placed on the thigh to allow for full access to the extremity if a proximal tibial bone–harvest site is needed for bone graft.

Surgical Technique

Once the patient is sterilely prepared and draped, a dorsal longitudinal incision is made overlying the navicular (**Figure 5**). The standard C-arm fluoroscopy can be used before incision for localization if the fracture fragment is visualized on prior radiographs. Care must be taken on incision to identify and protect the dorsal branches of the superficial peroneal nerve. Deep dissection identifies the extensor hallucis longus and the neurovascular bundle. These are gently retracted medially to expose the talonavicular joint capsule (**Figure 6**). The joint capsule is incised to provide adequate visualization of the articular surface.

Once the joint surface is evaluated for softening, defects, or arthritic change, an elevator or a No. 15 blade can often be helpful to delineate of the navicular stress fracture in the dorsal cortex. Once it is clearly identified, the fracture site must be débrided fibrous tissue, if present. If no defect is present, the fracture is temporarily affixed with two guide pins for 4.0-mm partially threaded cannulated screws (**Figure 7**). These are placed from a lateral to medial direction because the fracture often orients in a dorsal-medial to plantar-lateral direction, with the smaller fracture fragment more lateral.[1] The position of the guide pins is confirmed with fluoroscopy before placement of the screws (**Figure 8**).

If the patient presents with a long-standing navicular nonunion, or if a large defect is present after débridement of fibrous tissue in the fracture plane, an additional bone graft procedure may be required. In this situation, many options are available. Depending on surgeon preference, allograft or bone graft harvested from the distal or proximal tibia can fill the void. We have no preference for bone graft selection and have appreciated no clinical difference in outcome. The plan for fixation is similar once the defect is filled in the navicular.

Complications

The most frequent and concerning complication regarding this injury is delayed union or nonunion. The navicular bone is inherently at higher risk for nonunion because of the delicate vascular nature and the high shear stress across the articular surfaces.[1,3,6,7] Nonunions occur in the setting of both nonsurgical and surgical management. Most frequently, in patients treated nonsurgically, nonunions develop following an incomplete course of non–weight bearing. Khan et al[4] have shown that a navicular fracture that has progressed to nonunion following attempted activity modification can successfully be treated to union with non–weight bearing. The risk of navicular stress fracture nonunion is low if the initial fracture is amenable to nonsurgical management.[3,4,6]

Surgical intervention does not always guarantee a successful fracture union. It is difficult to compare outcomes, however, because those treated surgically are more often displaced or established nonunions. Three of the five patients treated surgically for established nonunions in the series of Khan et al[4] went on to recurrent nonunion. In a series of primary surgical interventions by Fitch et al,[5] 1 of 19 patients developed nonunions. Not only are these more displaced fractures that may have gone on to nonunion or malunion without surgical fixation, but the surgical procedure itself also can cause further vascular compromise to the bone, increasing the risk of nonunion. Both nonsurgical and surgical treatment protocols have a risk of nonunion. Although the risk appears small, symptomatic nonunion in the high-demand athlete requires additional surgery, further jeopardizing return to preinjury activity and the patient's future career.

In addition to nonunion, refracture is a risk following both surgical and nonsurgical treatment. Very little literature discusses the actual risk of recurrent navicular stress fracture. This is a rare event but can be quite devastating to the elite athlete. Burne et al[8] reported that 2 of 11 patients who developed a recurrent stress injury, and Saxena and Fullem[6] reported 2 of 13. These recurrent fractures require treatment and further immobi-

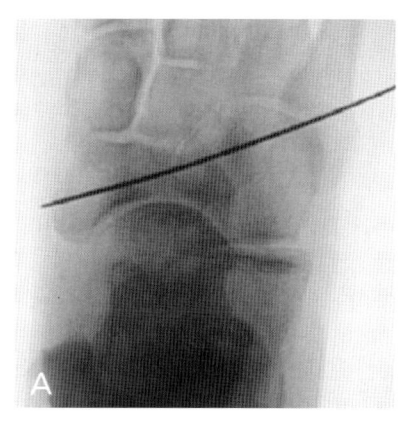

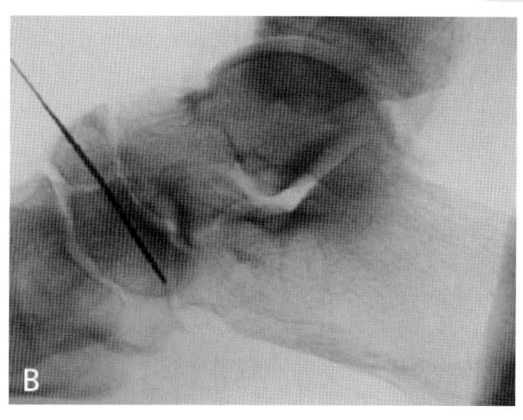

Figure 7 AP (**A**) and lateral (**B**) intraoperative fluoroscopic images demonstrate guide pin placement across the navicular perpendicular to the fracture line.

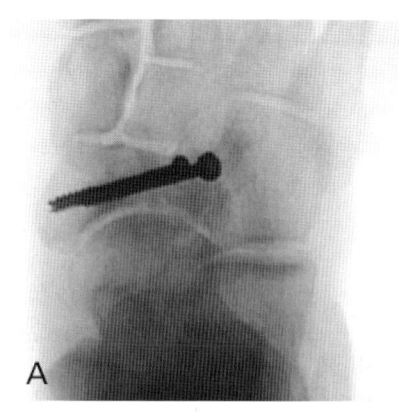

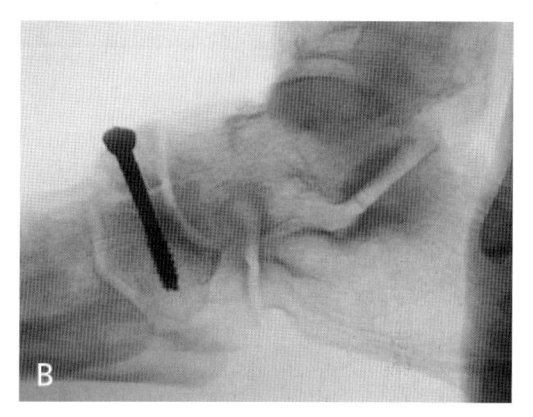

Figure 8 AP (**A**) and lateral (**B**) intraoperative fluoroscopic images confirm the placement of two 4.0-mm partially threaded cannulated screws.

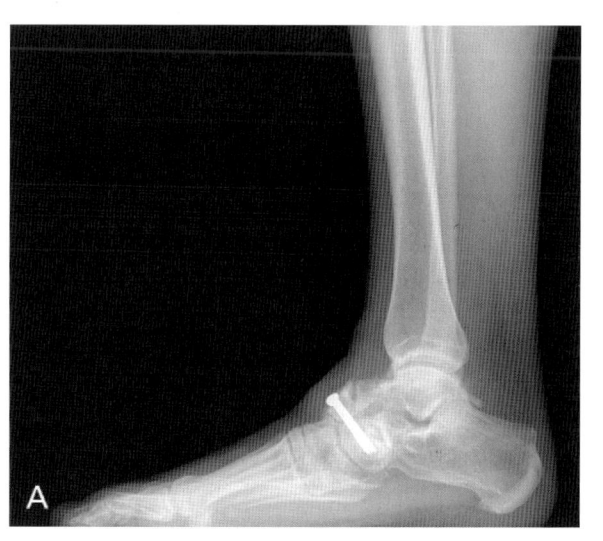

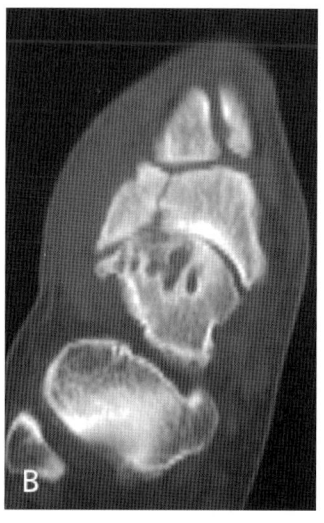

Figure 9 Lateral weight-bearing radiograph (**A**) and axial CT cut (**B**) show a navicular stress fracture nonunion following fixation, with the development of talonavicular arthritis.

lization. A patient who had inadequate nonsurgical treatment of an initial incomplete injury may be a candidate for a trial of strict non–weight-bearing immobilization. Otherwise, surgical repair should be offered to the patient to stabilize the fracture fragments. Some authors even propose initial surgical fixation of all stress fractures to reduce the risk of refracture on return to high-level athletics.[1,5]

In addition, both nonsurgically and surgically treated patients are at risk of developing symptomatic talonavicular arthritis (**Figure 9**). This is a rare long-term complication and is often a result of a chronic navicular nonunion. Unfortunately, limited options exist for definitive treatment of talonavicular arthritis, aside from arthrodesis. This is catastrophic for the elite athlete. Talonavicular arthrodesis eliminates 75% of subtalar motion. This is a salvage procedure performed for pain control. Following this, there are severe and unrecoverable limitations on athletic activities.

Postoperative Care and Rehabilitation

A variety of postoperative care protocols exist for these fractures. However, in our practice, if the stress fracture did not require additional bone grafting procedures, the patient will remain non–weight bearing for 6 weeks postoperatively but immobilization will be in a removable boot to allow the patient to work on motion of the ankle. Weight bearing progresses over the course of the next 2 to 4 weeks. Following that period, if the patient is still tender with palpation and has pain with ambulation, an additional CT scan of the foot will be performed to assess healing. After evaluation of the CT scan, there may be a continuation of restricted weight bearing until the fracture is completely united and symptoms are resolved.

We tend to transition from immobilization and progress weight bearing more slowly in patients who had a displaced navicular stress fracture or required additional bone grafting for a nonunion. Following surgical treatment, these patients will be placed in a cast for approximately 8 to 10 weeks before advancement of weight bearing and transition into a CAM (controlled ankle motion) walker. The cast is more protective and eliminates the shear force across the talonavicular joint that may contribute to difficult fracture healing. It is felt that the more severe the fracture, the longer the time required for recovery and advancement of activity.[6]

Once the decision is made to increase activities, the patient is allowed to progress weight bearing in a CAM walker and is ultimately weaned from the boot as the symptoms allow. This is over the course of 2 to 3 weeks. If further stiffness and weakness is an issue for the patient secondary to prolonged immobilization, physical therapy will be offered for assistance. Following union of the fracture and resolution of the symptoms, the patient is allowed to return to his or her preinjury activity level at 4 to 6 months. For the elite, high-demand athlete, some support the use of a preparticipation CT scan to confirm union of the stress fracture.[1,2,10] In a routine patient, follow-up CT scans are not recommended unless symptoms persist. The postinjury care and activity advancement should be based on clinical findings.[4]

Pearls

- The most important factor in the care of high-demand athletes with continuing foot pain is to maintain a high level of suspicion for navicular stress fractures. In the past, the incidence was reported to be 0.7%, but with the access and utilization of advanced imaging, the rate is more likely to be 14%.[3,4] Time is crucial when working with athletes, and a further delay in diagnosis only impairs the return to play.
- One of the most critical factors regarding the treatment of this fracture is clear disclosure of expectations to the patient. Although studies have shown no clear benefit of immediate surgical intervention, patients must be made aware that nonsurgical management may prolong the return to activity and that surgery may be required eventually if the fracture progresses to a nonunion. High-demand athletes must be forewarned that they will miss the season during treatment. This is often difficult for the treating physician to enforce due to external pressures, but inappropriate return to play will result in failure. These fractures can require 6 to 8 months for complete consolidation and the resolution of symptoms.
- After exposure of the stress fracture, we use two cannulated 4.0-mm partially threaded screws to affix the fracture. These are placed in a lateral to medial direction. This is important to note because the lateral piece is often much smaller. It may be difficult to secure the lateral piece from a medial starting point. Also, due to the size of the lateral piece, if a medial starting point is used, it may be impossible to have all the threads reach across the fracture site, limiting compression.
- Screw heads on the medial border can be prominent and cause irritation with shoe wear. If there is difficulty obtaining fixation with screws, precontoured, low-profile locking plates are available. This method is useful in the osteoporotic setting that can certainly occur following prolonged non–weight bearing. It is important to note that the use of locking plates does not alter the postoperative non–weight-bearing protocol.

References

1. Mann JA, Pedowitz DI: Evaluation and treatment of navicular stress fractures, including nonunions, revision surgery, and persistent pain after treatment. *Foot Ankle Clin* 2009;14(2):187-204.
2. Porter DA, Torma JK: Surgical technique for navicular stress fractures in athletes. *Tech Foot Ankle Surg* 2008;7(1):64-70.
3. Torg JS, Moyer J, Gaughan JP, Boden BP: Management of tarsal navicular stress fractures: Conservative versus surgical treatment: A meta-analysis. *Am J Sports Med* 2010;38(5):1048-1053.
4. Khan KM, Fuller PJ, Brukner PD, Kearney C, Burry HC: Outcome of conservative and surgical management of navicular stress fracture in athletes: Eighty-six cases proven with computerized tomography. *Am J Sports Med* 1992;20(6):657-666.
5. Fitch KD, Blackwell JB, Gilmour WN: Operation for non-union of stress fracture of the tarsal navicular. *J Bone Joint Surg Br* 1989;71(1):105-110.
6. Saxena A, Fullem B: Navicular stress fractures: A prospective study on athletes. *Foot Ankle Int* 2006;27(11):917-921.
7. Jones MH, Amendola AS: Navicular stress fractures. *Clin Sports Med* 2006;25(1):151-158, x-xi.
8. Burne SG, Mahoney CM, Forster BB, Koehle MS, Taunton JE, Khan KM: Tarsal navicular stress injury: Long-term outcome and clinicoradiological correlation using both computed tomography and magnetic resonance imaging. *Am J Sports Med* 2005;33(12):1875-1881.
9. Kiss ZS, Khan KM, Fuller PJ: Stress fractures of the tarsal navicular bone: CT findings in 55 cases. *AJR Am J Roentgenol* 1993;160(1):111-115.
10. Lee S, Anderson RB: Stress fractures of the tarsal navicular. *Foot Ankle Clin* 2004;9(1):85-104.

Chapter 81
Arthrodesis of the Hallux Metatarsophalangeal Joint

Chirag S. Patel, MD   Loretta Chou, MD

Patient Selection
Indications
First metatarsophalangeal (MTP) joint arthrodesis is commonly indicated for patients with hallux rigidus, hallux valgus with arthritis, failed surgeries of the hallux, neuromuscular conditions, inflammatory disease, and primary or secondary arthritis.[1] Hallux rigidus can be categorized into mild (grade 1), moderate (grade 2), and severe (grades 3 and 4) degenerative joint disease. First MTP joint arthrodesis is usually reserved for severe degenerative arthritis. First MTP joint arthrodesis is typically performed after nonsurgical treatment has failed. Initial treatment of early disease includes nonsteroidal anti-inflammatory medication, orthoses and shoe modification, taping, and occasional intra-articular steroid injection.[2]

Contraindications
Contraindications include active infection, certain malignant conditions, and nonarthritic conditions. Nonarthritic conditions include tenosynovitis of the flexor hallucis longus, osteochondral defect lesion, and pain referred to the hallux from other pathology.

Alternative Treatments
Resection arthroplasty, interposition graft arthroplasty, hemiarthroplasty, and total joint arthroplasty have been described as substitutes for arthrodesis of the first MTP joint. However, arthrodesis remains the gold standard of treatment. Gibson and Thomson[3] reported on a randomized controlled trial comparing arthrodesis and total joint arthroplasty. At 2-year follow-up, the group with arthrodesis had better pain ratings compared with the arthroplasty group. Stiffness continued to be a problem in the arthroplasty group, and there was a high rate (15.4%) of component loosening of the proximal phalanx.[3] Brewster[4] had similar results and concluded that arthrodesis had better results compared with total joint arthroplasty. Raikin and Ahmad[5] compared arthrodesis and metallic hemiarthroplasty and reported a 24% failure rate with hemiarthroplasty and a 4.8% revision rate. The hemiarthroplasty group had 57% good to excellent results compared with 81% for the arthrodesis group. The American Orthopaedic Foot & Ankle Society (AOFAS) rating was significantly better in the arthrodesis group. Brodsky et al[6] showed with a prospective gait analysis that patients have increased maximal ankle push-off power, increased single-limb support time, and decreased step width after first MTP joint arthrodesis. Thus, gait mechanics are not significantly altered and are likely improved from the preoperative diseased state.

Preoperative Imaging
Preoperative imaging consists of three weight-bearing views of the foot (AP, lateral, and oblique). In some cases, it is better to correct proximal pathology before distal pathology. Thus, when viewing imaging studies, it is important to not focus directly on the hallux but review the entire series of radiographs. However, a moderate amount of correction of the intermetatarsal angle (13° preoperative to 9.6° postoperative) can be achieved without a separate proximal osteotomy during first MTP joint arthrodesis.[7] Typical signs of osteoarthritis may be observed on radiographs: joint space narrowing, osteophytosis, sclerosis, and subchondral cysts. With severe deformity, joint subluxation or dislocation may be present (**Figure 1**). Radiographs are sufficient for preoperative planning. Noting the preoperative intermetatarsal angle, the hallux valgus angle, and the angle of inclination of the first metatarsal relative to the floor can be useful for planning and intraoperative correction (**Figure 1, B**). CT, MRI, or other imaging is typically not necessary for preoperative planning.

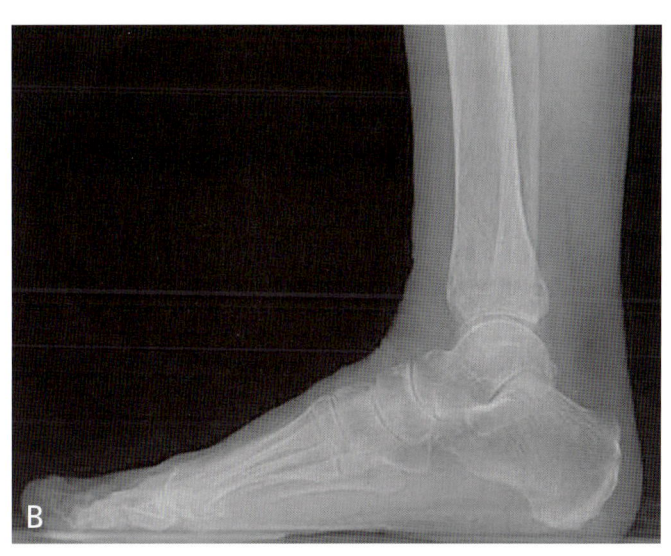

Figure 1 Preoperative weight-bearing AP (**A**) and lateral (**B**) radiographs of a right foot. The MTP angle is approximately 30°; the intermetatarsal angle is approximately 13°; and the inclination angle of the first metatarsal is approximately 30°. There are signs of first MTP joint arthritis as well: joint space narrowing, sclerosis, osteophytosis, and mild sclerosis. The MTP joint is also subluxated, and the metatarsal head is flattened.

Procedure
Special Equipment and Implants
A radiolucent table may be convenient in obtaining intraoperative imaging. A sterile Esmarch tourniquet may be used around the ankle. Mini-fluoroscopy or an image intensifier is helpful in assessing intraoperative deformity correction. A microsagittal saw or Hoke osteotomes are useful in preparing the MTP joint surfaces. Depending on bone size, a small fragment or a modular hand set can be used for lag fixation. Low-profile plates are typically used as fixation for MTP joint arthrodesis. Depending on the

---

Neither of the following authors nor any immediate family member has received anything of value from or owns stock in a commercial company or institution related directly or indirectly the subject of this chapter: Dr. Patel and Dr. Chou.

Section 6: Foot and Ankle

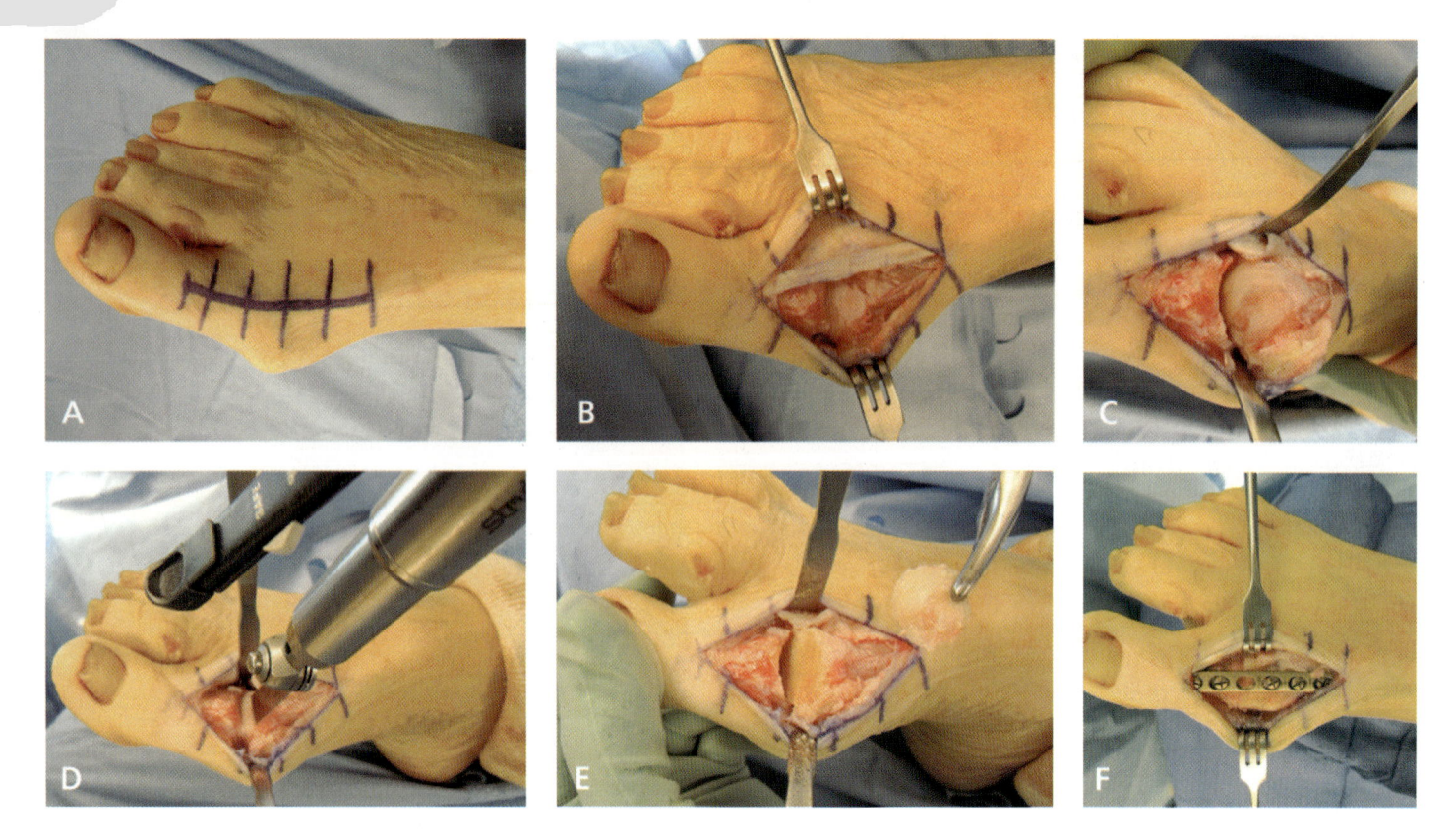

Figure 2 Intraoperative photographs demonstrate arthrodesis of the hallux metatarsophalangeal joint. **A,** Planned incision for the dorsal approach to the first MTP joint. **B,** The EHL tendon is exposed. **C,** The first MTP joint is exposed with hyperplantar flexion and the EHL tendon retracted laterally. The metatarsal head shows signs of severe arthritis—eburnation, loss of articular cartilage, and flattening of the convex surface. **D,** The first MTP joint is prepared using a flat-cut technique. A microsagittal saw is used to prepare the first metatarsal head. **E,** The first metatarsal head is cut and removed from the joint (It is shown held by a rongeur.). **F,** The first MTP joint has been prepared and fixed with a lag screw (not seen) and a plate-and-screw construct. Note that the hallux valgus is corrected.

technique, other special sets may be necessary.

Surgical Technique

In our preferred technique, the patient is positioned supine on the operating table. A local, regional, or spinal anesthetic in conjunction with sedation is sufficient for the procedure. General anesthesia can also be used if necessary. A thigh tourniquet can be used in patients with spinal or general anesthesia. However, an Esmarch ankle tourniquet is sufficient.

After the tourniquet is applied, a dorsal longitudinal incision is made over the MTP joint; alternatively, a medial midline approach may be used (**Figure 2, A**). Dissection is performed with Littler or tenotomy scissors to the capsule. The extensor hallucis longus (EHL) tendon can be mobilized and retracted laterally to aid in exposure (**Figure 2, B**). Care is taken not to damage any cutaneous nerve branches.

The capsule is incised sharply in line with the incision, and the MTP joint is exposed. The periosteum and capsule are incised in one layer and elevated sharply off the bone. Subperiosteal elevation is performed to expose the diaphysis of both bones (**Figure 2, C**). The joint is then prepared using a microsagittal saw or Hoke osteotomes (**Figure 2, D**). The cartilage is removed to the subchondral bone. Bony surfaces are prepared to obtain optimal positioning. The joint is aligned such that the MTP angle is no more than 15° valgus, the hallux is in neutral rotation, and the joint is approximately 20° dorsiflexed relative to the metatarsal (**Figure 2, E and F and Figure 3**). Pressure under the first metatarsal head increases with increased dorsiflexion. With decreasing dorsiflexion angle, the pressure under the first metatarsal head decreases but increases under the lesser toes, resulting in secondary metatarsalgia and callosities. The optimal dorsiflexion angle should be 20° to 25° relative to the first metatarsal.[8] Soft-tissue releases may be necessary to obtain acceptable correction.

After the joint is prepared, a Kirschner wire (K-wire) is used for provisional fixation. At this point, imaging can be used to confirm the alignment on AP and lateral projections. Next, a lag screw is used for compression and fixation. The screw trajectory is from distal medially to proximal laterally. An appropriate-size neutralization plate with bicortical screws is used for additional fixation. It is preferable to place three screws proximal and distal to the arthrodesis site; however, the proximal phalanx often can accommodate only two screws (**Figure 2, F and Figure 3**). The K-wire is removed. The capsule is repaired with a heavy absorbable suture in a simple interrupted manner. The skin is closed in interrupted fashion, and a compression dressing is placed.

Alternatively, ball-and-cup or cup-and-cone reamers can be used to prepare the metatarsal head and the base of the proximal phalanx. The articular cartilage and subchondral bone are removed on both sides of the joint. The proximal phalanx intramedullary canal is reamed with an end-cutting reamer. A guide pin is placed into the metatarsal head in the desired final position of the toe. A reamer is used to create a truncated cone that fits into the reamed proximal phalanx base. In a cadaveric study, Singh et al[9] compared the shortening between the flat cut and conical reaming technique (Refine Fusion Conical Reamer System, DePuy). The study showed no significant differences between the two techniques (7.1-mm flat cut versus 5.7-mm conical).

Chapter 81: Arthrodesis of the Hallux Metatarsophalangeal Joint

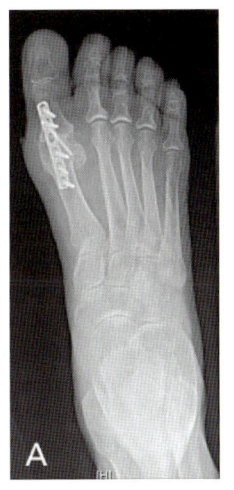

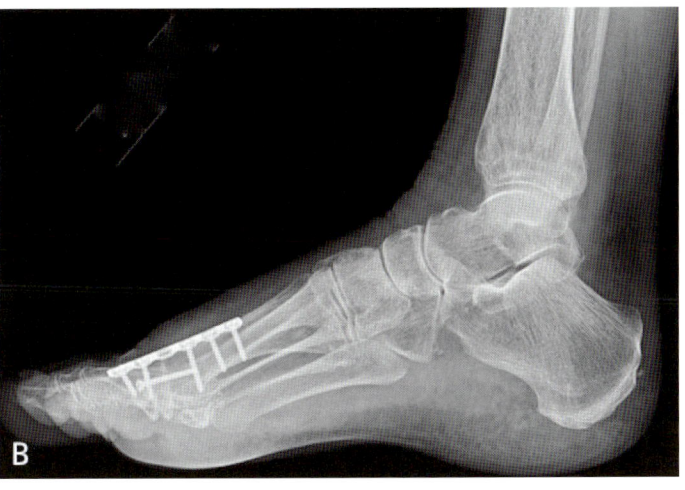

Figure 3 Postoperative AP (**A**) and lateral (**B**) radiographs show first MTP joint fusion with lag screw and plate construct with corrected MTP angle, intermetatarsal angle (approximately 9°), and dorsiflexion angle (approximately 10°). Note that the pulp of the hallux rests higher than the sole of the foot.

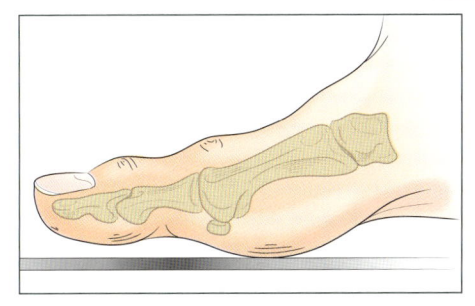

Figure 4 A flat x-ray plate can be useful in determining appropriate dorsiflexion. The plate should be parallel to the longitudinal axis of the distal and proximal phalanx on lateral projection when the foot is plantigrade. The toe pad should rest several millimeters off the plate in plantigrade position.

The ball-and-cup technique is similar. After the joint is exposed, a K-wire is placed into the metatarsal head, and an appropriate-size reamer is used to create a convex metatarsal head. Next, the K-wire is placed into the proximal phalanx base and an appropriate-size reamer is used to create a concave surface. The two surfaces are mated and aligned appropriately. After alignment, a K-wire is used to provisionally fix the MTP joint. In a prospective study with ball-and-cup preparation and plate-and-screw fixation (Accutrak congruent first MTP joint fusion system, Acumed), Bennett and Sabetta[10] reported a 98.7% fusion rate with only 3 of 230 feet having minor hardware problems. Likewise, Goucher and Coughlin[11] reported significantly improved pain and AOFAS scores (51 to 82) with an 8% nonunion rate for arthrodesis with ball-and-cup preparation (Hallu-Ream, Integra LifeSciences) and plate fixation.

There are many acceptable fixation techniques. An interfragmentary screw with or without a neutralization plate, plate alone, a single screw, two intersecting screws, headless screws, compression staples, and two threaded Steinmann pins crossing the interphalangeal joint and the MTP joint have been described as fixation techniques. An interposition graft may be necessary if lengthening is desired. Sharma et al[12] studied screw versus plate-and-screw fixation and concluded that there was no correlation between the type of fixation and time to fusion, patient satisfaction, or complication rate.

Complications

Complications with first MTP joint arthrodesis include nonunion, infection, hardware failure, hardware irritation, arthrosis of the interphalangeal joint, and malalignment. Persistent pain can be a sign of nonunion. If a painful nonunion persists, then revision of fixation with autograft or allograft bone may be necessary. Hope et al[13] investigated the necessity of revision of hallux MTP joint nonunion and concluded that hardware removal and débridement is a reasonable option following a failed arthrodesis.

Postoperative Care and Rehabilitation

The foot is placed in a postoperative shoe. The patient is allowed to bear weight through the heel and the lateral foot. In a retrospective review, Berlet et al[14] reported a 91.1% fusion rate at an average of 69 days with immediate weight bearing after first MTP joint fusion using crossed screws or a dorsal plate and screws alone. The dressing is removed on postoperative day 1 or 2. Radiographic evaluation is performed every 4 to 6 weeks until union is achieved. Radiographic union is typically seen approximately 10 to 12 weeks after surgery. If a delayed union is suspected, then the patient continues to wear the postoperative shoe until radiographic union is seen.

Pearls

Positioning the patient's foot near the edge of the bed allows easy access and maneuvering during the case. A bump under the hip can also aid with foot positioning during the case. Removing osteophytes before joint preparation allows better assessment of deformity correction. Hyperplantar-flexing the open joint can improve visualization and access to the metatarsal head and proximal phalanx. There are multiple preparation techniques as well as fixation methods that work. The underlying key to an arthrodesis is good fundamental technique. The bones must be prepared adequately. Compression must be achieved across the fusion site, and there must be sufficient fixation. For very sclerotic subchondral bone, an appropriate-size K-wire should be used to fenestrate the sclerotic area to allow for blood flow to the arthrodesis site. The hallux valgus angle should not be overcorrected into varus. A flat plate can be useful in determining appropriate dorsiflexion. The plate should be parallel to the longitudinal axis of the distal and proximal phalanx on lateral projection when the foot is plantigrade. The toe pad should rest several millimeters off the plate in plantigrade position.[14] In a retrospective review, Aas et al[15] reported a weak correlation between toe position and clinical outcome. They noted that a good estimate of the extension angle can be determined by the distance between a flat plate and the pulp of the distal phalanx (**Figure 4**). Additionally, care is taken not to impinge the hallux onto the second toe. Typically, there should be a 3- to 5-mm gap.[14] Repairing the capsule and the periosteal layer over the plate minimizes postoperative hardware irritation and toe swelling and improves bone healing. Compression dressing, elevation, and periodic icing can also minimize postoperative swelling.

References

1. Brodsky JW, Passmore RN, Pollo FE, Shabat S: Functional outcome of arthrodesis of the first metatarsophalangeal joint using parallel screw fixation. *Foot Ankle Int* 2005;26(2):140-146.

2. Marks RM: Arthrodesis of the first metatarsophalangeal joint. *Instr Course Lect* 2005;54:263-268.
3. Gibson JN, Thomson CE: Arthrodesis or total replacement arthroplasty for hallux rigidus: A randomized controlled trial. *Foot Ankle Int* 2005;26(9):680-690.
4. Brewster M: Does total joint replacement or arthrodesis of the first metatarsophalangeal joint yield better functional results? A systematic review of the literature. *J Foot Ankle Surg* 2010;49(6):546-552.
5. Raikin SM, Ahmad J: Comparison of arthrodesis and metallic hemiarthroplasty of the hallux metatarsophalangeal joint: Surgical technique. *J Bone Joint Surg Am* 2008;90(suppl, 2 pt 2):171-180.
6. Brodsky JW, Baum BS, Pollo FE, Mehta H: Prospective gait analysis in patients with first metatarsophalangeal joint arthrodesis for hallux rigidus. *Foot Ankle Int* 2007;28(2):162-165.
7. Pydah SK, Toh EM, Sirikonda SP, Walker CR: Intermetatarsal angular change following fusion of the first metatarsophalangeal joint. *Foot Ankle Int* 2009;30(5):415-418.
8. Bayomy AF, Aubin PM, Sangeorzan BJ, Ledoux WR: Arthrodesis of the first metatarsophalangeal joint: A robotic cadaver study of the dorsiflexion angle. *J Bone Joint Surg Am* 2010;92(8):1754-1764.
9. Singh B, Draeger R, Del Gaizo DJ, Parekh SG: Changes in length of the first ray with two different first MTP fusion techniques: A cadaveric study. *Foot Ankle Int* 2008;29(7):722-725.
10. Bennett GL, Sabetta J: First metatarsalphalangeal joint arthrodesis: Evaluation of plate and screw fixation. *Foot Ankle Int* 2009;30(8):752-757.
11. Goucher NR, Coughlin MJ: Hallux metatarsophalangeal joint arthrodesis using dome-shaped reamers and dorsal plate fixation: A prospective study. *Foot Ankle Int* 2006;27(11):869-876.
12. Sharma HK, Bhagat S, Deleeuw J, Denolf F: In vivo comparison of screw versus plate and screw fixation for first metatarsophalangeal arthrodesis: Does augmentation of internal compression screw fixation using a semi-tubular plate shorten time to clinical and radiologic fusion of the first metatarsophalangeal joint (MTPJ)? *J Foot Ankle Surg* 2008;47(1):2-7.
13. Hope M, Savva N, Whitehouse S, Elliot R, Saxby TS: Is it necessary to re-fuse a non-union of a hallux metatarsophalangeal joint arthrodesis? *Foot Ankle Int* 2010;31(8):662-669.
14. Berlet GC, Hyer CF, Glover JP: A retrospective review of immediate weightbearing after first metatarsophalangeal joint arthrodesis. *Foot Ankle Spec* 2008;1(1):24-28.
15. Aas M, Johnsen TM, Finsen V: Arthrodesis of the first metatarsophalangeal joint for hallux rigidus—optimal position of fusion. *Foot (Edinb)* 2008;18(3):131-135.

Chapter 82
Proximal and Distal First Metatarsal Osteotomies for Hallux Valgus

Christopher B. Hirose, MD   Michael J. Coughlin, MD

Patient Selection
Indications

We consider simultaneous proximal and distal first metatarsal osteotomies in patients who have clinically symptomatic moderate to severe hallux valgus deformities with congruent first metatarsophalangeal joints (**Figures 1** and **2**).

Radiographic findings include a first-second intermetatarsal angle greater than 13°, a distal metatarsal articular angle (DMAA) greater than 15°, and a congruent first metatarsophalangeal joint (**Figure 3**).

Congruent hallux deformities are uncommon. Piggott[1] noted a 9% occurrence (20 of 215 adult feet) of congruent first metatarsophalangeal joints, and Coughlin and Carlson[2] described a 2% prevalence (21 of 878) in adult feet.

Perhaps more important is the recognition of an increased DMAA angle. In a different Coughlin study, higher hallux valgus recurrence rates were found in those patients who had undergone distal soft-tissue realignment procedures but also had congruent first metatarsophalangeal joints.[3] When an already congruent joint is made incongruent, the proximal phalanx seeks its original position of congruency on the first metatarsal head, re-creating the hallux valgus deformity. Stiffness and pain can result. In contrast, with the distal first metatarsal closing-wedge osteotomy, the hallux valgus deformity is corrected by correcting the DMAA, keeping a congruent joint congruent.

We consider performing a triple osteotomy (adding a proximal phalangeal Akin osteotomy to the double first metatarsal osteotomy) in patients with hallux valgus interphalangeal deformities, in patients with significant rotational deformities, or in patients in whom we have performed a double first metatarsal osteotomy but a residual hallux valgus deformity remains. Both adult and juvenile deformities are considered for surgical treatment.[4] Although juvenile hallux valgus corrections have historically had high rates of failure, Smith and Coughlin[5] believe that these failures may have been due to an underappreciation of deformity. When all of the

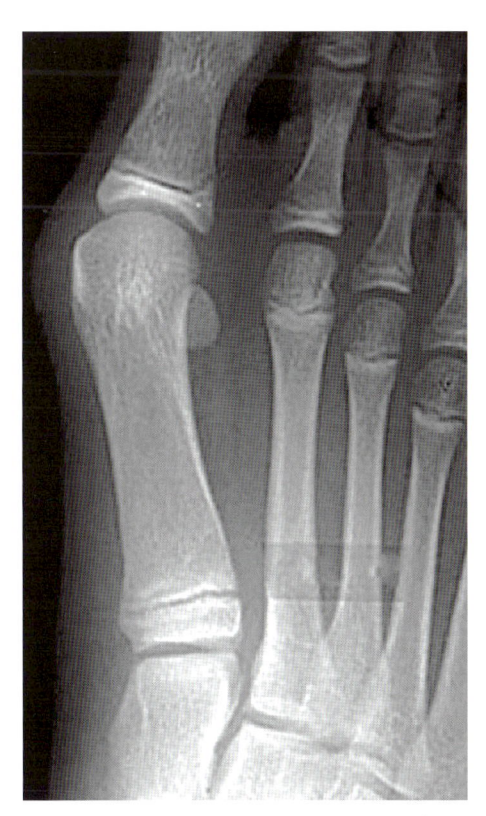

Figure 1 Preoperative AP radiograph of the foot of an adolescent shows a hallux valgus deformity with a congruent joint.

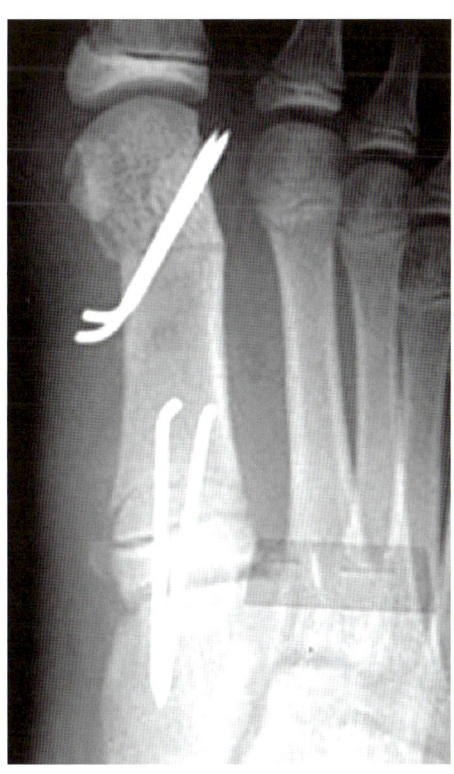

Figure 2 Postoperative AP radiograph shows proximal and distal first metatarsal osteotomies with correction of the distal metatarsal articular angle (DMAA).

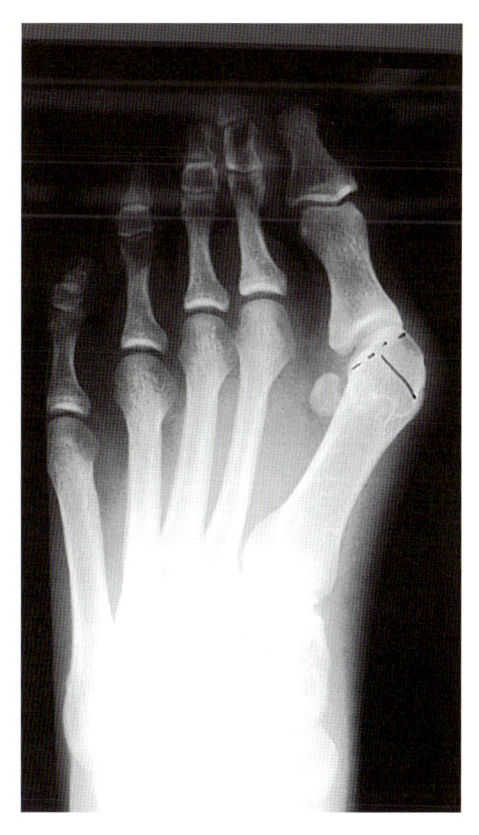

Figure 3 AP radiograph shows a severe DMAA.

Dr. Hirose or an immediate family member has stock or stock options held in Johnson & Johnson, Pfizer, and Stericycle and serves as a board member, owner, officer, or committee member of the North Pacific Orthopaedic Society. Dr. Coughlin or an immediate family member has received royalties from Integra LifeSciences, Tornier, and MMI; is a member of a speakers' bureau or has made paid presentations on behalf of Integra LifeSciences, SBI, MMI, and Tornier; serves as a paid consultant to or is an employee of SBI, Tornier, Integra LifeSciences, and MMI; has stock or stock options held in Tornier and MMI; has received research or institutional support from Tornier, SBI, and Integra LifeSciences; and has received nonincome support (such as equipment or services), commercially derived honoraria, or other non–research-related funding (such as paid travel) from SBI.

Section 3: Foot and Ankle

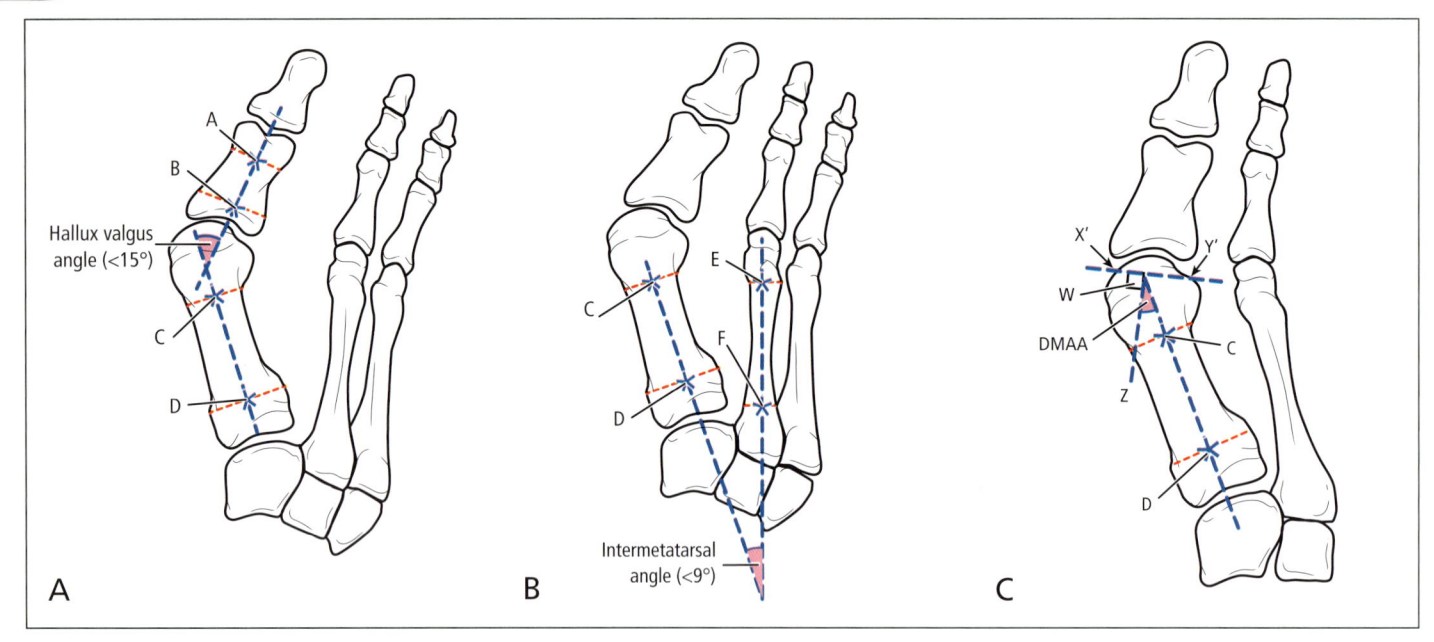

Figure 4 Illustrations show measurements that are made on preoperative radiographs to plan surgery for hallux valgus. **A,** Measuring the hallux valgus angle. A normal hallux valgus angle is less than 15°. A line (A) is drawn down the axis of the proximal phalanx and another line (B) is drawn down the axis of the first metatarsal. C and D are reference points midway between the medial and lateral cortex, at a point 1 cm from the end of the bone. **B,** Measuring the first-second intermetatarsal angle. A normal first-second intermetatarsal angle is less than 9°. E and F are reference points midway between the medial and lateral cortex, at a point 1 cm from the end of the bone. **C,** Measuring the distal metatarsal articular angle (DMAA). A normal DMAA is less than 6°. Line C–D delineates the longitudinal axis of the first metatarsal. X' and Y' are reference points of the medial and lateral edge of the articular surface. Line W–Z is drawn perpendicular to the line drawn between X' and Y'. The DMAA is the angle subtended by lines W–Z and C–D.

deformities are addressed and the DMAA is corrected with a distal closing-wedge metatarsal osteotomy, success rates are significantly higher. Coughlin[6] reported good or excellent results in 92% of 60 juvenile hallux valgus corrections.

Contraindications
When patients present with purely cosmetic concerns, arthritis of the first metatarsophalangeal joint, severe metatarsus adductus, spasticity, vascular insufficiency, active infections, or severe traumatic soft-tissue problems, we treat them nonsurgically.

Preoperative Imaging
Three weight-bearing radiographic views of the foot are obtained: AP, lateral, and oblique. The x-ray tube is centered over the tarsometatarsal joint and angled 15° toward the ankle joint, with a 1-m separation between the x-ray tube and the film. The hallux valgus angle (**Figure 4, A**), first-second intermetatarsal angle (**Figure 4, B**), distal metatarsal articular angle (**Figure 4, C**), and first metatarsophalangeal joint congruency (**Figure 5**) are measured and noted.

Procedure
Room Setup/Patient Positioning
We position the patient supine on a standard operating room table. A small bump is placed under the ipsilateral hip so that the foot points toward the ceiling. We place a mini C-arm fluoroscanner on the surgical side of the bed. An Esmarch tourniquet is wrapped around the ankle for exsanguination.

Special Instruments/Equipment/Implants
The following equipment should be on hand: a crescentic oscillating saw blade, a straight oscillating blade, a 3.5-mm solid small-fragment screw, and 0.062-in Kirschner wires (K-wires).

Video 82.1 Proximal and Distal First Metatarsal Osteotomy. Christopher B. Hirose, MD; Michael J. Coughlin, MD (6 min)

Surgical Technique
Distal Metatarsal Osteotomy
Attention is turned to the distal first metatarsal closing osteotomy to first correct the DMAA. We template hallux valgus deformities to resect a predetermined wedge of bone with the goal of correcting the DMAA to less than 6°. On average, a 4- to 6-mm wedge of bone is removed.[2] A longitudinal medial incision is made over the first metatarsal head, centered over the first metatarsophalangeal joint.

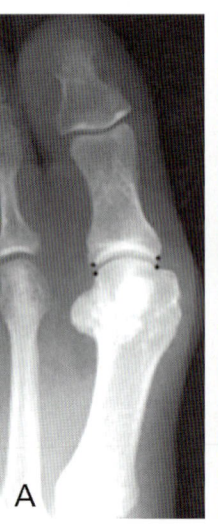

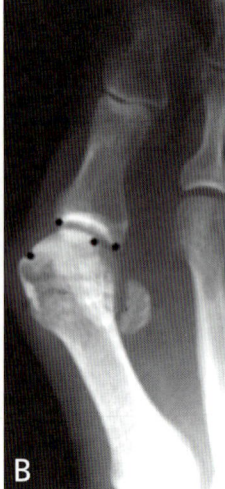

Figure 5 AP radiographs show a congruent (**A**) and an incongruent (**B**) first metatarsophalangeal joint.

Skin flaps are raised, and the dorsal medial cutaneous nerve is protected. An L-shaped capsulotomy is constructed, with the horizontal limb placed dorsally and the vertical limb placed proximally (**Figure 6, A**). This keeps the strongest portion of the capsule—the attachment to the proximal phalanx—intact.

The first metatarsophalangeal joint is then exposed (**Figure 6, B**). We routinely examine the cartilage of the first metatarsal head and that of the proximal pha-

Chapter 82: Proximal and Distal First Metatarsal Osteotomies for Hallux Valgus

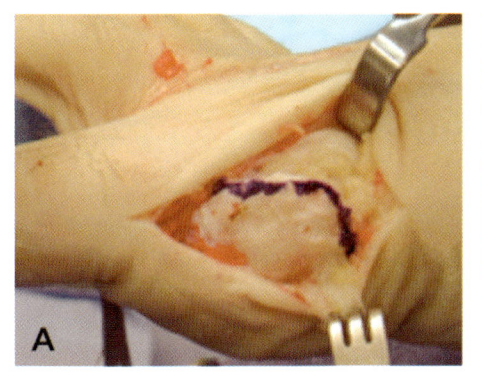

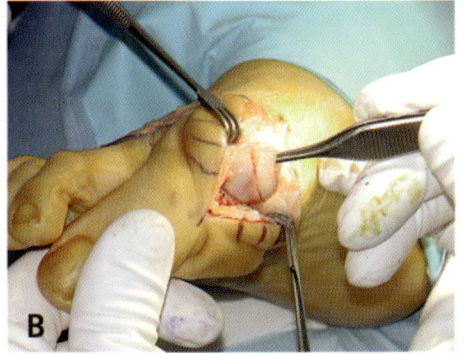

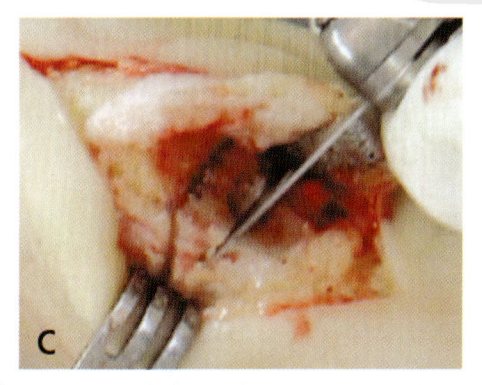

Figure 6 Intraoperative photographs demonstrate distal metatarsal osteotomy. **A,** The medial first metatarsophalangeal joint is shown with the capsulotomy outlined. **B,** The medial eminence of the cartilage of the first metatarsal head is resected. **C,** The medial wedge of bone is resected.

lanx for wear. The medial eminence is removed, keeping the saw blade parallel to the medial edge of the first metatarsal.

The saw blade is positioned at the metaphyseal-diaphyseal junction, 1.5 cm proximal to the first metatarsophalangeal joint and proximal to the sesamoids, to resect the medially based wedge of bone (**Figure 6, C**).

Reapproximating the proximal and distal fragments reduces the DMAA. The osteotomy is held in position with two 0.062-in K-wires, placed from dorsal distal to proximal plantar. The pins are cut below the skin, and the medial face of the first metatarsal head is then smoothed with the oscillating saw.

Proximal Metatarsal Osteotomy

A second incision is made over the proximal dorsal first metatarsal and is continued 3 cm distally, medial to the extensor hallucis longus tendon. In the coronal plane, a K-wire is placed into the medial cuneiform, perpendicular to the plane of the metatarsal heads, to serve as a reference for the position of the saw blade for the proximal metatarsal cut (**Figure 7, A**). A crescentic saw blade is positioned concave proximal, 1.0 cm distal to the metatarsal cuneiform joint (**Figure 7, B**).

From the lateral view of the foot, the blade is angled neither perpendicular to the axis of the first metatarsal nor perpendicular to the plantar surface of the foot, but halfway in between (**Figure 8**). In the coronal plane, the saw blade is kept parallel to the K-wire reference, so that when the first metatarsal is translated laterally, the plantar surface of the first metatarsal head remains in the same plane as a plane containing the second through fifth metatarsal heads.[7]

The osteotomy is made with a saline-cooled saw blade. The medial and lateral cortices are broken with a 0.25-in osteotome, and the first metatarsal is swung laterally so that the head is positioned over the sesamoids. The 0.25-in osteotome is routinely positioned over the lateral cortex of the proximal first metatarsal

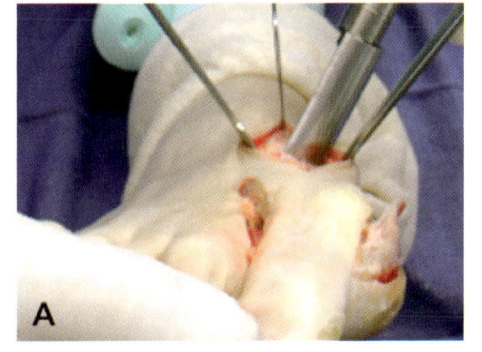

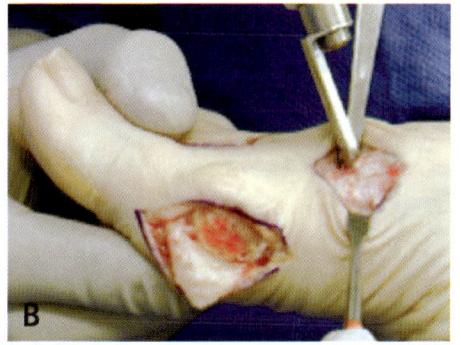

Figure 7 Intraoperative photographs show a proximal metatarsal osteotomy. **A,** A Kirschner wire is placed into the medial cuneiform, perpendicular to the plane of the metatarsal heads. **B,** The crescentic saw blade is oriented concave proximal, with the curve of the saw blade "smiling" when viewing the foot from distal to proximal.

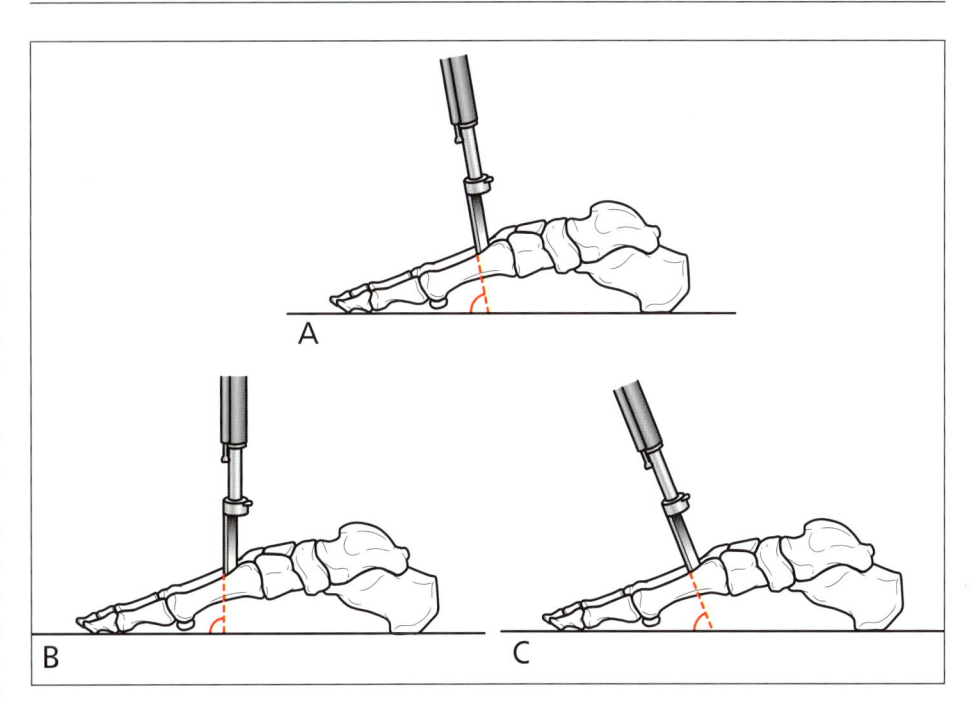

Figure 8 Illustration demonstrates proper saw blade orientation for proximal metatarsal osteotomy. The correct orientation (**A**) is neither perpendicular to the plantar surface of the foot (**B**) nor perpendicular to the long axis of the first metatarsal (**C**), but halfway between.

fragment to hold the proximal fragment in position as the surgeon swings the distal first metatarsal laterally. A 3.5-mm solid small-fragment screw and a 0.062-in K-wire are advanced obliquely across the

© 2013 American Academy of Orthopaedic Surgeons

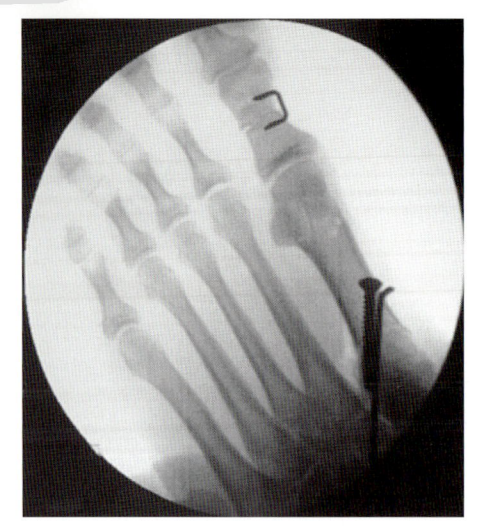

Figure 9 AP fluoroscopic view of the foot shows a 3.5-mm solid screw and a 0.062-in Kirschner wire securing the proximal crescentic osteotomy.

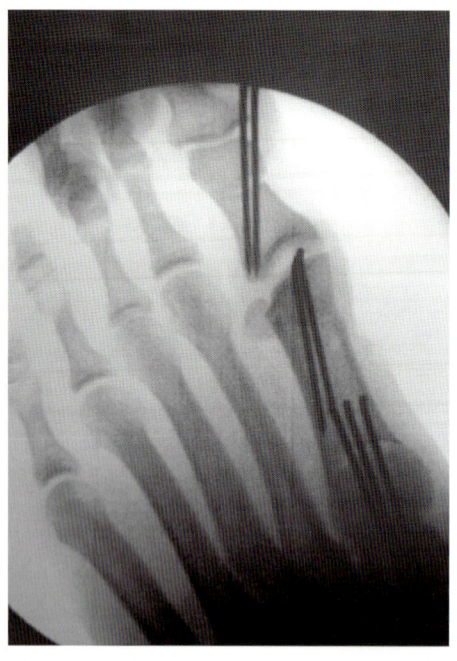

Figure 10 Fluoroscopic view of the foot of a patient with open physes shows a three–Kirschner wire fixation of the proximal crescentic osteotomy.

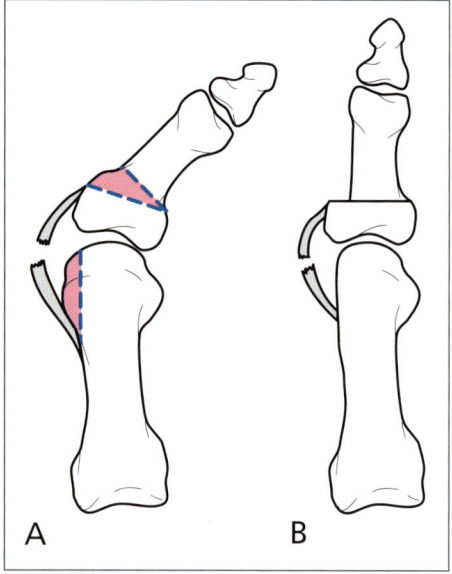

Figure 11 Illustration demonstrates an Akin proximal phalanx osteotomy. **A,** Preoperative wedge resection of the proximal phalanx and medial eminence resection of the first metatarsal. **B,** Postoperative reduction of the proximal phalanx.

osteotomy, starting 1 cm distal to the osteotomy (**Figure 9**).

In cases in which the physis is open, we recommend the use of three 0.062-in smooth K-wires and no screw (**Figure 10**).

When the quality of the bone is poor, we consider supplementing the screw with two longitudinal smooth K-wires placed from proximal medial to distal lateral in parallel fashion.[8]

The first metatarsophalangeal joint capsule is reapproximated and repaired with a 2-0 Vicryl suture (Ethicon) directed through a drill hole made from dorsal to plantar in the first metatarsal metaphysis. Both the horizontal and vertical limbs are repaired with interrupted suture. The hallux is held in neutral position and neutral rotation while the capsule is repaired, and the toe should remain in this position when the external forces holding the toe are released. If the hallux still drifts into valgus, or if there is a pronation deformity, an Akin osteotomy of the proximal phalanx is performed (**Figure 11**).

The distal medial incision is lengthened by 2 cm, and two small Hohmann retractors are placed deep to the extensor and flexor hallucis tendons. A saline-cooled saw blade is used to remove a 2- to 3-mm wedge of bone of the proximal phalanx at the proximal metaphyseal-diaphyseal junction, with effort made to keep the lateral cortex intact. The proximal phalanx is closed medially, derotated if necessary, and pinned with one or two 0.062-in K-wires placed from distal medial to proximal lateral across the osteotomy site. These pins are buried under the skin.

If continued deformity is present due to the strong pull of the adductor hallucis despite both proximal and distal first metatarsal and Akin osteotomies, we infrequently perform a distal soft-tissue release, as demonstrated in the video supplement. A main concern is osteonecrosis of the first metatarsal head. The reported incidence of osteonecrosis of the first metatarsal head with a distal first metatarsal osteotomy and distal soft-tissue release varies: Meier and Kenzora[9] reported a 20% incidence, whereas Peterson et al[10] noted an incidence of 1.7%.

A linear incision is made distal to the bifurcation of the deep peroneal nerve and is extended distally to the base of the first and second toes. The web space is entered and the conjoined tendon of the adductor hallucis is identified. A No. 15 blade is placed into the space between the lateral sesamoid and the first metatarsal head, releasing the metatarsal sesamoid ligament. The knife blade continues to be pushed distally toward the base of the proximal phalanx, and the conjoined tendon is released off the base of the proximal phalanx. The conjoined tendon is also released off the lateral edge of the lateral sesamoid. Two stay sutures are placed into the stump of the adductor tendon, and the tendon is sutured to the lateral first metatarsal head capsule.

All incisions are closed with an interrupted 3-0 monofilament suture. A forefoot spica gauze-and-tape dressing is wrapped around the hallux in the direction of supination while the hallux is held in neutral position (**Figure 12**).

A postoperative shoe is applied, and patients are allowed to bear weight on the heel. A cast may be applied if the patient proves to be noncompliant.

Complications

Postoperative complications of the double and triple osteotomies are rare. They include nonunion, dorsiflexion malunion of the proximal osteotomy, first metatarsal shortening, metatarsalgia, hallux varus, recurrence, and physeal arrest in adolescent patients. In the series by Coughlin and Carlson,[2] a hallux varus deformity developed in 1 of 21 feet, and a plantar flexion malunion developed at the distal first metatarsal osteotomy site in 1 of 21 feet. Although the average shortening of the first metatarsal was 6%, second metatarsal transfer lesions were rare, seen in 1 of 21 feet. In patients with open physes, none were noted to have had physeal arrest with smooth K-wire fixation.[2]

After first metatarsal distal osteotomies, degenerative changes of the first metatarsophalangeal joint as well as the metatarsal sesamoid articulations have been noted.[11]

There are also reports of dorsal malunion of the first metatarsal crescentic osteotomy due to loss of fixation. We consider using a dorsal medial plate fixation of the proximal crescentic osteotomy for

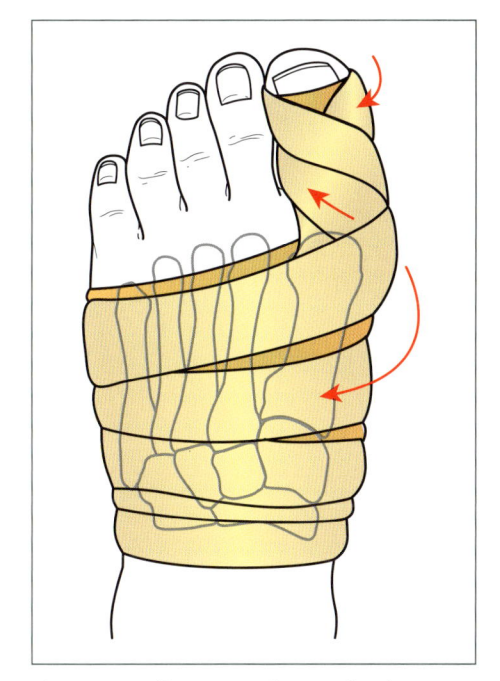

Figure 12 Illustration shows a forefoot spica dressing spiraled around the hallux in the direction of supination to counteract a pronated hallux valgus deformity.

revision cases, as this has proven to be a stronger construct in Sawbones models (Pacific Research Laboratories).[12]

Postoperative Care and Rehabilitation

The soft-tissue dressings are changed in 48 hours, and a new forefoot-hallux spica dressing is applied with 2-in Kling gauze and 0.5-in adhesive tape to hold the toe in neutral position. The dressings are changed every 10 days for 6 to 8 weeks to maintain the position of the hallux. We obtain the first series of three weight-bearing foot radiographs at 7 to 10 days postoperatively and adjust the forefoot-hallux spica dressing to fine-tune the position of the hallux. Sutures are removed at 3 weeks. Another series of three weight-bearing foot radiographs is obtained at week 6. If the osteotomies have healed, then the pins are removed in the office under local anesthesia and fluoroscopic guidance or intraoperatively as an outpatient. Patients are allowed to bear weight in a wide shoe or sandal. Range-of-motion exercises commence at 8 weeks following surgery.

Pearls

- We prefer the L-shaped capsulotomy over the first metatarsophalangeal joint, with the vertical limb placed proximally. Repairing the capsule is easily done by placing a vertically oriented drill hole through the first metatarsal metaphysis and repairing the capsule with an absorbable suture through the drill hole. If the degree of correction is not satisfactory, the repair is easily taken down and redone to place the hallux in the proper position.
- The proximal metatarsal crescentic osteotomy can be difficult. We find that placing the lateral edge of the saw blade so that it will cut through the proximal metatarsal cortex laterally helps to make a clean and reproducible cut. The blade is then translated through its natural curvature to cut the medial cortex. The osteotomy is then completed and opened with a 4-mm osteotome.
- To achieve the proper reduction of the first-second intermetatarsal angle, we place a 4-mm osteotome on the lateral cortex of the proximal portion of the first metatarsal to stabilize it while the distal fragment is shifted laterally. The osteotomy is provisionally pinned to check the correction under fluoroscopy and is readjusted before final fixation.

References

1. Piggott H: The natural history of hallux valgus in adolescence and early adult life. *J Bone Joint Surg Br* 1960;42:749-760.
2. Coughlin MJ, Carlson RE: Treatment of hallux valgus with an increased distal metatarsal articular angle: Evaluation of double and triple first ray osteotomies. *Foot Ankle Int* 1999;20(12):762-770.
3. Coughlin MJ: Hallux valgus in men: Effect of the distal metatarsal articular angle on hallux valgus correction. *Foot Ankle Int* 1997;18(8):463-470.
4. Petratos DV, Anastasopoulos JN, Plakogiannis CV, Matsinos GS: Correction of adolescent hallux valgus by proximal crescentic osteotomy of the first metatarsal. *Acta Orthop Belg* 2008;74(4):496-502.
5. Smith BW, Coughlin MJ: Treatment of hallux valgus with increased distal metatarsal articular angle: Use of double and triple osteotomies. *Foot Ankle Clin* 2009;14(3):369-382.
6. Coughlin MJ: Roger A. Mann Award: Juvenile hallux valgus. Etiology and treatment. *Foot Ankle Int* 1995;16(11):682-697.
7. Jones C, Coughlin M, Villadot R, Golanó P: Proximal crescentic metatarsal osteotomy: The effect of saw blade orientation on first ray elevation. *Foot Ankle Int* 2005;26(2):152-157.
8. Jung HG, Guyton GP, Parks BG, et al: Supplementary axial Kirschner wire fixation for crescentic and Ludloff proximal metatarsal osteotomies: A biomechanical study. *Foot Ankle Int* 2005;26(8):620-626.
9. Meier PJ, Kenzora JE: The risks and benefits of distal first metatarsal osteotomies. *Foot Ankle* 1985;6(1):7-17.
10. Peterson DA, Zilberfarb JL, Greene MA, Colgrove RC: Avascular necrosis of the first metatarsal head: Incidence in distal osteotomy combined with lateral soft tissue release. *Foot Ankle Int* 1994;15(2):59-63.
11. Bock P, Kristen KH, Kröner A, Engel A: Hallux valgus and cartilage degeneration in the first metatarsophalangeal joint. *J Bone Joint Surg Br* 2004;86(5):669-673.
12. Jones C, Coughlin M, Petersen W, Herbot M, Paletta J: Mechanical comparison of two types of fixation for proximal first metatarsal crescentic osteotomy. *Foot Ankle Int* 2005;26(5):371-374.

Chapter 83
Chronic Exertional Compartment Syndrome and Release

Emily A. Wagstrom, MD   Annunziato Amendola, MD   Brian R. Wolf, MD, MS

Patient Selection
Indications
The diagnosis of chronic exertional compartment syndrome (CECS) is made clinically. Patients with CECS are typically athletes participating in sports with a lot of running, but CECS can also be seen with jumping, cutting, and skating sports.[1] Patients with CECS typically present with pain that occurs following a certain amount of time exercising or after a certain intensity of exercise.[2-5] This leg pain typically dissipates with rest. CECS is often bilateral but can be unilateral, and it can occur without a distinguishable cause or inciting event. Patients are frequently asymptomatic at the time of examination.

The cause of pain and exact pathophysiology of CECS is unclear. However, it is thought that the leg muscle compartments, which are each confined by tight fascia, do not allow sufficient muscle expansion during exercise, leading to relative ischemia.[2] Pain symptoms result from muscle expansion and associated neurovascular function compromise due to elevated involved compartment pressures.

There are four muscle compartments in the leg: anterior, lateral, superficial posterior, and deep posterior. Each compartment contains one or more muscles and at least one neurovascular structure. The anterior compartment is the most commonly affected compartment, but it is not uncommon for multiple compartments to be involved.[2,4,6]

The diagnosis of CECS is typically confirmed using intracompartmental pressure measurement and the Pedowitz criteria.[6] Multiple devices for testing intracompartmental pressures are available, but all require needle insertion into the leg compartments. Pressure testing is done at rest and after exercising until symptoms occur. A video of postexercise testing can be seen in the video supplement. Testing is considered confirmatory of CECS if pre-exercise resting compartment pressure is equal to or greater than 15 mm Hg. Confirmatory pressures after exercise are 1-min postexercise pressure equal to or greater than 30 mm Hg, and/or 5-min postexercise pressure equal to or greater than 20 mm Hg. Surgical treatment is indicated if the patient has failed nonsurgical management, typically lasting 3 to 6 months, and desires to continue with the associated activity.[7,8]

Video 83.1 Intracompartmental Pressure Testing: Post-Exercise. Mary Lloyd Ireland, MD (22 s)

Contraindications
Compartment releases are contraindicated if compartment pressures are not confirmatory of a diagnosis of CECS.

Preoperative Imaging
Imaging is typically not useful for the diagnosis or management of CECS.

Video 83.2 Fasciotomy: Two-Incision Technique. Mary Lloyd Ireland, MD (2 min)

Procedure
The compartments to be released are determined using patient history of where the pain is located, as well as compartment pressure testing results. If the patient has bilateral symptoms, then bilateral procedures can be performed in the same surgical setting.

Anterior and Lateral Compartments
Our preference is to use a two-incision technique for release of the anterior and lateral compartments.[1,9] A video of the two-incision technique can be seen in the video supplement.

The anterior intermuscular septum (IMS) is superficially located, centered between the palpable anterior border of the tibia and the lateral border of the fibula. Two longitudinal incisions, each 3 cm in length, are placed along the IMS, located approximately midway between the subcutaneous anterior border of the tibia and the subcutaneous lateral border of the fibula. The distal incision is centered over the exit of the superficial peroneal nerve, approximately 10 cm from the ankle joint line. The proximal incision is centered 10 cm distal to the proximal fibula (**Figure 1**). The incisions are carried down full-thickness to the muscle fascia. Using blunt instrument and finger dissection, the plane is developed over the muscle fascia and under the subcutaneous adipose tissues between the two incisions, as well as proximally and distally toward the knee and ankle. One channel is made over each compartment to avoid making a large subcutaneous space and minimize the occurrence of postoperative fluid collection.

The superficial peroneal nerve and any branches are visualized through the distal incision (**Figure 2, A**) and protected throughout the procedure. The fascia around the nerve is released if deemed to be tight. A small longitudinal incision is then made into the anterior and lateral fascia 1 cm on either side of the IMS at both incisions (**Figure 2, B**). From the proximal incision, the anterior and lateral compartment fasciotomy is carried proximally (**Figure 2, C**). We prefer to use

---

Dr. Amendola or an immediate family member has received royalties from Arthrex and Arthrosurface; serves as a paid consultant to or is an employee of Arthrex and Zimmer; serves as an unpaid consultant to MTP Solutions; has stock or stock options held in Arthrosurface and MTP Solutions; and serves as a board member, owner, officer, or committee member of the American Board of Orthopaedic Surgery, the American Orthopaedic Society for Sports Medicine, and the International Society of Arthroscopy, Knee Surgery, and Orthopaedic Sports Medicine. Dr. Wolf or an immediate family member serves as a board member, owner, officer, or committee member of the American Orthopaedic Society for Sports Medicine and the Arthroscopy Association of North America. Neither Dr. Wagstrom nor any immediate family member has received anything of value from or has stock or stock options held in a commercial company or institution related directly or indirectly to the subject of this chapter.

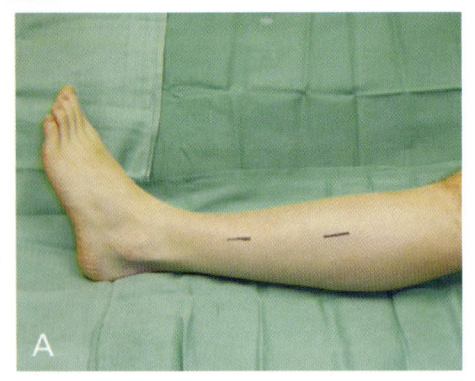

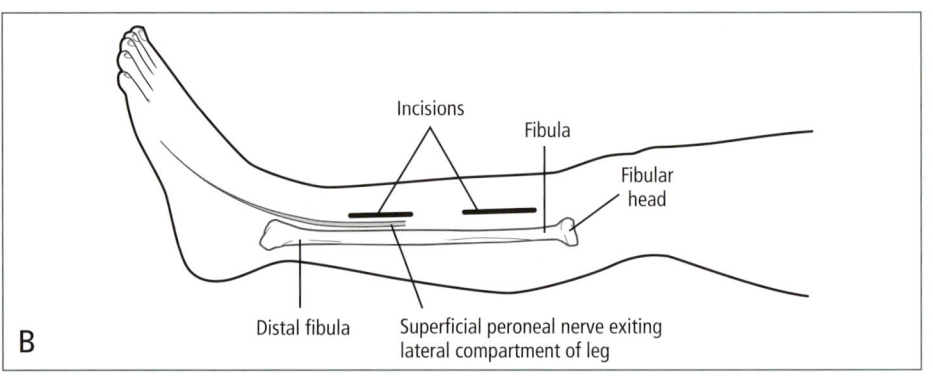

Figure 1 Photograph (**A**) and illustration (**B**) show skin markings for anterior and lateral compartment two-incision technique. (Panel A reproduced with permission from Bederka B, Amendola A: Leg pain and exertional compartment syndromes, in DeLee JC, Drez D, Miller MD, eds: *DeLee and Drez's Orthopaedic Sports Medicine: Principles and Practice*, ed 3. Philadelphia, PA, Saunders Elsevier, 2010, vol 2, pp 1857-1864.)

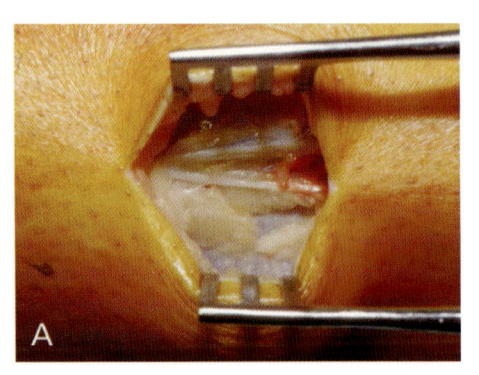

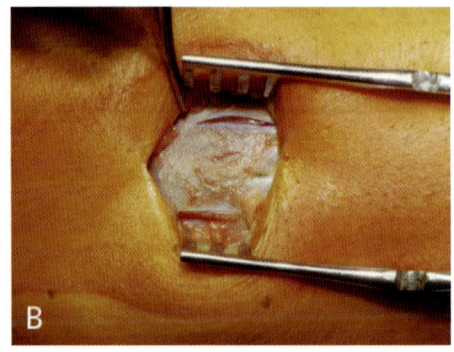

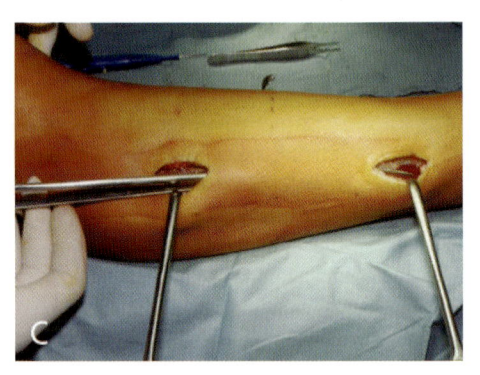

Figure 2 Intraoperative photographs show two-incision technique for anterior and lateral compartment releases. **A**, The superficial peroneal nerve is visualized in the distal lateral incision. **B**, The intermuscular raphe is seen between the fascial incisions. **C**, Fasciotomy is performed using long Metzenbaum scissors in a push-cut fashion. The nerve is visualized directly and protected in the distal incision. (Reproduced with permission from Bederka B, Amendola A: Leg pain and exertional compartment syndromes, in DeLee JC, Drez D, Miller MD, eds: *DeLee and Drez's Orthopaedic Sports Medicine: Principles and Practice*, ed 3. Philadelphia, PA, Saunders Elsevier, 2010, vol 2, pp 1857-1864.)

8- and 12-in Metzenbaum scissors, but a fasciotome may also be used. The distal incision is then used to carry the fasciotomies distally to the level of the superior extensor retinaculum. Using either proximal or distal incisions, the fasciotomies are connected under the skin bridge.

The two-incision technique offers several advantages, including easier access to the anterior and lateral compartment fascia adjacent to the IMS and confirmation of a complete fasciotomy. When using the two-incision technique, we recommend not proceeding with the fasciotomy until there is clear separation of the subcutaneous tissue from the fascia. This decreases the risk of injury to the subcutaneous structures, makes fasciotomy easier, and allows more comprehensive inspection to confirm complete fasciotomy.

Posterior Compartments

We prefer a single-incision technique for the release of the deep posterior and posterior tibialis compartments. A 10-cm incision is located 1 cm posterior to the posteromedial subcutaneous border of the tibia, centered at the distal insertion of the gastrocnemius muscle (**Figure 3, A**). It is important to identify the long saphenous nerve and vein, which are usually in the center of the field and are easily located on the posteromedial border of the tibia.

A small vertical incision is made at the osseofascial junction (**Figure 3, B**). The fascia is released distally to the level of the tibialis posterior tendon using Metzenbaum scissors and staying directly on the posterior border of the tibia. The surgeon's finger should follow the instrument to ensure a complete release. The release is then taken proximally. The soleus will then be encountered in the proximal one third of the tibia at the soleus bridge. Release of this stout structure must be complete, as it also represents the proximal confluence of the flexor hallucis longus and flexor digitorum longus fascia. This releases the deep posterior compartment.

A Cobb elevator or an osteotome is then used to release the tibialis posterior muscle off the tibia, completing the release of the tibialis posterior compartment (**Figure 3, C**). This effectively releases the deep posterior compartments. It is crucial to remain directly on the posterior aspect of the tibia throughout the release to ensure safety of the posterior tibial neurovascular bundle, which is posterior to the tibialis posterior and flexor digitorum longus. Verification of an adequate release by digital examination is of the utmost importance.

Prior to wound closure, it is important that the tourniquet be released and meticulous hemostasis be obtained to avoid seroma or hematoma formation. The subcutaneous tissues are closed and the skin is sutured using a subcuticular stitch. A sterile dressing and a compression bandage are applied.

Complications

Postoperative complications include hematoma (9%), anterior ankle pain (5%), superficial peroneal nerve injury (2%), and recurrence (2%).[10] Careful surgical technique minimizes the risk of most of these complications.

Postoperative Care and Rehabilitation

The patient is allowed to bear weight as tolerated immediately, using crutches as needed.[1] It is important to begin early

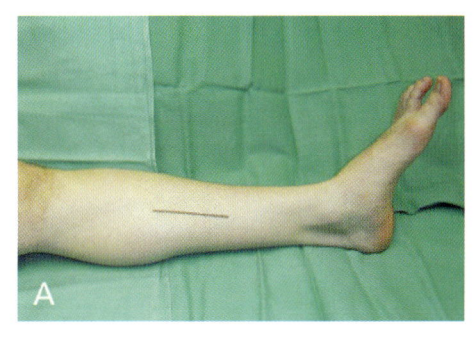

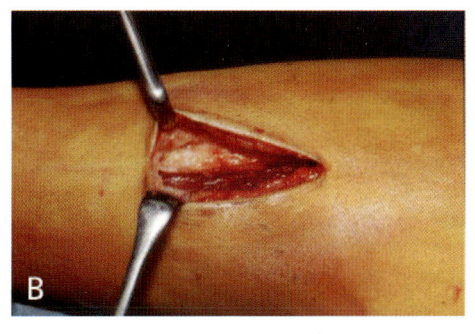

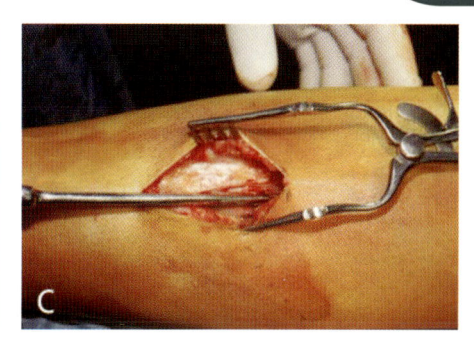

Figure 3 Posterior compartment releases. **A**, Photograph shows skin marking for posterior compartment releases. **B**, Intraoperative photograph shows the fascial incision. **C**, Intraoperative photograph shows the muscle fascia being taken directly off of the posteromedial border of the tibia. (Reproduced with permission from Bederka B, Amendola A: Leg pain and exertional compartment syndromes, in DeLee JC, Drez D, Miller MD, eds: *DeLee and Drez's Orthopaedic Sports Medicine: Principles and Practice*, ed 3. Philadelphia, PA, Saunders Elsevier, 2010, vol 2, pp 1857-1864.)

passive and active range-of-motion exercises to prevent postoperative fascial scarring.[2,3,11]

For the first 2 days after surgery, patients follow a RICE (rest, ice, compression, elevation) regimen, as well as anterior and posterior stretching (toe-pointing) three to five times per day.

Between days 3 and 14 after surgery, patients should perform aggressive anterior and posterior compartment stretches three times per day, increase the walking distance, and initiate stationary cycling once they have weaned themselves from the crutches.

At 2 weeks after surgery, the wounds are checked and a formal physical therapy regimen of stretching and functional return to sport-specific activity is begun.

Running may be implemented at 5 to 6 weeks postoperatively, with speed and agility drills added during the eighth week.[2,3,11] It is anticipated that athletes return to full sports participation by 3 months after surgery.

Pearls

- Most cases of CECS can be diagnosed by taking a careful and detailed history. Confirmation of the diagnosis with pressure testing is recommended in all cases.
- During surgery, great care must be taken to avoid injury to the superficial peroneal nerve and the saphenous structures.
- It is imperative to completely release involved compartments to avoid recurrence or incomplete resolution of symptoms.
- Hemostasis is very important to avoid fluid collection complications after surgery.
- Early rehabilitation after surgery is recommended for optimal and expedient outcomes.

References

1. Bederka B, Amendola A: Leg pain and exertional compartment syndromes, in DeLee JC, Drez D, Miller MD, eds: *DeLee and Drez's Orthopaedic Sports Medicine: Principles and Practice*, ed 3. Philadelphia, PA, Saunders Elsevier, 2010, vol 2, pp 1857-1864.
2. Blackman PG: A review of chronic exertional compartment syndrome in the lower leg. *Med Sci Sports Exerc* 2000;32(3, suppl):S4-S10.
3. Fraipont MJ, Adamson GJ: Chronic exertional compartment syndrome. *J Am Acad Orthop Surg* 2003;11(4):268-276.
4. Touliopolous S, Hershman EB: Lower leg pain: Diagnosis and treatment of compartment syndromes and other pain syndromes of the leg. *Sports Med* 1999;27(3):193-204.
5. Wilder RP, Sethi S: Overuse injuries: Tendinopathies, stress fractures, compartment syndrome, and shin splints. *Clin Sports Med* 2004;23(1):55-81, vi.
6. Pedowitz RA, Hargens AR, Mubarak SJ, Gershuni DH: Modified criteria for the objective diagnosis of chronic compartment syndrome of the leg. *Am J Sports Med* 1990;18(1):35-40.
7. Edwards PH Jr, Wright ML, Hartman JF: A practical approach for the differential diagnosis of chronic leg pain in the athlete. *Am J Sports Med* 2005;33(8):1241-1249.
8. Rorabeck CH, Bourne RB, Fowler PJ, Finlay JB, Nott L: The role of tissue pressure measurement in diagnosing chronic anterior compartment syndrome. *Am J Sports Med* 1988;16(2):143-146.
9. Rorabeck CH, Bourne RB, Fowler PJ: The surgical treatment of exertional compartment syndrome in athletes. *J Bone Joint Surg Am* 1983;65(9):1245-1251.
10. de Fijter WM, Scheltinga MR, Luiting MG: Minimally invasive fasciotomy in chronic exertional compartment syndrome and fascial hernias of the anterior lower leg: Short- and long-term results. *Mil Med* 2006;171(5):399-403.
11. Edwards P, Myerson MS: Exertional compartment syndrome of the leg: Steps for expedient return to activity. *Phys Sportsmed* 1996;24(4):31-46.

Video References

8.1 Ireland ML: *Intracompartmental Pressure Testing: Post-Exercise.* Lexington, KY, 2000.
8.2 Ireland ML: *Fasciotomy: Two-Incision Technique.* Lexington, KY, 2000.

Chapter 84
Transtibial Amputation

COL James R. Ficke, MD   MAJ Daniel J. Stinner, MD

Introduction

Whether necessitated by trauma, congenital anomaly, tumor, infection, or ischemia, transtibial amputations are commonly performed by orthopaedic surgeons. Burgess et al[1] initially described the benefits achieved using a myofascial posterior flap when providing distal coverage of the residual limb. This method was quickly popularized as a result of the successful application of this technique in patients with peripheral vascular disease.[1] However, the relatively short posterior flap by today's standards had its drawbacks, including retraction of the skin incision over the anterior tibia with atrophy of the residual limb, which may result in pressure sores and skin breakdown. This technique was later modified by Assal et al[2] to incorporate a longer and thicker posterior flap, with improved fixation of the flap to prevent the migration of the distal soft tissue.

The ideal bone length of the residual limb is 2.5 cm for every 30 cm of body height, which equates to approximately 12.5 to 17.5 cm.[3] Although the fibula is commonly sectioned approximately 1 cm proximal to the tibial cut in the standard transtibial amputation, this technique is modified when performing a bone-bridge synostosis of the residual limb.

Ertl[4] first reported on his bone-bridging technique in 1949. Since then, there have been various modifications of the procedure but very little available literature demonstrating objective outcomes in patients treated with this surgical technique.[5,6] Proponents of this procedure believe that the bone bridge allows the residual limb to be end-bearing or, at a minimum, allows the fibula to contribute in weight bearing, thus distributing the mechanical load of the residual limb. In addition, many supporters feel that it prevents discordant tibiofibular movement, referred to as chopsticking, which may be a source of pain in transtibial amputees.

Patient Selection

Patients who undergo a transtibial amputation are considered either ischemic or nonischemic. Patients in the nonischemic group are typically younger and healthier, with indications for amputation more likely being due to trauma, tumor, infection, or congenital deformities. Those with ischemic limbs likely have additional comorbidities that need to be assessed before surgical intervention. In addition, successful wound healing in this patient population can be dramatically improved through appropriate surgical technique using a long posterior flap.

When possible, preoperative assessment of healing potential should be performed. Ideally, patients undergoing a transtibial amputation should have an ankle-brachial index greater than 0.5, transcutaneous oxygen saturation on room air greater than 20 to 30 mm Hg, an albumin level greater than 2.5 g/dL, and an absolute lymphocyte count greater than 1,500/µL.[7,8] This preoperative assessment is important because 9% to 15% of transtibial amputations ultimately progress to a higher level of limb loss.[9,10]

Indications

General indications for a transtibial amputation include high-energy trauma, a dysvascular extremity, uncontrolled infection, tumor, congenital deformities/deficiencies, and chronic pain. Specific indications in trauma still are not clearly defined, as recent reports demonstrate equivalent function for amputations and limb salvage. There are no clear absolute indications that have validated outcomes. Furthermore, loss of plantar sensation should not be considered a current indication in the early trauma patient. Similarly, dysvascular patients considered for amputation are those who have nonreconstructible injuries or are not revascularization candidates. However, when considering the standard Burgess technique versus the bone-bridge synostosis, the current available data must be taken into account in the decision-making process.

Although the specific patient population that would most benefit from the bone-bridge synostosis has not been defined in the literature, available data do allow some generalizations. Gwinn et al[11] performed a retrospective analysis of 37 patients who underwent bone-bridge transtibial amputations in 42 extremities for lower extremity trauma to identify perioperative differences between those undergoing bone-bridge and non–bone-bridge amputations. Their results demonstrated increased surgical times in those undergoing bone bridging (179 minutes versus 112 minutes, $P < 0.0005$) and increased tourniquet times (115 minutes versus 71 minutes, $P < 0.0005$). Although they argue that the longer surgical and tourniquet time should not be considered a contraindication to performing a bone-bridge transtibial amputation in a young, healthy patient, these factors have been associated with increased complications in those undergoing other lower extremity surgery.[12,13]

Because of the increased surgical and tourniquet times associated with the bone-bridge synostosis technique,[11] we recommend that it be reserved for young, healthy, active individuals. In addition, those with fibular instability or disruption of the interosseous membrane may benefit from this technique as a primary or revision amputation.[5]

Contraindications

Patients with dysvascular limbs whose clinical workup as described previously does not meet the appropriate values that are predictive of successful wound healing[7,8] should undergo optimization before undergoing an amputation at this level or consideration of amputation at a higher level because a high rate of transtibial amputations ultimately progress to a higher level of amputation.

Procedure
Room Setup/Patient Positioning
The patient is placed supine on a standard operating room table. A small bump can

---

COL Ficke serves as a board member, owner, officer, or committee member of the American Orthopaedic Foot & Ankle Society, the American Academy of Orthopaedic Surgeons, the Society of Military Orthopaedic Surgeons, and the Airlift Research Foundation. MAJ Stinner serves as a board member, owner, officer, or committee member of the Society of Military Orthopaedic Surgeons and the Orthopaedic Trauma Association.

Section 6: Foot and Ankle

be placed under the surgical hip so that the patella is directed upward. A proximal thigh tourniquet is typically placed before surgical preparation and draping.

Radiographs should be readily available, with measurements from the joint line or the tibial tubercle to the proposed site of the tibial cut.

Special Instruments/Equipment/Implants

For a transtibial amputation, the following instruments and equipment should be on hand: a basic major orthopaedic instrument set, an oscillating saw, a drill, an amputation knife, silk free ties and stick ties (vessel clips if preferred), and a suction drain for wound closure, based on surgeon preference.

If bone-bridge synostosis using screw fixation is to be performed, a small or large fragment set may be required, depending on the screw size the surgeon intends to use for the bridge. A number of variations to this surgical technique have been described, and the appropriate bone-bridge fixation device must be available.[14] A chisel or an osteotome will be needed for this procedure, as well as an intraoperative C-arm fluoroscopy system.

Video 84.1 Transtibial Amputation. COL James R. Ficke, MD; MAJ Daniel J. Stinner, MD (5 min)

Surgical Technique

After positioning the patient, a pneumatic tourniquet is used. Exsanguination should be performed, except in a possible septic or neoplastic situation. Gravity can assist in minimizing the blood remaining within the distal limb before inflation. The tibial tubercle is marked and measurements are obtained from either the tubercle or the medial joint line to identify the desired level of the tibial resection. Next, the skin is marked at 1 cm distal to the projected tibial cut, perpendicular to the tibia from the posterior border of the tibia and lateral to the fibula when it can be palpated.

The video supplement includes a demonstration of the transtibial amputation and a demonstration of the bone-bridge technique. Although the video shows the rounded ends of the anterior skin incision drawn freehand, an alternative method to minimize redundant skin "dog ears" is to trace out the thumb hole of a hemostat at both ends of the anterior transverse skin incision (**Figure 1**). The posterior flap skin is then marked such that it is at least 1.5 times the length of the transverse cut. This is an extremely important determination because it permits an extended posterior flap at the completion of the procedure. The posterior skin flap should be distal to the palpable musculotendinous junction of the gastrocnemius. Rounding the corners at the distal end of the posterior skin flap also facilitates elimination of redundant skin at closure.

This entire circumference is then incised through the underlying fascia. When performing a bone bridge and preserving the periosteal flap of the anteromedial tibia, care is taken to not divide the proximal periosteum. A vertical skin incision can be directed over the anterior crest of the tibia to facilitate exposure for a long tibial periosteal flap. With division of the fascia, the deep and superficial peroneal nerves should be identified and resected sharply, using gentle traction. The anterior compartment musculature is sharply dissected at the most proximal wound exposure to minimize bulk and facilitate myodesis and skin closure. Alternatively, electrocautery can be used, which facilitates muscular hemostasis. Prior to deep muscular transection, the anterior tibial artery is identified, isolated, and ligated. A suture ligature for the anterior and posterior tibial arteries ensures vascular control.

Video 84.2 Bone Bridging in Transtibial Amputation. Marco A. Guedes de Souza Pinto, MD; Michael S. Pinzur, MD; Lew C. Schon, MD; Douglas G. Smith, MD (13 min)

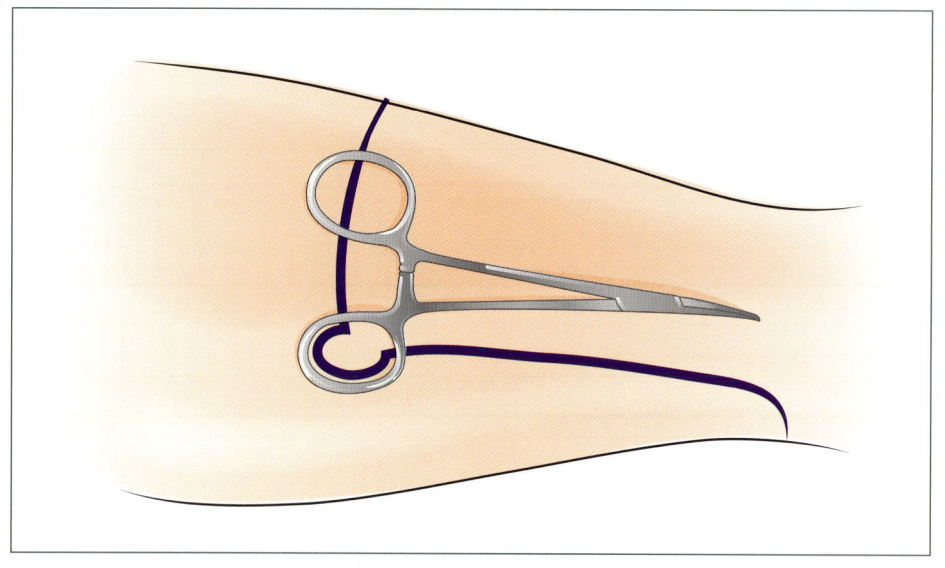

Figure 1 Illustration depicts a method to minimize redundant skin "dog ears."

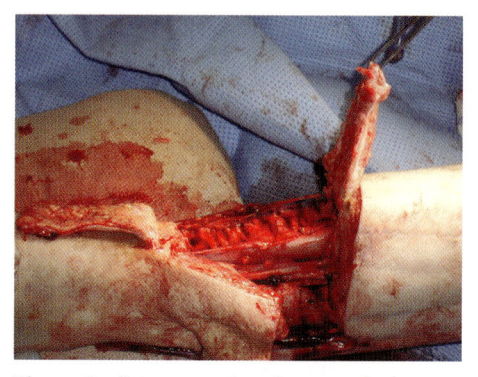

Figure 2 Intraoperative photograph shows elevation of the periosteal flap. Multiple small bone fragments can be seen.

Video 84.3 Periosteal Flap Development. COL James R. Ficke, MD; MAJ Daniel J. Stinner, MD (2 min)

At this point in the procedure, if a bone bridge is planned, the periosteal flap should be elevated using a single-beveled wide chisel (**Figure 2**). (The complete bone-bridging procedure can be seen in the video supplement.) The anterior and posterior margins of the anteromedial tibial periosteum are incised sharply for 8 to 10 cm distally, and the flap is raised with the bevel positioned superficially. A series of small bone fragments should be left attached to the periosteum. These fragments are not essential in the most proximal few centimeters where the periosteal sleeve overlies the end of the tibia. It is imperative to have enough periosteum to reach well past the lateral edge of the fibula. This flap is protected with a moist gauze sponge, and the remainder of the tibia is isolated using a curved periosteal elevator. The intraosseous membrane is divided, and the fibula is identified and prepared for osteotomy. For a standard amputation, the fibula is resected approximately 1 cm above the level of the tibial cut at a slightly proximal lateral angle. With a bone-bridge procedure, it is important to measure the interosseous distance (between the lateral tibia and the medial fibula; (**Figure 3**) and preserve this distance. The distal cut of the fibula would be this interosseous distance plus approximately 2 cm to inlay into the tibia distal to the tibial resection level. Tibial transection is then performed using a power saw with saline irrigation, followed by transection of the fibula at the appropriate length for the type of transtibial amputation being performed.

The posterior tibial muscle lies between the bone and the neurovascular bundle and provides working space to obtain vascular control. Therefore, when a tourniquet is used, a sharp amputation knife can be inserted and used to transect and taper the posterior soft tissue. The deep posterior compartment and often much of the soleus are removed at the level of the tibial bone cut to facilitate tension-free myodesis and skin closure. With the amputation knife, a smooth contour can be achieved and the gastrocnemius fascia preserved to facilitate solid myodesis. The tibial nerve is identified and dissected from adjacent vascular structures. It should be injected proximally with 1% lidocaine and then resected using a sharp scalpel under gentle tension to allow retraction proximal to the level of the bone cut. Suturing the tibial nerve is not necessary for hemostasis. The posterior tibial artery is identified and doubly ligated with a single suture ligature or vascular clip. Similarly, the tibial veins are ligated and the remaining deep posterior compartment resected to the level of the distal bone cut. At this point, the major vascular structures have been ligated and the tibial and peroneal nerves have been resected in the gastrocnemius, which is tapered to permit gentle tension myodesis.

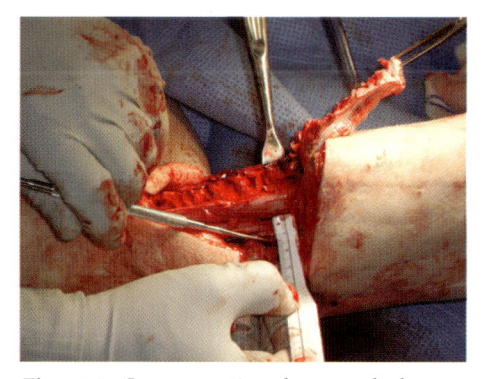

The tourniquet can now be released and meticulous muscular hemostasis obtained. An anterior tibial bone bevel must be performed to minimize prosthesis pressure and optimize socket comfort. The bevel should begin outside the medullary canal at an angle of approximately 45°. Sharp edges of the tibia should be rasped and rounded. The perimeter of the medullary canal should not be disrupted by the anterior bevel (**Figure 4, A**). The preparation for a bone bridge is described at the end of this procedure section.

Drill holes for a myodesis can be placed proximal to the level of the anterior bone bevel. Alternatively, direct suture to the anterior periosteum permits some mobility of the muscle flap. Saline irrigation removes most bone particulate matter; this is important to minimize heterotopic ossification. Myodesis is performed using a locking Krackow-style suture within the gastrocnemius aponeurosis and secured on the anterior tibia (**Figure 4, B**). Generally a No. 2 or No. 5 braided suture is used, although cases of sterile abscess formation can develop with inner core–type sutures. At this point, a small-diameter drain can be placed submuscularly, depending on surgeon preference. The borders of the gastrocnemius are secured to the proximal anterior fascia. Whenever possible, the extended posterior flap is overlaid onto the anterior skin to avoid placing a skin scar over the bony end of the residual limb (**Figure 4, C**).

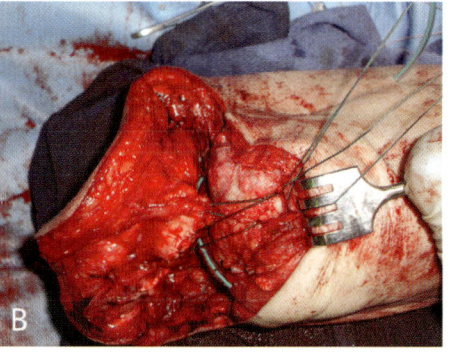

In most traumatic amputations, it is preferable to transect bone above the zone of injury. Occasionally, however, the bone and muscle are viable and the skin is not. If skin coverage is insufficient to retain adequate tibial bone length, then subsequent skin grafting can be performed. Generally, this is best performed as a staged procedure, following a period to enable wound-bed granulation.

Following secure myodesis and layered fascial closure, the skin is closed with interrupted tension-relieving or vertical mattress sutures (**Figure 5, A** and **B**). A standard postoperative dressing is placed, using gauze and cotton or abdominal padding with plaster splinting above the knee to minimize the development of a knee flexion contracture. There is no clear evidence of enhanced function with immediate postoperative prosthesis use or weight bearing. Perioperative antibiotics are routinely continued until drain removal, and a postoperative dressing is changed at 3 to 5 days.

Preparation for a Bone-Bridge Procedure

Following elevation of the anteromedial periosteal flap and tibial resection, the next step is to prepare the fibula, as demonstrated in the bone-bridging technique

Figure 3 Intraoperative photograph shows measurement of the intraosseous distance at the level of tibial transection in preparation for a bone-bridge procedure.

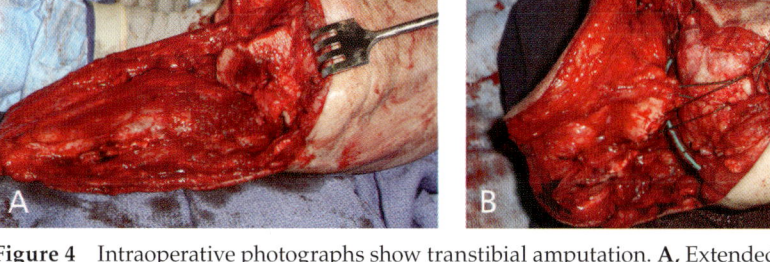

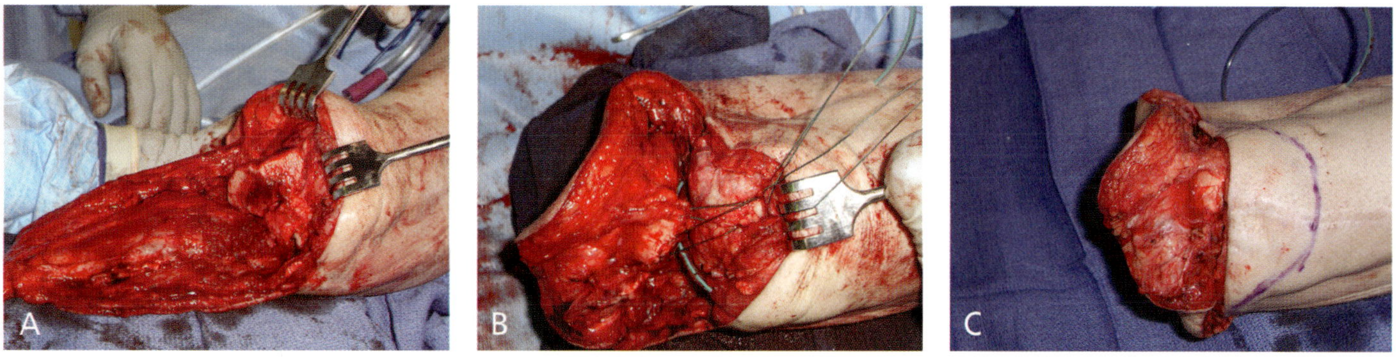

Figure 4 Intraoperative photographs show transtibial amputation. **A,** Extended posterior flap with tapered gastrocnemius. Note that the tibial bevel does not encroach on the medullary canal. **B,** Myodesis is achieved with large braided suture to bone. The periosteal flap can be seen underneath, and the submuscular drain is in place. **C,** The completed myodesisis. The posterior skin flap overlap is traced before suprafascial skin excision.

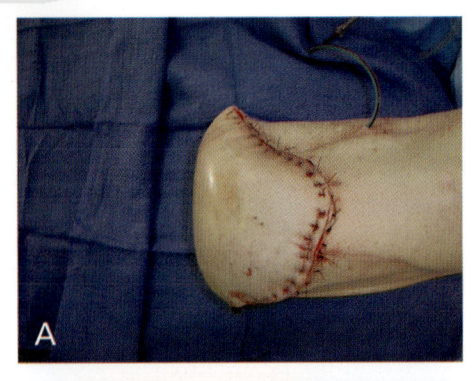

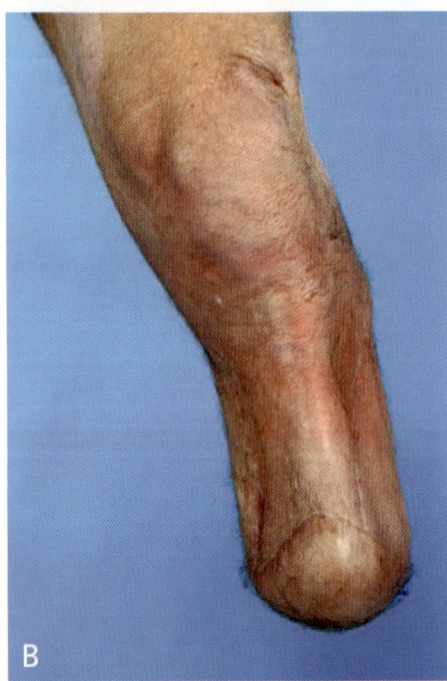

Figure 5 Photographs depict transtibial amputation. **A**, Postoperative wound appearance with interrupted mattress sutures. **B**, Transtibial amputation at 10-month follow-up. This patient had returned to full activity, including running.

video supplement. It is important to retain attachment of the peroneal musculature or at least the lateral periosteum of the fibula. The initial cut of the fibula is performed several centimeters distal to the tibial cut, which permits removal of the distal leg, hemostasis, and preparation of the gastrocnemius. The proximal fibular cut should be performed at the same level of the distal tibia. Elevation of the lateral periosteum at the level of this fibular cut and 1 cm distally enables a second cut, while retaining fibular soft-tissue attachments. A notch is cut in the posterior lateral tibia deep enough to completely house the fibula. At this point, it is important to ensure that the intraosseous distance is the same or slightly less than that measured before bone resection.

The bone bridge can be secured using nonabsorbable sutures through drill holes at the lateral and medial aspects or by a long 3.5-mm cortical screw inserted from the lateral aspect of the fibula through the intramedullary canal of the transverse fibula into the medial cortex of the tibia. Alternatively, a nonabsorbable suture anchor can be used. The previously prepared periosteal sleeve still attached to the anteromedial tibia is overlaid and sutured around the fibula. It is this sleeve that facilitates ossification of the bone bridge and the ultimate stability of the procedure.

Complications

Pain can present in many forms in this patient population. In addition to typical postoperative pain, patients can experience phantom limb pain, complex regional pain syndrome, or localized residual limb pain from prominent neuromata, limb-socket interface problems, or insufficient soft-tissue coverage.

One of the first goals in the initial postoperative period is edema control because edema can have a profound effect on wound healing. This is typically done with elevation, rigid dressings with soft compression, and eventual progression to elastic prosthetic shrinkers.

Following a transtibial amputation, knee flexion contractures must be prevented. Rigid dressings with the knee in extension help to prevent contractures. In addition, early prone positioning can help prevent hip flexion contractures before patient mobilizing.

Wound breakdown is more common in patients with vascular disease and diabetes but it can occur in any patient. Optimizing preoperative nutrition, ensuring meticulous intraoperative hemostasis, and initiating postoperative edema control should all be undertaken to minimize this risk.

Postoperative Care and Rehabilitation

Ultimately, the goals of rehabilitation following a transtibial amputation involve a return to function.[15] That functional level will be influenced greatly by the premorbid condition of the patient and the patient's desires following amputation.

Phase 1 (Week 1)

Focused summary: Bed-to-wheelchair mobility, range-of-motion exercises, edema control, knee immobilizer, transition to outpatient rehabilitation, and independent gait training with walker/crutches.

1. Wound management
   a. A sterile intraoperative dressing with a well-padded cast is applied, holding the knee in extension to prevent flexion contracture.
   b. Perioperative antibiotics are given until the drain is removed.
   c. Drain is removed at 48 hours, or earlier if minimal output.
   d. Dressing remains in place for the first week.

2. Rehabilitation goals
   a. Functional mobility/basic ambulation is achieved.
      i. Bed mobility
      ii. Transfers
      iii. Ambulation with assistive device
      iv. Wheelchair use as appropriate
   b. Baseline balance and conditioning are maintained/restored.
   c. Appropriate residual limb management/self-care is learned.

Phase 2 (Weeks 2–10)

Focused summary: Progress from wound healing, shrinkage of the residual limb, and simulated weight bearing to donning a new prosthesis, progressive weight bearing with a wheeled walker, walking on uneven surfaces, and navigating home environment successfully.

1. Wound management
   a. Sutures are removed. Timing is dependent on wound healing, but typically is done at week 3.
   b. Shrinker use is begun once wounds are closed, healed, and dry; no sutures or sterile adhesive strips should be used.
   c. Transition is made to liner when deemed appropriate by prosthetist.

2. Rehabilitation goals
   a. Appropriate exercises are performed independently.
      i. Strengthening
      ii. Core stability/lumbar stabilization
      iii. Balance
      iv. Cardiovascular conditioning
   b. Sufficient range of motion is gained to allow optimal gait training with use of prosthetic device.
   c. Independence with mobility and ambulation with appropriate assistive devices is achieved.
   d. Independence with residual limb care is achieved.

Phase 3 (Weeks 11–)

Focused summary: Return to an active lifestyle, advanced ambulation patterns, and vocational and sport-specific training.

1. Rehabilitation goals
   a. Weight-bearing and weight-shifting activities are progressed.
   b. Rehabilitation exercises are performed independently.
   c. Gait is normalized.
   d. Gait progresses to modified independence or independence with appropriate assistive device.
   e. Return to high-level/high-impact conditioning is achieved.
   f. Return to organized and individual sport activity is achieved.
   g. Return to vocation-specific training is achieved.

Pearls

- A hemostat loop can be used to trace a semicircle at each end of the anterior transverse skin incision. This facilitates closure that will reduce or prevent "dog ears."
- The deep medial longitudinal incision should be placed anterior to the long saphenous vein to permit venous clearance.
- The anterior compartment muscles should be cleared at or proximal to the tibial bone cut to reduce bulk anterolaterally. This is required for the bridge but also eases tension-free skin closure.
- When creating the periosteal layer for the bone bridge, a single-bevel chisel can be used to elevate attached bone chips. The bevel is placed up, and alternating wrist actions are used to create smaller malleable bone fragments attached to the periosteum.
- Vascular ligation requires suture ligature or a vascular clip to prevent the pulsatile disruption of simple ties—the "rubber band on a newspaper" effect.
- The bone ends should be rounded with a rasp to prevent potential sharp corners. A power saw held at an angle and pulled across the sharp surface is an effective power rasp. Care should be taken to make sure that the anterior bevel does not encroach into the medullary canal because this can resorb to leave two sharp corners.
- Braided single-component suture material should be used for myodesis. FiberWire (Arthrex) has been associated with sterile abscesses.[16]
- In preparing the sutures for myodesis, we make sure the material crosses the posterior gastrocnemius aponeurosis and is pulled tightly into the muscle tissue. The gastrocnemius and associated myodesis can later atrophy and leave the suture loose.

References

1. Burgess EM, Romano RL, Zettl JH, Schrock RD Jr: Amputations of the leg for peripheral vascular insufficiency. *J Bone Joint Surg Am* 1971;53(5):874-890.
2. Assal M, Blanck R, Smith DG: Extended posterior flap for transtibial amputation. *Orthopedics* 2005;28(6):542-546.
3. Canale ST, Beaty JH, eds: *Campbell's Operative Orthopaedics*, ed 11. Philadelphia, PA, Mosby Elsevier, 2008.
4. Ertl J: Uber amputationsstumpfe. *Chirurg* 1949;20:218-224.
5. Pinzur MS, Beck J, Himes R, Callaci J: Distal tibiofibular bone-bridging in transtibial amputation. *J Bone Joint Surg Am* 2008;90(12):2682-2687.
6. Dougherty PJ: Transtibial amputees from the Vietnam War. Twenty-eight-year follow-up. *J Bone Joint Surg Am* 2001;83-A(3):383-389.
7. Dickhaut SC, DeLee JC, Page CP: Nutritional status: Importance in predicting wound-healing after amputation. *J Bone Joint Surg Am* 1984;66(1):71-75.
8. Ng VY, Berlet GC: Evolving techniques in foot and ankle amputation. *J Am Acad Orthop Surg* 2010;18(4):223-235.
9. Dillingham TR, Pezzin LE, Shore AD: Reamputation, mortality, and health care costs among persons with dysvascular lower-limb amputations. *Arch Phys Med Rehabil* 2005;86(3):480-486.
10. Norgren L, Hiatt WR, Dormandy JA, et al; TASC II Working Group: Inter-society consensus for the management of peripheral arterial disease (TASC II). *Eur J Vasc Endovasc Surg* 2007;33(suppl 1):S1-S75.
11. Gwinn DE, Keeling J, Froehner JW, McGuigan FX, Andersen R: Perioperative differences between bone bridging and non-bone bridging transtibial amputations for wartime lower extremity trauma. *Foot Ankle Int* 2008;29(8):787-793.
12. Horlocker TT, Hebl JR, Gali B, et al: Anesthetic, patient, and surgical risk factors for neurologic complications after prolonged total tourniquet time during total knee arthroplasty. *Anesth Analg* 2006;102(3):950-955.
13. Konrad G, Markmiller M, Lenich A, Mayr E, Rüter A: Tourniquets may increase postoperative swelling and pain after internal fixation of ankle fractures. *Clin Orthop Relat Res* 2005;433:189-194.
14. Berlet GC, Pokabla C, Serynek P: An alternative technique for the Ertl osteomyoplasty. *Foot Ankle Int* 2009;30(5):443-446.
15. Gailey RS, Springer BA, Scherer M: Physical therapy for the polytrauma casualty with limb loss, in Pasquina PF, Cooper RA, eds: *Care of the Combat Amputee*. Falls Church, VA, Office of the Surgeon General, United States Army, 2009, pp 451-492.
16. Mack AW, Freedman BA, Shawen SB, Gajewski DA, Kalasinsky VF, Lewin-Smith MR: Wound complications following the use of FiberWire in lower-extremity traumatic amputations: A case series. *J Bone Joint Surg Am* 2009;91(3):680-685.

Chapter 85
Midfoot Amputations

Terrence M. Philbin, DO Bryan Witt, DO

Introduction

Historically, patients have viewed amputations as disfiguring and a failure of treatment instead of regarding them as the beginning of a healing process.[1-3] Advances in surgical techniques and prosthetic devices have initiated a reemergence of partial foot amputations[1,2] (**Figure 1**). Pedal amputations result in increased function, better cosmesis, improved lifestyle, and decreased energy consumption as compared with transtibial amputations.[2] Among the midfoot amputations, the most commonly performed is the transmetatarsal amputation; however, the Lisfranc and Chopart amputations are also considered viable options.[4]

In the United States, there are approximately 1.7 million people living with an amputation.[5] Moreover, an average of 133,235 amputations are performed yearly in the United States.[5] The vast majority of amputations (82%) are due to vascular conditions that are increasing in incidence.[5] Trauma- and congenital-associated amputations are the second and third most common causes of amputations, respectively.[5] Lower limb amputations account for 97% of all dysvascular amputations.[5] Over 50% of all lower extremity amputations are either transfemoral or transtibial; pedal amputations constitute 31% of lower extremity amputations.[5]

The transmetatarsal amputation was described by McKittrick in 1949 as a surgical option to treat pedal infections associated with diabetes mellitus.[1,2,6] This amputation is an alternative to the standard transtibial amputation and generally has a lower mortality rate, results in less energy expenditure with ambulation, and provides a distal weight-bearing stump.[1,2] Approximately 10,000 transmetatarsal amputations are performed yearly in the United States.[1,2] The amputation is described as a resection of the metatarsal bones at the midshaft level.

The Lisfranc amputation was developed in the 1800s by Lisfranc de St. Martin, a French surgeon during the Napoleonic war.[1,4] Lisfranc described this midfoot amputation as a disarticulation between the metatarsals and tarsal bones.[4]

The Chopart amputation was described by Chopart, a French surgeon in the late 1700s. This amputation is performed at a more proximal level in comparison to the Lisfranc and transmetatarsal amputations.[4] The Chopart amputation involves disarticulating the talonavicular and calcaneocuboid joints[1,2,4] (**Figure 2**).

Patient Selection
Indications

The primary indication for a midfoot amputation is extensive soft-tissue compromise of the forefoot that does not allow a more distal amputation.[1,4,7] These soft-tissue complications can be due to a variety of medical or traumatic events, including traumatic nonsalvageable forefoot injury (**Figure 3**), diabetes mellitus, Charcot neuroarthropathy, frostbite, peripheral vascular disease, bony neoplasm, osteomyelitis, soft-tissue infection, failed prior surgery, and intractable pain.[2,7-9]

Contraindications

Midfoot amputations are contraindicated in patients with vascular insufficiency at the level of the proposed amputation.[3,4,6-8] Inadequate perfusion to the amputated stump leads to poor wound healing, requiring another, more proximal amputation.[3,4,6-8] In addition, patients receiving a pedal amputation secondary to infection require an amputation that is proximal to the active site of infection.[3,7] Amputating below the level of infection may necessitate future surgery to completely eradicate the infection.[3,7] Furthermore, patients who are nonambulators, especially those being considered for a Chopart or Lisfranc amputation, should have a higher transtibial amputation.[4] Also, those patients who have any type of revascularization procedure to the lower extremity should wait at least 72 hours before proceeding with a pedal amputation.[7]

Preoperative Evaluation
Laboratory and Diagnostic Tests

The preoperative management of a patient undergoing pedal amputation often requires a multitude of laboratory and diagnostic tests. The underlying pathologic reason for amputation, whether traumatic, infectious, or vascular, will guide the surgeon's decision making with regard to preoperative planning. A multidisciplinary team approach, including representatives from internal medicine, cardiology, nephrology, vascular surgery, and wound management, among other health care professionals, is paramount for the most appropriate care of the pedal amputation patient.[1,8,10,11]

Prior to midfoot amputation, preoperative laboratory testing is completed, including an assessment of immune and nutritional status.[1,4,10,11] A complete blood count with differential is obtained to determine the presence or absence of acute infection.[11] A white blood cell count greater than 12,000 and increased polymorphonuclear leukocytes may indicate an infectious process.[8,11] The erythrocyte sedimentation rate and C-reactive protein level are nonspecific markers of inflammation.[11] These tests aid in the diagnosis of an infectious process such as osteomyelitis.[11] Moreover, the total lymphocyte count is used to determine the potential for wound healing.[11] A level greater than 1,500 is considered immunocompetent and is associated with a better healing prognosis.[1,6,9-11] Hemoglobin and hematocrit levels are assessed for the presence

---

Dr. Philbin or an immediate family member has received royalties from Orthohelix, Biomet, and Stryker; is a member of a speakers' bureau or has made paid presentations on behalf of DJ Orthopaedics, Pfizer, Biomet, Footmax, Orthohelix, and Stryker; serves as a paid consultant to or is an employee of Biomet, Orthohelix, Pfizer, DJ Orthopaedics, Lifenet, Amniox, and Stryker; has stock or stock options held in Orthohelix; has received research or institutional support from Biomet, DJ Orthopaedics, Pfizer, Biomimetic, and Artelon; and serves as a board member, owner, officer, or committee member of the Arthritis Foundation, the American Orthopaedic Foot & Ankle Society, the American Academy of Orthopaedic Surgeons Communications Cabinet, the American Osteopathic Academy of Orthopaedics Board, and the American Diabetes Association Central Ohio Board. Neither Dr. Witt nor any immediate family member has received anything of value from or owns stock in a commercial company or institution related directly or indirectly to the subject of this chapter.

Section 6: Foot and Ankle

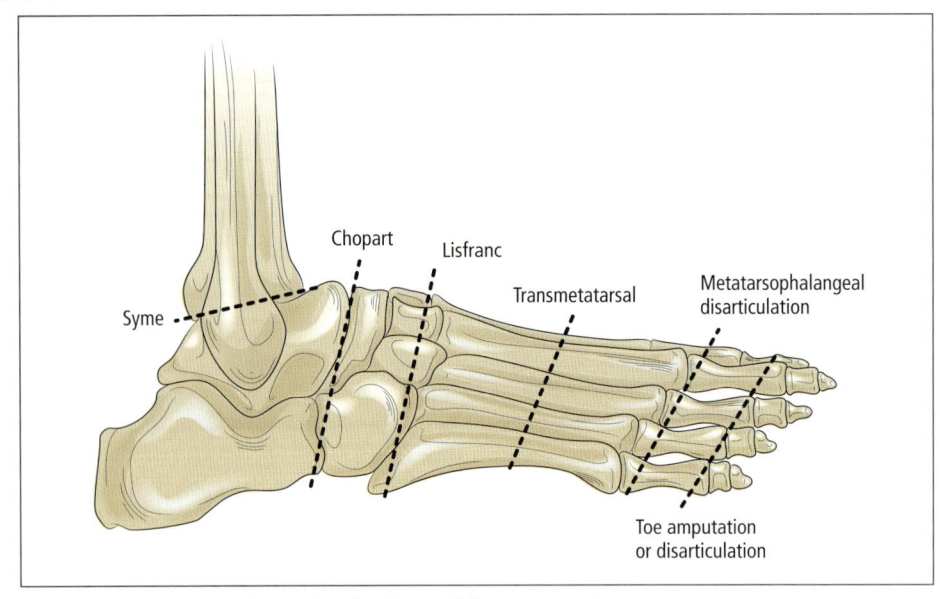

Figure 1 Illustration depicts levels of partial foot amputation.

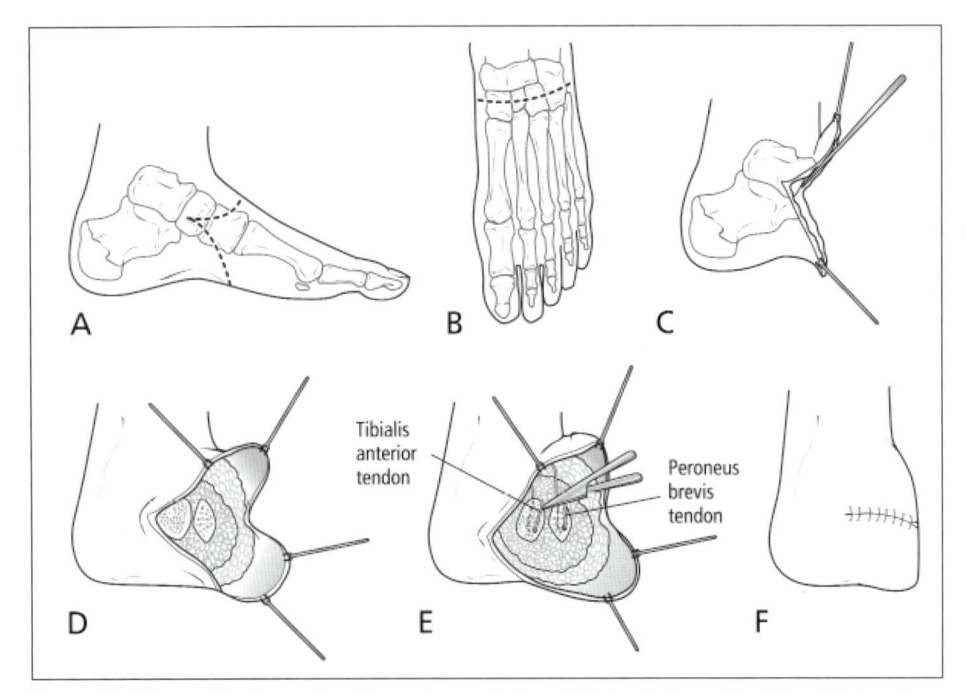

Figure 2 Illustration shows the Chopart amputation. **A,** Lateral view of incision. **B,** Dorsal view of incision. **C** and **D,** Dorsal and plantar flaps after resection of the distal foot. **E,** Transfer of the anterior tibialis tendon to the talar neck and transfer of the peroneus brevis tendon to the anterior calcaneus. **F,** Appearance of completed amputation after skin closure.

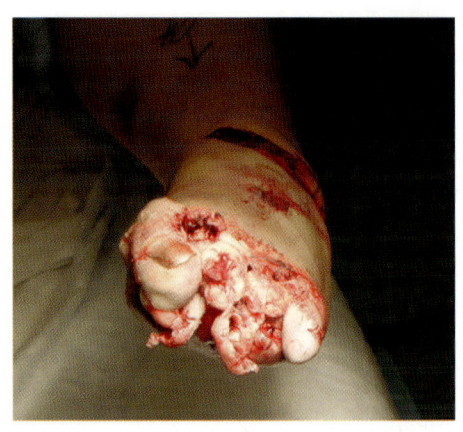

Figure 3 Photograph depicts a traumatic nonsalvageable forefoot injury. (Courtesy of Christopher Hyer, DPM, FACFAS, Orthopedic Foot and Ankle Center, Westerville, OH.)

of anemia.[11] Low hemoglobin and hematocrit levels are associated with poor tissue oxygenation and healing capacity.[9,11] Furthermore, serum albumin and protein levels are assessed preoperatively to determine the patient's healing capacity.[1,11] A serum albumin level greater than 3.0 g/dL and protein level greater than 6.0 g/dL are associated with improved wound healing.[1,6,8,10,11]

A comprehensive vascular examination is imperative for all patients undergoing a pedal amputation.[4,10,11] It is extremely important to assess the perfusion of the affected lower extremity to determine the appropriate level of amputation and healing capacity.[10,11] The vascular examination begins with assessing the peripheral pulses, including the dorsalis pedis and the posterior tibial.[10,11] In addition, capillary refill is assessed to determine digital perfusion. Furthermore, the patient's skin should be examined for atrophic changes as well as hair loss about the foot.[10,11] Nonpalpable peripheral pulses, sluggish capillary refill, atrophic skin changes, and loss of hair require further vascular examination.[10,11]

Noninvasive vascular studies, such as the ankle brachial index (ABI), can help determine the appropriate level of amputation and the postoperative healing potential.[1,6,10,11] An ABI less than 0.9 may indicate impaired peripheral vasculature; an ABI greater than 0.5 is associated with better potential for distal stump healing.[1,2,6,8,10] However, the ABI can be falsely normal in patients with noncompressible blood vessels.[10,11] High suspicion and more invasive testing are required in these individuals. The arterial Doppler ultrasound examination with waveforms is useful in determining arterial occlusive disease.[10,11] A monophasic waveform indicates arterial occlusive disease, whereas a triphasic waveform represents vascular patency.[10,11] Transcutaneous oxygen pressures can also be effective in determining the level of ischemia and the potential for wound healing.[1,4,6,10,11] A pressure less than 30 mm Hg is an indicator of limb ischemia and poor wound healing capacity.[1,2,6,8,10,11] Patients with abnormal noninvasive vascular studies require an invasive examination of the affected lower extremity vasculature.[10,11]

A vascular surgery consultation is warranted in patients with impaired noninvasive vascular studies.[1,2,4,10,11] The vascular surgeon will determine if invasive diagnostic testing or endovascular surgery is indicated before an amputation.[2,4,11] Digital subtraction angiography, magnetic resonance angiography, and CT angiography can determine the level of arterial occlusive disease.[11] If a specific arterial lesion is identified, surgical correction of the arterial occlusion is warranted.[11] This correction may allow the surgeon to perform a more distal amputation. However, if a revascularization procedure is performed, an amputation cannot be performed for at least 72 hours.[7,11]

552 © 2013 American Academy of Orthopaedic Surgeons

Imaging

All patients undergoing a pedal amputation require radiographic imaging for preoperative planning.[10,11] Three radiographic views, preferably weight-bearing, of the foot and ankle are important in the initial patient evaluation.[10] These radiographs are necessary to evaluate fractures involved in traumatic amputations (Figure 4) and identify bony neoplasms, congenital abnormalities, and infectious processes, such as gas within the soft tissues.[11] CT can further delineate pathologic processes seen on radiographs or detect bony or soft-tissue abnormalities not seen on plain radiographs, including bone sequestra, cortical destruction, and periosteal new bone formation representing an osteomyelitic process.[11] In addition, CT can identify bony tumors, occult fractures, and soft-tissue abscesses.[11] MRI aids in further delineating the extent of a bony neoplastic process or infectious involvement and is useful in determining the appropriate level of amputation[10,11] (Figure 5). Nuclear imaging is useful in identifying osteomyelitis, occult fractures, soft-tissue perfusion in frostbite, and an appropriate level of amputation.[11] The indium 111-labeled white blood cell scan is specific for diagnosing osteomyelitis.[10] Furthermore, combining the tagged white blood cell scan with a technetium Tc 99m scan adds greater accuracy in differentiating an infectious from a noninfectious process.[10]

Procedure

Room Setup/Patient Positioning

Midfoot amputations can be performed using regional, epidural, or general anesthesia.[6] After being anesthetized, the patient is placed in the supine position on the operating table with a bump underneath the hip of the affected side.[6] The foot and lower leg are sterilely prepared and draped in the usual fashion.[6] Prior to making an incision, a sterile marking pen is used to trace the skin incision to aid in the visualization of the dorsal and plantar skin flaps.[6] An ankle Esmarch bandage is used to exsanguinate the foot and ankle, except if an infectious process is suspected.[9] The same Esmarch is then used as an ankle tourniquet to maintain hemostasis, exercising caution to not use it over areas of vascular bypass grafts.[9]

Surgical Technique

Transmetatarsal Amputation

A dorsal skin incision is made, using a No. 10 blade scalpel, starting at the dorso-

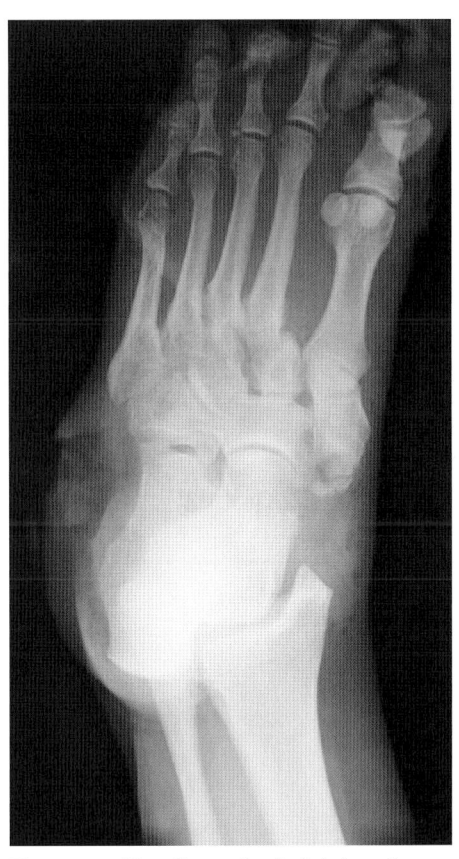

Figure 4 AP radiograph of a left foot shows a traumatic Lisfranc fracture-dislocation.

medial aspect of the foot at the midshaft level of the first metatarsal.[6] The incision is continued transversely across the dorsal aspect of the foot along the midshafts of the second, third, and fourth metatarsals.[6] The dorsal skin incision ends over the dorsolateral aspect of the midshaft area of the fifth metatarsal[6] (Figure 6, A). The medial incision starts from the medial edge of the dorsal incision and continues distally to the level of the first metatarsal head.[6] The lateral incision starts from the lateral edge of the dorsal incision and continues distally to the level of the fifth metatarsal head.[6] The medial and lateral incisions are curved plantarward, and a transverse skin incision is made across the plantar aspect of the foot along the metatarsal heads.[6]

The skin incision is continued deep, dissecting through the subcutaneous tissue to the level of muscle. The vasculature of the foot, including the dorsalis pedis artery, is identified and ligated to help maintain hemostasis.[4,6,8] Furthermore, branches of the peroneal and posterior tibial nerves are sharply transected as they are encountered along the dorsal and plantar surfaces of the foot, respectively. The nerves are allowed to retract back into the soft tissues to prevent a postoperative neuroma.[12] The exten-

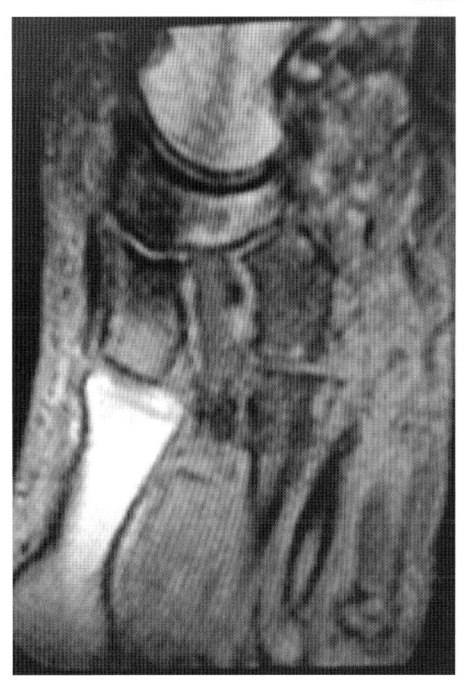

Figure 5 T2-weighted MRI depicts increased uptake of the first metatarsal bone associated with osteomyelitis.

sor and flexor tendons of the foot are pulled distally and transected sharply.[4,9] The tendons will retract proximal to the level of the skin incision.[4,9] The incision is continued sharply down to the metatarsal bones.[6] Full-thickness myocutaneous skin flaps are maintained to optimize wound healing.[1,4,6,9] To maintain a full-thickness plantar flap, an elevator is used to reflect the soft tissues from the metatarsals proximally to the level of the metatarsal shafts[4,6,8] (Figure 6, B). Upon completion, the dissection creates a "fishmouth" type incision.[4,8] The plantar flap created is longer than the dorsal flap, allowing the thick plantar skin to be pulled over the distal aspect of the stump, providing a better surface for weight bearing and load transfer.[1,4,6,8,9]

After the plantar and dorsal incisions are completed, the metatarsal shafts are resected using a small oscillating saw at the level of the dorsal skin incision[6] (Figure 6, C). The metatarsals are transected in a dorsal distal to plantar proximal direction.[1,6,9] Furthermore, the resected ends of the first and fifth metatarsal bones are beveled medially and laterally, respectively, to prevent the development of skin ulcerations.[6] Care is taken to preserve the peroneus brevis when transecting the fifth metatarsal.[8] Finally, the wound is copiously irrigated using pulse lavage or a bulb syringe.[4,6]

Prior to wound closure, the plantar flap is sharply debulked to allow for adequate

Section 6: Foot and Ankle

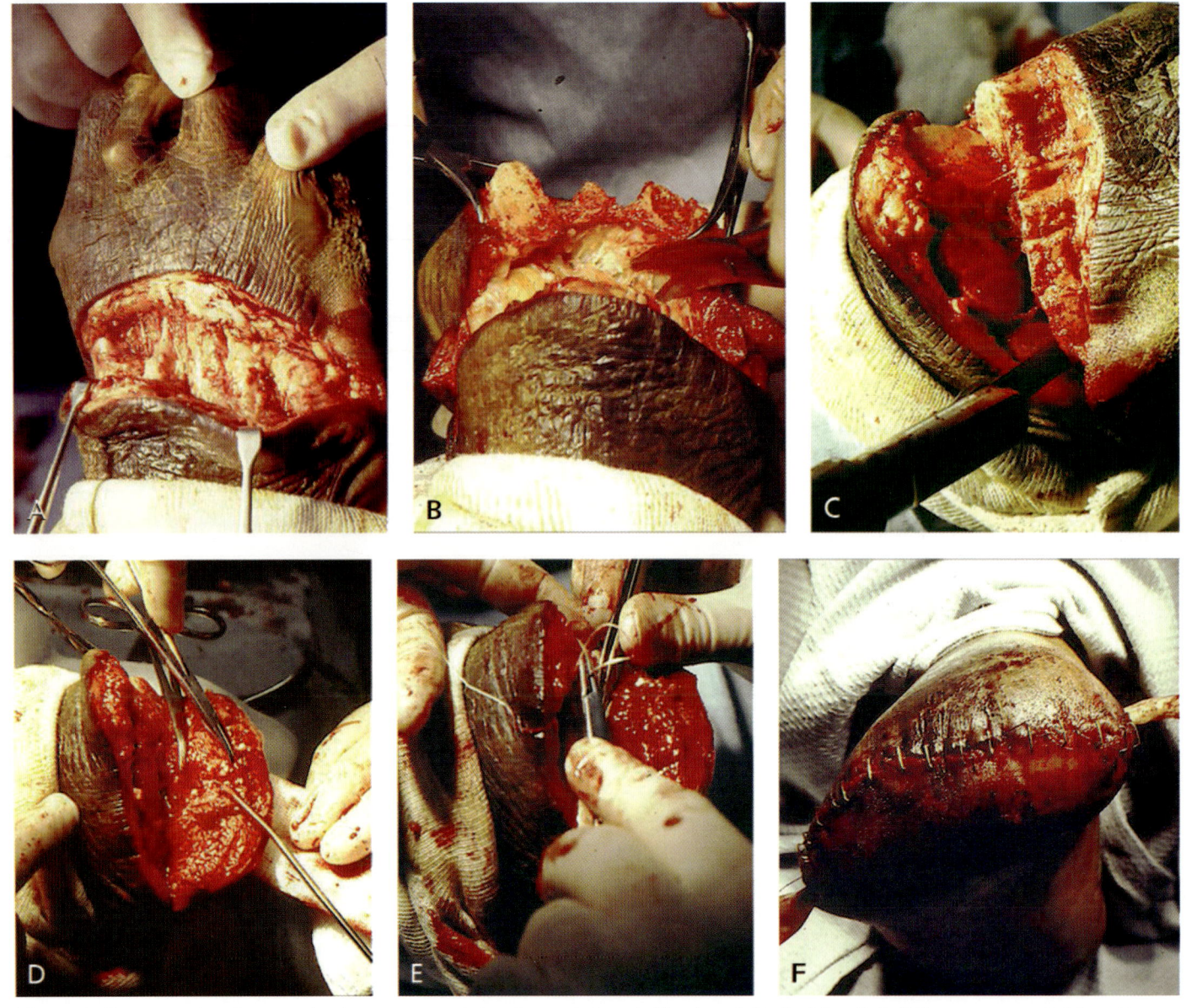

Figure 6 Intraoperative photographs show a transmetatarsal amputation. **A,** The dorsal skin incision. **B,** Soft tissues are resected from the plantar surface of the metatarsal bones to maintain a full-thickness myocutaneous flap. **C,** An oscillating saw is used to transect the metatarsal bones at the level of the midshaft in a dorsal distal to plantar proximal direction. **D,** The plantar flap is debulked to allow appropriate closure. **E,** The deep fascia is approximated using absorbable suture. **F,** The completed transmetatarsal amputation, with the skin approximated using skin staples. (Courtesy of Ronald M. Sage, DPM, FACFAS, Department of Orthopaedic Surgery and Rehabilitation, Loyola University Health System, Maywood, IL.)

closure[4,6,9] (Figure 6, D). Care is taken to prevent devascularization of the plantar flap by not removing an overabundance of subcutaneous tissue from the plantar surface of the foot.[4] After debulking the plantar flap, a drain may be placed within the wound if infection is suspected.[4,6] Then absorbable suture is placed to approximate the deep fascia[4,6] (Figure 6, E). The integument is approximated using 3-0 nylon horizontal mattress suture or skin staples[4,6] (Figure 6, F).

Lisfranc Amputation

At the level of the midfoot, a dorsal skin incision using a No. 10 blade scalpel is made starting on the dorsomedial aspect of the foot just distal to the first metatarsocuneiform joint.[6] The incision is continued transversely across the dorsal aspect of the foot.[6] The dorsal incision ends over the dorsolateral aspect of the foot distal to the fifth metatarsal base.[6] The medial incision is started from the medial edge of the dorsal incision just distal to the level of the first metatarsocuneiform joint, proceeding distally to the first metatarsal neck.[6] Likewise, the lateral incision is made starting from the lateral edge of the dorsal incision just distal to the fifth metatarsal base, proceeding distally to the fifth metatarsal neck.[6] The medial and lateral incisions are curved plantarward, and a transverse skin incision is made across the plantar aspect of the foot at the level of the metatarsal necks.[6]

The deep soft-tissue dissection proceeds as described in the previous section on transmetatarsal amputations.

After completing the plantar and dorsal incisions, the tarsometatarsal joints are visualized, and the metatarsals are disarticulated from the tarsal bones.[1,4,6] Initially, the first metatarsal is disarticulated from the medial cuneiform using sharp dissection.[1,6] The second metatarsal is then resected at the level of the medial and lateral cuneiform using a small oscillating saw.[4,6] The third and fourth metatarsals are then sharply disarticulated from the lateral cuneiform and the cuboid, respectively.[1,6] Finally, the fifth metatarsal is transected at the level of the metaphysis using a small oscillating saw.[1,4,6] By preserving the proximal portion of the fifth metatarsal, the peroneus brevis insertion and function are maintained.[1,6] All bony prominences are smoothed using a rongeur or bone rasp to prevent skin breakdown or ulcerations.[4] The wound closure is continued as described in the previous section on transmetatarsal amputations.

Chopart Amputation

At the level of the midfoot, a dorsal skin incision using a No. 10 blade scalpel is made, starting on the dorsomedial aspect of the foot just distal to the navicular tuberosity.[4,6] The skin incision is continued transversely along the dorsal surface of the foot.[4,6] The dorsal incision ends over the dorsolateral aspect of the foot at a point midway between the fifth metatarsal base and the lateral malleolus.[4,6] The medial incision is made starting from the medial edge of the dorsal incision just distal to the navicular tuberosity and is continued distally to the midshaft region of the first metatarsal.[4,6] Likewise, a lateral skin incision is made starting at the lateral edge of the dorsal incision at the point midway between the fifth metatarsal base and the lateral malleolus and is continued to the midshaft region of the fifth metatarsal.[4,6] At the midshaft level of the first and fifth metatarsals, the medial and lateral skin incisions are curved plantarward.[4,6] The plantar incision is continued transversely across the foot at the level of the midshaft region of the metatarsals[4,6] (Figure 2, A and B). The deep soft-tissue dissection proceeds as described in the section on transmetatarsal amputation; however, in the Chopart amputation, care must be taken to dissect and preserve the anterior tibialis and peroneus brevis tendons for later reattachment.[1,6,9]

After completing the plantar and dorsal incisions, the talonavicular and calcaneocuboid joints are visualized (Figure 2, C and D). The dorsal and plantar ligaments of the calcaneocuboid and talonavicular joints are sharply released.[6,9] The navicular and cuboid are disarticulated from the talus and calcaneus, respectively.[4,6] All bony prominences, especially the anterior process of the calcaneus and the dorsal talar head, are smoothed with a rongeur or bone rasp to prevent skin breakdown or ulcerations.[1,4] Furthermore, the articular cartilage is removed using a rongeur from the distal calcaneus and the talus, allowing for better adherence of the soft-tissue flap.[4] The anterior tibial and peroneus brevis tendons are reattached to the talus and calcaneus, respectively[1,4,6,9] (Figure 2, E). These foot dorsiflexors will help prevent the equinus deformity caused by the overpowering plantar-flexion force of the Achilles tendon.[3,9] The wound closure is continued as described in the section on transmetatarsal amputations.

Complications

The goal of a partial foot amputation is to achieve a well-healed distal stump that requires no additional revision surgeries.[1,3,12] Infectious, neurologic, and orthopaedic complications among others are devastating consequences associated with poor preoperative planning or surgical techniques.[3,4,12]

Postoperative infections are a devastating complication of midfoot amputation surgery.[4,12] Infections may occur because of nonsterile techniques during surgery or inadequate resection of infected soft and bony tissues.[12] Infections may lead to multiple subsequent surgeries, including repeat amputation at a more proximal level.[12]

Neurologic complications associated with partial foot amputations include stump neuromas and phantom limb pain.[12] Amputation stump neuromas are common complications of pedal amputations.[12] Extreme care must be used when handling nerves during these procedures.[12] The nerves are always transected sharply with a scalpel and retracted back into the soft-tissue stump, away from the weight-bearing surface.[12] Scissors are never used to transect nerves.[12] Phantom limb pain is commonly associated with midfoot amputations. In fact, nearly all patients with pedal amputations experience this symptom.[12] During the preoperative period, it is critical to counsel the patient regarding phantom limb pain.

Orthopaedic postoperative complications include skin ulcerations and muscle-tendon imbalance.[1-3,12] Skin breakdown and ulcerations stem from a failure to smooth bony prominences during the procedure, leading to increased contact pressures in those areas.[12] Excessive removal of subcutaneous tissue from the plantar flap creates a dysvascular stump, leading to skin breakdown and necrosis.[12] In addition, bony exostoses can form after midfoot amputations, resulting in increased contact pressures and areas of skin breakdown.[12] A soft-tissue imbalance of muscles and tendons about the foot results in postoperative foot deformities that cause increased contact stresses and problems appropriately fitting a pedal prosthesis.[6,12] The most common soft-tissue imbalance associated with midfoot amputations is an equinovarus deformity of the residual stump.[1-4,6,12] The equinovarus deformity is a result of the overpowering of the Achilles tendon in relation to the foot dorsiflexors.[3,12] Failure to identify the equinovarus deformity during surgery results in unacceptable positioning of the amputated stump.[1,3,4,12] To prevent an equinovarus deformity during midfoot amputations, an Achilles tendon lengthening procedure is performed.[1,3,4,6] Furthermore, failure to reattach the anterior tibialis tendon and the peroneus brevis tendon to the hindfoot during the Chopart amputation can also lead to an equinovarus deformity of the amputated stump.[1,3,6,12]

Postoperative Care and Rehabilitation

After the procedure and before the patient awakes from anesthesia, the patient is placed in a well-padded and molded posterior splint with the ankle in a neutral position.[4,9] This allows protection of the amputation site and provides immobilization for the Achilles tendon lengthening procedure if performed.[9] If used, the suction drain is removed on postoperative day 2 or when output is less than 10 to 20 mL over a 24-hour period.[4] Sutures are removed at 3 weeks or after wound healing is ensured.[4] The patient is kept non–weight bearing until the wound site at the distal stump is well healed.[8,9] After the stump wound is well healed, the patient can begin ambulating with a prosthetic device.[4]

The goal of the midfoot prosthesis is to provide the patient with a well-molded and well-fit prosthesis that allows ambulation with the least amount of energy expenditure.[2] The prosthesis must be designed to prevent skin breakdown and ulcerations by limiting contact stresses across the distal stump.[2] This process may take several weeks or months of working with a well-trained prosthetist to make the necessary modifications.

Patients with transmetatarsal amputations need a prosthesis that allows the foot to roll over the end of the shoe, decreasing the load across the residual stump during midstance and toe-off.[2] The prosthetic insert is composed of a Plastazote and polyethylene foam laminated together to form the insert.[2] The base of the insert is composed of cork and a viscoelastic polymer.[2] A toe filler is needed to replace the void in the shoe from the amputation.[2] The toe filler is typically composed of polystyrene foam.[2] Furthermore, a rocker-bottom shoe will help reduce stress across the distal stump.[2,13]

On occasion, patients may not tolerate a shoe insert and may need additional support to prevent the amputated stump from moving within the shoe.[2] An ankle-foot orthosis (AFO) can provide better stability to the distal stump and helps reduce the contact stress at the prosthesis-stump interface.[2,13] Other alternatives for patients with transmetatarsal amputations are the Chicago Boot, the Imler partial foot prosthesis, or the Lange partial foot prosthesis.[2,13] These devices were developed for more active patients.[2] The Lange partial foot prosthesis can be constructed with prefabricated toes to give a cosmetic appearance to the foot.[2] However, these prostheses are difficult to place on and take off the stump.[2] Patients with diabetes mellitus require special attention with regard to prosthetic management secondary to higher risks of skin ulcerations.[2] Diabetic patients require a full-length, rocker-bottom shoe with a total contact insert.[2]

Prosthetic devices for patients with Lisfranc amputations are similar to those with transmetatarsal amputations, with a few exceptions.[2,13] A longer toe plate and greater height added to the proximal portion of the prosthesis will distribute stress across a greater surface of the residual amputated stump.[2,13] Furthermore, a more proximally placed rocker bottom will also decrease stress across the distal stump.[2,13] A foreshortened shoe is another alternative for patients with a Lisfranc amputation; however, this prosthesis may be cosmetically unacceptable.[2] An AFO is a great prosthetic design for patients with a residual equinus deformity after a Lisfranc amputation.[2] The AFO will keep the residual limb at neutral dorsiflexion during heel strike, thus limiting the contact stress of the distal stump.[2]

Prosthetic devices for patients with Chopart amputations differ from those for the more distal Lisfranc and transmetatarsal amputations.[2] Because of the more proximal nature of the amputated stump, the patient will have a shorter lever arm, diminished push-off, and poor stability.[2,13] A full-length shoe with an AFO and prosthetic forefoot filler is a functional option for some amputees.[2,13] The AFO provides a stable ankle joint and a rigid lever within the shoe to promote weight transfer from heel to toe.[2,13] The forefoot filler is made of molded foam and is used to prevent distal collapse of the shoe and hold the distal stump in place.[2] An alternative design includes a posterior leaf-spring AFO with a custom insert and molded prosthetic forefoot filler.[2,13] Furthermore, by adding a rocker-bottom shoe, a decrease in the ground-reaction forces about the amputated stump is accomplished.[2] A foreshortened shoe may be an option for patients with diabetes mellitus.[2] For more active patients, a Lange partial foot prosthesis is used to allow greater ambulatory distances.[2,13]

Pearls

- Full-thickness myocutaneous skin flaps should be maintained to avoid wound complications.
- The creation of long plantar flaps allows the thick plantar skin to be pulled over the distal aspect of the stump to help prevent wound complications and allow a better weight-bearing surface.
- In a Lisfranc amputation, the proximal portion of the fifth metatarsal should be preserved to maintain the peroneus brevis insertion and function.
- During a Chopart amputation, the anterior tibialis and peroneus brevis tendons should be reattached to the talus and the calcaneus, respectively, to prevent an equinus deformity caused by the unopposed Achilles tendon.
- To prevent an equinovarus deformity of the stump, an Achilles tendon lengthening procedure may need to be performed.

References

1. Philbin TM, Berlet GC, Lee TH: Lower-extremity amputations in association with diabetes mellitus. *Foot Ankle Clin* 2006;11(4):791-804.
2. Philbin TM, Leyes M, Sferra JJ, Donley BG: Orthotic and prosthetic devices in partial foot amputations. *Foot Ankle Clin* 2001;6(2):215-228, v.
3. Schweinberger MH, Roukis TS: Soft-tissue and osseous techniques to balance forefoot and midfoot amputations. *Clin Podiatr Med Surg* 2008;25(4):623-639, viii-ix.
4. DeCotiis MA: Lisfranc and Chopart amputations. *Clin Podiatr Med Surg* 2005;22(3):385-393.
5. Dillingham TR, Pezzin LE, MacKenzie EJ: Limb amputation and limb deficiency: Epidemiology and recent trends in the United States. *South Med J* 2002;95(8):875-883.
6. Sanders LJ: Transmetatarsal and midfoot amputations. *Clin Podiatr Med Surg* 1997;14(4):741-762.
7. Wallace GF: Indications for amputations. *Clin Podiatr Med Surg* 2005;22(3):315-328.
8. Ng VY, Berlet GC: Evolving techniques in foot and ankle amputation. *J Am Acad Orthop Surg* 2010;18(4):223-235.
9. Brodsky J: Amputations of the foot and ankle, in Coughlin M, Mann R, Saltzman C, eds: *Surgery of the Foot and Ankle*, ed 8. Philadelphia, PA, Mosby Elsevier, 2007, pp 1369-1398.
10. Philbin T: The diabetic foot, in Pinzer M, ed: *Orthopaedic Knowledge Update: Foot and Ankle*, ed 4. Rosemont, IL, American Academy of Orthopaedic Surgeons, 2008, pp 273-290.
11. Cook KD: Perioperative management of pedal amputations. *Clin Podiatr Med Surg* 2005;22(3):329-341.
12. Sullivan JP: Complications of pedal amputations. *Clin Podiatr Med Surg* 2005;22(3):469-484.
13. Yonclas PP, O'Donnell CJ: Prosthetic management of the partial foot amputee. *Clin Podiatr Med Surg* 2005;22(3):485-502.

Spine

Section Editor
Andrew C. Hecht, MD

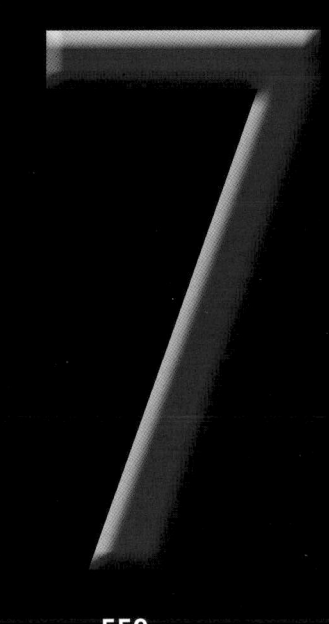

86 Anterior Cervical Diskectomy and Fusion 559
Howard S. An, MD; Thomas D. Cha, MD, MBA

87 Anterior Cervical Corpectomy and Fusion/Instrumentation 563
Daniel G. Kang, MD; Ronald A. Lehman, Jr, MD; K. Daniel Riew, MD

88 Posterior Cervical Foraminotomy 575
Kern Singh, MD; Steven J. Fineberg, MD; Matthew Oglesby, BA;
Jonathan A. Hoskins, MD; Vamshi Yelavarthi, BA

89 Posterior Cervical Laminectomy and Fusion 579
Sheeraz A. Qureshi, MD, MBA; Andrew C. Hecht, MD

90 Cervical Laminoplasty 585
Nikhil A. Thakur, MD; Brett A. Freedman, MD; John G. Heller, MD

91 Placement of Thoracic Pedicle Screws 591
Kevin W. Wilson, MD; Ronald A. Lehman, Jr, MD;
Lawrence G. Lenke, MD

92 Lumbar Microdiskectomy 601
Bradley Moatz, MD; P. Justin Tortolani, MD

93 Lumbar Laminectomy 607
Samuel M. Davis, MD; Scott D. Boden, MD

94 Instrumented Lumbar Fusion 611
Andrew J. Schoenfeld, MD; Christopher M. Bono, MD

95 Transforaminal Lumbar Interbody Fusion 617
Oliver O. Tannous, MD; Kelley Banagan, MD; Steven C. Ludwig, MD

96 Anterior Lumbar Interbody Fusion 625
Andrew Park, MD

Chapter 86
Anterior Cervical Diskectomy and Fusion

Howard S. An, MD   Thomas D. Cha, MD, MBA

Patient Selection

Anterior cervical diskectomy and fusion (ACDF), first described by Robinson and Smith[1] in the 1950s to treat radicular symptoms, has been a very successful procedure as evidenced by the frequency of its use. The clinical evaluation of patients with cervical degenerative disorders requires interpretation of patient symptoms, meticulous physical examination, and appropriate selection of diagnostic tests. A useful approach for the clinician is to categorize the symptoms and findings as axial neck pain, radiculopathy, myelopathy, or some combination of the three.

Indications

The indications for surgical intervention in cervical radiculopathy include: failure of a 3-month trial of nonsurgical treatment to relieve persistent or recurrent radicular arm pain with or without neurologic deficit, and the presence of a progressive neurologic deficit. Neuroradiographic findings must be consistent with the clinical signs and symptoms, and the duration and magnitude of symptoms must be sufficient to justify surgery.[2]

The surgical indications for the treatment of cervical myelopathy are not as well defined as they are for the treatment of radiculopathy. A patient with a mild, long-standing, and nonprogressive myelopathy without significant disability can be observed closely. Surgical intervention is recommended in the following situations: (1) progressive myelopathy, (2) moderate or severe myelopathy that is stable and of short duration (<1 year), and (3) mild myelopathy that affects routine activities of daily living. The age of the patient or severity of the disease is not a contraindication for surgery. It is imperative, however, that the patient understand that the goal of surgery is to prevent neurologic worsening, although most of the patient's neurologic function improves following surgical decompression.

Contraindications

Contraindications for the procedure include predominantly dorsal compression of the neural elements or isolated trauma to the posterior elements that is not amenable to anterior cervical spine surgery. In addition, severe soft-tissue destruction or anomalies of the anterior cervical spine (eg, postradiation) that preclude the anterior cervical approach are relative contraindications.

Preoperative Imaging

Several neuroradiologic imaging techniques are available to closely evaluate patients with cervical radiculopathy and myelopathy. Because each modality has its own inherent strengths and weaknesses, a combination of examinations is often required. Initial assessment begins with plain radiographic AP and lateral views. Oblique views are useful to evaluate bony narrowing of the foramina. Flexion-extension views are useful when instability is suspected or when evaluating the rigidity of sagittal plane deformity. Findings such as disk space narrowing, developmental canal stenosis, subluxations and malalignments, and vertebral osteophtye formation must be evaluated in the context of the patient's symptoms. Abnormal findings on plain radiographs may not identify the cause of the clinical picture; therefore, further correlative studies may be necessary before recommending specific treatment. Changes on plain radiographs may also confirm the clinical suspicion of typical degenerative disease and reassure the clinician and the patient that appropriate therapy is being followed.

MRI is the most sensitive modality for assessing the morphology of the spinal cord and its relation to the spinal canal as well as for providing direct information about nerve root or cord compression. MRI also shows intramedullary cord changes that may relate to disease prognosis. MRI is less sensitive in detecting foraminal stenosis, however, and does not demonstrate cortical margins as well as CT. CT scans with 45° oblique reconstruction views allow enhanced assessment of the neural foramina (**Figure 1**).

Myelography is occasionally used in the setting of unclear pathology and in patients with preexisting metal implants that would produce artifact in other modalities. A plain AP radiograph with water soluble myelography can demonstrate exiting nerve roots at the level of the pedicle or the typical filling defect seen with nerve root compression. The lateral view may show spinal cord compression by the disk or posterior vertebral osteophytes and/or hypertrophied ligamentum flavum. Afterward, CT can be done for three-dimensional depictions; however, as with myelography, neural compression by deformity of the dural sac or nerve roots can only be inferred, and the etiology of contrast blockade cannot be determined.

Rarely, electromyography/nerve conduction velocity (EMG/NCV) studies may be used to confirm suspected radiculopathy or to further evaluate symptoms with atypical findings. These tests may be most useful when attempting to differentiate root compression and a peripheral neuropathy. Nuclear medicine bone scanning, local diagnostic injections, diskography, and cerebrospinal fluid analysis have a limited role in the diagnostic process.

Dr. An or an immediate family member has received royalties from U & I; serves as a paid consultant to or is an employee of Smith & Nephew, Life Spine, Zimmer, Pioneer, Advanced Biologics, and Halozyme; has stock or stock options held in Pioneer, Spinal Kinetics, U & I, Anulex, and Articular Engineering; has received research or institutional support from Synthes, Baxter, Spinalcyte, Globus Medical, and the National Institutes of Health; has received nonincome support (such as equipment or services), commercially derived honoraria, or other non–research-related funding (such as paid travel) from Synthes and Rush University Medical Center; and serves as a board member, owner, officer, or committee member of the International Society for the Study of the Lumbar Spine, Spinal Kinetics, Pioneer, Medyssey, Advanced Biologics, and Articular Engineering. Neither Dr. Cha nor any immediate family member has received anything of value from or has stock or stock options held in a commercial company or institution related directly or indirectly to the subject of this chapter.

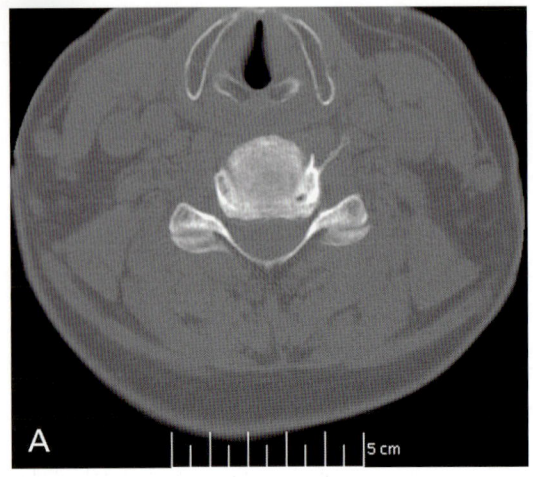

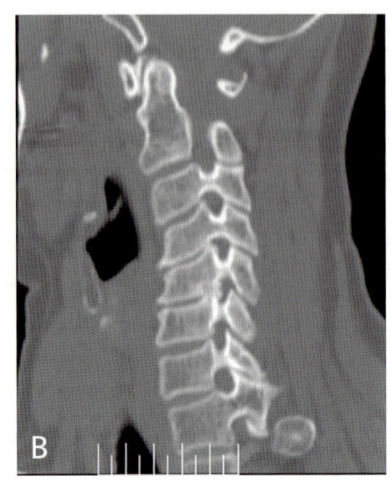

Figure 1 CT scans used to evaluate a patient before anterior cervical diskectomy and fusion. **A**, An axial cut through the C5-6 interspace demonstrates foraminal stenosis on the left side from osteophyte formation. **B**, An oblique CT reconstruction demonstrates the specific areas of bony overgrowth into the left C5-6 foramen.

Video 86.1 Anterior Cervical Diskectomy and Fusion With Plating. Howard S. An, MD; Thomas D. Cha, MD (7 min)

Procedure

Room Setup/Patient Positioning
The patient is positioned supine on a standard operating table with a head and foot that can be reversed to allow clearance for a fluoroscopy unit. A reverse Trendelenburg position can be used to reduce venous bleeding if needed. Halter or skeletal traction can be used to stabilize the head. We prefer to use Gardner-Wells tongs with 15 lb of weight to provide axial traction. The neck is then positioned slightly extended and in neutral rotation. The patient's arms are adducted to the side and the shoulders are gently pulled and secured with tape to aid in the radiographic identification of lower cervical spine levels, with care taken to avoid excessive traction that can result in a brachial plexus injury. The superficial anatomic landmarks for incision include the hyoid bone overlying C3, thyroid cartilage overlying the C4-5 interspace, and cricoid cartilage overlying the C6 level. It is important to prepare into the surgical field the sternal notch and midpoint of the chin as midline anatomic markers.

Special Instruments/Equipment/Implants
Magnification, with either surgical loupes or an operating room microscope, and lighting optimize visualization of anatomic structures.

Surgical Technique
Surgical exposure of the anterior aspect of the cervical spine is a relatively safe procedure; normal anatomic fascial planes are taken advantage of during the approach. The more cosmetically appealing transverse incision, which extends from midline to the middle of the sternocleidomastoid muscle, can be used to expose one to three levels. In the rare case that requires exposure of four or more levels, a longitudinal incision along the anterior border of the sternocleidomastoid muscle can be used. Historically, a left-sided approach has been advocated because of the more consistent course of the recurrent laryngeal nerve under the aortic trunk. A recent retrospective review demonstrated no differences between the rate of recurrent laryngeal nerve injury in right- or left-side approaches, however.[3]

After the skin incision, the anterior approach is performed by undermining the skin and subcutaneous tissue superiorly and inferiorly before dividing the platysma in line with the skin incision. The deep cervical fascia is divided between the strap muscles (medially) and the sternocleidomastoid muscle (laterally). Pushing the muscle belly of the sternocleidomastoid muscle medially allows easier detection of the medial edge of the muscle to determine the proper plane that is developed with blunt dissection through the pretracheal fascia. The superior, middle, and inferior thyroid arteries extend through the pretracheal fascia from the carotid artery to the midline, superficial to the C3 and C5 vertebrae and below the C6 vertebra, respectively. The intervening area provides a relatively avascular plane for dissection (**Figure 2, A**). The right recurrent laryngeal nerve ascends in the neck after passing around the subclavian vessels and courses medially and cranially at the C6-C7 level, often along with the inferior thyroid artery. The left recurrent laryngeal nerve ascends after curving around the aortic arch along the tracheoesophageal groove in a more midline and protected position.

Next, the carotid sheath is mobilized laterally and the trachea and esophagus are swept medially, which brings the exposure down to the prevertebral fascia. At this point, a localizing lateral radiograph should be taken, appreciating that the intervertebral disks are more prominent than the vertebral bodies. Once at the intended level, the longus colli muscles can be mobilized laterally with a Cobb elevator or curette (**Figure 2, B**).

Diskectomy is performed by sharply incising the anterior anulus and removing the anterior longitudinal ligament. At this point, we recommend using a burr to remove anterior osteophytes from the vertebral end plates and fashion a rectangular window to prepare for grafting as well as creating a working space to perform a thorough diskectomy. The diskectomy, which is performed using curets and rongeurs, should be performed to the uncovertebral joints laterally, which are recognized by the upcurving of the end plate at the uncus and to the posterior longitudinal ligament posteriorly, which can be recognized by the vertical orientation of its fibers. The posterior longitudinal ligament is removed in cases of myelopathy or extruded disk herniation. Direct decompression of the nerve root can be accomplished with a small Kerrison rongeur or curet, always working from lateral to medial.

Several techniques of anterior interbody fusion in the cervical spine have been described; they differ in graft configuration. We routinely use a tricortical iliac crest allograft and have published fusion rates equivalent to those of autograft with our technique.[4] The graft height should be 2 mm greater than the preexisting disk height, or a total height of at least 5 mm, to obtain adequate compressive strength and to enlarge the neural foramina. Overdistraction of the disk space by more than 4 mm in excess of the preexisting height may result in graft collapse and pseudarthrosis by overly increasing the graft load.[5] Disk space distraction is achieved with skull traction, laminar spreaders, vertebral screws, or a combination of these techniques. The end plates

Chapter 86: Anterior Cervical Diskectomy and Fusion

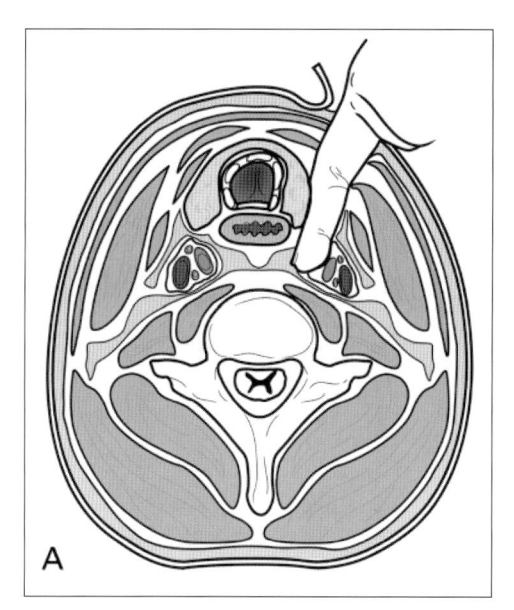

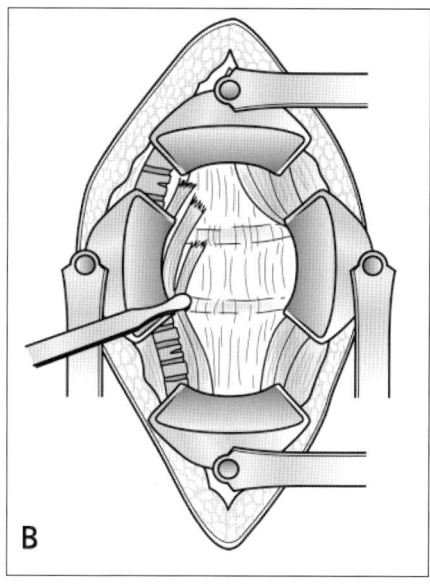

Figure 2 Illustrations show the surgical approach for anterior cervical diskectomy and fusion. **A,** The surgeon's finger demonstrates the plane through the deep cervical fascia (strap muscles medially, sternocleidomastoid laterally) and the pretracheal fascia (trachea/esophagus medially, carotid sheath laterally) down to the prevertebral fascia. **B,** Blunt elevation of the medial edges of the bilateral longus colli muscles exposes the intended disk space and adjacent vertebral bodies.

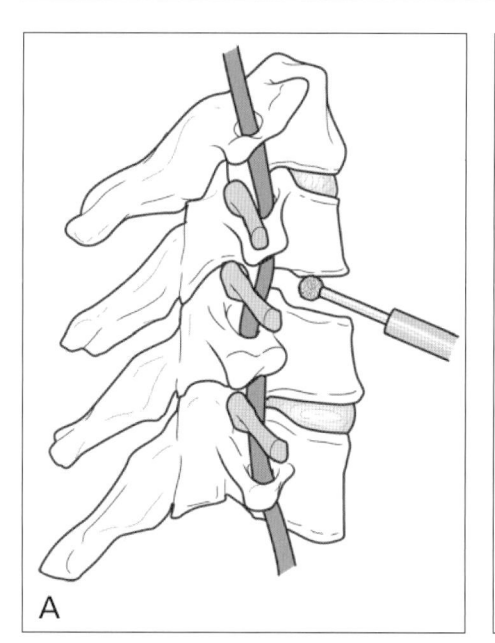

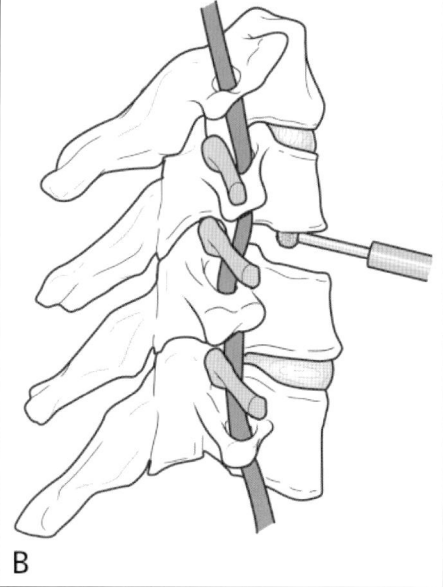

Figure 3 Illustrations demonstrate end plate preparation in a diskectomy. **A,** Following distraction by Caspar pins or a lamina spreader, a burr is used to smooth the superior and inferior end plates to create parallel surfaces. **B,** A 3-mm hole is created in the middle of the superior and inferior end plates. This can enhance vascularity and outflow of bone marrow cells while maintaining end plate structural integrity.

are burred to create a flat surface on both sides of the intervertebral space (**Figure 3, A**). Additionally, a 3- to 4-mm hole may be created in the middle of the end plates to promote vascularization of the graft (**Figure 3, B**). After the depth and width of the disk space have been measured, the tricortical graft (harvested from the anterior iliac region or allograft) is contoured to fit into the disk space and inserted with the leading cortical edge anteriorly and inset 2 mm beyond the vertebral bodies. The graft should be stable with compression following removal of all traction devices.

The technique of anterior plating begins with selection of an appropriately sized plate extending from the middle or proximal portion of the superior vertebra to the middle or distal portion of the inferior vertebra. The plate should make maximal contact with the anterolateral surface of the spine. A burr or rongeur can be used to remove osteophytes from the anterior aspect of the vertebra to create a smooth bed for the plate. The plate is fixed to the spine with screws. The angle of the screws is determined by biomechanical principles, with screws angled away from the graft providing increased rigidity in flexion and extension and a horizontal screw allowing the most resistance to pullout.[6] Newer instrumentation systems provide static or dynamic screw/plate interfaces or a mechanism to lock the screws to the plate to increase the overall rigidity of the construct.

Intraoperative imaging can confirm placement of the anterior cervical plate. The wound is closed, beginning with platysmal approximation and subcutaneous sutures. We routinely use a postoperative drain placed in the deep space for the first 24 hours. The wound is dressed with a sterile bulky dressing, and a soft collar is placed.

Complications
A recent retrospective review of patients undergoing one- to three-level primary anterior cervical diskectomy and fusion procedures for cervical spondylosis at one institution revealed the following complications and rates: mortality due to esophageal perforation (0.1%), postoperative dysphagia (9.5%), postoperative hematoma (5.6%), symptomatic recurrent laryngeal nerve palsy (3.1%), dural penetration (0.5%), esophageal perforation (0.3%), Horner syndrome (0.1%), instrumentation backout (0.1%), and superficial wound infection (0.1%).[7] The overall morbidity was 19.3% (196 of 1,015 patients).

Postoperative Care and Rehabilitation
Patients should continue to wear a soft-collar brace at all times except to shower for 1 to 2 weeks and should be in a monitored setting for the first 24 hours to observe for signs of respiratory compromise. Patients are encouraged to be up and out of bed beginning the evening of the surgery.

Pearls
- A 45° oblique reconstruction of a preoperative CT scan can allow excellent assessment of the neural foramina.
- Reverse Trendelenburg positioning of the bed can reduce venous bleeding.
- Adequate elevation of the longus colli muscles allows for proper deep retractor placement, assessment of the midline, and visualization of the uncovertebral joints for foraminal decompression.

© 2013 American Academy of Orthopaedic Surgeons

- The most appropriate graft thickness is approximately 2 mm larger than the preoperative disk space height, to allow foraminal distraction.
- Distraction of more than 4 mm can excessively load the graft, leading to graft collapse or pseudarthrosis.
- A central burr hole in the superior and inferior end plates increases vascularity to the interbody graft while maintaining end-plate structural integrity.
- To assess for esophageal perforation, diluted indigo carmine can be flushed through a nasogastric or orogastric tube at the level of the esophagus to check for extravasation into the surgical field.

References

1. Robinson RA, Smith GW: Anterolateral cervical disc removal and interbody fusion for cervical disc syndrome. *Bull Johns Hopkins Hosp* 1955;96:223-224.
2. Fischgrund J, Herkowitz H: Anterior surgical procedures for cervical spondylotic radiculopathy and myelopathy, in An HS, ed: *Surgery of the Cervical Spine*. Baltimore, MD, Williams & Wilkins, 1994, pp 196-212.
3. Beutler WJ, Sweeney CA, Connolly PJ: Recurrent laryngeal nerve injury with anterior cervical spine surgery risk with laterality of surgical approach. *Spine (Phila Pa 1976)* 2001;26(12):1337-1342.
4. Samartzis D, Shen FH, Goldberg EJ, An HS: Is autograft the gold standard in achieving radiographic fusion in one-level anterior cervical discectomy and fusion with rigid anterior plate fixation? *Spine (Phila Pa 1976)* 2005;30(15):1756-1761.
5. An HS, Evanich CJ, Nowicki BH, Haughton VM: Ideal thickness of Smith-Robinson graft for anterior cervical fusion: A cadaveric study with computed tomographic correlation. *Spine (Phila Pa 1976)* 1993;18(14):2043-2047.
6. Lim TH, Kim JG, Fujiwara A, et al: Biomechanical evaluation of diagonal fixation in pedicle screw instrumentation. *Spine (Phila Pa 1976)* 2001;26(22):2498-2503.
7. Fountas KN, Kapsalaki EZ, Nikolakakos LG, et al: Anterior cervical discectomy and fusion associated complications. *Spine (Phila Pa 1976)* 2007;32(21):2310-2317.

Chapter 87
Anterior Cervical Corpectomy and Fusion/Instrumentation

Daniel G. Kang, MD   Ronald A. Lehman, Jr, MD   K. Daniel Riew, MD

Patient Selection
Indications

Anterior cervical corpectomy and fusion (ACCF) is most commonly performed for cervical spondylosis, with symptoms of cervical radiculopathy, myelopathy, or a combination of both. Cervical spondylosis describes a wide spectrum of degenerative changes in the cervical spine that involve the intervertebral disk, vertebral body, uncovertebral joint, and facet joint. Cervical radiculopathy is described as nerve root compression that causes radiating pain from the neck into the upper extremity. Cervical nerve root compression occurs most commonly by herniation of intervertebral disk material, but it is also associated with loss of foraminal height due to chronic disk degeneration as well as osteophytes and facet hypertrophy.[1] Indications for surgical management include severe or progressive neurologic deficit or significant pain that fails to respond to nonsurgical treatment.

Cervical spondylotic myelopathy occurs as a result of the degenerative process with aging, but it is also commonly associated with ossification of the posterior longitudinal ligament (OPLL), hypertrophy of the ligamentum flavum, or a congenitally narrowed cervical canal.[2] Other causes of cervical spinal cord compression include trauma, instability, tumor, infection, epidural abscess, and kyphotic deformity.[3] Early surgical management is beneficial for most patients with severe or progressive myelopathy with concordant radiographic evidence of cord compression. For patients with nonprogressive mild to moderate myelopathy, however, no clearly established guidelines exist to dictate surgical management.[4] In our practice, we recommend surgery for nonprogressive myelopathy when myelopathic symptoms and long-tract signs are present, in combination with a Japanese Orthopaedic Association (JOA) score of less than 13 points and concordant radiographic evidence of cord compression. In addition, any patient with a cord signal change on MRI is recommended for surgery. The results of surgical management are generally better in patients who undergo decompression early rather than late, as prolonged compression can result in irreversible histologic and physiologic changes within the spinal cord.[5,6] Patients with mild myelopathy are occasionally offered a trial of observation with collar immobilization and activity modification; however, nonsurgical management is generally not successful in reversing or permanently preventing the stepwise progression of myelopathy.[5] The primary goal of ACCF is to decompress the spinal cord to prevent further neurologic deterioration and possibly reverse myelopathic symptoms. Secondary goals of ACCF include achieving successful fusion to stabilize abnormal motion segments to relieve spondylotic neck pain and correcting deformity, which may secondarily improve cord perfusion by decompressing obstructed spinal vessels.[5]

The major advantages of the anterior approach for cervical myelopathy and radiculopathy is the ability to directly decompress structures most commonly responsible for cord compression and nerve root impingement, including herniated disk material, osteophytes, and the posterior longitudinal ligament (PLL). In contrast to posterior approaches, anterior decompression can also indirectly relieve nerve root compression through re-establishing disk height and, subsequently, neuroforaminal height, as well as better correct kyphotic deformity and provide a fusion to address spondylotic neck pain.[5] Several techniques are used for anterior cervical decompression and fusion, and the optimal technique continues to be debated. Corpectomy is considered over multilevel diskectomy in the patient who has two or three affected levels, developmental stenosis demonstrating an osseous anterior-posterior canal diameter of less than 13 mm, significant fixed cervical kyphosis, large posterior osteophytes adjacent to the end plate, a free disk fragment that has migrated posterior to the vertebral body, or a significant component of spondylotic neck pain.[5] The corpectomy procedure is more technically challenging, but it allows better decompression of the intervertebral level than does anterior cervical diskectomy and fusion. This is mainly a result of the improved access and visualization afforded by taking down the vertebral body at the intervening segment. Additionally, the bone graft/interbody spacer needs to fuse to only two surfaces, versus the four fusion surfaces required to obtain an arthrodesis in a two-level anterior cervical diskectomy and fusion. In patients who have only retrodiskal compression, we prefer to leave the posterior cortex of the corpectomy body intact. This improves the torsional stability of the construct and helps to prevent intrusion of the graft into the canal. For problems in three or more levels, if at all possible we try to perform a corpectomy of one level and diskectomies at the remaining levels to preserve stability, as a corpectomy-diskectomy is less likely to extrude a graft or collapse than is a two-level corpectomy.

Contraindications

Contraindications to ACCF are limited and include general contraindications to surgery, such as hemodynamic instability after trauma or multiple medical comorbidities that would preclude safe anesthetic induction. Other contraindications include tracheoesophageal trauma that would not allow safe anterior cervical exposure.[3] Severe osteoporosis could

---

Dr. Lehman or an immediate family member serves as a board member, owner, officer, or committee member of the American Academy of Orthopaedic Surgeons, the North American Spine Society, the Cervical Spine Research Society, and the Scoliosis Research Society. Dr. Riew or an immediate family member has received royalties from Biomet, Medtronic Sofamor Danek, and Osprey; has stock or stock options held in Amedica, Benvenue Medical, Expanding Orthopedics, NexGen, Osprey, Paradigm Spine, PSD, Spinal Kinetics, Spineology, and VertiFlex; has received research or institutional support from Medtronic Sofamor Danek and Cerapedics; and serves as a board member, owner, officer, or committee member of the Korean American Spine Society, the Cervical Spine Research Society, AOSpine, the North American Spine Society, and the Scoliosis Research Society. Neither Dr. Kang nor any immediate family member has received anything of value from or owns stock in a commercial company or institution related directly or indirectly to the subject of this chapter.

also lead to progressive segmental kyphosis or graft subsidence, resulting in a failed fusion. A posterior approach is considered when posterior compression is a result of buckling of a hypertrophic ligamentum flavum or shingling of the laminae in a patient with hyperlordosis.[5] A posterior decompression procedure is also considered when there are three or more affected levels in a patient without significant kyphotic deformity or neck pain.[7,8] We prefer to perform anterior surgery whenever possible, however, because the risk of infection is lower, it allows for more direct decompression, and there is less postoperative pain.

Preoperative Imaging

Radiographic evaluation for patients with cervical spondylosis includes upright AP, lateral, and flexion-extension lateral plain radiographic views and, most typically, MRI. CT myelography may be necessary if MRI cannot be obtained or the images are difficult to interpret. Rarely, both MRI and CT myelography may be required.

Plain radiographs are useful in localizing pathologic levels of cord or nerve root compression, determining the degree of congenital cervical stenosis, assessing cervical sagittal alignment, and evaluating instability on flexion-extension lateral views.[4] MRI and CT myelography can confirm spinal cord and nerve root compression. MRI is noninvasive and provides excellent evaluation of neural structures, soft tissues, and disk herniation, but it provides limited bony visualization.[2] It is critical to check the preoperative MRI for the presence of an anomalous vertebral artery. The artery may lie ventral to the vertebral foramen above C7, in which case it can be injured while the longus colli is elevated. Alternatively, the artery may weave a tortuous course through the vertebral body, in which case it can be injured during the corpectomy.

If a patient cannot undergo MRI for medical reasons (eg, cardiac pacemaker, aneurysm clips) or if metal from prior cervical spine instrumentation would preclude adequate visualization because of artifact, then CT myelography is considered. CT myelography provides outstanding resolution of bony structures, osteophytes, and OPLL, as well as neural anatomy of nerve root and spinal cord compression.[4] Also, if high-quality MRI is performed but questions remain regarding bony anatomy, a noncontrast CT scan can be obtained to provide complementary information for surgical planning. We obtain a plain CT in select situations to determine: (1) fusion assessment in patients with previous operations; (2) presence of severe facet arthrosis that may not have neural compression but may do better with a fusion for relief of axial pain; (3) the presence of OPLL or ossification of the ligamentum flavum, and the extent to which diffuse idiopathic skeletal hyperostosis (DISH) may have autofused segments; and (4) the presence of autofused facets that can help to limit the number of levels requiring fusions. Evaluation of vascular structures, particularly the vertebral arteries, in cases of tumor involvement of the vertebral bodies or spinal cord may require preoperative angiography and embolization of a vascular tumor.[3]

Procedure
Patient Positioning

The patient is positioned supine on the operating table, with the arms tucked to the sides. A small bump or roll is placed between the scapulae; this extends the neck slightly and drops the shoulders. If iliac crest autograft is to be used, a small bump is placed underneath the hip. If a fibular strut autograft is to be used, a thigh tourniquet is placed with a bump underneath the ipsilateral hip. We use a Jackson flat top operating table. If there is excessive bleeding during the case, the table can be tilted to 10° to 20° of reverse Trendelenburg, allowing venous drainage and reducing bleeding.[9] We prefer to use intraoperative transcranial motor- and somatosensory-evoked potentials to monitor spinal cord activity. In cases of severe myelopathy, where evoked potentials may be unreliable or severe stenosis would compromise the spinal cord with neck extension, the anesthetic protocol includes awake, fiberoptic, or nasotracheal intubation. Additionally, our practice has evolved to use transient intravenous anesthesia to facilitate better motor-evoked potential readings. Additionally, 3-in silk tape is used to tape the head down to the table to limit rotation during surgery. Gardner-Wells tongs are applied to the head in cases of corpectomies of three or more levels (because Caspar pins are difficult to place for such lengths), with initial intraoperative traction of 15 lb of weight. Evoked potentials are again reviewed before proceeding. The application of Gardner-Wells tongs facilitates in-line traction and helps to stabilize the head and spine and control rotation during decompression and fusion. We tape the shoulders to the bottom of the operating table with 3-in silk tape. Care is taken to prevent overpulling the shoulders because a traction brachial plexopathy can result. To avoid this, and to ensure that we can pull on the arms to obtain radiographic visualization of the lower levels, we place a looped Kerlex gauze bandage roll (Covidien) on the wrists and place the other end at the foot of the table to pull during radiographs. The patient is then prepared and draped in the usual manner.[9]

Special Instruments/Equipment/Implants
Graft

We prefer to use freeze-dried allograft fibula or ulna for most cases. An appropriately sized allograft is selected at the beginning of the case. We try to choose one that will maximally fill the corpectomy defect. An appropriately sized graft should leave only about 5 to 7 mm of lateral wall. The width of the vertebral body can be determined on the axial MRI or CT images. Occasionally, we choose a fresh-frozen graft for better healing.

Operating Microscope

We typically perform anterior cervical corpectomy using an operating microscope, although loupe magnification with a fiberoptic headlight may be used based on surgeon preference. We believe the operating microscope provides several advantages over loupe magnification. First, the magnification on the operating microscope can be changed easily during particular portions of the case, such as during corpectomy and decompression, when magnification is increased, or with graft placement and instrumentation, when magnification is decreased. Furthermore, the magnification of the microscope is more powerful than standard loupe magnification. The operating microscope also enhances lighting and visualization because it has a perfectly coaxial light source and allows operating room personnel to observe the progress of the surgical procedure.[9] The operating microscope is especially helpful when a complication such as a dural tear is encountered because it allows the co-surgeon to provide meaningful assistance. The ability of the co-surgeon to assist on all other aspects of the case cannot be underestimated. With the use of loupes, only one surgeon can adequately look into the surgical wound.

The operating microscope is covered with a sterile microscope drape at the start of surgery. The microscope is then brought into the operating field after the disk space is localized with a lateral image. We prefer to use the operating microscope from the beginning of the deep exposure and will even close the wound with the microscope. This makes it possible to get a perfect closure and also allows trainees to practice suturing under the microscope, a skill that is required to close dural leaks. Modern microscopes have a long boom, allowing the head of the microscope to be brought in from the foot of the table on the side of the assisting surgeon. Once the microscope is in proper position, the covering of the eyepieces are torn off and the eyepieces are adjusted to accommodate eye width as well as refraction.[9]

Approach

We perform a Smith-Robinson anteromedial approach for exposure of the middle and lower cervical spine. We prefer a left-sided approach;[9] however, either a right- or left-sided approach to the anterior cervical spine may be selected based on surgeon preference, or the approach may be dictated by prior anterior cervical exposure. Anecdotally, some surgeons have suggested that right-sided approaches more commonly injure the recurrent laryngeal nerve (RLN) as a result of anatomic considerations. In a retrospective review, Beutler et al[10] found no increased incidence of RLN injury when comparing right- and left-sided approaches. The authors reviewed only 173 right-sided and 155 left-sided cases, however, and reported a 2.7% RLN palsy rate. Such numbers are too underpowered to make conclusions about injury to a nonrecurrent laryngeal nerve, which occurs only on the right side and in only approximately 1% of cases.

In cases of revision anterior cervical exposure, preoperative evaluation with a direct laryngoscopy by an otolaryngologist is necessary to identify residual vocal cord paralysis.[2] If vocal cord paralysis is present, the approach is performed on the same side as the previous surgery. If no evidence of paralysis is present, however, the opposite side may be approached to reduce the need to dissect through previous scar tissue or adhesions.

Landmarks for Incision

Palpation of surface landmarks is useful in deciding incision location.[2] The hyoid bone is in the midline at the lower border of the mandible, approximately at the level of C3. The thyroid cartilage overlies approximately the C4-5 intervertebral disk space; it is the first large protuberance palpable inferior to the hyoid bone. The cricoid cartilage and carotid tubercle are at the level of C6.[9] The level of the incision can also be approximated by examining a preoperative lateral image. The surgeon can check the radiographs to determine the location of the surgical level with respect to the distance between the angle of the mandible and the clavicle. This provides another rough estimation of where to make the incision.

Surgical Technique

The surgical procedure should be performed in a nearly identical, stepwise fashion each time. This makes it possible for the surgeon, assistant, and scrub nurse to learn the procedure quickly and improve efficiency each time the procedure is performed. Here we describe our current technique for doing a corpectomy. Innumerable variations are possible, and we continue to vary our technique nearly every year to refine it. Our current technique is certainly not likely to be the best. For the novice, however, it does help to memorize a step-by-step technique such as this one until enough experience is gained to allow for variations without compromising efficiency.

Video 87.1 Cervical Corpectomy Part I: Exposure, Diskectomy, and Initial Corpectomy. Daniel G. Kang, MD; Ronald A. Lehman, Jr, MD; K. Daniel Riew, MD (19 min)

Superficial Exposure

For a single-level corpectomy, a 3- to 4-cm transverse incision is made along the Langer lines, beginning just past the midline and extending to the medial border of the sternocleidomastoid (SCM) muscle. For a multiple-level corpectomy, the skin incision is extended farther across the midline and to the lateral border of the SCM muscle. The steps of exposure are as follows:

1. The skin incision is marked with a fine-tip marker. Vertical lines are drawn every centimeter to serve as landmarks during closure so that the skin edges are brought back evenly. The skin is infiltrated with a local anesthetic with epinephrine using a 25-gauge needle as superficially as possible, immediately after the drapes are on the patient. This allows the anesthetic to take effect for at least 5 minutes while the rest of the equipment is being placed on the patient and decreases superficial bleeding. We usually call for a localizing radiograph at this point, as it takes several minutes for the radiology technician to arrive.

2. After incising the skin with a #10 blade, we switch to electrocautery to incise the subcutaneous tissue and platysma, which is also divided transversely. We use the cautery to develop a plane about 1 cm cranially and caudally and then use finger dissection to create subplatysmal pouches (**Figure 1, A**). This must be performed with caution because of the location of the anterior jugular vein and numerous small superficial veins from the external jugular system. If these start to bleed, they can simply be cauterized. A small Weitlaner self-retraining retractor is placed.

3. We then incise the fascia in the interval between the strap muscles (sternohyoid and sternothyroid) and the SCM muscle using the cautery followed by Metzenbaum scissors (**Figure 1, B**). The interval is further developed with blunt finger dissection. The carotid pulse can be palpated deep to the SCM muscle, delineating the location of the carotid sheath laterally, and the trachea and esophagus are palpated medially. Blunt dissection is performed through this interval posteriorly toward the midline to the prevertebral fascia and longus colli muscle. An appendiceal retractor is used to provide exposure. The omohyoid, which is deep to the SCM muscle, may be either retracted medially with the trachea, or divided if necessary to improve exposure (**Figure 1, C**). Beginners often find themselves dissecting medial to the omohyoid muscle, especially when approaching the lower cervical levels. Getting stuck in the axilla of this muscle limits cranial exposure, so it should be identified before starting the deep dissection. The SCM muscle fascia should be kept intact

Section 7: Spine

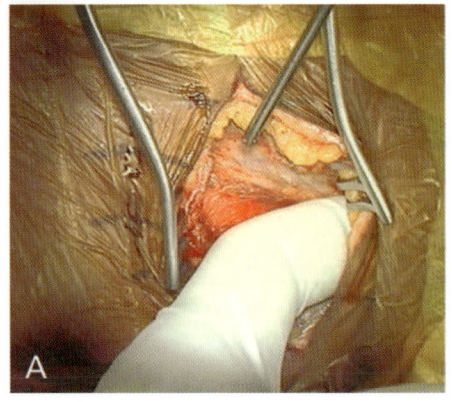

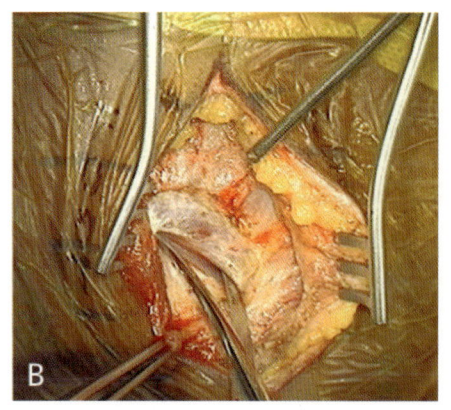

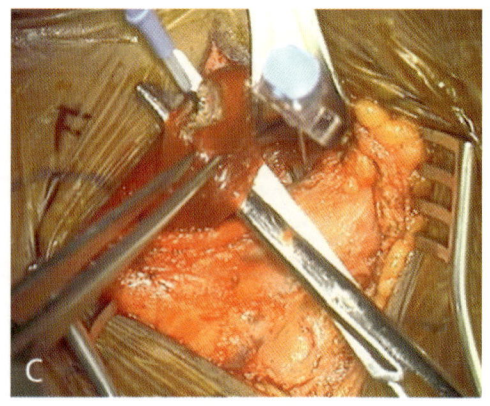

Figure 1 Intraoperative photographs show superficial exposure technique for anterior cervical corpectomy and fusion. **A,** Subplatysmal pouches are created 1 cm cranially and caudally using monopolar cautery and finger dissection. This should be performed with caution because of numerous small superficial veins. **B,** The fascia between the strap muscles (sternohyoid and sternothyroid) and the sternocleidomastoid (SCM) muscle is incised with monopolar cautery followed by Metzenbaum scissors. **C,** The omohyoid muscle, which is deep to the SCM muscle, is shown here elevated by the Metzenbaum scissors. It may be retracted medially with the trachea or divided if necessary to improve exposure.

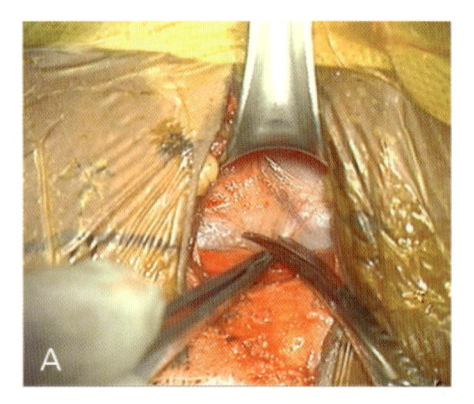

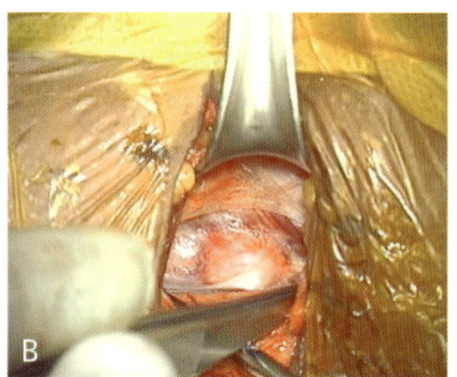

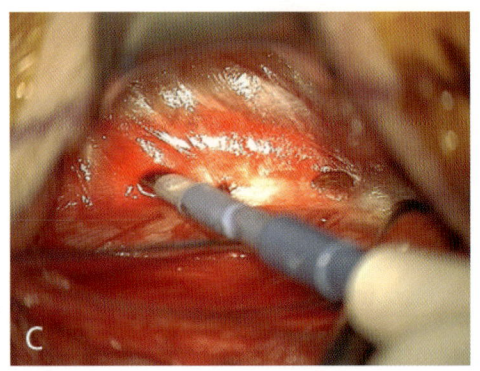

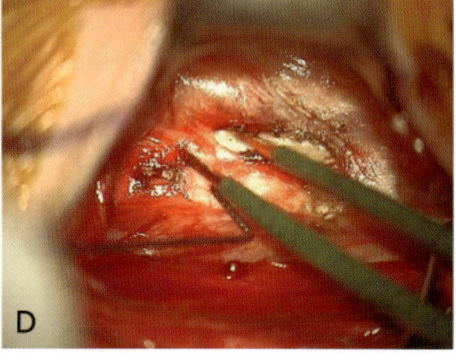

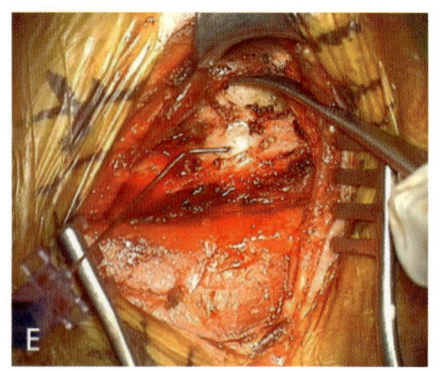

Figure 2 Intraoperative photographs show deep exposure technique for anterior cervical corpectomy and fusion. **A,** Metzenbaum scissors are used to make a small longitudinal incision within the prevertebral fascia. **B,** Forceps and scissors are crossed longitudinally to split the soft tissue along the midline to expose the longus colli muscle, anterior longitudinal ligament, intervertebral disk, and vertebral body. **C,** To help with centering the Caspar pins and plate later in the case, the midline between the longus colli in the vertebral bodies above and below each of the disk spaces is marked with monopolar cautery. **D,** The medial borders of the longus colli muscle are elevated in full-thickness flaps using bipolar cautery. **E,** The assistant elevates the longus with a Penfield No. 2 while the surgeon cauterizes any bleeders with the bipolar cautery.

to reduce bleeding and keep the plane of dissection out of the carotid sheath.[2,3] No efforts are made to specifically identify the RLN.[9]

Deep Exposure

4. The anterior vertebral bodies and longus colli should be easily palpated and visualized. The prevertebral fascia is divided longitudinally with scissors to expose the longus colli muscle, anterior longitudinal ligament, intervertebral disk, and vertebral body (**Figure 2, A** and **B**). Exposure of the C2 and C3 levels should be performed with caution, as the superior laryngeal and hypoglossal nerves may cross the plane of dissection and should be gently retracted along with the digastric and stylohyoid muscles. The inferior thyroid artery and vein are encountered at the C6 and C7 levels. They can be clamped and cauterized or, in most cases, gently retracted to obtain adequate exposure.[3]

5. By this time, the radiology technician has arrived, and a localizing image is obtained. If we are confident about the correct level, based on a combination of osteophytes and carotid tubercle, we place a 21-gauge spinal needle (bent at two right angles to prevent accidental puncture of the cord) into the disk space.

Chapter 87: Anterior Cervical Corpectomy and Fusion/Instrumentation

If there is any doubt regarding the correct level, we place a small clamp on the edge of the longus colli at the presumed level so as not to injure an uninvolved disk with a needle. The microscope is brought into the field and the remainder of the procedure is performed under magnification.

6. While waiting for the radiograph, we further enlarge the cranial-caudal extent of the deep dissection. This allows for better visualization and decreases the force required to retract the midline structures. For multilevel procedures, we partially retract the midline structures by packing a 4 × 4 sponge cranially and another caudally, to act as "soft" retractors. This distributes the force of retraction over a wider area. We then mark the midline between the longus colli in the vertebral bodies above and below each of the disk spaces with electrocautery (**Figure 2, C**). By marking this point before elevating the longus colli, it is much easier to center the Caspar pins and, later, the plate.

7. The preoperative MRI is checked for the presence of an anomalous vertebral artery that may lie on top of the vertebral foramen, or a tortuous one that meanders into the vertebral body.

8. We confirm three things on the localizing radiograph: we have the right level, the right patient has been exposed, and the neck is in correct alignment and not hyperextended or kyphotic.

9. The medial borders of the longus colli muscle are elevated in full-thickness flaps using bipolar cautery. Small vessels lie obliquely on top of the longus and perforate the muscle in the valley at the middle portion of the vertebral body. These vessels are cauterized on top of the longus, and then the space between the longus and the periosteum of the vertebral body is punctured with the bipolar and this area is cauterized. We continue all along the extent of the longus that is to be elevated (**Figure 2, D**). Because the sympathetic plexus lies superficially on the lateral aspect of the longus, lateral dissection (more than 6 to 7 mm) or cauterization on the ventral surface of the longus should be avoided. The assistant then elevates the longus with a Penfield No. 2 (**Figure 2, E**) while the surgeon cauterizes any bleeders with the bipolar cautery. The Penfield No. 2 safely dissects the longus in case there is an anomalous vertebral artery and also leaves the periosteum of the body intact, making it easier to cauterize the bleeder. If the periosteum has been burned off, then the bone-perforating bleeders can be waxed. The longus colli muscle is elevated laterally until the costal process of the vertebral body (ventral roof of the vertebral foramen) and the uncovertebral joints are exposed.[2] Posterior dissection at the disk spaces endangers the vertebral arteries, so we stay superficial to the level of the costal process.

10. Medial-lateral self-retaining retractors are placed under the developed longus colli muscle flaps. We use a three-pronged retractor, which stays under the longus better than smooth ones. If the exposure is inadequate, smooth cranial-caudal retractors are used until the Caspar pins are placed. Leaving these in for the duration of the operation may increase postoperative dysphagia.

11. The disk space and the surrounding anterior longitudinal ligament are outlined and incised with the cutting current of the monopolar cautery to expose any osteophytes and to accurately define the disk space (**Figure 3, A and B**). This allows for accurate placement of the Caspar pins. Then anterior osteophytes are removed with a Leksell rongeur and/or a burr (**Figure 3, C and D**) until the surface feels smooth to the touch.

12. The site is then irrigated.

13. Caspar pins are placed next (**Figure 3, E**). The previously marked midline (step 3) is used as a guide. A pair of bayonetted pickups works nicely as a soft-tissue retractor. The cranial pin is placed between 8 and 10 mm above the superior edge of the disk space. A distance of 8 mm allows for adequate end-plate preparation; 10 mm prevents violation of the next disk space. We prefer to do the following instead of using fluoroscopy. The caudal pin is placed 5 mm below the caudal edge of the disk space. Rather than measuring this with a ruler, we use a 5-mm suction tip as a guide. Both pins are directed parallel with the disk space to allow for good visualization and to prevent the caudal pin from perforating the next disk space. If the localizing radiograph demonstrates that the cervical alignment is too lordotic, we ask anesthesia personnel to place an adequately sized bump under the head before putting in the pins. If the alignment is kyphotic, then the bump is placed under the shoulder. Small alignment corrections can be made by placing the pins with the tips convergent or divergent to kyphose and lordose the segment, respectively.

14. The Weitlaner retractor is removed if this was not previously done. Failure to do this before putting the distractor on the Caspar pins will result in maceration of the skin with a poor cosmetic result. The Caspar distractor is placed. A left-sided distractor is used if the approach was on the left side; a right-sided distractor is used if the approach was on the right side.

Disk Removal

The steps for a single-level, C6 corpectomy are described here. The steps for multilevel corpectomies are essentially a duplication of the single-level procedure.

15. Diskectomy: The disks above and below the vertebral body are incised with a No. 15 blade (**Figure 4, A**). The sharp portion of the blade is 11 mm, so for small individuals, the surgeon should not plunge the knife deeper than the sharp edge. At the C5-6 disk space, the blade is placed into the midpoint of the disk and cut caudally until the blade hits the C6 end plate. Using a sawing up-and-down motion, the disk is cut off the C6 end plate and the blade is drawn laterally toward the surgeon until the curve of the uncinate is reached. The curve is followed cranially until the blade comes to rest against the C5 end plate. This defines the lateral extent of the disk space. This is repeated in the opposite direction, following the opposite uncinate up

Section 7: Spine

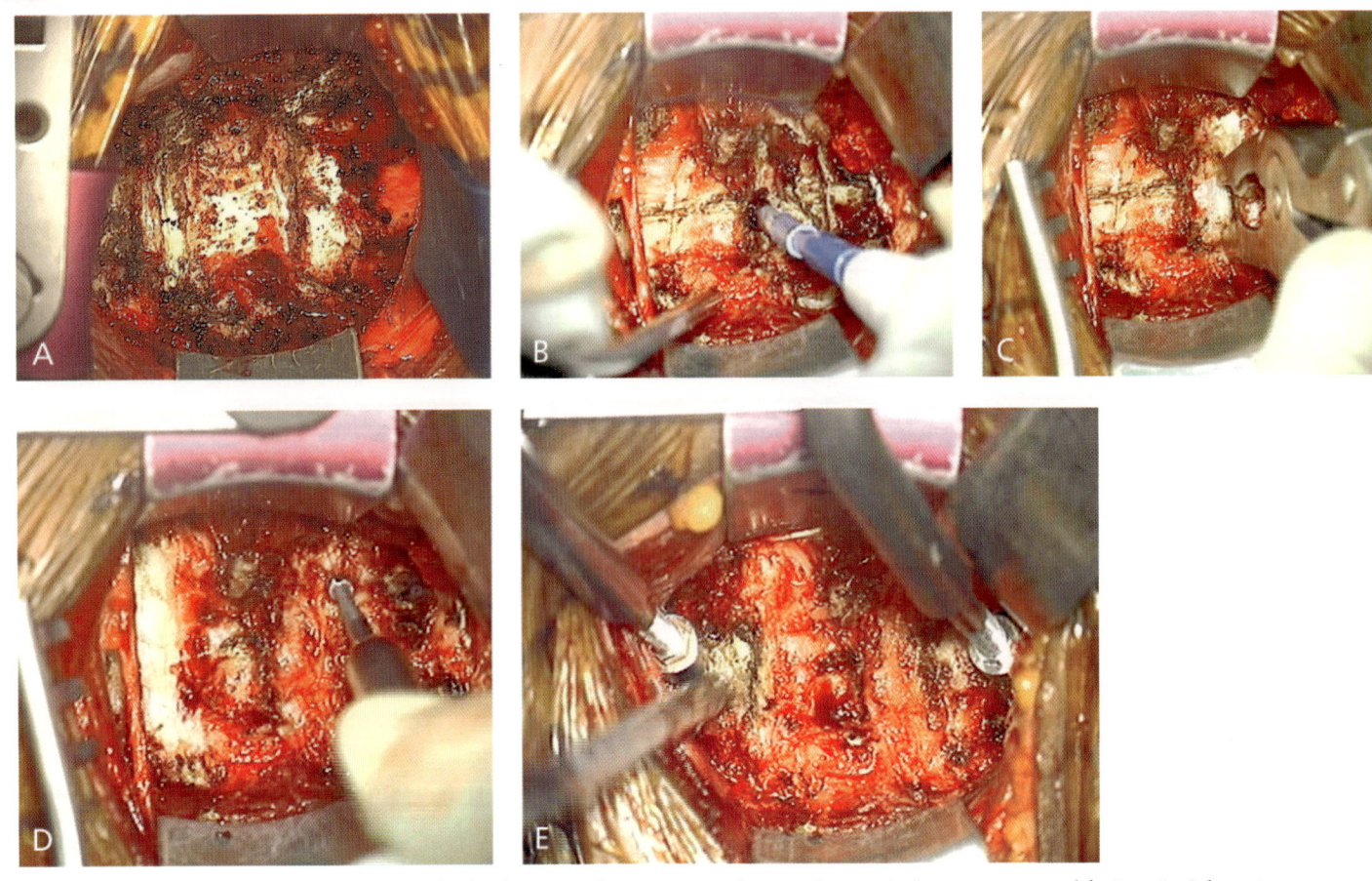

Figure 3 Intraoperative photographs show the final steps in deep exposure for anterior cervical corpectomy and fusion. **A**, Adequate visualization includes the vertebral body with the intervertebral disk above and below. **B**, Osteophytes and the disk space are accurately defined and outlined by incising the disk space and the surrounding anterior longitudinal ligament with the cutting current of the monopolar cautery. Anterior osteophytes are removed with a Leksell rongeur (**C**) and/or a burr (**D**) until the surface feels smooth to the touch. **E**, The Caspar pins are placed. Note the 5-mm suction tip used to gauge Caspar pin placement distance from the edge of the disk space.

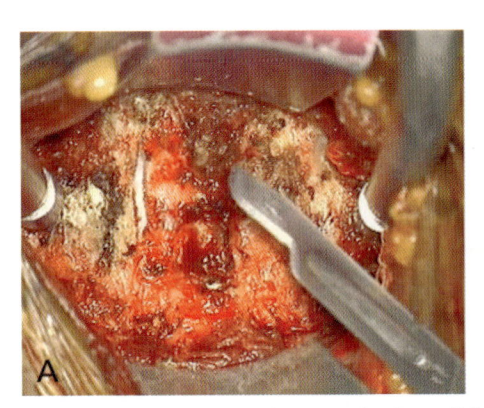

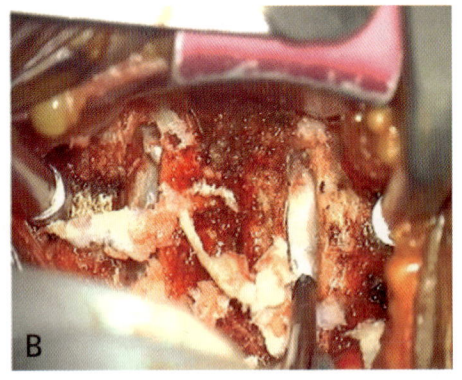

Figure 4 Intraoperative photographs show disk removal for anterior cervical corpectomy and fusion. **A**, Diskectomy is performed by incising the disk above and below the vertebral body with a No. 15 blade. **B**, The remaining disk material and cartilaginous end plate are scraped away using a microcuret.

to the C5 end plate. Starting at that point, the disk is cut off the C5 end plate. The assistant removes the disk with a pituitary, using two hands to prevent plunging past the disk space. The same steps are repeated to remove the C6-7 disk.

16. The largest microcuret (typically 5 mm) that will comfortably fit into the disk space is used to scrape the disk and cartilaginous end plate off the C6 end plate (**Figure 4, B**). This is done methodically, starting ventrally and slowly progressing dorsally until the subchondral bone is exposed. For the concave C5 end plate, it helps to turn the curet face up and slightly cranially and scrape from bottom up. We start from the contralateral side and slowly and methodically move toward the ipsilateral side. The assistant removes the debris with a pituitary. Next, the uncinates are cleaned of all disk material. The steps are repeated for the C6-7 disk space.

17. It is a good idea to move the retractor back and forth every 30 to 45 minutes to prevent constant pressure on one spot on the trachea and esophagus.

18. For the more delicate work of removing the posterior disk material, we switch to a 2- or 3-mm curet and remove the remaining disk at C5-6 until the PLL is exposed. This is repeated at C6-7. By decompressing to the PLL, the surgeon can judge the true depth of the corpectomy.

19. We irrigate and use the suction tube without a tip to vacuum up all disk fragments.

20. We then remove any remaining soft tissues and cartilage from the end plates with a burr.

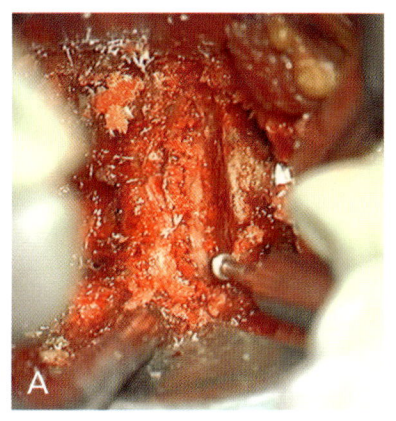

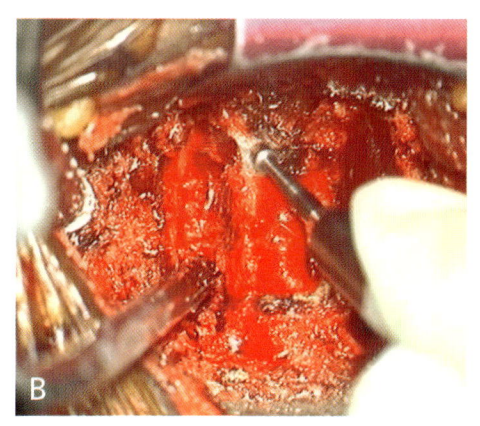

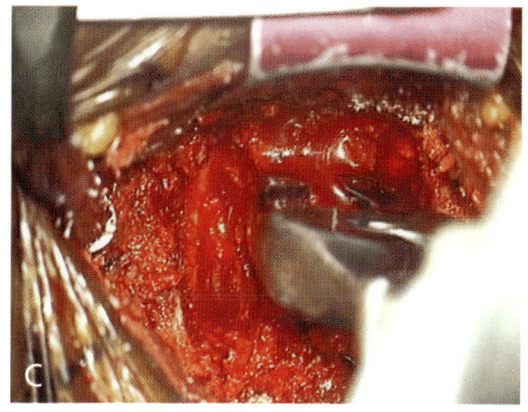

Figure 5 Intraoperative photographs show initial corpectomy for anterior cervical corpectomy and fusion. **A,** The ventral overhanging bone is removed using a high-speed burr. **B,** The width of the corpectomy is delineated by marking the lateral margins of the graft with monopolar electrocautery and then removing the cortical bone along these two lines with the burr. **C,** A large Leksell rongeur is used to harvest four relatively equal pieces of cancellous bone from the body of C6.

Initial Corpectomy

We use a 2-mm matchstick carbide-tipped burr that is more side-cutting than end-cutting. This allows the surgeon to place the tip of the burr on the PLL and remove the posterior osteophytes in a safe, efficient manner. The burr is safer than a Kerrison rongeur because the footplate of the rongeur is several millimeters thick, and requires impingement into the dura to adequately navigate the Kerrison rongeur under the posterior osteophytes. The uncovertebral joints serve as the most reliable reference to the lateral borders of the vertebral body and provide a pathway for decompression.[9] The surgeon must have a clear understanding of the lateral borders of the vertebral body and avoid being misled by the osteophytic changes along the anterior and lateral aspect of the disk spaces. Lateral vertebral osteophytes can easily be mistaken for the lateral vertebral body, causing the surgeon to remove bone overaggressively and endanger the vertebral artery.[3]

21. The first step in performing the corpectomy is to plane off the concave C5 end plate into a smooth surface (**Figure 5, A**). This is done by removing the ventral overhanging bone. The bone dust that results is collected using the spoon side of a Penfield No. 1 and saved for bone grafting.

22. To ensure that the graft will fit snugly against the lateral walls, we mark the corpectomy width by laying the graft on top of the vertebral body. We mark the lateral margins of the graft with electrocautery and then remove the cortical bone along these two lines with the burr (**Figure 5, B**). This delineates the width of the corpectomy.

23. We rapidly remove the cortical bone from the superior and inferior end plates and the ventral surface of C6 until bleeding cancellous bone is exposed. This should be done as rapidly as possible to minimize bleeding. With practice, it should not take more than 10 seconds.

24. A large Leksell rongeur is used to quickly harvest four relatively equal pieces of cancellous bone from the body of C6 (**Figure 5, C**). Usually, this will leave just the posterior cortex, along with approximately 2 mm of cancellous bone. If there is more than that, it can be removed with the Leksell rongeur or a burr. The removed cancellous bone is saved for later grafting. During the bone harvesting, there may be significant bleeding from the nutrient vessel in the center of the vertebral body, especially after the posterior cortex is exposed. It is imperative to continue with the corpectomy without stopping to obtain hemostasis. The cancellous bleeding can be coagulated with thrombin-soaked gelfoam or any hemostatic liquefied collagen product, followed by compression with a 1 × 1 cottonoid patty.

Video 87.2 Cervical Corpectomy Part II: Central Decompression, Foraminal Decompression, Fusion, and Instrumentation. Daniel G. Kang, MD; Ronald A. Lehman, Jr, MD; K. Daniel Riew, MD (35 min)

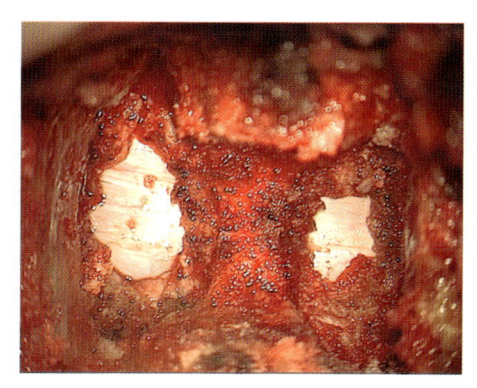

Figure 6 Intraoperative photograph shows the surgical area after central decompression for anterior cervical corpectomy and fusion. A burr was used to remove posterior osteophytes, and the posterior longitudinal ligament was thinned to a thickness of approximately 1 mm.

Central Decompression

25. The central decompression at the cephalad level (C5-6) is now performed using the burr. The key to using the burr safely and efficiently is learning how to keep it in one plane without going deeper or shallower while moving the burr. Using a medial-lateral motion, the burr is used to thin the PLL until it is about 1 mm thick. Keeping the burr exactly at this depth, it is gradually moved cranially and caudally until all osteophytes are removed. Caudally, the remaining cortex of C6 is removed until adequate decompression is achieved. In most cases where there is no OPLL or severe retrovertebral compression, at minimum a 5-mm band of this posterior

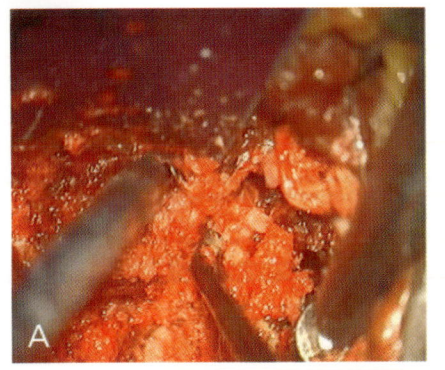

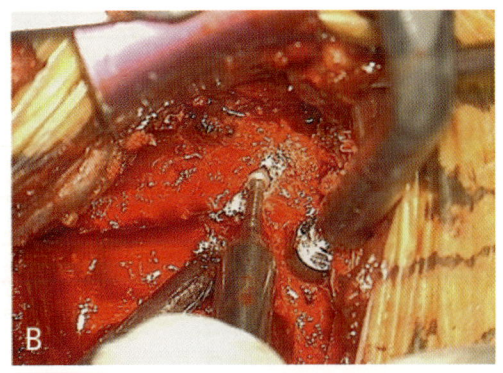

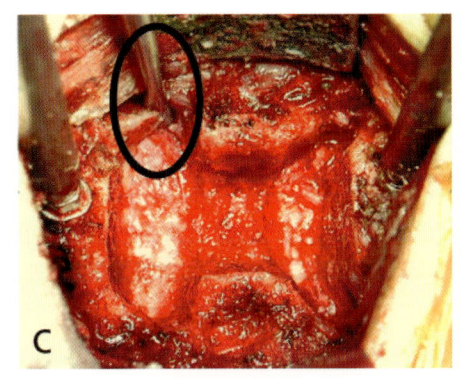

Figure 7 Intraoperative photographs show foraminal decompression and uncinate resection for anterior cervical corpectomy and fusion. **A,** A Penfield No. 4 is placed lateral to the uncinate to protect the vertebral artery, and a 2-mm curet is used to clean out and define the lateral border of the uncinate process. **B,** The lateral border of the decompression is established using the burr in an anterior-to-posterior direction, gradually moving farther and farther laterally until only about 1 to 2 mm of bone remains medial to the Penfield No. 2. **C,** Following a thorough foraminal decompression, all four foramina should be well visualized. A Penfield No. 2 (marked by the oval) points out the extent of the foraminal decompression at C6-7 on the right side.

wall can be left intact because its removal decreases torsional stability (**Figure 6**). In addition, it prevents graft intrusion into the canal.

26. Hemostasis is obtained with Surgiflo/Surgicel (Ethicon) or Floseal (Baxter Healthcare) and a cottonoid patty.

27. The C6-7 disk space is then decompressed in the same manner. If the patient has mild OPLL, then it can be thinned down with the same burr. A 1- or 2-mm curet can be used to remove any remaining bone that cannot be removed with the burr. If the OPLL is severe, it may involve the dura. For such cases, it is best to thin that area down until only about 1 to 2 mm of bone remains. The surrounding bone is then thinned until the ossified dura "floats" ventrally.

28. If there is a disk herniation, there may be a fragment behind the PLL. We inspect behind the PLL (which has been thinned down to about 1 mm) with a 2-mm curet and, if necessary, use it to tear the PLL to remove the trapped disk.

Foraminal Decompression and Uncinate Resection

If there is foraminal stenosis, it is addressed at this time.

29. Protecting the vertebral artery: The contralateral C5-C6 uncinate is cleaned out with a 2-mm curet to define its lateral border (**Figure 7, A**). A Penfield No. 4 is then placed lateral to the uncinate. Only about 5 mm of the tip should be buried because a deeper placement can impinge on the root. The Penfield No. 4 is tilted side to side to enlarge the space and then replaced with a Penfield No. 2. This usually causes bleeding, which is controlled with Surgiflo (Ethicon) and a small patty. This protects the vertebral artery and demarcates the outer border of the uncinate and any laterally projecting spurs. Now all the soft tissues in the uncinate are cleaned out with a pituitary.

30. The lateral border of the decompression is established with the burr. Because it is easy to "past point" (place the instrument deeper than the plane of dissection/interest) with a burr and hit an unintended object, it is best to burr in a plane that is parallel with a dangerous object such as the vertebral artery or nerve root. To establish the lateral border, burring in an anterior-to-posterior direction, we gradually move farther and farther laterally until only about 1 to 2 mm of bone remains medial to the Penfield No. 2 blade (**Figure 7, B**). The anterior-posterior burring excursion should be only about 8 to 10 mm, as the root becomes more ventral as it exits the foramen.

31. Decompressing the root: Now that the lateral margin of the decompression has been established, the root can be decompressed. We start medially, where the central decompression left off. The burr is placed on the PLL and, using a medial-lateral burring motion parallel with the nerve root, all foraminal osteophytes are carefully burred off. It is easier to remove the osteophytes projecting from C6 than those from C5 because C5 osteophytes extend more cranial than the disk space. Any remaining bone is removed with 1- and 2-mm microcurets. The decompression is complete when the surgeon can easily palpate the lateral margin of the C6 pedicle and there is no bone overlying the root. If there is severe uncinate hypertrophy, the laterally projecting spur can impinge on the root extraforaminally as it takes a ventral course. In such cases, the uncinate is resected by twisting the Penfield No. 2 to break off the thinned lateral uncinate. If it is too thick to break this way, the surgeon can thin it down further with the burr. Another option is to place a 2-mm curet in place of the Penfield No. 2 and gently lever laterally until the uncinate breaks off.

32. For the ipsilateral side, the same technique is used, but because the hand often gets in the way of adequate visualization, more care must be taken to prevent injury to the root. Until the surgeon becomes comfortable with using the burr in tight places, it may be worthwhile to move to the opposite side of the table to finish this foraminal decompression. With more experience, ipsilateral decompressions can be performed in the following manner. A No. 4 and a No. 2 Penfield are placed as for the opposite side. Alternatively, a 3-mm suction tip can be used. We start the burr at the ventral surface of the uncinate,

2 mm medial to the Penfield No. 2, and push in posteriorly about 8 to 10 mm to establish the lateral wall. Then we decompress the root as for the contralateral side. The C6-C7 foramina are decompressed in a similar manner. Following a thorough foraminal decompression, all four foramina should be well visualized (**Figure 7, C**).

End-Plate Preparation

33. The superior end plate of C7 is now carefully burred off to expose punctate bleeding bone. The caudal end plate of C5 also is freshened up until punctate bleeding is visualized.

34. The entire field is irrigated with copious amounts of antibiotic solution to remove bone dust and diskectomy debris.

Screw Sizing

35. Screws are placed into the disk level to determine the longest screw that can be used. The C5 screw should be started close to the end plate and angled cranially to keep it away from the graft. This keeps the plate as short as possible and away from the adjacent disk space. The head of the screw is held at the same depth as it will be when it is screwed into the plate. The screw tip should then touch the level of the dura. If screwed in straight, this would yield bicortical purchase, but as it is angled caudally, it just misses the deep cortex. For the caudal screw, we choose a screw that is 2 mm shy of the dura when the screw head is held at the same depth that it will be in the plate.

36. The retractor is relaxed to let the soft tissues recover while the corpectomy graft is sized and cut.

Graft

37. Sizing the bone graft: Following the corpectomy and foraminotomy, the size of the required bone graft is measured using cervical plates as templates. Because the plates come in various sizes, we find one that fits snugly into the corpectomy site after distracting the segment 2 to 3 mm. Using the plate as a template, we cut the graft. The caudal surface has an angled cut to match the 15° cranial tilt of the C7 superior end plate. The cranial surface is straight to minimally lordotic to match the vertical end plate of C5. Once the graft has been cut, we use it to size the shortest plate that will allow the screws to be 2 mm distal to the end of the graft.

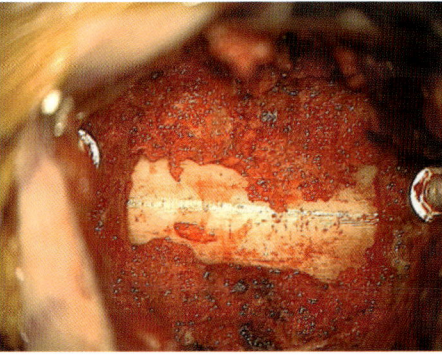

Figure 8 Intraoperative photograph shows bone graft in place for anterior cervical corpectomy and fusion. Bone dust and demineralized bone matrix have been used to fill the gaps and cover the graft.

38. The graft cavity is filled with bone dust, small bone fragments, and demineralized bone matrix. The retractor is then distracted again. The graft is then gently placed into the trough under Caspar distraction and tamped into place. Ideally, it should be countersunk 2 mm below the anterior cortex of the remaining vertebrae. Once the graft is positioned, the distraction through the Caspar pins is released to load the graft. An ideal graft should fit perfectly with no gaps between the graft and end plates.

39. Uncinate grafting: The uncinate area lateral to the graft is then burred to bleeding bone and the chunks of corpectomy bone are shaped and wedged tightly into these areas (**Figure 8**). The surgeon should avoid putting small pieces of bone graft from the corpectomy within the space lateral to the graft; these might migrate posteriorly into the root. Bone dust and demineralized bone matrix are used to fill any gaps and cover the graft.

Instrumentation

After placement of the strut graft, the shortest possible plate is selected that spans the length of the defect. This was done in step 37. We currently use a nonslotted plate with unicortical fixed-angle screws cranially and variable-angle screws caudally, allowing for dynamization and load-sharing of the graft but minimizing graft subsidence. We also routinely supplement two-level or greater corpectomies with posterior fixation.

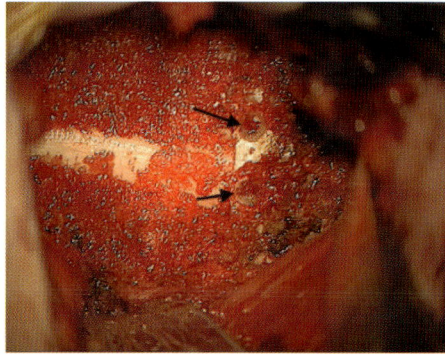

Figure 9 Intraoperative photograph shows instrumentation for anterior cervical corpectomy and fusion. For the cranial screws, a burr was used to create two shallow divots (arrows) 2 mm from the end plate to mark the location of the drill holes. The plate and two drill holes should be centered around the Caspar pin holes, which mark the midline.

40. We then call for a lateral radiograph, as it will take a few minutes for the radiology technician to respond.

41. The Caspar pins are removed, and the holes are filled with bone wax.

42. For the C5 screws, we use a burr to create two shallow divots 2 mm from the end plate to mark the location of the drill hole (**Figure 9**). The Caspar pin hole is used to center these holes.

43. If the plating system has a double-armed drill guide, we use it to drill the C5 holes, angled about 20° to 30° cranially.

44. Anterior osteophytes can cause the plate to be proud on the vertebral body, which decreases the depth of screw fixation and possibly increases the incidence of dysphagia. Therefore, before securing the plate, any osteophytes or prominences that were inadequately removed previously should be removed with the high-speed carbide burr to allow the plate to lie flat along the anterior aspect of the vertebral bodies.[2,3]

45. We then put the plate in and thread in the C5 screws about 90% of the way.

46. The double-armed drill guide is used to drill the C7 holes.

47. We screw in the C7 screws, then final-tighten the C5 screws. The plate tends to turn clockwise during final screw tightening, as the screw engages the plate. This can result in a tilted plate that is visible on AP radiographs. To prevent this, we countertorque the plate with a plate holder or a heavy needle driver.

48. The self-retaining retractor is removed, along with any sponge retractors that were used.

49. Final plate and screw placement is verified with a lateral radiograph. If the C7-T1 disk space was not visualized on the initial localizing radiograph, we pull down on the Kerlex gauze bandage roll while this image is obtained.

Closure

50. The site is irrigated.

51. We inspect for any bleeding using a handheld appendiceal retractor. The most common area for a postoperative hematoma is the edge of the longus colli. We place liquefied collagen (Surgiflo or Floseal [Baxter Healthcare] and Surgicel) along the medial borders of the longus colli. Any bleeders on the esophagus or at the tracheoesophageal groove are coagulated with hemostatic agents instead of electrocautery to prevent inadvertent injury to the RLN. We leave the hemostatic agents in the wound. The anterior structures of the neck, including the trachea, esophagus, and carotid sheath, are also closely inspected.

52. A 1/8-in Hemovac drain is placed through a separate stab hole such that all of the holes are 2 to 3 cm below any hemostatic agents to prevent clotting.

53. A layered closure is performed with a figure-of-8, interrupted 3-0 Monocryl suture (Ethicon) to approximate the platysma layer. The subcuticular tissue is approximated with interrupted, buried 5-0 Monocryl absorbable suture, followed by application of 0.25-in adhesive skin closure strips and sterile dressings.

54. Finally, we place a rigid collar with a firm plastic bivalved shell and removable padded liner.

Complications

In the immediate postoperative period, careful neurologic follow-up is performed. An evolving wound hematoma has the potential to obstruct breathing and swallowing, and a simple procedure to open the incision can provide rapid relief with drainage of the hematoma. Swallowing can be difficult for the first 2 to 3 days after retraction of the esophagus; this is generally caused by inflammation and edema. Swallowing difficulty (dysphagia) is the most common complication following anterior cervical spine surgery, with a reported incidence of 24%.[11] The etiology of postoperative swallowing problems is multifactorial, including esophageal denervation, soft-tissue swelling, and scar tissue formation.[11] For most patients, postoperative dysphagia improves with time, with one study reporting only 1.3% of patients with moderate or severe dysphagia by 24 months postoperatively.[12] As with dysphagia, most cases of postoperative dysphonia caused by RLN injury resolve with time. Reported rates for the early postoperative period range from 2% to 30%; persistent symptomatic vocal cord paresis ranges from 0.33% to 2.5%.[11]

Adverse events following anterior cervical spine surgery are categorized as intraoperative, early postoperative, and late postoperative. The most common and potentially serious complications include esophageal injury, vertebral artery injury, dural tear, spinal cord or nerve root injury, airway compromise, epidural hematoma, dysphagia, dysphonia, wound infection, and bone-graft dislodgment.[11] Esophageal injury is caused intraoperatively from inappropriate retractor placement, use of sharp-edged retractors, or inadvertent intraoperative trauma by a sharp instrument or high-speed burr.[11] The risk of deep cervical or mediastinal infection and secondary airway compromise makes these injuries serious and potentially life-threatening, but the reported incidence is low, ranging from 0.2% to 0.4%.[11] The rate of vertebral artery injury after anterior cervical spine surgery is 0.3%, with the most avoidable mechanism of injury, including excessively wide corpectomy as well as loss of the vertebral midline, leading to an off-center corpectomy.[11,13] The incidence of dural tear during anterior cervical spine surgery is reported to be 3.7%; however, patients undergoing revision anterior cervical spine surgery and those with OPLL are at increased risk of dural tear. In general, even with adequate dural repair, a lumbar cerebrospinal fluid drain is placed and the patient is placed in the upright position following surgery to reduce intraspinal cerebrospinal fluid pressure and prevent fistula formation.[11] The reported incidence of acute spinal cord injury following anterior cervical spine surgery ranges from 0.2% to 0.9%. Intraoperative neurologic monitoring with evoked potentials should be universally used for anterior cervical spine surgery, with other strategies to prevent iatrogenic spinal cord injury such as maintenance of systolic blood pressure above 80 mm Hg and awake intubation to prevent excessive cervical spine extension.[11]

Postoperative Care and Rehabilitation

If the retraction time exceeds 3 hours or if intubation was difficult, the patient remains intubated overnight in the intensive care unit, with extubation when the patient passes a cuff leak test. If the patient has severe dysphagia on the night of the surgery, 10 mg of dexamethasone is given intravenously. The head of the bed is elevated to above 30°. Antibiotic prophylaxis is continued until the drain is removed, which we do when the output is less than 20 mL over an 8-hour shift. Since we began using Surgicel and Surgiflo, this usually occurs within 8 hours and therefore we pull the drain and discharge most patients the morning after surgery. Ambulation is started the morning following surgery, and a progressive walking program is allowed 1 to 2 weeks after surgery. Patients are allowed to shower 1 day after surgery. Formal physical therapy is not necessary in most cases, and overhead lifting activities are generally restricted until a solid fusion is obtained. The cervical collar is worn most of the day and night for 6 weeks. It may be removed for a few hours each day, but the patient must be able to minimize neck motion.

Pearls

- Using Gardner-Wells tongs and taping the head to the table in proper orientation decrease the rotation of the head/spine during the surgery. This helps prevent asymmetric decompression and allows for proper implant/plate placement.

- The most common reasons for asymmetric corpectomy and injury to the vertebral artery are inadequate exposure (ie, lateral to the costal processes and defining the lateral aspect of the uncinate) and failure to maintain midline orientation.
- Creation of subplatysmal pouches during superficial exposure facilitates adequate exposure of up to six levels through a single transverse incision. The transverse incision is cosmetically more pleasing than a vertical or oblique incision.
- Improperly placed (ie, off-center) Caspar pins can induce a rotatory deformity during decompression and correction.
- The depth of the corpectomy is obtained by excising all disk material at the intervertebral interspace cephalad and caudad to the vertebral body being resected. This allows the surgeon to remove bone safely and efficiently down to the posterior cortex.
- A loose bone graft strut generally results from measuring the corpectomy site without traction on the spine.

References

1. Rhee JM, Yoon T, Riew KD: Cervical radiculopathy. *J Am Acad Orthop Surg* 2007;15(8):486-494.
2. Glattes RC, Taylor B, Riew KD: Controversies and perils: Anterior corpectomy or multilevel discectomy. *Tech Orthop* 2003;17(3):382-390.
3. Bae HW, Delamarter RB: Cervical vertebrectomy and plating, in Bradford DS, Zdeblick TA, eds: *Masters Techniques in Orthopaedic Surgery: The Spine*, ed 2. Philadelphia, PA, Lippincott Williams & Wilkins, 2004, pp 47-66.
4. Emery SE: Cervical spondylotic myelopathy: Diagnosis and treatment. *J Am Acad Orthop Surg* 2001;9(6):376-388.
5. Rao RD, Gourab K, David KS: Operative treatment of cervical spondylotic myelopathy. *J Bone Joint Surg Am* 2006;88(7):1619-1640.
6. Edwards CC II, Riew KD, Anderson PA, Hilibrand AS, Vaccaro AF: Cervical myelopathy: Current diagnostic and treatment strategies. *Spine J* 2003;3(1):68-81.
7. Cunningham MR, Hershman S, Bendo J: Systematic review of cohort studies comparing surgical treatments for cervical spondylotic myelopathy. *Spine (Phila Pa 1976)* 2010;35(5):537-543.
8. Mummaneni PV, Kaiser MG, Matz PG, et al: Cervical surgical techniques for the treatment of cervical spondylotic myelopathy. *J Neurosurg Spine* 2009;11(2):130-141.
9. Riew KD, McCulloch JA, Delamarter RB, An HS, Ahn NU: Microsurgery for degenerative conditions of the cervical spine. *Instr Course Lect* 2003;52:497-508.
10. Beutler WJ, Sweeney CA, Connolly PJ: Recurrent laryngeal nerve injury with anterior cervical spine surgery risk with laterality of surgical approach. *Spine (Phila Pa 1976)* 2001;26(12):1337-1342.
11. Daniels AH, Riew KD, Yoo JU, et al: Adverse events associated with anterior cervical spine surgery. *J Am Acad Orthop Surg* 2008;16(12):729-738.
12. Lee MJ, Bazaz R, Furey CG, Yoo J: Risk factors for dysphagia after anterior cervical spine surgery: A two-year prospective cohort study. *Spine J* 2007;7(2):141-147.
13. Burke JP, Gerszten PC, Welch WC: Iatrogenic vertebral artery injury during anterior cervical spine surgery. *Spine J* 2005;5(5):508-514.

Chapter 88
Posterior Cervical Foraminotomy

Kern Singh, MD   Steven J. Fineberg, MD   Matthew Oglesby, BA
Jonathan A. Hoskins, MD   Vamshi Yelavarthi, BA

Introduction
Decompressive procedures employed in the management of cervical radiculopathy have evolved in recent years. New advancements, such as the integration of minimally invasive techniques, offer an alternative to traditional open techniques. The concept behind minimally invasive techniques is to achieve symptom relief with the reduction in morbidity that is associated with traditional techniques. The posterior cervical foraminotomy can be executed using a minimally invasive approach to treat cervical radiculopathy. A prior study suggests that results from the procedure are comparable to that of a conventional open foraminotomy.[1]

Posterior cervical foraminotomy eliminates the risk of injuring structures in the anterior approach (ie, carotid artery, esophagus, recurrent laryngeal nerve).[2] In addition, the procedure does not require a fusion, does not destabilize the disk space, and is an easy approach to directly decompress the foramen.

An important limitation compared to the anterior approach is the inability to deal directly with pathology affecting the central aspect of the canal. Posterior procedures require more dissection of the large extensor spine muscle mass with a possible increase in postoperative neck pain.

The approach may be modified by undercutting of the spinous process to treat myelopathy; however, the relative efficacy and safety have not been demonstrated.[3]

Patient Selection
Indications
Cervical radiculopathy is frequently a result of an osteophyte, spondylosis, and/or lateral disk herniation compressing a nerve root in the neural foramen. Posterior cervical foraminotomy is appropriate for patients with persistent radiculopathy that correlates with findings on CT, MRI, and/or myelography and in whom nonsurgical management has failed. Patients with refractory radiculopathy after anterior cervical diskectomy and fusion are also indicated for posterior cervical foraminotomy.

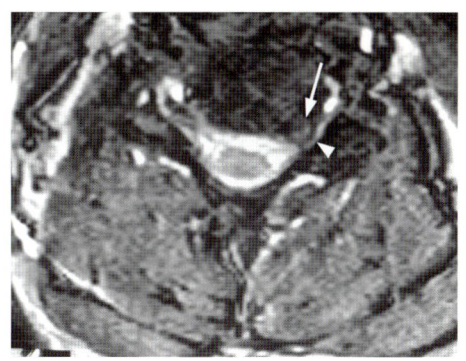

Figure 1 T2-weighted axial MRI shows a disk herniation (arrow) in the C5-6 neural foramen compressing the left C5-6 nerve root (arrowhead).

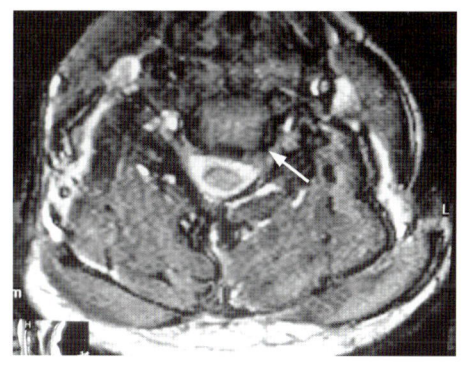

Figure 2 T2-weighted axial MRI shows severe compression of the left C5-6 nerve root (arrow) in the C5-6 neural foramen.

Contraindications
The spine surgeon must recognize the contraindications to performing posterior cervical foraminotomy. In the initial consultation, a thorough history and physical examination should be conducted, noting any signs or symptoms of a local skin infection, cervical myelopathy, significant kyphosis, or mechanical instability of the cervical spine. Evidence of spinal cord compression, significant disk herniation compressing the nerve root, and symptomatology not referable to the pathology visualized on imaging studies are contraindications to performing the procedure.

Preoperative Imaging
Routine preoperative imaging should consist of AP and lateral radiographs to assess cervical alignment. Dynamic flexion and extension views are also helpful to identify any instability that requires a fusion. MRI should also be obtained to evaluate the spinal cord and nerve roots for sites of compression (**Figures 1** and **2**). If MRI cannot be obtained, a CT myelogram may be performed instead.

Procedure
Room Setup/Patient Positioning
The procedure can be performed with the patient in the prone or seated position. After induction of general anesthesia, a three-pin Mayfield fixation is applied, fixing the head to the table in the prone position. A Wilson frame or similar bolsters are placed under the torso.

All possible neural compression points should be carefully protected and padded. The neck is extended, with care taken to avoid hyperextension. The chin is slightly tucked in a "military" posture that aids in the approach. Extreme flexion or extension of the neck should be avoided to prevent positioning the neck in a nonanatomic position. A reverse Trendelenburg position allows venous drainage and less bleeding during surgery.

A fluoroscopic C-arm is positioned under the drapes to allow visualization of the position of the retractors during the procedure. The shoulders should be taped down to allow better radiographic visualization of the neck. The knees are flexed to prevent distal migration of the patient.

Video 88.1 Open Cervical Foraminotomy. Kern Singh, MD; Steven J. Fineberg, MD; Matthew Oglesby; Jonathan A. Hoskins, MD; Vamshi Yelavarthi (3 min)

Surgical Technique
Open Posterior Cervical Foraminotomy
Instruments/Equipment
The open technique requires 1- or 2-mm thin-footed Kerrison rongeurs and a

---

Dr. Singh or an immediate family member has received royalties from Pioneer and Zimmer and serves as a paid consultant to or is an employee of DePuy, Stryker, and Zimmer. None of the following authors nor any immediate family member has received anything of value from or owns stock in a commercial company or institution related directly or indirectly to the subject of this chapter: Dr. Fineberg, Mr. Oglesby, Dr. Hoskins, and Mr. Yelavarthi.

Section 7: Spine

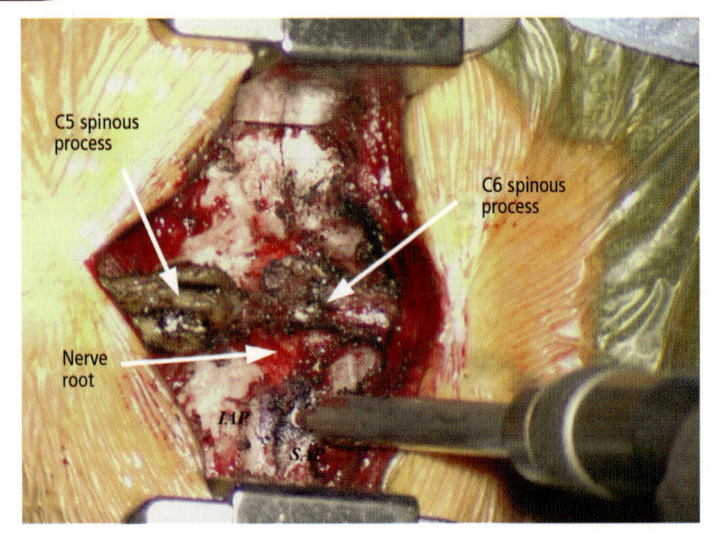

Figure 3 Intraoperative photograph demonstrates open posterior cervical foraminotomy. A high-speed burr is used to resect the medial third of the inferior articular process (IAP) of the cephalad vertebra.

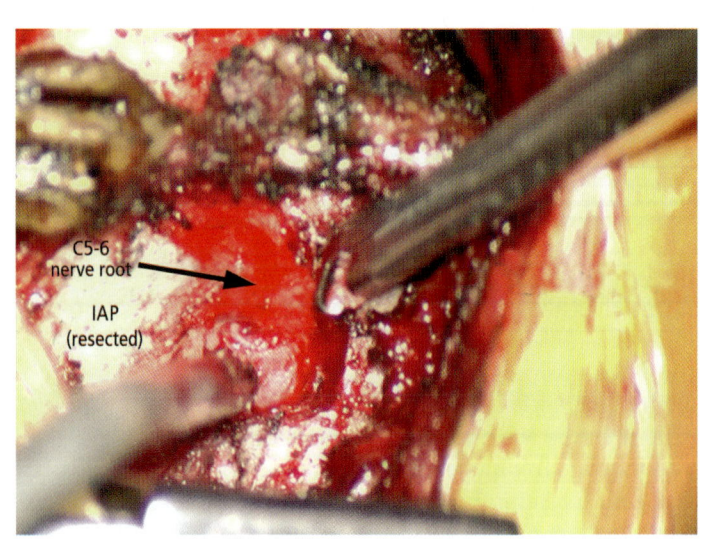

Figure 4 A Kerrison rongeur is used to excise the superior articular process (SAP) of the caudal vertebra. IAP = inferior articular process.

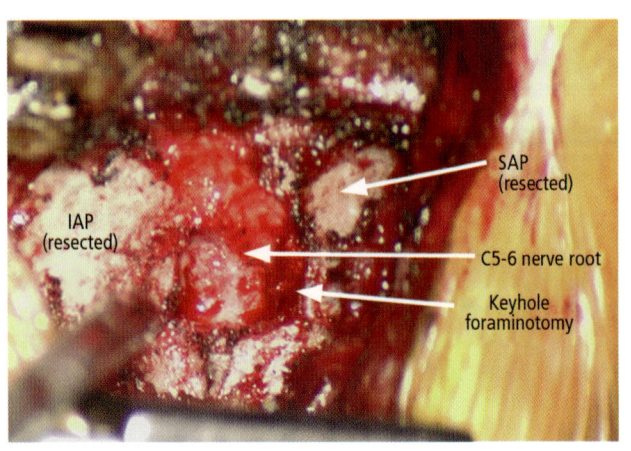

Figure 5 The nerve root is visualized in the keyhole foraminotomy. IAP = inferior articular process.

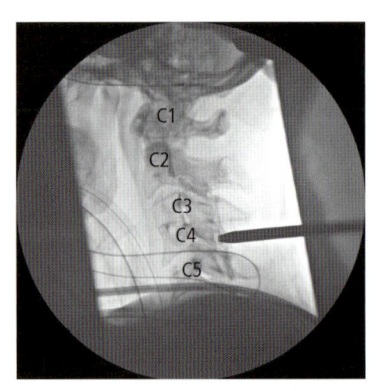

Figure 6 The initial tubular dilator is placed toward the facet joint under fluoroscopic guidance.

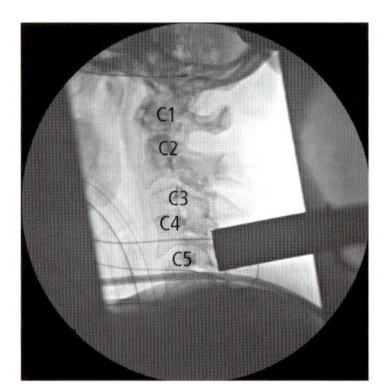

Figure 7 Sequential tubular dilators up to 18 mm are placed to create the working channel. Lateral fluoroscopic view shows the final dilator in place.

Video 88.2 Minimally Invasive Approach for Posterior Cervical Foraminotomy. Kern Singh, MD; Steven J. Fineberg, MD; Matthew Oglesby; Jonathan A. Hoskins, MD; Vamshi Yelavarthi (3 min)

2-mm round-tip burr or drill. Bovie electrocautery, self-retaining retractors, and a Cobb elevator should also be available for this procedure.

Exposure

A 2-cm incision is made slightly lateral (1.5 cm) to the midline. Electrocautery is used to carry the incision through the posterior fascia. Self-retaining retractors are placed to spread the paraspinal muscles. The muscle should be dissected to expose the medial half of the facet. Further dissection laterally is unnecessary and may destabilize the joint.

Foraminotomy

The inferior articular process (IAP) of the cephalad vertebra is identified. The medial third of the IAP and the inferior portion of the superior lamina are removed with a burr (**Figure 3**). The superior articular process (SAP) of the caudal vertebra is visualized. A Kerrison rongeur or a burr can be used to resect the SAP, exposing the exiting nerve root (**Figure 4**).

A keyhole foraminotomy is created with the nerve root visualized (**Figure 5**). Decompression should be performed until a nerve probe can easily be placed into the neuroforamen.

Closure

After completion of the decompression, the wound is irrigated with antibiotics and saline. The fascia is reapproximated, and the wound is closed in layers. The patient is returned to the supine position for extubation.

Minimally Invasive Posterior Cervical Foraminotomy

Instruments/Equipment

Fluoroscopy, a microscope, tubular dilators (up to 18 mm), a tubular retractor system, and Kirschner wires (K-wires) or a spinal needle are required for the minimally invasive technique. Bovie electrocautery, Kerrison rongeurs, and a 2-mm round-tip burr are also used, as in the open procedure.

Exposure

A lateral fluoroscopic image is used to identify the level in question; the placement of a spinal needle or a K-wire may assist in identifying the level. An incision is made slightly (0.5 cm) lateral to the midline. Electrocautery is used to carry

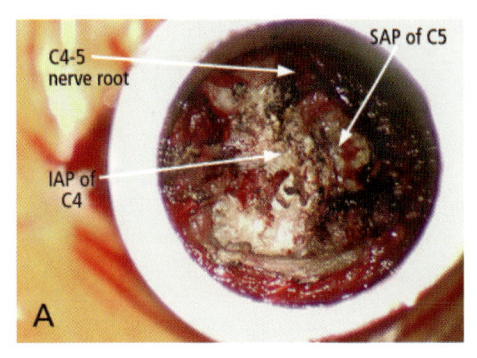

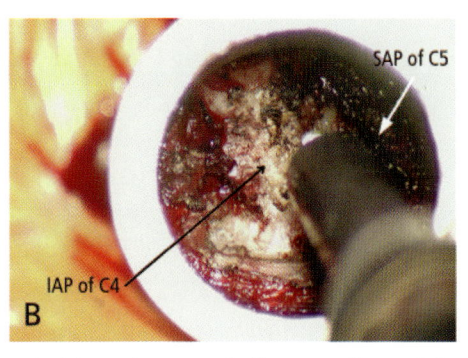

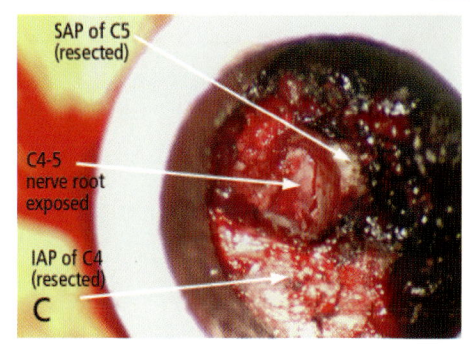

Figure 8 Photographs demonstrate posterior cervical foraminotomy. **A,** Exposure through the tubular retractor. The medial facet joint and inferior portion of the superior lamina are visualized in the surgical field. **B,** A high-speed burr is used to resect the medial third of the IAP of the cephalad vertebra. **C,** The IAP and SAP have been resected, and the nerve root is visualized. IAP = inferior articular process, SAP = superior articular process.

the incision through the posterior fascia. Under fluoroscopic guidance, sequential tubular dilators are placed at the medial facet joint to spread the paraspinal muscles (**Figures 6** and **7**).

Foraminotomy

Soft tissue is removed from the tubular retractor, and the medial half of the facet joint and inferior portion of the superior lamina are exposed (**Figure 8, A**). A burr is used to remove the medial one third of the IAP of the cephalad vertebra (**Figure 8, B**). Next, a burr or Kerrison rongeur is used to remove the SAP of the inferior vertebra. The nerve root is visualized exiting into the neuroforamen (**Figure 8, C**). A blunt nerve probe is placed into the neuroforamen, ensuring that complete decompression has been achieved.

Closure

After completion of the decompression, the wound is irrigated with antibiotics and saline. The retractors are removed, and a single stitch is placed in the fascia. The skin edges are anesthetized and then closed with absorbable sutures, and the patient is returned to the supine position.

Controversies

Minimally invasive posterior cervical foraminotomy has demonstrated clinical outcomes comparable with those of the traditional open approach. Critics of the minimally invasive technique suggest that visualization is compromised and is not worth the benefits of less tissue dissection.[4]

Complications

Some of the most common complications following foraminotomy include infection, durotomy, postoperative cervical instability, and persistent radiculopathy due to incomplete decompression.

Postoperative Care and Rehabilitation

Typically, a posterior cervical foraminotomy does not require postoperative immobilization. Patients are discharged home within a few hours of surgery.[5] No specific restrictions are necessary other than routine wound care. Patients may return to routine activities or work as soon as tolerated.

Pearls

- Posterior cervical foraminotomy is indicated in patients with cervical radiculopathy due to foraminal stenosis, posterolaterally herniated disks, or persistent symptoms after an anterior cervical fusion.
- Minimally invasive techniques have been developed to decrease tissue trauma and the morbidity associated with traditional open approaches.
- Foraminotomy is performed by resecting the IAP and the inferior lamina of the cephalad vertebra, followed by resection of the SAP of the caudal vertebra.
- Resection of more than 50% of the medial facet joint during a foraminotomy may result in subsequent segmental instability.
- The foraminotomy is complete when a blunt nerve probe is easily placed in the neuroforamen, ensuring adequate decompression.

References

1. Holly LT, Moftakhar P, Khoo LT, Wang JC, Shamie N: Minimally invasive 2-level posterior cervical foraminotomy: Preliminary clinical results. *J Spinal Disord Tech* 2007;20(1):20-24.
2. Jagannathan J, Sherman JH, Szabo T, Shaffrey CI, Jane JA: The posterior cervical foraminotomy in the treatment of cervical disc/osteophyte disease: A single-surgeon experience with a minimum of 5 years' clinical and radiographic follow-up. *J Neurosurg Spine* 2009;10(4):347-356.
3. Resnick DK: Posterior cervical foraminotomy and discectomy, in Wolfla CE, Resnick DK, eds: *Neurosurgical Operative Atlas: Spine and Peripheral Nerves.* New York, NY, Thieme, 2007, pp 82-86.
4. Epstein NE: Minimally invasive/endoscopic vs "open" posterior cervical laminoforaminotomy: Do the risks outweigh the benefits? *Surg Neurol* 2009;71(3): 330-331.
5. Adamson TE: Microendoscopic posterior cervical laminoforaminotomy for unilateral radiculopathy: Results of a new technique in 100 cases. *J Neurosurg* 2001;95(1, suppl):51-57.

Chapter 89
Posterior Cervical Laminectomy and Fusion

Sheeraz A. Qureshi, MD, MBA   Andrew C. Hecht, MD

Patient Selection

Cervical degenerative disease is the most common form of acquired disability in patients older than 50 years.[1] The most common clinical manifestations of degenerative changes in the cervical spine are neck pain, radiculopathy, and myelopathy. A combination of symptoms is not unusual. Patients who continue to be symptomatic despite an appropriate trial of nonsurgical management are indicated for surgical intervention.

Once the decision has been made to proceed with surgical management, a number of variables are taken into consideration to determine the optimal surgical approach. These variables include alignment of the cervical spine, number of levels involved, nature of the pathologic process, and surgeon preference.

In general, posterior approaches to decompress the cervical spine are chosen in patients with neutral to lordotic cervical alignment and more than two levels of compressive pathology. Certain pathologic processes, such as ossification of the posterior longitudinal ligament and intradural tumors, are preferentially treated through a posterior approach. In the presence of cervical kyphosis or if there is significant ventral compression of the spinal cord, anterior procedures should be considered before posterior decompressive procedures.

Options for central and foraminal decompression of the cervical spinal cord and nerves from a posterior approach include laminoplasty and laminectomy/fusion. Either procedure can be combined with foraminotomies to directly decompress the cervical nerve roots from a posterior approach. When cervical laminectomy is decided upon as the treatment of choice, we strongly recommend comcomitant posterior cervical fusion to prevent the extremely complicated and disabling complication of postlaminectomy kyphosis.[2]

Preoperative Imaging

We strongly recommend that all patients have standing AP, lateral, flexion, and extension radiographs prior to surgery. Plain radiographs can provide valuable information with regard to spinal alignment and the fixed or flexible nature of any preexisting spinal deformity. All patients should also have an MRI and CT scan or CT myelogram before surgery (**Figure 1**). CT scans are very helpful for surgical planning for the sizes of lateral mass screws and upper thoracic pedicle screws and for identifying any variations of the vertebral anatomy that may complicate placement of hardware. The surgeon should always take note of aberrant vertebral artery anatomy even though vertebral artery injury from posterior cervical subaxial instrumentation is extremely rare.

Video 89.1 Posterior Cervical Laminectomy and Fusion. Sheeraz A. Qureshi, MD, MBA; Andrew C. Hecht, MD (19 min)

Procedure
Room Setup/Patient Positioning

Posterior cervical laminectomy and fusion is performed with the patient under general endotracheal anesthesia. Although most patients tolerate standard intubation techniques, if an exacerbation of symptoms occurs with flexion or extension of the neck, or if there is severe spinal cord compression, the surgical team should strongly consider an awake fiberoptic intubation. The patient's symptoms should be discussed with the anesthesiologist so that a mutual decision can be made as to the best method of intubation. It is our practice to obtain spinal cord monitoring baselines—SSEP (somatosensory-evoked potentials) and MEP (motor-evoked potentials)—before placing the patient in the prone position.

General endotracheal anesthesia is induced with the patient on a Jackson table with flat board. It is important to remind the anesthesiologist that the tube cannot be secured with a tie around the head as this would be in the surgical field. The tube should be heavily taped in position, as any prepositioning ties will need to be removed once the patient is prone.

We use SSEP and MEP monitoring as well as intraoperative electromyography in all patients undergoing posterior cervical laminectomy and fusion. Although evidence is lacking that such monitoring improves outcomes, we believe that changes in motor or sensory potentials can be predictive of neurologic dysfunction. Malpositioned instrumentation can result in abnormal electromyographic activity if there is resultant nerve root irritation. In addition, most monitoring changes are due to blood pressure changes, and this monitoring can ensure that the appropriate mean arterial pressure is maintained during surgery. A bite block should be placed by the anesthesiologist when evoked potential monitoring is being used.

After general endotracheal anesthesia is induced and with the patient in the supine position, a Foley catheter is placed using standard sterile technique. Sequential compression devices are applied for prophylaxis against deep venous thrombosis, and evoked potential monitoring leads are placed. We obtain baseline potentials at this point.

After baseline potentials are obtained, Gardner-Wells tongs are applied in standard fashion below the equator of the skull and immediately above and just anterior to the pinnae. We prefer to use Gardner-Wells tongs because of their

---

Dr. Qureshi or an immediate family member has received royalties from Zimmer; is a member of a speakers' bureau or has made paid presentations on behalf of Medtronic, Stryker, and Zimmer; serves as a paid consultant to or is an employee of Stryker, Zimmer, and Medtronic; and serves as a board member, owner, officer, or committee member of the American Academy of Orthopaedic Surgeons, the Cervical Spine Research Society, the Musculoskeletal Transplant Foundation, and the North American Spine Society. Dr. Hecht or an immediate family member has received royalties from Zimmer; is a member of a speakers' bureau or has made paid presentations on behalf of Stryker and DePuy; serves as a paid consultant to or is an employee of Stryker, Zimmer, and Medtronic Sofamor Danek; has stock or stock options held in Johnson & Johnson; and serves as a board member, owner, officer, or committee member of the American Academy of Orthopaedic Surgeons and the Musculoskeletal Transplant Foundation.

simplicity and ability to be applied by a single operator. The pins of the Gardner-Wells tongs are tightened simultaneously until the indicator pin protrudes 1 mm. At this point, a pressure of 6 to 8 in-lb (13.6 kg) is achieved, which correlates with a pull-out strength of 60 to 120 lb. Twenty pounds of weight are then hung from the Gardner-Wells tongs for continuous in-line skull traction and maintenance of head position throughout the procedure. Bivector traction is occasionally used to place a slight extension moment on the skull after decompression.

Preparations are then made to perform a rotisserie turn using the Jackson table so that the patient can be positioned prone. A soft facial pillow is placed on the patient and pillows are positioned along the patient's lower extremities. The Jackson table with four posts (hip and thigh pads) and chest board is then placed on top of the patient and locked into position with care taken to provide as much compression on the patient as possible so that the patient is firmly held between the two frames (**Figure 2, A**). We then use four belts that are tightened around the two frames for additional support.

At this point, the entire team is positioned around the patient and the endotracheal tube is disconnected from the circuit. The rotational control on the Jackson table is released and the rotisserie turn is performed quickly with the surgeon at the head of the table (**Figure 2, B**). This is demonstrated in the video supplement. The rotational lock is once again applied and the endotracheal tube is reconnected. The belts are then removed and the flat board is disconnected from the frame of the Jackson table, leaving the patient in a prone position on the four-post frame with chest board and face pillow and head in traction provided by 20 lb of weight on the Gardner-Wells tongs. Evoked potentials are again checked to make sure that there has been no change during positioning. One member of the team should be assigned to hold each arm once the patient is prone and before the straps are released to make sure the arms do not fall before the arm boards are reattached to the table.

Upon confirmation that evoked potentials have remained stable, final positioning is completed. The patient's arms are held at the side of the body and allowed to rest comfortably on the arm supports of the Jackson table. If needed, gentle traction can be applied to the upper extremities through the shoulders (or skin) using silk tape. All bony prominences must be adequately padded.

After the patient is appropriately positioned, a fluoroscopy machine is brought into the lateral position and placed proximally, just above the surgical field. Our preference is to use a three-dimensional fluoroscopy unit so that intraoperative three-dimensional images can be obtained to more completely assess instrumentation.

The posterior hairline is shaved up to the occipital protuberance. This allows for maximal exposure if any intraoperative complications occur that require

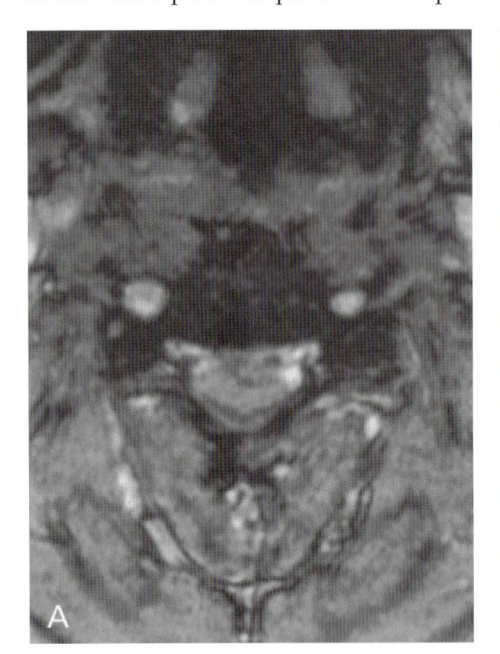

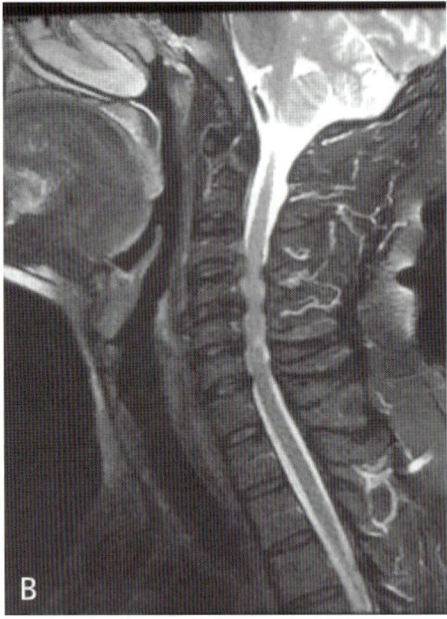

Figure 1 **A**, Axial T2-weighted MRI shows cervical spinal cord compression. **B**, Sagittal T2-weighted MRI shows multilevel cervical spinal cord compression.

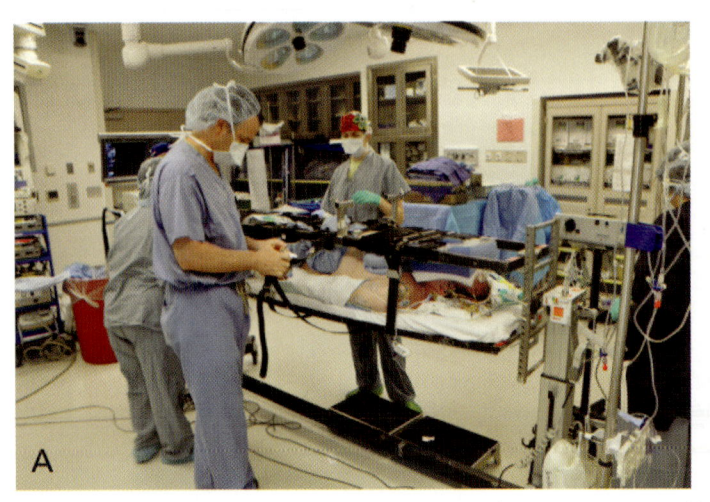

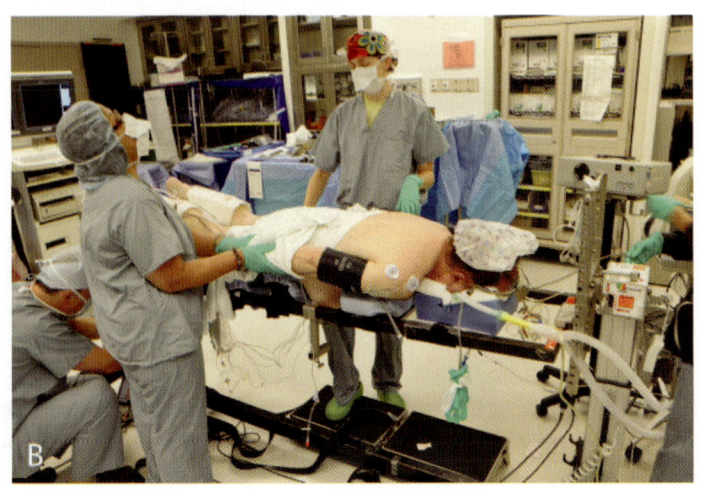

Figure 2 Photographs show patient positioning for posterior cervical laminectomy and fusion. **A**, The patient is placed supine on a Jackson table with a flat board. A four-post frame with chest board is placed over the patient and all pads and pillows are positioned appropriately in preparation for the rotisserie turn. **B**, After the rotisserie turn is completed, the flat board is removed and the patient is now in the prone position on the four-post frame.

proximal extension of decompression or fusion. Nonsterile waterproof plastic draping is applied to outline the surgical field. The skin is then prepared in sterile fashion using the surgeon's preparatory solution of choice.

Sterile draping is then applied. We place four blue towels over the previously applied nonsterile plastic draping. This is followed by sheets placed distally, proximally, and along either side of the patient. Sterile fluoroscopy drapes are then applied over either side of the fluoroscopy unit so that it can be a part of the sterile field and easily used throughout the case. An iodine-impregnated sticky drape is used to cover the exposed skin surface. This is followed by a U-shaped drape placed both distally and proximally as the final layer of draping.

Next, antibiotic prophylaxis is given. A time-out is always called with the attention of the entire team before the incision is made.

Special Instruments/Equipment/Implants
For this procedure, the following equipment should be on hand:
- Jackson table with flat board and four-post frame
- Gardner-Wells tongs with 20 lb of weight
- Insulated electrocautery and bipolar cautery
- Angled cerebellar retractors
- High-speed burr with non–end-cutting drill attachment
- Multiple angled curets
- Kerrison (1 mm through 3 mm) and Leksell rongeurs
- Lateral mass and pedicle fixation (screws, rods, end caps)

Surgical Technique
Exposure
A midline skin incision is used. The length and location of the incision can be determined using fluoroscopy. The skin and subcutaneous tissues are incised. It is important to control all bleeding as it occurs. Once the cervical fascia is exposed, it is incised in the midline and a subperiosteal dissection of the muscle is performed bilaterally using electrocautery. The exposure is performed to the lateral masses of the vertebrae that are going to be instrumented.

Self-retaining retractors are placed once adequate hemostasis is obtained. We prefer to use angled cerebellar retractors and relax them every 45 minutes to reduce the risk of muscle ischemia.

Confirming Surgical Level
After exposure is completed, an intraoperative fluoroscopic image is obtained to confirm appropriate surgical levels. Various techniques can be used to count and mark cervical levels. We use the C2 vertebra as our guide and count down from there. A Penfield 4 elevator is placed into an exposed facet joint and a fluoroscopic image is obtained. Facet joints are counted starting from C2-3 for confirmation of surgical level.

Instrumentation
Upon confirmation of appropriate surgical levels, attention is turned to instrumentation and decompression. Our practice is to first drill pilot holes for placement of all of the lateral mass screws bilaterally and then perform the laminectomy. If the cervicothoracic junction is going to be crossed, we place the T1 pedicle screws after the laminectomy and then finally place the lateral mass screws.

The optimal position for drilling and placement of lateral mass screws has been researched extensively. We use the technique recommended by An et al[3] (**Figure 3**). A 2-mm burr is used to make a small depression in the lateral mass 1 mm medial to the center to serve as an anchoring/starting point for the drill bit. A drill with a drill stop set at 12 to 14 mm, depending on the size of the lateral mass, is then set into the groove and a unicortical screw tract is created with the drill angled 30° lateral and 15° cephalad. We use unicortical screws, as these have been shown to have clinical results equivalent to bicortical screws and minimize the risk of injury to the neurovascular structures.[4] A ball-tipped probe is used to confirm the integrity of the screw tract. This is followed by tapping each screw tract to the same depth that it was drilled. If both cortices have been drilled, a depth gauge can be used to confirm the appropriate screw length.

Decompression
After all subaxial screw tracts are drilled, probed, and tapped, attention is turned to the laminectomy. A high-speed burr with a non–end-cutting attachment is used to create troughs bilaterally in the laminae just medial to the lateral masses. A non–end-cutting burr is preferred because it decreases the likelihood of injury to the underlying dura or spinal cord as the anterior cortex of the lamina is resected. Drilling is stopped frequently, and a Penfield 4 elevator is used to check the depth

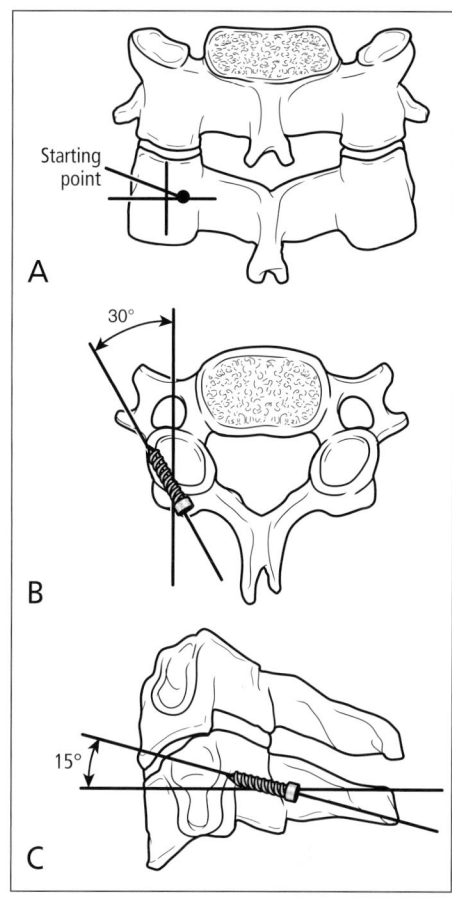

Figure 3 Illustrations depict the starting point (**A**), angulation (**B**), and final placement (**C**) of lateral mass screws using the An technique. Note that the starting point is just medial to the midpoint of the lateral mass and the screw is aimed from medial to lateral in the axial plane and from inferior to superior in the sagittal plane.

of the trough. Once the ligamentum flavum is reached, drilling is discontinued and a nerve hook is used to elevate the flavum, which is then resected using a 2-mm Kerrison rongeur.

Once the troughs have been completed through the anterior and posterior cortices of the laminae and the ligamentum flavum has been resected, Leksell rongeurs are used to grab the spinous processes of the most cephalad and caudal levels. Constant upward pressure is maintained on the laminae so that there is no compression on any part of the cervical spinal cord and any adhesions under the lamina are teased off as the lamina is removed en bloc. Evoked potential monitoring should be checked at this point, and the patient's mean arterial pressure should be maintained at its baseline to avoid an ischemic injury to the cord. Angled curets should be used to elevate the laminae sequentially from distal to proximal off the cervical spinal

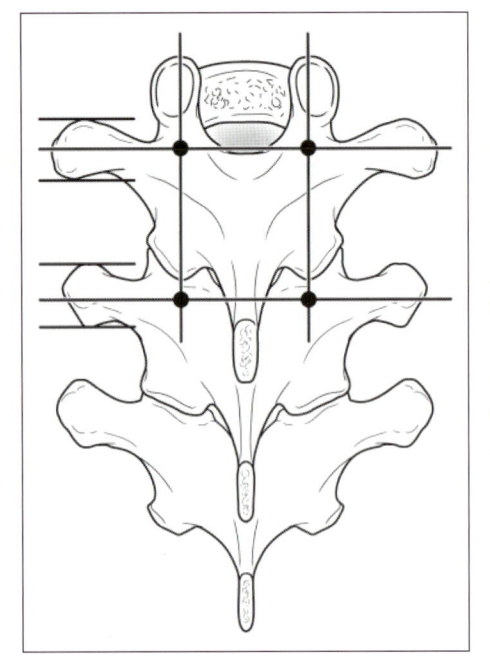

Figure 4 Illustration shows the starting points (black dots) for placement of thoracic pedicle screws. The points are lateral to a vertical line bisecting the facet joint along the upper one third of the transverse process.

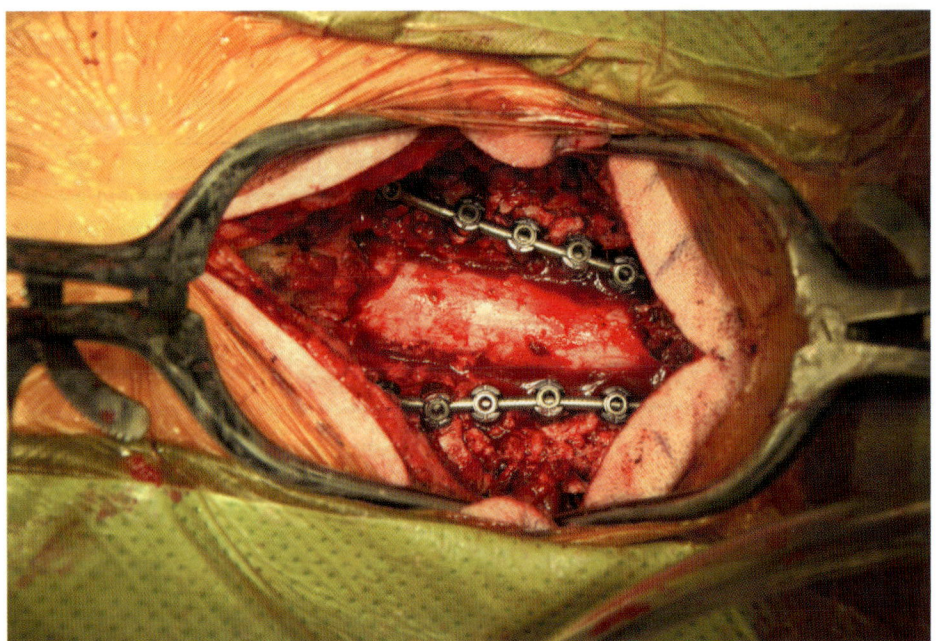

Figure 5 Intraoperative photograph shows the decompressed spinal cord following the removal of laminae. Lateral mass instrumentation is in place and interconnected using rods and end caps.

cord in an en bloc fashion. Meticulous hemostasis should be achieved using bipolar cautery and hemostatic agents.

Crossing the Cervicothoracic Junction

If the cervicothoracic junction is to be crossed, T1 pedicle screws are placed at this point. It is our practice to cross the cervicothoracic junction in all cases where a laminectomy and fusion would otherwise be taken to C7 because of the high rate of breakdown at this junctional segment.[5] A laminoforaminotomy is performed at T1 so that the medial border of the pedicle can be easily palpated. A 2- or 3-mm burr is then used to create a starting point located at the intersection of the midpoint of the transverse process and lateral pars (**Figure 4**). A pedicle blush may be noted, suggesting entrance into the cancellous bone of the pedicle. The appropriate amount of medialization changes from T1 to T3 (25° to 30°, to as low as 10°). A pedicle awl or gearshift helps make the tract within the pedicle. Palpation of the medial border of the pedicle can be used to assess the medial-lateral and cranial-caudal angulation of the pedicle. Conversely, the screw can be placed under live fluoroscopy. If a curved awl is used, it should be angled laterally for the first 15 mm to enter the body with the least risk of medial compromise. It should then be removed and a ball-tipped probe used to confirm the tract. The awl should then be reintroduced with the curvature aimed medially to enter the vertebral body. The tract is again palpated with the ball-tipped probe, and, upon confirmation, the tract is tapped. A 4.0-mm screw of appropriate length is placed bilaterally.

Lateral mass screws are then placed in the previously drilled tracts. We use 3.5-mm–diameter screws in the lateral masses with 4.0-mm screws available for rescue. Care must be taken in handling of all instrumentation because the spinal cord is now exposed. The wound is then irrigated with 1 to 2 L of saline solution. Plain radiographs or three-dimensional intraoperative imaging (if available) can then be obtained to confirm placement of hardware.

Fusion

Once all screws are in place, a high-speed burr is used to decorticate the facet joints and lateral aspects of the lateral masses to be fused bilaterally. Local bone from the laminectomy is used to achieve a biologic arthrodesis. Bone graft extenders such as demineralized bone matrix can be used, as can iliac crest bone graft, if the surgeon deems it necessary.

Closure

After all fusion, bone is packed into the appropriate areas, appropriately sized rods are placed into the screw heads, and end caps are placed and finally tightened (**Figure 5**). Meticulous hemostasis of the muscle should be obtained after removal of the retractors. A subfascial drain is placed. The muscle and fascia are closed in separate layers using a heavy interrupted absorbable suture (0 or 1). The subcutaneous tissue is closed with interrupted sutures of 2-0 absorbable material. The skin may be closed with subcuticular suture, skin staples, or both. It is our standard practice to use a topical skin adhesive over the final layer of suture.

Complications

Vascular Complications

Lateral mass screws can potentially injure the vertebral artery. This is most commonly seen with medial screw position because the foramen transversarium is located medial to the center of the lateral mass from C3 to C5. Thus, a lateral direction of screw placement is always recommended for lateral mass screws. In the review by Heller et al[6] of 654 lateral mass screws placed in 78 patients using a lateral trajectory, no vertebral artery injuries were reported. This is an exceedingly rare and reportable complication.

Neurologic Complications

Spinal cord injury is the most feared complication of cervical spine surgery. Fortunately, the likelihood of transient or permanent spinal cord injury is extremely low. The incidence of neurologic complications after cervical spine surgery is less than 1%, although the rate is slightly higher with posterior surgery than with an anterior approach. The greatest risk of injury to the spinal cord is most likely during removal of the laminae in the setting of severe cervical stenosis. We recommend elevating the patient's blood pressure in this setting to prevent an ischemic cord injury.

Nerve root palsies can occur postoperatively, most commonly within the first 3 postoperative days. A motor-dominant paralysis is most commonly seen and is most often unilateral. The fifth cervical nerve root is most frequently affected, followed by the sixth and seventh, but any root in the zone of decompression can be affected. Although the incidence of this complication varies, it is estimated to occur in 5% to 10% of patients. The mechanism of this complication is not understood, but theories of nerve root tethering due to posterior migration of the spinal cord as well as nerve root ischemia have been suggested. The prognosis is generally good. Treatment consists of observation and physical therapy, although some surgeons advocate early nerve root decompression. Prophylactic foraminotomies of the C5 root have not led to reliable prevention of C5 palsies.

Dural Injury

Hannallah et al[7] reported the prevalence of incidental durotomy during cervical spine surgery to be 1%. The authors found no difference in prevalence between anterior and posterior surgery. Because posterior durotomies tend to be more accessible than anterior ones, they should be repaired intraoperatively using suture or a patch and can be reinforced with fibrin glue. In repairs that are not watertight or in failed repairs, a lumbar subarachnoid drainage catheter should be used.

Postlaminectomy Kyphosis

Although cervical laminectomy is extremely effective in decompressing the neural elements, there is concern about the destabilizing nature of the procedure with resultant change in sagittal alignment of the cervical spine. The most concerning consequence of this is postlaminectomy cervical kyphosis, which results in sagittal plane imbalance, placing the spinal cord at risk. We therefore strongly recommend against laminectomy in the cervical spine without fusion. The treatment of postlaminectomy cervical kyphosis most commonly consists of anterior reconstruction followed by posterior stabilization.

Complications Associated With Lateral Mass Instrumentation

Complications associated with lateral mass instrumentation include screw impingement on the nerve root, vertebral artery injury, screw loosening, screw cut-out, and rod fracture. The rate of complication with newer instrumentation is unknown; however, in plate-screw constructs, the rate of single-level radiculopathy was found to be less than 2%.[8] In our series of lateral mass instrumentation assessed with intraoperative three-dimensional fluoroscopy, no patients had postoperative complications related to hardware.[9]

Postoperative Care and Rehabilitation

Postoperatively, patients are placed in a hard cervical collar for 6 weeks. Overhead activity is restricted for the same period. If external skin sutures or staples are used, they are removed 2 weeks postoperatively.

Pearls

- Draping the fluoroscopy unit into the field can save time and help with accurate placement of instrumentation.
- Subperiosteal dissection and attention to meticulous hemostasis facilitates perfect visualization of bony anatomy for proper placement of hardware and safe completion of laminectomy.
- Frequent release of self-retaining retractors can prevent ischemic injury to the paraspinal musculature.
- Evoked potential monitoring can indicate if a neurologic injury has occurred and can also be helpful in preventing neurologic issues related to positioning.
- Drilling and tapping lateral mass screw holes before laminectomy can help minimize drilling over the exposed neural elements.
- A watertight closure of the muscle and fascial layers along with use of subfascial drains is vital to prevent postoperative seroma formation and wound complications.

References

1. Law MD Jr, Bernhardt M, White AA III: Evaluation and management of cervical spondylotic myelopathy. *Instr Course Lect* 1995;44:99-110.
2. Park Y, Riew KD, Cho W: The long-term results of anterior surgical reconstruction in patients with postlaminectomy cervical kyphosis. *Spine J* 2010;10(5):380-387.
3. An HS, Gordin R, Renner K: Anatomic considerations for plate-screw fixation of the cervical spine. *Spine (Phila Pa 1976)* 1991;16(10, suppl):S548-S551.
4. Seybold EA, Baker JA, Criscitiello AA, Ordway NR, Park CK, Connolly PJ: Characteristics of unicortical and bicortical lateral mass screws in the cervical spine. *Spine (Phila Pa 1976)* 1999;24(22):2397-2403.
5. McGirt MJ, Sutter EG, Xu R, et al: Biomechanical comparison of translaminar versus pedicle screws at T1 and T2 in long subaxial cervical constructs. *Neurosurgery* 2009;65(6, suppl):167-172.
6. Heller JG, Silcox DH III, Sutterlin CE III: Complications of posterior cervical plating. *Spine (Phila Pa 1976)* 1995;20(22):2442-2448.
7. Hannallah D, Lee J, Khan M, Donaldson WF, Kang JD: Cerebrospinal fluid leaks following cervical spine surgery. *J Bone Joint Surg Am* 2008;90(5):1101-1105.
8. Deen HG, Birch BD, Wharen RE, Reimer R: Lateral mass screw-rod fixation of the cervical spine: A prospective clinical series with 1-year follow-up. *Spine J* 2003;3(6):489-495.
9. Hecht AC, Koehler SM, Laudone JC, Jenkins A, Qureshi S: Is intraoperative CT of posterior cervical spine instrumentation cost-effective and does it reduce complications? *Clin Orthop Relat Res* 2011;469(4):1035-1041.

Chapter 90
Cervical Laminoplasty

Nikhil A. Thakur, MD   Brett A. Freedman, MD   John G. Heller, MD

Patient Selection
Indications
Laminoplasty rapidly gained popularity in Japan for the treatment of cervical myelopathy due to ossification of the posterior longitudinal ligament (OPLL) and multilevel cervical spondylosis. That these innovations might originate in Japan stands to reason, given the high rates of OPLL and congenital cervical stenosis in that population.

Today, indications for laminoplasty have expanded to some degree. Laminoplasty remains the mainstay for treating cervical myelopathy due to OPLL and multilevel spondylosis involving three or more motion segments (**Figure 1**). Other indications include spinal cord decompression to salvage a failed anterior cervical decompression and fusion (ACDF) procedure, recurrent myelopathy due to adjacent segment disease after ACDF, and as a primary treatment of myelopathy in patients at increased risk for nonunions (eg, smokers and patients with metabolic bone disease). Laminoplasty is particularly well indicated in patients with developmentally narrow spinal canals (midbody AP diameter <12 mm) because spinal canal expansion directly treats the underlying primary pathology. This use should be particularly appealing because 50% of patients undergoing ACDF for cervical spondylotic myelopathy have relative (<13 mm) or absolute (<10 mm) developmental spinal canal stenosis.

Contraindications
Laminoplasty is relatively contraindicated in the following situations: (1) epidural fibrosis (eg, following infection or previous posterior spinal surgery), (2) large "hill-shaped" lesions of OPLL[1] that occupy more than 50% to 60% of the AP canal diameter, (3) axial neck pain as the patient's primary clinical symptom, and (4) fixed kyphosis (5° to 13°). Additional potential reasons to select an alternative procedure include morbid obesity and diabetes mellitus, which can result in a two- to eightfold increase in surgical-site infections, particularly with a posterior cervical approach. In addition, there are technical challenges related to positioning morbidly obese patients on the operating table and surgical exposure.

With regard to the overall alignment of the cervical spine, lordotic or straight spines have been reported to have statistically significantly higher functional recovery outcomes than kyphotic or sigmoid-shaped curves after laminoplasty.[2] Suda et al[2] recommended patients whose cervical spines range from lordotic to 13° or less of kyphosis as ideal candidates for laminoplasty if there is no cord signal change on the T2-weighted MRI. If there is cord signal hyperintensity on the T2-weighted MRI, then the upper limit of acceptable preoperative kyphosis is 5° or less. The presence of a lordotic alignment is not a prerequisite for performing a laminoplasty. This myth is born of misinterpretation of the literature over the years, which seems to have taken on a life of its own.

Types of Laminoplasty
The two major schools of laminoplasty derive from the Hirabayashi "open door" procedure and Kurokawa's "French door" technique. Other subsequently described techniques are variations on these themes. These techniques are illustrated in **Figure 2**. Most differ in how the surgeon secures the laminae in their new position or in how the exposure is made. Initially, hinges were either tethered open with suture or wire or propped open with bone grafts or other spacers, such as ceramic or polyethylene blocks. Recent innovations have adapted plates and screws to securely fix the laminae in place.

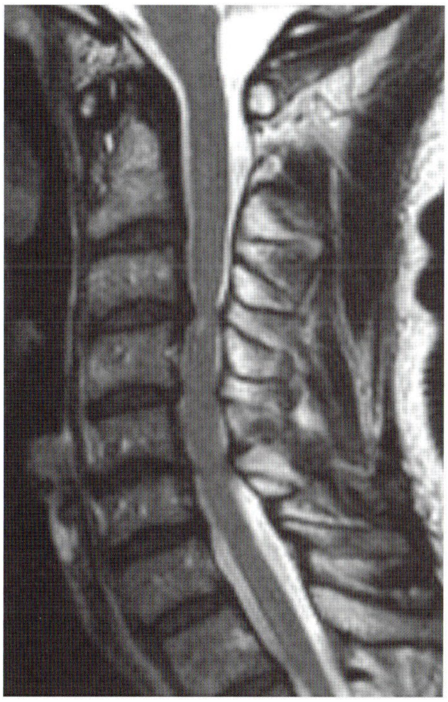

Figure 1 T2-weighted sagittal MRI demonstrates multilevel cervical stenosis secondary to spondylosis.

Preoperative Imaging
The preoperative diagnostic imaging workup should consist of plain radiographs of the cervical spine, including AP and neutral lateral radiographs (**Figure 3**). Flexion-extension views have been shown in some studies to be useful in determining the presence of instability, such as spondylolisthesis. Sakai et al[3] showed that the presence of a posterior spondylolisthesis resulted in significantly lower Japanese Orthopaedic Association recovery rates compared with anterior spondylolisthesis or no spondylolisthesis (which had equivalent outcomes).

The K-line (kyphosis line) concept was introduced by Fujiyoshi et al[4] as a tool to determine if laminoplasty could be used successfully in patients with OPLL. This tool can also be extended to address large ventral lesions or fixed kyphoses, which

---

Dr. Freedman or an immediate family member has received nonincome support (such as equipment or services), commercially derived honoraria, or other non–research-related funding (such as paid travel) from Medtronic. Dr. Heller or an immediate family member has received royalties from Medtronic; is a member of a speakers' bureau or has made paid presentations on behalf of Medtronic; serves as a paid consultant to or is an employee of Medtronic; has stock or stock options held in Medtronic; and serves as a board member, owner, officer, or committee member of the Cervical Spine Research Society. Neither Dr. Thakur nor any immediate family member has received anything of value from or has stock or stock options held in a commercial company or institution related directly or indirectly to the subject of this chapter.

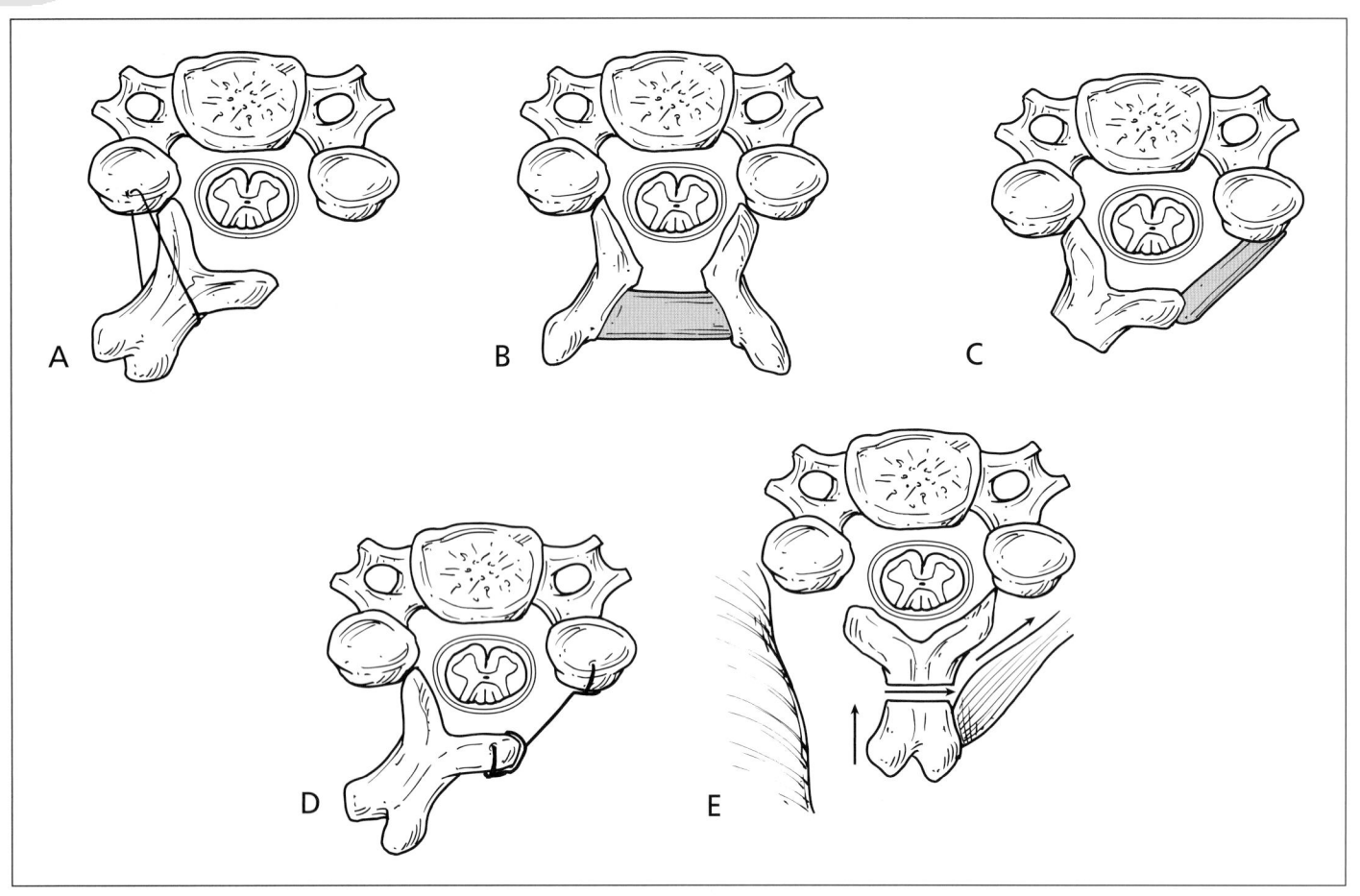

Figure 2 Illustrations depict common techniques used for cervical laminoplasty. **A,** Single-door laminoplasty. Sutures are placed through the spinous process to the articular capsule on the hinge side to hold the lamina elevated. **B,** Double-door laminoplasty. The spinous process is osteotomized in the midline and the two halves are pried open on laterally based hinges. Structural bone graft or a spacer fills the defect between the split spinous processes and prevents closure of the laminoplasty doors. **C,** Single-door laminoplasty with use of bone graft or a spacer to prop the door open. **D,** Single-door laminoplasty with use of a laminoplasty plate. **E,** Unilateral muscle-stripping approach; this approach is used to maintain the integrity of soft tissues on the contralateral side. The laminae on one side are exposed, with preservation of the nuchal, supraspinous, and interspinous ligaments. The spinous processes are osteotomized at their bases and are reflected to the intact side, allowing exposure of the posterior laminar bone. The arrows indicate the plane of the osteotomy and exposure.

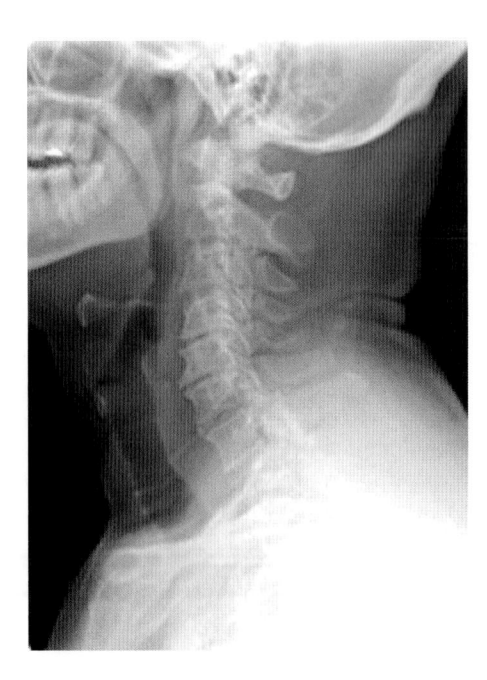

Figure 3 Neutral lateral radiograph of the cervical spine demonstrates multilevel cervical spondylosis/spondylolisthesis.

are often contraindications to laminoplasty. The K-line was defined as the line connecting the midpoints of the spinal canal at C2 and C7 on a lateral cervical radiograph.[4] A positive (+) K-line did not have an OPLL lesion crossing it, whereas a negative (−) K-line was present when the pathology extended dorsally beyond the line (**Figure 4**). In the (+) K-line group, the average neurologic recovery rate following laminoplasty was 66%, compared with 19% in the (−) K-line group.

An MRI study is useful in preoperative planning to determine which levels need to be included in the laminoplasty. Moreover, MRI allows the surgeon to determine if a C2 dome laminectomy should be included with the laminoplasty technique. Factors such as hypertrophied flavum, congenital stenosis, and cervical spine lateral architecture can result in impingement of the cord at the C2 level after laminoplasty due to cord drift-back and cause postoperative myelopathy.

The use of a CT study or a CT myelogram study is surgeon- and patient-specific. A CT scan gives the surgeon a more precise appreciation of the bone anatomy, including the presence of OPLL (**Figure 5**), ossified ligamentum flavum, or foraminal stenosis with osteophyte formation. Foraminal stenosis detected on CT and correlated with physical examination can be addressed during the surgical procedure, with a foraminotomy on the affected side. Myelography enhances structural detail, including details of patterns of compression and thickness and shape of lamina. At times, it is indicated when the MRI leaves some doubt as to the nature and extent of the pathology. A CT scan also helps determine the "occupation ratio" for a large ventral lesion (AP diameter of the lesion/AP diameter of the canal × 100). An occupation ratio of more than 50% to 60% is often considered a relative contraindication to laminoplasty. These additional anatomic details can

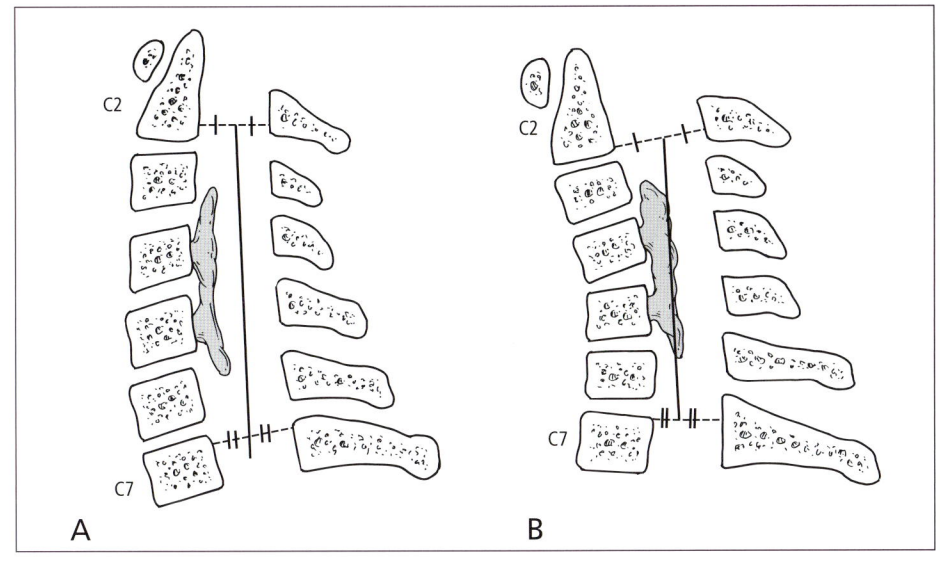

Figure 4 Illustration of the K-line concept. A positive (+) K-line (**A**) occurs when the compressive pathology ossification of the posterior longitudinal ligament remains ventral to the line. A negative (−) K-line (**B**) is defined by the pathology extending dorsally to or across the line.

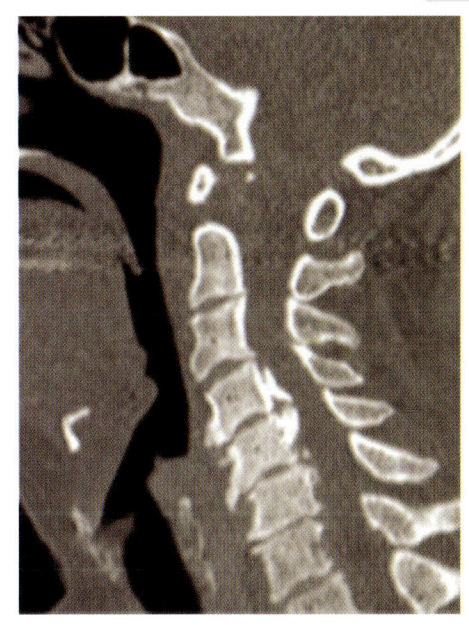

Figure 5 CT scan shows focal ossification of the posterior longitudinal ligament.

provide important tactical information to be used intraoperatively.

Procedure

Room Setup/Patient Positioning

Laminoplasty is performed with the patient in the prone position. We recommend that the patient's comfortable range of motion be assessed preoperatively so that the patient can be positioned in some flexion during surgery. The advantages to this include the following: (1) cervical extension may result in worsening of canal stenosis and cord compression, and (2) the procedure is technically easier because the overlap or "shingling" of the laminae is reduced (**Figure 6**). This also helps with the excessive skin folds present in some patients.

A Mayfield three-pin head holder is used to immobilize the cervical spine, as well as to protect the face and eyes. Longitudinal bolsters are placed on the lateral border of the chest to take pressure off the central chest and abdomen. Knees and ankles are flexed to reduce lower extremity neural tension. We do not routinely tape the shoulders. However, tape may be used to shift the redundant soft tissues when needed in obese patients. A reverse Trendelenburg position is used to decrease venous pressure, thereby decreasing intraoperative blood loss.

Special Instruments/Equipment/Implants

Monitoring of somatosensory-evoked potentials (SSEPs) is generally recommended during laminoplasty procedures for myelopathy. In our opinion, the routine use of motor-evoked potentials (MEPs) is open to discussion. We tend to recommend monitoring electromyograms when foraminotomies are added to the surgical plan. Neuromonitoring may also serve to identify potentially significant episodes of hypotension or decreases in spinal cord perfusion. In both of these circumstances, early detection of a potential problem allows for rapid intervention and neurologic protection. Moreover, we prefer to use an arterial catheter for continuous monitoring of the mean arterial pressure, which is kept at a suitable level by whatever means necessary.

Roh et al[5] reported the largest series of patients undergoing cervical spine procedures with SSEP monitoring. They found that degradation of SSEPs from baseline was seen in 17 (2.1%) of 809 patients, which prompted intervention with prevention of neurologic sequelae in 15 of these 17 patients (88%). The authors noted that monitoring may also help identify brachial plexopathies associated with positioning (eg, taping down the shoulders), particularly in obese individuals.[5]

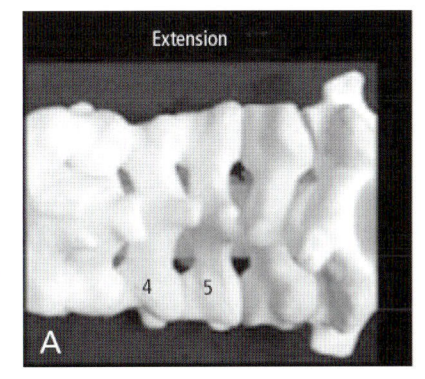

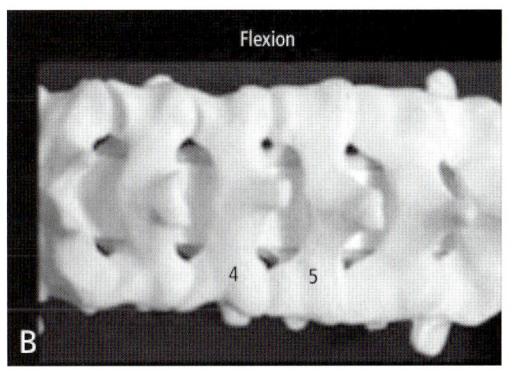

Figure 6 Posterior view of cervical spine model shows shingling of laminae in extension (**A**) versus flexion (**B**). (Courtesy of John Rhee, MD, Atlanta, GA.)

The use of MEPs has been shown to be beneficial in cervical spine surgery as an adjunct to SSEPs. A recent article demonstrated that MEPs were more sensitive to changes associated with cervical myelopathy than SSEPs during intraoperative monitoring[6] and can be useful during laminoplasty. However, they are more susceptible to technical issues, and the lack of neuromuscular blockade required by MEPs creates its own set of safety issues for patients.

Surgical Technique

We prefer an open-door laminoplasty technique, as originally described by Hirabayashi. Because only two troughs are required, it is a bit more time-efficient than a French-door procedure. However,

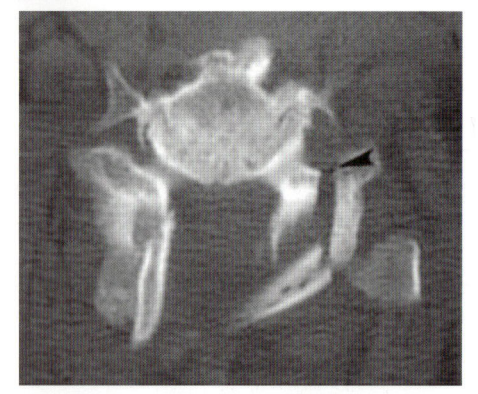

Figure 7 Axial CT scan of the cervical spine shows the lateral laminoplasty trough (arrowhead) violating the facet and extending into the transversarium foramen.

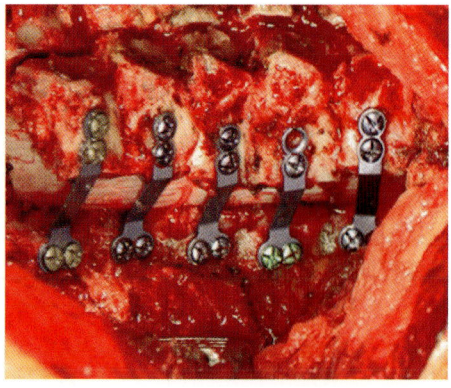

Figure 8 Intraoperative photograph shows an open-door laminoplasty from C3-C7, fixed rigidly with segmental plate fixation.

the open-door laminoplasty can be associated with more lateral epidural bleeding than the French-door procedure. In addition, it is easier to perform supplemental foraminotomies on the open side of a Hirabayashi-style operation than it is to do so with French-door procedures.

Intraoperatively, the hinge and open side troughs are made at the lamina–lateral mass junction. Often, this corresponds to an inflection point where the two structures merge. However, the landmarks may either be indistinct or obscured by facet arthrosis. Correlation with a preoperative CT scan can be quite helpful. The troughs are created using a high-speed burr with the surgeon's tip of choice. The depth of the trough, which need not be any more than approximately 4 mm, should also be assessed frequently during preparation. If the surgeon goes too lateral and deep, there is a potential risk of damage to the vertebral artery (**Figure 7**). Excessive removal of bone medially can result in an inadequate decompression.

The open-side trough should be made first. It is important to exercise caution with the burr until the ligamentum flavum is visualized at the inferior half of the lamina. The remaining cranial opening can be completed either with a burr or with the curet and a Kerrison rongeur. We recommend a 3-mm round diamond burr for this last step, unless the surgeon is highly experienced with more aggressive tips. Bipolar cautery should be used to coagulate and divide the plexus of veins as the laminoplasty is opened. These veins arborize dorsally from the longitudinal veins that course over the nerve roots in the lateral spinal canal. The surgeon should try to coagulate them a few millimeters dorsal to their branch point because they are easier to control if a short stump of the vein remains on the longitudinal vein.

On the hinge side of the laminoplasty, the placement of the trough is the same. The burr should be used to remove the dorsal cortical bone and the underlying cancellous bone. The inner cortical layer is thinned until a stiff hinge is fashioned. Excessive bone removal will result in a floppy hinge, which may displace into the canal and cause either root or cord impingement.

We use a laminoplasty plate to rigidly fix the laminae in their open position (**Figure 8**). It is not necessary to employ additional bone grafts with these plates. Doing so adds technical difficulty and expense without clinical benefit. In a study looking at plate-only laminoplasty in 54 patients, Rhee and Basra[7] reported a 93% hinge healing rate at 1 year, with no loss of fixation or premature closure in any patient. No revision surgery was required in any patient, and canal expansion was maintained in the unhealed group (4 patients, 7%) as well.

Complications

Infection
Wound infections with laminoplasty are reported to be around 3% to 4%, which is similar to other posterior cervical procedures. Perioperative antibiotics and good surgical technique, including watertight fascial closure, can minimize infection rates. The addition of a separate drain for a thick subcutaneous layer can also be beneficial.

Neck Pain
Historically, postoperative axial neck pain has been reported to occur in up to 40% of patients at 10-year follow-up.[8] The sources for axial neck pain have been thought to include facet joint injury, deep extensor muscle denervation, detachment of C2 and/or C7 muscles, detachment of the nuchal ligament, and prolonged postoperative external immobilization.[9]

In the past few years, several studies have looked at maintaining muscle and nuchal ligament insertions on C2 and C7. Hosono et al[10] reported significantly improved axial pain in the postoperative period among patients who underwent a C3-C6 laminoplasty versus the traditional C3-C7 laminoplasty. The C3-C6 group reported a 5.4% incidence of axial neck pain compared with 29% of patients who were symptomatic after C3-C7 laminoplasty ($P = 0.015$). Given that both groups had equivalent neurologic improvements, the inclusion of the C7 level in a posterior laminoplasty ought to be avoided when possible. Sakaura et al[11] also reported a 3.2% rate of axial neck pain in a 5-year prospective follow-up of patients who had a C3-C6 laminoplasty but no significant difference in neck pain when detaching the muscle insertions at C3-C6 versus maintaining these insertions. Others have found that early active range of motion after surgery may play as important a role as any other measures in reducing pain and stiffness.

Postoperative Kyphosis and Loss of Motion
The incidence of postoperative kyphosis is lower than reported with a laminectomy and ranges from 0% to 22% in the literature. In the uncommon event of significant postoperative kyphosis developing, poor neurologic recovery and late neurologic deterioration can manifest in patients.[12] One possible etiology for the loss of lordosis and subsequent kyphosis is attributed to the detachment of the semispinalis cervicis from its insertion at C2.[13] Sakaura et al[14] found that by preserving C2 and C7 muscle attachments, lordosis was equally maintained in patients with or without C3-C6 muscle detachment. Maeda et al[15] demonstrated that postoperative kyphotic deformity occurred in stiffer spines, whereas lordosis was maintained in flexible cervical spines after laminoplasty. Maeda et al[15] concluded that maintaining range of motion postoperatively prevented stiffness and subsequent kyphotic deformity and recommended using a soft collar for only 1 week after surgery. We share this observation.

Hence, the data suggest that when possible, preserving muscle attachments to the C2 and the C7 laminae may play a role in reducing axial pain and preventing the development of postoperative kyphosis. We routinely do not use any cervical orthoses in the postoperative management of these patients. All of our patients are encouraged to pursue unrestricted active range of motion as soon as tolerated and also start isotonic exercises 6 weeks postoperatively.

Laminar Closure: Restenosis

Laminar closure has been reported with a wide variety of laminoplasty techniques. Matsumoto et al[16] reported a 34% lamina reclosure rate when using early active range of motion after the traditional Hirabayashi suture method to perform the laminoplasty. However, Matsumoto et al[16] observed no significant changes in outcomes in short-term follow-up. In a 5-year follow-up of the same cohort, Matsumoto et al[17] reported that, although not statistically significant, the recovery rates tended to decline in the closure group compared with the nonclosure group. Matsumoto et al[17] recommended considering the use of more rigid laminar fixation methods, such as plates and screws, to prevent laminar closure.

Motor Root Palsy

The incidence of motor root palsies after laminoplasty has been reported to be 5% to 12%, with the C5 nerve root being most commonly involved. Although the issue of motor root palsy was brought to light within the laminoplasty literature, such nerve root events are not unique to this operation. This complication has been reported to occur in similar frequency with other cervical myelopathy procedures, including laminectomy, laminectomy and fusion, and ACDF.[7] This calls into question whether the issue is a by-product of the treatment or the disease itself.

Several theories have been proposed for this complication. The C5 nerve root is thought to be most susceptible because it typically exits at the apex of a lordotic curve and often has a short course that makes it vulnerable during excessive posterior cord migration. However, posterior cord migration cannot explain why this also occurs with anterior decompression operations. Other potential causes include reperfusion injury, C4-C5 neuroforaminal stenosis, and C3-C4 central stenosis.

In a review of 630 patients who underwent anterior or posterior based cervical procedures, 42 patients (6.7%) reported a postoperative C5 palsy.[18] Of these patients, the incidence was highest for laminectomy and fusion (9.5%), followed by corpectomy with posterior fusion (8.4%), corpectomy only (5.1%), and laminoplasty (4.8%). These findings certainly bring into question the theory of excessive cord drift-back with a short course for the C5 nerve root.

Clinically, patients most often exhibit weakness of the deltoid and biceps muscles. A minority can experience sensory dysfunction and radicular symptoms. Nonetheless, it is generally a painless onset of weakness. These signs and symptoms generally manifest 2 to 3 days after surgery, but they can appear at any time from immediately after surgery to 2 months postoperatively. Nassr et al[18] reported the time to maximum recovery ranging from 1 week to 2 years, with a mean time of 21 weeks. Residual motor deficits were lowest in the laminoplasty group (0%) and highest in the laminectomy and fusion group (27.3%).

Postoperative Care and Rehabilitation

Postoperative care consists of typical postoperative surgical wound management. We do not recommend any brace or collar wear because it impedes early active range of motion, which is strongly encouraged. Prolonged immobilization of any sort risks increased axial pain, loss of range of motion, and possible kyphosis. Active neck and shoulder conditioning begins with isotonic exercises 6 weeks after surgery. In the interim, patients are encouraged to engage in daily nonimpact aerobic conditioning, such as walking or stationary cycling. The latter is more practical for those with significant preoperative gait problems.

Follow-up consists of a clinical assessment with static radiographs at 6 weeks. Isotonic exercises are initiated at that time and progressed as tolerated. Lateral flexion-extension radiographs are obtained at 3-month intervals thereafter until the patient has reached maximal neurologic improvement, which is to be expected by about 1 year after surgery. As demonstrated by Rhee and Basra,[7] hinges are fairly reliably healed by 6 months. Thereafter, provided there are no instability patterns on the dynamic radiographs, patients are free to engage in any activities, including most sports.

Pearls

- Cervical lordotic alignment is not a prerequisite to laminoplasty.
- The K-line concept is a useful tool in selecting patients. A (+) K-line correlates with a significantly higher neurologic recovery rate.
- Neuromonitoring can help identify intraoperative neurologic changes. Electromyograms are often used when foraminotomies are also being performed.
- The surgeon should preserve as much of the muscle insertion at C2 as possible and avoid including C7, if this does not compromise the degree of spinal cord decompression.
- We recommend using plates to keep the lamina open, without using graft.
- Immediate active range of motion without the use of collars is important in preventing postoperative axial pain, stiffness, and kyphosis.

References

1. Iwasaki M, Okuda S, Miyauchi A, et al: Surgical strategy for cervical myelopathy due to ossification of the posterior longitudinal ligament: Part 1. Clinical results and limitations of laminoplasty. *Spine (Phila Pa 1976)* 2007;32(6):647-653.

2. Suda K, Abumi K, Ito M, Shono Y, Kaneda K, Fujiya M: Local kyphosis reduces surgical outcomes of expansive open-door laminoplasty for cervical spondylotic myelopathy. *Spine (Phila Pa 1976)* 2003;28(12):1258-1262.

3. Sakai Y, Matsuyama Y, Inoue K, Ishiguro N: Postoperative instability after laminoplasty for cervical myelopathy with spondylolisthesis. *J Spinal Disord Tech* 2005;18(1):1-5.

4. Fujiyoshi T, Yamazaki M, Kawabe J, et al: A new concept for making decisions regarding the surgical approach for cervical ossification of the posterior longitudinal ligament: The K-line. *Spine (Phila Pa 1976)* 2008;33(26):E990-E993.

5. Roh MS, Wilson-Holden TJ, Padberg AM, Park JB, Daniel Riew K: The utility of somatosensory evoked potential monitoring during cervical spine surgery: How often does it prompt intervention and affect outcome? *Asian Spine J* 2007;1(1):43-47.

6. Haghighi SS, Mundis G, Zhang R, Ramirez B: Correlation between transcranial motor and somatosensory-evoked potential findings in cervical myelopathy or radiculopathy during cervical spine surgery. *Neurol Res* 2011;33(9):893-898.

7. Rhee JM, Basra S: Posterior surgery for cervical myelopathy: Laminectomy, laminectomy with fusion, and laminoplasty. *Asian Spine J* 2008;2(2):114-126.

8. Wada E, Suzuki S, Kanazawa A, Matsuoka T, Miyamoto S, Yonenobu K: Subtotal corpectomy versus laminoplasty for mul-

tilevel cervical spondylotic myelopathy: A long-term follow-up study over 10 years. *Spine (Phila Pa 1976)* 2001;26(13):1443-1447, discussion 1448.

9. Hosono N, Sakaura H, Mukai Y, Yoshikawa H: The source of axial pain after cervical laminoplasty—C7 is more crucial than deep extensor muscles. *Spine (Phila Pa 1976)* 2007;32(26):2985-2988.

10. Hosono N, Sakaura H, Mukai Y, Fujii R, Yoshikawa H: C3-6 laminoplasty takes over C3-7 laminoplasty with significantly lower incidence of axial neck pain. *Eur Spine J* 2006;15(9):1375-1379.

11. Sakaura H, Hosono N, Mukai Y, Iwasaki M, Yoshikawa H: Medium-term outcomes of C3-6 laminoplasty for cervical myelopathy: A prospective study with a minimum 5-year follow-up. *Eur Spine J* 2011;20(6):928-933.

12. Liu G, Buchowski JM, Bunmaprasert T, Yeom JS, Shen H, Riew KD: Revision surgery following cervical laminoplasty: Etiology and treatment strategies. *Spine (Phila Pa 1976)* 2009;34(25):2760-2768.

13. Takeuchi K, Yokoyama T, Aburakawa S, Itabashi T, Toh S: Anatomic study of the semispinalis cervicis for reattachment during laminoplasty. *Clin Orthop Relat Res* 2005;436:126-131.

14. Sakaura H, Hosono N, Mukai Y, Fujimori T, Iwasaki M, Yoshikawa H: Preservation of muscles attached to the C2 and C7 spinous processes rather than subaxial deep extensors reduces adverse effects after cervical laminoplasty. *Spine (Phila Pa 1976)* 2010;35(16):E782-E786.

15. Maeda T, Arizono T, Saito T, Iwamoto Y: Cervical alignment, range of motion, and instability after cervical laminoplasty. *Clin Orthop Relat Res* 2002;401:132-138.

16. Matsumoto M, Watanabe K, Tsuji T, et al: Risk factors for closure of lamina after open-door laminoplasty. *J Neurosurg Spine* 2008;9(6):530-537.

17. Matsumoto M, Watanabe K, Hosogane N, et al: Impact of lamina closure on long-term outcomes of open-door laminoplasty in patients with cervical myelopathy: Minimum 5-year follow-up study. *Spine (Phila Pa 1976)* 2012;37(15):1288-1291.

18. Nassr A, Eck JC, Ponnappan RK, Zanoun RR, Donaldson WF III, Kang JD: The incidence of C5 palsy after multilevel cervical decompression procedures: A review of 750 consecutive cases. *Spine (Phila Pa 1976)* 2012;37(3):174-178.

Chapter 91
Placement of Thoracic Pedicle Screws

Kevin W. Wilson, MD   Ronald A. Lehman, Jr, MD   Lawrence G. Lenke, MD

Patient Selection
Indications

Thoracic pedicle screw fixation in spinal disorders has gained an increasingly larger acceptance because of its well-recognized advantages in achieving stable three-column fixation and improved control of three-dimensional deformities. Thoracic pedicle screw fixation is commonly and safely used for instrumented fusion constructs in the treatment of degenerative disorders, traumatic injuries, and deformities, but a thorough knowledge of the thoracic spine anatomy and surrounding structures is required.[1-4] Thoracic pedicle screws are indicated for the stabilization of spinal segments after neural decompression for fracture, tumor, or infection or after correction of kyphotic or scoliotic deformities.

Contraindications

Contraindications to elective pedicle screw fixation are similar to those for other instrumentation procedures of the spine. As with any surgical procedure involving implants, the patient should be free from signs and symptoms of infection. Metal allergies can be a consideration. The ability to place pedicle screws and salvage options should be considered when preoperative images are reviewed for severely deformed, hypoplastic, or absent pedicles at the level of the planned instrumentation. Relatively few contraindications exist to surgical stabilization of unstable thoracic spine trauma; however, medically unstable or underresuscitated patients should be stabilized before undergoing a prolonged procedure in the prone position with expected blood loss. Severe osteoporosis is a relative contraindication. Inadequate screw purchase as a result of low bone mineral density may be addressed with screw augmentation techniques, such as polymethylmethacrylate screw augmentation.[5]

Preoperative Imaging

Preoperative AP and lateral radiographs are imperative for surgical planning (Figure 1). CT can be obtained to evaluate the pedicle size and the anatomy of deformities. Pedicle dimensions can be evaluated on AP and lateral radiographs if the surgeon is mindful of the plane of the x-ray beam. The most accurate assessment of pedicles is made in the true frontal plane. Assessment of pedicles of rotated levels may be nearly impossible on plain radiographs. If, at any level, the pedicle size appears to be too small to accept a 5-mm screw, or the plain radiography examination is insufficient, CT may be used to provide accurate evaluation of the levels to be instrumented. It is our experience, however, that CT scans occasionally are fraught with inadequacies when used to estimate the true size of a pedicle. A detailed understanding of the three-dimensional anatomy of the vertebral body/pedicle is of the utmost importance. A thorough knowledge of the curve magnitude, length of fixation construct, and pedicle size will optimize surgical time. Pedicles in the midthoracic spine have the smallest width in patients of all ages, and the pedicles at the apices of the concavity of a scoliotic curve typically are smaller than those on the convex side. In one report of 30 patients with adolescent idiopathic scoliosis, thoracic pedicle size varied from 4.0 to 8.2 mm.[6] Typically, screws 80% to 115% of the size of the outer pedicle diameter can be inserted safely through gradual plastic deformation—a technique known as pediculoplasty—with a probe and bone tap. Pediatric pedicles possess greater inherent viscoelastic potential for pedicle expansion than do pedicles in adults.

Procedure
Room Setup/Patient Positioning

The patient is placed prone on a radiolucent four-poster frame or OSI table (Orthopedic Systems) with a spine top, which consists of an open-frame design with

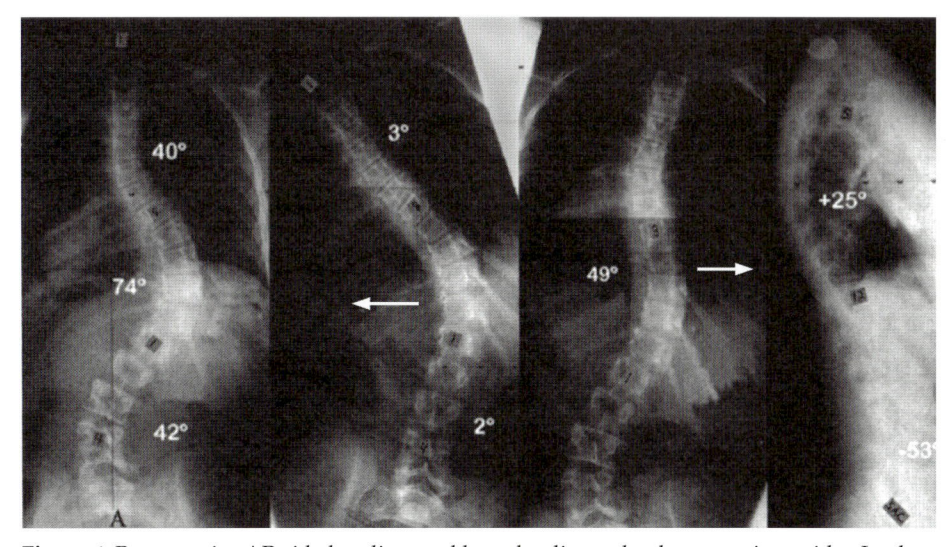

Figure 1 Preoperative AP, side-bending, and lateral radiographs show a patient with a Lenke type 1AN curve with only 34% side-bending flexibility. (Adapted with permission from Lehman RA, Lenke LG, Keeler KA, et al: Operative treatment of adolescent idiopathic scoliosis with posterior pedicle screw-only constructs: Minimum three-year follow-up of one hundred fourteen cases. *Spine [Phila Pa 1976]* 2008;33[4]:1598-1604.)

Dr. Lehman or an immediate family member serves as a board member, owner, officer, or committee member of the American Academy of Orthopaedic Surgeons, the North American Spine Society, the Cervical Spine Research Society, and the Scoliosis Research Society. Dr. Lenke or an immediate family member has received royalties from Medtronic; has received research or institutional support from DePuy and Axial Biotech; and serves as a board member, owner, officer, or committee member of the Scoliosis Research Society. Neither Dr. Wilson nor any immediate family member has received anything of value from or has stock or stock options held in a commercial company or institution related directly or indirectly to the subject of this chapter.

Section 7: Spine

positioning pads to support the prone patient, to facilitate intraoperative imaging, maintain adequate sagittal alignment, and minimize pressure on the anterior thorax or abdomen. During prone positioning, it is important to ensure that the patient is moved down toward the foot of the operating table as much as possible. This allows the arm boards to be positioned as close to the head of the operating table as possible; otherwise, the surgeon has difficulty standing while gaining access to place the screws in the proximal thoracic spine. We typically place the legs in a sling to promote systemic venous return. Hyperkyphosis of the proximal thoracic segments can make it difficult to gain the correct sagittal trajectory when placing screws in the proximal thoracic spine. Additionally, the skull and paraspinal muscles in the lateral aspect of the wound can interfere with probe trajectory, which is convergent in the upper thoracic spine. Halo skull traction can be considered, if necessary, to facilitate flexing the patient's neck to reduce the kyphotic angle for easier screw placement (**Figure 2**).

Neuromonitoring, including somatosensory-evoked potentials and motor-evoked potentials, should be used to monitor the spinal cord during screw insertion and correction maneuvers. Real-time spontaneous electromyography (EMG) monitoring of thoracic nerve roots T6 through T12 through the rectus abdominis musculature adds a layer of safety, and triggered EMG can be used to confirm screw placement.

Special Instruments/Equipment/Implants

Fluoroscopic and computer-generated image–guided techniques have been developed to improve pedicle screw placement accuracy[7]; however, their use typically requires additional resources and may require longer surgery time, theoretically increasing blood loss and the opportunity for infection. In time, advancements in technology may improve placement accuracy and patient outcomes, but details of these techniques are beyond the scope of this chapter. The foundations of pedicle screw placement are understanding the anatomy and developing the skill and tactile sense to navigate pedicle tracts, which can be done with techniques and instruments available to most spine surgeons. Freehand insertion of screws, without the use of intraoperative radiographic guidance or tracking, appears to be safe and reliable and is described in this chapter.[8] The thoracic gearshift probe and flexible ball-tipped pedicle-sounding device are critical components of the pedicle screw instrumentation set.

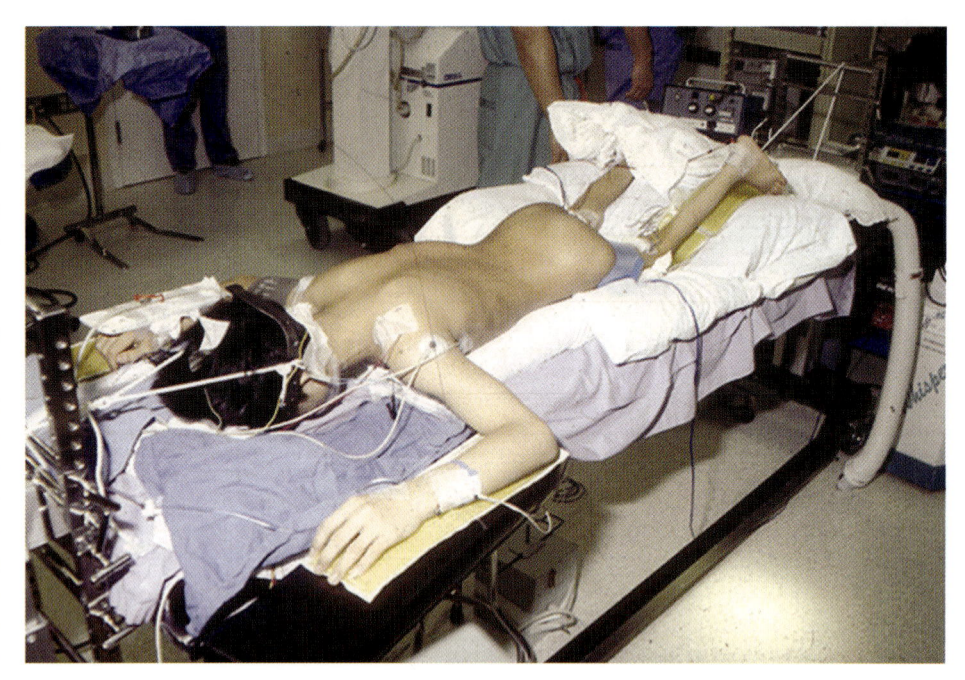

Figure 2 Photograph depicts a halo skull traction setup with the patient on the spine table.

For pediatric and adult deformity cases, it is important to have a variety of screw sizes available, as dictated by preoperative planning. In the immature spine, the pedicle widths are smaller and increase with age. A significant decrease is seen in the width of the concave pedicles compared with the convex side in patients with thoracic scoliosis. The instrumentation sets should contain pedicle screws ranging in diameter from 4 to 7 mm, in 0.5-mm increments. Lengths should range from 25 mm for small-diameter screws to 55 mm for large-diameter screws. Monoaxial screw heads have a lower profile, which is conducive to the superficial thoracic spine and allows better manipulation of the spine during derotation maneuvers. Additionally, these screws are less expensive than their multiaxial counterparts. Polyaxial screws may be helpful for rod placement after curve correction because their ability to vary the angle of the screw head allows better seating of the rod to the screw. More recently, uniaxial screws have become available; these screws combine the benefits of the monoaxial and multiaxial screw heads. They are locked in the axial plane to allow for vertebral column derotation but permit variance in the cephalocaudad direction, resulting in easier seating of the rod.

Surgical Technique
Incision and Exposure

The extent of the skin incision is marked, from the highest planned instrumented vertebra to the lowest. The incision should be a straight, vertical line connecting these two points to ensure a straight incision after the scoliosis is corrected. For short-segment procedures, levels should be confirmed using surface anatomy landmarks with fluoroscopic confirmation. In deformity or scoliosis procedures, the neutral vertebrae are selected carefully at both ends of the curve. Exposure typically involves an incision from the spinous process above the most cranial vertebra to the spinous process of the most caudal vertebra in the segment to be instrumented. For an expeditious approach, the anesthesia team should paralyze the patient pharmacologically to facilitate exposure of the soft tissues. Muscle paralysis allows for better retraction of the paraspinal muscles during dissection and reduces muscle contraction during unipolar cautery, thereby reducing blood loss. Additionally, pharmacologically induced hypotension further aids in reducing blood loss. The anesthesiologist should be reminded to reverse the paralysis before instrumentation, to avoid its interfering with electrophysiologic monitoring.

The surgeon carries the dissection along the midline and carefully dissects subperiosteally laterally to the tips of the transverse processes (**Figure 3**). Meticulous exposure of the posterior elements is

Chapter 91: Placement of Thoracic Pedicle Screws

required to place thoracic pedicle screws successfully. In an immature spine, the dorsal spinous process epiphysis can be bluntly scraped away to provide an obvious periosteal edge. The posterior elements are exposed by staying strictly subperiosteal to reduce bleeding. Bovie electrocautery is used as the periosteum is scraped laterally to the tips of the transverse processes, bilaterally. Next, a wide facetectomy is performed. The facetectomy facilitates access for the starting point, allows for facet fusion, provides local bone graft via the resected facet to facilitate fusion, and allows the spine to become more flexible to facilitate better correction. Using an osteotome, the inferior 3 to 5 mm of the inferior facet is removed, and the exposed cartilage is scraped from the top of the superior facet surface to enhance the fusion bed for intra-articular arthrodesis.

Starting Point and Trajectory

A good starting level is the most neutrally rotated and most distal instrumented vertebra. By working in successive levels from caudal to cephalad in the thoracic spine, with an appreciation for the general trends of the starting points, fine adjustments may be made to the trajectory of each screw based on the screw position of the previous level or contralateral pedicle. The starting points can be grouped according to their location (**Figure 4**). The T1 through T3 and T12 starting points are at the midpoint of the transverse process in the vertical direction and 2 mm lateral to the midpoint of the facet. This is known as the superior facet rule (**Figure 5**). The starting points for T4, T5, and T11 lie at the proximal third of the transverse process and 2 mm lateral to the midpoint of the facet. The T6 and T10 starting points lie along the ridge, or confluence, of the cephalad aspect of the lamina, whereas the vertical starting points of T7 through T9 lie at the junction of the facet and lamina.

In our own surgical experience, we have noted a reliable and unique anatomic structure known as the ventral lamina. The ventral lamina is formed by the roof of the spinal canal that becomes confluent laterally with the medial aspect of the pedicle wall (**Figure 6**). An increased understanding of its three-dimensional structure and relationships has improved our ability to place screws safely in pedicles previously thought impossible, or too difficult, to instrument. A consistent anatomic relationship exists between the

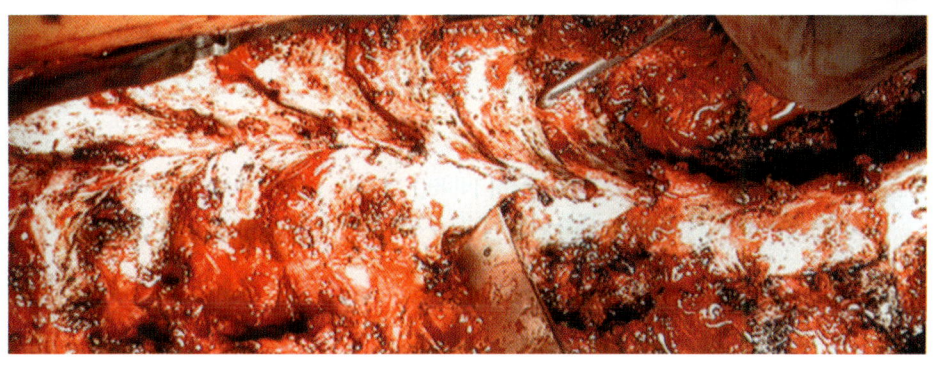

Figure 3 Intraoperative photograph shows the posterior elements of the spine exposed to the edge of the transverse processes bilaterally. The inferior facets are removed with a 0.5-in straight osteotome (down to T10) or rongeur (below T10). Articular cartilage is removed from the dorsal side of the superior facet of the inferior vertebra using a small curet. (Reproduced with permission from Kim YJ, Lenke LG, Bridwell KH, Cho YS, Riew KD: Free hand pedicle screw placement in the thoracic spine: Is it safe? *Spine [Phila Pa 1976]* 2004;29[3]:333-342.)

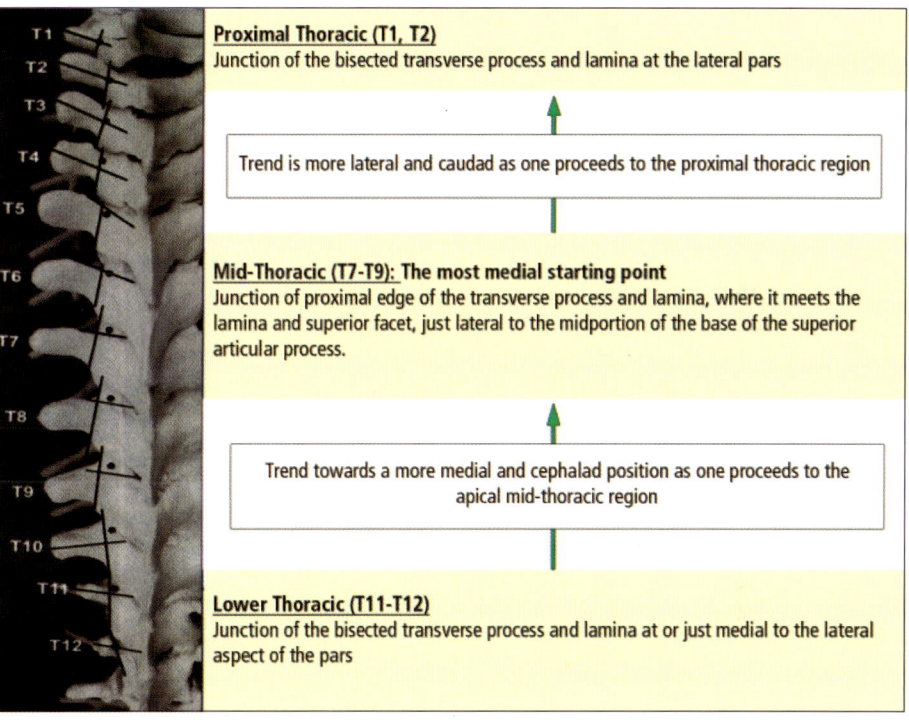

Proximal Thoracic (T1, T2)
Junction of the bisected transverse process and lamina at the lateral pars

Trend is more lateral and caudad as one proceeds to the proximal thoracic region

Mid-Thoracic (T7-T9): The most medial starting point
Junction of proximal edge of the transverse process and lamina, where it meets the lamina and superior facet, just lateral to the midportion of the base of the superior articular process.

Trend towards a more medial and cephalad position as one proceeds to the apical mid-thoracic region

Lower Thoracic (T11-T12)
Junction of the bisected transverse process and lamina at or just medial to the lateral aspect of the pars

Figure 4 Illustration shows pedicle screw starting points using a 3.5-mm acorn-tipped burr. The posterior elements are burred to create a posterior cortical breach approximately 5 mm in depth. (Adapted with permission from Kim YJ, Lenke LG, Bridwell KH, Cho YS, Riew KD: Free hand pedicle screw placement in the thoracic spine: Is it safe? *Spine [Phila Pa 1976]* 2004;29[3]:333-342.)

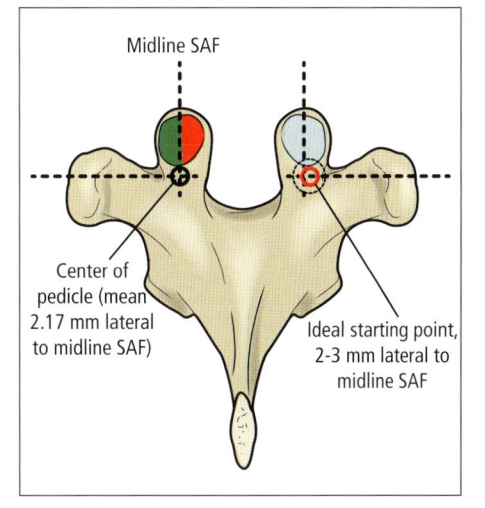

Figure 5 Illustration of the posterior view of the vertebra depicts the ideal starting point for a thoracic pedicle screw as determined using the superior facet rule, according to which the screw should not start medial to the midpoint of the superior articular facet (SAF). The medial aspect of the facet is shown in red. In the diagram, the midline of the SAF is marked by the vertical dashed line. The red circle demarcates the ideal starting point. The dotted circle depicts the outline of the pedicle. According to the superior facet rule, the optimal starting point should be 2 to 3 mm lateral to the SAF midline, allowing placement of the screw in the center of the pedicle and avoiding penetration of the canal.

© 2013 American Academy of Orthopaedic Surgeons

ventral lamina and the superior articular facet (SAF) at all thoracic levels, except at T12 because of its transitional nature. The ventral lamina can be used as a reliable guide for the starting point in pedicle screw placement. Taking advantage of the fact that the medial cortical wall is thicker than the lateral wall and that the ventral lamina consistently is medial to the midpoint of the SAF, the medial cortical wall can be used as a guide for the path of the pedicle screw while avoiding the feared medial cortical breach. We recommend that the starting point for the placement of pedicle screws be 2 to 3 mm lateral to the midpoint of the SAF.

After the starting point is identified, a dorsal cortical pilot hole is made with a high-speed burr. The intrapedicular cancellous bone may provide a pedicle blush, signaling the entrance at the base of the pedicle, although smaller pedicles may not blush because of limited cancellous bone.

Lehman et al[9] described the anatomic and straight-forward approaches to screw trajectory (**Figure 7** and 8). For the anatomic trajectory, the screw pathway follows the anatomic axis of the pedicle, which is angled 15° to 22° caudad in the sagittal plane. The straight-forward approach uses the sagittal trajectory that parallels the superior end plate of the vertebral body. A 39% increase in maximum insertional torque and a 27% increase in pullout strength have been demonstrated with the straight-forward approach; therefore, it is recommended for most patients.[9] The anatomic approach should be reserved for salvage purposes.

It is important to understand vertebral level and curve-specific anatomic differences. Idiopathic scoliosis is associated with distinctive intervertebral deformity. The convexity of the curve tends to allow a more reliable and safe placement of pedicle screws with a relatively larger pedicle diameter and a wider epidural space. The pedicles on the concave side, however, often are shorter, dysplastic, and more sclerotic, and are located near the spinal cord. The width of the epidural space is less than 1 mm at the thoracic apical vertebral levels on the concave side but is between 3 and 5 mm on the convex side.[10] This makes anatomic sense, because the spinal cord is "draped" over the concavity of the curve.

Taking time to appreciate the rotation and pedicle orientation is critical to orienting the probe correctly. It is important to realize that the anatomic orientation of the pedicles in relation to each vertebral body does not change, but rotation between levels changes drastically. The apical concave pedicles of severe curves may require the plane of orientation and hand position to be almost parallel to the floor.

Gearshift Probing

The thoracic gearshift probe is used to find the cancellous soft spot at the entrance of the pedicle (**Figure 9**). In the thoracic spine, the concavity of the gearshift is directed laterally. Probing of the pedicle should proceed with smooth and consistent movements. Any sudden shift or advancement signals pedicle wall or vertebral body violation and should be investigated immediately to avoid complications. During probing, the nondominant hand is used to brace the gearshift to prevent sudden advancements. The anterior and lateral vertebral body cortices are most susceptible to penetration by the gearshift probe.

The curve of the gearshift should be pointed laterally on entrance to avoid medial wall penetration. The 2-mm tip should "fall" through the cancellous inner portion of the pedicle, even if it is quite small. We carefully sink the probe to a depth of 15 to 20 mm (beyond the medially located spinal canal), being mindful of the trajectory and the level-specific pedicle anatomy. The gearshift is removed, and the tip is rotated 180°,

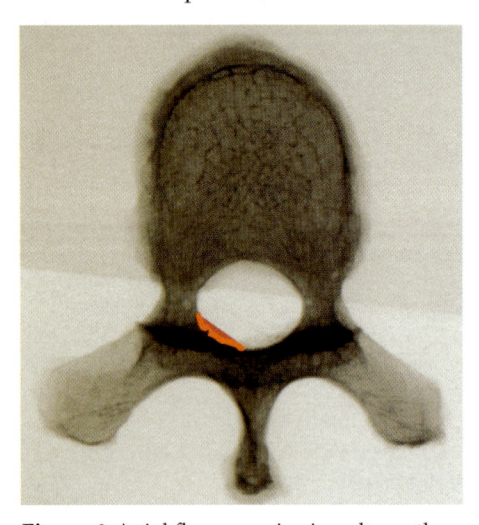

Figure 6 Axial fluoroscopic view shows the dissected thoracic vertebra with the ventral lamina outlined in red. As shown here, the ventral lamina forms the roof of the spinal canal and is confluent with the medial pedicle wall.

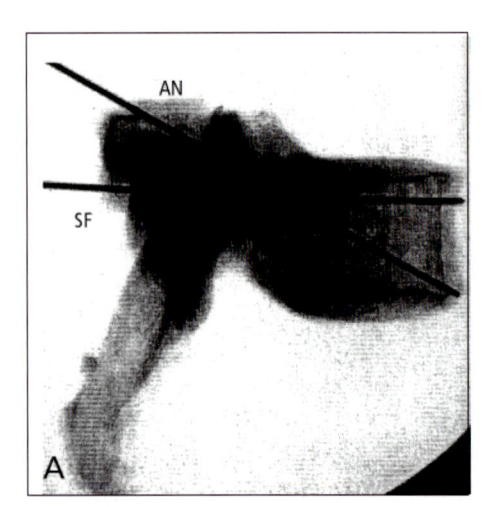

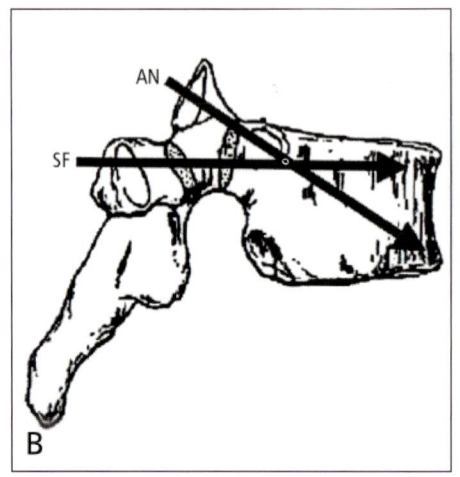

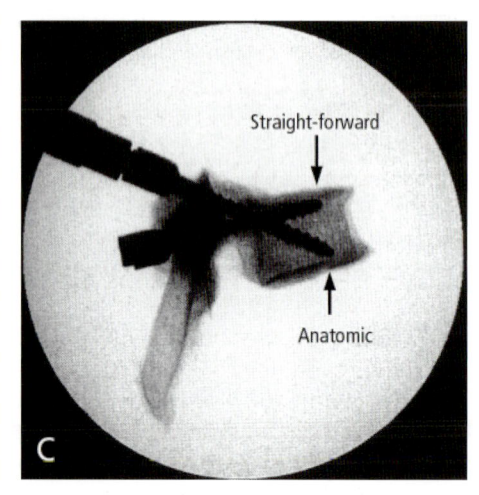

Figure 7 The anatomic (AN) and straight-forward (SF) approaches to screw trajectory for thoracic pedicle screws. **A,** Lateral fluoroscopic view shows the placement of Kirschner wires using both the SF and AN trajectories. **B,** Illustration of the lateral aspect of a vertebra shows the SF and AN trajectories. **C,** Lateral fluoroscopic image shows the thoracic pedicle screw placement using the SF and AN trajectory techniques. (Adapted with permission from Lehman RA, Polly DW, Kuklo TR, Cunningham B, Kirk KL, Belmont PJ Jr: Straight-forward versus anatomic trajectory technique of thoracic pedicle screw fixation: A biomechanical analysis. *Spine [Phila Pa 1976]* 2003;28[18]:2058-2065.)

Chapter 91: Placement of Thoracic Pedicle Screws

Level	Thoracic Pedicle Screw Starting Points- Anatomic Trajectory Cephalo-Caudad Starting Point	Medial-Lateral Starting Point	Level	Thoracic Pedicle Screw Starting Points- Anatomic Trajectory- Sagittal Inclinations Cephalo-Caudad Starting Point	Medial-Lateral Starting Point
T1	Inferior 1/3 Facet	Midpoint Facet	T1	Inferior 1/3 Facet	Midpoint Facet
T2	Inferior 1/3 Facet	Midpoint Facet	T2	Inferior 1/3 Facet	Midpoint Facet
T3	Inferior 1/3 Facet	Midpoint Facet	T3	Inferior 1/3 Facet	Midpoint Facet
T4	Inferior 1/3 Facet	Midpoint Facet	T4	Inferior 1/3 Facet	Midpoint Facet
T5	Midpoint Facet	Midpoint Facet	T5	Midpoint Facet	Midpoint Facet
T6	Midpoint Facet	Midpoint Facet	T6	Midpoint Facet	Midpoint Facet
T7	Midpoint Facet	Midpoint Facet	T7	Midpoint Facet	Midpoint Facet
T8	Midpoint Facet	Midpoint Facet	T8	Midpoint Facet	Midpoint Facet
T9	Midpoint Facet	Midpoint Facet	T9	Midpoint Facet	Midpoint Facet
T10	Midpoint Facet	Midpoint Facet	T10	Midpoint Facet	Midpoint Facet
T11	Midpoint Facet	Midpoint Facet	T11	Midpoint Facet	Midpoint Facet
T12	Midpoint Facet	Midpoint Facet	T12	Midpoint Facet	Midpoint Facet

Figure 8 Starting points for the straight-forward (black) and anatomic (white) pedicle screw trajectories. Dorsal (**A**) and sagittal (**B**) starting points for the anatomic and straight-forward trajectories are shown in models of the spine. **C**, Lateral radiograph of a model shows the full extent of both trajectories. AN = anatomic; SF = straight-forward. (Adapted with permission from Lehman RA, Polly DW, Kuklo TR, Cunningham B, Kirk KL, Belmont PJ Jr: Straight-forward versus anatomic trajectory technique of thoracic pedicle screw fixation: A biomechanical analysis. *Spine [Phila Pa 1976]* 2003;28[18]:2058-2065.)

to point medially. Then, we carefully reenter the same tract at the base of the pedicle and follow it medially, advancing the tip of the gearshift into the body of the vertebra. The ultimate depth averages 40 to 45 mm in the lower thoracic region, 35 to 40 mm in the midthoracic region, and 30 to 35 mm in the proximal thoracic region in adolescents and most adults. The gearshift probe is removed and the hole is visualized to ensure that only nonpulsatile blood is present, not cerebrospinal fluid. Excessive bleeding may be a signal of epidural bleeding from medial wall perforation.

Pedicle Sounding

A flexible ball-tipped sounding probe allows tactile investigation of the pedicle tracts (**Figure 10**). The medial, lateral, superior, and inferior aspects of the tract are palpated to ensure the continuity of the four walls. Next, the probe is advanced carefully to the floor of the tract, the anterior cortex of the vertebral body. The proximal 10 to 15 mm of the channel represents the isthmus of the pedicle and should be palpated carefully. Most pedicle wall perforations are located in the isthmus. If a perforation is identified, we remove the sounding device and use the gearshift probe to redirect the tract in a new and more appropriate direction.

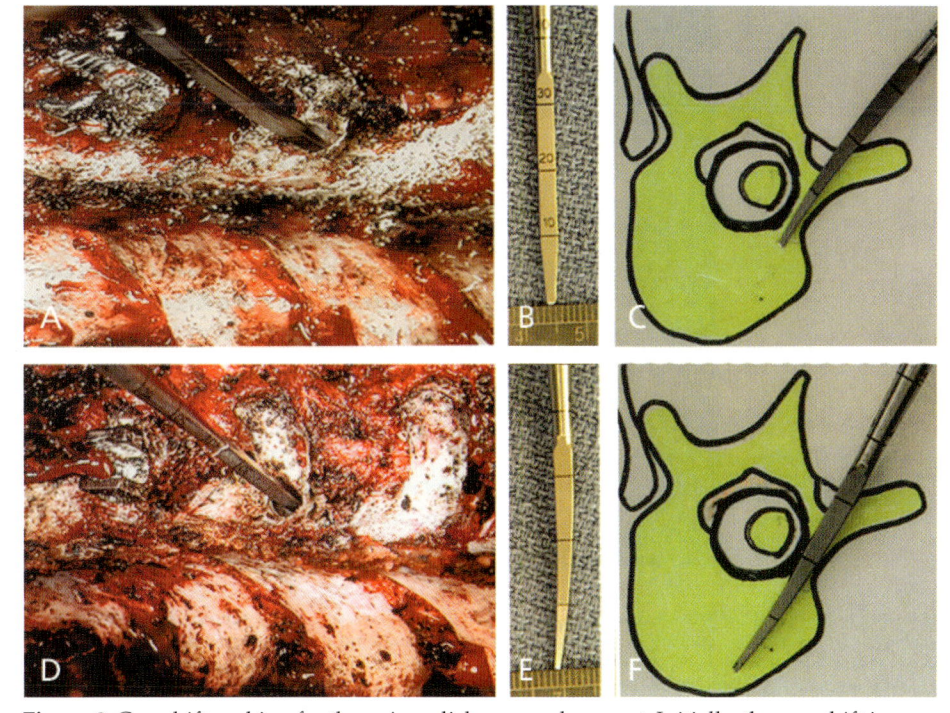

Figure 9 Gearshift probing for thoracic pedicle screw placement. Initially, the gearshift is directed laterally to a depth of 20 mm, the approximate depth of the pedicle, to diminish the likelihood of medial pedicle perforation. **A**, Intraoperative photograph demonstrates the probe placement with the curve directed laterally. **B**, Standard probes are graduated to gauge the depth of penetration. **C**, Axial diagram shows the curve of the probe directed laterally. Then, the gearshift is removed and redirected medially. The nondominant hand is used to brace the gearshift and prevent sudden advancements. **D**, Intraoperative photograph shows the probe placement with the curve directed medially. **E**, Lateral view of the probe shows the typical curve and graduations. **F**, Axial diagram shows the medially directed curve of the probe. (Reproduced with permission from Kim YJ, Lenke LG, Bridwell KH, Cho YS, Riew KD: Free hand pedicle screw placement in the thoracic spine: Is it safe? *Spine [Phila Pa 1976]* 2004;29[3]:333-342.)

© 2013 American Academy of Orthopaedic Surgeons

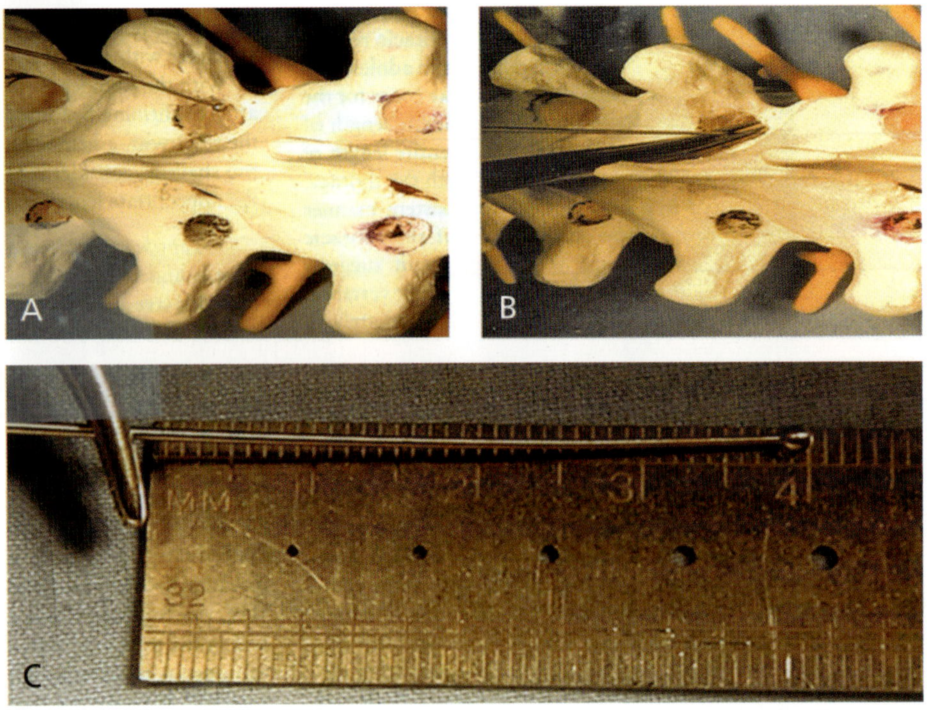

Figure 10 Photographs demonstrate palpation and pedicle length measurement. **A,** All four walls of the pedicle tract floor are palpated using the ball-tipped probe to ensure intrapedicular placement. With the probe fully inserted, the probe is clipped with a hemostat at the level of the lamina (**B**), and the tract length is measured to determine pedicle screw length (**C**). (Adapted with permission from Kim YJ, Lenke LG, Bridwell KH, Cho YS, Riew KD: Free hand pedicle screw placement in the thoracic spine: Is it safe? *Spine [Phila Pa 1976]* 2004;29[3]:333-342.)

Even in the most experienced hands, the positive predictive value of sounding approximates 82%.[11] The probe is placed fully into the pedicle until it abuts the bottom of the vertebral body, and a tonsil hemostat is used to clamp the probe to allow proper measurement of the cord length of the tract.

Tapping, Repalpation, and Screw Placement

After confirmation of pedicle integrity, the sounding probe is removed. The pedicle tract is tapped with a tap that is 0.5 to 1 mm smaller in diameter than the planned screw diameter (**Figure 11, A**). Undertapping of the pedicle results in a significantly higher insertion torque than tapping "line to line."[12] If resistance is encountered, a smaller tap size should be attempted. Then the tapped tract should be evaluated using the flexible ball-tipped sounding probe, which should be able to palpate the bony ridges of each of the four walls (**Figure 11, B**). The floor of the tract should be confirmed once again. With the probe in contact with the floor, a hemostat can be clamped on the probe at the entrance of the pedicle tract to measure screw length. The accuracy of the screw length can be compared with preoperative measurements, known anatomic parameters, and adjacent screws. Patient size and screw trajectory will affect screw length. Lateral trajectories often shorten the screw tract.

The screw is inserted slowly by hand, being mindful of the trajectory marked by the handle of the previously inserted pedicle probe (**Figure 11, C**). The viscoelastic expansion of the pedicle walls should be optimized with the slow, deliberate insertion of the screw. The goal is to fit the maximum diameter and length of screw without compromising bone integrity.

Confirmation of Intraosseous Screws

It is helpful to obtain intraoperative AP and lateral radiographs to assess the screw trajectories before proceeding with rods or deformity correction (**Figure 12, A and B**). Fluoroscopy also can be used and has the advantage of adjusting to a true coronal image to assess each screw. Symmetric placement should be verified throughout the coronal and sagittal planes. The sagittal image should show parallel orientation with the superior end plate and no penetration of screw tips beyond the anterior vertebral body cortex. Intraoperative plain radiography has been shown to be accurate when compared with CT, and approximately 1% to 2% of pedicle screws are readjusted or removed as a result of intraoperative radiographic findings[13] (**Figure 12, C**). If the length or trajectory of any screw does not appear to correlate with adjacent screws, the screw should be removed so that tract integrity can be confirmed with the ball-tipped probe.

Additionally, EMG assessment can be used to further validate screw position. Triggered EMG responses through the screw are recorded with real-time monitoring of the thoracic nerve roots through the rectus abdominis musculature, which is valid for T6 through T12. For thoracic pedicle screws, a triggered EMG threshold of less than 6.0 mA should signal the possibility of a medial pedicle wall breach by a screw and prompt investigation of the pedicle tract.[14] Moreover, when stimulating a pedicle screw, if the electrical response is less than 65% of the average of all previously stimulated screws, the surgeon is obligated to remove the screw and repalpate the tract.

The discovery of a pedicle wall breach should prompt an attempt at salvage of that vertebral level. The lateral wall is up to three times thinner in most cases; as a result, it is the most common area of breach. If a lateral breach is suspected, the gearshift probe is redirected carefully to a more medial trajectory. The decision to replace or discard the screw is based on the repeated pedicle wall palpation, the position of the screw on radiographs, and surgeon assessment of screw purchase during placement. If any doubt exists about proper screw placement, the surgeon should remove the screw and reassess. If doubt remains, the surgeon should leave the screw out and skip the level or substitute a laminar hook at that level. Bone wax can be used to halt bleeding from an abandoned probe hole.

When all screws are in satisfactory position, additional corrective and bone grafting procedures can take place. This is followed by final instrumentation.

Closure

After thoroughly irrigating the entire extent of the wound, the deep fascia can be reapproximated using 1-0 absorbable suture. Deep and superficial drains typically are placed. Deep dermal approximation is performed with buried, interrupted, 2-0 absorbable suture. Final skin approximation may be performed

Chapter 91: Placement of Thoracic Pedicle Screws

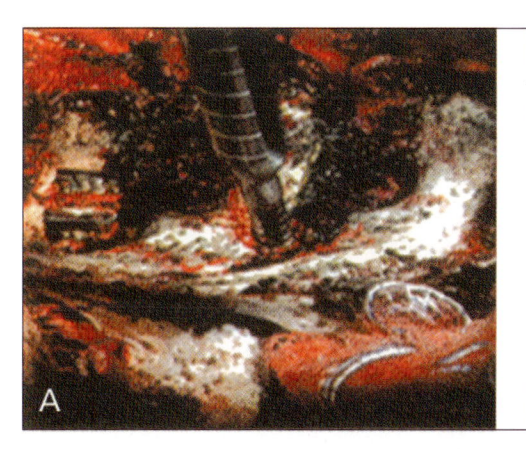

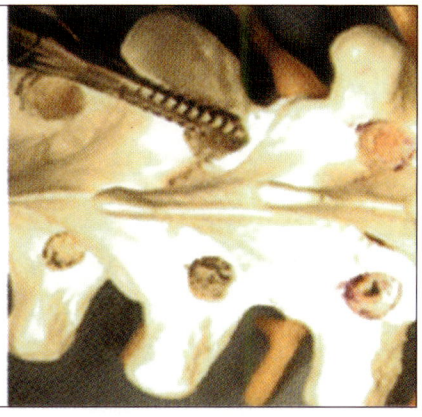

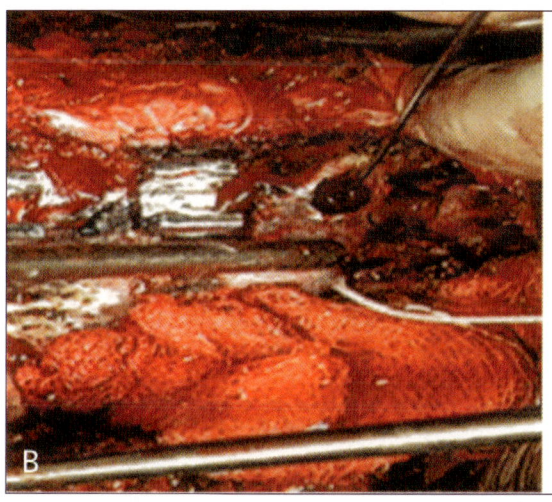

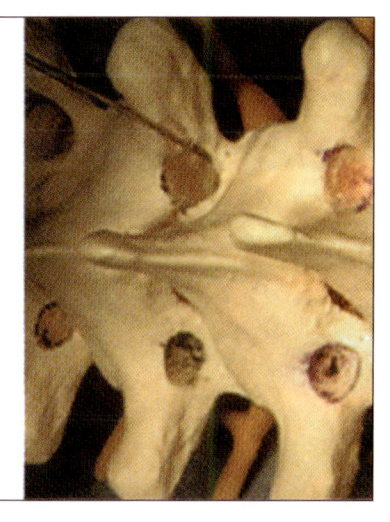

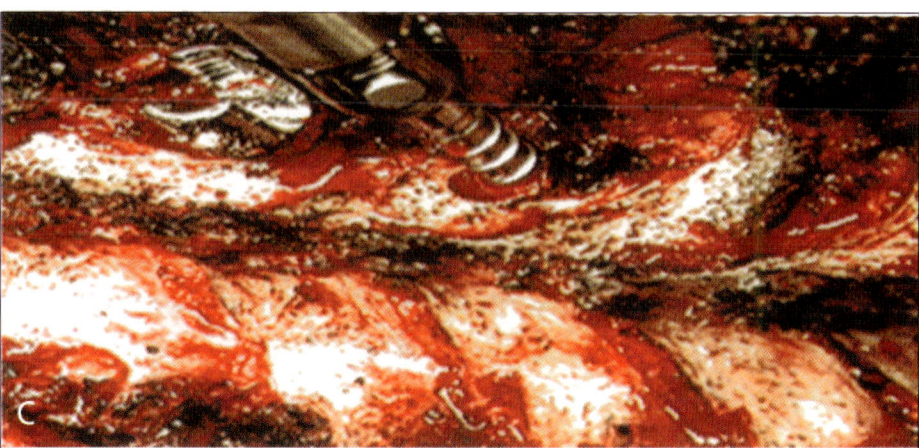

Figure 11 Tapping, repalpation, and slow screw placement. **A,** The pedicle is undertapped 0.5 mm smaller than the intended screw diameter, as shown intraoperatively (left) and in a model (right). **B,** The pedicle tract is repalpated with the ball-tipped probe, as shown intraoperatively (left) and in a model (right). **C,** The screw is placed very slowly to maximize the viscoelastic expansion of the pedicle tract. Careful attention must be paid to screw height to facilitate rod placement later. (Adapted with permission from Kim YJ, Lenke LG, Bridwell KH, Cho YS, Riew KD: Free hand pedicle screw placement in the thoracic spine: Is it safe? *Spine* [Phila Pa 1976] 2004;29[3]:333-342.)

with running subcuticular 3-0 absorbable monofilament. Adhesive strips can supplement the closure. Liquid topical skin adhesive may be used to provide a moisture barrier, which may be advantageous for incisions in patients with poor bowel or bladder control.

Complications

Compared with lumbar pedicle screws, thoracic pedicle screws have a relatively increased risk of neurovascular complications because of the smaller pedicle size. Current complication rates are published from large spine centers with fellowship-trained surgeons, and learning curves have proven significant in several cadaveric and clinical studies. The most common complication associated with thoracic pedicle screws is screw malposition (**Figure 13**). It should be noted that the juxtapedicular technique (in-out-in) and the placement of thoracic pedicle screws in the costovertebral junction are viable options to obtain fixation in the thoracic spine. Furthermore, it has been shown that slightly medial (2 mm) or lateral (6 mm) violations have little clinical or anatomic consequence.[15]

In a systematic review of the use of pedicle screws in pediatric spinal deformity, a reported 4.2% malposition rate was found among 4,570 screws.[15] When standard postoperative CT scans were obtained routinely to evaluate screw position, the rate of malposition increased to 15.7%, but less than 1% of these patients required reoperation for misplaced or loose screws. This systematic review did not demonstrate any major permanent catastrophic neurologic or vascular injury caused by screw misplacement. The reasons for reoperation included an asymptomatic intrathoracic screw causing pleural effusion, transient paraparesis due to a medial breach and epidural hematoma, 3-mm anterior penetration of the anterior vertebral body without evidence of vascular injury, medial pedicle breach greater than 4 mm without neurologic deficit, fixation failure with and without loss of correction, early pedicle fracture in a monosegmental construct, and asymptomatic aortic abutment in 1 patient. Three studies (5,370 screws total) reported intraoperative pedicle fracture, with an incidence of 0.50% per screw inserted. Dural leaks have been reported after screw placement in three studies, at a rate of 0.35% per screw inserted. Only 10 superficial infections and 10 deep infections were reported in the same 12 studies, in a total of 1,045 patients.[15] Aortic abutment was noted in 6 of 8,147 screws in 8 studies reporting this finding. Pseudarthrosis was reported in a single case among 192 patients across 5 studies specifically reporting this complication. The highest reported incidence of screw pullout was 0.67%, and loosening was observed in 38 (0.54%) of 6,972 pedicle screws across 8 studies. Screw breakage was reported in a single case.[15]

A thorough understanding of the three-dimensional pedicle anatomy, spatial orientation of each vertebral level, and angle

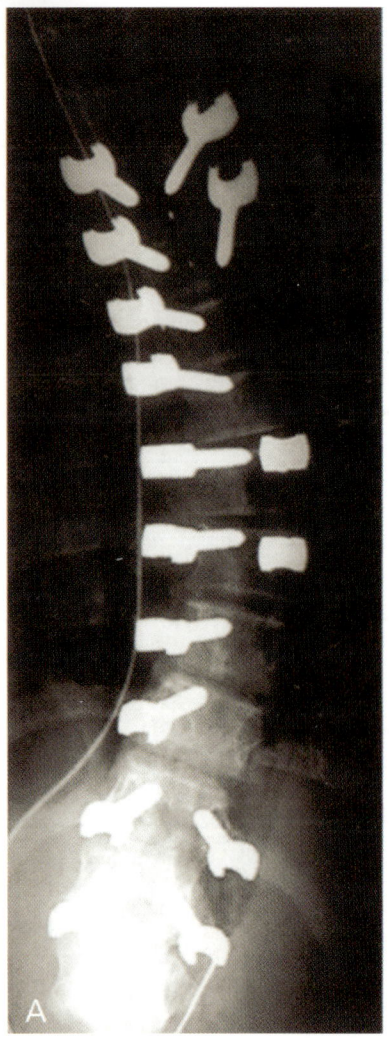

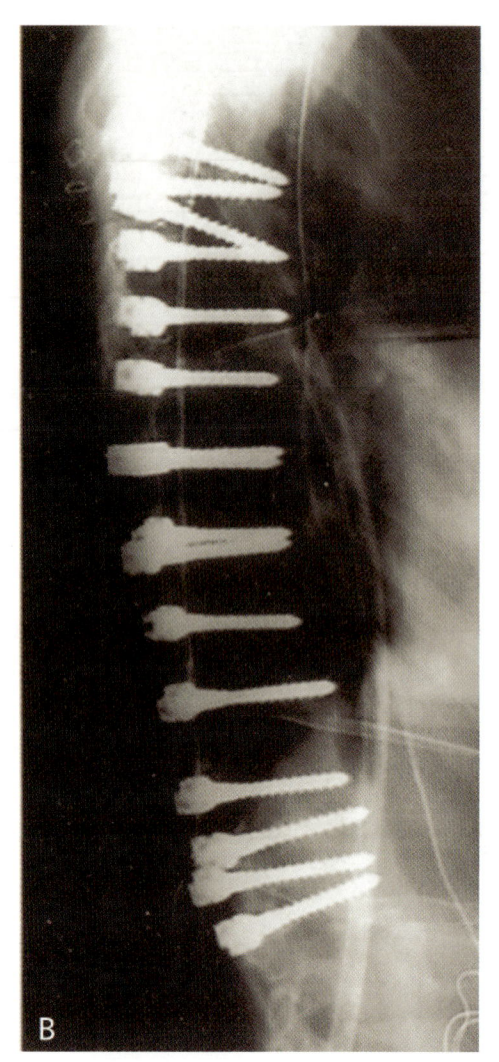

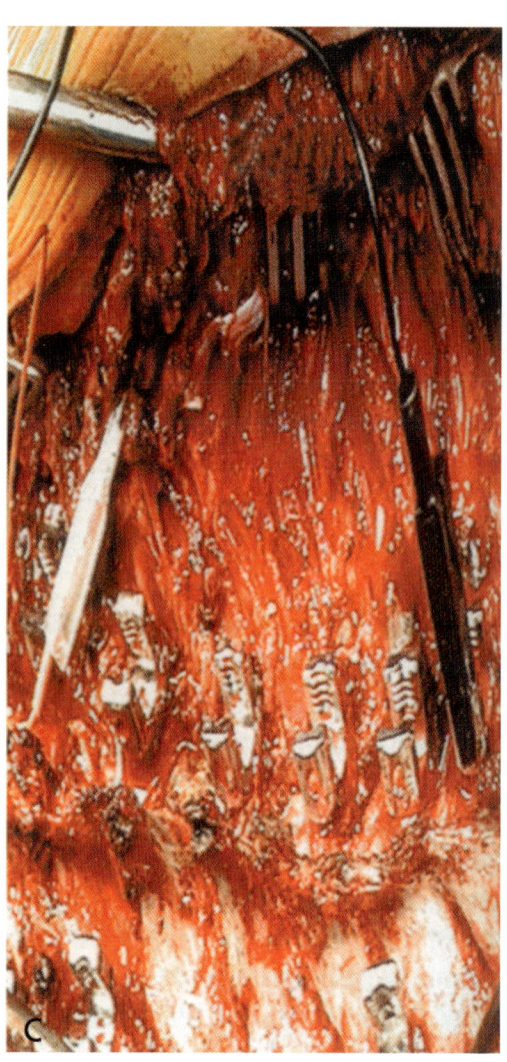

Figure 12 Confirmation of intraosseous screw placement. AP (**A**) and lateral (**B**) radiographs are obtained after all screws are placed. **C,** Intraoperative photograph depicts the triggered electromyographic testing of the screws. Thoracic screws from T6 to T12 can be monitored with the rectus abdominis muscles. (Adapted with permission from Kim YJ, Lenke LG, Bridwell KH, Cho YS, Riew KD: Free hand pedicle screw placement in the thoracic spine: Is it safe? *Spine [Phila Pa 1976]* 2004;29[3]:333-342.)

of trajectory required for each pedicle will prevent complications related to screw malposition, which is directly related to fixation failure. Strict adherence to a stepwise approach to placing an appropriately sized screw for optimal fit and fill of the pedicle in the correct trajectory will lead to safe placement of thoracic pedicle screws and excellent fixation.

Postoperative Care and Rehabilitation

Standard wound management, pain control, and physical therapy for mobilization and transfer training are used. The routine is dictated by the indication for the pedicle screws. In most deformity cases, patients are encouraged to get out of bed as early as the first postoperative day, depending on hemodynamic status. Drains usually remain until the output is less than 30 mL per 8 hours for a 24-hour period, typically 48 to 72 hours maximum. Diet usually is restricted to clear liquids until the return of bowel sounds or the passage of flatus, as a precaution against postoperative ileus. Postoperative weight-bearing AP and lateral radiographs are obtained before discharge to assess spinal alignment and position of the instrumentation.

Pearls

- The surgeon should adhere to the superior facet rule to avoid medial penetration. The starting point should be 2 mm lateral to the midpoint of the superior facet.[16]
- A wide inferior facetectomy will improve visualization of the superior facet for anatomic landmarks of the starting points, allow greater deformity correction, provide local bone graft, and create a greater surface area for fusion.
- To optimize screw diameter, pediculoplasty should be considered. A better fit and fill are obtained if cautious tapping and screw insertion are used, to take advantage of the plastic deformation and slow expansion of the pedicle.[16]
- The ability to accurately detect the presence or absence of a pedicle tract violation and location of the breach, if present, depends on the surgeon's level of training. Probing the pedicle tract before placement of the pedicle screws in the thoracic spine likely is a learned skill that improves with repetition and experience.[11]
- Most screw purchase strength variability among pedicle screws can be explained by regional differences in bone mineral density at the bone-screw interface.[17] Successful surgeons begin to appreciate screw purchase at the time of insertion.

References

1. Suk SI, Lee SM, Chung ER, Kim JH, Kim SS: Selective thoracic fusion with segmen-

Chapter 91: Placement of Thoracic Pedicle Screws

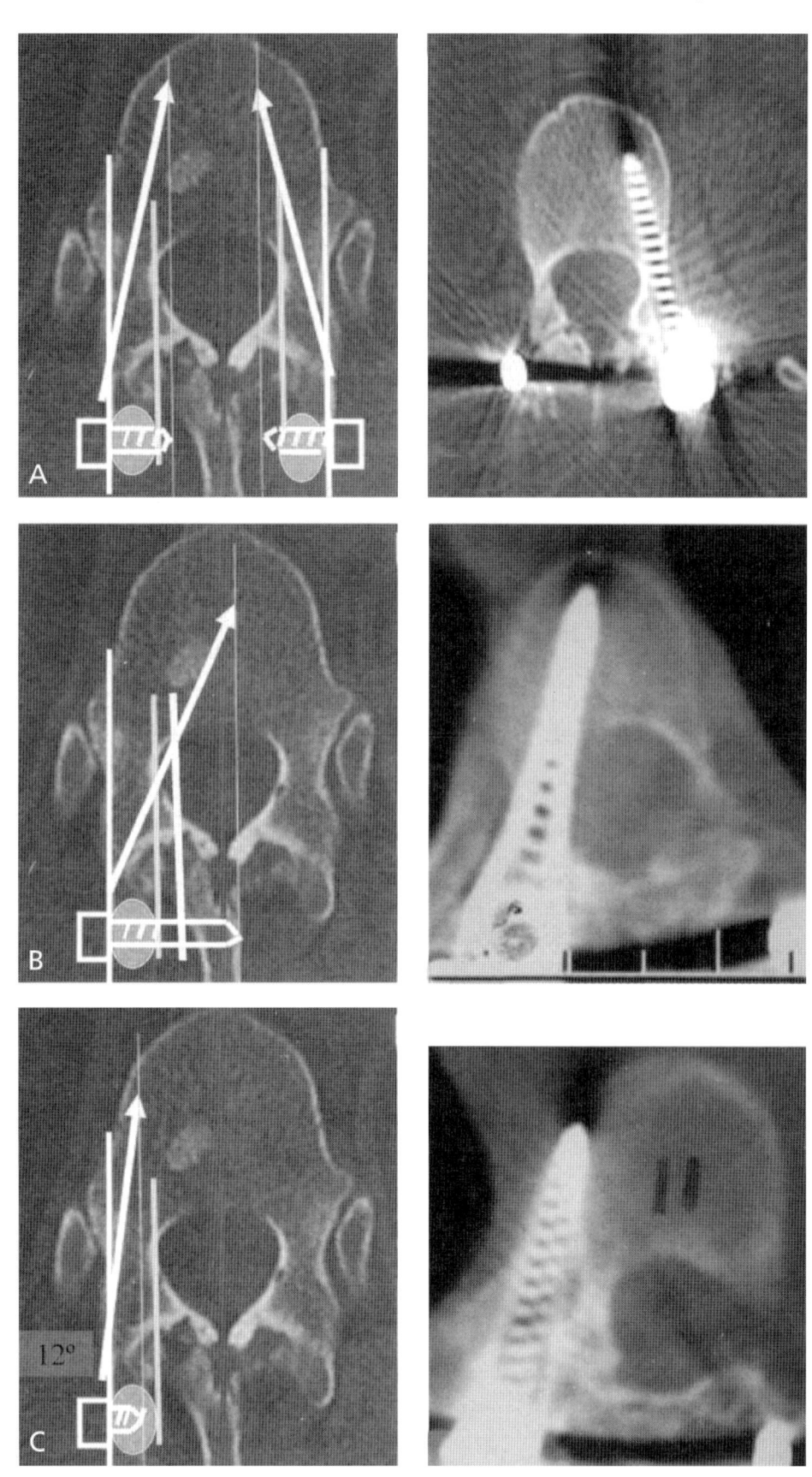

Figure 13 Preoperative (left) and postoperative (right) axial CT scans demonstrate thoracic pedicle screw trajectories. The vertical white lines demarcate the boundaries of the pedicle, or the lateral and medial cortices. The arrow on the left image corresponds to the final screw trajectory seen on the postoperative image on the right. **A,** The screw axis lies between the outer cortices of the pedicle wall. **B,** A medial breach: the axis of the screw violates the medial cortex. **C,** A lateral breach: the axis of the screw violates the lateral cortex. (Adapted with permission from Lehman RA, Lenke LG, Keeler KA, Kim YJ, Cheh G: Computed tomography evaluation of pedicle screws placed in the pediatric deformed spine over an 8-year period. Spine [Phila Pa 1976] 2007;32[24]:2679-2684.)

tal pedicle screw fixation in the treatment of thoracic idiopathic scoliosis: More than 5-year follow-up. *Spine (Phila Pa 1976)* 2005;30(14):1602-1609.

2. Kuklo TR, Lenke LG, O'Brien MF, Lehman RA Jr, Polly DW Jr, Schroeder TM: Accuracy and efficacy of thoracic pedicle screws in curves more than 90 degrees. *Spine (Phila Pa 1976)* 2005;30(2):222-226.

3. Liu S, Li H, Liang C, et al: Monosegmental transpedicular fixation for selected patients with thoracolumbar burst fractures. *J Spinal Disord Tech* 2009;22(1):38-44.

4. Lehman RA Jr, Lenke LG, Keeler KA, et al: Operative treatment of adolescent idiopathic scoliosis with posterior pedicle screw-only constructs: Minimum three-year follow-up of one hundred fourteen cases. *Spine (Phila Pa 1976)* 2008;33(14):1598-1604.

5. Chang MC, Liu CL, Chen TH: Polymethylmethacrylate augmentation of pedicle screw for osteoporotic spinal surgery: A novel technique. *Spine (Phila Pa 1976)* 2008;33(10):E317-E324.

6. O'Brien MF, Lenke LG, Mardjetko S, et al: Pedicle morphology in thoracic adolescent idiopathic scoliosis: Is pedicle fixation an anatomically viable technique? *Spine (Phila Pa 1976)* 2000;25(18):2285-2293.

7. Kotani Y, Abumi K, Ito M, et al: Accuracy analysis of pedicle screw placement in posterior scoliosis surgery: Comparison between conventional fluoroscopic and computer-assisted technique. *Spine (Phila Pa 1976)* 2007;32(14):1543-1550.

8. Kim YJ, Lenke LG, Bridwell KH, Cho YS, Riew KD: Free hand pedicle screw placement in the thoracic spine: Is it safe? *Spine (Phila Pa 1976)* 2004;29(3):333-342.

9. Lehman RA Jr, Polly DW Jr, Kuklo TR, Cunningham B, Kirk KL, Belmont PJ Jr: Straight-forward versus anatomic trajectory technique of thoracic pedicle screw fixation: A biomechanical analysis. *Spine (Phila Pa 1976)* 2003;28(18):2058-2065.

10. Liljenqvist UR, Allkemper T, Hackenberg L, Link TM, Steinbeck J, Halm HF: Analysis of vertebral morphology in idiopathic scoliosis with use of magnetic resonance imaging and multiplanar reconstruction. *J Bone Joint Surg Am* 2002;84-A(3):359-368.

11. Lehman RA, Potter BK, Kuklo TR, et al: Probing for thoracic pedicle screw tract violation(s): Is it valid? *J Spinal Disord Tech* 2004;17(4):277-283.

12. Kuklo TR, Lehman RA Jr: Effect of various tapping diameters on insertion of thoracic pedicle screws: A biomechanical analysis. *Spine (Phila Pa 1976)* 2003;28(18):2066-2071.

13. Kim YJ, Lenke LG, Cheh G, Riew KD: Evaluation of pedicle screw placement in

the deformed spine using intraoperative plain radiographs: A comparison with computerized tomography. *Spine (Phila Pa 1976)* 2005;30(18):2084-2088.

14. Raynor BL, Lenke LG, Kim YJ, et al: Can triggered electromyograph thresholds predict safe thoracic pedicle screw placement? *Spine (Phila Pa 1976)* 2002;27(18):2030-2035.

15. Hicks JM, Singla A, Shen FH, Arlet V: Complications of pedicle screw fixation in scoliosis surgery: A systematic review. *Spine (Phila Pa 1976)* 2010;35(11):E465-E470.

16. Lehman RA Jr, Lenke LG, Keeler KA, Kim YJ, Cheh G: Computed tomography evaluation of pedicle screws placed in the pediatric deformed spine over an 8-year period. *Spine (Phila Pa 1976)* 2007;32(24):2679-2684.

17. Deckelmann S, Schwyn R, Van der Pol B, Windolf M, Heini PF, Benneker LM: DensiProbe Spine: A novel instrument for intraoperative measurement of bone density in transpedicular screw fixation. *Spine (Phila Pa 1976)* 2010;35(6):607-612.

Chapter 92
Lumbar Microdiskectomy

Bradley Moatz, MD   P. Justin Tortolani, MD

Patient Selection
Indications

Lumbar microdiskectomy is indicated in patients with a symptomatic lumbar intervertebral disk herniation (IDH) that is refractory to a reasonable trial of nonsurgical treatment.[1,2] Well-suited patients present with leg pain, or "sciatica," that follows a clear-cut radicular pattern. A thorough history and physical examination can predict the level of the IDH before confirmatory imaging studies are obtained. Oral corticosteroids, nonsteroidal anti-inflammatory drugs, physical therapy, and lumbar epidural steroid injection at the level of the IDH or affected nerve root are nonsurgical measures that are commonly used to manage pain and loss of function.[1] Progressive loss of motor function (eg, footdrop) that interferes with the patient's quality of life represents the strongest indication for surgery. Intractable pain despite nonsurgical treatment is the most common indication for microdiskectomy.

Contraindications

Lumbar microdiskectomy is contraindicated for patients in whom no evidence of an IDH is present on imaging studies. Particular attention should be paid to patients who present with a painless footdrop because the differential diagnosis for this entity is extensive: peroneal nerve palsy, tertiary syphilis, diabetic mononeuropathy, fascioscapulohumeral dystrophy, stroke, multiple sclerosis, and amyotrophic lateral sclerosis. These entities should be considered when evaluating patients with a paucity of findings present on MRI. Greater trochanteric pain syndrome (GTPS) is a common cause of radiating leg pain that can mimic an L5 radiculopathy based on the location of pain in the gluteus and lateral thigh.[3] Importantly, GTPS is not characterized by radiation of pain below the proximal calf, and other neurologic symptoms (eg, numbness, tingling, motor weakness) and signs (loss of reflexes) are absent.

Preoperative Imaging

Closed MRI represents the gold standard for identification of the location and size of a suspected herniated nucleus pulposus (HNP).[4] Sagittal T2-weighted sequences (**Figure 1, A**) provide accurate identification of the level of the disk herniation as well as the degree of foraminal encroachment. In certain cases, it is possible to determine whether the disk herniation is subligamentous and whether it has migrated cephalad or caudad within the spinal canal. Axial T2-weighted sequences (**Figure 1, B**) allow the surgeon to determine whether the HNP is central, paramedian, subarticular, or far lateral. In the case of a far lateral HNP, the axial T1-weighted images may demonstrate the HNP in better clarity because the fat outside the canal (high signal intensity) contrasts well with the low-signal-intensity disk material. Plain radiographs should be obtained before surgery to evaluate for deformity (scoliosis or spondylolisthesis) or a spina bifida occulta, which may not be evident on MRI obtained in the supine position.

Video 92.1 Lumbar Microdiskectomy. Bradley Moatz, MD; P. Justin Tortolani, MD (30 min)

Procedure
Room Setup/Patient Positioning

The patient is placed prone on a Jackson table (**Figure 2, A**) and all bony prominences are padded well. The face and head are suspended in a padded holder, which allows clear visualization of the eyes, nose, and endotracheal tube. The knees are flexed and the legs are padded with memory foam pillows. Once the patient is positioned, the table is brought into the jackknife position (**Figure 2, B**). This reduces the lumbar lordosis and facilitates exposure of the disk by increasing the interlaminar distance. The C-arm is then brought into the lateral position (**Figure 2, C**) and is draped out of the sterile field once the skin is prepared. **Figure 3** shows the placement of the operating room equipment and personnel.

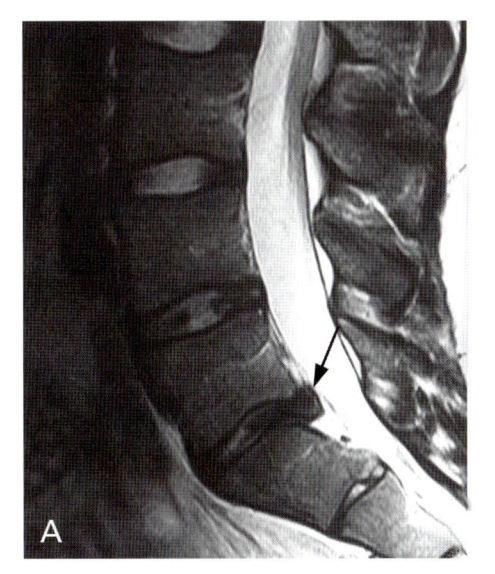

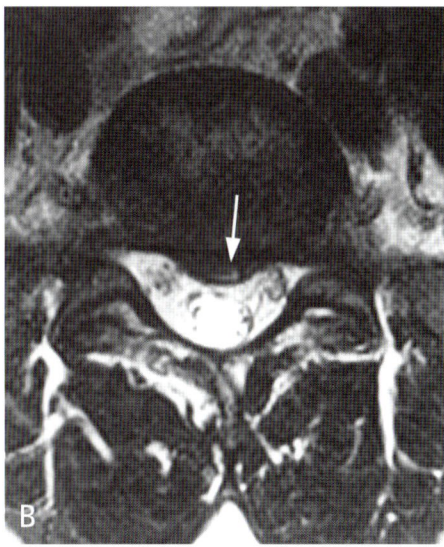

Figure 1 T2-weighted MRIs of a 21-year-old athlete who presented with left S1 radiculopathy. **A,** Sagittal image demonstrates an L5/S1 disk herniation. **B,** Axial image demonstrates the left paramedian location (arrow).

Dr. Moatz or an immediate family member has received nonincome support (such as equipment or services), commercially derived honoraria, or other non–research-related funding (such as paid travel) from Globus Medical and Vertebral Technologies. Dr. Tortolani or an immediate family member has received royalties from Globus Medical; is a member of a speakers' bureau or has made paid presentations on behalf of Globus Medical; serves as a paid consultant to or is an employee of Globus Medical and Integra LifeSciences; and has received research or institutional support from Globus Medical.

Section 7: Spine

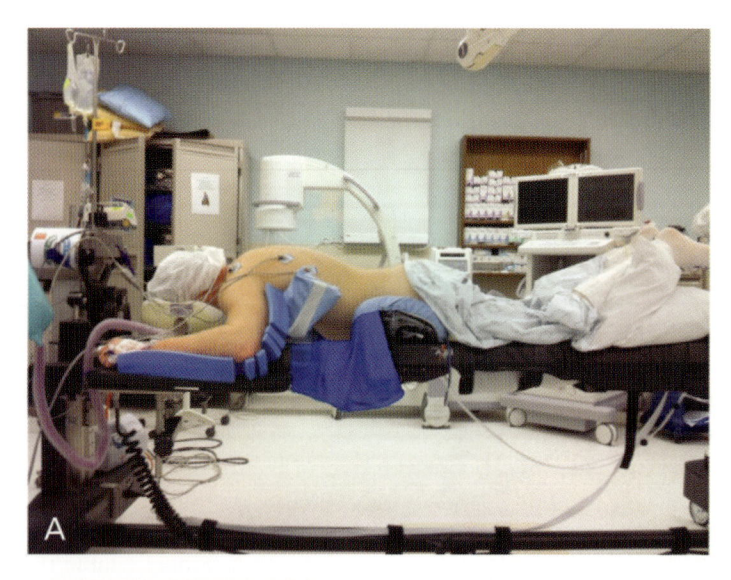

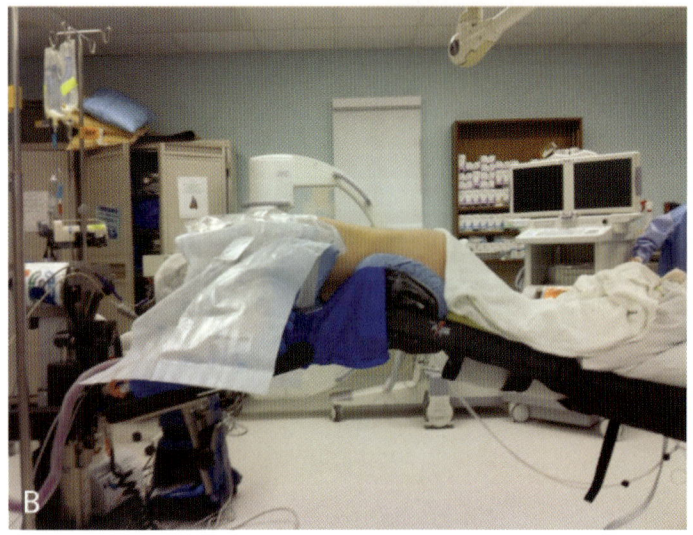

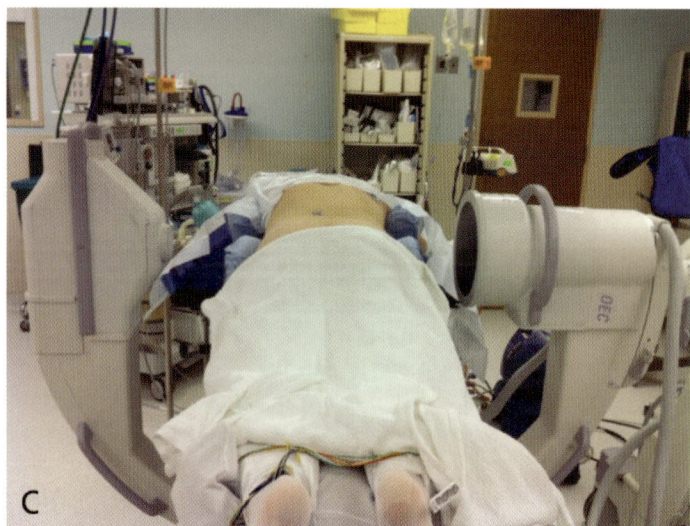

Figure 2 Photographs demonstrate patient positioning and setup for lumbar microdiskectomy. **A,** The patient is positioned prone on the Jackson table, with all bony prominences well padded. **B,** The patient is positioned prone, with the Jackson table in the jackknife position to increase interlaminar distance. **C,** The C-arm in position for lateral imaging of the lumbar spine.

Special Instruments/Equipment/Implants

The tools needed to successfully perform a lumbar diskectomy include a C-arm fluoroscope, a surgical microscope, and an adjustable Jackson table.

Surgical Technique for Lumbar Microdiskectomy

Preparation

Once the patient is prepared and draped, the midline is identified by palpation of the coccyx and sacrum distally and the lumbar spinous processes proximally. The iliac crest is palpated on the sides of the patient and serves as a guide to the L4 vertebral level. Using this anatomic guide, a spinal needle is inserted off the midline and directed toward the disk of interest. A lateral fluoroscopic image is obtained to visualize this marker, thereby confirming the best location for the skin incision (**Figure 4**).

Exposure

After infiltration of the dermis and subcutaneous fat with 0.5% bupivacaine with epinephrine, a 3-cm skin incision is made directly midline, centered over the disk of interest. Dissection is carried down to the level of the deep fascia, and a single cerebellar retractor is inserted to retract the subcutaneous fat and skin. A vertical incision is then made in the lumbodorsal fascia, just lateral to the midline, on the side of the disk herniation. Using an Army-Navy retractor alternating in the superior and inferior aspect of the wound allows the surgeon to create a fascial incision that is longer than the skin incision, if needed. The lumbodorsal musculature is then subperiosteally detached from the posterior elements over the interspace of interest. For an L4-5 disk herniation, the surgeon exposes the spinous process and lamina of L4 to the level of the pars interarticularis proximally and the spinous process and lamina of L5 to the level of the pars interarticularis distally. Care is taken to avoid cutting any muscle at this stage. Our preference is to simply detach the musculotendinous attachments to the tip of the spinous processes and interspinous ligaments. Once this is accomplished, a laterally directed sweeping motion with a 1.5-cm Cobb curet allows the surgeon to retract the muscles over the L4-5 facet joint capsule.

A Kocher clamp is then secured to the inferior edge of the cephalad lamina, and a lateral fluoroscopic image is obtained to check that the exposed level is correct (**Figure 5**). Once the appropriate level is confirmed, a Taylor retractor is placed lateral to the exposed facet. This allows excellent visibility of the deep surgical field, is essentially atraumatic, and ensures that no muscle will creep into the surgical field during the remainder of the procedure. The tip of the Taylor retrac-

Chapter 92: Lumbar Microdiskectomy

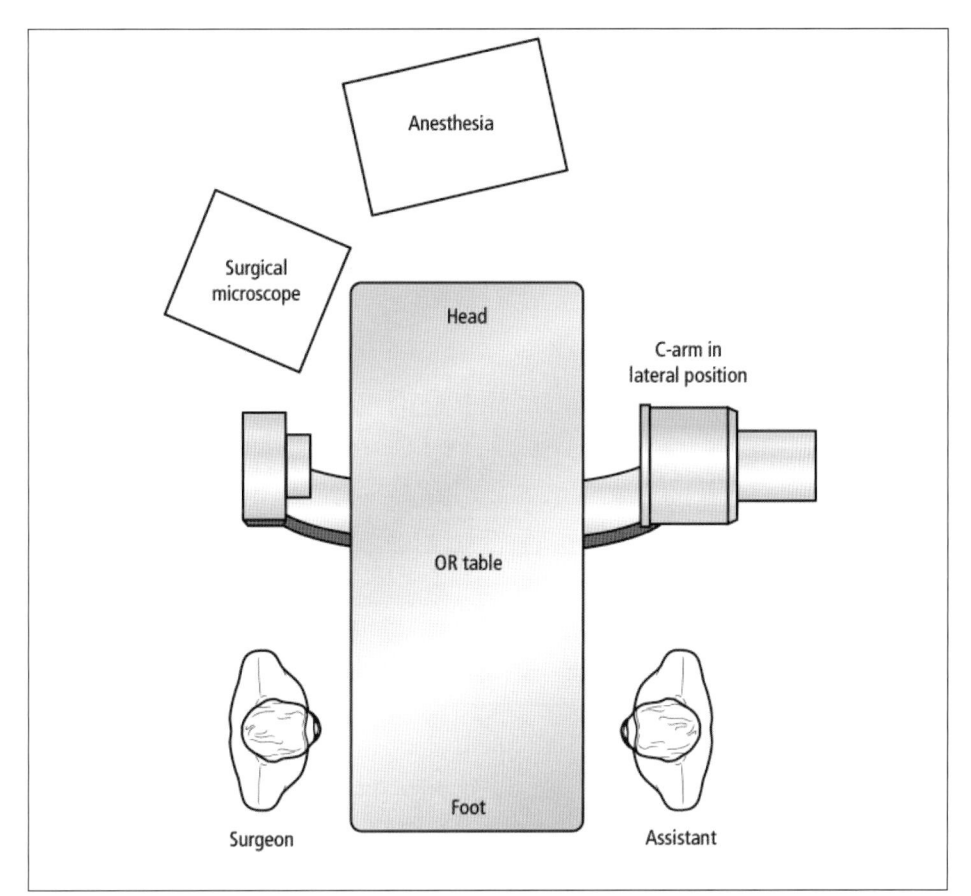

Figure 3 Illustration depicts the placement of the operating room equipment and personnel for lumbar microdiskectomy.

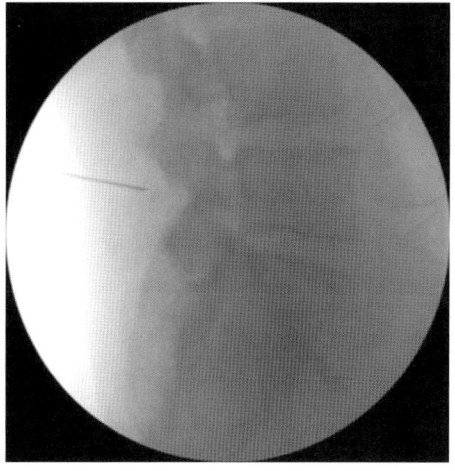

Figure 4 Intraoperative lateral fluoroscopic image of the lumbar spine shows a spinal needle pointing to the level of the disk herniation (L5-S1).

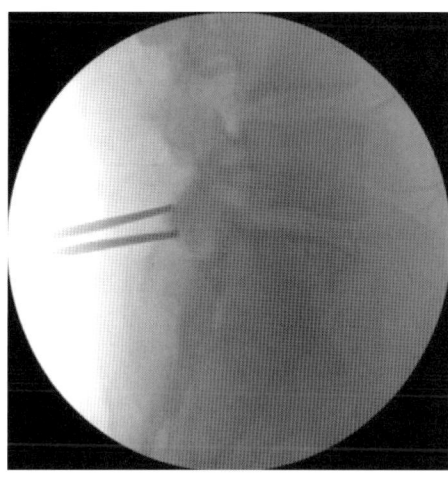

Figure 5 Intraoperative lateral fluoroscopic image of the lumbar spine shows a Kocher clamp placed on the inferior lamina of L5, thereby confirming the correct surgical level for L5-S1 microdiskectomy.

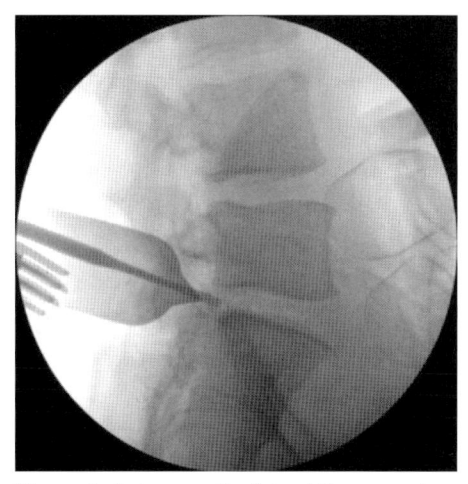

Figure 6 Intraoperative lateral fluoroscopic image shows the lumbar spine after the Taylor retractor has been positioned around the lateral aspect of the L5-S1 facet joint. The pointed tip of the Taylor retractor points to the level of the diskectomy. A Penfield 4 is placed along the posterior aspect of the L5-S1 as a final confirmation of the desired surgical level.

tor and a Penfield 4 can also be used as an additional check of the spinal level on fluoroscopy (**Figure 6**). The Taylor retractor is tamped gently to seat the tip around the facet joint. Once positioned, the Taylor retractor is held in position by looping a gauze bandage around the free (handle) end of the Taylor retractor and the surgeon's foot. Although our preference is to use the Taylor retractor, other deep, self-retaining retractors such as the McCulloch can be used effectively, based on surgeon preference.

Decompression

Once the exposure is complete, a surgical microscope is brought into the field. An angled size 2 curet is used to create a plane between the ligamentum flavum and the lamina of the cephalad vertebra. A high-speed burr is then used to thin the laminar bone for subsequent hemilaminotomy. The laminotomy window should extend cephalad from the interspace to the level of the pars interarticularis of the superior vertebra and caudad from the interspace to the superiormost 3 mm of the inferior lamina. We extend the laminotomy laterally to the medial edge of the facet joint complex (**Figure 7**). With the ligamentum flavum serving as a protective barrier over the dura, a 45° Kerrison punch is used to remove the remaining bone and complete the laminotomy. The ligamentum flavum generally can be removed en bloc by dissecting it free from the medial edge of the facet. An angled 2-0 microcuret may be helpful at this stage to release the adhesions between the facet joint capsule and the ligamentum flavum. Once this is accomplished, the medial 3 mm of the facet is resected with the Kerrison punch. A foraminotomy is then performed by angling the Kerrison punch out the foramen of the traversing nerve root. Any remaining ligamentum flavum can be removed with a pituitary rongeur.

Once the dura is visualized clearly, a Penfield 4 is used to identify the lateral edge (shoulder region) of the traversing nerve root. Epidural bleeding can be controlled with a combination of bipolar cautery and thrombin-soaked gel foam gauze. With the Penfield 4, the traversing nerve is mobilized gently toward the midline, revealing the underlying disk space. A nerve root retractor is then placed around the nerve root, holding it toward the midline. The bipolar cautery is useful in coagulating epidural vessels directly over the disk herniation.

© 2013 American Academy of Orthopaedic Surgeons

603

Section 7: Spine

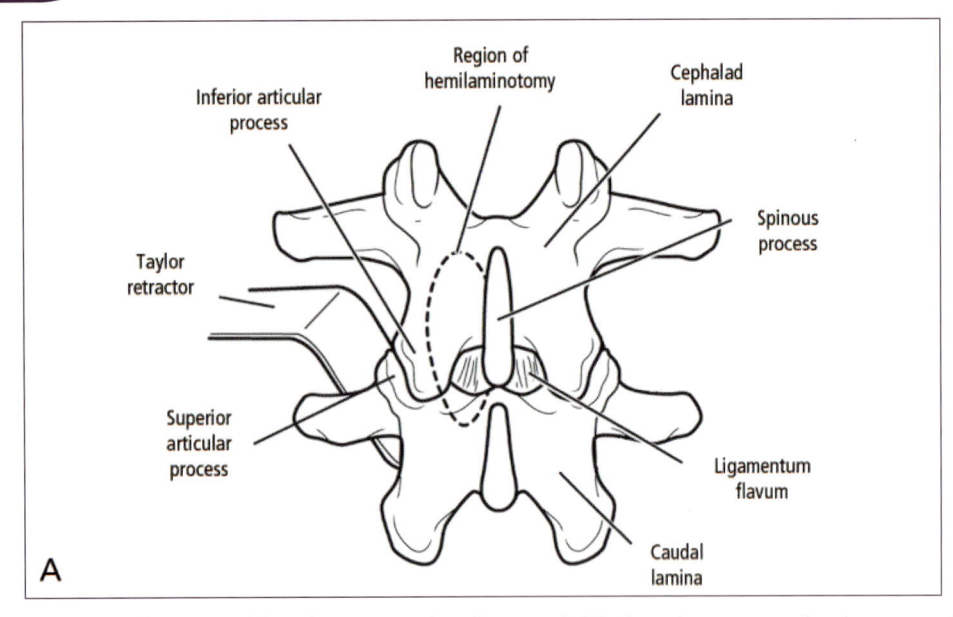

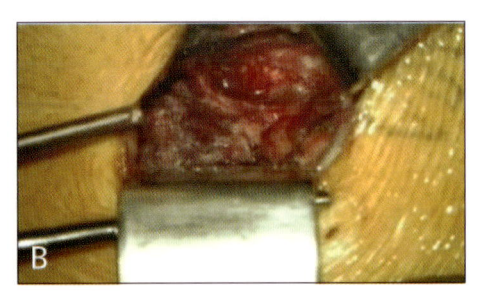

Figure 7 Illustration (**A**) and intraoperative photograph (**B**) show the exposure for decompression for lumbar microdiskectomy.

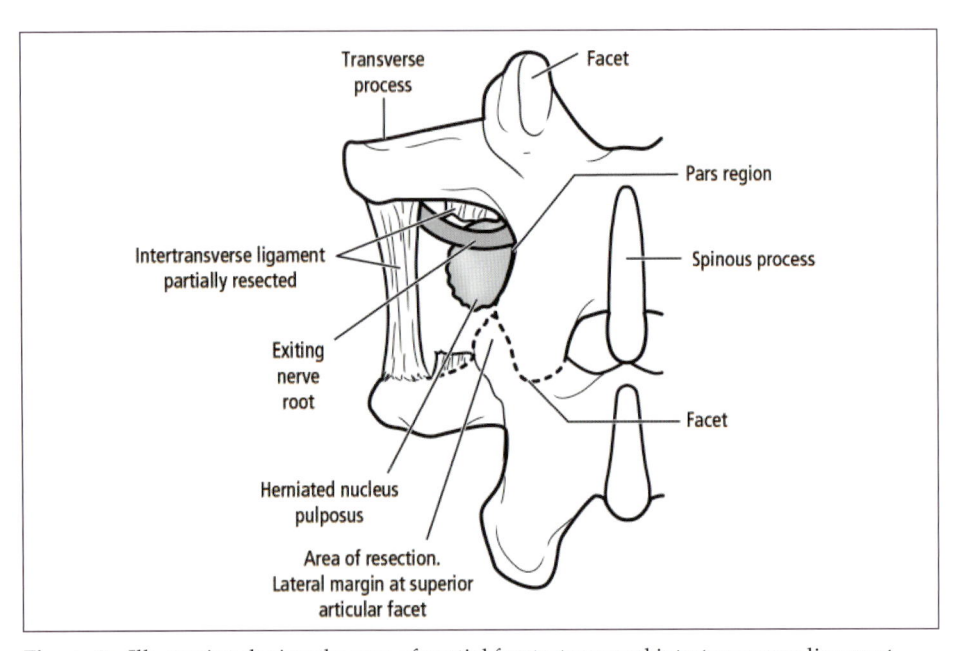

Figure 8 Illustration depicts the area of partial facetectomy and intertransverse ligament resection for access to a far lateral disk herniation.

After localization of the correct level with fluoroscopy, the skin incision is made two fingerbreadths lateral to the midline and continued to the intermuscular septum between the multifidus and longissimus muscles. Subperiosteal dissection to the transverse process just cephalad to the disk herniation is continued using electrocautery and/or a Cobb dissector. The transverse process and associated facet joint are used as anatomic landmarks to ensure the correct level of surgery.

A Gelpi retractor can be helpful at this stage to retract the lumbar musculature laterally, away from the lateral border of the superior articular process of the facet joint at the level of the disk herniation. Radiography is then performed to confirm the correct level. With the 4-mm Kerrison rongeur, partial resection of the lateral margin of the superior facet is performed to assist in disk exposure. The intertransverse ligament is identified and removed as needed to expose the exiting nerve root (**Figure 8**). This generally is performed in a medial-to-lateral direction. The most common technical error with this approach is not having enough medial exposure. The disk herniation itself should be identified medial to the nerve root. Medial dissection into the pars interarticularis may be necessary to ensure complete nerve decompression.

A far-lateral herniation almost always displaces the nerve root superiorly because the pedicle below blocks any inferior migration, and the nerve root usually is displaced superiorly by the disk fragment. The free fragment of disk material usually is found medial and inferior to the exiting root. Extensive distal dissec-

Once the disk herniation is completely exposed, a No. 15 blade is used to create an incision directly over the disk herniation. For smaller, contained herniations without a large annular defect, a vertical slit incision may be all that is required. We prefer to use a slit incision because this affords potentially faster healing of the anulus with enhanced outcomes.[5] In this case, as soon as the anulus is incised, the low-viscosity nuclear material is aspirated easily into the suction tip. For higher viscosity herniations, a micropituitary rongeur may be required for complete removal. Several additional passes with the micropituitary rongeur into the disk space help to ensure that no additional loose disk fragments are left behind. Alternatively, the surgeon also can use an angled microcuret placed into the disk space to dislodge any remaining fragments.

Closure
Closure is performed in layered fashion with absorbable No. 1 Vicryl suture (Ethicon) in the deep fascia, followed by 2-0 Vicryl in the subcutaneous tissue. The skin can be closed with subcuticular suture, staples, or a topical skin adhesive, based on surgeon and patient preference.

Surgical Technique for Far-Lateral Microdiskectomy
In the less common situation of a far-lateral HNP, the most direct access is via a paramedian muscle-splitting approach.

tion should only be attempted with care because the lumbar vasculature enters the lower foramen and the dorsal primary nerve root exits from the distal aspects of the nerve root.

Once the offending disk is identified and removed, the wound is flushed with normal saline both for the removal of loose fragments and to dilute any chemically irritating mediators of inflammation from the nucleus pulposus. The retractors are removed, and the wound is closed in layered fashion with the use of 0 Vicryl for the fascial layer and 2-0 Vicryl for the subcuticular closure.

Complications

Complications following lumbar microdiskectomy are relatively rare. The most feared and devastating complication, cauda equina syndrome, can occur in circumstances of excessive epidural bleeding or with large recurrent disk herniations. For this reason, bipolar cautery and gel foam should be used to ensure minimal bleeding at the time of wound closure. No consensus on this exists in the literature, but we do not restart anticoagulation medications until at least 48 hours postoperatively. In patients considered to be at high risk for bleeding, a subfascial drain can be inserted before wound closure. Less dramatic neurologic complications such as nerve root injury can occur from excessive nerve root retraction during the diskectomy. Care should be taken to retract the nerve root only to the extent necessary to remove the herniation. In our experience, making the largest possible laminotomy window reduces the amount of nerve retraction required.

If a dural tear occurs, it should be closed primarily in watertight fashion with 4-0 Nurolon suture (Ethicon). Additional dural sealants or placement of a fat graft over the dura may serve to reinforce the dural closure. In cases requiring closure of the dura, patients should be admitted and kept flat for 24 to 48 hours to reduce hydrostatic pressure on the repair site.

Epidural fibrosis should be suspected in patients presenting with new and unremitting radicular pain several weeks to months following the microdiskectomy. The exact cause is unknown; patients may present with nonmechanical pain that is not relieved by rest. Although evidence for this is lacking, we believe that placing a small amount of fat (harvested from the subcutaneous region) over the dura and exiting nerve root may reduce the risk of this complication. Although not truly a complication of microdiskectomy, recurrent radicular pain may occur in patients with a recurrent disk herniation after a period of being pain free.[6] In contrast to the symptoms of epidural fibrosis, these symptoms generally are triggered by activity, whereas knee and hip flexion provide relief. An MRI with gadolinium contrast will help the surgeon distinguish a recurrent disk herniation from epidural fibrosis.

Surgical-site infection following microdiskectomy is exceedingly rare with appropriate perioperative antibiotic administration. To further reduce this risk, we delay surgery in patients with known active infections in other regions, such as the skin, urinary tract, lungs, and teeth, even if they are under treatment for such infection.

Postoperative Care and Rehabilitation

Generally, patients are discharged 3 to 4 hours following lumbar microdiskectomy with oral opiate medications, stool softeners, and a muscle relaxant because many patients will report muscle spasms for the first several days following surgery.[7] Patients are encouraged to pursue normal activities of daily living, with the exception of waist bending and twisting and upper body lifting of more than 10 lb for the first 3 weeks. Isometric core and lower extremity exercises and hamstring flexibility routines are provided for patients to perform once per day at home for the first 3 weeks.[8] A formal outpatient physical therapy program is initiated at 3 weeks following surgery for continued core and progressive lower body strength and flexibility training. Patients are restricted from sports activities for 3 months following surgery. Return to work and driving is individualized to the patient's unique circumstances. We recently have instituted a "prehab" program whereby patients can practice and understand their postoperative care and rehabilitation before surgery.

Pearls

- Ascertaining the correct side and level of the IDH to be removed cannot be overemphasized. We strive to double-check the level and side of the herniation on MRI before obtaining consent for the procedure.
- The surgical "time out" serves as a second check. Fluoroscopic images obtained with the spinal needle pointing to the disk and with the Kocher clamp on the cephalad lamina serve as third and fourth checks.
- The tip of the Taylor retractor and the use of a Penfield 4 can be used as fifth and sixth checks of the spinal level with intraoperative fluoroscopy.
- If the disk herniation is not visualized on exposure, before performing the diskectomy, the surgeon should once again confirm that the surgical level and side are correct. The traversing nerve root should be retracted laterally (rather than medially, as described previously), thereby exposing the axilla of the nerve root. We have been pleasantly surprised in several circumstances to find the IDH to be located in the axilla of the nerve root.
- For microdiskectomy at the L5-S1 level, the surgeon should look for the presence of a spina bifida occulta on preoperative images to prevent inadvertent surgical plunging into the spinal canal and dura during the exposure.
- For a far-lateral disk procedure, we make sure to obtain true AP and lateral fluoroscopic views for planning the incision.
- Sometimes tilting the table away from the surgeon improves visualization into the foramen and the area that is lateral to the pedicle.
- Excessive retraction of the dorsal ganglion must be avoided because it can lead to postoperative radiculitis.
- The nerve root usually is displaced superiorly because the underlying pedicle blocks any inferior disk migration.

References

1. Weinstein JN, Lurie JD, Tosteson TD, et al: Surgical versus nonoperative treatment for lumbar disc herniation: Four-year results for the Spine Patient Outcomes Research Trial (SPORT). *Spine (Phila Pa 1976)* 2008;33(25):2789-2800.
2. Lurie JD, Tosteson AN, Tosteson TD, et al: Reliability of magnetic resonance imaging readings for lumbar disc herniation in the Spine Patient Outcomes Research Trial (SPORT). *Spine (Phila Pa 1976)* 2008;33(9):991-998.
3. Carragee EJ, Han MY, Suen PW, Kim D: Clinical outcomes after lumbar discectomy for sciatica: The effects of fragment type and anular competence. *J Bone Joint Surg Am* 2003;85(1):102-108.
4. Tortolani PJ, Carbone JJ, Quartararo LG: Greater trochanteric pain syndrome in patients referred to orthopedic spine specialists. *Spine J* 2002;2(4):251-254.

5. Carragee EJ, Spinnickie AO, Alamin TF, Paragioudakis S: A prospective controlled study of limited versus subtotal posterior discectomy: Short-term outcomes in patients with herniated lumbar intervertebral discs and large posterior anular defect. *Spine (Phila Pa 1976)* 2006;31(6):653-657.

6. Wera GD, Marcus RE, Ghanayem AJ, Bohlman HH: Failure within one year following subtotal lumbar discectomy. *J Bone Joint Surg Am* 2008;90(1):10-15.

7. Singhal A, Bernstein M: Outpatient lumbar microdiscectomy: A prospective study in 122 patients. *Can J Neurol Sci* 2002;29(3):249-252.

8. Newsome RJ, May S, Chiverton N, Cole AA: A prospective, randomised trial of immediate exercise following lumbar microdiscectomy: A preliminary study. *Physiotherapy* 2009;95(4):273-279.

Chapter 93
Lumbar Laminectomy

Samuel M. Davis, MD   Scott D. Boden, MD

Patient Selection
Lumbar spinal stenosis refers to a reduction in the size of the lumbar canal due to narrowing in the central canal, the lateral recess, or both. Patients with lumbar stenosis may present with radicular symptoms or reports of neurogenic claudication and classically report back, buttock, or posterior leg pain that worsens with standing and walking.

Indications
The ideal surgical candidate is one who has had a dedicated course of nonsurgical care (ideally, 3- to 6-month minimum) but has not gained satisfactory relief of pain, has a progressive neurologic deficit, or has severe impairment of activities of daily living. Nonsurgical treatments include weight loss, smoking cessation, physical therapy, and injections. A thorough nonsurgical management plan is particularly appropriate and necessary for patients with nontraditional symptoms and/or discordant history, imaging, and physical examination findings. After failed nonsurgical treatment, surgical decompression of the stenotic areas is usually indicated. Patients should also be evaluated for spondylolisthesis or instability because these conditions often require arthrodesis in addition to decompression.

Contraindications
A contraindication for laminectomy alone without arthrodesis might be severe degenerative disk changes in the face of concomitant low back pain.[1] The risk of perioperative complications increases with increasing age, so the elderly patient with multiple comorbidities may not be an appropriate candidate for surgical intervention. The risks and benefits should be discussed with the patient and/or his or her family in a shared decision-making process.

Preoperative Imaging
Preoperative imaging should include weight-bearing AP, lateral, and flexion-extension views of the lumbar spine. The images must be scrutinized closely for evidence of spondylolisthesis or instability. Additionally, the spine should be evaluated for osteophytes, asymmetric disk collapse, lateral listhesis, scoliosis, and any bony destruction because these findings may warrant additional workup or surgical procedures. Additional imaging should include MRI, MRI plus CT, or myelogram/CT, depending on the need to highlight neurologic compression and define bony anatomy. For example, a straightforward case of lumbar spinal stenosis can be sufficiently evaluated with a high-quality MRI (**Figure 1**). On the other hand, if the MRI quality is poor and/or pedicle screws are planned, then a myelogram/CT scan may be the best study. Finally, if the MRI is of good quality but pedicle screws are planned, then a plain CT may help define the bony anatomy. Although MRI is most helpful for visualization of the neural elements and soft tissues, CT is best to visualize bony pathology, such as ossification of the ligamentum flavum or abnormal pedicular anatomy.

Procedure
Room Setup/Patient Positioning
The patient can be positioned prone on a Jackson table, a regular operating room table with a bolster under the anterior superior iliac spines and the chest, or a Wilson frame, which allows the abdomen to hang freely, minimizing intra-abdominal venous pressure. The Wilson frame is beneficial because it creates more kyphosis within the lumbar spine, thus making the decompression a little easier, but it may not be as desirable if an arthrodesis is planned. Additional positions include the 90/90 position on an Andrews frame, which is also known as the knee-chest position. The advantage of the 90/90 position is that it decreases intra-abdominal venous pressure, which in turn decreases epidural venous pressure; however, it may also be associated with a higher frequency of complications related to positioning, including compartment syndrome.[2] Regardless of the specific table used, the abdomen should be free to allow for secondary decompression of the epidural venous plexus.

After positioning, the back should be prepared in a routine sterile fashion. A surgical timeout is performed. All members of the surgical team participate in identification of the patient and the surgical site as well as confirmation of the surgical procedure and preoperative antibiotic administration.

The level(s) to be operated on may be localized percutaneously by one of several methods. We prefer the insertion of two needles near the level estimated by palpation of the iliac crests. The marking needles should be placed slightly off the midline to avoid inadvertent dural puncture. A cross-table lateral radiograph can then be used to approximate the location of the desired incision. The surgical level should be confirmed with a marker or clamp placed directly on a bony structure once the spine is fully exposed to minimize the chance of wrong-level surgery.

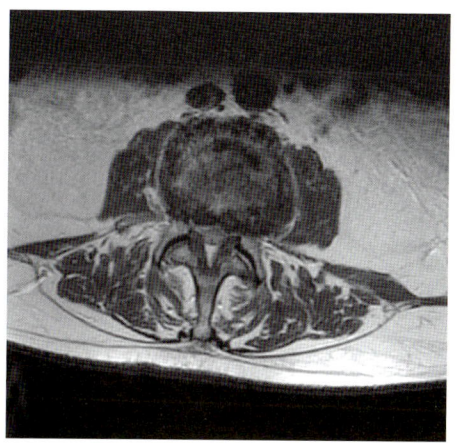

Figure 1 Axial T2-weighted MRI of the lumbar spine shows both central and lateral recess stenosis. Note the left facet arthropathy, as evidenced by the high signal intensity in that area.

Dr. Boden or an immediate family member has received royalties from Osteotech and Medtronic and serves as a board member, owner, officer, or committee member of the American Orthopaedic Association, the Eastern Orthopaedic Association, and the International Society for Study of the Lumbar Spine. Neither Dr. Davis nor any immediate family member has received anything of value from or has stock or stock options held in a commercial company or institution related directly or indirectly to the subject of this chapter.

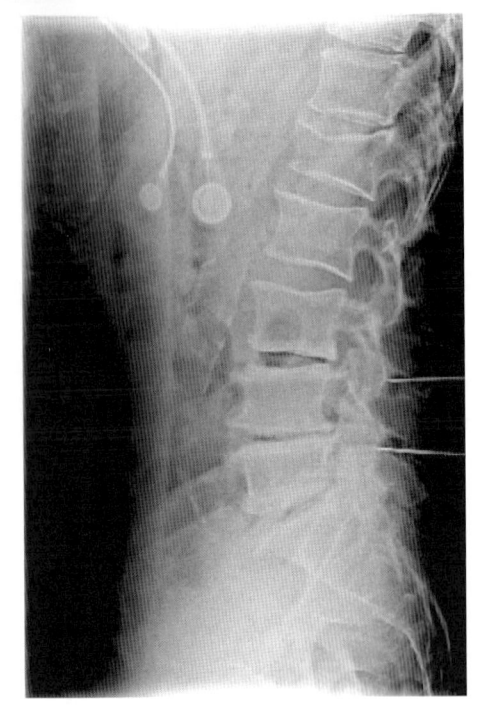

Figure 2 Intraoperative lateral radiograph shows spinal needles pointing toward the L3-4 and L4-5 disk spaces, the levels to be decompressed.

Surgical Technique

Incision and Exposure

A midline incision is made. Two Wheatlander self-retaining retractors are placed, and the Bovie monopolar electrocautery device is used to dissect through the subcutaneous tissues down to the level of the lumbodorsal fascia. The fascia should be clearly delineated in the midline and no farther laterally than needed to avoid creation of dead space. Clear identification of the fascial layer is done primarily to permit accurate reapproximation during closing to achieve a watertight fascial closure. The spinous process(es) of interest is identified based on the percutaneous localizing needles or an intraoperative lateral radiograph with a marker on a bony landmark. Subperiosteal dissection is undertaken down to the level of the lamina. In an average-size patient, inserting cerebellar retractors for retraction may be useful. In a very large patient, a larger hinged self-retaining retractor may be used. The facets of the level(s) of interest are exposed, taking care not to violate the joint capsule. If uncertainty remains with regard to which level is exposed, the level(s) to be decompressed are accurately identified by inserting two spinal needles into the exposed facets and obtaining an intraoperative lateral radiograph (**Figure 2**). The facets of interest should be marked with an indelible marking pen. The radiograph is evaluated, and the level is confirmed.

Soft-tissue exposure for decompression should proceed to the lateral aspect of the facet without violating the capsule. The lateral aspect of the pars interarticularis should also be clearly visible. This is critical to avoid excessive thinning of the pars, which places it at risk for iatrogenic fracture.

Decompression

Decompression of the lumbar spine is accomplished in three distinct stages. Stage 1 is the central decompression; stage 2 includes decompression of the lateral recess; and stage 3 involves decompression of the neuroforamina.[1]

Central Decompression

The Leksell rongeur is used to remove the interspinous ligament (**Figure 3, A**). The spinous process overlying the disk space to be decompressed is removed with a Horsley bone cutter (**Figure 3, B**). The surgeon continues using the Leksell rongeur to remove the outer cortex of the lamina at the inferior half, using the ligamentum flavum for natural protection of the neural elements (**Figure 3, C**). Once sufficiently thinned, the inner cortex of lamina is removed with Kerrison rongeurs. A small, curved Epstein curet is used to separate the ligamentum flavum from the remaining lamina (**Figure 3, D**), creating a space for the Kerrison rongeur to work safely. Bone is excised rostrally until epidural fat is exposed, at the upper border of the ligamentum flavum (**Figure 3, E**). Excision of bone cephalad to the superior margin of the ligamentum flavum places the dura at risk for inadvertent laceration because it has no protection here. The use of small cottonoid sponges can help protect the dura while the surgeon continues to remove bone rostral to the ligamentum flavum. The medial border of the facet joint may be removed with Kerrison rongeurs or a small osteotome. A Penfield dissector No. 3 is passed between the ligamentum flavum and the dura mater to create a working space and ensure there are no dural adhesions (**Figure 3, F**). In the case of epidural adhesions, a small curet or elevator is used to separate the ligamentum flavum from the dura. The curet works better for this purpose because of its broader surface, which lessens the risk of a dural tear. The completed central decompression should remove the entire lamina and all of the ligamentum flavum (**Figure 3, G**).

Lateral Recess Decompression

A Woodson elevator is used to identify the space between the remaining ligamentum flavum and the lateral recess and also those areas therein that need to be decompressed. An appropriately sized Kerrison rongeur is used to safely enter this space and remove the impinging structures (**Figure 4**). A cottonoid patty is inserted over the dura for protection. Alternatively, a 10- to 12-French suction tip or a Penfield dissector No. 3 can be used to retract the dural sac and make access to the lateral recess safer. The back of the Kerrison rongeur always remains flush with the dura to prevent inadvertent durotomy. The thicker the Kerrison rongeur footplate, the greater the safety margin to prevent redundant dura from becoming caught in the jaws of the rongeur; thus the largest Kerrison that can fit into the space without compression of the neural elements is usually the best choice. Excision of bone proceeds to the medial border of the pedicle; however, the medial facetectomy is limited to less than 50% of the total surface area to prevent iatrogenic instability.

Foraminal Decompression

The final stage is decompression of the neuroforamina. This space is probed with an angled Frazier dural elevator to identify impinging structures (**Figure 5, A**). A Kerrison rongeur is used to remove osteophytes from the superior articular process, and the trajectory of the rongeur, when used in this area, is in line with the nerve root (**Figure 5, B**). A Penfield dissector No. 4 is used to gently manipulate the nerve root to confirm that it is freely mobile.

Closure

The wound is irrigated with normal lactated Ringer solution or antibiotic-impregnated solution. Final epidural and intramuscular hemostasis is obtained with the use of bipolar and monopolar electrocautery, respectively. A medium Hemovac drain is inserted, exiting the wound at the cephalad end. The lumbodorsal fascia is identified and carefully reapproximated using No. 1 Vicryl suture (Ethicon) placed in a figure-of-8 fashion. The fascial closure is inspected for any areas of compromise. A second layer, directly above the lumbodorsal fascia, is reapproximated in a similar fashion in overweight patients to aid closure of dead space. The immediate subdermal layer is reapproximated with inverted,

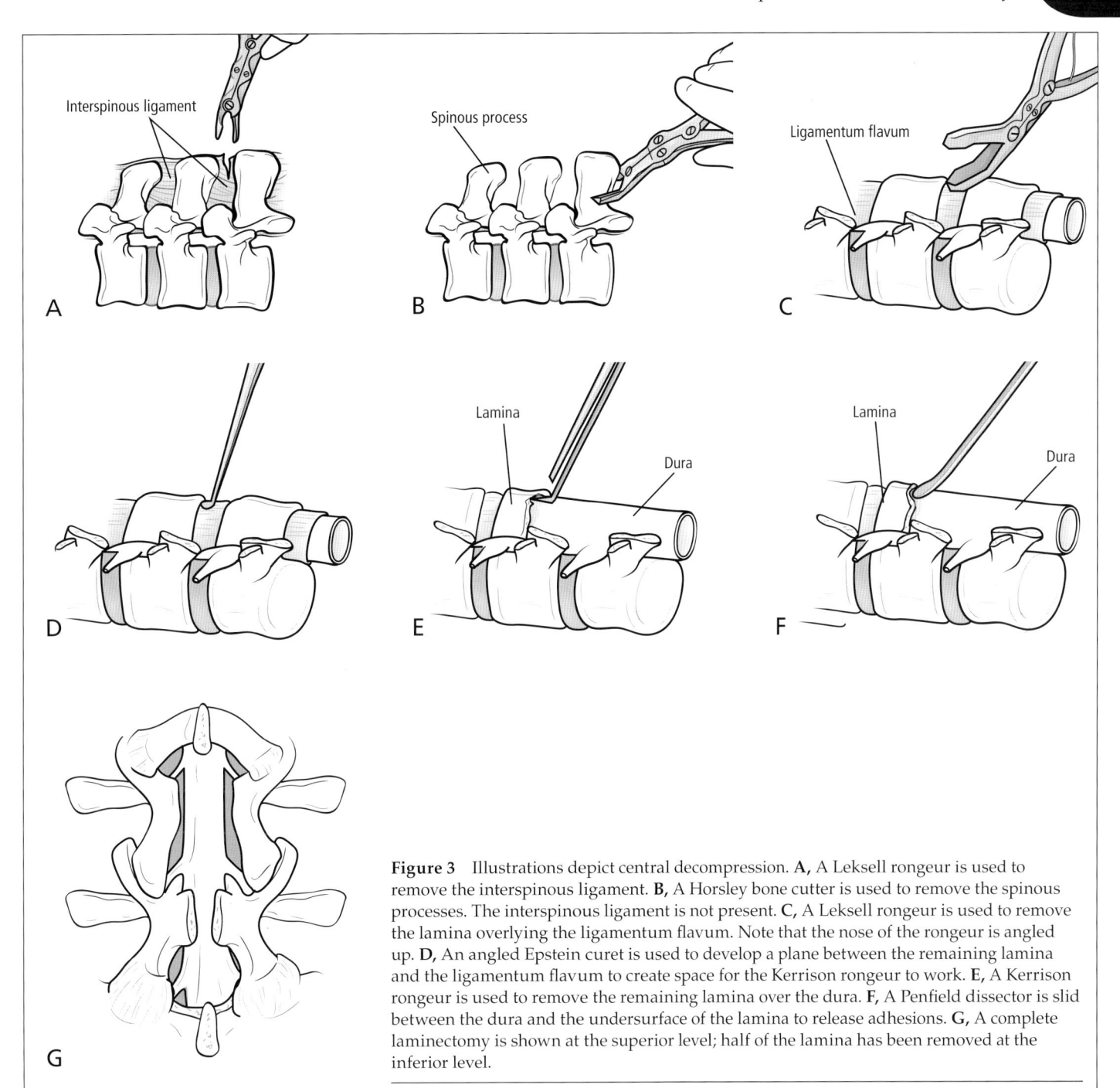

Figure 3 Illustrations depict central decompression. **A**, A Leksell rongeur is used to remove the interspinous ligament. **B**, A Horsley bone cutter is used to remove the spinous processes. The interspinous ligament is not present. **C**, A Leksell rongeur is used to remove the lamina overlying the ligamentum flavum. Note that the nose of the rongeur is angled up. **D**, An angled Epstein curet is used to develop a plane between the remaining lamina and the ligamentum flavum to create space for the Kerrison rongeur to work. **E**, A Kerrison rongeur is used to remove the remaining lamina over the dura. **F**, A Penfield dissector is slid between the dura and the undersurface of the lamina to release adhesions. **G**, A complete laminectomy is shown at the superior level; half of the lamina has been removed at the inferior level.

interrupted stitches using 2-0 Vicryl suture. The skin is closed with 3-0 or 4-0 Monocryl suture (Ethicon) in a running subcuticular fashion. Topical skin adhesive is applied and, once dry, the wound is dressed with 4 × 4 gauze sponges and soft cloth surgical tape. Alternatively, the wound is covered with benzoin and adhesive strips.

Complications

Complications specific to lumbar laminectomy include postoperative neurologic deficits, cerebrospinal fluid leaks and fistulas, facet and/or pars fractures, and infection. In general, the mortality rate ranges from 1% to 3%, depending on patient age and presence of comorbidities.[3,4] Studies often document a higher morbidity rate in elderly patients undergoing spine surgery compared with the rate in younger patients. There have been recent reports, however, of acceptably low complication rates in this older patient population that would support spinal surgery in this group.[5-8] Li et al[5] recently reported on the rates of complications after reviewing a large series of elderly patients who underwent lumbar laminectomy. They found that the in-hospital mortality rate was 0.17% and the overall complication rate was 12.17%. The most common complications were postoperative hematoma (5.2%) and nonspecific renal complications (2.8%). They also found that mortality and complication rates increased with age and the presence of comorbidities. Patients older than 85 years with three or more comorbidities were found to have a complication rate of 18.9% and a mortality rate of 1.4%. Patients older than 85 years with no comorbidities had a lower complication rate (14.7%) and mortality rate (0.22%).[5]

In lumbar spine surgery, the rate of durotomy is between 1% and 17%.[9] Any durotomy found at the time of surgery should be repaired. Primary closure with 5-0 or 6-0 Prolene (Ethicon) is preferred when possible. For larger defects, the surgeon can consider using a muscle

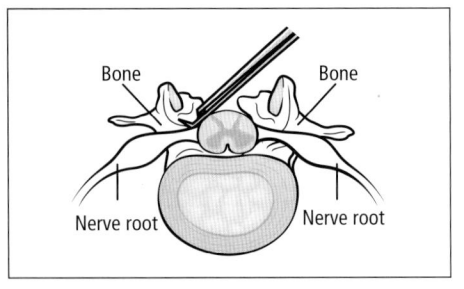

Figure 4 Illustration depicts lateral recess decompression. A Kerrison rongeur is used to remove bone and ligamentum flavum from the lateral recess.

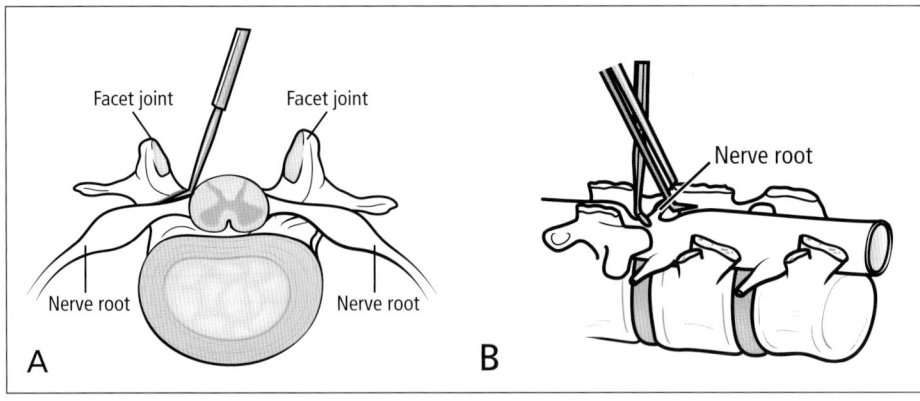

Figure 5 Illustrations depict foraminal decompression. **A,** A Frazier dural elevator is used to palpate the foraminal space to assess stenosis. **B,** A Kerrison rongeur is used to remove bone from within the foraminal space. Note that the Kerrison rongeur is angled in the same direction as the nerve root.

or a fascial graft. Other adjuncts such as DuraGen patches (Integra), fibrin glue, and subarachnoid lumbar drains are considered for tears not amenable to primary closure. Patients are generally kept flat in bed for 48 hours to allow the durotomy to seal, but this time frame may be adjusted depending on the severity of the tear and/or the integrity of the repair. Patients are also generally kept in a supine position in bed, but lying on the side or prone may encourage less egress of fluid through the durotomy site and thus hasten healing.

Postoperative Care and Rehabilitation

All patients receive postoperative antibiotics for 24 hours. A patient-controlled anesthesia (PCA) pump is often used for pain control. Patients begin to transfer from bed to chair at 24 to 48 hours postoperatively, as pain dictates. On postoperative day 1, the drain is removed (depending on the amount of drainage) as well as the Foley catheter. The PCA is discontinued, and the patient is transitioned to oral medications for pain control. Physical therapists provide assistance with overall gait and mobility. Most patients who have an uncomplicated single-level laminectomy go home on postoperative day 1. Those who undergo multilevel decompressions may stay for an additional day, depending on their ability to mobilize and/or the drain output. Bracing is not routinely used. Patients are allowed to shower 3 to 5 days after discharge but are not allowed to take baths or soak (eg, pool, sauna). They are instructed to avoid any bending, lifting, and twisting for 6 weeks, which coincides with their first postoperative visit.

Pearls

- Confirmation of the correct surgical level should be performed before starting any portion of the decompression.
- Care should be taken to avoid violation of the facet capsule to avoid iatrogenic arthrosis or instability.
- The pars interarticularis should be exposed to safely decompress the level of interest.
- A potential space should always be created between the bone and the ligamentum flavum to allow safe passage of the Kerrison rongeur.
- The use of cottonoid sponges can protect the dura from the Kerrison rongeur once the ligamentum flavum has been removed.
- Care should be taken to carefully release adhesions to avoid inadvertent durotomy.
- Decompression at the level of interest should proceed to the medial border of the pedicle.
- Visualization of the shoulder of the nerve root ensures that the entry zone to the foramen is adequately decompressed.
- When performing the foraminotomy, the Kerrison rongeur should work parallel to the trajectory of the nerve root.

References

1. Hanley EN, Patt JC: Surgical management of lumbar spinal stenosis, in Herkowitz HN, Garfin S, Eismont FJ, Bell GR, Balderston RA, eds: *Rothman-Simeone: The Spine*, ed 5. Philadelphia, PA, Saunders, 2006, pp 1015-1024.
2. Singh K, Samartzis D, Biyani A, An HS: Lumbar spinal stenosis. *J Am Acad Orthop Surg* 2008;16(3):171-176.
3. Atlas SJ, Keller RB, Wu YA, Deyo RA, Singer DE: Long-term outcomes of surgical and nonsurgical management of lumbar spinal stenosis: 8 to 10 year results from the Maine Lumbar Spine Study. *Spine (Phila Pa 1976)* 2005;30(8):936-943.
4. Galiano K, Obwegeser AA, Gabl MV, Bauer R, Twerdy K: Long-term outcome of laminectomy for spinal stenosis in octogenarians. *Spine (Phila Pa 1976)* 2005;30(3):332-335.
5. Li G, Patil CG, Lad SP, Ho C, Tian W, Boakye M: Effects of age and comorbidities on complication rates and adverse outcomes after lumbar laminectomy in elderly patients. *Spine (Phila Pa 1976)* 2008;33(11):1250-1255.
6. Best NM, Sasso RC: Outpatient lumbar spine decompression in 233 patients 65 years of age or older. *Spine (Phila Pa 1976)* 2007;32(10):1135-1140.
7. Cassinelli EH, Eubanks J, Vogt M, Furey C, Yoo J, Bohlman HH: Risk factors for the development of perioperative complications in elderly patients undergoing lumbar decompression and arthrodesis for spinal stenosis: An analysis of 166 patients. *Spine (Phila Pa 1976)* 2007;32(2):230-235.
8. Deyo RA, Cherkin DC, Loeser JD, Bigos SJ, Ciol MA: Morbidity and mortality in association with operations on the lumbar spine: The influence of age, diagnosis, and procedure. *J Bone Joint Surg Am* 1992;74(4):536-543.
9. Saxler G, Krämer J, Barden B, Kurt A, Pförtner J, Bernsmann K: The long-term clinical sequelae of incidental durotomy in lumbar disc surgery. *Spine (Phila Pa 1976)* 2005;30(20):2298-2302.

Chapter 94
Instrumented Lumbar Fusion

Andrew J. Schoenfeld, MD   Christopher M. Bono, MD

Patient Selection

Transpedicular (pedicle) screws gained wide popularity in the United States through the efforts of Steffee et al,[1] and since the late 1980s, their indications and use have expanded substantially.[2-4] Pedicle screws are anchored within the corticocancellous core of the vertebral pedicle. This anatomic region offers the strongest point of fixation within the spine and affords pedicle screws a biomechanical advantage over other instrumentation techniques such as hooks, wires, or anterior vertebral body screws.[2,5-7] Several investigations have shown that the use of pedicle screw fixation enhances arthrodesis rates in the lumbar spine.[2-4] It is an important component of more modern surgical techniques, such as transforaminal lumbar interbody fusion, all-posterior correction of idiopathic scoliosis, minimally invasive treatment of fractures, and posterior dynamic stabilization.

Indications

Transpedicular instrumentation may be indicated in any situation in which a lumbar fusion will be performed.[4] Common spinal conditions that are treated using instrumented lumbar fusion include stenosis with spondylolisthesis, spinal tumors, fractures, deformity, iatrogenic instability, and recurrent disk herniations.[1-5]

Contraindications

Absolute contraindications to pedicle screw fixation are anatomic variations that render the pedicle too small to safely accept the smallest available diameter pedicle screw and congenital absence of the pedicle. A relative contraindication is the presence of a tumor or other destructive bone lesion that would not adequately support a screw. Patients with profound osteoporosis are at increased risk of screw loosening, loss of fixation, and construct failure.

Preoperative Imaging

Ideally, patients who are selected for a lumbar fusion procedure should have plain radiographs and an MRI or CT scan. At minimum, MRI or CT is required to assess the pedicle dimensions. Plain radiographs are most useful to assess spinal alignment. Rotational deformities must be appreciated because these can affect the degree of medialization of the screw path. Hyper- or hypolordosis must also be noted because this will affect the sagittal alignment of the screw path.

In the lumbar spine, the optimal starting point for a pedicle screw can be identified by the intersection of two orthogonal lines: a horizontal line that bisects the transverse process, and a vertical line along the medial aspect of the pars interarticularis (**Figure 1**). These anatomic landmarks should be visualized on the AP view preoperatively.

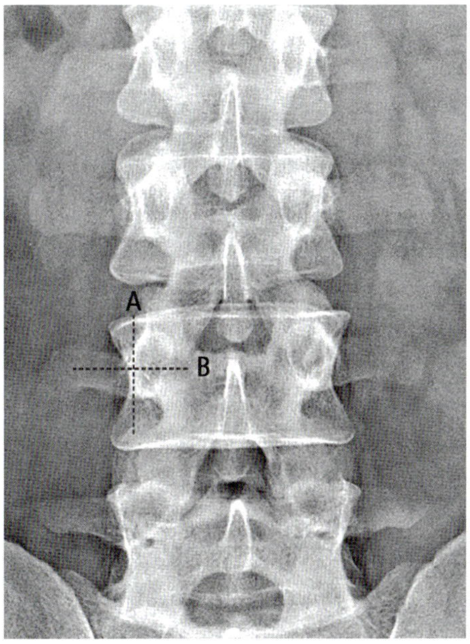

More precise preoperative planning can be achieved using axial MRI or CT images. Factors that may prevent the safe insertion of pedicle screws, such as dysplastic or absent pedicles, aberrant nerve roots, or dural ectasia, are best appreciated in these images. Axial images should be routinely used to measure the pedicle diameters and approximate screw lengths at the proposed instrumented levels (**Figure 2, A**). Screw length can be measured preoperatively by measuring from the posterior aspect of the superior articular process to a desired depth within the vertebral body (**Figure 2, B**). The smallest transverse width of the pedicle should be used to determine pedicle screw diameter. The pullout strength of the pedicle screw is dependent on the interface between the cortical bone of the pedicle and the screw threads.[6,7] Therefore, it is not advisable to undersize the screws. Screws with a slightly larger width may be used as "rescue" screws in the setting of a compromised screw tract. Careful, slow insertion will allow the cortical walls of the tract to accommodate screws with a moderately larger width. There is no good evidence, however, that supports the routine use of larger width pedicle screws in conventional tracts that have not been otherwise compromised. Approximate screw sizes for each vertebral level and side are transcribed on a preoperative template paper that can be brought to surgery.

Figure 1 The appropriate starting point for pedicle screw insertion can be identified on an AP radiograph. Line A extends along the medial aspect of the pars interarticularis; line B bisects the transverse process. The intersection of these two lines indicates an appropriate starting point for screw insertion.

Dr. Schoenfeld or an immediate family member serves as a board member, owner, officer, or committee member of the American Academy of Orthopaedic Surgeons. Dr. Bono or an immediate family member has received nonincome support (such as equipment or services), commercially derived honoraria, or other non–research-related funding (such as paid travel) from Harvard Clinical Research Institute and Intrinsic Therapeutics and serves as a board member, owner, officer, or committee member of the American Academy of Orthopaedic Surgeons, the International Society for the Advancement of Spinal Surgery, and the North American Spine Society.

Disclaimer: Some authors are employees of the U.S. federal government and the United States Army. The opinions or assertions contained herein are the private views of the authors and are not to be construed as official or reflecting the views of William Beaumont Army Medical Center, the Department of Defense, or the United States government.

Section 7: Spine

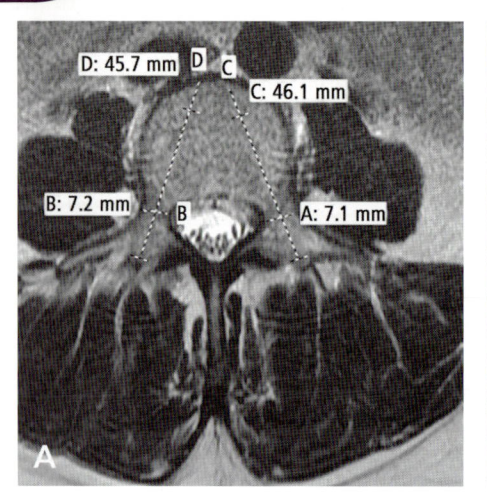

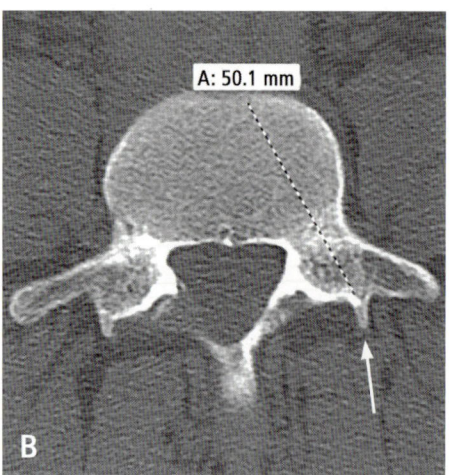

Figure 2 Preoperative images used to plan pedicle screw placement. **A,** Axial MRI shows the templating used to determine the appropriate size of pedicle screws. The widths (lines A and B) and lengths (lines C and D) are determined for pedicle screws bilaterally. **B,** Axial CT scan shows how the accessory process (arrow) can be used as an anatomic landmark for the screw insertion site.

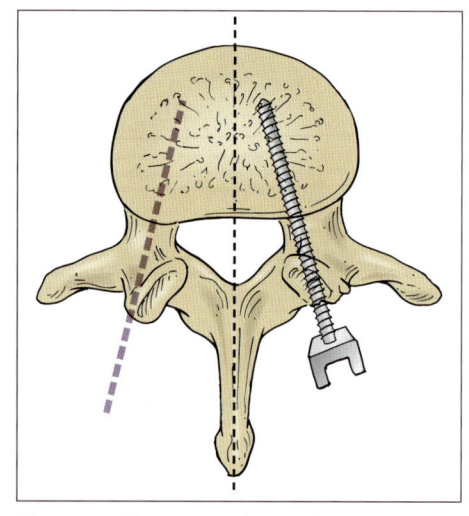

Figure 3 Illustration shows the proper trajectory for pedicle screw insertion within the vertebral body. Note that the screw tip does not cross the midline.

Video 94.1 Lumbar Laminectomy. Howard S. An, MD; Dino Samartzis, BS; Ashok Biyani, MD (4 min)

Procedure

Room Setup/Patient Positioning

Proper positioning of the patient is critical. The patient should be placed prone on a well-padded radiolucent table appropriate for spinal surgery. We prefer a Jackson four-poster surgical frame with a chest pad and supports for the iliac crest and thighs. The abdomen should hang free to reduce intra-abdominal pressure, thereby decompressing the Batson plexus and minimizing epidural bleeding during a decompression procedure. Additional padding should be placed under the knees and along the anterior legs to avoid pressure points. The shoulders should be abducted and the elbows flexed no more than 90° on well-padded arm boards. The anterior shoulder should be properly bolstered if needed to prevent brachial plexus stretch. A head positioner should maintain the neck in a neutral position, avoid pressure around the eyes, and allow access to the endotracheal tube.

Once proper positioning has been ensured, all wires, lines, and catheters should be secured to the frame of the operating table. This allows the C-arm to move about the patient with less risk of inadvertently dislodging a critical monitor or access mechanism. The operating table should be placed in the center of the room, with the anesthesia station located at the head. The surgeon and assistant stand on opposite sides of the patient. The fluoroscopic imaging system can be placed in an appropriate position where the operating surgeon can easily see the images. The preoperative template paper may be secured to the image viewer for ease of consultation.

Before the patient is prepared and draped, we make sure that adequate fluoroscopic views can be obtained. Minor adjustment of the patient's rotation on the table can yield a better AP view of the surgical levels. In addition, the lateral view can be used to mark the levels of the pedicles to be instrumented and thus help determine the incision size.

Special Instruments/Equipment/Implants

Pedicle screws are inserted by first preparing a tract (**Figure 3**). Starter awls, taps, and depth gauges can be used during this process and are usually provided in the pedicle screw manufacturer's instrumentation set. With the screw in place, a rod is secured to each with a "blocker" or set screw. The set screws are final tightened using the manufacturer's torque-limiting driver, which avoids undertightening or stripping of the set screw.

Some surgeons find it useful to have a burr available for instrumentation cases. A larger (5-mm) burr can be used to define the lateral edge of arthritic facet joints to appropriately visualize the starting point for the pedicle screws. A larger burr is also effective for removing the posterior cortical bone at the insertion site to better visualize the cancellous bone of the pedicle. A large burr is also the most common tool used to decorticate bone in the area of the fusion bed.

If desired, electrophysiologic monitoring can be used to assess nerve root activity during the procedure and test pedicle screws for aberrant placement.[8,9] Triggered electromyography (EMG) performed by stimulating the pedicle screw after it has been inserted yields a threshold at which the adjacent lumbar nerve root is stimulated. High thresholds, typically greater than 10 mA, are needed if the screw is contained in bone and are thus indicative of a well-placed screw.[4,8,9] Moderate thresholds (5 to 9 mA) suggest that a breach of the pedicle wall may be present but the screw is not contacting the nerve; low thresholds (< 5 mA) suggest that the screw is in direct contact with the nerve. If there is a discrepancy in the threshold reading, the EMG probe can be used to directly stimulate a nerve root to obtain a baseline reading for comparison.[4]

Video 94.2 Spinal Fusion. Howard S. An, MD; Dino Samartzis, BS; Ashok Biyani, MD (7 min)

Surgical Technique

A midline incision is made to perform a standard posterior approach to the lumbar spine (**Figure 4**). Alternative incisions can be used, such as bilateral paraspinous incisions, if the midline structures are to be maintained. The length of the skin incision can be minimized by using lateral fluoroscopy to assist in plotting an incision that extends from the spinous pro-

612 © 2013 American Academy of Orthopaedic Surgeons

Chapter 94: Instrumented Lumbar Fusion

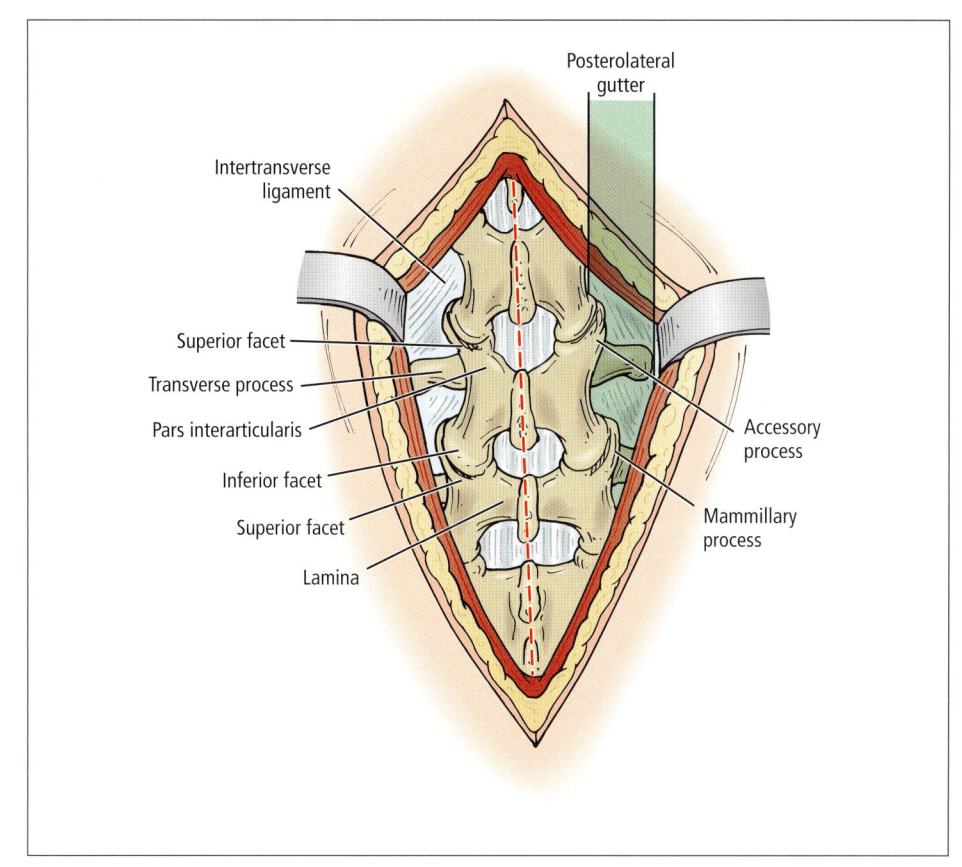

Figure 4 Illustration shows the relevant anatomy of the posterior elements of the lumbar spine for lumbar fusion using pedicle screws. The dashed red line indicates the approximate site of the surgical incision.

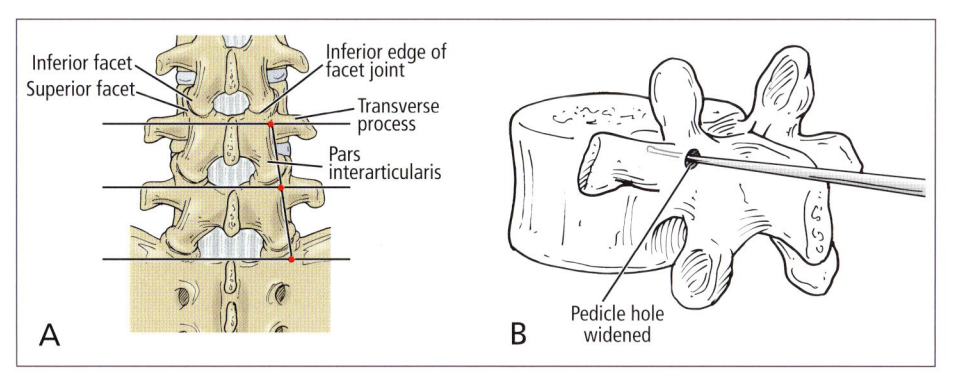

Figure 5 Illustrations demonstrate the technique for inserting pedicle screws. **A,** The appropriate starting points (red dots) of pedicle screws within the lumbar spine are shown. **B,** The proper path for cannulating the lumbar pedicle and the tract for screw insertion is shown.

First, the starting point is located by identifying the junction between a horizontal line bisecting the transverse process and a vertical line running along the superior articular process (**Figure 5, A**). The medial aspect of the pars can also be used as a guide post, as discussed previously (**Figure 1**). This point usually corresponds to the inferolateral aspect of the facet joint. In some patients, an accessory process may be present (**Figure 4**) that can be a useful landmark for the screw insertion site. Because of the unique anatomy of the S1 vertebra, the appropriate starting point for an S1 pedicle screw is at the junction of the sacral ala and the inferolateral aspect of the S1 superior articular process, which once again roughly corresponds to the inferolateral aspect of the facet joint. Not uncommonly, the facet joints are hypertrophic, which can obscure the appropriate starting point for pedicle screws. In such cases, the osteophytes can be removed to allow accurate localization.

With the site identified, the cortex of the bone must be entered. This can be performed using a rongeur, a start awl, or a small (3-mm) burr. Our preference is to use a burr guided by an AP fluoroscopic view. Generally, a blush of bleeding from the underlying cancellous bone will be encountered upon entry into the pedicle. Next, the pedicle finder is inserted to create the screw tract.

Using lateral fluoroscopy, the pedicle finder is slowly advanced under manual control through the pedicle and into the vertebral body (**Figure 5, B**). During this process, the finder should be angled medially about 10° to 15° until the tip reaches the posterior portion of the vertebral body. Once at this level, more aggressive medial angulation can be applied. Steady but yielding resistance should be felt during insertion. Increasing resistance can indicate abutment with a cortical border. Sudden "give-way" can suggest penetration of a cortical boundary and should also prompt repositioning and image confirmation. Barring these hindrances, the probe is advanced to the desired depth within the vertebral body, usually near the junction of the anterior and middle thirds. Bicortical pedicle screw placement is generally not advisable, except in the case of screws placed into the S1 vertebral body. The length of the screw is judged using laser markings on the finder.

The pedicle finder is then removed, and the screw tract is assessed with a ball-tipped probe. It is carefully advanced

cess of the vertebral level above the most cranial vertebra to the spinous process of the caudal instrumented level. The paraspinal musculature is stripped subperiosteally with the use of electrocautery. Care should be taken to avoid injury to the facet joint capsules until the desired levels of fusion have been confirmed intraoperatively. Dissection lateral to the facet capsules enables exposure of the relatively deep transverse processes. Exposure is complete once the transverse processes, pars interarticulari, laminae, facet joints, and spinous processes in the zone of fusion are adequately exposed. If any decompression is indicated, we like to perform it at this stage; however, some surgeons prefer to instrument first and then perform decompression.

Pedicle screw insertion can be performed with or without live image guidance. At a minimum, plain radiographs should be obtained in sterile fashion after instrumentation has been placed to check its orientation. Live image guidance can range from simple fluoroscopy to more sophisticated computerized image registry. We prefer to use orthogonal fluoroscopic images during screw insertion.

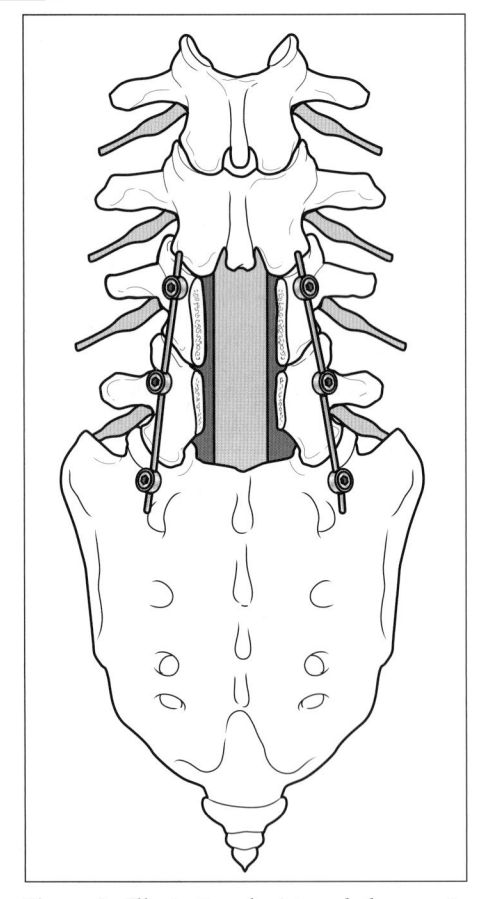

Figure 6 Illustration depicts rod placement for pedicle screw fixation. The proper placement of connector rods within the pedicle screw heads is shown.

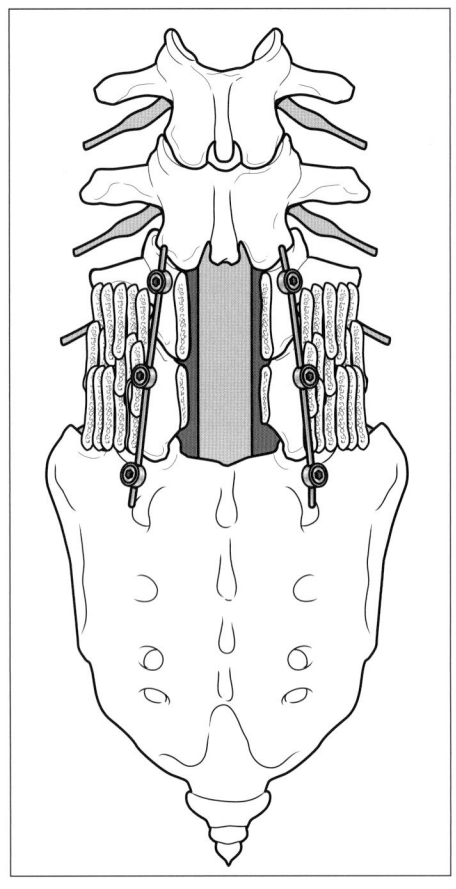

Figure 7 Illustration demonstrates the appropriate final appearance of a posterolateral instrumented lumbar fusion construct following bone graft placement.

through the tract and used to confirm four intact "walls" (superior, inferior, lateral, and medial cortices within the pedicle) and a solid "floor" (end point within the vertebral body). If a cortical violation is identified, a new pedicle tract should be created following a more appropriate trajectory. If desired, the screw tract can be tapped at this time. Tapping may not be necessary in all patients and has been shown to decrease screw pullout strength in osteoporotic bone.[6,7] We prefer to undertap the screw hole.

The screw length is judged intraoperatively, but the screw width is determined preoperatively by measurements made on axial CT or magnetic resonance images. Once the appropriately sized screw is inserted into the prepared tract, its position can be confirmed using AP and lateral fluoroscopic views. On a perfect AP view, the screw tip should not cross the midline. On a perfect lateral view, the screw should be confined within the bony borders of the pedicle. If desired, EMG stimulation may be used at this time to assess thresholds as described previously.[8,9]

After all screws have been satisfactorily inserted and their orientation confirmed radiographically, flexible rod templates can be used to estimate the appropriate size of the longitudinal member (ie, rod). In most instances, 5.5- or 6.0-mm titanium rods are used. Larger diameter rods create a stiffer construct, which can be useful in certain instances (eg, deformity, tumor, trauma). However, stress shielding of the arthrodesis site may also potentiate pseudarthrosis. Stainless steel rods are more rigid than their titanium counterparts; however, they cannot be coupled with titanium pedicle screws and are less resistant to bacterial colonization. Although an adequately sized, precut, precontoured rod can be used in most short constructs, rods may also be cut to size and bent to provide a more custom fit. An appropriately sized rod should extend beyond the margins of the cephalad and caudad pedicle screw heads by no more than 2 to 3 mm to avoid impingement on the facet joints of the adjacent nonfused levels (**Figure 6**).

Next, the rod is fixated to the screw heads by inserting set screws. These must be final tightened using the specific manufacturer's torque-limiting devices. During final tightening, an antitorque sleeve is placed over the pedicle screw head to counteract rotational forces to the construct. This is particularly important in patients with osteopenic bone. Final radiographs are obtained to confirm the position and alignment of the construct. The use of "cross-links," or coupler connections, can further enhance the biomechanical rigidity of an instrumented construct. This may be useful in the setting of osteoporotic or osteopenic bone, where there is a concern regarding the purchase of the pedicle screws. Such devices, however, are not routinely used in short-segment constructs (ie, those spanning three lumbar levels or less).

Next, preparation of the fusion bed and bone graft placement is performed. Some authors prefer to decorticate the transverse processes before screw insertion because the screw heads somewhat obscure visualization. At a minimum, the transverse processes and facet joints within the zone of fusion should be decorticated. All cartilage should be removed from within the facet joints in the fusion zone. If the midline structures are still present, the laminae and spinous processes can also be decorticated. A generous amount of bone graft is then placed along these surfaces (**Figure 7**).

At this time, the wound is copiously irrigated and adequate hemostasis is confirmed. A subfascial drain can be placed. The wound is closed in multilayer fashion, with particular attention paid to achieving a tight reapproximation of the lumbar fascia. Simple buried, interrupted sutures are used to close the subcutaneous layers. A running subcuticular absorbable suture, staples, or a running locked nylon suture may be used to definitively close the skin. A sterile dressing is applied, and the patient is transferred to a hospital bed.

Complications

Despite their utility, pedicle screws have been shown to increase the potential for complications compared with stand-alone decompression or uninstrumented fusion.[2,5] Complications specific to transpedicular instrumentation include nerve root impingement from misplaced screws, fracture of the pedicle, dural tear, and injury to the great vessels.[5,8,10-12] Moreover, suboptimal screw placement may not be as biomechanically strong and could potentiate increased risk of failure.

Successful insertion of pedicle screws requires an intimate three-dimensional understanding of spinal anatomy.

Overall, the risk of complications following instrumented spinal fusions has been reported to be in the range of 10% to 20%.[3,5,8,10-12] This risk may be higher in complex cases such as spinal deformity, revision surgery, or instances of tumor. The risk of neural compromise is greater for screws that breach the medial or inferior pedicle wall.[8,10,13] Inferior pedicle wall breaches in the lower lumbar spine are at greater risk of nerve root impingement than those that occur at more cephalad levels.[13]

In a review of 424 pedicle screws inserted using fluoroscopic guidance in 102 patients, Amato et al[10] reported a misplacement rate of 5%, with an additional 3% of screws demonstrating pedicle wall violation. The direction of misplacement was most commonly lateral, and only two patients sustained nerve root injury from the misplaced screws. Although some authors have reported a misplacement rate closer to 2%,[8] the meta-analysis performed by Kosmopoulos and Schizas[14] returned an average rate of 9% for transpedicular screw misplacement in a combined series of more than 37,000 screws.

Several authors have hypothesized that most misplaced screws, especially those involving a breach in the lateral pedicle wall, do not result in symptoms or damage to adjacent structures.[8,10,13] In a series of 226 patients undergoing posterior fusion procedures, Krishna et al[12] reported a 7% incidence of neuralgia (16 patients), but the condition was found to result from screw misplacement in only two instances. In the study by Amato et al,[10] fewer than 10% of patients with misplaced screws were symptomatic. Similarly, Foxx et al[11] documented that among 182 patients, 33 of 680 pedicle screws were in contact with a major vascular structure, including the aorta, iliac artery, and iliac veins. In most instances, the offending screw was at L5 or S1. None of the screws appeared to have penetrated the blood vessels, however, and no clinically relevant sequelae were reported.

Postoperative Care and Rehabilitation

Patients who undergo lumbar instrumented spinal fusion may remain in the hospital for approximately 3 days after the procedure. Ambulation is encouraged on postoperative day 1, if not earlier. The Foley catheter is discontinued as soon as the patient is able to stand or sit at the side of the bed. Prophylactic postoperative antibiotics are continued for 24 hours after surgery. The subfascial drain is maintained until the output is less than 30 cm³ per shift, which most commonly occurs by the morning of the second postoperative day. The surgical dressing is changed on the second postoperative day unless it is soiled or saturated before that time. Standing AP and lateral radiographs are obtained once the patient has ambulated and is able to bear weight comfortably (Figure 8).

Individuals are restricted from heavy lifting, vigorous twisting at the waist, and flexion at the waist according to surgeon preference. Our practice is to recommend avoiding these activities for 12 weeks after fusion. Clinical and radiographic follow-up after surgery usually occurs at 2 weeks, 3 months, 6 months, and 1 year.

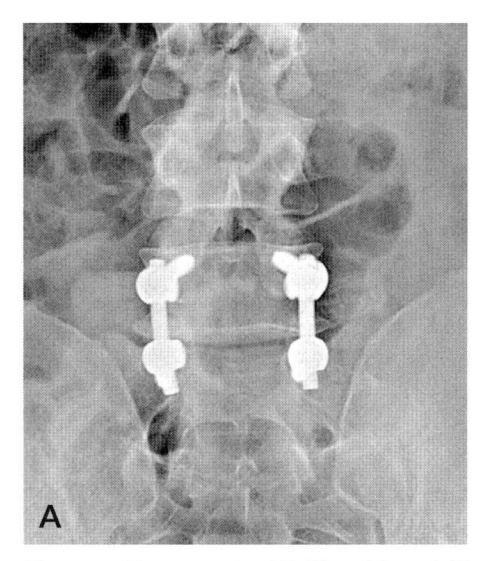

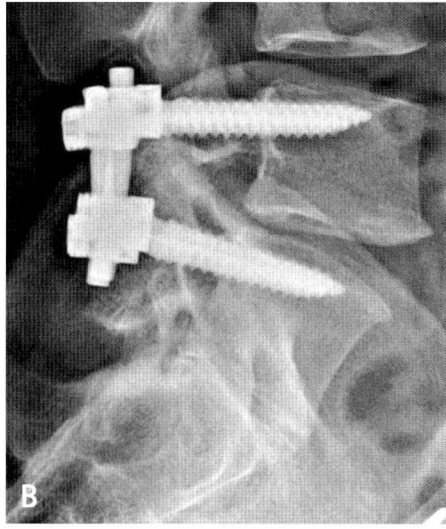

Figure 8 Postoperative AP (**A**) and lateral (**B**) radiographs of a patient who underwent an instrumented L5-S1 fusion for dynamic instability. The images demonstrate correct positioning of the pedicle screws as they should appear on AP and lateral radiographs.

Pearls

- Performing the same surgical step at multiple screw insertion sites (ie, consecutively preparing all screw tracts with the pedicle finder before proceeding with tapping or screw insertion) can be time efficient.
- Failure of the pedicle screw driver to maintain a medial trajectory following screw insertion may indicate a laterally misplaced screw.
- If the position of a screw is questionable, the C-arm can be used to "rainbow" over the pedicle tube so that the beam is in line with the exact trajectory of the pedicle. If the pedicle screw has been placed correctly, the resultant image will show the screw as a bull's-eye within the cortical ring of the pedicle. A similar maneuver can also be performed prior to screw insertion, using a ball-tipped probe.
- Preparation of the fusion bed may be easier if performed before rod or screw insertion.
- Failure to confirm a satisfactory pedicle screw tract with the ball-tipped probe increases the risk of screw misplacement and damage to adjacent structures.
- Damaging facet joints or the facet capsule in regions of the spine not included within the fusion can increase the potential for adjacent segment degeneration.
- Inadequate surgical exposure inhibits successful preparation of a fusion bed and also increases the risk of screw misplacement.
- If osteophytes over hypertrophic facet joints are not resected, the starting point is more difficult to identify, and the risk of screw misplacement can be increased.

References

1. Steffee AD, Biscup RS, Sitkowski DJ: Segmental spine plates with pedicle screw fixation: A new internal fixation device for disorders of the lumbar and thoracolumbar spine. *Clin Orthop Relat Res* 1986;203:45-53.
2. Zhang HY, Kim DH: Transpedicular screw fixation, in Kim DH, Henn JS, Vaccaro AR, Dickman CA, eds: *Surgical Anatomy and Techniques to the Spine*. Philadelphia, PA, Saunders, 2006, pp 239-245.

3. Fritzell P, Hägg O, Wessberg P, Nordwall A; Swedish Lumbar Spine Study Group: 2001 Volvo Award Winner in Clinical Studies: Lumbar fusion versus nonsurgical treatment for chronic low back pain. A multicenter randomized controlled trial from the Swedish Lumbar Spine Study Group. *Spine (Phila Pa 1976)* 2001;26(23):2521-2534.

4. Glassman SD, Carreon L, Dimar JR: Outcome of lumbar arthrodesis in patients sixty-five years of age or older: Surgical technique. *J Bone Joint Surg Am* 2010;92(suppl 1, pt 1):77-84.

5. Esses SI, Sachs BL, Dreyzin V: Complications associated with the technique of pedicle screw fixation: A selected survey of ABS members. *Spine (Phila Pa 1976)* 1993;18(15):2231-2239.

6. Carmouche JJ, Molinari RW, Gerlinger T, Devine J, Patience T: Effects of pilot hole preparation technique on pedicle screw fixation in different regions of the osteoporotic thoracic and lumbar spine. *J Neurosurg Spine* 2005;3(5):364-370.

7. Chatzistergos PE, Sapkas G, Kourkoulis SK: The influence of the insertion technique on the pullout force of pedicle screws: An experimental study. *Spine (Phila Pa 1976)* 2010;35(9):E332-E337.

8. Kim YW, Lenke LG, Kim YJ, et al: Free-hand pedicle screw placement during revision spinal surgery: Analysis of 552 screws. *Spine (Phila Pa 1976)* 2008;33(10):1141-1148.

9. Clements DH, Morledge DE, Martin WH, Betz RR: Evoked and spontaneous electromyography to evaluate lumbosacral pedicle screw placement. *Spine (Phila Pa 1976)* 1996;21(5):600-604.

10. Amato V, Giannachi L, Irace C, Corona C: Accuracy of pedicle screw placement in the lumbosacral spine using conventional technique: Computed tomography postoperative assessment in 102 consecutive patients. *J Neurosurg Spine* 2010;12(3):306-313.

11. Foxx KC, Kwak RC, Latzman JM, Samadani U: A retrospective analysis of pedicle screws in contact with the great vessels. *J Neurosurg Spine* 2010;13(3):403-406.

12. Krishna M, Pollock RD, Bhatia C: Incidence, etiology, classification, and management of neuralgia after posterior lumbar interbody fusion surgery in 226 patients. *Spine J* 2008;8(2):374-379.

13. Söyüncü Y, Yildirim FB, Sekban H, Ozdemir H, Akyildiz F, Sindel M: Anatomic evaluation and relationship between the lumbar pedicle and adjacent neural structures: An anatomic study. *J Spinal Disord Tech* 2005;18(3):243-246.

14. Kosmopoulos V, Schizas C: Pedicle screw placement accuracy: A meta-analysis. *Spine (Phila Pa 1976)* 2007;32(3):E111-E120.

Video Reference

94.1 Adapted from An HS, Samartzis D, Biyani A: Video: *Lumbar Spinal Stenosis: Laminoplasty.* Rosemont, IL, American Academy of Orthopaedic Surgeons, 2003.

94.2 Adapted from An HS, Samartzis D, Biyani A: Video: *Lumbar Spinal Stenosis: Laminoplasty.* Rosemont, IL, American Academy of Orthopaedic Surgeons, 2003.

Chapter 95
Transforaminal Lumbar Interbody Fusion

Oliver O. Tannous, MD   Kelley Banagan, MD   Steven C. Ludwig, MD

Introduction

Transforaminal lumbar interbody fusion (TLIF) was first described by Harms and Rolinger[1] in 1982. The approach they introduced allows the surgeon to access the intervertebral disk space with relative ease and safety. Similar to posterior lumbar interbody fusion, TLIF provides the surgeon with the ability to fuse a spinal segment anteriorly and posteriorly through a single posterior procedure.[2] This approach eliminates the morbidity and potential complications of anterior fusion, including iliac vessel damage, deep venous thrombosis secondary to vessel retraction, and retrograde ejaculation from hypogastric plexus injury.[3]

The transforaminal approach also provides several advantages over the direct posterior approach. TLIF allows the surgeon to access the disk space through a single unilateral posterior approach. This allows preservation of the contralateral lamina and spinous process, which creates a larger surface area to achieve a concomitant posterolateral fusion. Additionally, a transforaminal approach to the disk space exposes the neural foramen for direct decompression and eliminates the need to retract the thecal sac, reducing the risk of incidental durotomy, permitting access to more cephalad lumbar levels, and minimizing risk of injury to the conus medullaris and spinal cord. This approach is also favored in revision cases in which epidural fibrosis is sometimes present.

The intervertebral disk space is an ideal environment for obtaining bony fusion, largely because of the compressive forces of the anterior column and the abundant blood supply provided by the surgically prepared end plates. In the human spine, 80% of the mechanical load is transmitted through the vertebral body and 20% is transmitted through the posterior elements. With a standard posterolateral fusion, the fusion bed is placed under tensile forces as compared with the interbody fusion, in which the forces are under compression, thus rendering interbody fusion advantageous in many clinical scenarios. TLIF combined with posterolateral instrumentation and fusion, however, achieves fusion rates greater than 90% and clinical outcomes comparable to those achieved with anterior lumbar interbody fusion combined with posterolateral instrumentation and fusion.[3-5] With a combined TLIF and posterolateral technique, patients benefit from results similar to those achieved through a single unilateral approach, with less blood loss and avoidance of the morbidity associated with the anterior approach.

Patient Selection
Indications
TLIF is ideal for treating lumbar spine deformity and degenerative disk disease because interbody fusion restores disk space height and lordosis, indirectly decompressing the neural foramen and achieving sagittal balance. The indications for TLIF include isthmic spondylolisthesis (grades I and II), foraminal intervertebral disk herniations, recurrent disk herniations, degenerative disk disease causing mechanical back pain with or without radiculopathy, postlaminectomy spondylolisthesis, postlaminectomy kyphosis, and lumbar coronal or sagittal plane deformities.

Contraindications
Despite its many advantages, TLIF is not indicated for every patient. Contraindications for TLIF include severe osteopenia, in which setting the implant and/or graft material might subside into the end plates of the superior and inferior vertebral bodies. Patients with bleeding disorders are at risk of developing an epidural hematoma as a result of the facetectomy, which is crucial to performing this procedure and can cause substantial bleeding. TLIF is also relatively contraindicated in patients with an active infection, either local or systemic.

Preoperative Imaging
Figure 1, A and **B,** are preoperative AP and lateral radiographs, respectively, of a 54-year-old woman with a history of intractable left-greater-than-right lower extremity radiculopathy. At the time of initial evaluation, radiographs revealed an L4-L5 spondylolisthesis. **Figure 1, C** shows a preoperative sagittal CT scan of the same patient. The patient underwent posterior decompression, fusion, and TLIF at the L4-L5 level.

Procedure
Room Setup/Patient Positioning
After induction of general anesthesia, the patient is turned prone on a Jackson table. Care is taken to pad all bony prominences, including the anterior superior iliac spines and the elbows. The abdomen is freed of compression to relieve intra-abdominal pressure throughout the procedure. Neuromonitors are placed on the lower extremities in a lumbar dermatomal distribution. Throughout the procedure, the anesthesiologist keeps the patient in a relatively hypotensive state to help reduce blood loss. Neuromonitoring and fluoroscopic technicians must be available throughout the case.

Special Instruments/Equipment/Implants
- Pedicle screw system
- Structural interbody spacer options: titanium cages, polyetheretherketone cages, structural machined allograft, poly-L/D-lactide resorbable spacer
- Bone graft materials
- C-arm
- Neuromonitoring equipment
- Bipolar cautery, straight osteotome, Kerrison and Leksell rongeurs, straight and curved curets and pituitaries, disk space shavers, disk space dilators, disk space trials, a high-speed burr

---

Dr. Banagan or an immediate family member serves as a paid consultant to or is an employee of Spinal Dimensions. Dr. Ludwig or an immediate family member has received royalties from DePuy and Globus Medical; is a member of a speakers' bureau or has made paid presentations on behalf of DePuy and Synthes; serves as a paid consultant to or is an employee of DePuy, Globus Medical, and Synthes; has stock or stock options held in Globus Medical and Alphatec Spine; and serves as a board member, owner, officer, or committee member of the Cervical Spine Research Society. Neither Dr. Tannous nor any immediate family member has received anything of value from or has stock or stock options held in a commercial company or institution related directly or indirectly to the subject of this chapter.

Section 7: Spine

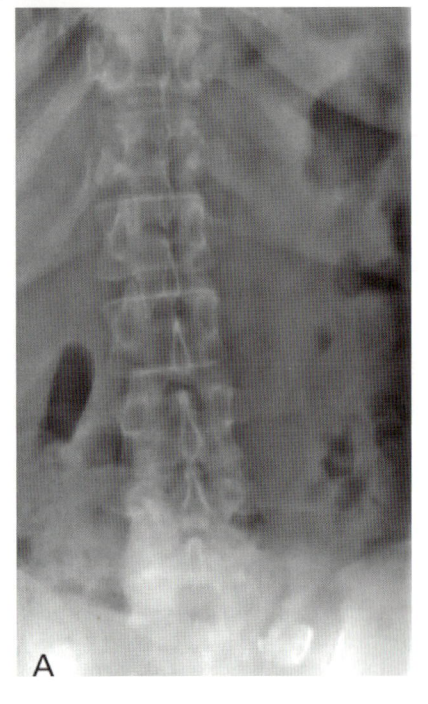

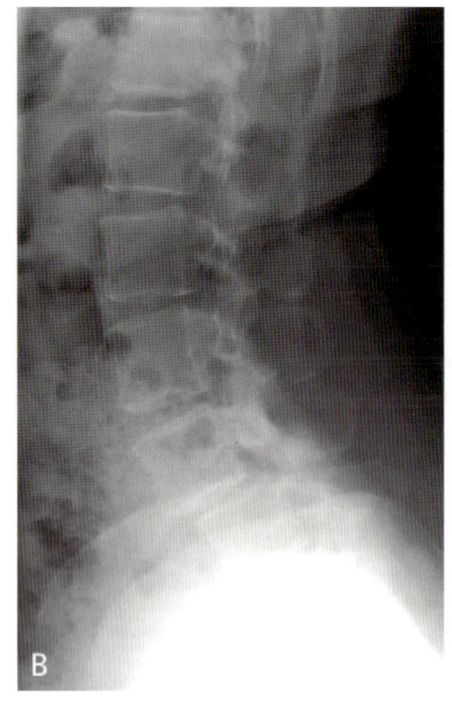

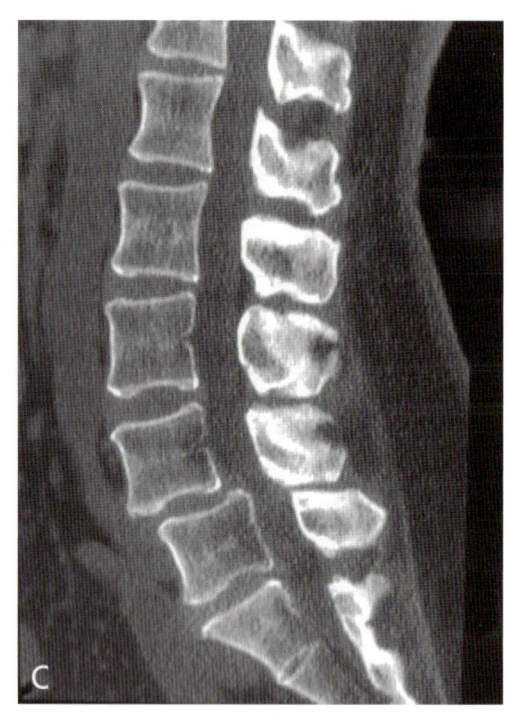

Figure 1 Preoperative images of a 54-year-old woman who presented with reports of worsening back pain and lower extremity radiculopathy reveal L4-L5 spondylolisthesis. **A,** AP radiograph. **B,** Lateral radiograph. **C,** Sagittal CT scan.

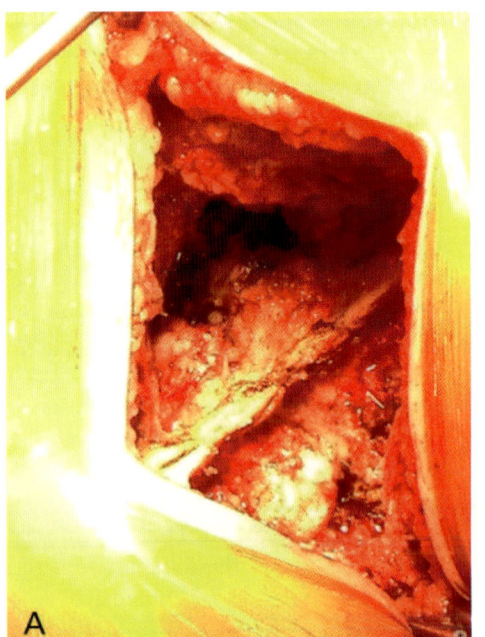

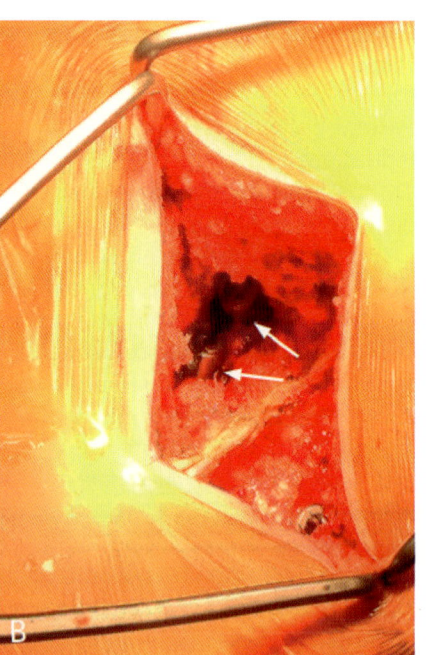

Figure 2 Intraoperative photographs of a transforaminal lumbar interbody fusion (TLIF). **A,** A standard midline dissection is made through the skin and subcutaneous tissues, exposing the transverse processes of the involved level. **B,** Pedicle screws are placed at the indicated levels (arrows) prior to creating a working TLIF window.

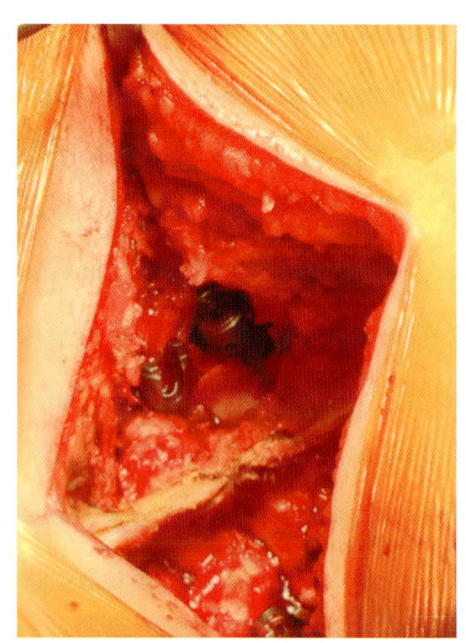

Figure 3 Intraoperative photograph shows the TLIF window created to access the disk space.

Surgical Technique
Open TLIF
Once the patient is positioned and prepared in a sterile fashion, the lumbar level(s) of interest are marked with the use of fluoroscopic visualization. The surgeon can choose to perform the TLIF on the side with the greatest clinical and/or radiographic pathologic abnormality. A standard midline incision is created through the skin and subcutaneous tissues. The dissection is continued in a standard subperiosteal manner, which might include the transverse process of the involved levels (**Figure 2, A**). Once dissection is achieved, pedicle screws are placed at the indicated level(s) (**Figure 2, B**). Next, a window is created to access the disk space (**Figure 3**). The inferior articular facet of the cephalad vertebra and the superior articular facet of the caudal vertebra are resected. To achieve resection, a straight osteotome is used to create a partial laminotomy in the inferior lamina of the cephalad vertebra (**Figure 4, A**); the pars interarticularis is then transected and the inferior facet of the vertebra above is removed (**Figure 4, B**). Kerrison and Leksell rongeurs are used to resect the superior articular facet of the caudal vertebra (**Figure 4, C**). This bone is saved to be used as local autologous bone graft.

Chapter 95: Transforaminal Lumbar Interbody Fusion

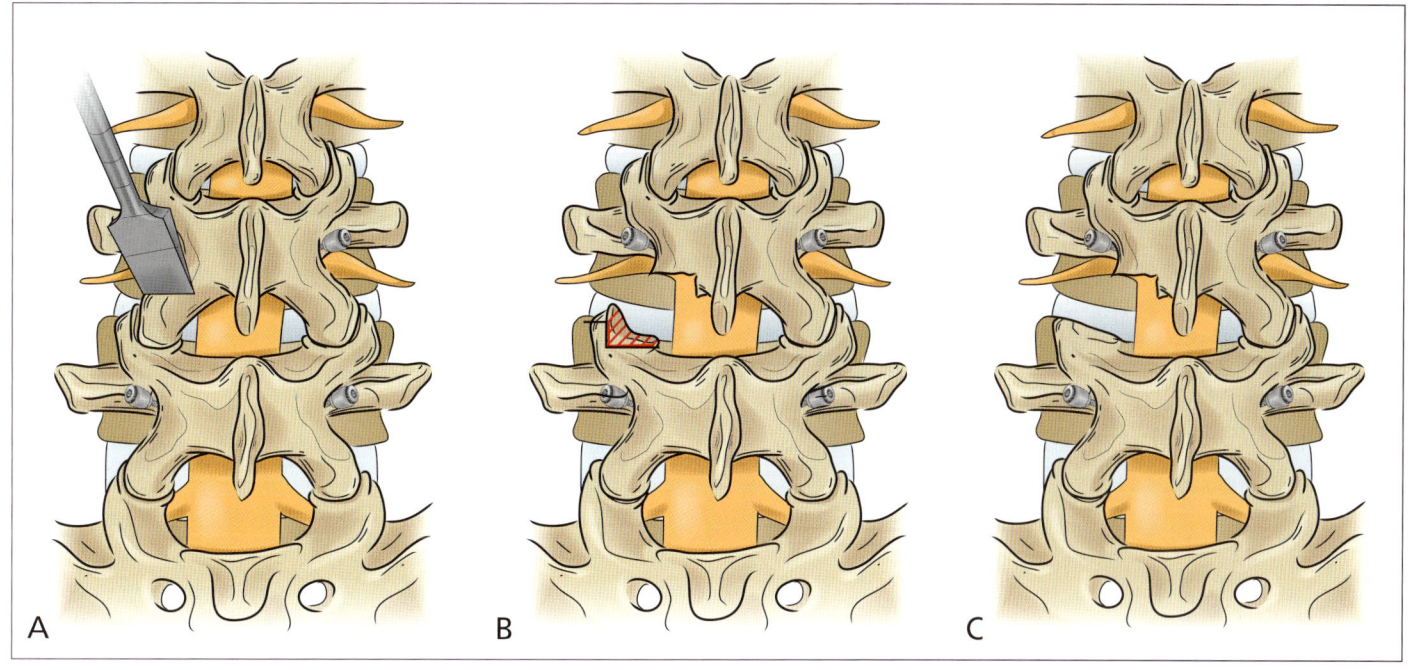

Figure 4 Illustrations show a laminotomy during a TLIF. **A,** A straight osteotome is used to create a partial laminotomy in the inferior lamina of the cephalad vertebra. **B,** The pars interarticularis of the vertebra above is transected and the inferior facet is removed. **C,** The superior articular facet of the caudal vertebra is resected, allowing a window of access to the intervertebral disk.

Once the working window is created, the exiting nerve root is decompressed, and completion of the facetectomy allows for the traversing nerve root to be visualized and freed up. Bipolar cautery is applied to bleeding epidural vessels, and a nerve root retractor is placed medially to protect the dural sac. The advantage of the transforaminal approach is that minimal retraction of the dural sac is needed. Exposure of the disk space is achieved with a Penfield dissector. A large boxcut annulotomy is created in the disk space to begin a thorough and complete diskectomy.

The diskectomy is initiated with straight pituitary rongeurs and curets (Figure 5, A) and is continued with angled pituitaries and curets (Figure 5, B) to access the contralateral disk space. Disk and cartilage material is carefully removed from the superior and inferior end plates with straight and angled curets. Sequential dilators and shavers can be used to open up the disk space and facilitate a complete diskectomy (Figure 6).

Once the end plates are prepared, a lamina spreader can be used to help distract at the spinous processes. Alternatively, additional distraction force can be applied to the pedicle screws (Figure 7).

Once serial dilation has achieved the desired fit, a trial implant is inserted and tamped anteriorly and medially. The fit of the trial implant is confirmed with tactile feedback and radiographically. The

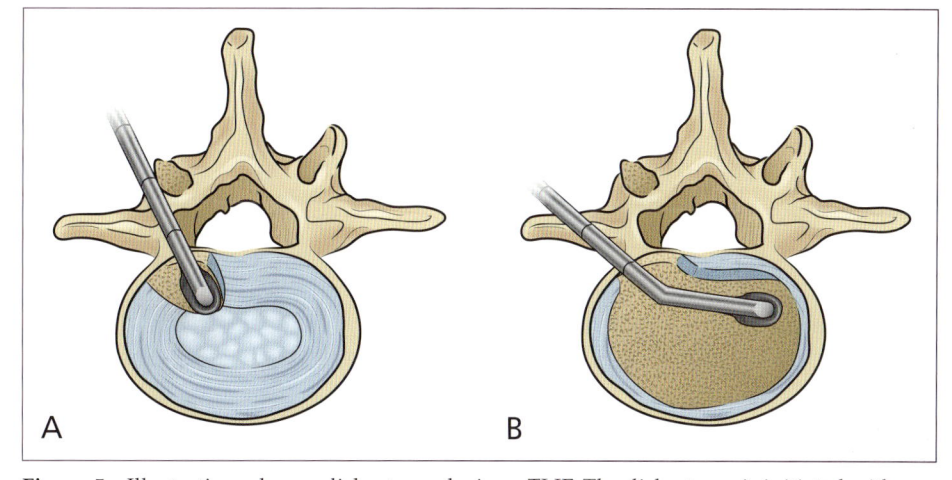

Figure 5 Illustrations show a diskectomy during a TLIF. The diskectomy is initiated with straight curets (**A**) and is continued with angled curets (**B**) to access the contralateral disk space.

trial is then removed, and the implant is tamped into the anterocentral aspect of the disk space (Figure 8). This positioning optimizes the load-sharing capacity of the implant and helps restore lumbar lordosis.

If pedicle screws were not inserted at the start of the procedure, they are inserted at this point. Rods are then placed, and compression is applied to compress the interbody graft and to improve the lumbar lordosis. Final tightening of the implants is performed, and radiographic confirmation of appropriate implant and graft placement is assessed (Figure 9). The surrounding bone is decorticated with a high-speed burr to form a fusion bed. Depending on the clinical scenario, the surgeon might choose to perform an intertransverse process fusion. The foramen and canal are probed to verify that no free bone is present. The wound is irrigated, and bone graft is placed meticulously about the fusion bed. Finally, wound drains are placed and the wound is closed.

Minimally Invasive TLIF

The indications for minimally invasive TLIF are similar to those for the open technique. The success of the minimally invasive procedure is in part a function

© 2013 American Academy of Orthopaedic Surgeons

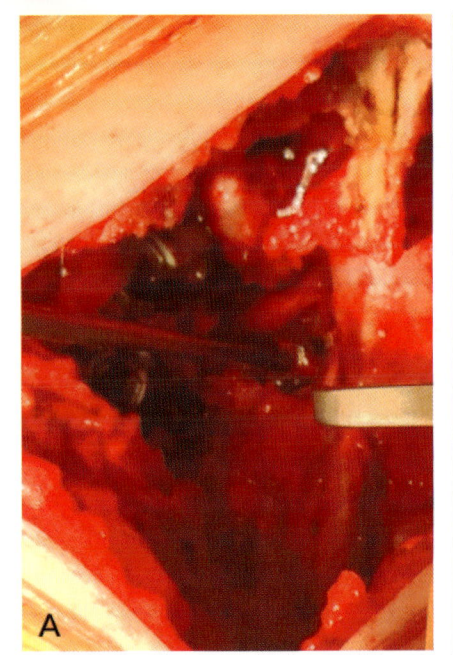

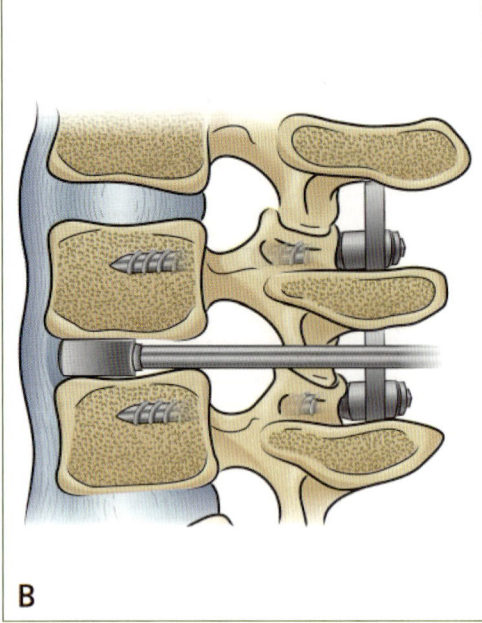

Figure 6 Sequential dilators are used to distract the disk space and facilitate the performance of a complete diskectomy during a TLIF. Intraoperative photograph (**A**) and illustration (**B**) show insertion of a dilator into the disk space.

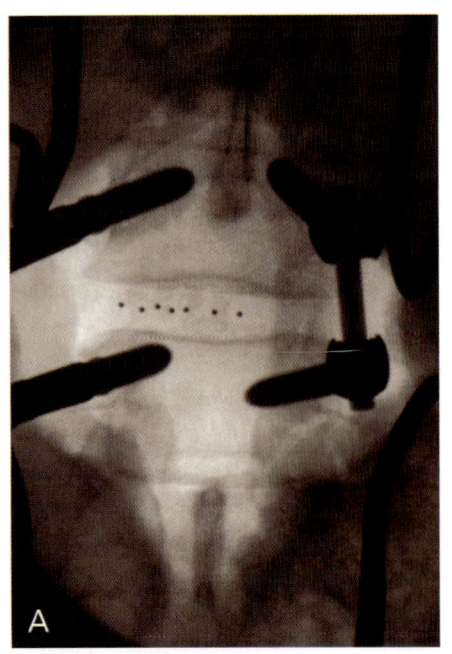

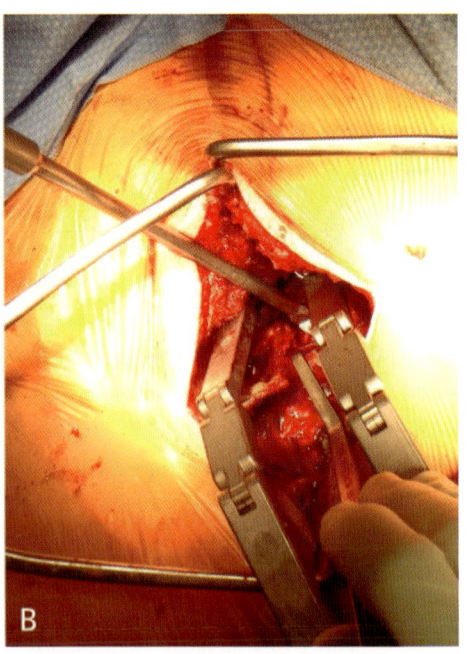

Figure 7 Images demonstrate distraction being applied to the pedicle screws to facilitate the insertion of the implant into the anterior central aspect of the disk space. **A**, Fluoroscopic image of the patient in Figure 1. **B**, Intraoperative photograph.

of the surgeon's experience and comfort with the technique, which requires a steep learning curve.

Under fluoroscopic guidance, a 2- to 5-cm incision is made approximately 4 to 5 cm lateral to the midline and centered over the facet joint. A guidewire is inserted, aiming toward the facet with a lateral-to-medial vector. Bleeding is controlled with electrocautery. Serial dilators are passed over the guidewire, and a 22- to 26-mm–diameter tube is inserted directly over the facet complex. Once this is achieved, a microscope or illuminated tube and loupe combination is used for the remainder of the procedure. The remaining steps of the procedure are similar to those of the open technique.

Minimally Invasive Versus Open TLIF

During the past decade, the minimally invasive technique of TLIF has gained increasing popularity around the world, as evidenced by the increasing number of studies published during the past several years. The minimally invasive technique has several purported benefits over the open technique, including less blood loss, the need for fewer postoperative transfusions, less postoperative back pain, quicker time to ambulation, a briefer hospital stay, and significantly fewer surgical-site infections.[6,7] These benefits are credited to the significantly less extensive and traumatic dissection required.[6,8]

One study that conducted a literature review of 10 minimally invasive TLIF procedures and 20 open TLIF procedures calculated a cumulative incidence of surgical-site infection of 0.4% in minimally invasive TLIF cases versus 4.0% of open TLIF cases.[7] As with any minimally invasive technique, however, a learning curve is associated with minimally invasive TLIF. In one study of 86 cases, the authors described a significant decrease in surgical time and blood loss between the first third and latter two thirds of their patient cohort, resembling a logarithmic curve approaching a steady state after the first 30 cases.[8] Interestingly, the authors state that a plateau in operating room time was reached long after the surgeons achieved proficiency, which they attribute to the additional learning curve of the surgical team, including scrub nurses, assistants, and fluoroscopic technicians.[8]

Complications

The TLIF procedure has become increasingly popular since its original description in 1982, as has the minimally invasive TLIF during the past decade. Several complications associated with TLIF, however, have been described. They include infection, durotomy, pseudarthrosis, postoperative radiculopathy, symptomatic pedicle screw malposition, migration of the interbody spacer, ileus, and epidural hematoma.[4,5,9-13]

Infection

The overall average infection rate associated with TLIF is reported to be 3.3% (range, 0% to 9%).[4,9-13] In almost all cases in which the infection was not a superficial site infection, surgical irrigation, débridement, and long-term antibiotics administered intravenously were indicated.

Incidental Durotomy

The rate of incidental durotomy is reported to be between 0% and 20%, with an average of 4.8%.[4,10,13] In one series of 531 open TLIF procedures, the authors found that durotomy is 1.75 times more likely to occur during a revision lumbar procedure; this is attributed to the scar tissue that forms around the dura.[10]

Hematoma
The reported postoperative epidural hematoma rate is 3% to 4%.[12,13] In all reported cases, revision surgery was required to address this complication.

Postoperative Radiculopathy
Postoperative radiculopathy is reported at an average rate of 5.3% (range, 0% to 14%).[4,12,13] This is defined as new-onset pain or muscle weakness in a dermatomal distribution. In one study of 119 TLIF procedures, postoperative radiculopathy occurred in 14% of the cases in which recombinant human bone morphogenetic protein–2 (rhBMP-2) was used within the intervertebral space, compared with 3% of the cases in which iliac crest autograft was used.[12] Interestingly, within the rhBMP-2 group, the authors found that the rate of radiculopathy diminished 75% when a hydrogel sealant was used to seal the annulotomy.[12]

Pseudarthrosis
In a meta-analysis of studies reporting fusion rates of open versus minimally invasive TLIF techniques, the authors calculated an overall pseudarthrosis rate of 9% for the open technique and 5% for the minimally invasive method.[5] The authors were unable to perform subgroup analysis regarding fusion enhancers because of the lack of data and homogeneity across studies; however, they noted that bone morphogenetic protein (BMP) was used in 12.2% of open TLIF cases versus 50% of minimally invasive TLIF cases.[5] These data suggest BMP has an enhancing effect on interbody and posterolateral fusion. In one study in which the pseudarthrosis rate was 23%, the authors attributed the aberrantly high rate to a learning curve effect, specifically vertebral endplate preparation technique and type of interbody implant used.[11] They reported a 40% pseudarthrosis rate with split femoral ring allograft compared with 7.5% with milled semilunar allograft.[11]

Pedicle Screw Malposition
Although symptomatic pedicle screw malposition is a rare complication in the hands of an experienced surgeon, the rate is reported to be between 1.4% and 2.1% in three large series.[10,12,13] In all cases, patients underwent revision surgery for screw removal.

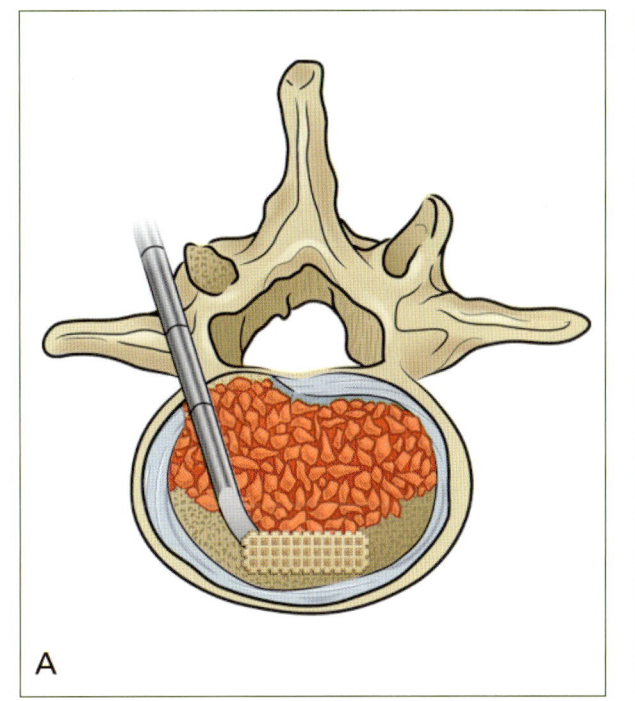

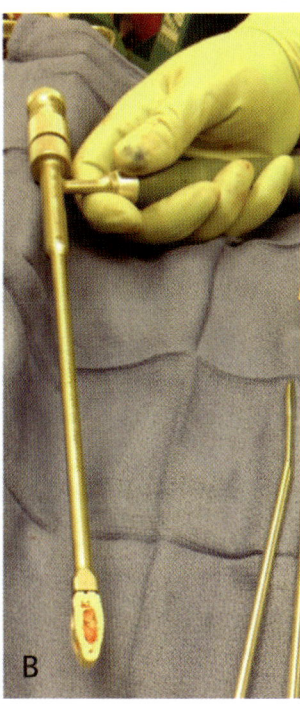

Figure 8 Placement of the TLIF implant. **A,** Illustration shows the TLIF implant being tamped into the anterocentral aspect of the disk space. The remainder of the intervertebral space is filled with bone graft. **B,** Photograph shows the interbody implant with interposed bone graft, attached to the inserter.

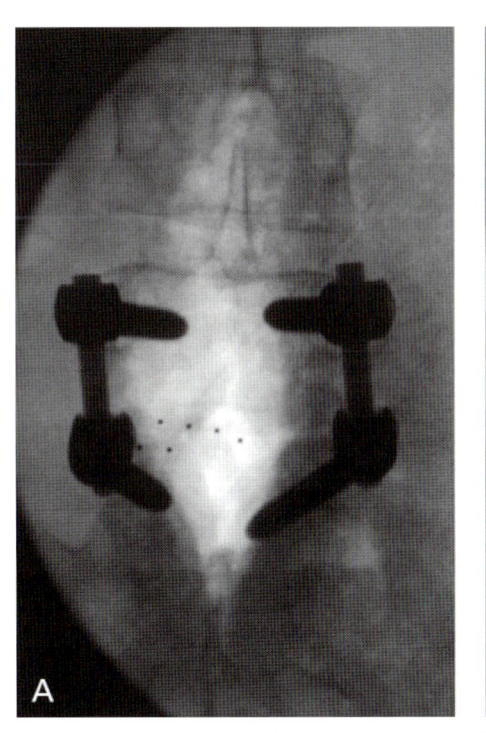

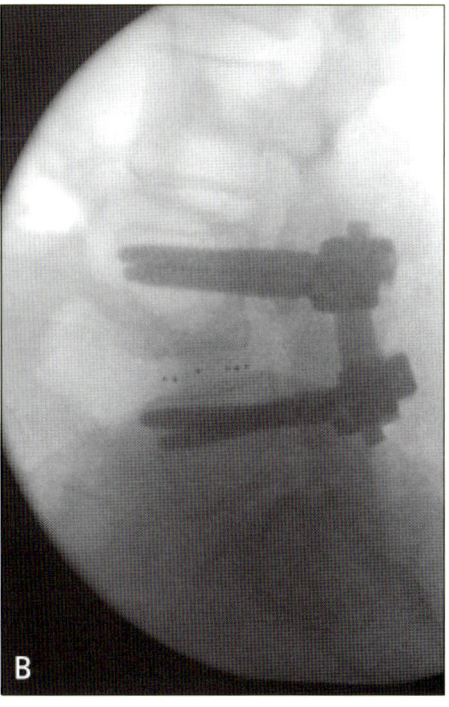

Figure 9 Intraoperative fluoroscopic images of the patient in Figures 1 and 7 obtained after implant placement for transforaminal lumbar interbody fusion. **A,** AP view confirms screw and interbody placement. The interbody is represented by the dots visible within the disk space. **B,** Lateral view.

Interbody Spacer Migration
Intervertebral implant migration or symptomatic graft extrusion is a rare but serious complication. Most series that report complications associated with TLIF do not note implant migration. Such underreporting likely occurs because most implant migration is asymptomatic. In one large series, migration of the interbody spacer occurred in 1.9% of the cases (10 patients).[10] Nine of ten patients underwent revision surgery; most of the patients presented with new-onset radicular symptoms in the distribution of the

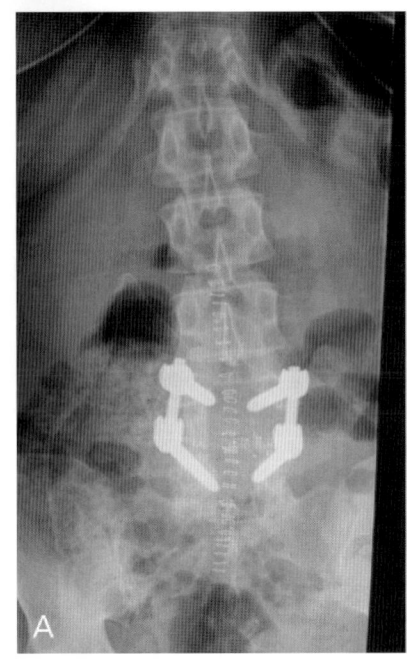

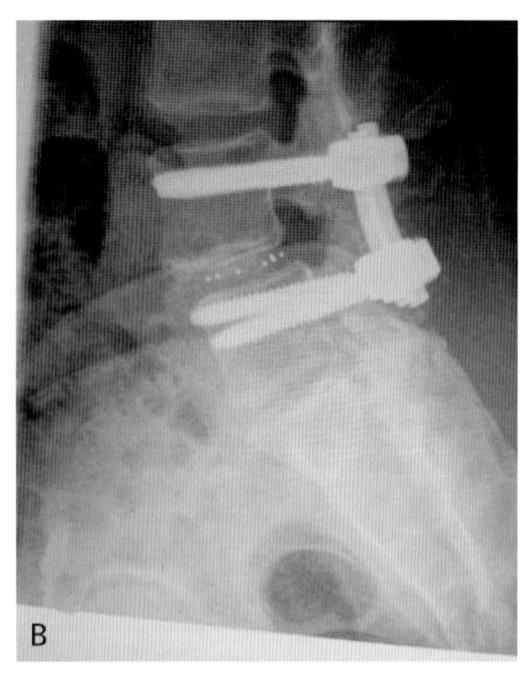

Figure 10 Postoperative standing AP (**A**) and lateral (**B**) radiographs of the 54-year-old patient in Figures 1, 7, and 9 who underwent TLIF and posterolateral fusion for the treatment of L4-L5 spondylolisthesis, associated stenosis, and resultant lower extremity radiculopathy.

cage migration. Many factors are related to this complication, including interbody preparation, implant selection, and implant placement.[9]

Ileus

The incidence of postoperative ileus with a TLIF approach has been reported to be 3%.[4,12] This is significantly lower than the rate reported with an anterior approach.[3]

Postoperative Care and Rehabilitation

Immediate mobilization of the patient postoperatively is encouraged. Standing AP and lateral radiographs are obtained before the patient is discharged (**Figure 10**). During the patient's hospitalization, physical and occupational therapists are consulted to teach the patient the proper ways of bending, lifting, and turning. The patient is instructed to ambulate as much as possible to improve aerobic conditioning. No restrictions are assigned regarding stair climbing. No postoperative bracing is required. Patients are allowed to drive when they feel they can appropriately react to the road and are no longer receiving narcotics. Postoperative outpatient physical therapy is implemented at 6 weeks postoperatively. All restrictions regarding activities are typically lifted at the 3-month postoperative visit. Patients are followed both clinically and radiographically for a minimum of 1 year or until confirmation of fusion has been obtained.

Pearls

- Care must be taken to free the ligamentum flavum from the lamina, especially during revision cases in which significant fibrosis is present.
- Care must be taken not to violate the pedicles above or below the level(s) of interest during this exposure. The Kerrison rongeur is used to resect the pars interarticularis. A high-speed cutting burr is used to thin down the bony elements.
- Care must be taken to protect the exiting nerve root in the foraminal zone. The dorsal root ganglion is present in this region and can be iatrogenically damaged.
- The annulotomy must not be performed before achieving complete visualization of both the exiting and traversing nerve roots.
- Thorough preparation of the end plates is critical. This will ensure the absence of disk material within the fusion bed and enhance the fusion potential.
- A thorough end-plate preparation must be performed without violating the subchondral bone of the end plate. This can lead to subsidence of the implant, nonunion, and the development of segmental kyphosis.
- One must be mindful not to violate the anterior anulus to avoid anterior migration of the cage, bone graft, and iatrogenic damage to the great vessels.
- The surgeon must distract cautiously on the spinous processes, as this can cause iatrogenic fractures in osteopenic patients. Similar care is warranted when distracting the pedicle screws, as this can cause loosening and loss of fixation.
- The surgeon must be mindful not to insert bone graft into the foramen when performing an intertransverse process fusion, especially on the TLIF side.

Acknowledgment

We thank senior editor and writer Dori Kelly, MA, for invaluable assistance with the manuscript and figures.

References

1. Harms J, Rolinger H: A one-stager procedure in operative treatment of spondylolistheses: Dorsal traction-reposition and anterior fusion [German]. *Z Orthop Ihre Grenzgeb* 1982;120(3):343-347.
2. Cole CD, McCall TD, Schmidt MH, Dailey AT: Comparison of low back fusion techniques: Transforaminal lumbar interbody fusion (TLIF) or posterior lumbar interbody fusion (PLIF) approaches. *Curr Rev Musculoskelet Med* 2009;2(2):118-126.
3. Herkowitz HN, Garfin SR, Eismont FJ, Bell GR, Balderston RA: *Rothman-Simeone The Spine*, ed 6. Philadelphia, PA, Saunders, 2011.
4. Potter BK, Freedman BA, Verwiebe EG, Hall JM, Polly DW Jr, Kuklo TR: Transforaminal lumbar interbody fusion: Clinical and radiographic results and complications in 100 consecutive patients. *J Spinal Disord Tech* 2005;18(4):337-346.
5. Wu RH, Fraser JF, Härtl R: Minimal access versus open transforaminal lumbar interbody fusion: Meta-analysis of fusion rates. *Spine (Phila Pa 1976)* 2010;35(26):2273-2281.
6. Shunwu F, Xing Z, Fengdong Z, Xiangqian F: Minimally invasive transforaminal lumbar interbody fusion for the treatment of degenerative lumbar diseases. *Spine (Phila Pa 1976)* 2010;35(17):1615-1620.
7. Parker SL, Adogwa O, Witham TF, Aaronson OS, Cheng J, McGirt MJ: Postoperative infection after minimally invasive versus open transforaminal lumbar interbody fusion (TLIF): Literature review and cost analysis. *Minim Invasive Neurosurg* 2011;54(1):33-37.
8. Lee JC, Jang HD, Shin BJ: Learning curve and clinical outcomes of minimally invasive transforaminal lumbar interbody fusion: Our experience in 86 consecutive cases. *Spine (Phila Pa 1976)* 2012;37(18):1548-1557.
9. Chrastil J, Patel AA: Complications associated with posterior and transforami-

nal lumbar interbody fusion. *J Am Acad Orthop Surg* 2012;20(5):283-291.
10. Tormenti MJ, Maserati MB, Bonfield CM, et al: Perioperative surgical complications of transforaminal lumbar interbody fusion: A single-center experience. *J Neurosurg Spine* 2012;16(1):44-50.
11. Faundez AA, Schwender JD, Safriel Y, et al: Clinical and radiological outcome of anterior-posterior fusion versus transforaminal lumbar interbody fusion for symptomatic disc degeneration: A retrospective comparative study of 133 patients. *Eur Spine J* 2009;18(2):203-211.
12. Rihn JA, Patel R, Makda J, et al: Complications associated with single-level transforaminal lumbar interbody fusion. *Spine J* 2009;9(8):623-629.
13. Villavicencio AT, Burneikiene S, Bulsara KR, Thramann JJ: Perioperative complications in transforaminal lumbar interbody fusion versus anterior-posterior reconstruction for lumbar disc degeneration and instability. *J Spinal Disord Tech* 2006;19(2):92-97.

Chapter 96
Anterior Lumbar Interbody Fusion

Andrew Park, MD

Introduction

The anterior lumbar interbody technique for fusion of the lower lumbar spine is being performed with increasing frequency. As surgeons become more familiar and more comfortable with this approach, more clinical scenarios traditionally approached via a posterior surgical technique may be handled with an anterior procedure. Lumbar levels from L2 to the sacrum can be accessed via a single retroperitoneal approach in most instances. The anterior lumbar approach presents significant advantages in long deformity constructs, which extend down to the sacrum or pelvis. The caudal level of long spine reconstructions is more likely to develop a pseudarthrosis. This is particularly true of the L5-S1 level.

One significant advantage of the anterior technique is its high fusion rate compared with posterolateral intertransverse fusion. This is particularly true for the L5-S1 level.[1,2] In addition, the correction of coronal plane deformity and the graft surface area is substantially greater through an anterior interbody technique.

Patient Selection
Indications

The anterior lumbar approach for spinal fusion is most often performed at L4-L5 and L5-S1. Most commonly, a single-level fusion is done through a retroperitoneal approach. Alternative approaches include transabdominal and laparoscopic; however, both of those approaches are associated with a higher frequency of postoperative complications. Most notable among the disadvantages are prolonged postoperative ileus, a higher incidence of bowel injury, and a higher incidence of retrograde ejaculation in male patients.

The indication most commonly leading to surgery at a single level in the lower lumbar spine is lumbar disk degeneration with low back pain. Other conditions for which an anterior approach may be considered include diskitis/osteomyelitis, nonunion of a posterior fusion procedure, spinal deformity surgery, recurrent disk herniation, total disk replacement/revision, fractures, and tumor surgery.

Contraindications

The primary contraindication to an anterior lumbar surgical approach is in a revision setting, in particular at L4-L5. The interspace at L5-S1 may be approached from the opposite side from the index approach in most cases without a significantly increased risk of vascular injury. A direct lateral approach to the interspaces above L5-S1 may be a safer alternative to revision anterior surgery.

Prior to consideration of a revision anterior lumbar exposure, alternative techniques to address the spinal pathology should be considered. Those approaches may include a direct lateral approach or a posterior approach to avoid the vascular risks associated with revision anterior retroperitoneal exposure. Morbid obesity may be considered a relative contraindication to anterior lumbar surgery.

Diagnosis

For the purposes of this chapter, degenerative disk disease will be the focus. This diagnosis is most commonly encountered at L4-L5 and L5-S1. Multilevel disease is also commonly seen in the lower lumbar spine. The patient will typically present with a long-standing history of low back pain, usually with occasional exacerbations over a period of many years. After the failure of nonsurgical treatment, including physical therapy, activity modification, and nonsteroidal anti-inflammatory medications, surgical treatment may be an appropriate consideration.

Preoperative Imaging

Plain radiographs typically demonstrate height loss on the lateral view (**Figure 1**). Although instability on flexion-extension views may be coexistent with the degenerative disk, this is relatively uncommon.

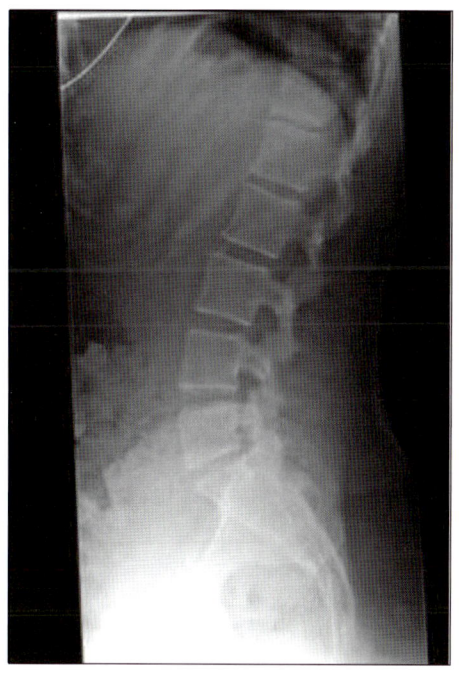

Figure 1 Lateral radiograph shows a loss of disk space height at L5-S1.

The surgeon must beware of spondylolysis affecting the involved motion segment because this may impact the need for additional fixation in the surgical decision making. A vacuum disk sign may also be seen on either standing, recumbent, or flexion-extension radiographs.[3,4]

MRI changes may include loss of disk space height, loss of signal intensity in the nucleus pulposus of the intervertebral disk on T2-weighted images, posterior disk bulge on axial imaging, and possibly Modic end-plate changes affecting the inferior end plate of the superior vertebrae and the superior end plate of the inferior vertebrae (**Figure 2**). Nerve root compression may also be seen on axial imaging affecting the central canal, the subarticular recess, or the far lateral zone of the neural foramen.[5]

Other diagnostic maneuvers may include diskography and postdiskography imaging. This area continues to be the subject of considerable debate regarding its utility and relevance to surgical decision making. Diskography also introduces variability in techniques and in interpretation of the results. Even the inclusion of a control level is debated based on the theoretical potential for creating

---

Dr. Park or an immediate family member is a member of a speakers' bureau or has made paid presentations on behalf of Zimmer; serves as a paid consultant to or is an employee of Zimmer, Ulrich, and Osteomed; serves as an unpaid consultant to Difusion; has received research or institutional support from DePuy; and has stock or stock options held in Difusion.

Section 7: Spine

accelerated disk degeneration at the control level.

Procedure
Room Setup/Patient Positioning

The surgical procedure should be performed on an operating table that allows for intraoperative fluoroscopic imaging (**Figure 3**). I prefer either a flat Jackson OSI table (**Figure 4**) or a Jackson Axis OSI table (**Figure 5**; Mizuho OSI). The Axis table allows for flexion or extension of the table to create more or less lumbar lordosis during the procedure (**Figure 6**). This may be of potential benefit in deformity cases or in a severely collapsed disk space. Another alternative would be the use of an inflatable arterial line cuff under the lower lumbar spine as a bolster to increase lumbar lordosis during the procedure. If this option is selected, access to the cuff's inflation should be checked before beginning the procedure.

Patient positioning on the operating room table should be done with great care and precision to ensure that there is no rotation of the pelvis or torso and that the patient is appropriately padded. The arms may be placed to the side or over the chest (**Figures 4** through **6**). Placing the arms over the chest allows the C-arm to stay in the surgical field in the lateral position for periodic imaging without the need for multiple drapes. This will improve the sterile technique by reducing the number of sterile drapes over the C-arm while switching from the AP to lateral imaging planes.

Special Instruments/Equipment/Implants

The surgical approach may be done with either a self-retaining retractor system or handheld retractors. Surgeon preference (usually dictated by the exposing surgeon) determines which retractor system is used. The Bookwalter self-retaining retractor system (DePuy) or Balfour retractors (V. Mueller) are commonly used at my institution. Handheld vein retractors for management of the inferior vena cava and the abdominal aorta or the iliac vessels are critical to performing this procedure. The retractors shown in **Figure 7** are the type that I prefer. This retractor is available in 6-in and 8-in sizes.

Intradiskal distractors are also quite helpful to distract the disk space open during disk removal. Typically, distractors of various sizes from 7 mm to 15 mm in 1-mm increments are used to maintain distraction of the disk space while

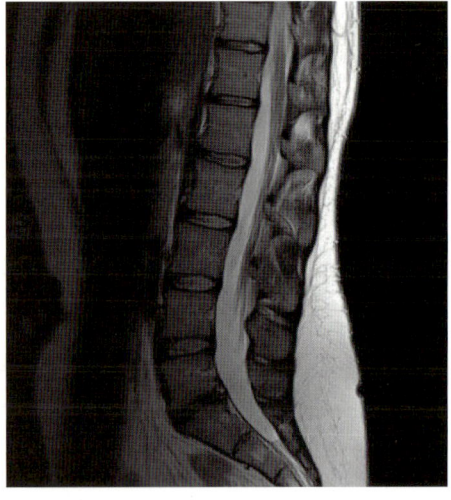

Figure 2 Sagittal T2-weighted MRI demonstrates typical changes associated with a symptomatic lumbar degenerative disk.

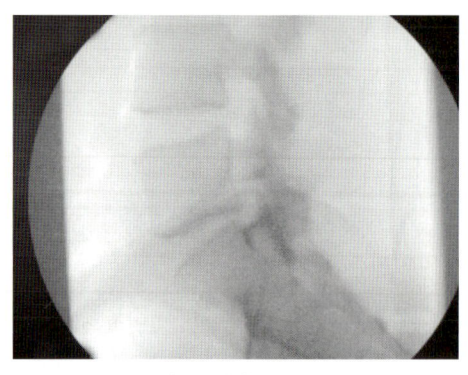

Figure 3 True lateral fluoroscopic image demonstrates disk collapse at L5-S1.

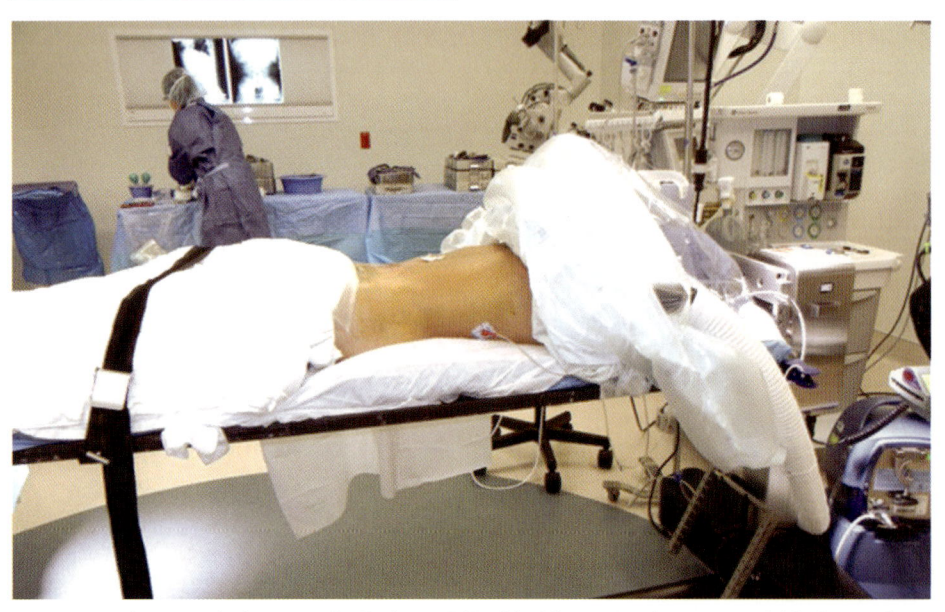

Figure 4 Photograph depicts a flat Jackson OSI table. The patient's arms are folded over the chest to allow intraoperative fluoroscopy in the lateral plane.

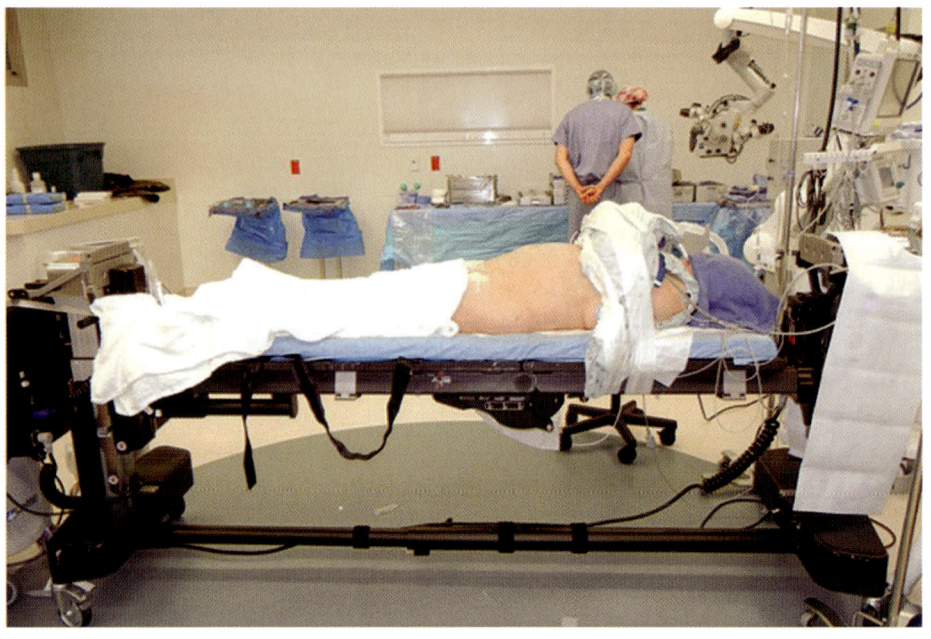

Figure 5 A Jackson Axis OSI table in the flat position.

© 2013 American Academy of Orthopaedic Surgeons

Chapter 96: Anterior Lumbar Interbody Fusion

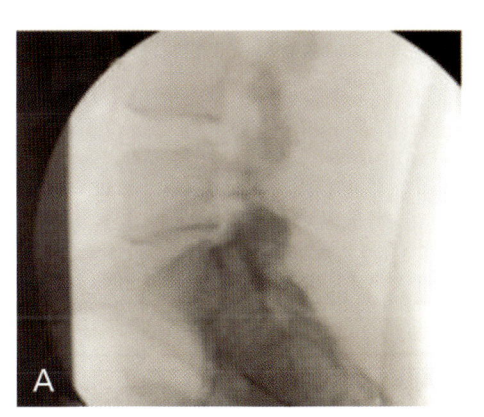

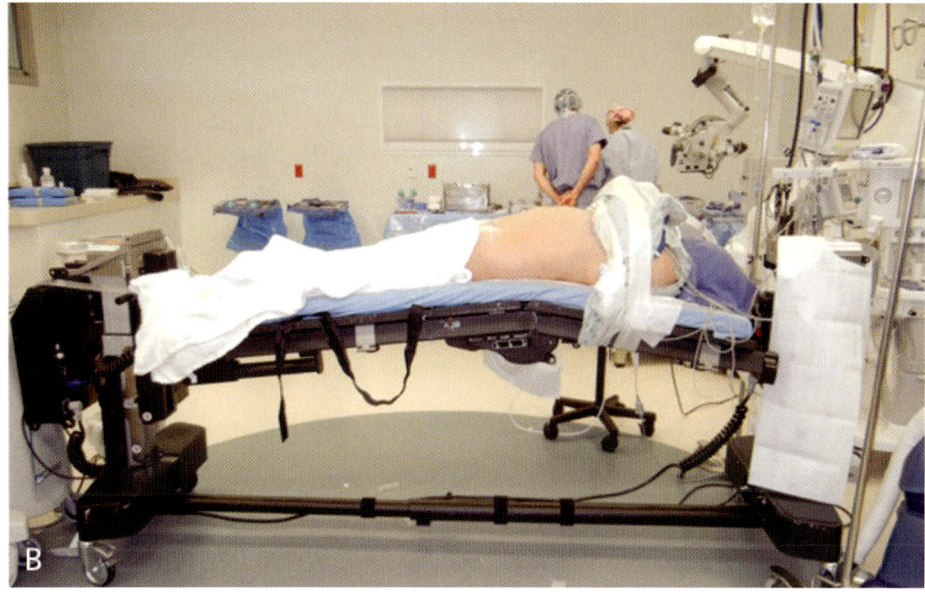

Figure 6 Note the increased lordosis at L5-S1 as seen on a lateral fluroscopic image (**A**) with extension of the operating table using the extension function of the Axis table (**B**).

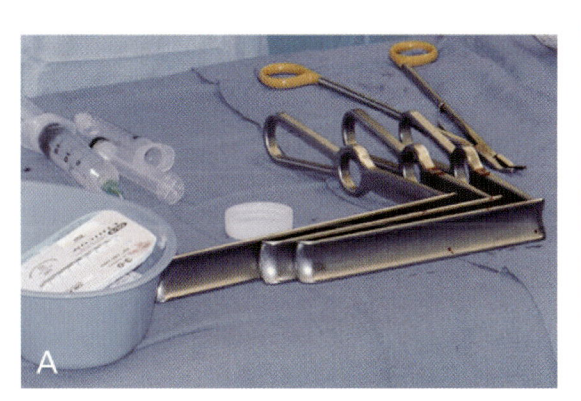

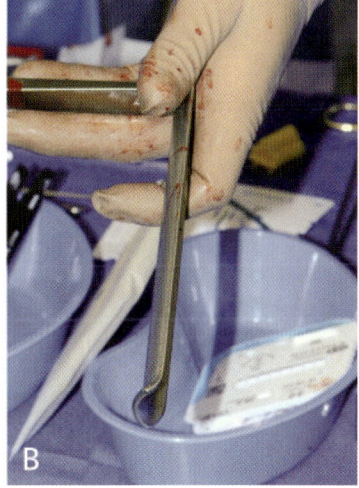

Figure 7 Photographs of the instruments used for anterior lumbar interbody fusion. **A,** Handheld vascular retractors of various lengths. **B,** Note the gentle curve at the tip of the vein retractor to assist with retraction and visualization.

working to remove the disk material. My preferred method is to alternate the disk space distractors from right to left while working the opposite side. This allows sequential dilation of the disk space while facilitating visualization of the side opposite the disk distractor.

Surgical Technique

Once the patient is positioned, images may be obtained with the C-arm to confirm that there is no significant rotation of the targeted disk space. This also may be helpful in localization of the surgical incision (**Figure 8**). Direct access to the disk space in the plane of the disk space is required for the insertion of most anterior lumbar interbody devices.

Anterior spinal exposures may be done through relatively small incisions and should be quick and relatively bloodless procedures. Experienced surgeons should be able to perform a one- or two-level exposure safely in 10 to 15 minutes. The spine is approached through a midline vertical fascial incision, even if the skin is cut transversely. The literature describes other approaches, including oblique and paramedian fascial incisions. It is my opinion that these are more difficult because the spine is a midline structure, and general and vascular surgeons are most familiar with the midline fascial incision.

Once the disk space is exposed, both AP and lateral images should be obtained to confirm the surgical level and establish the midline of the disk space. The midline should be marked on the disk space (**Figure 9**) or on the vertebral body to be used later as an internal reference point for placing the implant in a central location within the disk space.

Many different interbody devices exist that may accomplish the objective of reconstructing the interspace and achieving a solid fusion. Some devices have integrated fixation designed into the implant. Others may be used alone or in conjunction with supplemental fixation. One type of cage used is shown in **Figure 10**.

Complications

Exposure-related complications include injury to vascular structures, bowel injuries, or retrograde ejaculation. Additional complications may include thrombophlebitis, pulmonary embolism, incisional hernia, and prolonged ileus.

Management of the vascular structures is the most critical component of the surgical exposure. The assistance of a general or vascular surgeon who is familiar with the type of exposure and visualization needed to safely perform the diskectomy and reconstruction may be helpful. The L5-S1 interspace is generally easier and safer to expose than the L4-L5 level. At L5-S1, it may be preferable to do the exposure from the right side through a retroperitoneal plane. This allows L4-L5 to be exposed in a subsequent procedure from the left side. To expose L4-L5 or multiple levels, generally a left-sided approach is preferred to ligate the iliolumbar vein, which is typically a left-sided structure.

© 2013 American Academy of Orthopaedic Surgeons

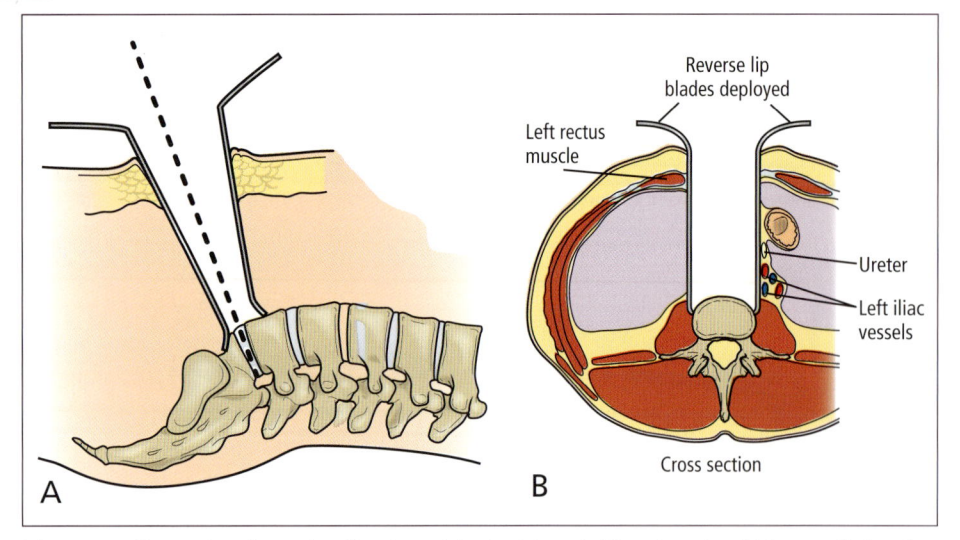

Figure 8 Illustration shows localization of the incision. **A,** The view should be parallel to the disk space of the surgical level. The retroperitoneal plane may be approached from either the right or the left side and allows full exposure of the disks while retracting the great vessels. **B,** Illustration shows a left-sided approach. The retractors should not be depressed too firmly, or compression of the neurologic structures within the psoas muscle could result in a neurologic deficit following surgery.

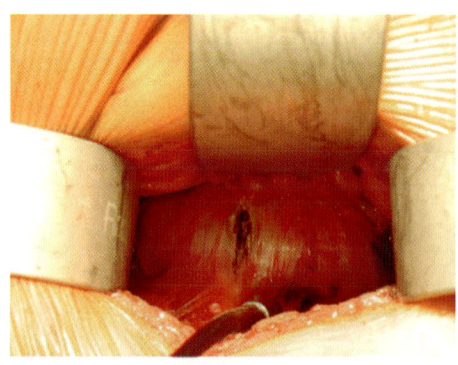

Figure 9 Intraoperative photograph shows the marking of the midline of the disk space. This is important for providing a reference point when placing the final implant.

Some authors have suggested that a right-sided retroperitoneal approach may be done for any level from L2 through the sacrum.[6] They have also proposed that the incidence of retrograde ejaculation is less frequent through a right-sided approach because the dissection of the left side superior hypogastric plexus is a sensitive structure.

Bowel injuries are very uncommon with a retroperitoneal approach. It is more common when doing the exposure transperitoneally. Bowel injuries are most frequent through a laparoscopic approach, especially when combined with a threaded interbody device, because visualization may be impaired.[7]

The incidence of retrograde ejaculation has recently been the subject of considerable debate. The historical literature supports that the incidence is primarily exposure related. The highest frequencies are seen in laparoscopic and transperitoneal approaches (10% to 15%) and least often seen in retroperitoneal exposures (1.5%).[8,9] The routine use of monopolar electrocautery also appears to increase the incidence of this complication compared with bipolar electrocautery. The impact of bone morphogenetic protein–2 (BMP-2; Infuse, Medtronic) on the incidence of retrograde ejaculation is uncertain. Recent reports have implicated that Infuse may be associated with an increased incidence of this complication.[10,11] However, the precise mechanism of this relationship is not understood at this time. Considerations include the possibility that Infuse may have some unintended reaction with the autonomic nervous system in the vicinity of the anterior lumbar spine.

Deep venous thrombosis and pulmonary embolism are unfortunate complications seen with anterior exposures. The incidence of deep venous thrombosis has been reported in the range of 3% to 5%. Pulmonary embolism occurs in less than 1% to 2% of patients.[12-14]

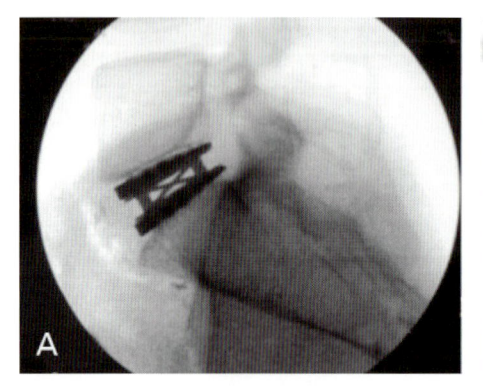

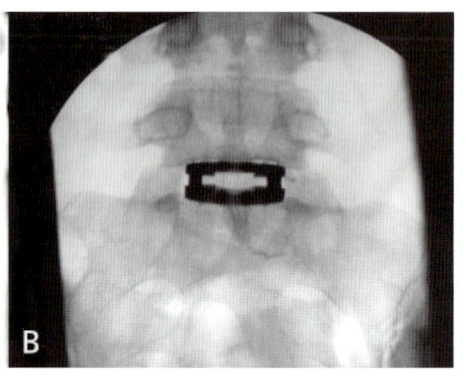

Figure 10 Postoperative lateral (**A**) and true AP (**B**) fluoroscopic images show an interbody cage in place. This particular cage is constructed of titanium and comes in four pieces: superior and inferior end-plate devices and two lateral struts. The cage is constructed in situ within the disk space for nontraumatic insertion and expansion of the disk space. Proper imaging is essential to ensure appropriate placement of the reconstructive device.

Postoperative Care and Rehabilitation

Patients may be mobilized either on the day of surgery or the following day with physical therapy. The use of an external brace may be at the discretion of the operating surgeon. Once the patient's mobility allows, the indwelling Foley catheter may be removed.

Following surgery, clear liquids may be started once bowel sounds return. Advancing diet to solid foods is typically allowed with the return of flatus. Most patients with single-level surgery are able to return to a normal diet by postoperative day 1 or 2.

Pearls

The key to safely performing an anterior lumbar fusion is management of the iliolumbar vasculature. Visualization of the vascular structures and gentle retraction of the vessels is required to effectively expose the disk space for the diskectomy and reconstruction. Relaxation of vascular retraction should be done several times during the procedure to prevent thrombosis of arterial structures.

During the diskectomy, it is very helpful to use temporary disk space distractors. This allows improved visualization and helps approximate for trialing implants. Many different implants and/or bone-graft options may be used for the spine reconstruction with excellent outcomes.

References

1. Burkus JK, Gornet MF, Schuler TC, Kleeman TJ, Zdeblick TA: Six-year outcomes of anterior lumbar interbody arthrodesis with use of interbody fusion cages and recombinant human bone morphogenetic protein-2. *J Bone Joint Surg Am* 2009;91(5):1181-1189.
2. Brau SA: Mini-open approach to the spine for anterior lumbar interbody fusion: Description of the procedure, results and complications. *Spine J* 2002;2(3):216-223.
3. Anderson DG, Sayadipour A, Shelby K, Albert TJ, Vaccaro AR, Weinstein MS: Anterior interbody arthrodesis with percutaneous posterior pedicle fixation for degenerative conditions of the lumbar spine. *Eur Spine J* 2011;20(8):1323-1330.
4. Strube P, Hoff E, Hartwig T, Perka CF, Gross C, Putzier M: Stand-alone anterior versus anteroposterior lumbar interbody single-level fusion after a mean follow-up of 41 months. *J Spinal Disord Tech* 2011;25(7):362-369.
5. Kim JS, Choi WG, Lee SH: Minimally invasive anterior lumbar interbody fusion followed by percutaneous pedicle screw fixation for isthmic spondylolisthesis: Minimum 5-year follow-up. *Spine J* 2010;10(5):404-409.
6. Edgard-Rosa G, Geneste G, Nègre G, Marnay T: Midline anterior approach from the right side to the lumbar spine for interbody fusion and total disc replacement: A new mobilization technique of the vena cava. *Spine (Phila Pa 1976)* 2012;37(9):E562-E569.
7. Than KD, Wang AC, Rahman SU, et al: Complication avoidance and management in anterior lumbar interbody fusion. *Neurosurg Focus* 2011;31(4):E6.
8. Burkus JK, Sandhu HS, Gornet MF, Longley MC: Use of rhBMP-2 in combination with structural cortical allografts: Clinical and radiographic outcomes in anterior lumbar spinal surgery. *J Bone Joint Surg Am* 2005;87(6):1205-1212.
9. Sasso RC, Burkus JK, LeHuec JC: Retrograde ejaculation after anterior lumbar interbody fusion: Transperitoneal versus retroperitoneal exposure. *Spine (Phila Pa 1976)* 2003;28(10):1023-1026.
10. Carragee EJ, Hurwitz EL, Weiner BK: A critical review of recombinant human bone morphogenetic protein-2 trials in spinal surgery: Emerging safety concerns and lessons learned. *Spine J* 2011;11(6): 471-491.
11. Carragee EJ, Mitsunaga KA, Hurwitz EL, Scuderi GJ: Retrograde ejaculation after anterior lumbar interbody fusion using rhBMP-2: A cohort controlled study. *Spine J* 2011;11(6):511-516.
12. Wood KB, Devine J, Fischer D, Dettori JR, Janssen M: Vascular injury in elective anterior lumbosacral surgery. *Spine (Phila Pa 1976)* 2010;35(9, suppl):S66-S75.
13. Garg J, Woo K, Hirsch J, Bruffey JD, Dilley RB: Vascular complications of exposure for anterior lumbar interbody fusion. *J Vasc Surg* 2010;51(4):946-950.
14. Fantini GA, Pappou IP, Girardi FP, Sandhu HS, Cammisa FP Jr: Major vascular injury during anterior lumbar spinal surgery: Incidence, risk factors, and management. *Spine (Phila Pa 1976)* 2007;32(24):2751-2758.

Pediatric Orthopaedics

Section Editor
Henry G. Chambers, MD

97 Closed and Open Reduction of Supracondylar Humerus Fractures 633
David L. Skaggs, MD; Paul D. Choi, MD; Cordelia Carter, MD

98 Reduction and Fixation of Lateral Condyle Fractures of the
Distal Humerus 641
Neeraj M. Patel, MD, MPH, MBS; John M. Flynn, MD

99 Intramedullary Fixation of Radial and Ulnar Shaft Fractures in
Skeletally Immature Patients 647
Maya E. Pring, MD; Hilton P. Gottschalk, MD; Henry G. Chambers, MD

100 Incision and Drainage of the Septic Hip 653
Benjamin J. Shore, MD, FRCSC; Mininder S. Kocher, MD, MPH

101 Percutaneous in Situ Fixation of Slipped Capital Femoral Epiphysis . . . 657
Randall T. Loder, MD

102 Fixation of Pediatric Femur Fractures 663
Ernest L. Sink, MD

103 Femoral Derotation Osteotomy in Adolescents and Young Adults 673
Harish S. Hosalkar, MD

104 Surgical Reduction and Fixation of Tibial
Spine Fractures in Children 677
Eric Wall, MD

105 Treatment of Clubfoot Using the Ponseti Method 683
Blaise Alexander Nemeth, MD, MS; Kenneth J. Noonan, MD

106 Treatment of Tarsal Coalitions 689
Scott J. Mubarak, MD

107 Lower Extremity Surgery in Children With Cerebral Palsy 695
Nirav K. Pandya, MD; Henry G. Chambers, MD

Chapter 97

Closed and Open Reduction of Supracondylar Humerus Fractures

David L. Skaggs, MD   Paul D. Choi, MD   Cordelia Carter, MD

Introduction

Supracondylar humerus fractures are among the most common orthopaedic injuries of childhood, comprising roughly two thirds of all fractures involving the elbow in children. With an estimated annual incidence of 177 in 100,000 patients, as reported by Houshian et al[1] in a recent Danish study, supracondylar humerus fractures represent a significant proportion of the injuries presenting to the emergency department for urgent orthopaedic care. It is therefore essential that the treating orthopaedist be armed with the proper tools for appropriate management of this common injury.

Supracondylar humerus fractures most frequently occur in children aged 3 to 10 years, with an average age of 6.7 years reported in the literature.[2] The mechanism of injury typically involves a fall onto the outstretched upper extremity, with the vast majority of fractures resulting from a fall with the arm held in an extended or hyperextended position. Nearly 98% of all supracondylar humerus fractures are of this extension type, with the remaining 2% to 3% representing the much rarer flexion-type supracondylar fracture.

The most widely used classification system for supracondylar humerus fractures is that of Gartland, first described in 1959.[2] This system, as originally conceived, describes type I fractures as nondisplaced, with neither medial-lateral fracture displacement nor rotational malalignment. In the type I fracture, the anterior humeral line intersects the middle third of the capitellum on the lateral radiographic view, and the Baumann angle is normal (10° to 26°) on the AP view. In some cases, the only radiographic evidence of a type I fracture may be the presence of the posterior fat pad sign. Type II fractures are moderately displaced, with the extended distal fragment hinging on the intact posterior humeral cortex. Fractures that are completely displaced without any cortical contact are classified as type III. Type III fractures demonstrate varying degrees of rotational malalignment and may have significant comminution with associated soft-tissue injuries and disruption of the periosteal hinge. Finally, a modification to the Gartland classification system has been made by Leitch et al,[3] who proposed the addition of a type IV fracture. This type of supracondylar fracture is multidirectionally unstable with complete incompetence of the periosteal hinge; as a result, the distal fracture fragment may be displaced into either a flexed or extended position.

Patient Evaluation

Initial assessment of the child with a supracondylar humerus fracture includes both clinical and radiographic evaluations. Physical examination involves inspection of the soft tissues of the arm, looking for evidence of surgical emergencies, including open fracture or compartment syndrome. Puckering of the skin anteriorly may be present and is associated with penetration of the brachialis by the proximal fracture fragment, which then engages the deeper layers of the dermis. Ecchymosis anteriorly in the antecubital fossa is indicative of significant underlying soft-tissue injury and should be considered a "red flag" for a possible evolving compartment syndrome (**Figure 1**).

The adjacent bones and joints should be evaluated for the presence of concomitant injuries; importantly, combined forearm and elbow injuries place the patient at a higher risk for developing compartment syndrome. Following inspection of the skin and soft tissues, the presence and strength of a radial pulse should be noted along with an assessment of hand perfusion. A warm, pink hand may be considered well perfused, whereas a cool, white or blue-tinged hand is considered poorly perfused. Careful sensorimotor examination of the median, anterior interosseous, ulnar, radial, and posterior interosseous nerves is essential because traumatic neurapraxia is quite common. In a recent meta-analysis of 5,148 pediatric patients with displaced supracondylar humerus fractures, Babal et al[4] identified traumatic nerve injuries at a rate of 11%. These authors confirmed the results of earlier studies, reporting that the anterior interosseous nerve (AIN) is the most frequently affected nerve in extension-type fractures. In their series, 34% of all traumatic neurapraxias associated with displaced extension-type supracondylar fractures involved the AIN. They additionally noted that flexion-type fractures were associated with an overall higher rate of traumatic neurapraxia than extension-type fractures as well as with a vastly higher rate of injury to the ulnar nerve; 91% of traumatic nerve injuries in patients with flexion-type fractures involved the ulnar nerve.

Radiographic evaluation is routinely performed in the emergency setting, with AP and lateral views of the elbow being standard. As described previously, the normal radiographic appearance of the pediatric elbow includes an anterior

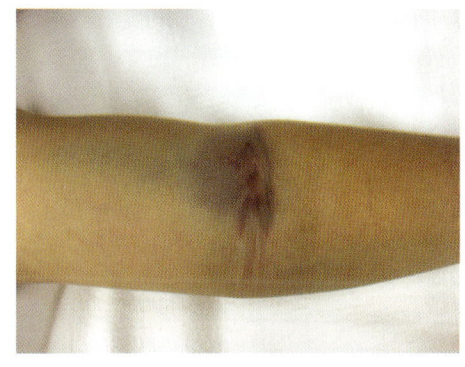

Figure 1 Photograph depicts ecchymosis of the antecubital fossa with associated puckering of the skin anteriorly in a child with a supracondylar humerus fracture. This is a red flag for significant underlying soft-tissue injury.

Dr. Skaggs or an immediate family member has received royalties from Biomet and Medtronic; is a member of a speakers' bureau or has made paid presentations on behalf of Medtronic, Stryker, and Biomet; serves as a paid consultant to or is an employee of Medtronic, Stryker, and Biomet; and serves as a board member, owner, officer, or committee member of the Pediatric Orthopaedic Society of North America, the Growing Spine Study Group, and the Scoliosis Research Society. Dr. Choi or an immediate family member is a member of a speakers' bureau or has made paid presentations on behalf of Stryker and serves as a paid consultant to or is an employee of Stryker and Integra. Dr. Carter or an immediate family member serves as a paid consultant to or is an employee of Arthrex.

Section 8: Pediatric Orthopaedics

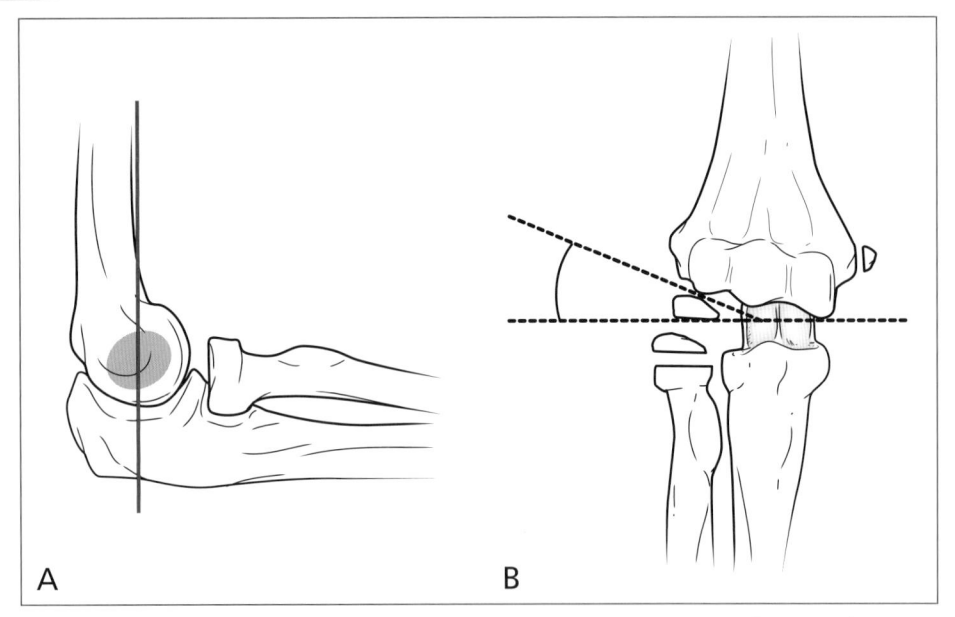

Figure 2 Illustrations show normal radiographic angles for the pediatric elbow. **A**, The anterior humeral line—a line drawn adjacent to the anterior humeral cortex on a true lateral view of the elbow—should intersect the capitellum in its central third. **B**, The Baumann angle is defined as the angle formed by the intersection of a line drawn perpendicular to the long axis of the humeral shaft with a line drawn parallel to the lateral humeral condylar physis. A Baumann angle greater than 10° is generally considered acceptable.

humeral line that intersects the capitellum on the lateral view and a Baumann angle between 10° and 26° (**Figure 2**). Decreases in this angle are associated with varus angulation of the fracture. Comminution of the medial column should raise concern for varus angulation, and fractures with medial comminution typically require surgical treatment. Although radiographs of the contralateral elbow may be useful for purposes of comparison, they are not usually required. Finally, standard orthogonal views of the adjacent bones and joints should be strongly considered to evaluate for "floating elbow" fracture patterns and other associated injuries, especially if concomitant injury cannot be ruled out by physical examination.

Nonsurgical Management
Most authors agree that the treatment of type I supracondylar humerus fractures is immobilization in a long-arm cast for 3 weeks. Although it is tempting to place the elbow in maximal flexion to optimize fracture reduction, increasing amounts of elbow flexion have been associated with obliteration of the radial pulse and elevated compartment pressures, especially in fractures with more displacement and associated soft-tissue injury.[5,6] For type I injuries, we recommend placement of a long-arm cast with the elbow positioned in less than 90° of flexion and the forearm in neutral rotation.

Although some centers continue to advocate for the closed management of type II fractures, there is good evidence that late complications of cast immobilization—including loss of reduction, delayed surgery, poor clinical outcomes, and increased forearm compartment pressures—do occur. By contrast, in a recent review of 189 type II consecutive supracondylar fractures treated surgically with closed reduction and percutaneous pin fixation, there were no reported instances of anesthesia-related complication or loss of fracture reduction.[7] Clinical outcomes, as judged by the Flynn criteria, were uniformly good, with 187 of 189 patients having a good or excellent result and the remaining two patients having with a fair outcome. We noted a 2% infection rate and a 0.5% rate of reoperation (performed for a pin-tract infection). Based on these data, we believe that the benefits of closed reduction and percutaneous fixation for type II fractures outweigh the perceived risks of surgical intervention, and we routinely treat this type of fracture surgically. With regard to type III and IV supracondylar humerus fractures, there is little debate that surgical treatment is warranted.

Procedure
Room Setup/Patient Positioning
Once in the operating room, the patient is positioned supine on the operating table, general endotracheal anesthesia is administered, and a prophylactic dose of antibiotic is given. A short radiolucent arm board is applied to the operating table. In smaller patients, the head may be placed between the arm board and the operating table so that the elbow is far enough onto the arm board to facilitate fluoroscopic imaging and the head is not in danger of being pulled off the table during traction maneuvers. The patient is secured to the table with a safety strap. The bed is then turned 30° to 45°, so that the affected arm is positioned away from the anesthesiologist; this creates a larger working space for the surgeon and his or her assistant. The C-arm is positioned parallel to the bed and enters the surgical field from the foot of the bed; this machine, too, requires sterile surgical draping. The C-arm monitor is positioned directly across the table from the surgeon to allow direct viewing while placing pins. The arm is prepped to the shoulder in the usual sterile fashion, and the arm is draped free.

Surgical Technique
In most cases, surgery begins by attempted closed reduction of the fracture. This is performed by applying axial traction to the arm, with countertraction applied at the axilla by an assistant. The elbow is held in 20° to 30° of flexion during this maneuver to avoid tethering of the anterior neurovascular structures over the proximal spike of the fracture. The forearm may be alternately pronated and supinated to determine which position achieves the most fracture stability. In general, a posteromedially displaced fracture is associated with an intact medial periosteal hinge, which may be maximally tensioned with pronation of the forearm (**Figure 3**). Conversely, fractures that are displaced posterolaterally may be more stable with supination of the forearm, although this is variable.[8] Dynamic fluoroscopy alternating between forearm pronation and supination may be especially useful in determining the optimal position of the forearm for addressing varus/valgus malalignment of the fracture and ultimately the stability of the reduction. Medial-lateral fracture translation may also be addressed at this time by direct manipulation of the distal fragment.

Fracture Reduction
The reduction maneuver itself consists of pressure directed volarly on the tip of the olecranon using the surgeon's thumb(s) to lever the distal fragment anteriorly as

Chapter 97: Closed and Open Reduction of Supracondylar Humerus Fractures

the arm is slowly flexed to approximately 130° (Figure 4). A clunk may be heard and/or felt following attempted reduction, and an immediate increase in the passive flexion of the elbow is typically observed. If the fingers cannot touch the shoulder following the reduction maneuver, this may be an indication that there is residual extension at the fracture site and the fracture is not reduced.

Following the reduction maneuver, the fracture alignment is evaluated using multiple fluoroscopic views. On the lateral view, if the anterior humeral line crosses the capitellum, this is acceptable. On the AP view, the Baumann angle should be greater than 10°. Finally, internal and external oblique views of the distal humerus should be obtained to demonstrate the alignment of the medial and lateral humeral columns (Figure 5). Once adequate fracture reduction is confirmed, the hyperflexed elbow is wrapped with a sterile elastic bandage to effortlessly maintain fracture reduction and allow full attention to be given to pin placement.

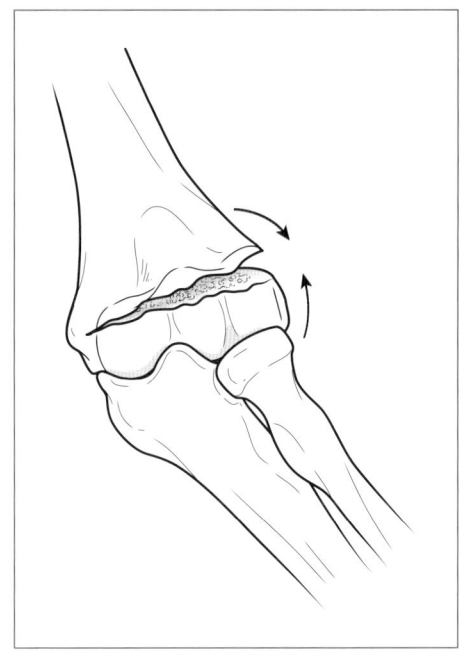

Figure 3 A posteromedially displaced fracture frequently has an intact periosteal hinge medially. Pronation of the forearm may facilitate fracture reduction in this setting by closing the periosteal hinge, with correction of varus angulation.

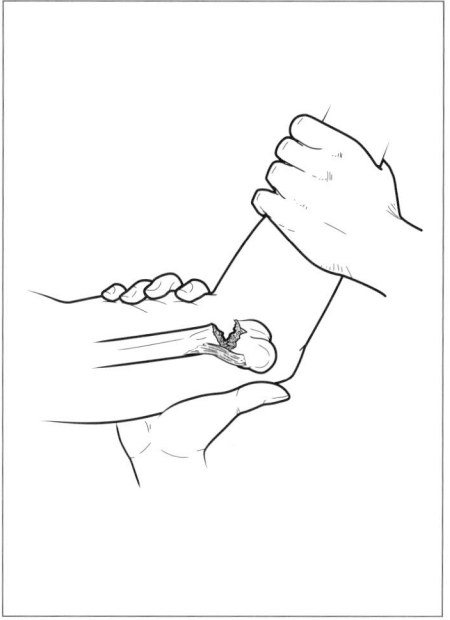

Figure 4 The reduction maneuver is performed by first applying axial traction to the patient's slightly flexed arm (with countertraction applied in the axilla by an assistant) and then levering the posteriorly displaced distal fragment back into place as the elbow is brought into flexion.

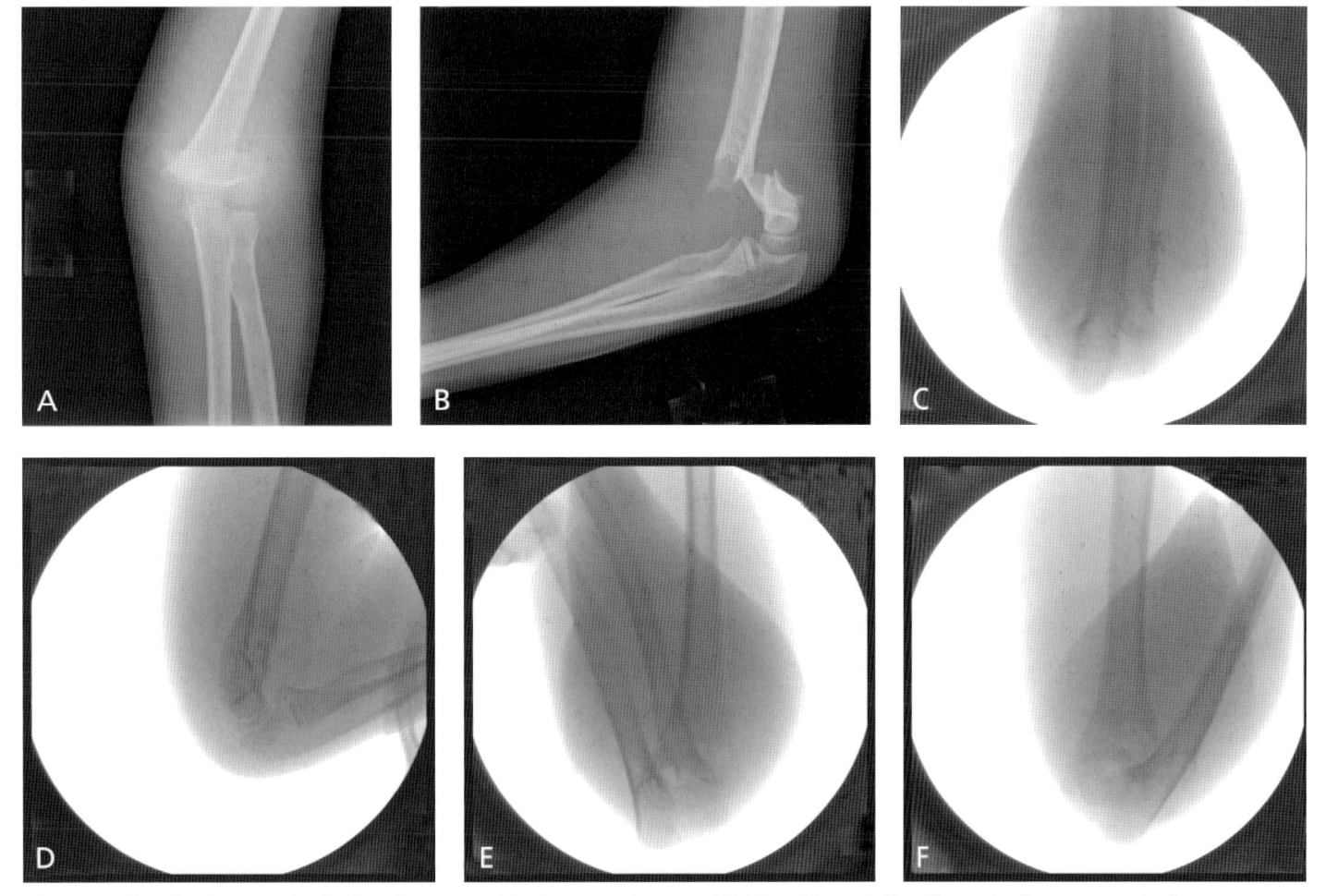

Figure 5 Closed reduction of a displaced supracondylar humerus fracture. AP (**A**) and lateral (**B**) radiographs demonstrate the fracture. Intraoperative AP (**C**) and lateral (**D**) fluoroscopic views of the same elbow following fracture reduction. Intraoperative internal (**E**) and external (**F**) oblique fluoroscopic views of the same fracture demonstrate acceptable alignment of the medial and lateral humeral columns. (Courtesy of Children's Orthopaedic Center, Los Angeles, CA.)

© 2013 American Academy of Orthopaedic Surgeons

If adequate fracture reduction cannot be achieved in a closed manner, the brachialis muscle may be torn, with the proximal fracture fragment buttonholed through it. Often, this is associated with anterior dimpling of the skin, significant ecchymosis, and a palpable fracture spike anteriorly. The "milking" maneuver has been described for this situation by Peters et al[9] and is performed as follows. First, the anterior musculature of the arm is grasped as proximally as possible with countertraction applied in the axilla by an assistant. Pressure is then applied to the anterior musculature in a proximal-to-distal direction as the muscles are "milked" distal to the proximal spike of the fracture. Release of the brachialis muscle from the fracture fragment may be accompanied by a palpable "pop," with improvement of the anterior dimpling. Fracture reduction may then be achieved by closed means. In their review of eight patients with otherwise irreducible supracondylar humerus fractures and clinical evidence of fracture displacement into the anterior soft tissues, Peters et al[9] reported success with fracture reduction by closed means following application of the milking maneuver with good long-term outcomes in all eight patients.

In some cases, the supracondylar humerus fracture may not be adequately reduced using closed means, or there is a "rubbery" end point to the reduction. In these instances, one must consider that the anterior neurovascular structures (typically the brachial artery and the median nerve) are interposed in the fracture site, and an open reduction to explore and release these tethered structures is indicated (**Figure 6**).

Fracture Fixation

In the vast majority of cases, adequate fracture reduction will be achieved in a closed fashion, and percutaneous fixation can be performed in the following manner: First, one or two folded sterile towels are placed beneath the affected elbow, effectively raising it off the table and facilitating the introduction of pins. Several 0.062-in Kirschner wires (K-wires) or, for larger patients, 2.0-mm Steinmann pins should be opened and available. A K-wire is held free and then placed onto the patient's skin at the level of the lateral humeral condyle. A Jones view of the elbow should be used to evaluate the pin trajectory; the goal is to capture either the lateral column or the central column of the distal humeral fragment with the first pin and engage two humeral cortices, thereby ensuring good bony purchase in both the proximal and distal fragments. When the starting point and anticipated trajectory for the K-wire are deemed satisfactory, the K-wire may be advanced manually through the skin and into the cartilaginous lateral humeral condyle, akin to placing a pin into a pincushion. Pin position on the AP and lateral views may be rechecked by fluoroscopy, and the K-wire is then advanced under power, feeling penetration of two bony cortices with the pin. Of note, advancing the K-wires across the olecranon fossa, in which case four cortices will be felt, is an acceptable option. Placement of K-wires across the olecranon fossa limits elbow extension while the pins are in place but potentially provides enhanced stability of the construct by increasing cortical purchase. We do this routinely. In the same percutaneous fashion using fluoroscopic guidance, the second (and third, if desired) pins can be placed divergent from or parallel to the first pin, using a second lateral-entry point. Pins that cross at the fracture site or converge proximally should be avoided (**Figure 7**).

Importantly, technical errors in pin placement account for the overwhelming majority of cases in which pin fixation is lost. In their review of 279 surgically treated displaced supracondylar humerus fractures, Sankar et al[10] identified eight patients in whom pin fixation had been lost between the time of surgery and the first postoperative visit, a 2.9% rate of hardware failure. These authors noted that all eight failures were associated with Gartland type III fractures, and seven of these had two lateral-entry pins placed for fixation. In each case of hardware failure, a specific technical error was identified, including type A, failure to engage both fragments with two pins or more; type B, failure to achieve bicortical fixation with two pins or more (it is better for the pins to be a little long than a little short); and type C, failure to achieve adequate pin separation (>2 mm) at the fracture site.

Once two pins are placed and their configuration on the AP image has been deemed acceptable, the shoulder is externally rotated 90° to evaluate the appearance of the fracture on the lateral image. The surgeon must ensure that there is

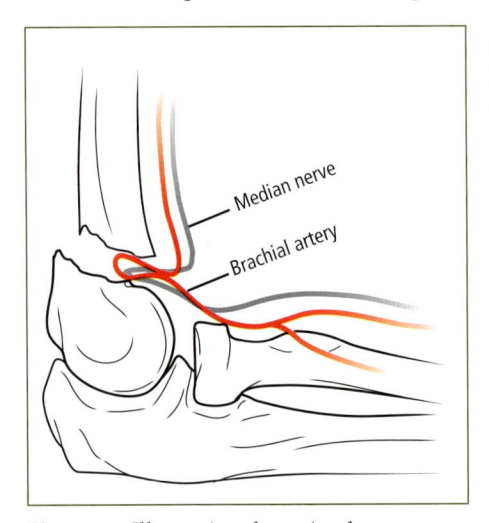

Figure 6 Illustration shows inadequate reduction of a supracondylar humerus fracture. The inability to achieve adequate fracture reduction may be associated with interposition of the anterior neurovascular structures within the fracture site.

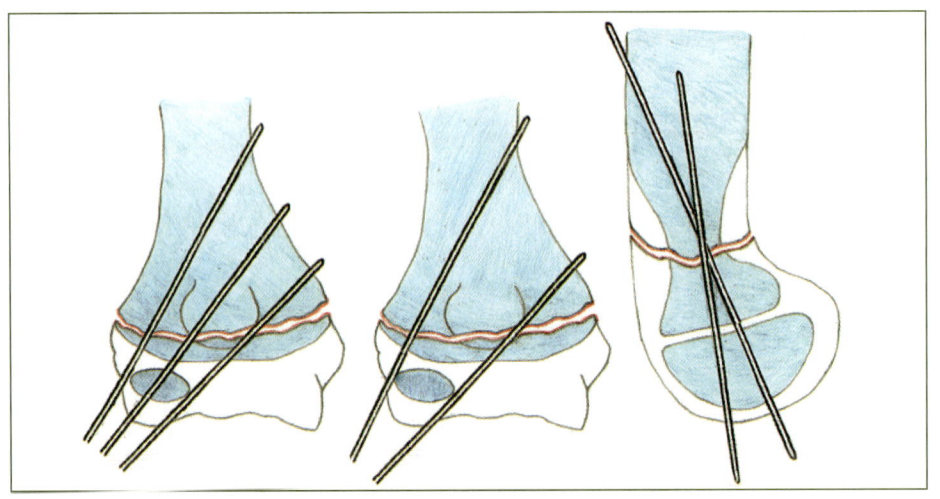

Figure 7 Illustration shows pin configuration for fixation of a supracondylar humerus fracture. Two or three pins may be placed in either a parallel or divergent manner, taking care to engage at least two columns of the humerus and to achieve adequate pin spread (>2 mm) at the fracture site. Convergently placed pins should be avoided. (Reproduced with permission from Skaggs DL, Cluck MW, Mostoli A, Hynn JM, Kay RM: Lateral-entry pin fixation in the management of supracondylar fractures in children. *J Bone Joint Surg Am* 2004;86[4]:702-707.)

adequate fixation in the distal fragment on this view. Of note, having a slightly anterior-to-posterior trajectory of the pins as they are advanced across the proximal fragment may maximize bony purchase by going through the capitellum (Figure 8).

Following pin placement, the stability of the fracture should be evaluated by performing dynamic fluoroscopic stress views of the elbow in both the sagittal (flexion-extension stress) and coronal (varus-valgus stress) planes. If there is any uncertainty about the stability of the construct, an additional pin should be placed. Once construct stability is confirmed, final fluoroscopic images should be taken, including AP (with the elbow in extension), lateral, and internal and external oblique views. One helpful technique is to save the image showing fracture reduction at its worst, to aid in evaluating films performed at follow-up visits, should there be there concern over loss of reduction.

Dressing and Casting

Once adequate reduction and fixation have been achieved, the pins are bent to an angle of 90°, 1 cm from their entry into the skin; the pins are then cut to a length of 1 to 1.5 cm. Sterile dressings should then be applied in a way that protects the skin from the pins and accommodates the significant soft-tissue swelling that is often present. This can be achieved by making a slit in a square of sterile felt and placing it beneath the pins. Strips of 0.5-in–thick sterile foam may then be placed over the dorsal and volar aspects of the arm and overwrapped loosely with sterile cotton undercast padding; no circumferential dressings should be placed underneath the foam. This allows room for postoperative swelling and obviates the need to split the cast. Finally, a long-arm cast is loosely applied with the arm held in 60° to 70° of flexion and the forearm neutrally positioned, after ensuring that the radial pulse is present in this position (Figure 9).

Lateral-Entry Versus Medial-Entry Pins

There is good evidence in the literature to support the use of lateral-entry–only pin constructs. In 2001, Skaggs et al[11] reported retrospectively on 281 displaced (Gartland type II and III) supracondylar humerus fractures treated with either lateral-entry–only pin fixation or a crossed-pin construct. When the authors looked specifically at iatrogenic ulnar nerve palsy in this patient population, they found a 4.9% rate of injury to the ulnar nerve that was associated in every case with the placement of a medial-entry pin. In this patient series, even exposure of the medial-entry pin site through a small incision before pin placement did not infallibly prevent ulnar nerve injury.

In a subsequent study, Skaggs et al[12] reviewed 124 consecutive supracondylar fractures treated with lateral-entry pin fixation alone. In this patient population, they reported no clinical loss of elbow motion, loss of fracture reduction, iatrogenic nerve palsy, need for additional surgery, or cubitus varus deformity. The authors concluded that for even the most unstable supracondylar humerus fractures, adequate fracture stability can be achieved using only lateral-entry pins, thus decreasing the risk of iatrogenic ulnar nerve palsy.

Although lateral-entry constructs have become increasingly popular, medial-entry pins may also be used for fixation—especially in cases with excessive lateral

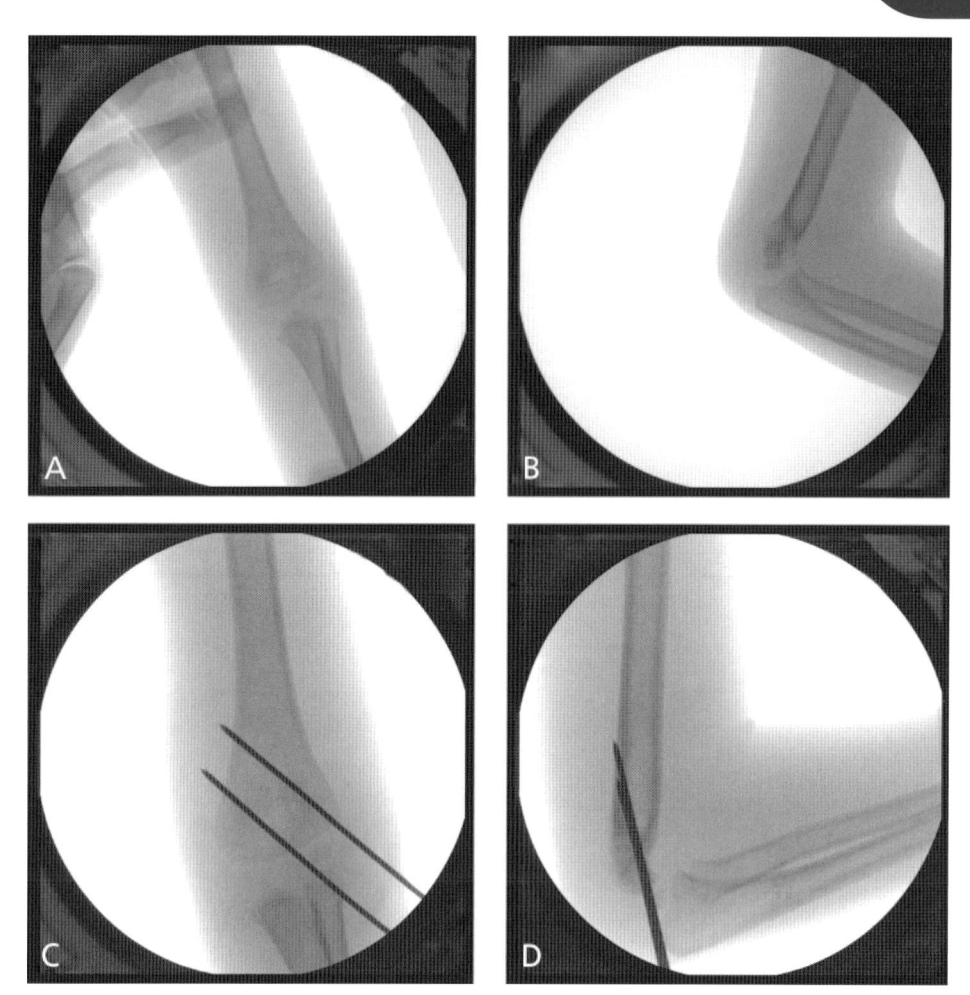

Figure 8 Intraoperative AP (**A**) and lateral (**B**) fluoroscopic views show a typical type II supracondylar humerus fracture. Intraoperative AP (**C**) and lateral (**D**) fluroscopic views show pin placement following fracture reduction and fixation. Note the slight anterior-to-posterior trajectory of the pins on the lateral view. (Courtesy of Children's Orthopaedic Center, Los Angeles, CA.)

comminution or extremely distal fracture lines, where adequate purchase laterally in the distal fragment is not easily obtained. If placement of a medial pin is undertaken, it should be placed after the first lateral-entry pin so that the elbow can be extended without displacing the fracture; positioning the arm in relative extension prevents the ulnar nerve from subluxating anteriorly over the medial epicondyle and being speared by an advancing K-wire. The authors use medial pins in less than 1% of fractures.

Special Situations
Flexion-Type Fractures

An uncommon variant of the supracondylar humerus fracture, the flexion-type fracture, must be recognized and appropriately treated in a timely fashion. Mahan et al[13] recently published their 10-year experience with flexion-type supracondylar fractures using a cohort of patients with extension-type injuries treated at the same institution during the same time period as a control group.

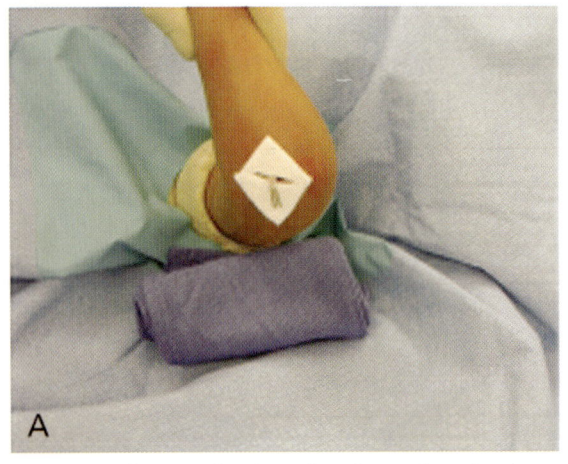

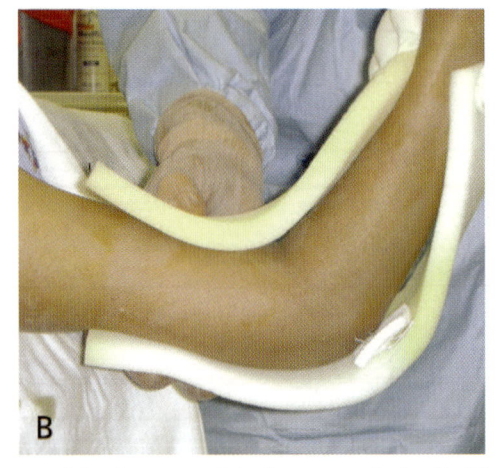

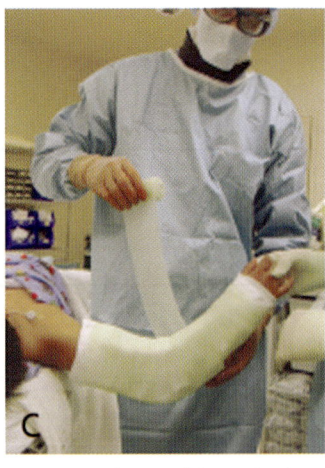

Figure 9 Photographs show dressing and casting for supracondylar fractures of the humerus. **A,** Sterile felt squares may be used to protect the skin. Petrolatum gauze mesh strips or sterile gauze may also be used for this purpose. **B,** In cases of significant swelling, strips of sterile foam may be placed volarly and dorsally on the skin and then overwrapped loosely with sterile cotton undercast padding. **C,** A long-arm cast is loosely applied, with the elbow in roughly 70° of flexion. (Reproduced with permission from Skaggs D: Closed reduction and pinning of supracondylar humerus fractures, in Tolo VT, Skaggs DL, eds: *Master Techniques in Orthopaedic Surgery: Pediatrics.* Philadelphia, PA, Lippincott Williams & Wilkins, 2008, p 12.)

They found that the 58 patients with flexion-type fractures differed from the control group in several ways. Patients with flexion-type injuries were significantly older (7.5 years versus 5.8 years, on average), were significantly more likely to have preoperative ulnar nerve symptoms requiring decompression, and were significantly more likely to require an open reduction of the fracture than their extension-type counterparts by a factor of three. Despite these findings, closed reduction is still possible in most cases. In terms of the surgical approach to fracture reduction and fixation, the flexion-type fracture differs from the extension-type fracture in one significant aspect: reduction is performed with the elbow positioned in relative extension.

Type IV Fractures

For fractures that are multidirectionally unstable (Gartland type IV), the recommended reduction maneuver is slightly different. As described by Leitch et al,[3] the fracture is first confirmed to be multidirectionally unstable by demonstrating both flexion and extension of the distal fragment on lateral fluoroscopic views. Unlike stable fractures, which are treated by immediate fracture reduction, for multidirectionally unstable fractures these authors recommend first placing two 0.062-in K-wires into the lateral aspect of the distal fracture fragment before fracture reduction and then using AP and lateral fluoroscopic imaging to confirm adequate pin placement and anticipated pin trajectory.

Fracture reduction is attempted initially in the coronal plane. Direct manipulation of the fracture fragments to correct varus and valgus malalignment as well as any major rotational deformity is employed with the elbow held in relative extension. AP views of the elbow are obtained in this position. Once adequate alignment in the coronal plane is established, the C-arm is rotated 90° to a lateral position, and the deformity in the sagittal plane is addressed by passive flexion or extension of the elbow; direct anterior-posterior translation of the fracture fragments may also be useful. Manual pressure on the medial and/or lateral humeral condyles is used to correct residual rotational deformity. After fracture reduction is confirmed on the lateral fluoroscopic view, the pins may be advanced across the fracture site—in an anterior-to-posterior direction as described previously for type II and III fractures—and the C-arm is again rotated to provide an AP view. One or more additional pins are frequently placed to ensure adequate stability of the construct.

Open Fractures

Open reduction of a pediatric supracondylar humerus fracture is at times necessary. Indications for open reduction include open fracture, neurovascular injury warranting exploration, failure to achieve or maintain a closed reduction secondary to interposed soft tissues at the fracture site or severe soft-tissue swelling, and loss of previously present neurologic or vascular function following closed reduction. Although various approaches to the elbow have been described for the open treatment of supracondylar humerus fractures (eg, lateral, medial, posterior, and combined approaches), we prefer the anterior approach.[14,15]

After positioning and draping in the previously described fashion, a sterile tourniquet is placed as high on the arm as possible without immediate inflation. A 3-cm incision is made transversely in the anterior cubital fossa, at the level of the natural flexion crease. The incision begins just medial to the palpable biceps tendon and is extended laterally. A No. 15 blade is used to go through the skin, followed by blunt dissection of the subcutaneous tissue beneath. Care is taken to dissect well lateral to the biceps tendon and its distal aponeurosis to ensure that the neurovascular structures that run just medial to it—the brachial vein, brachial artery, and median nerve—are not damaged. The median nerve and brachial artery may be tightly tented over the proximal fracture fragment. Not infrequently, the proximal fracture fragment is buttonholed anteriorly through the brachialis muscle, and this rent in the soft-tissue envelope may be exploited to provide direct access to the fracture site. Fracture hematoma is evacuated with a combination of suction and saline lavage.

The fracture site, once cleaned, is inspected for interposed soft tissues. The placement of retractors into the surgical wound while examining the fracture site should be done with care to prevent direct or indirect injury to nearby neurovascular structures. Interposed tissues may include joint capsule, periosteum, muscle fibers (brachialis, common flexor, and triceps muscle interposition have all been described), and neurovascular structures, including the radial nerve, the median nerve, and the brachial artery. These are gently freed from the fracture site as necessary. Of note, soft-tissue interposition is fairly common and should be considered a primary cause of irreducibility in the supracondylar humerus fracture. In their report of 61 children with Gartland type III fractures treated with open reduction and percutaneous fixation through an anterior approach, Ay et al[14] noted that the proximal fracture fragment was buttonholed through the brachialis muscle in 46% of cases, and the anterior joint capsule was interposed in the fracture fragments in 33% of cases.

In the same report, Ay et al[14] noted a 5% to 10% rate of traumatic nerve palsy preoperatively; in each case of traumatic neurovascular injury, the affected nerve at the time of open surgery was found to be tethered anteriorly (AIN palsy) or kinked anterolaterally (radial nerve palsy). Surgical release of the incarcerated nerve from the fracture site was reliably associated with full neurologic recovery within 3 months of surgery.

Vascular compromise is not infrequently associated with displaced supracondylar humerus fractures, with an estimated 10% to 20% of children presenting with a pulseless limb. Often, fracture reduction results in return of the radial pulse, although a small subset of patients will require open exploration of the vessels. If there is any doubt regarding the integrity of the neurovascular structures surrounding the elbow, they may be formally explored by extending the transverse incision in a lazy-S fashion for approximately 5 cm both proximally (along the medial aspect of the biceps brachii) and distally (along the medial border of the brachioradialis).

Once the approach to the humerus is successfully made and the fracture fragments are mobilized, attention is turned to fracture reduction. This is typically achieved through direct manipulation of the fracture fragments and often consists of pressure applied posteriorly to the proximal fracture fragment with the distal fragment stabilized. Palpable cortical step-offs medially and laterally are indicative of residual rotational malalignment and should be reduced if possible. However, once the soft tissues are removed from the fracture site, the reduction is often less stable than when reduced closed; the surgeon should expect some "fiddling" and be patient. Fracture reduction is followed by percutaneous pin fixation, adhering to the concepts described previously.

Postoperative Care and Rehabilitation

A minority of children with minimal swelling and minimal risk for compartment syndrome may be discharged to home with appropriate parental education on elevation and early warning signs requiring a return to the emergency department. Most children will be admitted to the hospital for observation and serial neurovascular checks. Once the surgeon is certain that an evolving compartment syndrome is not present and the neurovascular examination is stable, the child may be discharged home, with routine follow-up scheduled for 1 week after surgery. At this visit, AP and lateral views of the elbow in cast are obtained, and care is taken to ensure that the neurovascular examination is stable and that signs of pin-site infection, such as worsening pain, malodorous drainage, and fevers, are not present. Cast immobilization is continued, and the next routine follow-up generally is scheduled for the third postoperative week. At this visit, new radiographs are obtained out of the cast, and the pins are removed in the office. Generally, a return to regular activities of daily living is expected at this visit, with restrictions placed on activities that would place the patient at risk for a fall and refracture through the healing bone. Physical therapy is not routinely ordered because parents are trained to perform gentle range-of-motion exercises. Patients return for a range-of-motion check at 6 to 8 weeks postoperatively and are generally allowed to return to full activities at that time. Repeat radiographs are not typically obtained once healing has been demonstrated unless there is a concern about a loss of elbow motion or persistent elbow pain.

Pearls

- Some authors recommend using the C-arm itself as the operating table; however, this setup is inadequate for obtaining lateral views by rotation of the machine (useful for unstable type IV fractures) and inadequate for fractures that require open reduction.
- To achieve and maintain adequate reduction:
  - Consider using a sterile elastic bandage to hold the reduction with the elbow hyperflexed while pins are placed.
  - Check internal and external oblique views to evaluate medial and lateral columns.
  - Remember that the two most important criteria for assessing reduction are a Baumann angle >10° and the anterior humeral line intersecting the capitellum.
  - Save the worst fluoroscopic view intraoperatively to be used as a comparison later in the office.
  - Recognize that if a gap remains at the fracture site after reduction, or there is a rubbery feel, interposition of neurovascular structures may be present, and the surgeon should proceed with open reduction.
- Technical errors in pin placement can be avoided by
  - Engaging medial and lateral columns just proximal to the fracture.
  - Achieving bicortical fixation with each pin.
  - Maximizing pin spread at the fracture site.
  - Ensuring bony purchase in the distal fragment (by not starting too posteriorly or too near the lateral edge).
  - Avoiding pins crossing at the fracture site because they function essentially as one pin.
- Persistent instability or inadequate fixation can be recognized by performing stress views of the fracture in both the AP and lateral planes.
- For medial-entry pins, neurovascular structures are protected by extending the elbow during pin placement to prevent anterior subluxation of the ulnar nerve and iatrogenic injury.
- Careful attention must be paid to the soft tissues and the neurovascular status of the arm by
  - Avoiding tight circumferential dressings.
  - Considering the use of sterile foam to allow for swelling in the cast.
  - Avoiding elbow flexion >70° in the postoperative cast.
  - Rechecking the radial pulse after fracture reduction.

References

1. Houshian S, Mehdi B, Larsen MS: The epidemiology of elbow fracture in children: Analysis of 355 fractures, with special reference to supracondylar humerus fractures. *J Orthop Sci* 2001;6(4):312-315.

2. Kasser JR, Beaty JH: Supracondylar fractures of the distal humerus, in Beaty JH, Kasser JR, eds: *Rockwood and Wilkins' Fractures in Children*. Philadelphia, PA, Lippincott Williams & Wilkins, 2006, pp 543-589.

3. Leitch KK, Kay RM, Femino JD, Tolo VT, Storer SK, Skaggs DL: Treatment of multidirectionally unstable supracondylar humeral fractures in children: A modified Gartland type-IV fracture. *J Bone Joint Surg Am* 2006;88(5):980-985.

4. Babal JC, Mehlman CT, Klein G: Nerve injuries associated with pediatric supracondylar humeral fractures: A meta-analysis. *J Pediatr Orthop* 2010;30(3):253-263.

5. Mapes RC, Hennrikus WL: The effect of elbow position on the radial pulse measured by Doppler ultrasonography after surgical treatment of supracondylar elbow fractures in children. *J Pediatr Orthop* 1998;18(4):441-444.

6. Battaglia TC, Armstrong DG, Schwend RM: Factors affecting forearm compartment pressures in children with supracondylar fractures of the humerus. *J Pediatr Orthop* 2002;22(4):431-439.

7. Skaggs DL, Sankar WN, Albrektson J, Vaishnav S, Choi PD, Kay RM: How safe is the operative treatment of Gartland type 2 supracondylar humerus fractures in children? *J Pediatr Orthop* 2008;28(2):139-141.

8. Omid R, Choi PD, Skaggs DL: Supracondylar humeral fractures in children. *J Bone Joint Surg Am* 2008;90(5):1121-1132.

9. Peters CL, Scott SM, Stevens PM: Closed reduction and percutaneous pinning of displaced supracondylar humerus fractures in children: Description of a new closed reduction technique for fractures with brachialis muscle entrapment. *J Orthop Trauma* 1995;9(5):430-434.

10. Sankar WN, Hebela NM, Skaggs DL, Flynn JM: Loss of pin fixation in displaced supracondylar humeral fractures in children: Causes and prevention. *J Bone Joint Surg Am* 2007;89(4):713-717.

11. Skaggs DL, Hale JM, Bassett J, Kaminsky C, Kay RM, Tolo VT: Operative treatment of supracondylar fractures of the humerus in children: The consequences of pin placement. *J Bone Joint Surg Am* 2001;83(5):735-740.

12. Skaggs DL, Cluck MW, Mostofi A, Flynn JM, Kay RM: Lateral-entry pin fixation in the management of supracondylar fractures in children. *J Bone Joint Surg Am* 2004;86(4):702-707.

13. Mahan ST, May CD, Kocher MS: Operative management of displaced flexion supracondylar humerus fractures in children. *J Pediatr Orthop* 2007;27(5):551-556.

14. Ay S, Akinci M, Kamiloglu S, Ercetin O: Open reduction of displaced pediatric supracondylar humeral fractures through the anterior cubital approach. *J Pediatr Orthop* 2005;25(2):149-153.

15. Koudstaal MJ, De Ridder VA, De Lange S, Ulrich C: Pediatric supracondylar humerus fractures: The anterior approach. *J Orthop Trauma* 2002;16(6):409-412.

Chapter 98
Reduction and Fixation of Lateral Condyle Fractures of the Distal Humerus

Neeraj M. Patel, MD, MPH, MBS   John M. Flynn, MD

Patient Selection

Fractures of the lateral condyle of the humerus typically occur as a result of a fall, either on an outstretched hand or from a height. Classically, these injuries are categorized as Milch type I fractures if they pass through the ossific nucleus of the capitellum or Milch type II fractures if they pass medial to the capitellum and into the trochlear groove.[1] Treatment depends more on the extent of displacement than on location, however[2] (Figure 1).

Nonsurgical treatment with a long-arm cast is adequate for nondisplaced or minimally displaced fractures (<2 mm). Surgery is recommended for fractures with greater than 2 mm of displacement or fragment rotation. Closed reduction with percutaneous pinning may be appropriate for minimally displaced fractures (2 to 4 mm) when a perfect intra-articular reduction can be obtained. Open reduction and internal fixation is recommended for fractures that are unstable or significantly displaced (>4 mm).[3,4]

Preoperative Imaging

When a lateral condyle fracture is suspected, AP, lateral, and internal oblique radiographs should be obtained (Figure 2). The oblique view is particularly valuable in determining maximum displacement and for following the fractures after closed or open treatment. Careful examination of multiple radiographic views is necessary to assess any potential rotational displacement. Of note, the size of the fracture fragment is typically larger than is visualized on plain radiographs because of its cartilaginous component. Hinging of the condylar fragment into the joint space might be difficult to determine radiographically for some minimally displaced fractures. In such situations, MRI or magnetic resonance arthrography can be considered to assess for disruption of the articular surface. Treatment decisions can typically be made with radiographs, however, so these other modalities are not commonly used because of their cost and because they frequently require patient sedation.[5]

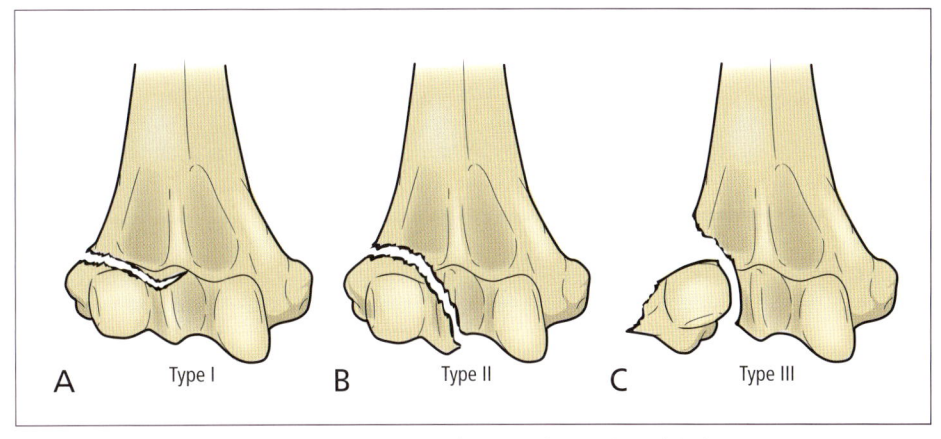

Figure 1 Illustrations show the Milch classification of lateral condyle fractures. **A,** Type I: displaced less than 2 mm with no violation of the articular surface. **B,** Type II: displaced 2 mm or more with no violation of the articular surface. **C,** Type III: displaced 2 mm or more with disruption of the articular surface.

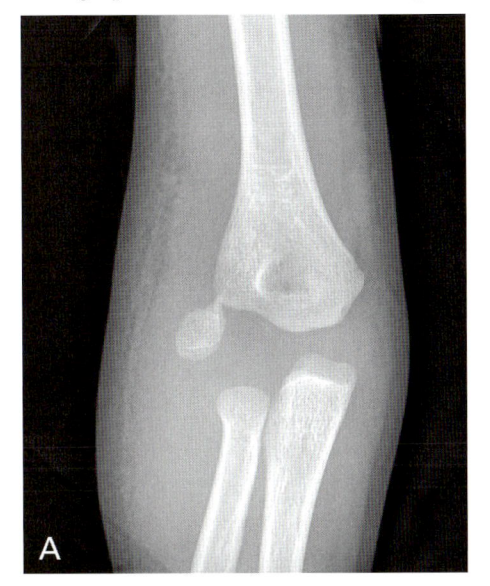

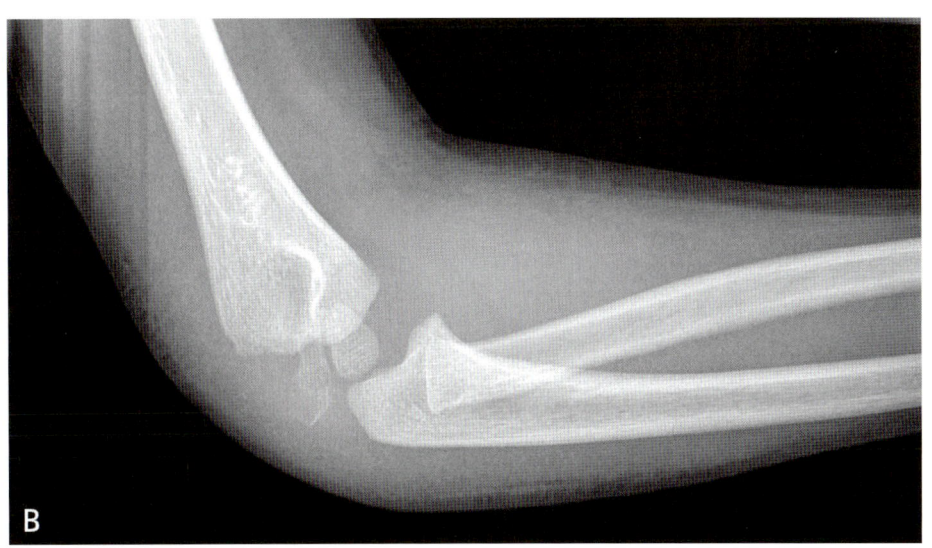

Figure 2 AP (**A**) and lateral (**B**) radiographs show a lateral condyle fracture in the right arm of a 5-year-old patient.

Dr. Flynn or an immediate family member has received royalties from Biomet and serves as a board member, owner, officer, or committee member of the Pediatric Orthopaedic Society of North America, the Scoliosis Research Society, and the American Academy of Orthopaedic Surgeons. Neither Dr. Patel nor any immediate family member has received anything of value from or has stock or stock options held in a commercial company or institution related directly or indirectly to the subject of this chapter.

Section 8: Pediatric Orthopaedics

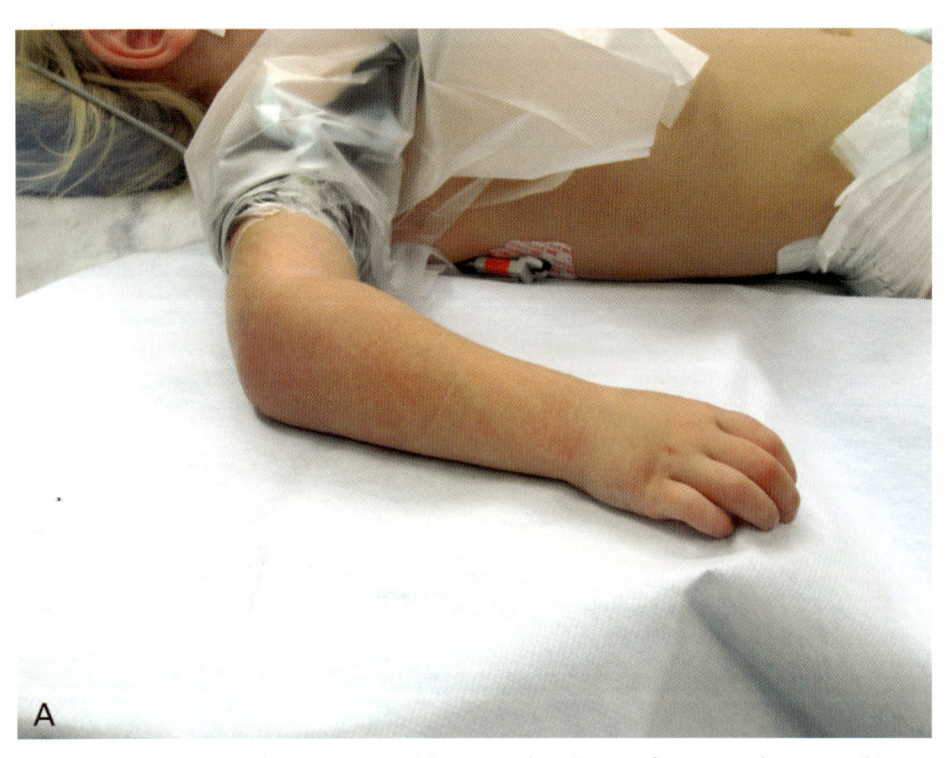

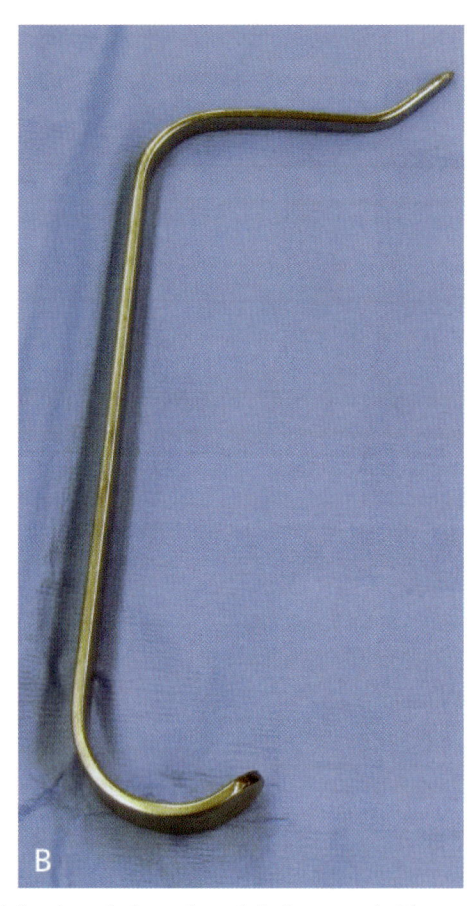

Figure 3 Photographs show patient positioning and equipment for open reduction and internal fixation of a lateral condyle fracture. **A,** The arm is shown on a hand table and with a tourniquet in place. **B,** A small right-angle retractor; this may be used to raise anterior soft tissues.

Procedure
Special Instruments/Equipment/Implants
A fluoroscopic unit is valuable for intraoperative imaging. A tourniquet is valuable for creating a bloodless field, improving visualization, and assessing joint surface congruity (**Figure 3, A**). A pin driver is required to place pins, typically 0.062-in Kirschner wires (K-wires). For open reduction, a small right-angle retractor and a towel clip are useful (**Figure 3, B**). Alternatively, a compression screw can be used in an older child with a larger bony portion of the condylar fragment. A splint or cast is necessary for postoperative immobilization.

Surgical Technique
Closed Reduction and Percutaneous Pinning
Fracture stability can be evaluated under anesthesia with varus stress radiographs and arthrography. After closed reduction is performed, two divergent pins are used for percutaneous fixation, using the same pattern as that for fixation of supracondylar fractures. The first wire is introduced into the lateral condyle from distal-lateral to proximal-medial to engage the condylar fragment. A second wire is placed similarly and diverges from the first at the fracture site (**Figure 4**). Once satisfactory reduction and fixation are achieved, the wires are cut and bent 90° outside the skin. Nonadherent fine-mesh gauze infused with a blend of petrolatum with 3% bismuth tribromophenate is wrapped around the base of the wires to prevent the wires from migrating under the skin, preventing motion at the skin-wire interface and the subsequent risk of pin infection. With a long-arm cast or splint, the elbow is immobilized in 80° of flexion with the forearm in neutral position.

Open Reduction and Internal Fixation
A lateral Kocher-type incision is made, with approximately 2 to 3 cm of the incision proximal to the elbow joint and 1 to 2 cm of the incision distal to it. The incision is positioned slightly anterior, which allows for better visualization and pin placement posterior and distal to the incision rather than entering through the incision itself (**Figure 5**). As the incision is carried through the subcutaneous tissue, a shallow surgical interval is noted between the brachioradialis and the lateral condyle of the humerus. Most of the dissection has already been done by the fracture itself. Evacuation of the fracture hematoma will improve fracture visualization, as will any potential tears through the aponeurosis of the brachioradialis. Of note, the vascular supply of the lateral condyle epiphysis originates in the soft tissues on the posterior aspect of the fractured condyle. Therefore, it is important to avoid stripping of the posterior tissues from the fracture fragment. Exposure is considered adequate once the medialmost aspect of the fracture can be assessed anteriorly (**Figure 6, A**).

A small right-angle retractor can be used to lift the anterior soft tissues for direct visualization of the articular surface without excessive stretching. When the fracture site and elbow joint have been assessed by visualization and palpation, one wire is drilled through the skin and into the fracture fragment, penetrating just enough to see that it is in the center of the fragment. The fracture is then reduced into perfect anatomic position and confirmed visually. This first wire is then driven across the distal humerus, engaging the medial cortex (**Figure 6, B**). After the anatomic reduction is confirmed radiographically, the second pin is placed

Chapter 98: Reduction and Fixation of Lateral Condyle Fractures of the Distal Humerus

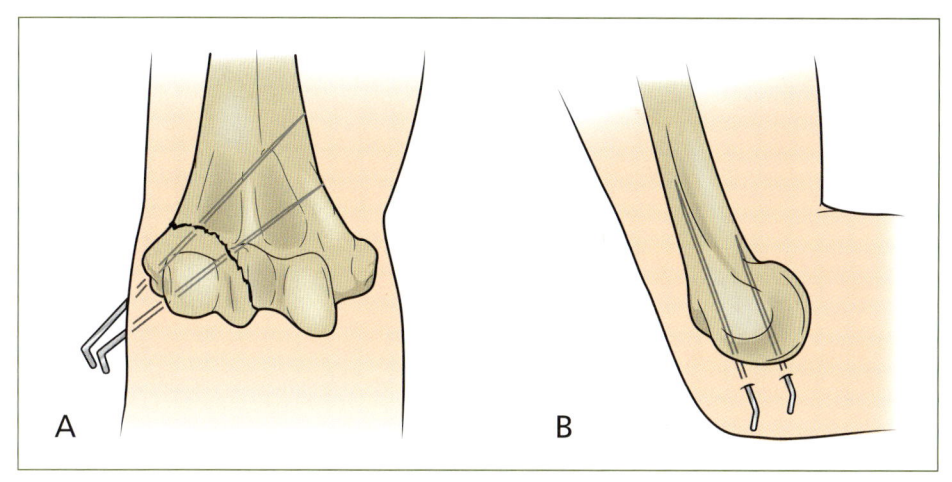

Figure 4 Illustrations of the anterior (**A**) and lateral (**B**) aspects of the elbow demonstrate optimal pin placement for a lateral condyle fracture.

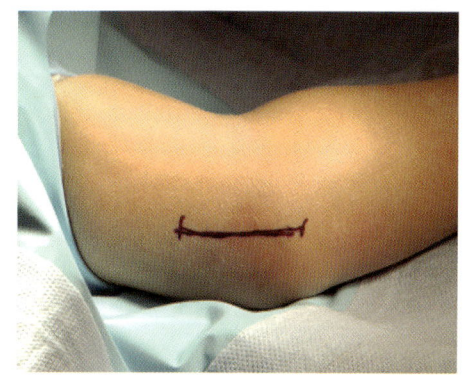

Figure 5 Photograph shows the planned incision for open reduction and internal fixation of a lateral condyle fracture marked on the skin. A lateral Kocher-type incision is used, keeping it slightly anterior so that the pins may be placed posterior and distal to it.

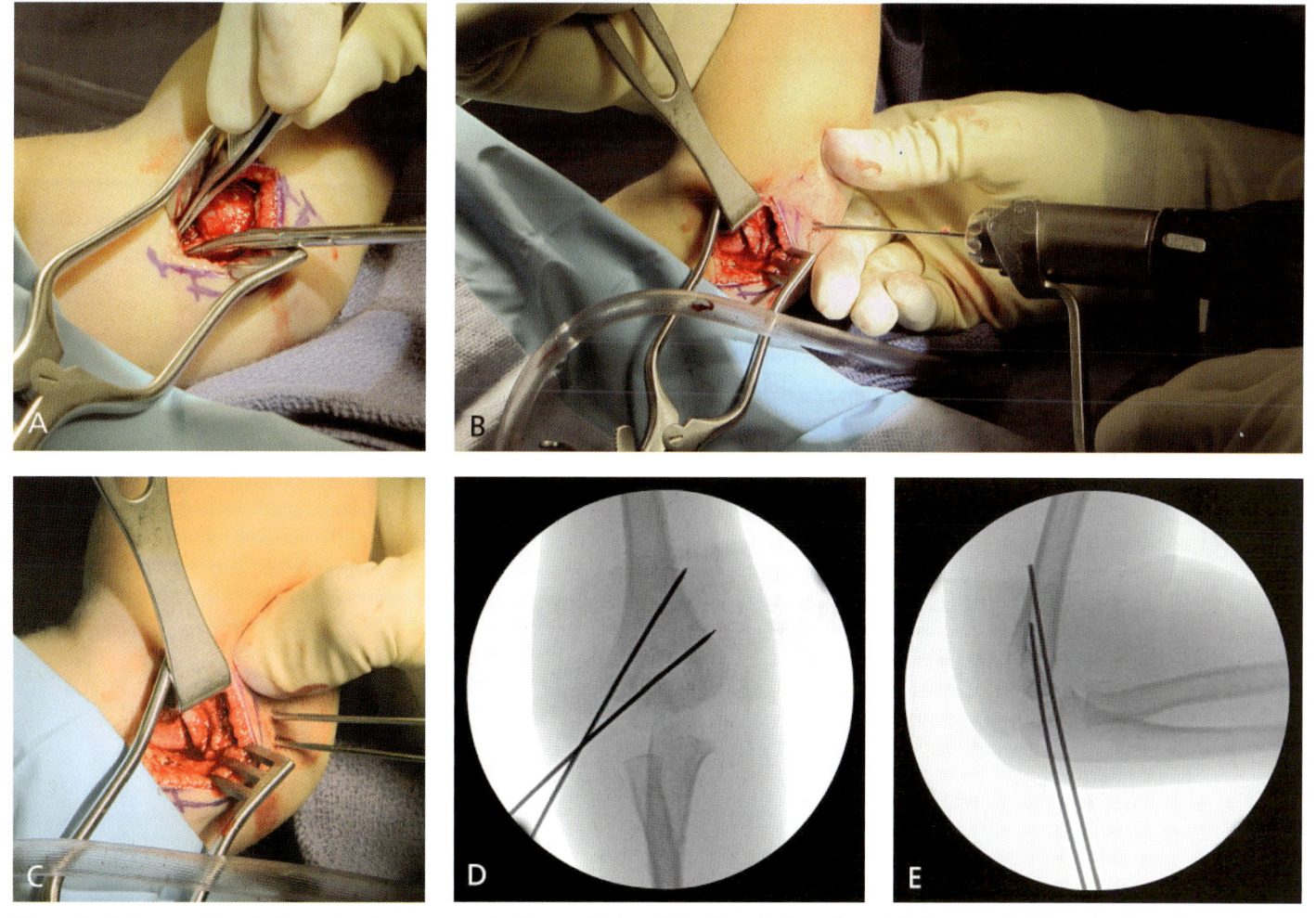

Figure 6 Intraoperative photographs show open reduction and internal fixation of a lateral condyle fracture. **A,** Dissection is performed anteriorly, with special care taken to avoid stripping of the posterior soft tissues. **B,** The first wire is inserted through the lateral aspect of the fracture fragment. **C,** Two divergent wires are placed through the fracture site. AP (**D**) and lateral (**E**) intraoperative fluoroscopic images demonstrate divergent pin placement.

in a divergent fashion (**Figure 6, C**), engaging a large portion of the fracture fragment, crossing the fracture line, and engaging the medial cortex. There is no problem if one or both wires go through the olecranon fossa. Reduction is verified fluoroscopically. Fluoroscopy is then used to confirm reduction and pin placement with gentle stressing (**Figure 6, D** and **E**). Additional pins are required if satisfactory fixation is not achieved. When possible, the periosteal flap should be sutured because this may decrease the risk of postoperative bone spur formation.

The wires may then be cut and bent at 90° if they are to be left outside the skin. Sterile felt or the petrolatum blend gauze

© 2013 American Academy of Orthopaedic Surgeons

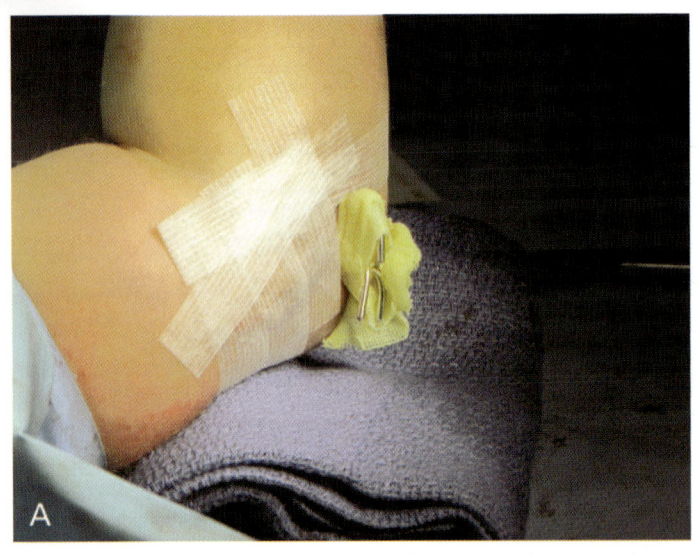

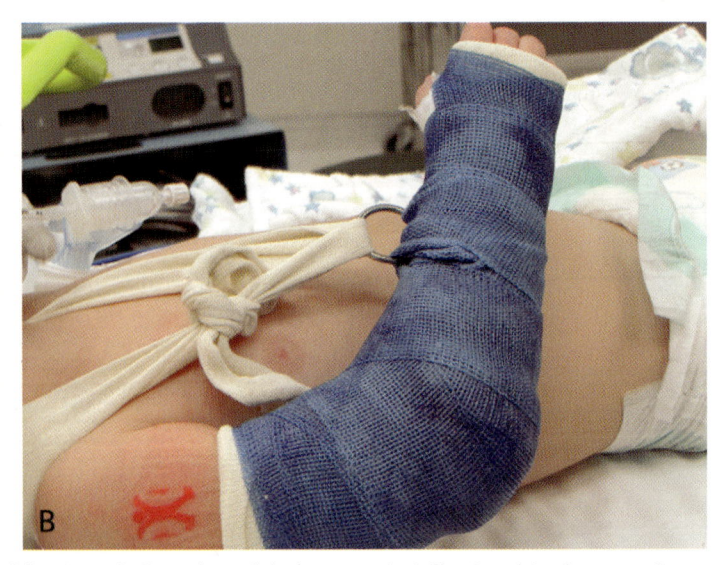

Figure 7 Photographs show an elbow after open reduction and internal fixation of a lateral condyle fracture. **A,** Adhesive skin closure strips have been applied, and fine-mesh gauze infused with a petrolatum blend has been placed between the skin and the cut ends of the wires. **B,** The elbow is immobilized in a long arm cast at 80° of flexion.

may be placed between the skin and the cut end of the wire to lessen postoperative skin irritation. Some surgeons prefer that the wires be cut as short as possible, bent, and left beneath the skin. Although this method may decrease the risk of pin-tract infection, it necessitates an additional surgery for removal.

Resorbable pins (1.5 mm) can be used for fixation instead of K-wires, although this is not our preferred method. If this method is chosen, the fracture must first be reduced and temporarily pinned with guidewires. Once the guidewires are confirmed fluoroscopically, they are replaced by resorbable pins of appropriate length, with any excess length cut and removed.

If an older patient is found to have a large condylar fragment, compression screws may be used for fixation. This technique has potential disadvantages, however. The compressive threads may disrupt growth in younger patients, or the screw head may become symptomatic, requiring a return to the operating room for removal. Therefore, this method is typically used only in delayed unions or nonunions.

The wound is irrigated and closed in routine fashion with absorbable sutures and adhesive skin closure strips, and a sterile dressing is applied (**Figure 7, A**). Finally, the elbow should be immobilized in 80° of flexion with the forearm positioned neutral in a cast or a posterior splint (**Figure 7, B**).

Complications

Osteonecrosis may occur as a result of the injury or from excessive intraoperative stripping of soft tissue from the posterior aspect of the fracture fragment, which disrupts lateral epiphyseal blood flow. The risk of posterior or lateral bone spurs may be diminished by suturing of the periosteal flap during surgery. Delayed union, malunion, and nonunion are more common in nonsurgical cases, but they may occur in surgical patients. Delayed union may require prolonged casting of up to 12 weeks; malunion and nonunion usually require additional surgery. Other potential complications include wound infection, pin-tract infection, growth arrest, stiffness, and tardy ulnar nerve palsy.

Postoperative Care and Rehabilitation

A long arm cast is applied. Casts can be bivalved in the operating room in the context of significant swelling. The patient returns for the first follow-up 4 weeks after surgery, and radiographs are taken with the cast off but the pins in. As long as there is some initial callus (usually seen posteriorly), the pins are removed, and a new cast is placed for the final 2 weeks of immobilization. Six weeks of overall mobilization are recommended after open reduction and internal fixation of the lateral condyle fracture in a child. After the second cast is removed, at 6 weeks after surgery, the patient is instructed to begin gentle range-of-motion exercises. Physical therapy is rarely necessary following treatment of a lateral condyle fracture, but it can be considered if range of motion about the elbow fails to improve within 4 weeks of treatment.

Pearls

- Posterior dissection should be avoided because it may disrupt the lateral epiphyseal vascular supply and result in osteonecrosis of the fracture fragment.
- Divergent, bicortical pins prevent loss of fixation.
- Gentle stressing of the fracture under fluoroscopy before closure can help to evaluate the quality of reduction and fixation. If the fracture is still unstable, additional pins or suture should be applied.
- The risk of postoperative bone spurs may be decreased by closure of the periosteum.
- Placement of felt or fine-mesh gauze infused with a petrolatum blend between the skin and the cut ends of the wires can lessen postoperative skin irritation and swelling.
- Open anatomic reduction should generally be avoided in patients who present 3 or more weeks after the initial injury. In these patients, the soft-tissue stripping required for anatomic reduction risks devascularization of the fragment and disruption of the significant healing and remodeling that have already occurred. This then increases the risk of growth arrest, decreased range of motion, tardy ulnar nerve palsy, osteonecrosis, and valgus deformity.

References

1. Milch H: Fractures and fracture-dislocations of the humeral condyles. *J Trauma* 1964;4:592-607.

2. Weiss JM, Graves S, Yang S, Mendelsohn E, Kay RM, Skaggs DL: A new classification system predictive of complications in surgically treated pediatric humeral lateral condyle fractures. *J Pediatr Orthop* 2009;29(6):602-605.

3. Jakob R, Fowles JV, Rang M, Kassab MT: Observations concerning fractures of the lateral humeral condyle in children. *J Bone Joint Surg Br* 1975;57(4):430-436.

4. Sullivan JA: Fractures of the lateral condyle of the humerus. *J Am Acad Orthop Surg* 2006;14(1):58-62.

5. Bhandari M, Tornetta P, Swiontkowksi MF; Evidence-Based Orthopaedic Trauma Working Group: Displaced lateral condyle fractures of the distal humerus. *J Orthop Trauma* 2003;17(4):306-308.

Chapter 99
Intramedullary Fixation of Radial and Ulnar Shaft Fractures in Skeletally Immature Patients

Maya E. Pring, MD   Hilton P. Gottschalk, MD   Henry G. Chambers, MD

Patient Selection

Pediatric radial and ulnar shaft fractures are treated differently than similar fractures in adults. Adult forearm fractures are commonly fixed with plates and screws to maintain alignment and allow early mobilization to prevent stiffness. Plates and screws are not commonly used in the skeletally immature patient, for the following reasons: They disrupt the periosteal blood supply and fracture hematoma, which may alter the healing potential, and they create a stress riser both while the plate is in place and once it is removed, which leads to increased risk of repeat fracture as children return to regular activities. Pediatric fractures heal much more quickly and have remodeling potential, so anatomic alignment is not always necessary; furthermore, because children rarely have difficulty with stiffness, early mobilization is not as important as it is with adults.[1,2] Intramedullary (IM) fixation is a minimally invasive and relatively safe method of fixing pediatric forearm fractures that are not amenable to routine casting. This technique minimizes soft-tissue disruption and scarring and allows for easy implant removal.

Indications

Radial and ulnar shaft fractures are among the most common injuries seen in any pediatric emergency department.[1,2] Both-bone forearm fractures can be sustained through a variety of mechanisms, from simple falls onto the outstretched arm to higher energy falls sustained in contact sports or wheeled activities such as skateboarding, motorcycle riding, and all-terrain vehicle riding. Simple both-bone forearm fractures in children and adolescents usually can be treated in a closed fashion with reduction and casting.[1-3] If the fracture is open (**Figure 1**) or if an adequate closed reduction cannot be obtained or maintained in a cast, IM fixation can stabilize and maintain reduction with minimal soft-tissue disruption and scarring.[2-5] The implants are easily removed with minimal downtime once the fracture is healed. Fractures with associated compartment syndrome that require fasciotomies are also best stabilized with IM implants to avoid the need for a cast or anything that may increase compartment pressures.[5] A patient with multiple

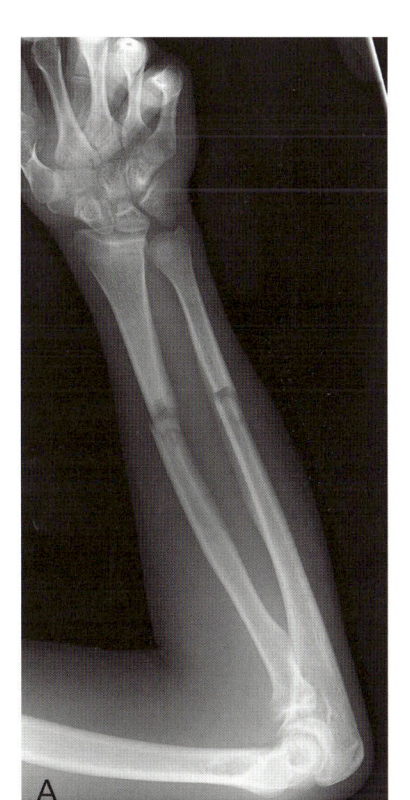

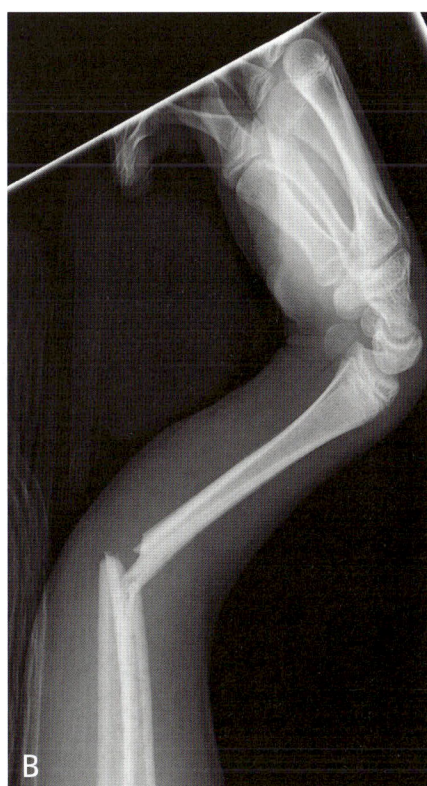

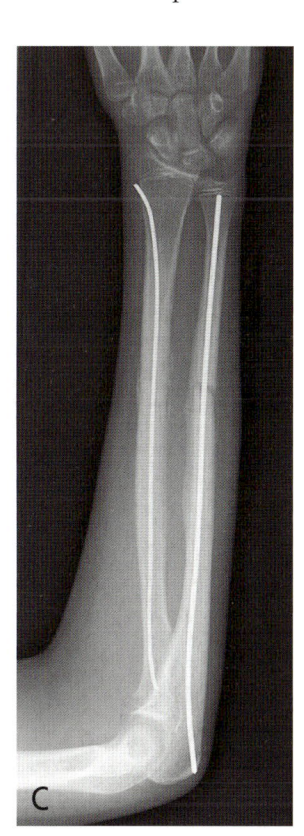

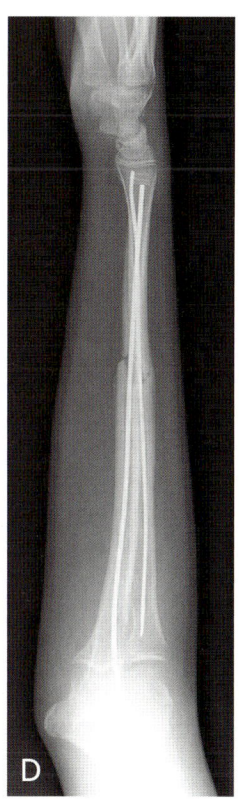

Figure 1 Radiographs of a patient who sustained an open both-bone forearm fracture. Preoperative PA (**A**) and lateral (**B**) views. PA (**C**) and lateral (**D**) views obtained after intramedullary nail fixation.

Dr. Pring or an immediate family member serves as a board member, owner, officer, or committee member of the American Academy for Cerebral Palsy and Developmental Medicine and the Pediatric Orthopaedic Society of North America. Dr. Gottschalk or an immediate family member serves as a paid consultant to or is an employee of Biogen Idec and has stock or stock options held in Biogen Idec. Dr. Chambers or an immediate family member serves as a paid consultant to or is an employee of Allergen, Merz Pharmaceuticals, and OrthoPediatrics and serves as a board member, owner, officer, or committee member of the American Academy of Orthopaedic Surgeons, the American Academy for Cerebral Palsy and Developmental Medicine, and the Pediatric Orthopaedic Society of North America.

Table 1 General Guidelines for Acceptable Values in Both-Bone Forearm Fractures[a]

Age	Acceptable Angulation	Acceptable Translation	Acceptable Rotation
Younger than 9 years	≤15°	Bayonet	≤45°
9 years or older with >2 years of growth remaining	≤10° for proximal fractures ≤15° for distal fractures	100%	≤30°

[a]Data from Noonan KJ, Price CT: Forearm and distal radius fractures in children. *J Am Acad Orthop Surg* 1998;6(3):146-156.

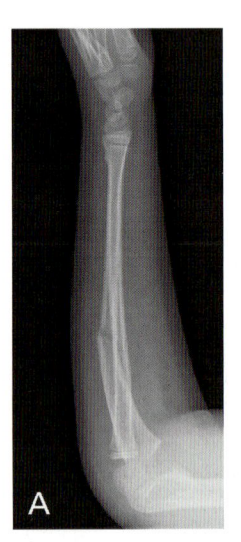

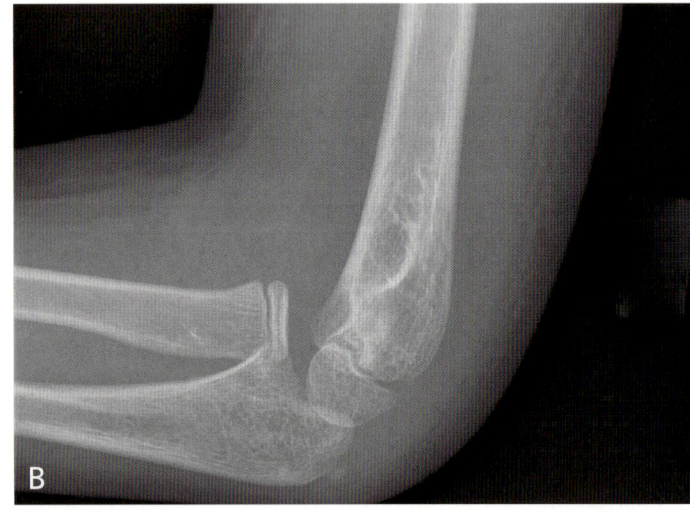

Figure 2 Radiographs demonstrate the importance of imaging adjacent joints. **A**, Lateral radiograph of forearm shows an ulnar shaft fracture and a distal radial buckle fracture. **B**, Dedicated lateral radiograph of the same patient's elbow shows a Monteggia variant and a dislocation of the proximal radiocapitellar joint.

fractures who would be significantly disabled if not able to use the arm may also benefit from IM stabilization of the forearm fracture.

Acceptable reduction is different at different ages. In young children, fractures have a high potential for remodeling; the closer children get to skeletal maturity, the less likely fractures are to remodel. Distal fractures also have significantly more remodeling potential than proximal fractures.[2,5] Fractures are more likely to remodel when closer to the physis and in the plane of motion (dorsal or volar angulation at the wrist). Rotational deformity is unlikely to remodel, so a loss of pronation and supination, even in young children, can create a long-term functional deficit.[1,2] Even though angulation and displacement are described on AP and lateral views, the actual fracture angulation and displacement are always in a single plane, and the magnitude of the deformity is at least as great as that seen on each view.[2] General guidelines for acceptable values in treating radial and ulnar shaft fractures are presented in **Table 1**; however, all of the factors described previously need to be considered when making the decision to proceed with surgery versus allowing the fracture to heal with slight malunion and the expectation that remodeling will occur and function will be near normal.

Contraindications
IM fixation in children younger than 5 years has been reported,[4] but given the high potential for remodeling in this population, there is very little role for IM fixation in this age group. On the other end of the pediatric age spectrum, in skeletally mature patients, the implants discussed in this chapter may not be rigid enough to maintain anatomic alignment, and as there is minimal remodeling potential, other methods of fixation, such as plates and screws, should be considered.[5] Contraindications to IM fixation include intra-articular fractures, significantly comminuted fractures, and fractures with gross contamination. If significant comminution is present, it is difficult to maintain the length of the bone with an IM implant. This can lead to shortening of one bone, which may disrupt the distal and/or proximal radioulnar joints. Also, it is difficult to get good fixation of distal/metaphyseal radius fractures with an IM implant.[6] Proximal radius fractures (even radial neck fractures) can be reduced and stabilized with an appropriately contoured implant as long as the patient is close enough to skeletal maturity that crossing the physis with the implant is not a concern.

Preoperative Imaging
Diagnostic imaging includes AP and lateral radiographs of the forearm and dedicated views of the wrist and the elbow to ensure that the proximal radioulnar joint (PRUJ) and the distal radioulnar joint (DRUJ) are intact.[1,2] A Monteggia fracture (ulnar fracture with dislocation of the radiocapitellar joint) (**Figure 2**) or a Galeazzi fracture (radial fracture with dislocation of the DRUJ) is easily missed if the joints above and below the fracture are not carefully examined radiographically. The dislocation may occur far from the fracture and be missed by a radiograph centered on the deformity.

Video 99.1 Distal Forearm Fractures: Both-Bone Forearm Fracture Intramedullary Nailing: Step 1. Kelly D. Carmichael, MD; Chris English, MD (25 min)

Procedure
Room Setup/Patient Positioning
When setting up the operating room, it is important to organize the room so that the C-arm can easily be brought in and out of the field without disrupting the surgery. The monitor should be positioned so that the surgeon does not have to turn his or her head to see the monitor. The arm is positioned on a radiolucent arm board perpendicular to the operating table (**Figure 3**).

Special Instruments/Equipment/Implants
A variety of commercially available flexible implants can be used, both titanium

Chapter 99: Intramedullary Fixation of Radial and Ulnar Shaft Fractures in Skeletally Immature Patients

(more flexible) and stainless steel (more rigid); these come with a prebent tip to make passage down the IM canal easier. The surgeon will still need to contour the rod to maximize stability at the fracture site.[3,7] For younger children, Kirschner wires (K-wires) can be used in the same fashion, but more contouring is required. When planning which size implant or K-wire to use, the narrowest portion of the IM canal should be measured on the radiograph, and the surgeon should plan to fill 60% to 80% of the canal diameter with the IM implant.[3,6-8] No reaming is done, and the implant does not need to fill the canal.

Surgical Technique

Some controversy exists as to which bone to reduce first. Some authors recommend starting with the easiest fracture first because this may lead to an acceptable reduction and stability of the other bone.[2,7] We recommend starting with the bone that is going to be more difficult to reduce first, usually the radius.[3,8] Once one bone is stabilized, it may be more difficult to reduce a bone that is significantly shortened or angulated, especially if there is significant swelling. Because the ulna is subcutaneous along its length, it is usually easier to manipulate; therefore, it is often better to fix the ulna after the radius has been aligned and fixed. The surgeon need not worry about reducing the fractures until the first implant has been inserted and passed to the fracture site. The implant can then be used as a tool to assist with fracture reduction.

Fixing the Radius

The implant should be precontoured to reproduce the dorsal radial bow. The easiest way to do this is to lay the implant on the forearm with the tip curved toward the bicipital tuberosity and then mark the actual bone length and the point where the maximal bow on the implant is desired. Then a contouring tool is used to create a smooth, gentle curve from the tip to the point where the implant will exit the bone (**Figure 4**). A slight S-shaped bend at the exit point will help with later rotation, when the implant is being used to re-create the radial bow.

The radial implant is placed retrograde, starting distally but at least 1.5 cm proximal to the distal radial physis, to avoid injury to the physis and the perichondrial ring. The importance of protecting the growth potential of the distal radius makes fixing distal metaphyseal radius

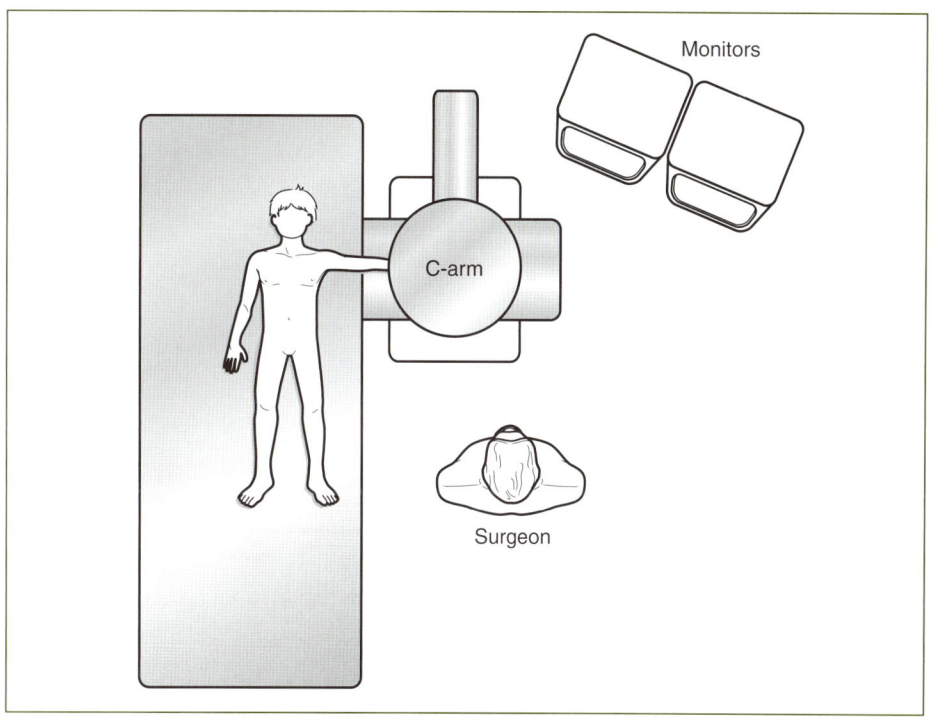

Figure 3 Illustration shows the operating room setup for intramedullary fixation of a forearm fracture.

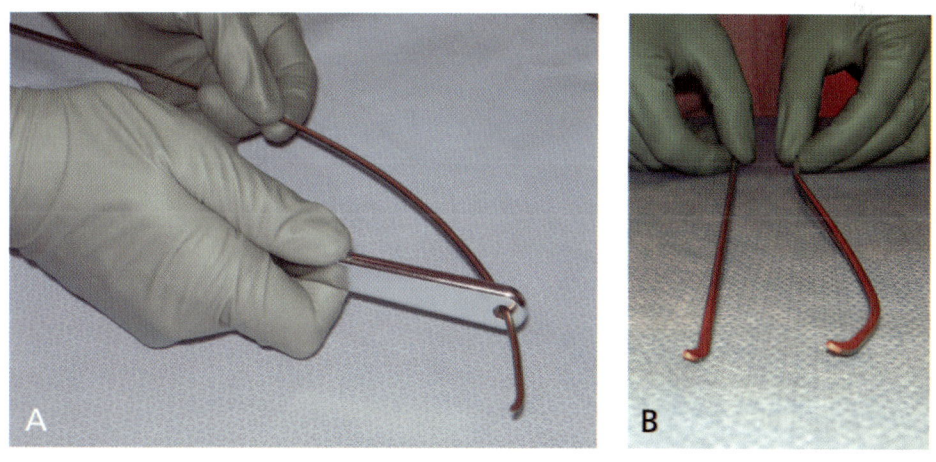

Figure 4 Photographs show precontouring of the intramedullary implant for the radius in a both-bone forearm fracture. **A,** A contouring tool is used to create a smooth, gentle curve from the tip to the point where the implant will exit the bone. **B,** A slight S bend is created at the exit point. This will help with later rotation when using the implant to re-create the radial bow.

fractures with this technique difficult; a different method, such as percutaneous K-wire fixation, should be considered for distal metaphyseal radius fractures.[8] A small incision (<1.5 cm) is made on the dorsal-radial side of the distal radius, taking care to protect and avoid the superficial radial nerve.[2-5,7,8] If this nerve is injured during the approach, drilling, or implant insertion, the patient will have an area of decreased sensation on the dorsal-radial side of the wrist and the thumb. The interval between the extensor pollicis brevis and the extensor carpi radialis longus (first and second compartments) or the interval between the extensor carpi radialis brevis and the extensor pollicis longus (second and third compartments) can be used (**Figure 5**). Care should be taken not to have a prominent implant tip under a tendon because tendon rupture caused by IM implants has been reported.[4,5]

The surgeon should bluntly dissect down to bone and then use a drill bit slightly larger than the implant to be inserted to create the entry point through one cortex of the radius.[3] The entry site should be at the proximal end of the incision to allow easy passage of the implant. A drill guide is used to avoid wrapping the soft tissues, including the superficial

© 2013 American Academy of Orthopaedic Surgeons

Section 8: Pediatric Orthopaedics

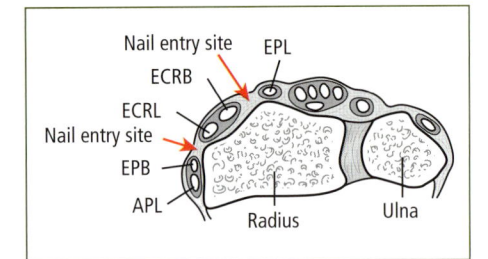

Figure 5 Illustration shows a cross section of the forearm. The interval between the extensor pollicis brevis (EPB) and the extensor carpi radialis longus (ECRL) or the interval between the extensor carpi radialis brevis (ECRB) and the extensor pollicis longus (EPL) can be used as starting points in the radius. APL = abductor pollicis longus.

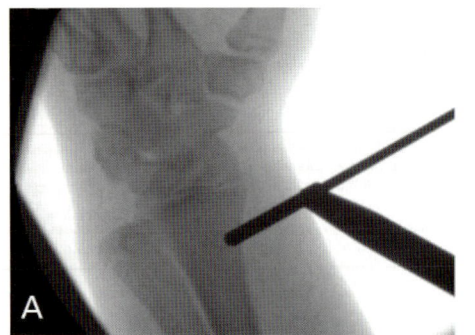

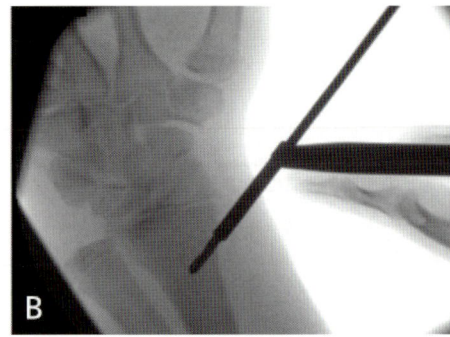

Figure 6 Fluoroscopic images of a forearm with a both-bone fracture show drilling for the nail entry site for intramedullary fixation of the radius. **A,** A drill guide is used to prevent wrapping up soft tissue while the drill is started perpendicular to the bone. **B,** After breaching the first cortex, the surgeon continues spinning the drill bit and angles the tip toward the elbow to create an oblong entry site through only one cortex.

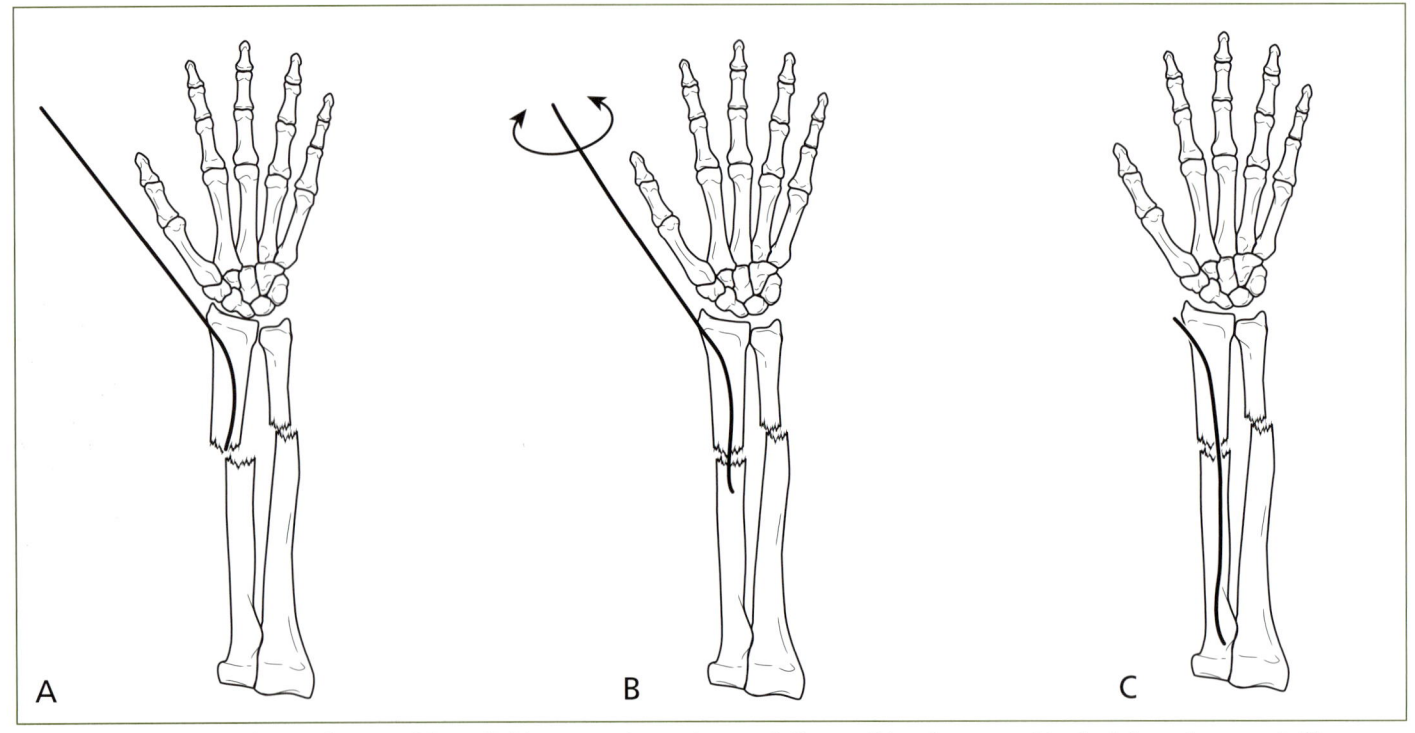

Figure 7 Illustrations show reduction of the radial fracture using an intramedullary nail in a forearm with a both-bone fracture. **A,** The implant is advanced to the fracture site. **B,** The implant is rotated to allow passage into the proximal fragment. **C,** The implant is used as a lever to manipulate the distal fragment to the proximal fragment. The implant tip can be used to "catch" the canal of the proximal fragment.

radial nerve, around the drill (**Figure 6**). The surgeon starts with the drill perpendicular to the bone; once one cortex has been opened, rather than insert the drill any farther, the surgeon continues spinning it and angles the drill tip toward the elbow to create an oblong entry site through only one cortex.[3,7] If both cortices are breached by the drill, passage of the implant will be more difficult. The drill is then removed, and the precontoured implant tip is inserted into the distal radius. With a slight rocking motion, the implant is advanced down the canal to the fracture site.

At this point, the radial fracture will need to be reduced. Manual traction and manipulation is often enough, but if reduction is difficult, the implant is passed slightly out of the distal fragment; the implant can be used as a lever to manipulate the distal fragment to the proximal fragment, and the implant tip can be used to "catch" the canal of the proximal fragment (**Figure 7**). Multiple passes of the implant that miss the proximal fragment can cause soft-tissue disruption and bleeding, which increases the risk of compartment syndrome.[2,4,5] If closed methods are not adequate or multiple unsuccessful attempts have been made a small incision should be made at the fracture site (along the line from the radial styloid to the bicipital tuberosity—the Henry approach), and the fracture can be reduced under direct visualization. Fasciotomies should be considered if the swelling is concerning for impending compartment syndrome.

Once the implant tip is inside the proximal fragment, it can be worked up the canal, stopping just before the proximal radial physis. The implant is rotated to reestablish the dorsal-radial bow.[3,7-9] Tamping the tip into the bicipital tuberosity gives good stability. The implant is then pulled away from the entry site (without creating a bend) and cut approximately 1 cm from the bone, allowing the implant to snap back and rest against the bone.[3] If it is cut properly, there will be no need to tamp it into the bone any farther. The surgeon should leave enough protruding from the bone to allow easy removal once

Chapter 99: Intramedullary Fixation of Radial and Ulnar Shaft Fractures in Skeletally Immature Patients

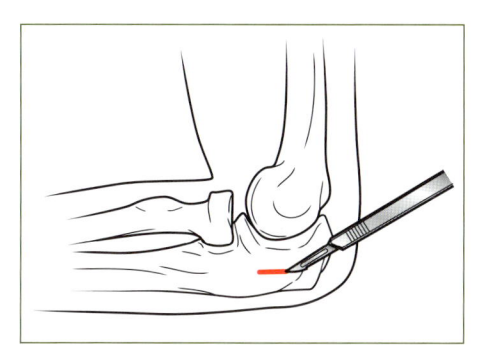

Figure 8 Illustration shows the incision for the nail entry site for intramedullary fixation of the ulna.

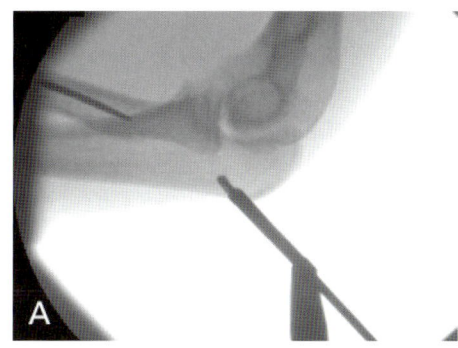

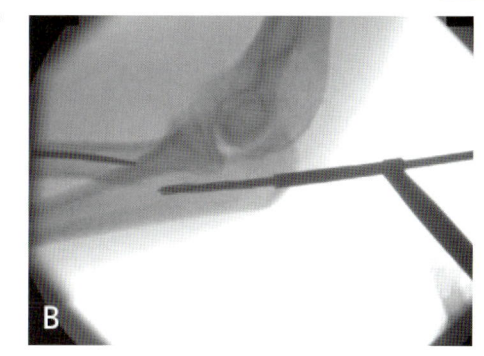

Figure 9 Fluoroscopic images show drilling for the nail entry site for intramedullary fixation of the ulna in a both-bone fracture of the forearm. **A,** Using a drill guide, the drill tip is placed midway between the joint and the posterior aspect of the olecranon. **B,** The surgeon drills through one cortex only; then, with the drill tip spinning but not advancing, the drill bit is angled toward the wrist in line with the ulna.

the bone has healed, but not so much that it will erode through the soft tissues after skin closure.

Fixing the Ulna

The ulnar implant does not need much precontouring, as the ulna is naturally straight, but if K-wires are used, the tip can be bent a little so that the implant will bounce off the far cortex when entering and then advance down the IM canal. This slight bend also helps get the implant across the fracture and into the distal fragment.[3,8] Commercial implants have a bend at the tip and typically do not need further contouring.

The ulna is approached proximally; a small incision (~1 cm) is made on the lateral side of the olecranon midway between the joint and the posterior border of the olecranon and 2 to 3 cm distal to the tip of the olecranon (**Figure 8**). It is important to be on the lateral side because the ulnar nerve lies on the medial side of the olecranon.[2,3,7] Incision can be taken down directly to bone and through the periosteum. Our technique is to insert the drill tip, gently feel the joint and the posterior aspect of the olecranon, and then place the drill midway between these two spots, perpendicular to the bone. We drill through one cortex only; then, with the drill tip spinning but not advancing, the drill bit is angled toward the wrist in line with the ulna (**Figure 9**).

The implant is then passed to the fracture site and the fracture is reduced. Because the ulna is subcutaneous along its length, closed manipulation is usually adequate to align the fracture fragments. If reduction cannot be easily obtained, a small incision is made at the fracture site, along the subcutaneous border, to allow reduction under direct visualization. The tip of the implant can be turned to hook it inside the distal piece even if alignment is not anatomic; as the implant advances into the distal fragment, it will help correct any malalignment. The implant should be passed just to the distal ulnar physis but not across it. The implant can then be cut approximately 1 cm from the entry point into the bone. The cut end should lie flat against the olecranon and not irritate the patient.

Closure and Casting

Skin is closed over both implants, typically with an absorbable suture. It is important to confirm that the forearm has full pronation and supination. Correct rotational alignment is achieved when the radial styloid and the bicipital tuberosity are on opposite sides (radial styloid lateral and bicipital tuberosity medial) with the forearm supinated[2] (**Figure 10**).

The forearm can then be splinted or casted to allow soft-tissue healing. In younger children, casting is preferred because the risk of stiffness is minimal and a cast slows them down a little to prevent reinjury. Flexible implants by design do not provide rigid fixation. There will be some micromotion at the fracture site during healing; discomfort can be minimized with a cast. A splint or a univalve cast should be used for the first week to allow for some soft-tissue swelling. Patients should be monitored overnight, as there is a risk of compartment syndrome following IM fixation of both-bone forearm fractures. After 3 to 4 weeks, there is usually adequate healing to remove immobilization and start gentle motion.[2,3]

Complications

As the use of IM fixation for pediatric both-bone forearm fractures has become more popular, complications associated with the technique have been reported. These include superficial infections around the entry site, skin irritation at the entry site, fracture displacement after implant removal, hardware migration, loss of reduction, refracture, tendon rupture, nerve injury, decreased range of

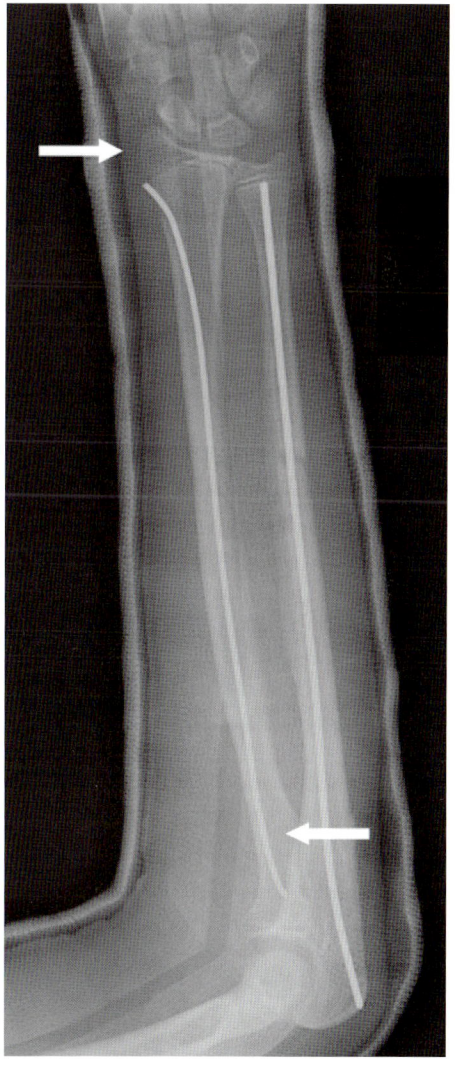

Figure 10 PA radiograph obtained following intramedullary fixation of a both-bone forearm fracture shows appropriate rotational alignment. With the forearm supinated, the radial styloid is lateral (upper arrow) and the bicipital tuberosity is medial (lower arrow).

© 2013 American Academy of Orthopaedic Surgeons

motion, muscle entrapment, delayed union/nonunion, and compartment syndrome.[4-7] Although compartment syndrome is rare in pediatric both-bone forearm fractures, multiple passes with IM nails/rods can increase the risk for soft-tissue damage and subsequent compartment syndrome. Thus, we have adopted the "three-pass rule": We recommend making a small incision over the fracture site for direct visualization and to ease passage of the implant if three unsuccessful attempts have been made to pass the implant across the fracture.[4,5,7]

Postoperative Care and Rehabilitation

In skeletally immature children, implants are usually removed 6 to 9 months after surgery if there is evidence of complete healing on radiographs.[3,7,9] If the implants are left in longer, bone can grow over the tip of the implant, making removal difficult. The two incisions along the distal radius and proximal ulna can be reopened. Again, it is important to protect the superficial radial nerve, which is close to the distal radial incision. Each implant tip can be grabbed with a pair of vice-grip pliers or an implant removal tool if at least 1 cm was left protruding from the bone when the implants were inserted. If the implant was cut too short or was tamped into the bone, or if the implant was left in too long and bone grew over the tip, it will be necessary to remove enough bone to expose the implant and grip it. If such bone removal is done, it is prudent to use a cast or splint postoperatively to prevent fracture through the weakened area until it has healed. If the implants are easily removed without removing additional bone, there will be a small stress riser at the point where the implant was removed from the bone; however, because this is in metaphyseal bone, it tends to heal quickly, and immobilization after removal is not necessary.[3,6,9]

Pearls

- Dedicated views of the wrist and the elbow should be obtained to ensure that the PRUJ and the DRUJ are intact.
- In general, a 2-mm–diameter nail can be used in children younger than 10 years, and a 2.5-mm nail can be used in patients 10 years and older.[3]
- Correct contour of the implant is key. The terminal tip (3 mm) of the radial nail should be bent to approximately 40° to allow for easy passage of the nail in the canal, and the implant should have a gradual curve of 30° with the apex at the fracture site.[3,7]
- The ulnar nail requires only minimal prebending (<10°), which allows for three-point fixation once inside the canal.
- If the tip is curved too much on either nail, this can lead to "binding" in the canal and may necessitate decreasing the terminal bend or even using a smaller diameter nail.
- Multiple passes should be avoided. If needed, a small incision can be made over the fracture site to remove entrapped muscle and facilitate placement of the implant.

References

1. Rodríguez-Merchán EC: Pediatric fractures of the forearm. *Clin Orthop Relat Res* 2005;432:65-72.
2. Noonan KJ, Price CT: Forearm and distal radius fractures in children. *J Am Acad Orthop Surg* 1998;6(3):146-156.
3. Garg NK, Ballal MS, Malek IA, Webster RA, Bruce CE: Use of elastic stable intramedullary nailing for treating unstable forearm fractures in children. *J Trauma* 2008;65(1):109-115.
4. Flynn JM, Jones KJ, Garner MR, Goebel J: Eleven years experience in the operative management of pediatric forearm fractures. *J Pediatr Orthop* 2010;30(4):313-319.
5. Yuan PS, Pring ME, Gaynor TP, Mubarak SJ, Newton PO: Compartment syndrome following intramedullary fixation of pediatric forearm fractures. *J Pediatr Orthop* 2004;24(4):370-375.
6. Slongo TF: Complications and failures of the ESIN technique. *Injury* 2005;36(suppl 1):A78-A85.
7. Lascombes P, Prevot J, Ligier JN, Metaizeau JP, Poncelet T: Elastic stable intramedullary nailing in forearm shaft fractures in children: 85 cases. *J Pediatr Orthop* 1990;10(2):167-171.
8. Schmittenbecher PP: State-of-the-art treatment of forearm shaft fractures. *Injury* 2005;36(suppl 1):A25-A34.
9. Reinhardt KR, Feldman DS, Green DW, Sala DA, Widmann RF, Scher DM: Comparison of intramedullary nailing to plating for both-bone forearm fractures in older children. *J Pediatr Orthop* 2008;28(4):403-409.

Video Reference

99.1 Carmichael KD, English C: Distal Forearm Fractures: Both-Bone Forearm Fracture Intramedullary Nailing: Step 1. *Orthopaedic Knowledge Online Journal* 2004;2(7).

Chapter 100
Incision and Drainage of the Septic Hip

Benjamin J. Shore, MD, FRCSC   Mininder S. Kocher, MD, MPH

Patient Selection

The diagnosis of pediatric septic arthritis of the hip can be elusive and can create significant anxiety for the treating orthopaedic surgeon. Septic arthritis must be considered when treating a child with an atraumatic history who refuses to bear weight on the affected extremity. The differential diagnosis is extensive, and differentiation between septic arthritis and transient synovitis in a child with an acutely irritable hip can be very challenging. Furthermore, delay in diagnosis of a septic hip can be detrimental to long-term outcomes.[1-3]

Septic arthritis of the hip most commonly affects children younger than 4 years. In this age group, a thorough patient history is helpful in making the diagnosis. Parents and patients will often describe a history of progressive hip pain and increasing reluctance to bear weight or use the affected leg. In addition, parents may describe a recent illness or note that the child may be having flu-like symptoms, such as general malaise and fever. There may also be a remote history of trauma, which is often noncontributory. The neonatal patient will be most challenging to identify because often the presentation is subtle, with no increase in fever or inflammatory markers. A high index of suspicion should be held if a neonate demonstrates pseudoparalysis or irritability of a particular limb.

If an effusion is present, the hip will be held in a position of flexion and obligate external rotation, to reduce intracapsular pressure. Rotation of the hip is poorly tolerated, but the degree of discomfort is related to the duration of the infection. Palpation of an effusion is not possible in most cases.

Preoperative Imaging/Testing

A standard AP pelvic radiograph is useful to rule out other causes of limp, such as slipped capital femoral epiphysis, bone neoplasm, chronic osteomyelitis, and Legg-Calvé-Perthes disease. Greater than 2 mm of side-to-side difference from the medial part of the femoral head to the medial part of the acetabulum is diagnostic of an effusion.[1] Ultrasound of the hip is now a common modality for diagnosing the presence of an effusion and, in some centers, a diagnostic aspiration can be completed simultaneously. Important diagnostic blood work includes a complete blood cell count, including differential, erythrocyte sedimentation rate (ESR), C-reactive protein (CRP) level, Lyme titer (depending on geographic region), blood culture, and antistreptolysin O titer.

Kocher et al[4] have described a clinical prediction rule for the differentiation between septic arthritis and transient synovitis of the hip that is based on four independent, multivariate predictors of septic arthritis of the hip: a history of fever (temperature >39.5°C), non–weight bearing, ESR greater than 40 mm/h, and a serum white blood cell count greater than 12,000 cells/mm^3 (>12.0 × 10^9/L). More recently, Caird et al[5] demonstrated the utility of an elevated CRP level (>20 mg/L) as a fifth independent predictor in diagnosing septic arthritis. At the authors' institution, a combination of Kocher's criteria and CRP level is used to help make the diagnosis of septic arthritis. In addition to these predictors, an aspiration of the hip joint (either in the radiology suite or the operating room) can be diagnostic. A well-accepted definition of septic arthritis is a joint aspirate with a white blood cell count greater than 50,000 cells/mm^3 (50.0 × 10^9/L). Conversely, a joint aspiration with a white blood cell count under 25,000 cells/mm^3 (25.0 × 10^9/L) has been universally accepted to reflect an inflammatory process, such as transient synovitis. Aspirations that reveal a white blood cell count between 25,000 and 50,000 cells/mm^3 are more challenging for the orthopaedic surgeon; in these situations, a combination of clinical examination, inflammatory markers, and aspiration results helps guide the surgeon in decision making. At our institution, when the diagnosis is still uncertain, MRI of the affected joint is performed to help differentiate between septic arthritis and osteomyelitis of the proximal femur or the acetabulum.

Kocher's criteria for differentiating a septic hip have been applied at other institutions with variable results.[2-4] This has led authors to conclude that using a clinical prediction algorithm to differentiate between septic arthritis and transient synovitis has improved overall care for children. Despite these excellent prediction rules, the ultimate decision for surgical incision and drainage should be based on clinical judgment.

Procedure

Room Setup/Patient Positioning

The patient is positioned supine on a radiolucent operating room table. A small bump is placed under the ipsilateral hip to elevate it approximately 25°. In a small child, it may be easier if both lower extremities are draped free in sterile material. Square draping the hip should be avoided because it may be helpful for the surgeon to move the hip during the procedure.

Special Instruments/Equipment/Implants

If the diagnosis is still uncertain and no aspiration has been performed, then a long 22-gauge spinal needle is used to aspirate the hip. A portable fluoroscopy unit is helpful to confirm the location. A small amount of radiopaque dye can be injected into the joint to confirm position. Most of the of surgical dissection is performed bluntly with deep right-angle retractors and a Cobb elevator. At the end of the case, a drain or, Penrose catheter is left in the hip joint to decompress.

Dr. Shore or an immediate family member serves as a board member, owner, officer, or committee member of the American Academy of Cerebral Palsy and Developmental Medicine and the Pediatric Orthopaedic Society of North America. Dr. Kocher or an immediate family member has received royalties from Biomet; serves as a paid consultant to or is an employee of Biomet and OrthoPediatrics; has stock or stock options held in Fixes 4 Kids and Pivot Medical; and serves as a board member, owner, officer, or committee member of the American Academy of Orthopaedic Surgeons, the American Orthopaedic Society for Sports Medicine and the Pediatric Orthopaedic Society of North America.

Section 8: Pediatric Orthopaedics

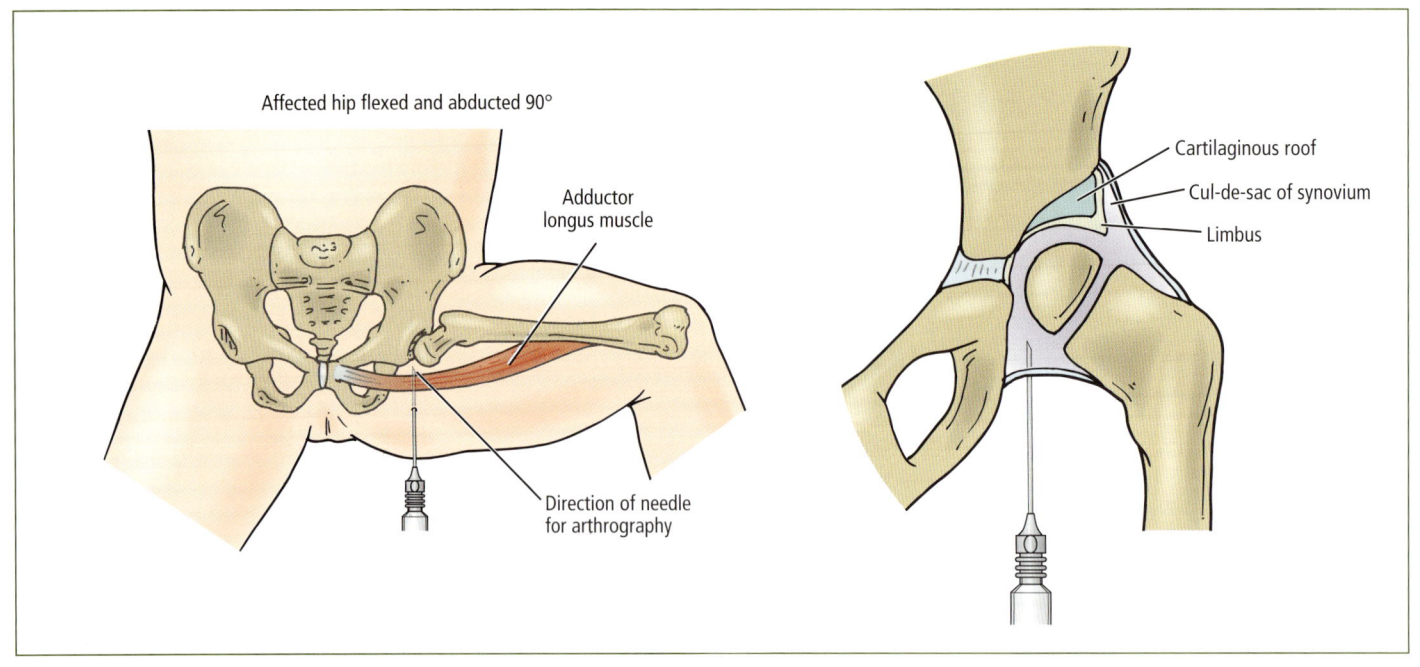

Figure 1 Illustration depicts hip aspiration with the relevant anatomic structures shown.

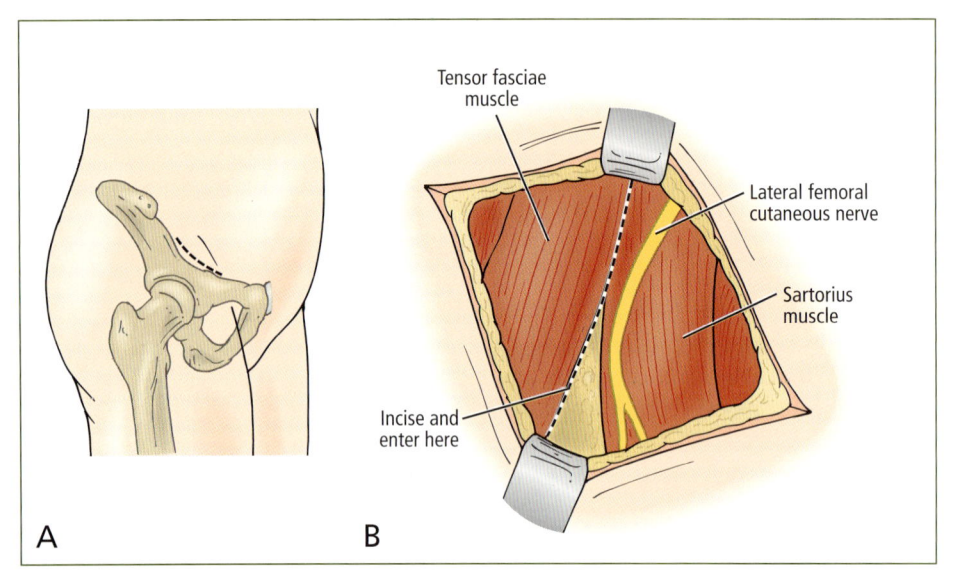

Figure 2 Illustrations show the skin incision and superficial dissection for drainage of a septic hip. **A,** The incision is centered over the anterior inferior iliac spine in line with a skin crease of the anterior hip. **B,** The superficial interval between the tensor fasciae latae and sartorius muscles. The surgeon should try to keep the lateral femoral cutaneous nerve medially with the sartorius if possible when accessing the deeper interval.

Surgical Technique

Hip Aspiration

The preferred position for aspiration of the hip is the "frog-leg" position of abduction and with the spinal needle (18- or 20-gauge) placed inferior to the adductor longus tendon and directed toward the ipsilateral nipple at a 45° angle relative to the floor. Fluoroscopy is used to confirm direction. A small amount (2 to 4 cm^3) of Optiray 320 (ioversol) dye is mixed in a 1:1 ratio with sterile saline and is injected to ensure that the needle is in the correct intra-articular position (**Figure 1**).

Incision and Drainage

A standard anterior skin incision is made in line with the skin crease of the anterior hip (made by flexing the hip to 90°). The incision is slightly more transverse, approximately 1 to 2 cm below the palpable crest of the anterior superior iliac spine (ASIS). The incision should be centered on the hip joint, which lies just inferior to the anterior inferior iliac spine (AIIS; **Figure 2**).

Sharp dissection is performed through the skin and subcutaneous tissue, with meticulous hemostasis using electrocautery. The first internervous interval to be identified is that between the sartorius (femoral nerve) muscle and the tensor fasciae latae (TFL; superior gluteal nerve) muscle. The lateral femoral cutaneous nerve (LFCN) of the thigh crosses this interval and needs to be identified and protected at all times during surgical exposure (**Figure 2, B**). Often, the interval can be palpated by placing the hip in a position of abduction and external rotation. Careful dissection is facilitated with Metzenbaum scissors at this level until the interval is identified and the nerve is protected. The course of the LFCN is variable, but often it will exit from medial to the ASIS running along the sartorius and then cross the interval to lie with the TFL approximately 4.5 cm distal to the ASIS.[6] In the distal portion of this interval lie branches of the lateral femoral circumflex vessel, which form the anterior circumflex vessels. To facilitate exposure of the deeper interval, the lateral femoral circumflex vessels may need to be coagulated without increased risk of osteonecrosis to the femoral head. The main blood supply to the femoral head comes from the lateral retinacular vessels, which branch off the medial femoral circumflex vessel posteriorly (**Figure 3**).

Once the superficial interval between the sartorius and the TFL is identified and developed, the direct head of the rectus femoris tendon must be identified. The direct head of the rectus femoris tendon will insert onto the AIIS and sometimes will be covered in a layer of fat and fibrous tissue in the setting of an infected hip. At the proximal extent of the direct head lies the indirect head, which will divide and travel out laterally to insert at the junction between the acetabulum and the hip joint capsule. In this deeper layer of dissection, blunt dissection with a Cobb elevator is often enough to facilitate the appropriate deep exposure. The direct head of the rectus femoris muscle is retracted medially to reveal the capsular iliacus and deep capsule of the hip joint. In the setting of infection, this layer often is fairly indurated and inflamed, and it is difficult to identify the plane between the capsular iliacus muscles and the hip joint capsule. A Cobb or peanut retractor can be used to sweep the soft tissues off the capsule and prepare for arthrotomy. If the surgeon is uncertain of the location, simple internal and external rotation of the hip will illustrate the proper position of the hip joint. In rare cases, when access to the hip capsule is limited, ligation of the reflected head of the rectus has the potential to facilitate greater exposure of the hip capsule (**Figure 4**).

Once the capsule has been cleared off, a square window of capsule is removed. The size of the capsular window varies (1 to 2 cm) depending on the size of the child, but the arthrotomy must be large enough to facilitate a thorough irrigation and débridement as well as placement of a drain at the end of the case. Aerobic and anaerobic cultures should be taken at the time of the arthrotomy, including two samples for Gram stain and cell count. The hip joint should be irrigated until all purulent material has been removed, which often involves movement of the hip joint to facilitate irrigation posteriorly. We routinely do not drill the metaphysis of the femoral neck unless there is clinical suspicion of concurrent osteomyelitis.

Prior to closure, the stability of the joint should be assessed. In very young children (under 18 months), arthrotomy of the hip can create inadvertent hip instability. After irrigation and débridement, careful dynamic examination by placing the hip in extreme positions of adduction and extension will demonstrate instability. If instability is identified, treatment with a postoperative spica cast for 3 weeks is sufficient. A drain is placed into the hip joint and brought out through the skin incision. The capsule and deep tissue are left open, and the superficial tissues are closed in layers with an absorbable suture. A light dressing is applied, and the Penrose drain is discontinued after approximately 48 hours.

Complications

Few complications exist for irrigation and débridement. The most common complications are associated with delays in diagnosis and definitive surgical care, resulting in osteonecrosis and destruction

Figure 3 Illustrations demonstrate neurovascular hip joint anatomy. **A,** The lateral femoral circumflex vessels lie anteriorly and may need to be ligated during deep exposure. **B,** This posterior view of the hip joint illustrates the medial femoral circumflex vessels, which provide most of the blood supply to the femoral head.

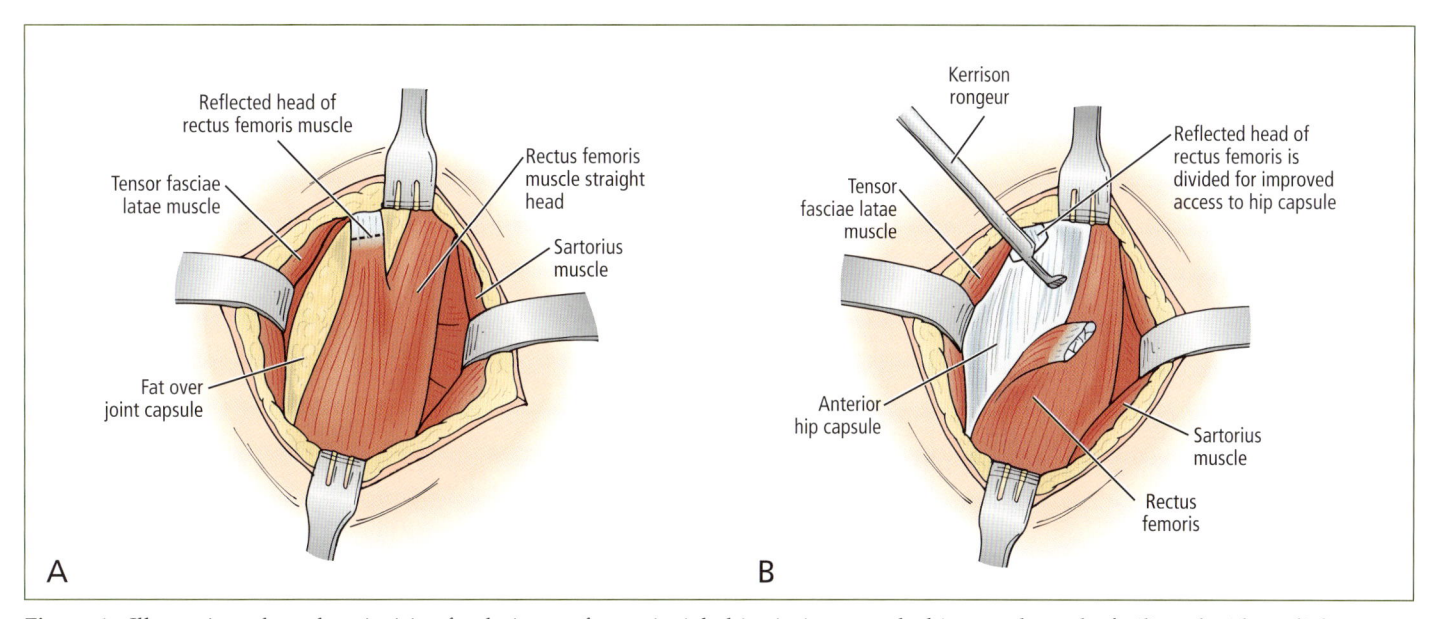

Figure 4 Illustrations show deep incision for drainage of a septic right hip. **A,** Access to the hip capsule can be facilitated with medial retraction of the direct head of the rectus femoris tendon. To increase access to the hip joint, the reflected head of the rectus femoris tendon may be released. **B,** With the reflected rectus tendon tenotomized, a small window is made in the anterior capsule to facilitate irrigation and débridement.

of the femoral head, capital growth arrest, and resultant limb-length discrepancy. Painful neuroma from damage to the LFCN occurs rarely.

Postoperative Care and Rehabilitation

Intravenous antibiotics are initiated after the hip has been débrided in the operating room. The duration of antibiotics follows the clinical practice guidelines used at Boston Children's Hospital.[7] If the patient demonstrates clinical signs of improvement (decreased fever, swelling, and hip joint irritability) after 72 hours of intravenous antibiotics and the patient is negative for methicillin-resistant *Staphylococcus aureus* (MRSA), then transition to oral antibiotics will occur. The patient will remain on oral antibiotics for 21 days, with weekly follow-up to ensure continued clinical improvement. If, within the first 48 hours, the patient does not defervesce, has increasing inflammatory markers, and continues to have persistent pain with hip range of motion, then repeat irrigation and débridement is indicated.

During the postoperative period, the drain is left in place for 48 hours, after which it is discontinued. Physical therapy is encouraged in the early postoperative period. The patient is to remain non–weight bearing for 6 weeks postoperatively. In rare instances, when a child is very young and instability of the hip is appreciated at the time of surgery, postoperative spica casting is instituted.

Pearls

- A timely and accurate diagnosis is critical. Differentiation between transient synovitis and septic arthritis can be made with the help of a thorough history, physical examination, and laboratory tests. The hip is aspirated when in doubt.
- Although inflammatory arthritis can occasionally present as an acutely irritable hip with an aspirate of greater than 50,000 white blood cells/mm^3, it is better to err on the side of surgical drainage because a delay in treatment is often associated with devastating complications, such as growth disturbance, joint destruction, and systemic illness.
- After surgical débridement of the hip has been performed for the treatment of suspected septic arthritis, a patient should demonstrate clinical improvement, with improved hip range of motion, loss of fever, decreasing CRP level, and overall decrease in symptoms. If a patient does not respond well to incision, drainage, and antibiotics, then the surgeon must consider MRSA or a different organism/etiology. It is important to follow cultures and sensitivities closely and collaborate with infectious disease services frequently. MRSA bone and joint infections are often more difficult to treat, requiring multiple surgical procedures. Associated proximal femoral or pelvic osteomyelitis and abscesses of the pelvis and iliopsoas should be considered in these scenarios. MRI is an accurate adjuvant modality to investigate for these associated conditions.

References

1. Betz RR, Cooperman DR, Wopperer JM, et al: Late sequelae of septic arthritis of the hip in infancy and childhood. *J Pediatr Orthop* 1990;10(3):365-372.
2. Luhmann SJ, Jones A, Schootman M, Gordon JE, Schoenecker PL, Luhmann JD: Differentiation between septic arthritis and transient synovitis of the hip in children with clinical prediction algorithms. *J Bone Joint Surg Am* 2004;86-A(5):956-962.
3. Sultan J, Hughes PJ: Septic arthritis or transient synovitis of the hip in children: The value of clinical prediction algorithms. *J Bone Joint Surg Br* 2010;92(9):1289-1293.
4. Kocher MS, Zurakowski D, Kasser JR: Differentiating between septic arthritis and transient synovitis of the hip in children: An evidence-based clinical prediction algorithm. *J Bone Joint Surg Am* 1999;81(12):1662-1670.
5. Caird MS, Flynn JM, Leung YL, Millman JE, D'Italia JG, Dormans JP: Factors distinguishing septic arthritis from transient synovitis of the hip in children: A prospective study. *J Bone Joint Surg Am* 2006;88(6):1251-1257.
6. Ropars M, Morandi X, Huten D, Thomazeau H, Berton E, Darnault P: Anatomical study of the lateral femoral cutaneous nerve with special reference to minimally invasive anterior approach for total hip replacement. *Surg Radiol Anat* 2009;31(3):199-204.
7. Kocher MS, Mandiga R, Murphy JM, et al: A clinical practice guideline for treatment of septic arthritis in children: Efficacy in improving process of care and effect on outcome of septic arthritis of the hip. *J Bone Joint Surg Am* 2003;85(6):994-999.

Chapter 101
Percutaneous in Situ Fixation of Slipped Capital Femoral Epiphysis

Randall T. Loder, MD

Introduction

Slipped capital femoral epiphysis (SCFE) is an adolescent hip disorder defined as a posterior and inferior slip of the proximal femoral epiphysis relative to the metaphysis. However, the relationship of the epiphysis and its articular surface relative to the acetabulum is not altered, and the movement is better defined as an anterior and superior slip of the proximal femoral metaphysis (neck) relative to the epiphysis. The technique of internal fixation is much easier to comprehend when this is understood.

The vast majority (>95%) of SCFEs are stable.[1] A child with a stable SCFE is able to walk, with or without crutches; a child with an unstable SCFE is unable to walk, with or without crutches. The prognosis for a child with a stable SCFE is very good, with an incidence of osteonecrosis approaching zero. The prognosis for a child with an unstable SCFE is guarded due to the increased risk of osteonecrosis, which may be up to 50%.

A child with a stable SCFE has a history of intermittent limp for several weeks to months. It may or may not be associated with thigh, knee, or groin pain. Hip pain is variably present, often resulting in diagnostic delay. Physical examination demonstrates a loss of internal rotation and spontaneous external rotation with hip flexion. Abduction and flexion are usually decreased, especially in more severe cases (>50°). In the long-standing case, shortening of the lower extremity with varying degrees of thigh atrophy is noted; the parents will also describe a gradually increasing external rotation gait and limb-length discrepancy.

Patient Selection

Any child with a stable SCFE and open physes needs treatment. Without stabilization, progression is highly likely. The goals of treatment are to (1) prevent further slipping until physeal closure; (2) avoid complications, primarily osteonecrosis and chondrolysis; and (3) maintain adequate hip function. Four main treatments have been described:

Dr. Loder serves as an unpaid consultant to OrthoPediatrics.

(1) internal fixation, (2) epiphysiodesis, (3) proximal femoral osteotomy, and (4) spica cast immobilization. Today, most authors advocate an in situ fixation with a single screw for any mild or moderate stable SCFE. The initial treatment of severe SCFE is more controversial. Primary osteotomy has been advocated by some to improve joint mechanics, motion, and hip function. However, the incidence of complications is higher with osteotomy than in situ fixation, so most surgeons recommend in situ fixation as the primary treatment for severe SCFE. In situ fixation allows the synovitis to subside, which will in itself result in improved motion. After complete physeal closure (usually 1 or 2 years later), the child's functional limitations, gait pattern, and pain can be more leisurely assessed. A decision regarding the need for osteotomy can then be made after a thorough discussion of the risks and benefits with the child and parents.

Circumstances for bilateral pinning (ie, prophylactic fixation of the opposite hip) include patients with underlying endocrinopathies (hypothyroidism, renal insufficiency, growth hormone supplementation) and the very young child (open triradiate cartilage and/or age younger than 9 years in girls or 11 years in boys).

Preoperative Imaging

In a stable SCFE, the diagnosis is confirmed with AP and lateral pelvis radiographs (**Figure 1**); both views are needed because an early SCFE is often seen only on the lateral view. Both hips should always be visualized, as the incidence of simultaneous bilateral SCFE may approach 20%. Either frog-lateral or cross-table lateral radiographs may be used. Proponents of the cross-table lateral view argue that the variability in positioning for the frog-lateral view due to the limitation of hip motion inaccurately represents the SCFE. The frog-lateral view can also theoretically convert a stable SCFE to an unstable SCFE. Proponents of the frog-lateral view argue that the lateral epiphyseal-shaft angle, commonly used to assess slip magnitude, is measured on the frog-lateral view. It is also the view on which many of the preoperative osteotomy plans are dependent. Comparisons between literature series are also possible with this view due to its common use.

Slip magnitude is best measured using the epiphyseal-shaft angle.[2] This angle is measured on the frog-lateral pelvis radiograph (**Figure 2**). A line is drawn between the anterior and posterior tips of the epiphysis at the physeal level; a line is then drawn perpendicular to this epiphyseal line. A line is next drawn along the midaxis of the femoral shaft. The epiphyseal-shaft angle is the angle formed by the intersection of the perpendicular line and the femoral shaft line. It is measured for both hips, and the magnitude of slip displacement is the angle of the involved hip minus the angle of the contralateral normal hip. Using this angle, SCFEs can be classified as mild (<30°), moderate (30° to 50°), or severe (>50°). In the case of bilateral SCFEs, 10° to 12° is used as the normal hip angle.

Video 101.1 Single Screw Fixation for Slipped Capital Femoral Epiphysis. David D. Aronsson, MD (5 min)

Procedure

The most common technique for in situ single central fixation of a stable SCFE uses a cannulated screw system.[3-8] Unless there are extremely extenuating circumstances, only stainless steel (never titanium) screws should be used. Titanium screws have a much higher complication rate if screw removal is ever needed (eg, breakage, stripping of the head, inability to remove the screw). A single screw is placed into the center of the epiphysis in both the AP and lateral planes. In the stable SCFE, there is never a need for two screws.

Either a fracture table or a radiolucent table can be used. I prefer a fracture table, although there has been no demonstrable difference between the two table types.[9,10]

Room Setup/Patient Positioning

The patient is positioned supine on a fracture table, so that the image intensifier can be moved rather than the lower extremity. If the hospital has the luxury

Section 8: Pediatric Orthopaedics

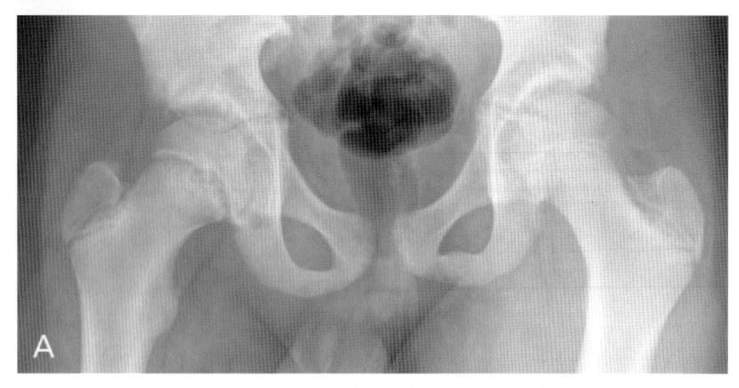

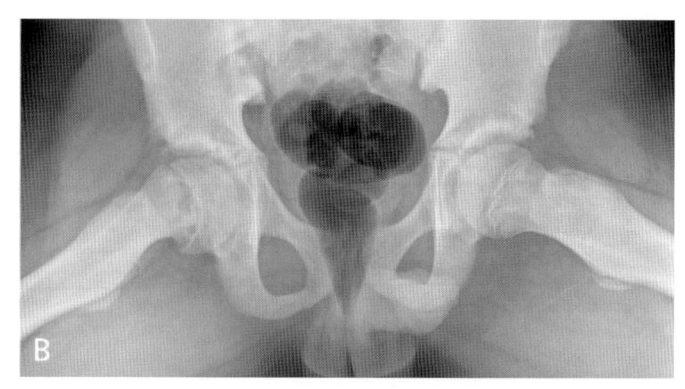

Figure 1 Preoperative AP (**A**) and frog-lateral (**B**) radiographs show a left SCFE in an 11-year, 11-month-old boy. (Reproduced from Loder RT, Aronsson DD, Weinstein SL, Breur GJ, Ganz R, Leunig M: Slipped capital femoral epiphysis. *Instr Course Lect* 2008;57:473-498.)

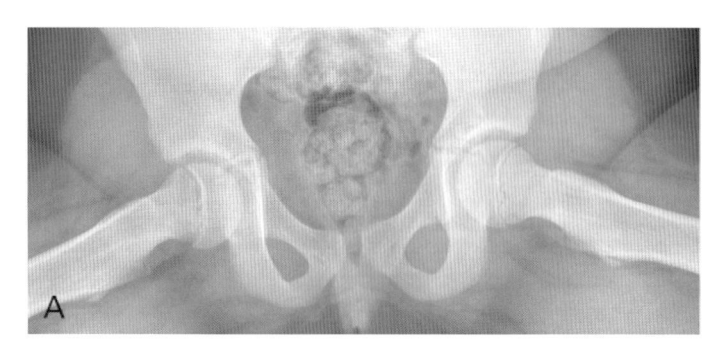

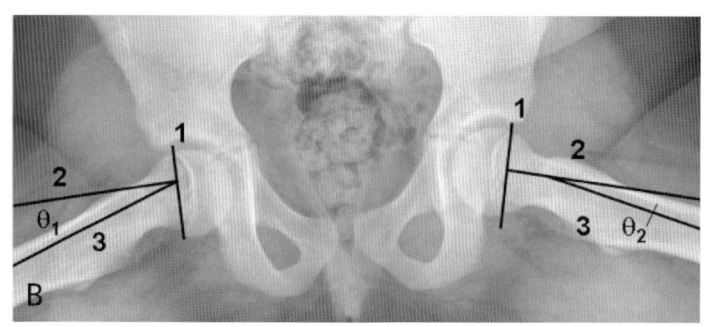

Figure 2 The lateral epiphyseal-shaft angle of Southwick is measured on the frog-lateral radiograph. **A**, Frog-lateral radiograph of a 9-year-old girl with a mild right SCFE. **B**, Line 1 is drawn between the anterior and the posterior physis; line 2 is perpendicular to line 1; line 3 is an axial line along the shaft of the femur. The angle defined by the intersection of lines 2 and 3 is the lateral epiphyseal-shaft angle (θ). The slip angle is calculated by subtracting the lateral epiphyseal-shaft angle of the normal hip from the slip side. In this example, the angle on the right hip (θ_1) created by lines 2 and 3 is 20°, and on the left hip the angle (θ_2) is 7°. Thus, the SCFE magnitude is 20° − 7°, or 13° (a mild SCFE). (Reproduced from Loder RT, Aronsson DD, Weinstein SL, Breur GJ, Ganz R, Leunig M: Slipped capital femoral epiphysis. *Instr Course Lect* 2008;57:473-498.)

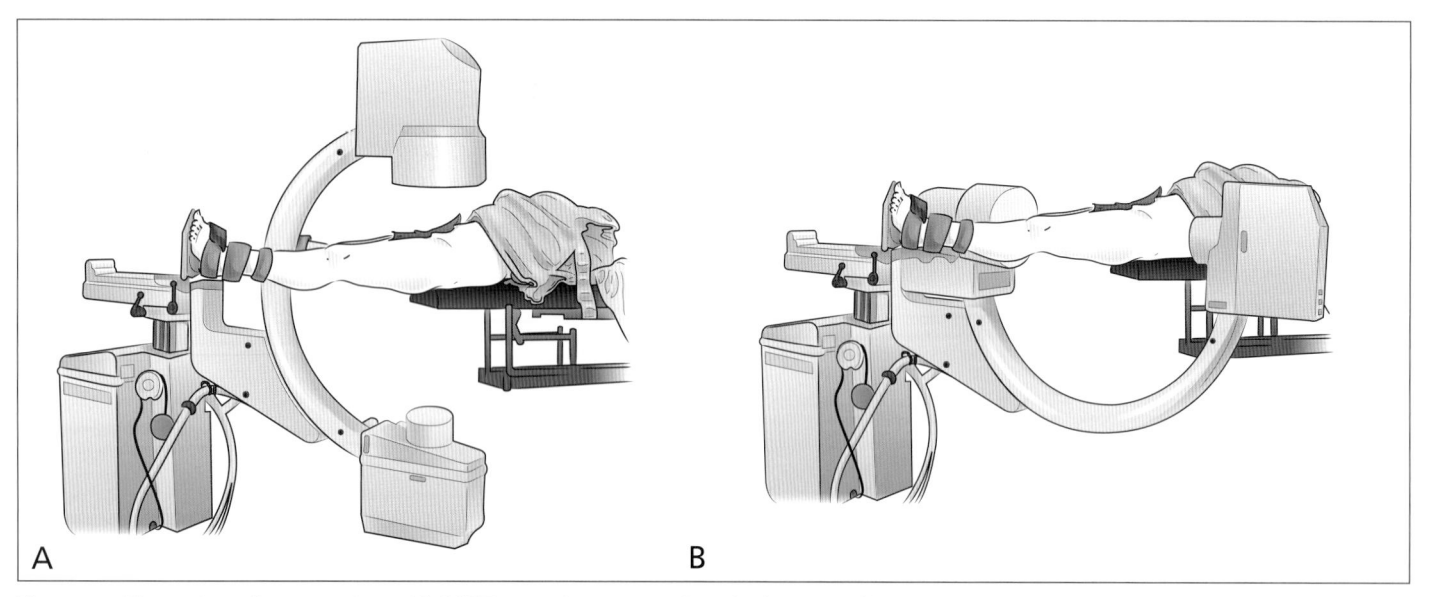

Figure 3 Illustrations show a patient with SCFE properly positioned on the fracture table. **A**, The AP position of the fluoroscope. **B**, The cross-table lateral position of the fluoroscope.

of two image intensifiers, simultaneous biplanar fluoroscopy can be used. Care must be taken when transporting the patient onto the fracture table that no reduction maneuvers are performed and forceful traction is not applied to the lower extremity. The fracture table is used only as a "positioning device," allowing the involved limb to lie comfortably in its natural position of rotation. The opposite limb is placed into abduction with the hip extended, and the image intensifier is moved into position between the two lower extremities.

Prior to surgical draping, the ability to obtain adequate AP and cross-table lateral images is confirmed (**Figure 3**). A guide pin is then placed onto the skin overlying the proximal femur, and an AP image is obtained. The pin is positioned in the center of the epiphysis and perpendicular to the physis. A line is drawn on the skin to record this guide pin position in the AP projection (**Figure 4, A**). A similar skin line is drawn for the lateral image (**Figure 4, B**), again positioning the pin so that it is in the center of the epiphysis and

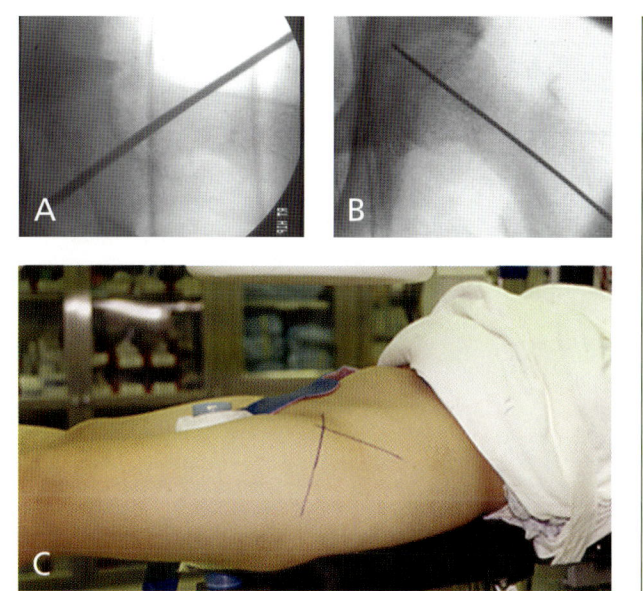

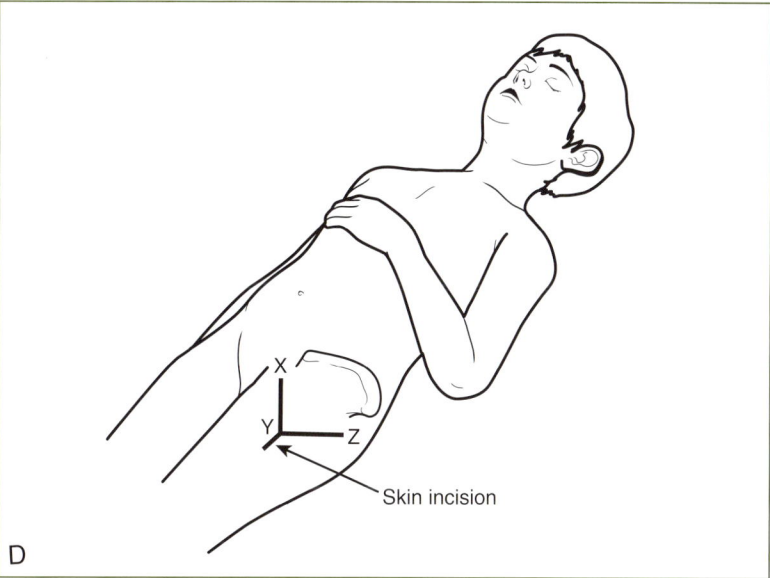

Chapter 101: Percutaneous in Situ Fixation of Slipped Capital Femoral Epiphysis

Figure 4 A guide pin is placed onto the skin overlying the hip such that the pin is positioned in the center of the epiphysis and perpendicular to the physis in both the AP and lateral images. **A,** Intraoperative fluoroscopic images show the guide pin over the hip on the skin and the correct position of the pin relative to the epiphysis—in the center and perpendicular to the physis on both the AP (**A**) and (**B**) lateral images. **C,** Photograph shows the skin lines. **D,** Illustration shows the skin lines drawn to record the position of the guide pin; the incision is made at the intersection of the skin lines. X = anterior line, Y = lateral line, Z = skin incision. (Adapted from Loder RT, Aronsson DD, Dobbs MB, Weinstein SL: Slipped capital femoral epiphysis. *Instr Course Lect* 2001;50:555-570.)

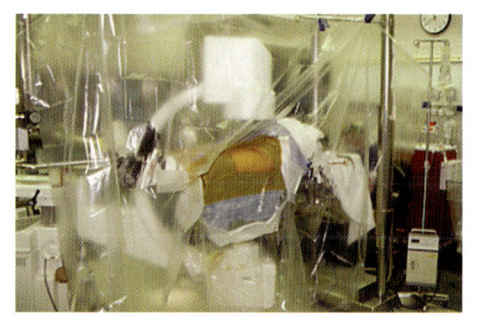

Figure 5 Photograph depicts draping of the patient using a transparent "shower curtain" type of drape.

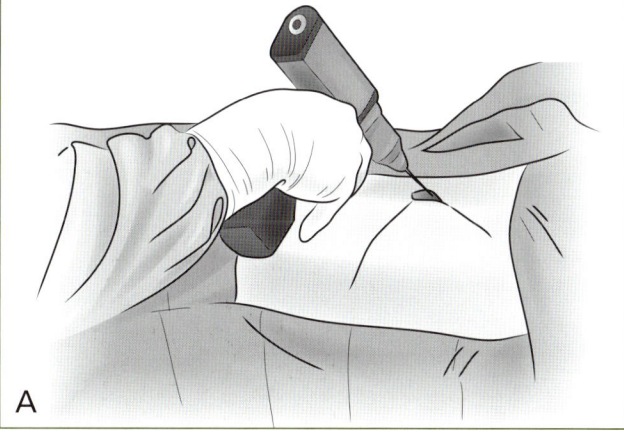

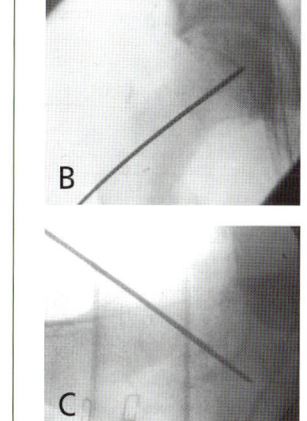

Figure 6 **A,** Illustration shows the guide pin for the cannulated screw being inserted after a small incision is made at the intersection of the skin marking lines. Note that the guide pin follows the trajectory of both skin marking lines. Intraoperative fluoroscopic views demonstrate the guide pin advanced across the physis and in the center of the epiphysis perpendicular to the physis in both the AP (**B**) and (**C**) lateral projections.

perpendicular to the physis. With a SCFE, the epiphysis is posteriorly displaced relative to the femoral neck, and the guide pin in the lateral projection angles from anterior to posterior. This is opposite to that of a femoral neck fracture, where it angles from posterior to anterior. Thus, the two skin lines intersect on the anterolateral aspect of the thigh (**Figure 4, C and D**); as the slip becomes more severe, the intersection point becomes more anterior. Because of the retroversion of the posteriorly displaced epiphysis in SCFE, the osseous entry point of the guide pin is on the anterior aspect of the femur. In mild SCFEs, it is often at the anterior intertrochanteric line; in severe SCFEs, it moves up onto the anterior femoral neck.

Surgical Technique

The anterolateral portion of the thigh is prepped and draped. I prefer to use a transparent "shower curtain" type of isolation drape (**Figure 5**) with multiple Kocher clamps on the base of the drape as weights; this allows movement of the image intensifier in both the AP and lateral projections without violating surgical field sterility. The guide pin is then introduced through the skin at the intersection of the skin lines (**Figure 6**); it may be introduced either through a stab wound or a small 1- to 2-cm incision. I make a 1- to 2-cm incision, incise the fascia lata (this can also be done in the obese child), and then bluntly dissect down to the femoral neck and hip capsule with a finger, following the previously drawn skin lines. This helps prepare the path for the guide pin and ensures that the femoral artery is not in the way in a severe SCFE. Incising the fascia lata also allows adjustment of the guide pin angle without tethering the pin on the tight fascia lata; a tight fascia lata can often result in bending of the pin when trying to reposition it because the fascia lata tethers it, resulting in bending.

The guide pin is advanced onto the anterolateral cortex of the femur, keeping the drill and the guide pin aligned according to the skin lines. Once the guide pin contacts the femoral cortex, its point of entry and angular direction are confirmed in both the AP and lateral projections. When satisfied that the entry point and the direction of the guide pin are correct, the guide pin is carefully advanced

Section 8: Pediatric Orthopaedics

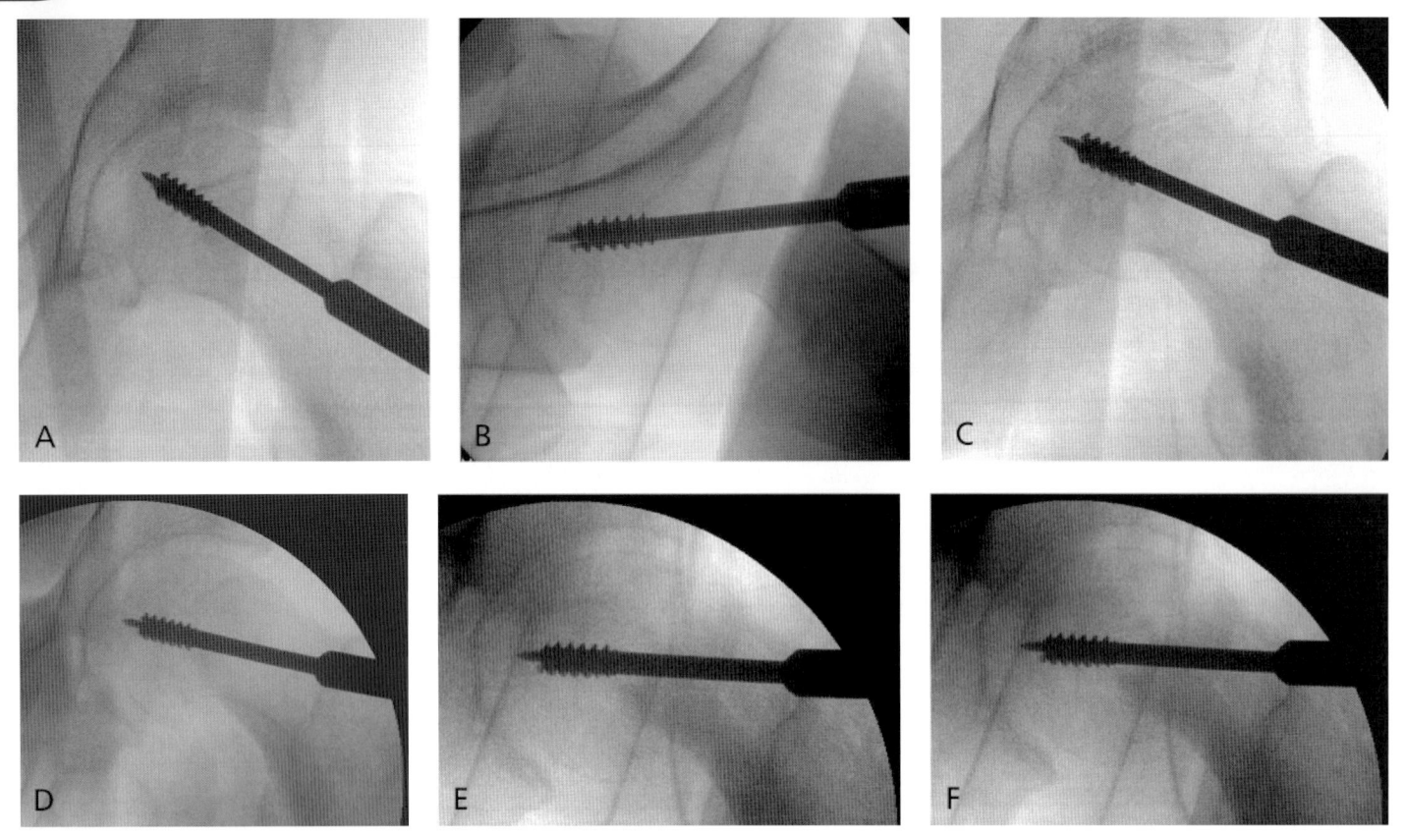

Figure 7 Fluoroscopic images show screw insertion. **A** and **B,** A cannulated screw is inserted after drilling and tapping the hole over the guide pin. **C** through **F,** Incremental fluoroscopic images obtained approximately every 20° from the AP to the lateral position document that the tip of the cannulated screw is in the epiphysis in all views.

into the femoral neck, with the angle of entry frequently checked on both the AP and lateral images. Ideally, there should be only one entry point into the femoral cortex; extra holes act as stress risers, increasing the risk of postoperative fracture. The guide pin should not be advanced across the physis until it is certain that the pin will enter the center of the epiphysis perpendicular to the physis in both the AP and lateral projections (**Figure 6, B** and **C**). After the pin has crossed the physis, the tip should be advanced to the proper depth which should be no closer than 5 mm from the subchondral bone; any permanent pin position less than 5 mm from the subchondral bone increases the risk of joint penetration. This depth is determined on the lateral projection. Care should also be taken to ensure that the pin is not in the superior quadrant of the femoral head because this position may jeopardize the epiphyseal blood supply.

When the pin is in the appropriate position, screw length is determined by either placing another guidewire of identical length along the intraosseous guidewire and measuring the difference or using the appropriate measuring device for the cannulated screw system being used. A cannulated screw is then inserted in routine fashion after drilling and tapping. The screw should be at least 6.5 mm in diameter. While drilling and tapping, close monitoring of the guide pin is necessary to ensure that it does not break, does not penetrate the joint and enter the abdominal cavity, and does not withdraw from the femoral neck.

After the screw has been inserted (**Figure 7, A** and **B**), the guide pin is removed and confirmation that the screw tip does not penetrate the joint is obtained. This can be done by one of several techniques: (1) moving the limb in multiple directions in both AP and lateral views to confirm that it does not penetrate the joint, (2) the approach-withdraw phenomenon, and (3) intraoperative arthrography through the cannulated screw.

My approach is a variation of technique 1. Images of the hip are obtained every 20° while moving from an AP to a lateral projection, ensuring that the screw tip is no closer than 5 mm to the subchondral bone of the epiphysis (**Figure 7, C** through **F**). If it is, then the screw needs to be either backed off or replaced with a shorter one. After confirmation of appropriate screw position and depth, the incision is closed.

Complications

As mentioned previously, the screw must be of appropriate length to adequately engage the epiphysis without penetrating the joint. Joint penetration may result in chondrolysis (**Figure 8**). Guide pin breakage within the bone is a serious complication. If it happens before the cannulated screw has been placed, the point of breakage must first be determined. If it is broken at the level of the bone cortex where the pin enters the femoral cortex, then it may be retrievable by removing a small amount of the cortical bone surrounding it and grasping it with a pin remover, needle-nose vise grips, or some other device. This obviously necessitates increasing the incision size. If it breaks deep within the bone, then the only option is to position another guide pin, which will not likely be in the ideal position. It is best to prevent pin breakage by ensuring that the cannulated drill follows the exact same trajectory as the guide pin, without levering/angling on the pin by the drill. Levering/angling allows the drill to cut and notch the guide pin, resulting in subsequent breakage. Automatic grip/release drill chucks can also result in pin notching (**Figure 9**). For this reason, I prefer to use a standard Jacobs chuck

Chapter 101: Percutaneous in Situ Fixation of Slipped Capital Femoral Epiphysis

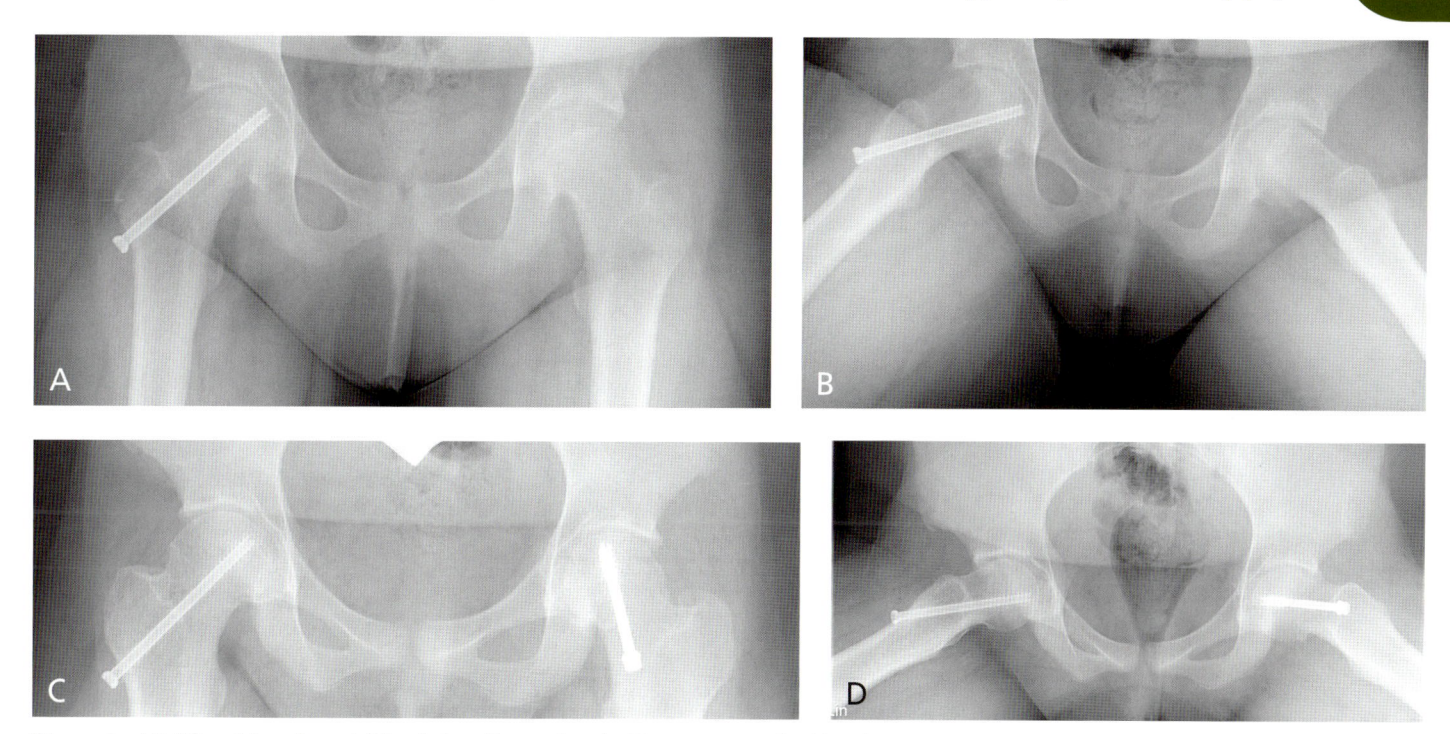

Figure 8 AP (**A**) and frog-lateral (**B**) pelvic radiographs of a 13-year, 6-month-old girl who had previously undergone in situ fixation for a right SCFE. Note the protrusion of the screw into the joint space and the joint space narrowing, indicative of chondrolysis. Also note the opposite left SCFE. The right screw was slightly withdrawn, and in situ fixation of the left SCFE was performed. At age 15 years and 5 months, AP (**C**) and frog-lateral (**D**) radiographs demonstrate physeal closure of both hips and improvement in the joint space narrowing of the right hip. (Reproduced from Loder RT, Aronsson DD, Weinstein SL, Breur GJ, Ganz R, Leunig M: Slipped capital femoral epiphysis. *Instr Course Lect* 2008;57:473-498.)

and tighten the guide pin in the standard manner.

If multiple guide pin entry points are required before the ideal pin position is achieved, then the empty guide pin entry holes are stress risers in the femur, which can result in a fracture.[11,12] This is especially true if the guide pin entry hole is at or distal to the level of the lesser trochanter.

Postoperative Care and Rehabilitation

Permanent radiographs are obtained either in the operating room before awakening the patient or in the postanesthesia care unit (**Figure 10**). If satisfactory, then toe-touch weight bearing is immediately allowed.[4,8] Discharge is often the same evening for a morning surgery, or the next day for an afternoon surgery. I recommend toe-touch weight bearing for 4 to 6 weeks; however, many children have no postoperative discomfort, so it is not uncommon to see them return for their first postoperative visit 1 to 2 weeks later carrying their crutches. At the first postoperative visit, the incision is checked and radiographs are obtained to ensure no change in fixation. The next visit is 4 to 6 weeks after surgery; radiographs are also obtained. Both AP and frog-lateral radiographs of the pelvis should

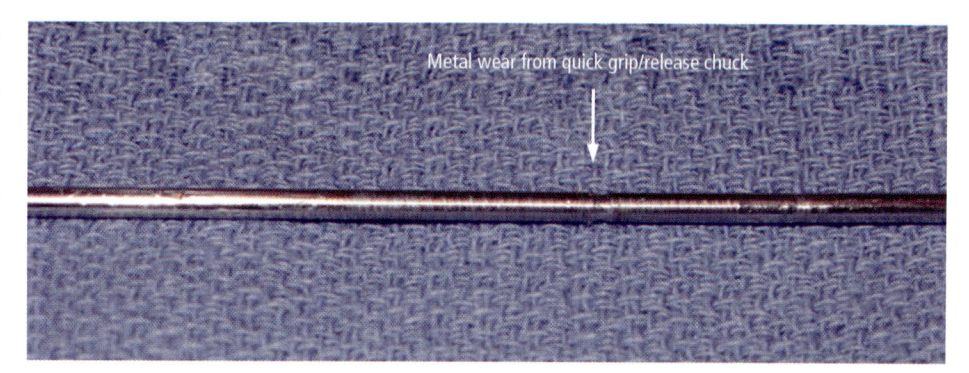

Figure 9 Photograph shows the notching of a guide pin from a cannulated screw set caused by an automatic grip/release chuck.

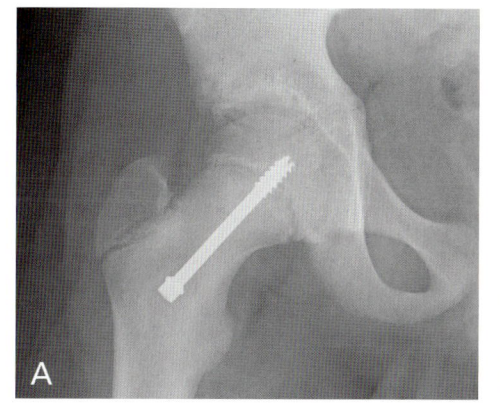

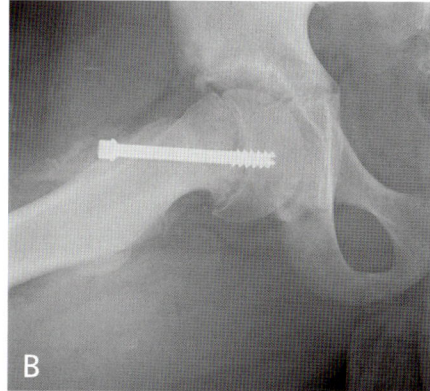

Figure 10 Postoperative radiographs of the patient in Figure 1 demonstrate ideal screw position in the center of the epiphysis perpendicular to the physis in both AP (**A**) and frog-lateral (**B**) projections. (Reproduced from Loder RT, Aronsson DD, Weinstein SL, Breur GJ, Ganz R, Leunig M: Slipped capital femoral epiphysis. *Instr Course Lect* 2008;57:473-498.)

be obtained so as to follow the opposite hip. After this time, normal activities are allowed except for running, jumping, or contact sports.

The child and parents need to be counseled to return immediately if there is any pain or loss of motion in either hip. Otherwise, return visits every 3 or 4 months are made, with repeat AP and frog-lateral radiographs of the pelvis, until complete physeal closure.[13] After physeal closure, all physical activities are allowed.

Screw removal is controversial. The morbidity and complications for screw removal are much greater than for insertion (incision, surgical time, blood loss, fracture risk). Most surgeons presently do not recommend screw removal for SCFE.[14]

Pearls

- The surgeon must be able to obtain good AP and lateral fluoroscopic images before prepping and draping.
- It is very important to not lever on the guide pin during insertion through the fascia lata and onto the bone; levering will frequently bend the pin, which can result in advertent cutting of the pin when drilling over it. Such cutting of the pin can occur either flush with the bone or, worse yet, inside the bone.
- Ideally, there should only be one pass of the guidewire; more passes create stress risers in the bone and increase the risk of postoperative fracture.
- The surgeon must be able to visualize the tip of the screw in multiple planes before closure.

References

1. Loder RT, Richards BS, Shapiro PS, Reznick LR, Aronson DD: Acute slipped capital femoral epiphysis: The importance of physeal stability. *J Bone Joint Surg Am* 1993;75(8):1134-1140.
2. Southwick WO: Osteotomy through the lesser trochanter for slipped capital femoral epiphysis. *J Bone Joint Surg Am* 1967;49(5):807-835.
3. Koval KJ, Lehman WB, Rose D, Koval RP, Grant A, Strongwater A: Treatment of slipped capital femoral epiphysis with a cannulated-screw technique. *J Bone Joint Surg Am* 1989;71(9):1370-1377.
4. Aronson DD, Carlson WE: Slipped capital femoral epiphysis: A prospective study of fixation with a single screw. *J Bone Joint Surg Am* 1992;74(6):810-819.
5. Lindaman LM, Canale ST, Beaty JH, Warner WC: A fluoroscopic technique for determining the incision site for percutaneous fixation of slipped capital femoral epiphysis. *J Pediatr Orthop* 1991;11(3):397-401.
6. Nguyen D, Morrissy RT: Slipped capital femoral epiphysis: Rationale for the technique of percutaneous in situ fixation. *J Pediatr Orthop* 1990;10(3):341-346.
7. Morrissy RT: Slipped capital femoral epiphysis technique of percutaneous in situ fixation. *J Pediatr Orthop* 1990;10(3):347-350.
8. Ward WT, Stefko J, Wood KB, Stanitski CL: Fixation with a single screw for slipped capital femoral epiphysis. *J Bone Joint Surg Am* 1992;74(6):799-809.
9. Blasier RD, Ramsey JR, White RR: Comparison of radiolucent and fracture tables in the treatment of slipped capital femoral epiphysis. *J Pediatr Orthop* 2004;24(6):642-644.
10. Carney BT, Talwalkar V, Grothaus M, Levine J: Comparison of fracture versus radiolucent table in the treatment of slipped capital femoral epiphysis. *Iowa Orthop J* 2006;26:33-36.
11. Baynham GC, Lucie RS, Cummings RJ: Femoral neck fracture secondary to in situ pinning of slipped capital femoral epiphysis: A previously unreported complication. *J Pediatr Orthop* 1991;11(2):187-190.
12. Canale ST, Azar F, Young J, Beaty JH, Warner WC, Whitmer G: Subtrochanteric fracture after fixation of slipped capital femoral epiphysis: A complication of unused drill holes. *J Pediatr Orthop* 1994;14(5):623-626.
13. Loder RT, Aronson DD, Greenfield ML: The epidemiology of bilateral slipped capital femoral epiphysis: A study of children in Michigan. *J Bone Joint Surg Am* 1993;75(8):1141-1147.
14. Loder RT, Feinberg JR: Orthopaedic implants in children: Survey results regarding routine removal by the pediatric and nonpediatric specialists. *J Pediatr Orthop* 2006;26(4):510-519.

Chapter 102
Fixation of Pediatric Femur Fractures

Ernest L. Sink, MD

Patient Selection

A wide variety of options are currently available for the management of femoral fractures in children and adolescents. Surgical stabilization is the treatment of choice for pediatric femur fractures in children older than 5 years. Surgical fixation allows a more rapid return to school and lower costs compared with traction and casting.[1,2] The surgeon has several options available for fixation, each of which yields satisfactory results when used properly. The surgeon who manages femoral fractures in children and adolescents must select the technique that is most appropriate for the individual patient. As long as proper technique is used, more than one acceptable option may be appropriate.

The method used depends on many factors, including fracture location, fracture pattern, patient size, and surgeon preference. Flexible elastic nailing is successful for most stable diaphyseal (middle 60% of the femur) fractures.[3,4] Elastic nails are more challenging to use in distal or proximal diaphyseal fractures and in comminuted or long oblique fracture patterns. Studies have shown a higher complication rate when titanium elastic nails are used to stabilize comminuted and long oblique "length-unstable" fractures.[5,6] Therefore, different methods of stabilization, such as external fixation, trochanteric-entry rigid nails, and submuscular bridge plating, have been implemented in length-unstable fractures to achieve greater stability. A recent study[7] compared the complications of surgical management in two cohorts. In one cohort, the investigators limited the use of elastic nails in unstable fractures, instead using submuscular plating and rigid trochanteric nails predominately; a subsequent significant decrease in complications was noted.

Three techniques for femoral fixation are described in this chapter: submuscular plating, elastic intramedullary nailing, and lateral trochanteric–entry nailing. Submuscular plating is suitable for patients with unstable femoral fractures or proximal and distal fractures in patients aged 5 years to skeletal maturity. In general, elastic intramedullary nails are ideal for stable diaphyseal femur fractures in patients aged 5 to 11 years. Lateral trochanteric–entry nails are better suited for children 12 years of age and older, when the proximal femoral diaphyseal diameter is large enough to accommodate the nails. They can be used in both stable and unstable fractures.

Submuscular Plating

Plate osteosynthesis is a proven method of stabilizing pediatric fractures.[8-12] This technique traditionally required a large exposure and significant soft-tissue disruption. The use of submuscular bridge plating for comminuted femur fractures allows rigid stabilization, minimally invasive techniques, avoidance of osteonecrosis, and stabilization of the diaphyseal/metaphyseal junction. Descriptions of the technique and its success have been published.[13,14] The following section describes this technique, which has simplified the management of unstable pediatric femur fractures.

Indications

The fractures most amenable to submuscular plating are comminuted or long oblique length-unstable pediatric femur fractures in patients aged 5 years to skeletal maturity. The technique also is reliable for proximal and distal-third femur fractures. Enough intact femur must be available to accommodate at least two screws in the proximal or distal diaphyseal region. With the increasing use of trochanteric-entry nails, the indications for submuscular plating might be further narrowed to unstable fracture patterns in patients who are too small or too young for trochanteric-entry nails (ages 5 to 12 years).

Preoperative Imaging

All patients should be evaluated for other injuries, specifically injuries to the ipsilateral hip and knee. The necessary radiographs are good AP and lateral views of the affected femur. The ipsilateral femoral neck and knee joint also should be visualized on these views or imaged separately. Although a true definition of an "unstable" pediatric femur fracture does not exist, a comminuted or very long oblique fracture generally is considered unstable (**Figure 1**).

Procedure

Room Setup/Patient Positioning

The patient is positioned supine on a fracture table. A provisional reduction is obtained with boot traction. Length and rotation are obtained with the traction; final alignment can be performed with the plate fixation described later. Once the patient is positioned on the fracture table, the unaffected leg is extended carefully and abducted to obtain a true lateral fluoroscopic image of the femur for planning screw placement. Alternatively, the unaffected leg may be flexed on a well-leg holder. A radiolucent table without traction may be used if adequate assistance is available to maintain traction. Care must be taken while obtaining provisional fixation to account for rotation. In comminuted fractures, rotation is the most difficult parameter to assess.

Special Instruments/Equipment/Implants

In our initial description of the procedure, my colleagues and I recommended a long, narrow 4.5-mm plate.[14] This plate is readily available and is easy to contour, and percutaneous screw placement is forgiving. Currently, many manufacturers offer pediatric submuscular femoral plates; some include an anterior bow and locking technology. The specific plate chosen is based on the surgeon's preference. The locking plate technology may be most important in osteopenic patients or in very proximal or distal fractures, where little room is available for screws. In my experience, a nonlocking stainless steel plate achieves enough stability in pediatric patients. In the series we reported, no plate failures or nonunions were noted.[14] The locking plate may require a

---

Dr. Sink or an immediate family member serves as a paid consultant to or is an employee of Pivot and serves as a board member, owner, officer, or committee member of the Pediatric Orthopaedic Society of North America.

longer surgical time because percutaneous screw placement is less forgiving. Using nonlocking screws assists in the reduction of the fracture. Therefore, if a locking plate is used, a combination of locking and nonlocking screws is needed to reduce the femur to the contoured plate. Self-tapping screws are used to facilitate percutaneous insertion and to limit the soft-tissue injury that may occur with tapping. Percutaneous screw fixation is easier with 4.5-mm screws because the screw heads are larger, and a 4.5-mm plate has the advantage of stronger fixation. In smaller children, a long, narrow 3.5-mm plate may be used; however, a 4.5-mm plate fits most femurs.

The plate length chosen will have approximately 10 to 16 holes, and the length will vary with fracture location and patient size. The plate commonly spans from just below the greater trochanteric apophysis to the metaphysis of the distal femur. The plate should be long enough to accommodate three screws proximal to and three screws distal to the fracture; however, in a proximal or a distal fracture, two screws may be adequate, particularly if they are locking screws. A table plate bender contours the plate to the lateral femur with a slight bend proximally and distally to accommodate the proximal and distal metaphyses. It is important to note that the final femoral varus/valgus alignment will match that of the plate; thus, it is critical to contour the plate as close to the native anatomy of the lateral femur as possible. The usual method of checking the contour is to place the precontoured plate on the anterior thigh and use the AP view on the C-arm to shadow the lateral cortex. The contralateral femur also may be used as a template. In my experience, no significant (>5°) misalignment has occurred as a result of misjudged contouring.

Surgical Technique

A 3- to 5-cm incision is made over the distal lateral thigh through the tensor fascia to expose the distal obliquely oriented fibers of the vastus lateralis muscle (**Figure 2, A**). Blunt dissection is performed deep to the distal muscle fibers to dissect the plane between the vastus lateralis and the periosteum of the lateral femur (**Figure 2, B and C**). Then the plate is slowly tunneled proximally in this plane (**Figure 3, A through C**). Care is taken to keep the plate on the lateral femur as it is advanced proximally past the fracture to the region of the greater trochanteric apophysis. The plate may be more difficult to pass along the lateral femur past the fracture. The surgeon may correct this by pulling the plate back and redirecting it. The C-arm also may aid the surgeon in plate advancement (**Figure 3, D through H**).

Once the plate is fully advanced, it should sit comfortably on the lateral fe-

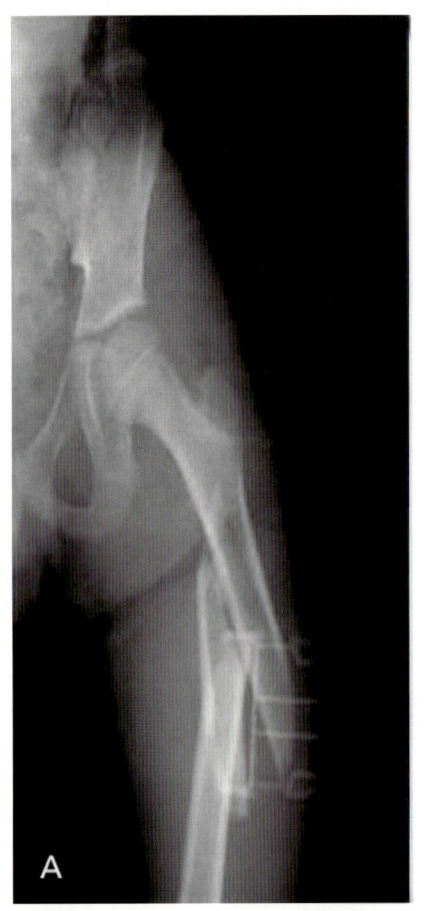

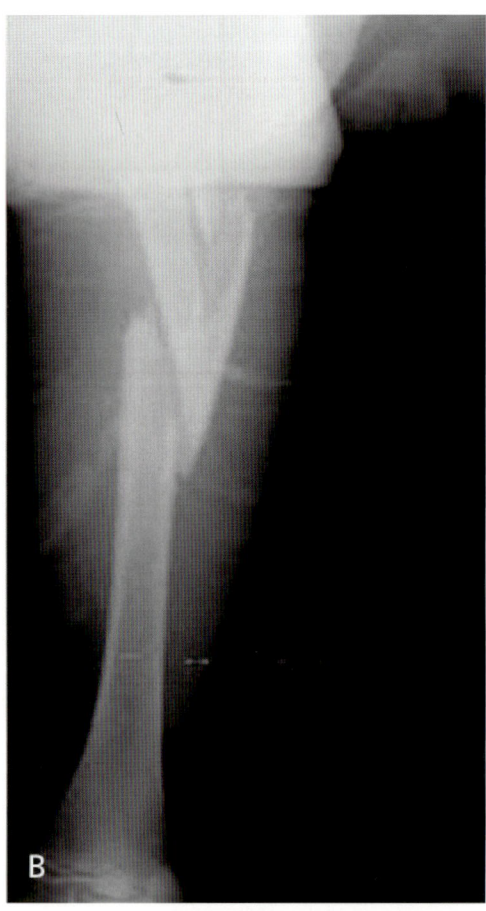

Figure 1 Preoperative AP (**A**) and lateral (**B**) radiographs of a 7-year-old child with an unstable femur fracture suitable for submuscular plating.

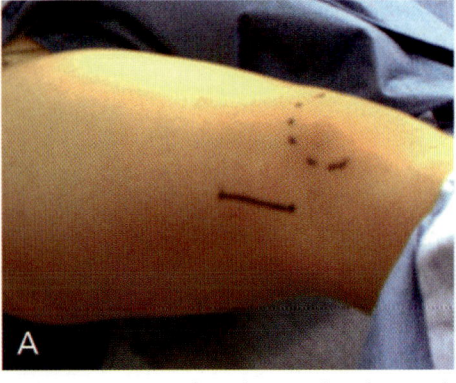

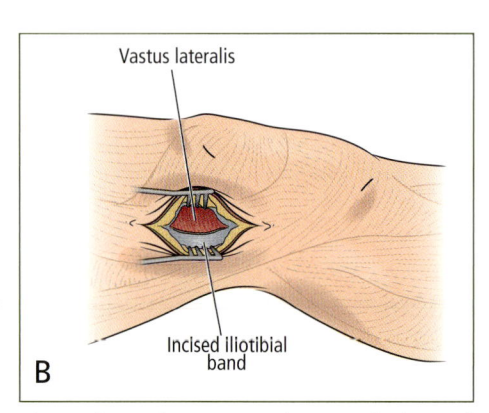

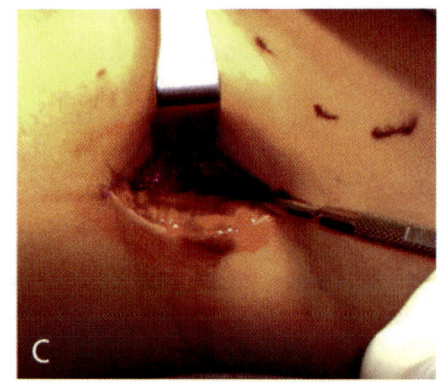

Figure 2 Incision for submuscular plating of a pediatric femur fracture. **A**, Photograph shows the location of the lateral incision and the landmark marked on the skin. **B**, Illustration indicates the approach through the iliotibial band to expose the distal oblique fibers of the vastus lateralis. **C**, Intraoperative photograph shows blunt dissection deep to the distal aspect of the vastus lateralis to access the subvastus plane, where the plate will be inserted.

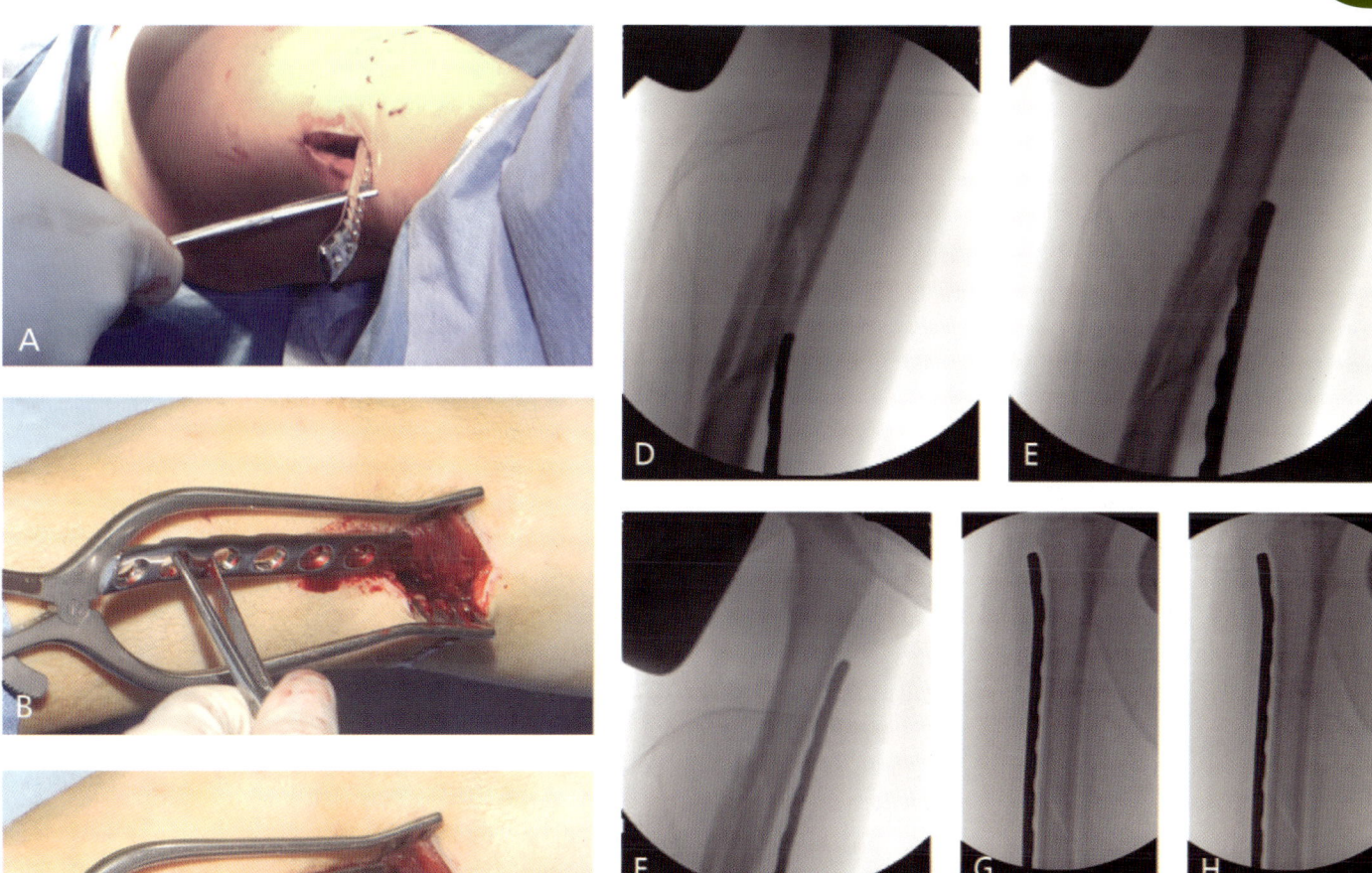

Chapter 102: Fixation of Pediatric Femur Fractures

Figure 3 Intraoperative photographs (**A** through **C**) and fluoroscopic images (**D** through **H**) show tunneling of the plate through the plane between the vastus lateralis and the periosteum of the lateral femur.

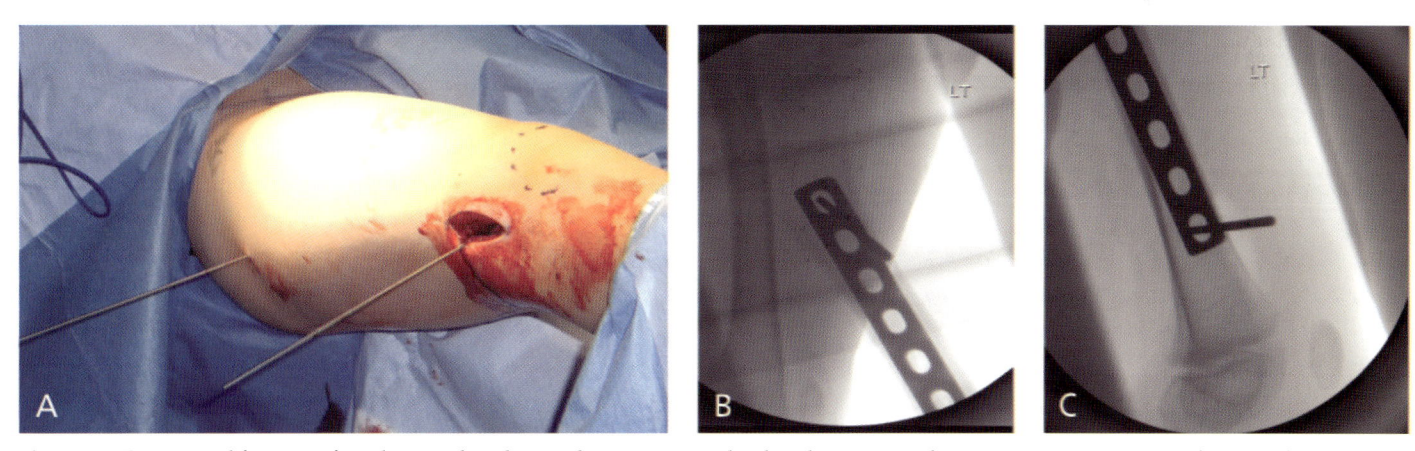

Figure 4 Provisional fixation of a submuscular plate with percutaneously placed K-wires is shown in an intraoperative photograph (**A**) and on fluoroscopic images at the proximal (**B**) and distal (**C**) ends of the plate.

mur. AP and lateral images are obtained to ensure that the plate is in good position in both planes and that the femoral length is restored. The plate is provisionally fixed to the femur with 2-mm Kirschner wires (K-wires) placed in the most proximal and distal screw holes (**Figure 4**). If the fracture is "sagging" in the lateral plane, the femur can be lifted in an anterior direction while a K-wire is placed through the plate to engage the femur in this region. A K-wire also can be used to adjust the anterior-posterior position of the plate on the lateral image (**Figure 4, B**). A long plate and correct screw placement are important for construct stability. The principle of pin placement in external fixation is used for screw placement. One screw should be placed close to both the proximal and distal limits of the fracture. The remaining screws are spread as far apart as possible because maximal screw spread improves construct stability. Three screws proximal to and three screws distal to the fracture are recommended. Occasionally, there may be room for only two screws in the very proximal and distal fracture; this may still be adequate with a long plate or adjunctive use of locking screws. The first

© 2013 American Academy of Orthopaedic Surgeons

Section 8: Pediatric Orthopaedics

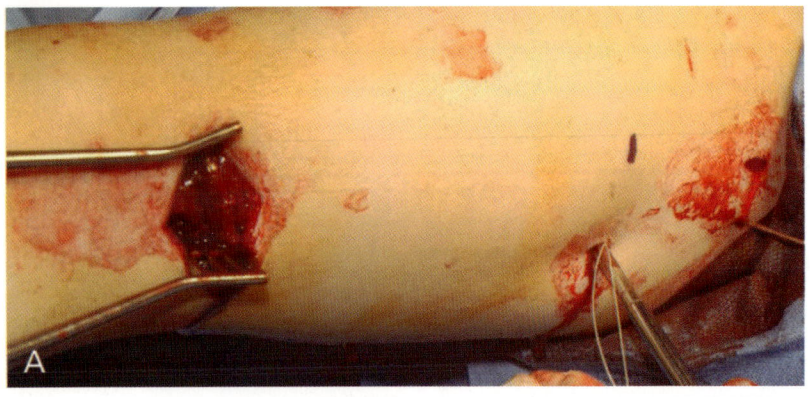

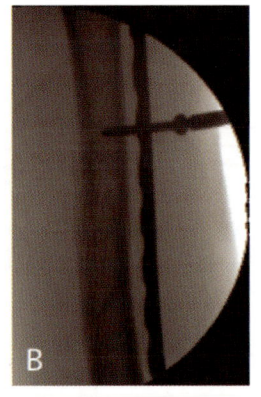

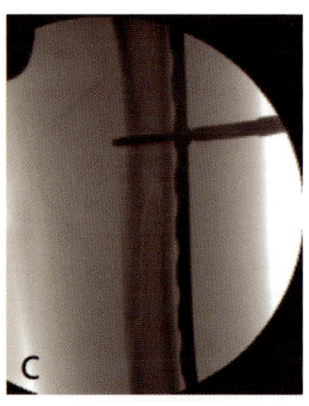

Figure 5 Intraoperative photograph (**A**) and fluoroscopic images (**B** and **C**) demonstrate the reduction of the femur to the precontoured plate with percutaneous screw placement in a pediatric femur fracture. (Panel A is reproduced with permission from Sink EL, Hedequist D, Morgan SJ, Hresko T: Results and technique of unstable pediatric femoral fractures treated with submuscular bridge plating. *J Pediatr Orthop* 2006;26[2]:177-181.)

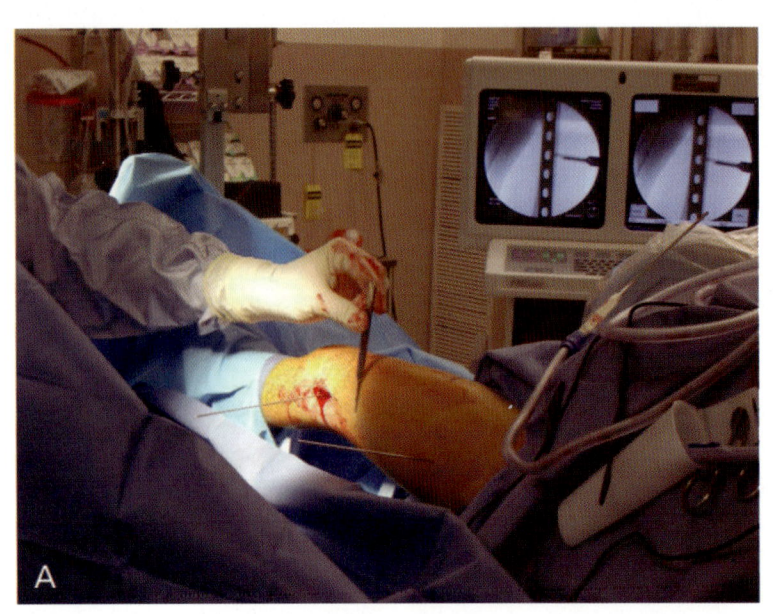

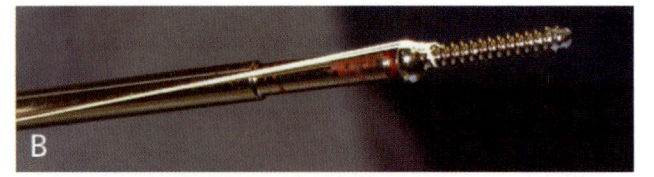

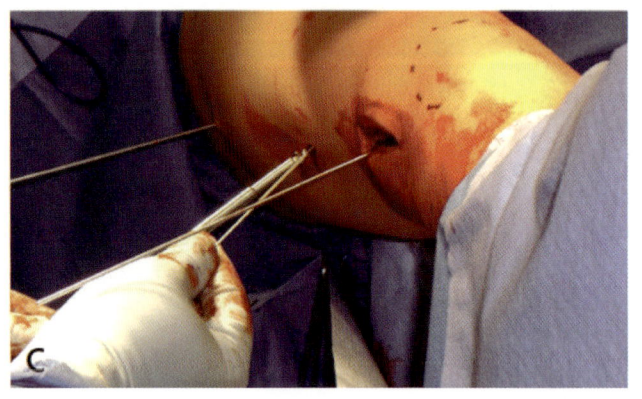

Figure 6 Percutaneous screw placement for submuscular plating of a pediatric femur fracture. **A,** Photograph shows the screws inserted using the "perfect circles" technique. **B,** Photograph shows a Vicryl tie attached to the screw to prevent losing the screw in the soft tissue. **C,** Intraoperative photograph shows the percutaneous screw insertion. (Panel A is reproduced with permission from Sink EL: Submuscular plating of femoral shaft fractures, in Flynn JM, Wiesel SW, eds: *Operative Techniques in Pediatric Orthopaedics*. Lippincott, Williams & Wilkins, Philadelphia, PA, 2010.)

screw should be placed where the femur is farthest from the plate, thus acting as a reduction screw. As the screw engages the far cortex, the femur will be reduced to the precontoured plate (**Figure 5**). The fracture is "bridged," and no attempt is made to place a screw across the fracture fragments, nor is the fracture exposed; the soft-tissue sleeve is left undisturbed around the fracture.

Accurate percutaneous screw placement is obtained as follows. Screws are placed using the "perfect circles" technique. Using a fluoroscopic image in the lateral plane, a No. 15 blade is placed on the skin over the hole and rotated horizontal to the beam through the skin, tensor fascia, and vastus fascia. Using a freehand technique, a 3.2-mm drill is placed in this small incision and its location in the desired hole is confirmed with fluoroscopy. The hole is then drilled through both cortices. The length of the screw is approximated by placing the depth gauge on the anterior thigh as the image is rotated to the AP view to obtain the approximate screw length. A 0-Vicryl suture (Ethicon) is tied around the 4.5-mm fully threaded cortical screw head so it will not be lost in the soft tissue. The screw is then placed through the plate and across the femur. As the screw engages the femur, it will reduce the femur to the precontoured plate (**Figure 6**). The Vicryl ties are cut and the incisions are closed. A soft dressing is applied.

Complications

Few complications have been reported for submuscular plating. One incident of plate failure was reported when a 3.5-mm titanium plate was used. This complication has not been reported with stainless steel and 4.5-mm plates. Refracture after plate removal is a potential concern. One case of this has been reported in the literature; the authors of the study believe the plate was removed too early.[13]

The potential for malunion can be minimized with accurate plate contouring. Nonunion has not been reported. Rotational malalignment, secondary to the comminuted and often proximal characteristics of the fractures treated with submuscular plating, is the greatest risk. Particularly in younger children, in whom version can be quite variable, plating the leg in traction in the correct rotation can be challenging. Using fluoroscopy to evaluate fracture geometry and examine the alignment of the contralateral leg and diaphyseal width of the ipsilateral leg preoperatively will help to assess rotation.

Postoperative Care and Rehabilitation

I often place patients in a knee immobilizer for early comfort with mobilization. No casting is required in the early postoperative period. Active knee range of motion is encouraged as comfort allows. Patients are not allowed to bear weight until bridging callus is seen, usually at 6 to 10 weeks.

If plate removal is chosen, this is done at around 6 months. If the plate is removed closer to 1 year postoperatively or even later, it may be too difficult to remove percutaneously because of tissue and bone ingrowth. In my experience, I have been able to remove the plate through the same percutaneous incisions in every case. Once the screws are removed using image guidance, a dull Cobb elevator is slid along the outer part of the plate to free the surrounding tissue. With the sharp end directed away from the bone, the Cobb elevator is advanced between the plate and the bone, thus freeing the plate. Once the plate is completely freed, it can be removed from the distal incision where it was advanced. After plate removal, patients may bear weight as tolerated but are kept from sports activities for 6 weeks.

Pearls

- Submuscular bridge plating is best for comminuted or long oblique pediatric femur fractures.
- For rigid stabilization, the plate should span from the greater trochanteric apophysis to the distal femoral metaphysis.
- A 4.5-mm stainless steel plate should be precontoured to accommodate the bend of the proximal and distal metaphyses. The plate is placed on the anterior aspect of the thigh before insertion, using fluoroscopy to shadow the lateral cortex and confirm the contour.
- The first nonlocking screw should be placed at the margin of the fracture, where the femur is farthest from the plate. Once the screw engages the far cortex, the femur will reduce to the plate.
- The surgeon should obtain as much screw spread as possible for the remaining screws to increase stability.
- An absorbable suture is tied around the screw head before percutaneous insertion so the screw will not disengage from the screwdriver in the soft tissue.

Elastic Intramedullary Nailing

Flexible or elastic intramedullary nails have the advantage of being appropriate for the small, young child without risking damage to the trochanter, the femoral neck, or the vascular supply to the femoral head. This method of internal fixation is best for transverse or stable fracture patterns in patients ages 5 to 11 years (**Figure 7**). Flexible nails are less stable in heavier (> 50 kg), older (> 11 years) children and for comminuted fractures.[6,7,15-17]

Procedure

Room Setup/Patient Positioning

The patient positioning when elastic intramedullary nails are used is identical to that for submuscular plating. Some surgeons may elect to use only a radiolucent table without traction as long as adequate assistance is available to maintain traction. The surgeon should have access to both the medial and lateral knee.

Special Instruments/Equipment/Implants

Various flexible elastic nails are available. The implant chosen is based on the surgeon's preference. New types of flexible nails that allow proximal and distal locking are currently being developed to help

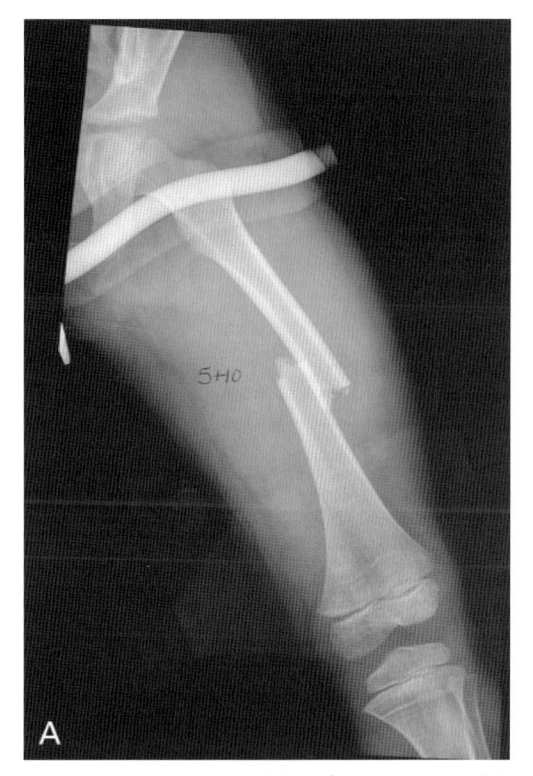

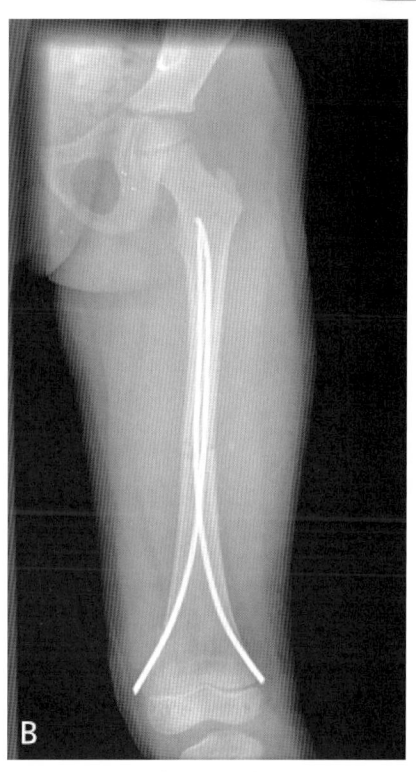

Figure 7 Preoperative (**A**) and postoperative (**B**) radiographs show fixation of a transverse femur fracture in a child using flexible intramedullary nails.

manage unstable fractures. Elastic intramedullary nails are made of stainless steel or titanium. The titanium models are readily available and are easy to insert, but the increased stability associated with the stainless steel models may be more beneficial in unstable fractures.[18,19]

Flexible rods are commonly inserted retrograde from the distal femoral metaphysis toward the proximal end of the femur. Two C-shaped nails, one inserted medially and one laterally, usually provide sufficient stability when three-point intramedullary contact is obtained. Other options for insertion include a unilateral approach distally, inserting one C-shaped nail and one S-shaped nail. When the fracture is very distal, nails may be introduced proximally in the region of the greater trochanter. Additional nails may be added for stability. Whether using titanium or elastic nails, the nail diameter chosen should be the largest diameter possible for the specific femoral diameter—at least 40% of the canal diameter. Therefore, two nails would fill at least 80% of the canal diameter. The two nails should be of the same diameter to prevent deformation once the nails are inserted. Both nails should be precontoured into a gentle C shape to maximize the stability of the fracture. Newer nails are of standard length and are cut in situ to the correct length. Ideally, the lateral nail should extend to the level of

Section 8: Pediatric Orthopaedics

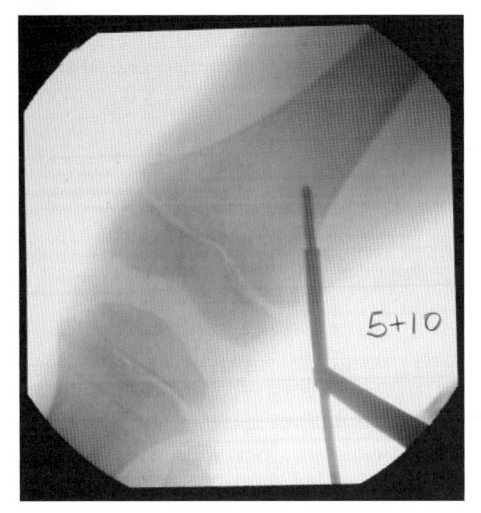

Figure 8 Fluoroscopic image shows the insertion point for a flexible intramedullary nail.

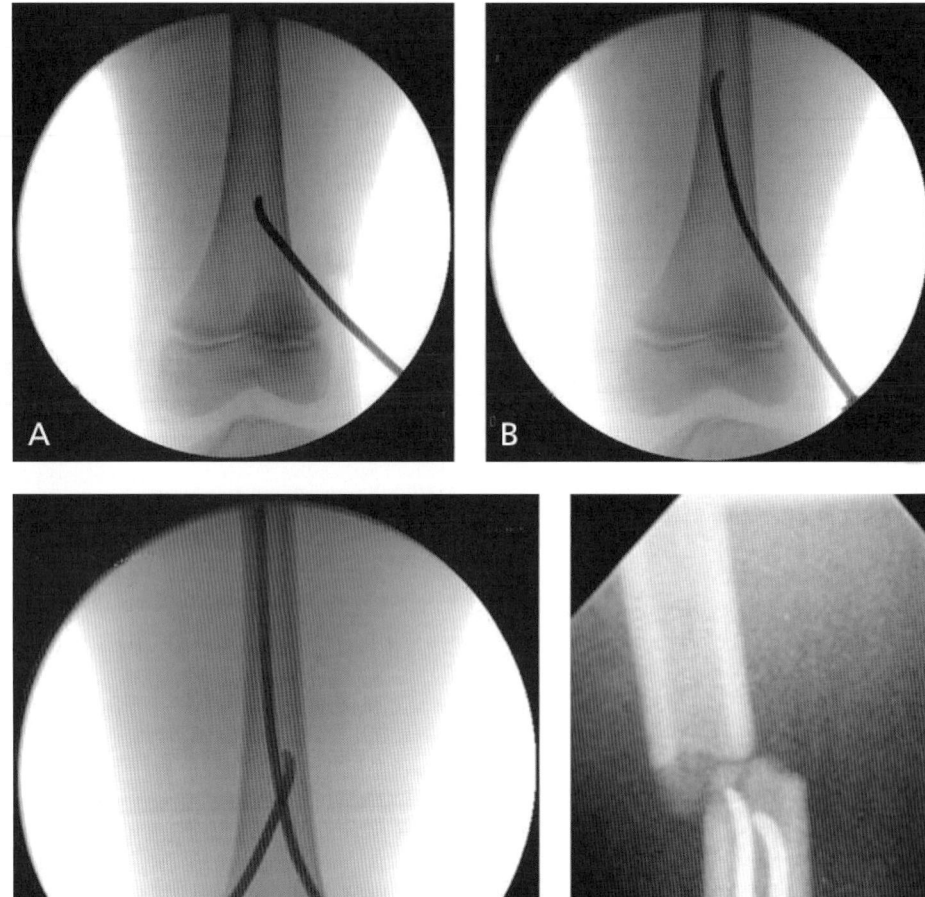

Figure 9 Fluoroscopic images demonstrate sequential insertion of the lateral and medial flexible intramedullary nails for a pediatric femur fracture. **A,** Insertion of the lateral nail. **B,** Advancement of the lateral nail. **C,** Placement of the medial nail. **D,** Both nails are inserted to the fracture site.

the greater trochanter and the medial nail into the base of the femoral neck. Assuming a midshaft diaphyseal fracture, if both nails reach above the level of the lesser trochanter, the fixation will be adequate.

Surgical Technique

The most commonly used insertion points for nails are medial and lateral at the top of the distal metaphyseal flare of the medial and lateral condyles. Nails inserted in these locations bind against the flare of the metaphysis proximal to the epiphysis, giving another point of fixation and minimizing any prominence. Nails that are started too low may back out or be prominent, which is one of the more common complications associated with this procedure.

An incision is made on the lateral side of the leg extending from approximately the superior pole of the patella to approximately two fingerbreadths above the superior pole of the patella. The fascia lata is incised, and the vastus lateralis muscle is retracted dorsally to expose the periosteum of the upper flare of the metaphysis. The position of the entry point is confirmed with fluoroscopy. Using a 4.5-mm drill bit, an oblique drill hole is made in the cortical bone of the metaphysis at an angle similar to that of the metaphyseal flare (**Figure 8**). This angle facilitates nail insertion and advancement into the diaphysis and helps avoid cracking of the opposite cortex when the rod is inserted. The insertion point on the medial side is made in the same manner, by elevating the vastus medialis muscle. A ridge of bone is present on the medial flare, and the drill hole should be made on the anterior aspect of this ridge to avoid an inadvertent posterior position.

In many cases, the fracture fragments will not be reduced perfectly, making it more difficult to pass the nails into the proximal fragment. Furthermore, if one nail is inserted completely past the fracture, the ability to manipulate the fracture into a more anatomic alignment with the nail tips will be difficult. Therefore, I recommend inserting and advancing the medial and lateral nails sequentially to the level of the fracture before crossing the fracture (**Figure 9**). The order of nail insertion is the surgeon's preference. I prefer to insert the lateral nail before the medial nail. Viewing with the image intensifier demonstrates which nail will be the easiest to drive across the fracture site. The first nail is advanced just proximal to the fracture and then rotated as needed to achieve the best fracture reduction (**Figure 10**). Motion of the proximal fragment demonstrates that the nail is in the fragment. At this point, the second nail can be advanced past the fracture and rotated as needed to further reduce the fracture. It is important to not advance the first rod too far past the fracture site until the second rod has passed the fracture site. If the first rod is advanced too far, it will shift the fragments and make passing of the second rod difficult or impossible. Traction is released. The nails are rotated so that the C contour bows out, and then they are advanced to their full length. The entire femur is viewed with the image intensifier to ensure that the fracture is reduced and not distracted and that the nails are properly positioned.

In rare instances that require further stability, it is possible to insert a third nail. This is accomplished most easily if the third nail is inserted before either of the other two nails is fully advanced. The insertion of the third nail has the advantage of providing extra rotational and slip stability by filling the canal and enhanc-

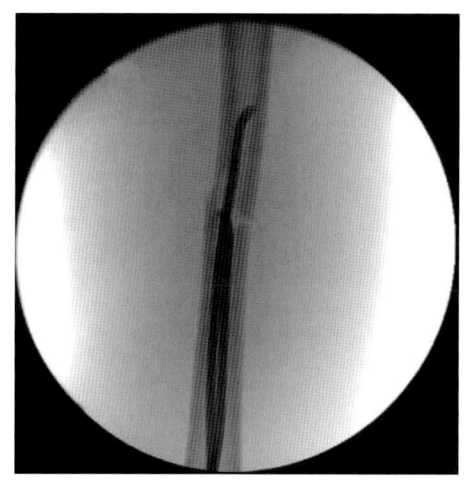

Figure 10 Fluoroscopic image shows that one nail has been advanced initially into the canal proximal to the fracture. The nail can be rotated to reduce the fracture prior to the second nail advancement.

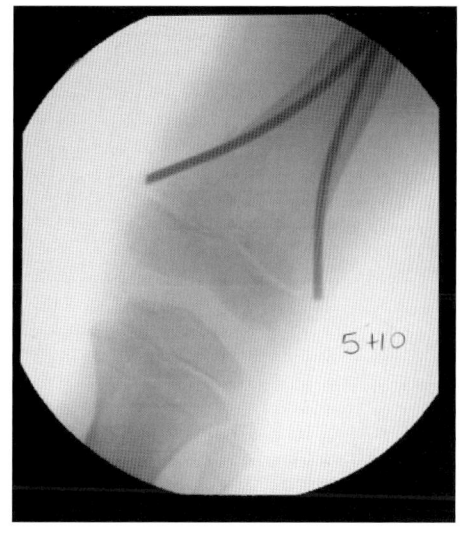

Figure 11 Fluoroscopic image shows the correct position of the elastic intramedullary nails, against the flare of the metaphysis proximal to the epiphysis so they are not prominent.

ing cortical contact. The surgeon should confirm that the third nail does not result in bending of the femur; this has been described with different diameter nails.

The nails are cut outside the skin. The final advancement is then performed with the bone tamp provided in the set. A lateral image of the femoral neck ensures that a nail does not exit the posterior metaphysis or femoral neck. The nails should rest against the flare of the metaphysis 1 to 2 cm outside of the cortex, just above the level of the physis, so they are not prominent (**Figure 11**). The nails should not be bent away from the bone. Nail removal remains possible with a small length of nail left outside the canal.

After insertion of the nails, the wounds are closed and a soft dressing is applied. A knee immobilizer may be used for postoperative comfort. In rare instances, a supplemental spica cast may be applied; however, if stability is a concern, other methods of fixation should be considered.

Complications

Many studies discuss the complications of elastic nailing.[6,7,17] Most complications pose no potential for long-term morbidity. The most common are nail prominence and pain. To lessen the incidence of nail prominence, nails should be cut short proximal to the level of the physis and should not be bent away from the metaphysis. Fracture site shortening has been described, particularly in more unstable fracture patterns and in patients older than 11 years. Limiting the use of elastic nails to more stable fracture patterns reduces the risk of shortening. A potential for malunion also exists, predominately in more proximal and distal fractures. Adhering to the principles of using the largest diameter nail possible, using similar-size nails with a bend opposite to each other, cutting the nails short, and using them in stable fractures in the middle 60% of the femur will reduce the incidence of potential complications.

Pearls

- Stable fractures in the middle 60% of the femur in patients aged 5 to 11 years are most suitable for elastic nailing.
- The largest nail diameter possible is used. The nails are prebent, and both nails should fill at least 80% of the canal diameter.
- Nail insertion through an oblique drill hole at the upper portion of the metaphyseal flare will facilitate proper positioning of the nail.
- Both nails should be advanced to the fracture site before crossing the fracture.
- The nail that requires less manipulation to cross the fracture should be advanced first and rotated to align the fracture anatomically. Then the second rod should be passed, before both rods are advanced to the upper femur.
- The nails should be cut short so they rest against the metaphysis and proximal to the epiphysis.

Trochanteric Intramedullary Fixation

Two devices used for intramedullary fixation are rigid nails and flexible unreamed nails. Rigid nails are ideal for adults because they can be locked proximally and distally to control shortening and rotation. The use of reamed rigid nails introduced through the piriformis fossa has been associated with a few incidences of osteonecrosis of the femoral head in children and adolescents, however. Rigid nails in children younger than 13 years have also been associated with growth disturbance with femoral neck deformity, including coxa valga and thinning of the femoral neck.[20] For these reasons, I do not recommend introducing rigid, reamed nails through the piriformis fossa unless the proximal femoral physis is completely closed. Various trochanteric-entry nails are commercially available for pediatric femur fractures. Trochanteric-entry nails are inserted lateral to the tip of the greater trochanter, theoretically providing a reduced risk of osteonecrosis and proximal femoral deformity.[20,21] The protocol at my institution for lateral trochanteric–entry nails indicates their use in patients older than 11 years with stable or unstable fractures in which the intramedullary canal and proximal femur are large enough to accept the nail.

Procedure

Surgical Technique

Patients are positioned either on the fracture table as described previously or on a radiolucent table. Many of the technical details rely on the manufacturer of the nail. Many new trochanteric-entry nails now are available for pediatric femur fractures with the benefits of minimal dissection and stable fixation. Trochanteric-entry nails are inserted lateral to the tip of the greater trochanter, theoretically providing less risk of osteonecrosis and proximal femoral deformity (**Figure 12, A**). An incision is made proximal to the tip of the greater trochanter. The tensor fascia is opened, and blunt dissection is performed in line with and through the fibers of the gluteus maximus to give access to the lateral trochanter. The most important point of the technique is to make sure the guidewire and the opening reamer are lateral to the tip of the greater trochanter. The guidewire should be centered in the flat area between the tip of the greater trochanter and the distal aspect of the greater trochanteric apophysis (**Figure 12, B**). The most technically challenging aspect of the procedure is correct placement of the guidewire. It should be placed in a way that does not violate the lateral cortex and does not create a pedestal near the lesser trochanter that makes advancement of the nail difficult. It is best to angle the guidewire to the middle of the femur at the level of the lesser trochanter. Good AP and lateral fluoroscopic images assist with accurate placement. Once the guidewire is in place, the opening reamer is used. The guidewire is then advanced past the fracture to the distal femur, stopping proximal to the distal femoral physis.

As mentioned previously, the next steps—reaming, choosing nail length and diameter, and determining the location of the locking screws—depend on the particular nail manufacturer. Rarely, the surgeon may decide it is necessary to place the proximal locking screw into the femoral neck. In this situation, the version of the femoral neck should be considered because femoral anteversion is often greater in skeletally immature children than in adults. It is recommended to use both a proximal and a distal locking screw. Postoperatively, a soft dressing is placed. Patients often can bear weight, at least partially, as tolerated and progress to full weight bearing within 6 weeks.

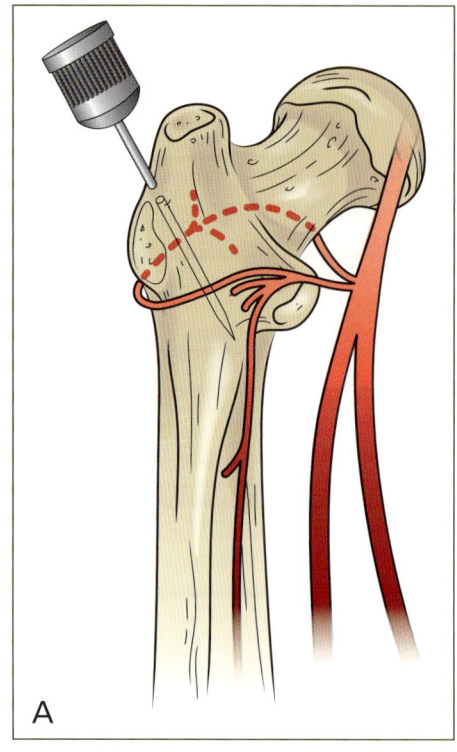

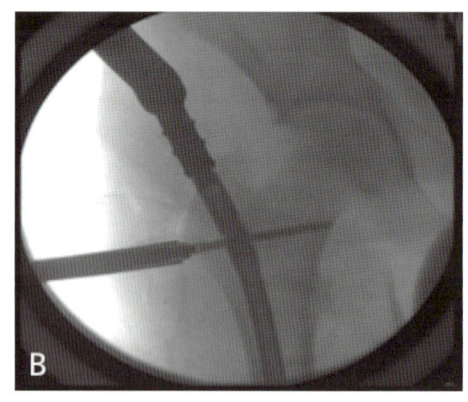

Figure 12 Trochanteric intramedullary fixation. Illustration (**A**) shows the insertion point for trochanteric-entry nails. Fluoroscopic image (**B**) depicts the position of the lateral trochanteric–entry nail guidewire insertion.

Complications

A theoretical risk for nonunion exists, but this is extremely rare in this age group. Implant irritation may occur at the greater trochanter or the screws distally. Finally, there is a remote risk of osteonecrosis of the femoral head, although the lateral entry site was developed to avoid this complication.

Pearls

- Trochanteric-entry nails are suitable for children 12 years of age and older with a stable or unstable fracture, unless the child is much smaller than is usual for that age (< 50 kg).
- Guidewire placement is critical. The surgeon should start lateral to the tip of the greater trochanter and aim the guidewire for the center of the femur at the level of the lesser trochanter.

References

1. Flynn JM, Luedtke LM, Ganley TJ, et al: Comparison of titanium elastic nails with traction and a spica cast to treat femoral fractures in children. *J Bone Joint Surg Am* 2004;86-A(4):770-777.
2. Buechsenschuetz KE, Mehlman CT, Shaw KJ, Crawford AH, Immerman EB: Femoral shaft fractures in children: Traction and casting versus elastic stable intramedullary nailing. *J Trauma* 2002;53(5):914-921.
3. Flynn JM, Hresko T, Reynolds RA, Blasier RD, Davidson R, Kasser J: Titanium elastic nails for pediatric femur fractures: A multicenter study of early results with analysis of complications. *J Pediatr Orthop* 2001;21(1):4-8.
4. Heinrich SD, Drvaric DM, Darr K, MacEwen GD: The operative stabilization of pediatric diaphyseal femur fractures with flexible intramedullary nails: A prospective analysis. *J Pediatr Orthop* 1994;14(4):501-507.
5. Sink EL, Gralla J, Repine M: Complications of pediatric femur fractures treated with titanium elastic nails: A comparison of fracture types. *J Pediatr Orthop* 2005;25(5):577-580.
6. Luhmann SJ, Schootman M, Schoenecker PL, Dobbs MB, Gordon JE: Complications of titanium elastic nails for pediatric femoral shaft fractures. *J Pediatr Orthop* 2003;23(4):443-447.
7. Sink EL, Faro F, Polousky J, Flynn K, Gralla J: Decreased complications of pediatric femur fractures with a change in management. *J Pediatr Orthop* 2010;30(7):633-637.
8. Caird MS, Mueller KA, Puryear A, Farley FA: Compression plating of pediatric femoral shaft fractures. *J Pediatr Orthop* 2003;23(4):448-452.
9. Eren OT, Küçükkaya M, Kabukçuoğlu YS, Balci V, Kuzgun U: [Plate fixation of closed femoral shaft fractures in adolescents]. *Acta Orthop Traumatol Turc* 2002;36(2):124-128.
10. Fyodorov I, Sturm PF, Robertson WW Jr: Compression-plate fixation of femoral shaft fractures in children aged 8 to 12 years. *J Pediatr Orthop* 1999;19(5):578-581.
11. Kregor PJ, Song KM, Routt ML Jr, Sangeorzan BJ, Liddell RM, Hansen ST Jr: Plate fixation of femoral shaft fractures in multiply injured children. *J Bone Joint Surg Am* 1993;75(12):1774-1780.
12. Ward WT, Levy J, Kaye A: Compression plating for child and adolescent femur fractures. *J Pediatr Orthop* 1992;12(5):626-632.
13. Kanlic EM, Anglen JO, Smith DG, Morgan SJ, Pesántez RF: Advantages of submuscular bridge plating for complex pediatric femur fractures. *Clin Orthop Relat Res* 2004;426:244-251.
14. Sink EL, Hedequist D, Morgan SJ, Hresko T: Results and technique of unstable pediatric femoral fractures treated with submuscular bridge plating. *J Pediatr Orthop* 2006;26(2):177-181.
15. Moroz LA, Launay F, Kocher MS, et al: Titanium elastic nailing of fractures of the femur in children: Predictors of complications and poor outcome. *J Bone Joint Surg Br* 2006;88(10):1361-1366.
16. Narayanan UG, Hyman JE, Wainwright AM, Rang M, Alman BA: Complications of elastic stable intramedullary nail

fixation of pediatric femoral fractures, and how to avoid them. *J Pediatr Orthop* 2004;24(4):363-369.

17. Ho CA, Skaggs DL, Tang CW, Kay RM: Use of flexible intramedullary nails in pediatric femur fractures. *J Pediatr Orthop* 2006;26(4):497-504.

18. Wall EJ, Jain V, Vora V, Mehlman CT, Crawford AH: Complications of titanium and stainless steel elastic nail fixation of pediatric femoral fractures. *J Bone Joint Surg Am* 2008;90(6):1305-1313.

19. Rathjen KE, Riccio AI, De La Garza D: Stainless steel flexible intramedullary fixation of unstable femoral shaft fractures in children. *J Pediatr Orthop* 2007;27(4):432-441.

20. Raney EM, Ogden JA, Grogan DP: Premature greater trochanteric epiphysiodesis secondary to intramedullary femoral rodding. *J Pediatr Orthop* 1993;13(4):516-520.

21. Keeler KA, Dart B, Luhmann SJ, et al: Antegrade intramedullary nailing of pediatric femoral fractures using an interlocking pediatric femoral nail and a lateral trochanteric entry point. *J Pediatr Orthop* 2009;29(4):345-351.

Chapter 103
Femoral Derotation Osteotomy in Adolescents and Young Adults

Harish S. Hosalkar, MD

Introduction

Femoral malrotation is a common cause of intoeing gait and patellofemoral malalignment in the pediatric, adolescent, and occasionally even the young adult population. Although most patients have spontaneous resolution of malrotation during the growing years,[1-5] the problem does persist in others, some of whom will go on to require surgical intervention during adolescence.[6-8]

We describe a technique for femoral derotation osteotomy over an intramedullary nail and provide some tips for technical ease. This procedure provides a safe and reliable method to correct femoral malrotation in adolescents and young adults with a rigid intramedullary nail.[9-12]

Patient Selection
Indications
This surgical technique is indicated for symptomatic femoral anteversion in adolescents (>12 years of age) presenting with intoeing gait, rotationally malunited femoral fractures that have failed to remodel with time, and patellofemoral malalignment with femoral malrotation.

Contraindications
Relative contraindications include patients younger than 10 years (potential risk to trochanteric physis), a femoral canal less than 8 mm wide (technical challenge), and extreme obesity.

Preoperative Imaging
We obtain standardized AP radiographs of the pelvis, full-length standing alignment radiographs of the lower extremities, and a torsional profile (our current preferred method is the MRI torsional profile). CT can be used in centers where an MRI torsional profile is not available or feasible.

Procedure
Room Setup/Patient Positioning
Prior to prepping and draping of the affected limb, it is essential to ensure that there is adequate space for the image intensifier. In view of the instrumentation sets as well as the length of the guidewire being passed around, it is important to perform this procedure in an operating room that is large enough and has adequate room for the table, instruments, imaging, and personnel.

The drapes separating the surgical field from the anesthesia personnel should be high enough (intravenous poles are used) so that the intramedullary nail guidewire does not risk becoming contaminated during the processes of reaming and nailing.

Derotational femoral osteotomy over an antegrade intramedullary nail can be performed with the patient in either the supine or the lateral decubitus (our preferred) position. Additionally, the procedure can be performed on a fracture table or a radiolucent flat-top table. A radiolucent flat-top table offers the advantages of easier and faster setup, ease of imaging, and the potential for multiple surgeries to be performed simultaneously (eg, concomitant tibial derotational osteotomy in complex malalignment syndrome).

Our preference is to use Stulberg hip positioners (Innomed) rather than a beanbag for lateral positioning. The procedure discussed in this chapter is performed with the patient in the lateral position. We describe the procedure using a lateral trochanteric entry system.

Surgical Technique
The entire limb is prepped in a standard fashion from the iliac crest to the toes. A small (<5 cm) incision is made over the tip of the greater trochanter in line with the femoral shaft. The fascia and abductor muscles are split longitudinally to expose the proximal trochanter. The trochanter is most prominent in the lateral position, thus making exposure easier. The anterior and posterior margins of the trochanter are palpated, and care is taken to protect the posterior vessels.

Video 103.1 Femoral Derotation Osteotomy in Adolescents and Young Adults. Harish S. Hosalkar, MD (7 min)

An awl or guide pin (we prefer the awl) is then placed in the starting position for the lateral entry antegrade nail, roughly 10° lateral to the tip of the trochanter. If a guide pin is used, its position can be confirmed under fluoroscopic guidance. When a guide pin is used, an additional step of preparing the proximal femur with a cannulated drill is necessary.

A flexible, ball-tipped guidewire is now inserted into the canal, and its position in the canal is confirmed with the image intensifier. Care should be taken to avoid violating the distal femoral physis in those patients with an open physis distally. After confirming the guidewire's position in the distal femur, the length and size of the nail are determined.

If reaming is desired, canal reaming is initiated with the smallest end-cutting reamer and progressed up to the desired width. The guidewire must be stabilized when backing the reamer from the canal. For derotation osteotomies, we ream the distal fragment 1 mm more than the nail diameter and the proximal fragment at least 2 mm more than the diameter to allow for nail accommodation in the altered morphology of the canal after derotation.

The osteotomy site is now determined with fluoroscopic guidance. We prefer the subtrochanteric region so that the osteotomy is sufficiently distal to the proximal locking screw and the distal part of the nail still has enough tract through the isthmus of the femur to achieve a stable nail placement and canal fit distally.

Once the osteotomy site is determined, a small (<5 cm) incision is made along the lateral aspect of the thigh and careful dissection is performed down to the femur. The iliotibial band and vastus lateralis fascia are handled with care to allow for good repair at the conclusion of the procedure. Care is taken to coagulate any perforating vessels along the posterior aspect of the femur. The periosteum is

---

Dr. Hosalkar or an immediate family member is a member of a speakers' bureau or has made paid presentations on behalf of Synthes; serves as a paid consultant to or is an employee of Allergan and Synthes; and has stock or stock options held in GlaxoSmithKline, Johnson & Johnson, and Pfizer.

incised, and retractors are placed around the femur subperiosteally to provide sufficient exposure of the planned osteotomy site.

Two unicortical drill holes are made with a 3.2-mm drill bit for marking the rotational alignment in the proximal as well as distal fragment, taking care to make the distal hole at least 2 cm from the planned osteotomy site. The proximal hole is made along the lateral aspect of the femur, and the distal hole is offset anteriorly or posteriorly by the appropriate distance (using the drill bit in the hole to estimate the angle) such that rotation of the distal fragment brings this hole in line with the proximal hole (**Figure 1, A**). We prefer the drill hole technique over a saw cut or proximal/distal Kirschner wire placement technique.

The guidewire is removed. The osteotomy is performed with an oscillating saw, taking care to place the cut exactly perpendicular to the femur and avoiding any bending or rotational torque moment until the cut is complete to prevent spike formation, obliquity, or spiraling of the cut.

Once the osteotomy is complete, the guidewire is again placed in the canal, and position and length are reconfirmed. The intramedullary nail is inserted and advanced in the proximal fragment while making sure that the osteotomy is not distracted, and the nail is advanced distally, with care taken not to penetrate the distal femoral physis.

Appropriate derotation (usually external rotation) of the distal femur is now accomplished and confirmed with the position of the previously made alignment drill holes (**Figure 1, B**). A 4.5-mm fully threaded cortical screw (we usually use a 16-mm screw, which is saved in the set) is placed through the previously made distal alignment hole that was created with a 3.2-mm drill bit as a temporary holding screw. This screw engages one of the grooves on the surface of the nail and locks the nail in the canal and to the bone in this rotated position during the rest of the procedure (**Figure 2**).

With the nail in position, locking screws are placed. Proximal locking is usually performed using the guide on the nail insertion handle. We prefer to use the locking screw placed obliquely from the greater trochanter toward the lesser trochanter and avoid the one going into the femoral neck.

We prefer to place the proximal locking screw first, before the temporary holding screw is placed. Distal locking screws are usually placed using the perfect circles technique. With the nail secured in position, the insertion handle is removed. Our preference is to place an end cap (for ease of nail removal at a later date if needed).

At this point, we remove the temporary holding screw (**Figure 3**). Final nail position and osteotomy alignment are confirmed using fluoroscopic image intensification. The surgical wounds at the nail entry site, the osteotomy site, and the sites of the proximal and distal locking screws are closed in layers.

Sterile dressings and a compression wrap are applied. We place the limb in a knee immobilizer for support and do not routinely use cast immobilization for these cases. Full-length AP and lateral radiographs of the affected limb are obtained postoperatively.

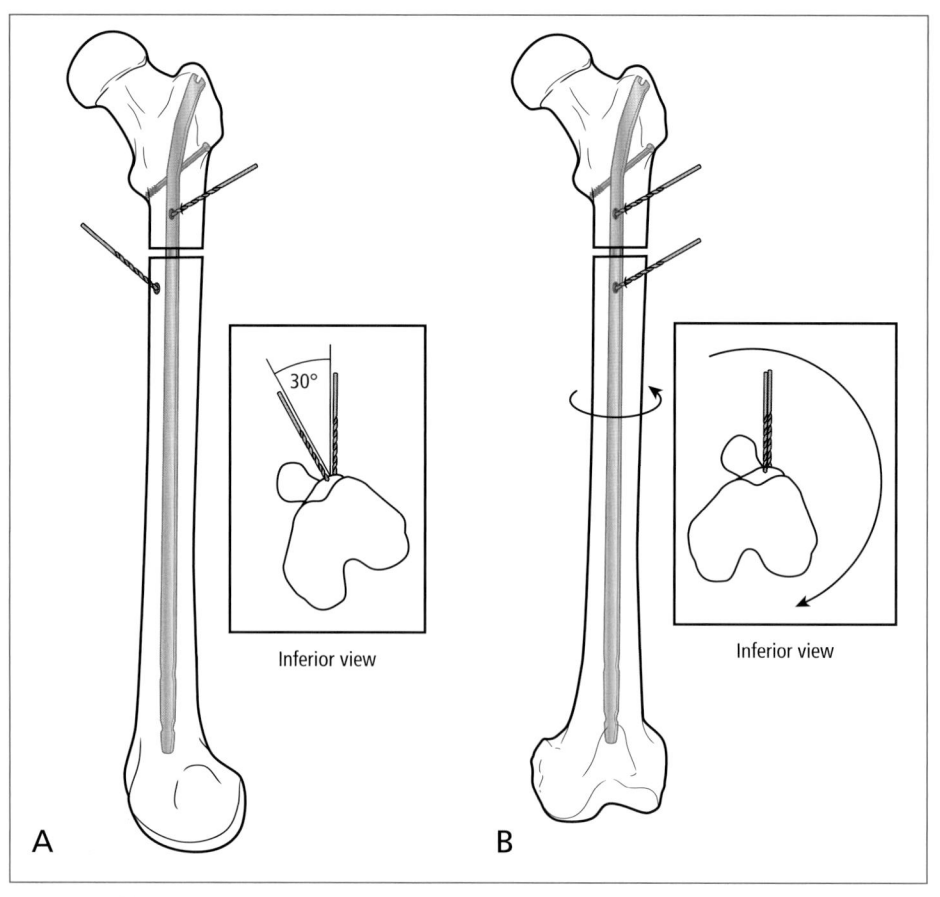

Figure 1 Illustrations show technique for alignment of the distal femur in femoral derotation osteotomy. **A,** Two unicortical drill holes are made such that rotation of the distal fragment will bring the distal hole in line with the proximal hole. **B,** Derotation is performed, aligning the proximal and distal drill holes.

Complications

Complications of femoral derotation osteotomy include inadequate rotation/malposition, distraction at the osteotomy leading to delayed union or nonunion, infection/osteomyelitis, damage to the trochanteric physis or the distal femoral physis, osteonecrosis of the femoral head related to damage during dissection or an inappropriate entry point, nerve palsy, compartment syndrome and vascular deficit, and symptomatic painful hardware.

Postoperative Care and Rehabilitation

Our patients use a knee immobilizer for 1 week, with crutch walking as soon as they can tolerate it (postoperative day 1 or 2).

Patients are toe-touch weight bearing for 2 weeks and partial weight bearing (20% to 50%) for the next 4 weeks, followed by weight bearing as tolerated.

The first postoperative visit is at 10 days to 2 weeks to check wound healing, followed by one at 6 weeks (with radiographs).

Our rehabilitation regimen includes isometric quadriceps and ankle pump exercises starting immediately after surgery (postoperative day 0); knee range-of-motion exercises starting after 2 weeks; quadriceps strengthening starting at 4 weeks; and hip abductor strengthen-

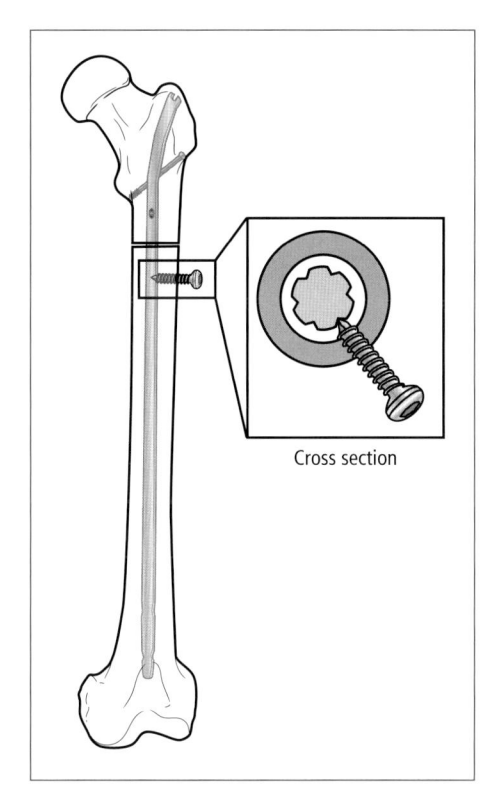

Figure 2 Illustration shows the screw placed through the distal drill hole, engaging one of the grooves on the surface of the nail and locking the nail in this rotated position.

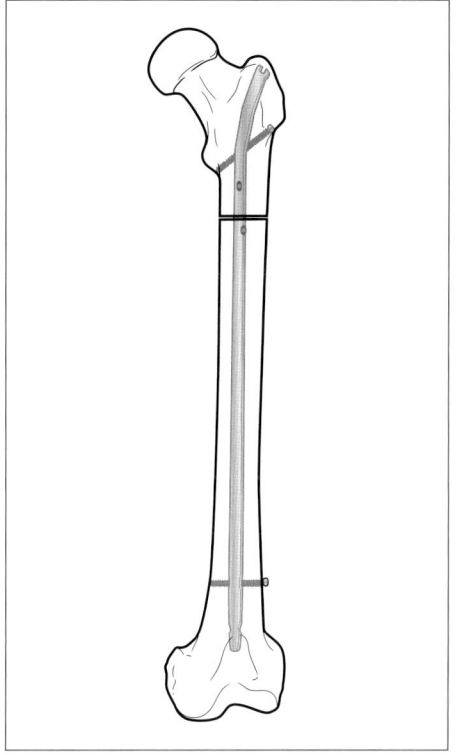

Figure 3 Illustration shows the distal locking screw in place. The screw that was used to hold the rotation of the fragment has been removed.

ing and hamstring and iliotibial band stretching starting at 6 weeks.

Patients are allowed weight bearing as tolerated or full weight bearing from 6 weeks. Full release to sports is not cleared before 12 weeks (and solid radiographic healing with 5/5 muscle strength in the lower extremity).

Pearls

- Femoral subtrochanteric diaphyseal osteotomy over an intramedullary nail provides a safe and reliable method to correct femoral malrotation in adolescents and young adults.
- Adequate exposure and identification of the correct entry point while safely protecting the posterior soft tissues and vascularity is extremely important.
- The surgeon should avoid violating the distal femoral growth plate and penetrating the distal anterior cortex while reaming or with the subsequent nail placement.
- Differential reaming is important to accommodate the canal mismatch and translation that happens after derotation.
- Intraoperative confirmation that the rotation is maintained, especially during the process of distal locking, is important. The temporary screw helps maintain the position during this process.
- Early mobilization should be encouraged, and progressive weight bearing may be started following wound healing in 2 weeks.

References

1. Crane L: Femoral torsion and its relation to toeing-in and toeing-out. *J Bone Joint Surg Am* 1959;41(3):421-428.
2. Engel GM, Staheli LT: The natural history of torsion and other factors influencing gait in childhood: A study of the angle of gait, tibial torsion, knee angle, hip rotation, and development of the arch in normal children. *Clin Orthop Relat Res* 1974;99:12-17.
3. Fabry G, Cheng LX, Molenaers G: Normal and abnormal torsional development in children. *Clin Orthop Relat Res* 1994;302:22-26.
4. Kling TF Jr, Hensinger RN: Angular and torsional deformities of the lower limbs in children. *Clin Orthop Relat Res* 1983;176:136-147.
5. McSweeny A: A study of femoral torsion in children. *J Bone Joint Surg Br* 1971;53(1):90-95.
6. Delgado ED, Schoenecker PL, Rich MM, Capelli AM: Treatment of severe torsional malalignment syndrome. *J Pediatr Orthop* 1996;16(4):484-488.
7. Bruce WD, Stevens PM: Surgical correction of miserable malalignment syndrome. *J Pediatr Orthop* 2004;24(4):392-396.
8. Gordon JE, Pappademos PC, Schoenecker PL, Dobbs MB, Luhmann SJ: Diaphyseal derotational osteotomy with intramedullary fixation for correction of excessive femoral anteversion in children. *J Pediatr Orthop* 2005;25(4):548-553.
9. Keeler KA, Dart B, Luhmann SJ, et al: Antegrade intramedullary nailing of pediatric femoral fractures using an interlocking pediatric femoral nail and a lateral trochanteric entry point. *J Pediatr Orthop* 2009;29(4):345-351.
10. Gordon JE, Swenning TA, Burd TA, Szymanski DA, Schoenecker PL: Proximal femoral radiographic changes after lateral transtrochanteric intramedullary nail placement in children. *J Bone Joint Surg Am* 2003;85(7):1295-1301.
11. Hosalkar H, Pandya NK, Cho RH, Glaser DA, Moor MA, Herman MJ: Intramedullary nailing of pediatric femoral shaft fracture. *J Am Acad Orthop Surg* 2011;19(8):472-481.
12. Momberger N, Stevens P, Smith J, Santora S, Scott S, Anderson J: Intramedullary nailing of femoral fractures in adolescents. *J Pediatr Orthop* 2000;20(4):482-484.

Chapter 104
Surgical Reduction and Fixation of Tibial Spine Fractures in Children

Eric Wall, MD

Patient Selection
Indications
Tibial spine fractures that are displaced 3 mm or more circumferentially require surgical reduction and fixation. Mildly displaced fractures, especially those that are hinged posteriorly, may be manipulated into an acceptable position of less than 3 mm anterior elevation. In the emergency department or the office, the knee effusion is aspirated and the joint is injected with approximately 10 mL of local anesthetic. A radiograph is taken with the knee in full extension with the ankle on a bolster to document that the displaced fracture has reduced into acceptable position of less than 3 mm of displacement. Then the knee is casted in near full extension. It is likely that the notch impinges on the fragment and pushes it into position. Fractures with minimal displacement can be casted directly. Nonsurgical treatment of tibial spine fractures can have excellent results.[1] Loss of full knee extension and joint laxity, nonunion, extension loss, meniscal entrapment, and reinjury can complicate the nonsurgical care of these fractures.[2,3] Minimally displaced type I Meyers and McKeever fractures respond well to nonsurgical treatment, but type II and III fractures have better outcomes with fixation.[4]

Open reduction and internal fixation of tibial spine fractures, despite good long-term outcomes,[5] has been supplanted by arthroscopic reduction and fixation with similarly good outcomes.[6] Fixation of a cadaver-simulated tibial spine fracture with three reinforced No. 2 sutures was found to be stronger than a single 4-mm cannulated screw.[7] In a bovine knee, fixation with suture or bioabsorbable pins showed more motion than a metal or bioabsorbable screw.[8] Screw and suture fixation can be placed entirely within the epiphysis, which minimizes the risk of growth disturbance.[9] Suture fixation is less likely to cause notch impingement or require removal than screw fixation.

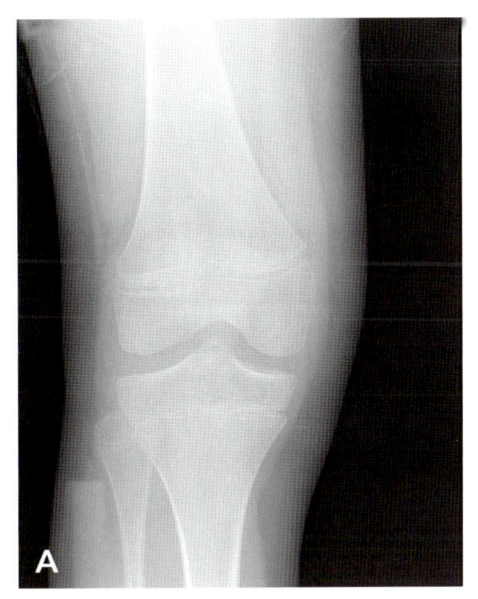

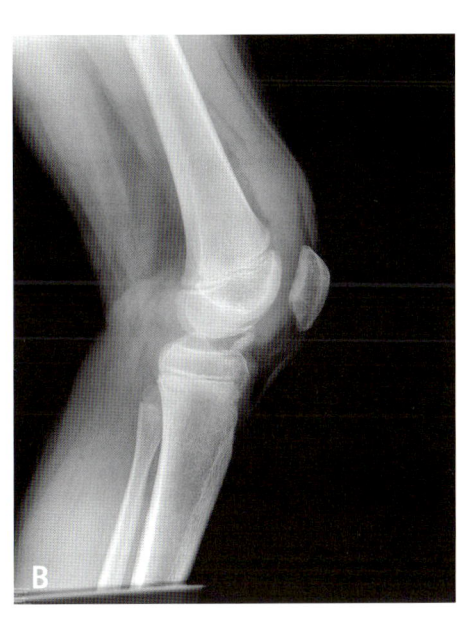

Figure 1 AP (**A**) and lateral (**B**) radiographs of a displaced type III tibial spine fracture. The lateral view usually most clearly demonstrates tibial spine fracture displacement and fragment size.

Contraindications
Although controversial, because of the risk of arthrofibrosis,[10] I recommend that surgical treatment be delayed until the hemarthrosis has resolved and the patient has regained most knee motion (>90° arc of motion). This is similar to most anterior cruciate ligament (ACL) reconstruction preoperative protocols ("prehab"). During this waiting period, the patient may be fully weight bearing and should wean out of a brace/immobilizer and undergo physical therapy before surgery. Surgical delay of 2 to 3 weeks improves arthroscopic visualization because the hemarthrosis will have largely resolved. The fracture does not heal during this waiting period because of its intra-articular location.

Preoperative Imaging
Plain radiographs, especially the lateral view, should be scrutinized to assess fracture displacement and fracture comminution, which is less suitable for screw fixation (**Figure 1**). Meniscal entrapment and meniscal tears can be identified preoperatively on MRI to help plan the procedure and estimate surgical time, and a CT scan or MRI can show true fracture displacement and any comminution of the epiphyseal bed into which the fracture will be fixed. The lateral radiograph (**Figure 2, A**) does not show the significant epiphyseal comminution that is apparent on an MRI (**Figure 2, B**). In this case, screw purchase restricted to the tibial epiphysis would be tenuous. Screw purchase across the growth plate into the metaphysis would be preferred.

Procedure
Room Setup/Patient Positioning
It is essential to position the patient's knee on the table so that a clear intraoperative lateral radiograph can be obtained. For suture fixation, the knee can be positioned in about 20° of flexion on top of the table by elevating the knee holder under the thigh. Cannulated screw fixation is facilitated with the knee at 60° to 90° of flexion, usually off the end of the table. The opposite leg can be placed in a well-padded hemilithotomy holder (well-leg holder), or the leg can be padded and abducted off the opposite lateral side of

---

Dr. Wall or an immediate family member serves as a paid consultant to or is an employee of OrthoPediatrics; serves as an unpaid consultant to SpineForm and Stryker; has received non-income support (such as equipment or services), commercially derived honoraria, or other non–research-related funding (such as paid travel) from SpineForm; and serves as a board member, owner, officer, or committee member of the Pediatric Orthopaedic Society of North America.

Section 8: Pediatric Orthopaedics

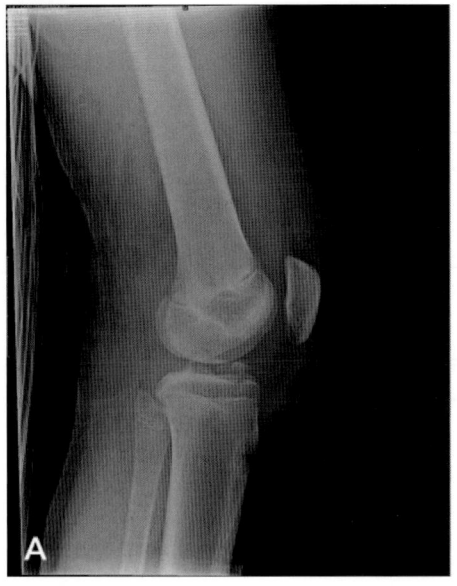

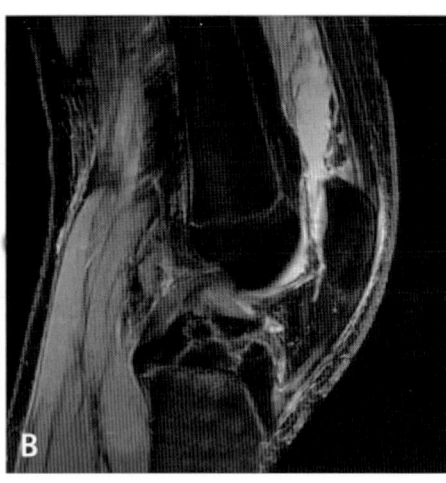

Figure 2 Images show a displaced type III tibial spine fracture in a 13-year-old boy; this fracture is amenable to screw fixation. **A,** Lateral radiograph. **B,** MRI shows that the displaced tibial spine fragment is large enough to fix with a screw and washer, but the rest of the tibial epiphysis has multiple fracture lines. In this case, epiphyseal screw fixation would be tenuous, and metaphyseal fixation is needed for secure screw purchase, which will allow early postoperative knee motion.

the table. It is helpful if the fluoroscopy C-arm can give an unobstructed view of the knee during fixation to document adequacy of reduction and the fixation device position.

Special Instruments/Equipment/Implants

For suture fixation, the following instruments and equipment should be on hand: No. 2 reinforced braided nonabsorbable suture, a suture lasso, an ACL tibial drill guide and guide pin, a microfracture pick, an arthroscopic curet, a Hewson suture passer, a standard fracture set with 3.5-mm drill guide, 30° and 70° arthroscopes, and an arthroscopy shaver.

Screw fixation will require a 4.0- or 4.5-mm cannulated screw/washer, a curet, an arthroscopy shaver, a microfracture pick, a Kirschner wire (K-wire) set, and nonabsorbable suture to tag the washer.

Surgical Technique

The following eight steps apply to both arthroscopic suture fixation and screw fixation:

1. The tourniquet is inflated to improve visualization during a potentially bloody procedure.
2. Arthroscopy starts with irrigation of any remaining hemarthrosis. The knee joint should be rinsed with saline several times through the arthroscope cannula before placing the arthroscope. An accessory outflow portal can be used if necessary.
3. The clot is shaved and curetted from the fracture crater that usually traverses the medial compartment. A portion of the anterior fat pad is resected to provide unobstructed visualization of the anterior fracture line (**Figure 3, A**).
4. The anterior horn of the medial meniscus is identified, as well as its transition into the transverse intermeniscal ligament, which can be entrapped beneath the tibial spine fracture.[11]
5. The lateral compartments are inspected for a meniscal tear. The lateral fracture line is usually not visible in the lateral compartment and may be covered by the anterior horn of the lateral meniscus.
6. The anterior tibial spine is elevated and the clot is shaved from beneath the spine (**Figure 3, B**). This is the longest portion of the procedure.
7. At this point, I reduce the tibial spine fracture, which is usually hinged posterolaterally. The anterior horn of the lateral meniscus is frequently attached to the tibial spine fracture fragment, and it covers the lateral fracture line, which is usually impossible to visualize after reduction. The tibial spine and the attached lateral meniscus need to be reduced anatomically to avoid impingement.[12,13] The anterior portion of the spine fracture is drawn in an anterior, medial, and distal direction until the well-visualized medial compartment fracture line is anatomic (**Figure 3, C**).
8. If the medial meniscus is entrapped, I pull the meniscus forward out of the fracture with an arthroscopic probe during final reduction. Reduction should be confirmed with lateral view arthroscopy and fluoroscopy.

Suture Fixation

The following seven steps apply only to suture fixation. **Figure 4** shows an AP and lateral view of a fragmented tibial spine fracture that is well suited to suture fixation and would be difficult to secure firmly with a screw.

1. Using an ACL tibial guide, the first tibial guide pin is started just medial to the patellar tendon in the tibial epiphysis. The pin is aimed so that it hits the anterolateral crater rim (**Figure 5**). The second guide pin is placed more medially up through the epiphysis to hit the crater on its anterior medial rim. This will create two all-epiphyseal bone tunnels, as depicted in **Figure 6, A** and **B**. A 10-mm-long horizontal skin incision is made between the two pins down to the tibial epiphysis, being careful not to disturb the proximal tibial growth plate.
2. A standard fracture drill guide is placed over the guide pin; the pin is then withdrawn and exchanged with a Hewson suture passer in each tibial drill hole (**Figure 6, C**).
3. Using a suture lasso, a reinforced No. 2 suture is passed through the first Hewson suture passer, then through the most distal ACL where it inserts into the spine fracture fragment, and finally through the second Hewson passer on the other side of the fracture (**Figure 6, D**). This is repeated with the second reinforced suture.
4. The reinforced sutures are drawn down through the tibial epiphysis with each Hewson passer (**Figure 6, E**).
5. With the knee at about 30° of flexion, the fracture is reduced with a microfracture pick, and the four ends of the two reinforced sutures are pulled tight. The sutures are tied and knot-

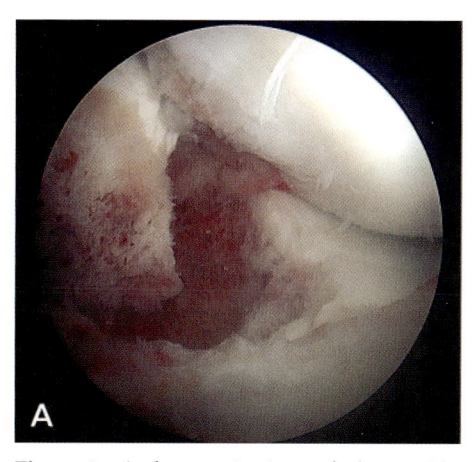

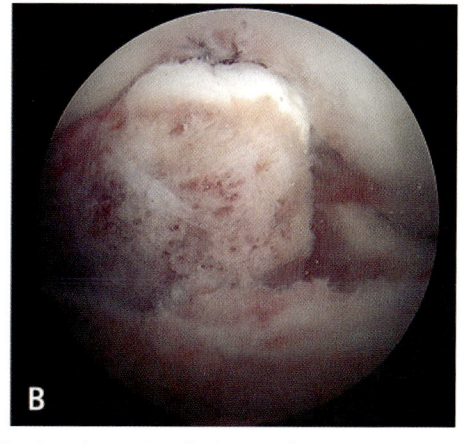

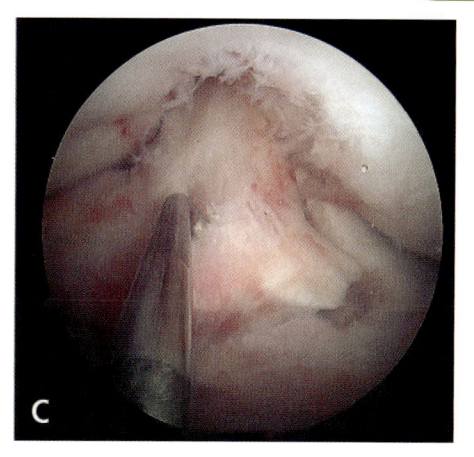

Chapter 104: Surgical Reduction and Fixation of Tibial Spine Fractures in Children

Figure 3 Arthroscopic views of a knee with a displaced type III tibial spine fracture (same patient as depicted in Figure 1) show the notch and the medial compartment. **A,** The fracture fragment is displaced in a lateral and proximal direction. The crater extends into the medial compartment. **B,** The fracture fragment is displaced superiorly into the notch to allow clot removal from the fracture. **C,** An arthroscopic probe is seen reducing the fracture fragment inferiorly and medially into the crater.

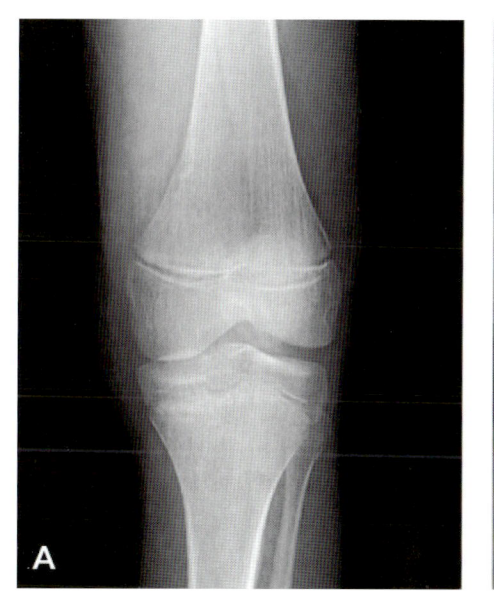

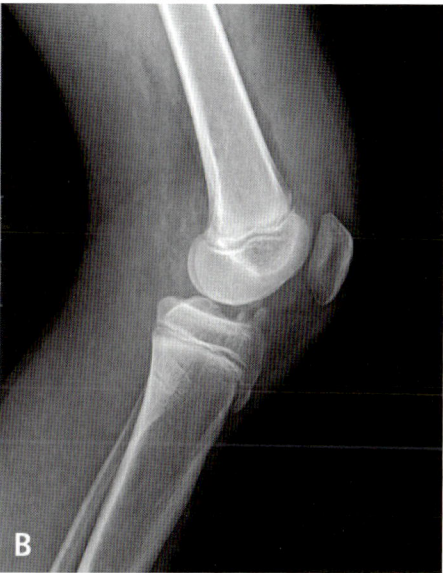

Figure 4 AP (**A**) and lateral (**B**) views of a comminuted tibial spine fracture.

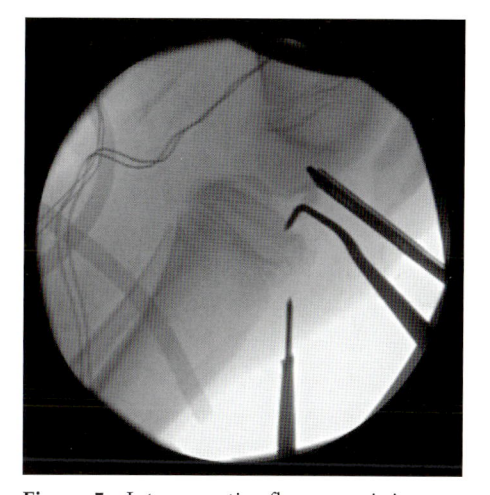

Figure 5 Intraoperative fluoroscopic image shows a tibial tunnel anterior cruciate ligament guide used to place a guidewire into the anterior rim of the fracture crater without passing through the growth plate (all-epiphyseal).

ted on the anterior tibial epiphyseal surface (**Figure 6, F**). The surgeon may need to pull the entrapped medial meniscus or the transverse meniscal ligament anteriorly from under the fracture with an arthoscopic probe during the final reduction maneuver.

6. Knee stability is tested, and the fracture fixation strength is tested though a full range of motion. Ideally, fixation should be secure enough to allow immediate range of motion of the knee. **Figure 7** shows the fracture depicted in **Figure 1, B** anatomically reduced into a position that remains stable after stress testing.

7. Adhesive skin closure strips are placed over the arthroscopic portals, and the tibial suture tunnel incision is sutured closed.

Cannulated Screw Fixation

Cannulated screw fixation is best suited for tibial spine fractures that have a large bony spine fragment attached to the ACL, as viewed on a lateral radiograph (**Figure 2, A**), a CT scan, or an MRI (**Figure 2, B**). The following five steps apply only to screw fixation:

1. An accessory portal for screw insertion is made directly medial to the equator of the patella with the knee at 60° to 90°.

2. A guide pin for a 4.0- or 4.5-mm cannulated screw is placed through the medial parapatellar portal down into the fracture fragment. Care must be taken to ensure that the guidewire is not touching the femoral condyle because subsequent drilling and screw placement will scuff the condylar cartilage. The fracture is reduced with a microfracture awl, and the guide pin is advanced into the fragment. The guide pin is placed about 5 mm posterior to the anteromedial edge of the fracture fragment. If the bone is solid, the fracture fragment (only) is predrilled over the guide pin before placing the screw with a 3.2-mm cannulated drill. It may be helpful to temporarily hold the fracture in the reduced position with a 0.062-in K-wire placed in a position that will not interfere with the guide pin or the cannulated screw.

3. A cannulated depth gauge is used to expand the soft tissue around the guide pin and measure screw length, which is usually 22 mm if it is not

© 2013 American Academy of Orthopaedic Surgeons

679

Section 8: Pediatric Orthopaedics

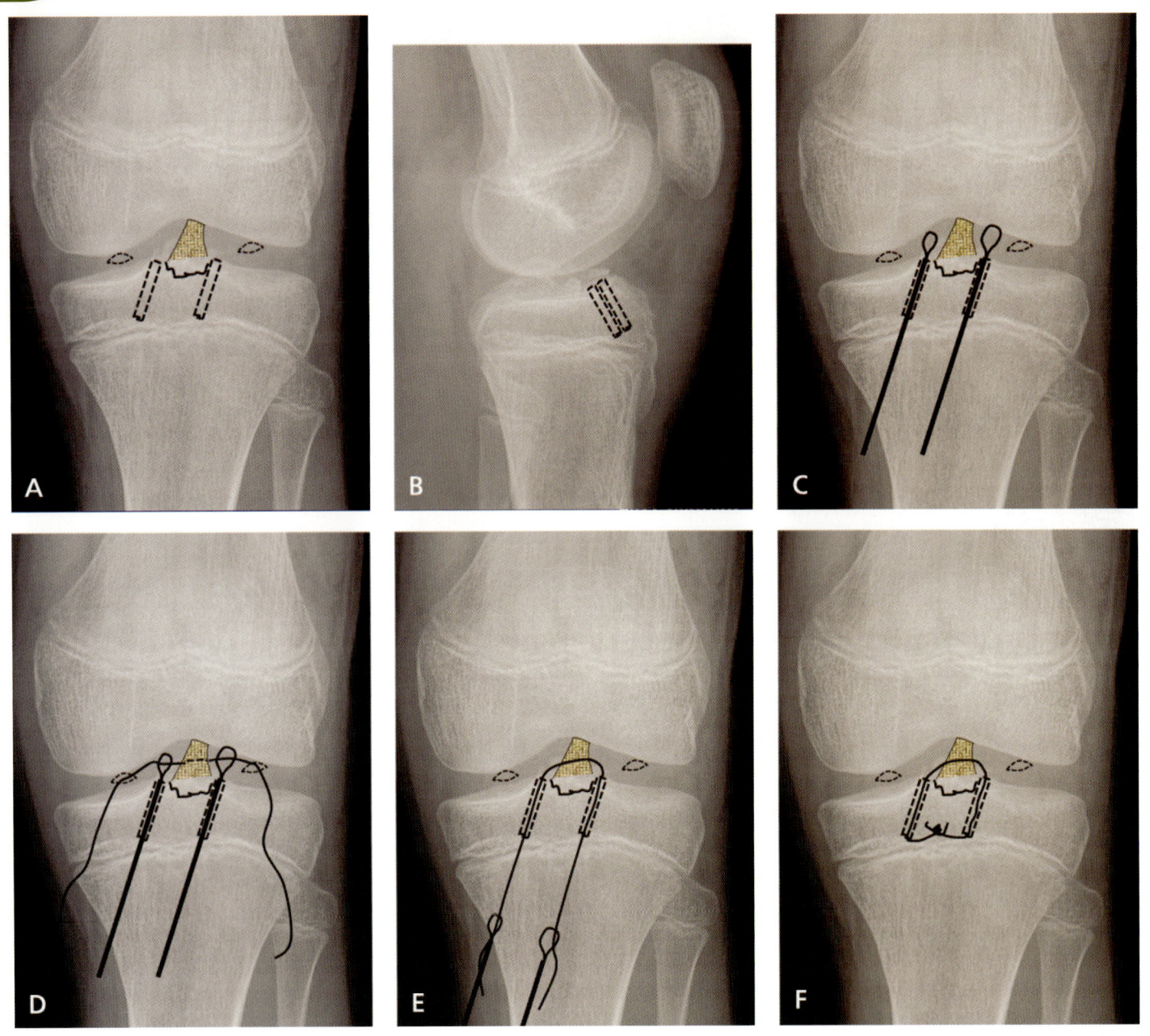

Figure 6 AP (**A**) and lateral (**B**) radiographs show two epiphyseal tunnels drilled percutaneously with an anterior cruciate ligament (ACL) guide and a guide pin anteromedial and anterolateral to the fracture. Tunnels are placed only in the epiphysis, with both tunnels medial to the patellar tendon. **B**, Lateral view that shows the same two epiphyseal bone tunnels from a different angle. **C**, Hewson suture passers are placed up through the tibial tunnels using a drill guide so the tunnel is not lost in the soft tissue during the guide pin–to–Hewson passer exchange. **D**, Reinforced suture is placed with a 90° suture passer through both Hewson suture passers and the ACL at its insertion into the tibial fracture fragment. **E**, Reinforced suture is drawn down into the tunnels with the Hewson passers and exits at the tibial skin incision. **F**, Sutures are tied securely over a bone bridge in the epiphysis.

crossing the growth plate. A long thread or fully threaded screw with a washer is used. If bone purchase is weak, a larger diameter screw should be used, or the screw should be placed across the growth plate into the tibial metaphysis (**Figure 8**). Care should be taken to ensure that the screw or guide pin does not overpenetrate the posterior wall of the proximal tibia, which can put the popliteal vessels at risk. Lateral view fluoroscopy can underestimate the protrusion of the screw or guide pin. As the cortex is approached, the knee is rotated 30° internally and externally to make sure the true position of the device tip relative to the tibial posterior cortex is caught. Any screw that crosses the open proximal tibia growth plate must be removed approximately 8 weeks later to avoid growth arrest. The screw head can also cause notch impingement, and a small notchplasty may be necessary. Proper screw placement is confirmed with arthroscopy (**Figure 9**) and fluoroscopy.

4. Tying a nonabsorbable suture around the washer and leaving a 2-cm tail aids in identifying and removing the screw and the washer arthroscopically at a later date. Parikh[14] has described an alternative technique for arthroscopic washer removal.

5. Adhesive skin closure strips are placed over the arthroscopic portals, and the accessory midpatellar portal, which is slightly larger, is sutured.

Open Surgical Fixation

Open fixation of tibial spine fractures may be necessary if the fracture fails to reduce with arthroscopic treatment. The

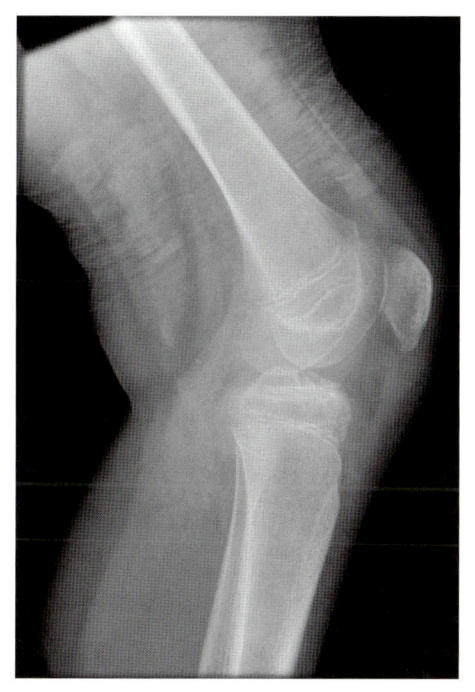

Figure 7 Postoperative lateral radiograph shows the tibial spine reduced into position after the placement of two reinforced sutures.

Figure 8 Postoperative fluoroscopic image shows anatomic reduction of the fracture with secure fixation to the posterior metaphyseal cortex. Notice that the guide pin starts just medial to the patella at its equator. Caution must be exercised to avoid overpenetrating the posterior metaphyseal cortex with the guide pin or the screw, which could cause serious neurovascular injury.

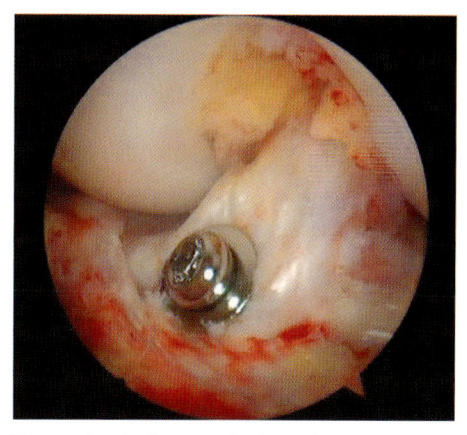

Figure 9 Arthroscopic view shows an anatomically reduced and securely fixed tibial spine fracture with screw. With secure fixation, the patient may start immediate range-of-motion exercises to avoid stiffness and arthrofibrosis.

best approach is usually through a medial parapatellar incision because the fracture is usually most displaced on its anteromedial aspect. Because of the deep, tight working area, the use of a headlight is strongly recommended. Army-Navy or Langenbeck retractors are used for tissue retraction. Visualization is improved by partially removing the the fat pad and the synovium that overlies the fracture. The fragment is usually much deeper than expected. Care must be taken not to injure the medial meniscus during the deep incision into the capsule. Fixation should be similar to that described for the arthoscopic suture and screw techniques.

Complications

Knee stiffness secondary to arthrofibrosis is a rare and perilous complication of arthroscopic treatment of tibial spine fractures. This risk may be minimized by delaying surgical fixation until the patient regains motion and the effusion resolves, similar to arthofibrosis prevention with ACL tear surgery. Patients who do not regain 5° to 90° motion by 3 to 4 weeks after surgery should undergo a very gentle manipulation under anesthesia. If any significant resistance to motion is present, an arthroscopic lysis of adhesions is performed before manipulation. This should minimize the risk of distal femur growth plate fracture, which is a pitfall. Adhesions within the joint can become adherent to the joint surface. A blunt joker elevator can be used to initially open up a space within the joint in which to place the arthroscope. A rotary shaver is then used to carefully remove the adhesions from the articular surface, allowing gentle manipulation. An epidural, continuous passive motion, and aggressive physical therapy can be used to maintain and improve motion after the lysis of adhesions and manipulation under anesthesia. Loss of full extension and joint laxity can be asymptomatic complications of surgical treatment.[15,16]

Postoperative Care and Rehabilitation

Every effort should be made to obtain secure fixation of the fracture with either two No. 2 reinforced sutures or with a 4.0-/4.5-mm cannulated screw and washer. To avoid postoperative stiffness, the patient should move the knee after 3 days of rest. I have the patient start physical therapy on postoperative day 3 with toe-touch weight bearing. I do not restrict active or passive motion. I have patients wean out of the brace within 1 week. I allow full weight bearing at about postoperative week 6.

Pearls

- Due to the risk of arthrofibrosis, surgical treatment should be delayed until the hemarthrosis has resolved and the patient has regained most knee motion (>90° arc of motion). If the patient has not achieved 90° of knee flexion or more than 5° of knee extension by 3 to 4 weeks postoperatively, consider arthroscopic lysis of adhesions followed by a knee manipulation under anesthesia. Knee manipulation alone may cause a distal femur growth plate fracture.
- In the suture fixation technique, during the step when the ACL tibial guide pin is exchanged for the Hewson suture passer, a fracture drill guide is placed over the guide pin before the exchange to maintain the alignment of the bone tunnel to ease passage of the suture passer into the tibial bone tunnels.
- For screw fixation, it may be helpful to hold the fracture in the reduced position with a 0.062-in K-wire placed in a position that will not interfere with the guide pin or the cannulated screw.
- If the meniscus or the intra-meniscal ligament is entrapped in the fracture, it should be pulled anteriorly out of the fracture with an arthroscopic probe during the final reduction step of the procedure.
- Care must be taken to ensure that the guidewire is not touching the femoral condyle because subsequent drilling and screw placement will scuff the cartilage.
- In my experience, approximately 50% of the time the epiphysis alone will not support screw fixation, and the screw must cross the growth plate and gain purchase in the tibial metaphysis.
- Both screw and suture fixation need to be very secure to allow early motion exercises, which may minimize the risk of arthrofibrosis and stiff-

ness. Overpenetrating the posterior metaphyseal cortex with the guide pin or the screw must be avoided; this could cause serious neurovascular injury. Multiple lateral fluoroscopic views should be obtained in slightly different degrees of rotation to confirm that the pin and screw are not too long on any view.
- Placing a nonabsorbable reinforced suture around the washer aids in its arthroscopic retrieval at a later date.

References

1. Wilfinger C, Castellani C, Raith J, Pilhatsch A, Höllwarth ME, Weinberg AM: Nonoperative treatment of tibial spine fractures in children: 38 patients with a minimum follow-up of 1 year. *J Orthop Trauma* 2009;23(7):519-524.

2. Willis RB, Blokker C, Stoll TM, Paterson DC, Galpin RD: Long-term follow-up of anterior tibial eminence fractures. *J Pediatr Orthop* 1993;13(3):361-364.

3. Vargas B, Lutz N, Dutoit M, Zambelli PY: Nonunion after fracture of the anterior tibial spine: Case report and review of the literature. *J Pediatr Orthop B* 2009;18(2):90-92.

4. Tudisco C, Giovarruscio R, Febo A, Savarese E, Bisicchia S: Intercondylar eminence avulsion fracture in children: Long-term follow-up of 14 cases at the end of skeletal growth. *J Pediatr Orthop B* 2010;19(5):403-408.

5. Rademakers MV, Kerkhoffs GM, Kager J, Goslings JC, Marti RK, Raaymakers EL: Tibial spine fractures: A long-term follow-up study of open reduction and internal fixation. *J Orthop Trauma* 2009;23(3):203-207.

6. Perugia D, Basiglini L, Vadalà A, Ferretti A: Clinical and radiological results of arthroscopically treated tibial spine fractures in childhood. *Int Orthop* 2009;33(1):243-248.

7. Bong MR, Romero A, Kubiak E, et al: Suture versus screw fixation of displaced tibial eminence fractures: A biomechanical comparison. *Arthroscopy* 2005;21(10):1172-1176.

8. Mahar AT, Duncan D, Oka R, Lowry A, Gillingham B, Chambers H: Biomechanical comparison of four different fixation techniques for pediatric tibial eminence avulsion fractures. *J Pediatr Orthop* 2008;28(2):159-162.

9. Vega JR, Irribarra LA, Baar AK, Iñiguez M, Salgado M, Gana N: Arthroscopic fixation of displaced tibial eminence fractures: A new growth plate-sparing method. *Arthroscopy* 2008;24(11):1239-1243.

10. Vander Have KL, Ganley TJ, Kocher MS, Price CT, Herrera-Soto JA: Arthrofibrosis after surgical fixation of tibial eminence fractures in children and adolescents. *Am J Sports Med* 2010;38(2):298-301.

11. Siparsky PN, Kocher MS: Current concepts in pediatric and adolescent arthroscopy. *Arthroscopy* 2009;25(12):1453-1469.

12. Ahn JH, Yoo JC: Clinical outcome of arthroscopic reduction and suture for displaced acute and chronic tibial spine fractures. *Knee Surg Sports Traumatol Arthrosc* 2005;13(2):116-121.

13. Lowe J, Chaimsky G, Freedman A, Zion I, Howard C: The anatomy of tibial eminence fractures: Arthroscopic observations following failed closed reduction. *J Bone Joint Surg Am* 2002;84(11):1933-1938.

14. Parikh SN: Arthroscopic removal of a cannulated screw and washer from the knee joint. *Orthopedics* 2010;33(9):675.

15. Park HJ, Urabe K, Naruse K, Aikawa J, Fujita M, Itoman M: Arthroscopic evaluation after surgical repair of intercondylar eminence fractures. *Arch Orthop Trauma Surg* 2007;127(9):753-757.

16. Kocher MS, Foreman ES, Micheli LJ: Laxity and functional outcome after arthroscopic reduction and internal fixation of displaced tibial spine fractures in children. *Arthroscopy* 2003;19(10):1085-1090.

Chapter 105
Treatment of Clubfoot Using the Ponseti Method

Blaise Alexander Nemeth, MD, MS   Kenneth J. Noonan, MD

Patient Selection
Indications
The Ponseti method is appropriate for treating all types of clubfoot. Ponseti casting may be used even in patients with teratologic clubfoot caused by spina bifida, arthrogryposis, or other syndromes.[1,2] Furthermore, children older than 2 years and those with a history of surgically treated clubfoot may be treated with Ponseti casting to minimize the extent of surgery or even prevent further surgery.[3,4]

Contraindications
There are no absolute contraindications to attempting Ponseti casting, although the benefit of casting to an individual patient must be considered. Delaying casting until the patient's condition improves may be prudent in premature infants; in infants with certain medical conditions, such as neonatal jaundice or poor feeding/growth; or in patients with unstable cardiorespiratory status.

Evaluation
Clubfoot deformity has four components: cavus, forefoot adductus, hindfoot varus, and equinus (**Figure 1**). Patients should be thoroughly examined for underlying etiologies, especially neurologic or muscular disorders.

In a patient with idiopathic clubfoot, it is not necessary to obtain radiographs of the feet before proceeding with casting. Forced dorsiflexion lateral images may be helpful later in the casting process, immediately before deciding whether or not percutaneous Achilles tenotomy is necessary (**Figure 2**).

Talipes equinovarus may be identified on prenatal ultrasonography as early as gestational week 12, although the false-positive rate is approximately 20%. More than 50% of infants with prenatally identified clubfoot are born with associated anomalies, primarily neurologic, cardiac, or other musculoskeletal disorders.[5]

Procedure
Room Setup/Patient Positioning
Casting is typically performed with the patient lying supine on the table, with the parents at the head of the patient to provide comfort measures (eg, bottle feeding, toys, singing). The patient's feet are at the edge of the side or foot of the table. Two practitioners are required: one to hold the patient's toes and the other to apply the cast. Older patients may sit upright in a parent's lap or at the edge of the table for application of the lower-leg portion of the cast and then recline into a supine position for extension to a long-leg cast.

The percutaneous Achilles tenotomy that is typically performed at the end of the casting process to achieve adequate dorsiflexion may be performed with the patient under local anesthesia in clinic, under conscious sedation, or under general anesthesia. Positioning is similar to that for cast application, with the difference that under anesthesia, the anesthesiologist or sedation specialist, rather than the parents, is positioned at the head of the patient to control the airway.

Special Instruments/Equipment/Implants
For the typical patient, plaster cast material is preferable to fiberglass. In large children who are difficult to control or who are very strong, fiberglass may be used to reinforce the plaster.

For tenotomy, some practitioners use a standard No. 11 or No. 15 blade; we prefer a 5100 or 6900 eye blade.

Sterilized cotton padding is used to dress the wound and pad under the cast following the tenotomy.

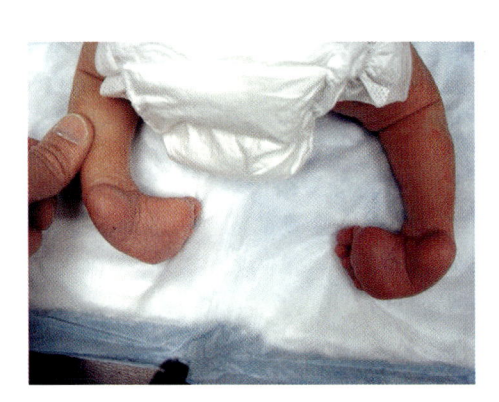

Figure 1 Clinical photograph of an infant with idiopathic clubfoot demonstrates the characteristic deformities of cavus, metatarsus adductus, hindfoot varus, and equinus.

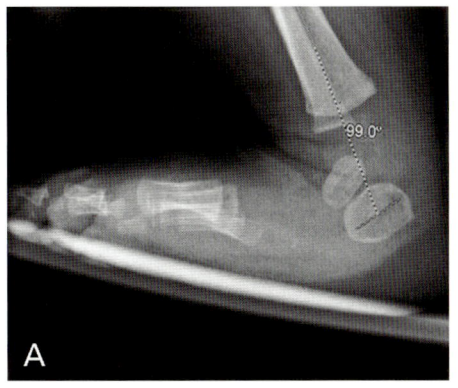

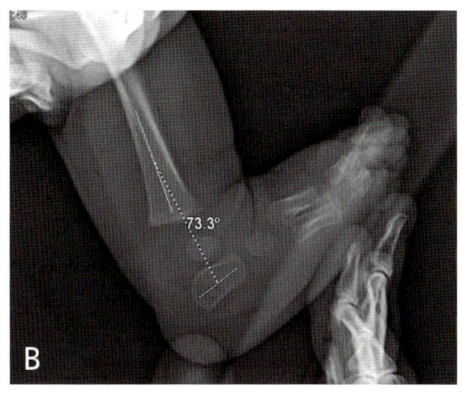

Figure 2 Forced dorsiflexion lateral radiographs of two different clubfeet before percutaneous Achilles tenotomy. **A,** Apparent dorsiflexion due to midfoot breach is seen, with persistent calcaneal pitch in equinus of 9°; a percutaneous Achilles tenotomy was performed. **B,** True dorsiflexion of greater than 15° is present, as evidenced by the normal calcaneal pitch; a percutaneous Achilles tenotomy was not performed, and the patient was placed directly into a foot abduction brace.

Dr. Nemeth or an immediate family member has received nonincome support (such as equipment or services), commercially derived honoraria, or other non–research-related funding (such as paid travel) from Biomet. Dr. Noonan or an immediate family member has received royalties from Biomet; serves as a paid consultant to or is an employee of Biomet; has received research or institutional support from Biomet; and serves as a board member, owner, officer, or committee member of the Pediatric Orthopaedic Society of North America.

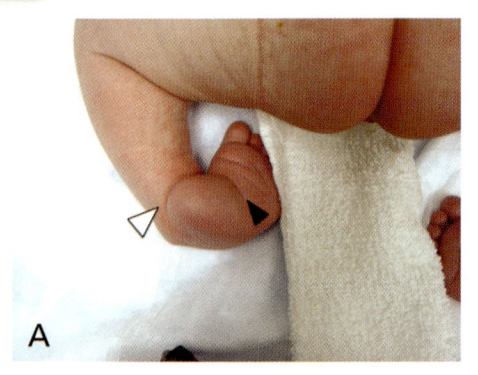

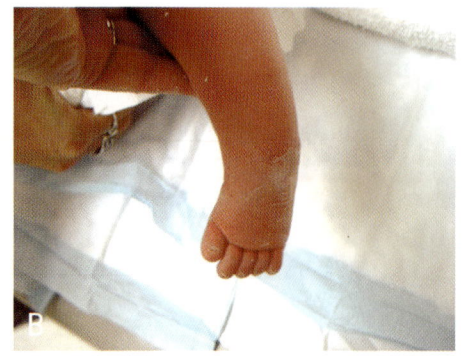

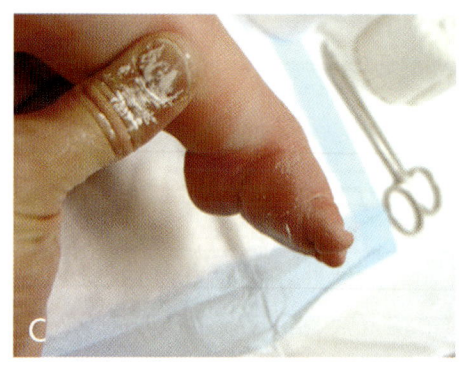

Figure 3 Clinical photographs show complex clubfoot. **A,** At birth, a deep plantar crease (black arrowhead) and posterior crease (white arrowhead) are present. **B,** After two casts, retraction of the great toe (**B**) and pronounced cavus deformity (**C**) are evident.

Video 105.1 Treatment of Congenital Clubfoot. Ignacio V. Ponseti, MD (24 min)

Surgical Technique
Serial Casting

First, the foot is stretched. One hand is used to abduct the foot (the right hand for the right foot, the left hand for the left foot), with the index finger placed along the medial aspect of the foot and the third, fourth, and fifth fingers supporting the plantar aspect of the foot. The contralateral hand is placed with the index finger behind the lateral malleolus and the thumb over the lateral head of the talus. Care is taken not to apply counterpressure over the lateral portion of the calcaneus because this will prevent correction of the deformity through the subtalar joint, the key to Ponseti correction.[6]

For the first casting, the first ray should be elevated to correct the cavus deformity. During all subsequent sessions, the first ray should remain elevated, keeping all the metatarsals aligned. This will prevent regeneration of the cavus deformity and rotation of the talus under the tibia as the foot is abducted.

After the foot has been stretched, a cast is applied to maintain the foot in the position of maximum stretch without overstretching. Starting at the toes, the lower leg is wrapped with two or three layers of cotton padding over the fingers of the practitioner who is holding the toes. Plaster is applied in two or three layers while the foot is held in the same manner as during stretching (supporting the foot against counterpressure over the lateral head of the talus, although persistent pressure should be avoided so as to not cause pressure sores). With the foot held with an abduction moment across the talar head, the cast is meticulously molded around the malleoli and posteriorly above the calcaneus.

The short-leg cast is then extended into a long-leg cast, up to the groin, with the knee flexed at 90°. In larger or stronger children, an anterior splint of four layers of plaster is applied over the knee during circumferential casting to provide additional strength but minimize bulk in the popliteal fossa.

Cast material should be trimmed away from around the toes dorsally and along both sides, leaving a plate under the toes, to allow full dorsiflexion but maintain stretch of the toe flexors. The dorsal edge should not be trimmed proximal to the web space of the toes because a tourniquet effect may occur, inducing swelling of the foot.

For complex and teratologic clubfeet, a posterior splint may be applied behind the lower leg and under the foot during casting, and the knee should be flexed 110° to 120° to prevent pulling back in the cast.[7]

Casts are changed weekly, although more frequent changes are possible.[8] Typically, four to six casts are required to achieve full correction.

Once the foot has reached 60° to 70° of abduction relative to the sagittal plane and if there is less than 15° of dorsiflexion, a percutaneous Achilles tenotomy is performed to correct the remaining equinus deformity. The final cast is applied with the foot in the position of maximum dorsiflexion obtained following the tenotomy and maximum abduction. If the practitioner believes the foot is adequately corrected and may not need a tenotomy, a lateral radiograph of the foot in maximum dorsiflexion should be obtained; 15° of dorsiflexion should be present without midfoot breach (**Figure 2**).

Complex Clubfoot

As treatment progresses, changes in the foot morphology may arise that lead to the characterization of a complex clubfoot. Following the first or second cast, the clinician may notice that the foot is swollen, red, irritated, and difficult to cast. The patient may have a history of cast slippage or skin sores. The swollen foot will have a persistent plantar crease (**Figure 3, A**), the great toe may start to retract (**Figure 3, B**), and the cavus deformity will remain pronounced (**Figure 3, C**). At this point, recognition of a complex clubfoot is important because modifications to the casting technique are necessary.[7] If the clinician fails to recognize this and forces the abduction, metatarsus abductus will result. If complex clubfoot is recognized earlier, attempts to obtain 70° of abduction should be abandoned, and efforts should be focused on stretching the plantar and posterior contracture. The foot is stretched and held using the fingers of both hands. The thumbs of both hands are placed under the metatarsal heads, dorsiflexing the foot against counterpressure applied by both index fingers over the dorsum of the talar neck (**Figure 4**). The middle fingers are used to mold behind the malleoli and above the calcaneus posteriorly.[7] A posterior splint is applied behind the lower leg and under the foot. The knee should be flexed 110° to 120° to prevent pulling back in the cast (**Figure 5**).

A percutaneous Achilles tenotomy is performed once the cavus is corrected and the foot has been abducted 40°. Further abduction usually only deforms the foot rather than providing additional correction[7] (**Figure 6**).

Four to eight casts may be required to achieve correction.

Teratologic Clubfoot

Casting is performed according to the Ponseti technique, using the modifications described earlier for complex clubfoot as necessary if retraction of the great toe or accentuation of the cavus deformity is noted. Percutaneous Achilles tenotomy is performed once 40° to 60° of abduction has been obtained.

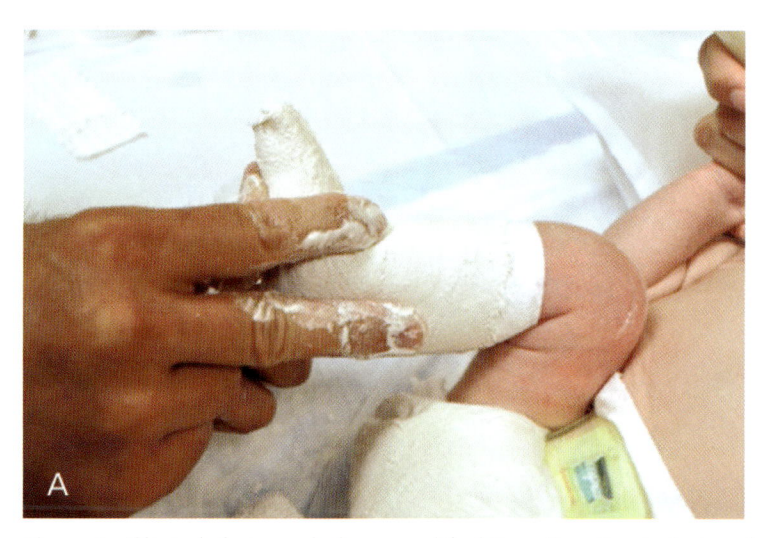

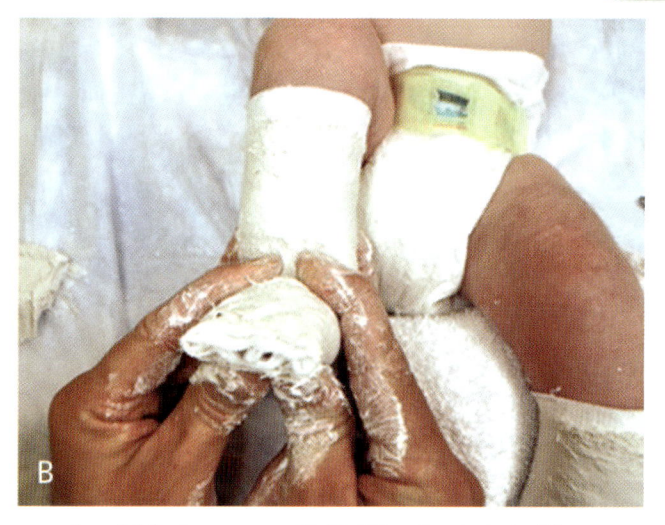

Figure 4 Clinical photograph shows modified Ponseti casting technique for a complex clubfoot as seen medially (**A**) and anteriorly (**B**).

Percutaneous Achilles Tenotomy

Once the foot has reached the appropriate degree of abduction (40° for complex clubfoot, 60° to 70° for idiopathic clubfoot, 40° to 60° for teratologic clubfoot), a percutaneous Achilles tenotomy is indicated if the foot does not dorsiflex sufficiently (5° for complex clubfoot, 10° for teratologic clubfoot, 15° for idiopathic clubfoot). A forced dorsiflexion lateral radiograph helps to differentiate true ankle dorsiflexion from apparent dorsiflexion due to midfoot breach, although it is always preferable to err on the side of performing the tenotomy (**Figure 2**).

If the tenotomy is performed under local anesthesia, either topical lidocaine cream or an injection of lidocaine is administered. Topical anesthetic should be placed at least 20 minutes before the procedure. If injecting lidocaine, a minimal amount (<0.05 mL) should be injected to prevent obscuring palpation of the tendon margins. In some cases, it may be preferable to administer local anesthetic into the tenotomy site after the procedure.[9]

The tenotomy site is prepared in a sterile manner. An assistant holds the leg with the knee flexed 90° and the foot in dorsiflexion under light tension; excessive tension may obscure the tendon.

The blade is inserted from a medial approach, immediately anterior to the Achilles tendon, 1 to 1.5 cm above the insertion of the Achilles on the calcaneus. A common pitfall is to fail to recognize that the insertion of the Achilles tendon is more proximal because of calcaneal elevation and thus the tenotomy site is more proximal. The blade should be inserted parallel to the tendon, taking care to avoid the posterior tibialis artery. This artery lies anterior to the tendon, behind the medial malleolus, and may be the only artery supplying the foot.[10] Once the blade tip passes the lateral aspect of the Achilles tendon, the blade is turned 90° to make contact with the tendon (**Figure 7, A**). Alternatively, the blade may be inserted at a 45° angle to the skin with the blade pointing posteriorly, toward the tendon. Once the blade has been inserted deeply enough to transect the tendon, the handle is lifted anteriorly, bringing the blade into contact with the tendon (**Figure 7, B**).

The tendon is then transected in an anterior-to-posterior direction, taking care not to pull the blade through the tendon (and then potentially through the overlying skin); instead, the clinician's contralateral finger or thumb is used to push the tendon through the blade. Cutting the tendon in this manner, as opposed to drawing the knife through the tendon, helps avoid inadvertent skin and tendon penetration. An increase in dorsiflexion of 15° to 20° should be obtained (less in the complex/teratologic clubfoot), and a "pop" is often noted. A defect should be palpable in the tendon.

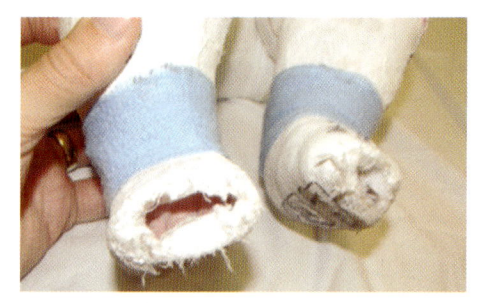

Figure 5 Clinical photograph shows retraction of the foot within the cast in a patient with spina bifida. Note that the toes are no longer visible beyond the distal end of the cast.

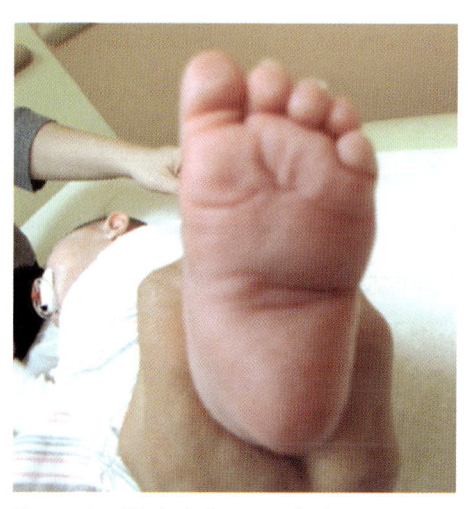

Figure 6 Clinical photograph shows overabduction of the forefoot and iatrogenic deformity caused by abduction of a complex clubfoot beyond 40°. This deformity will correct if the shoe is maintained at 40° of abduction during bracing.

Pressure is applied to stop any bleeding, and the leg is cleansed with sterile water to remove any sterilizing solution that may cause chemical irritation of the infant's skin. After residual bleeding has ceased, the lower leg is wrapped with sterile cotton padding and a short-leg plaster cast is applied while the foot is held in maximum dorsiflexion and abduction.

The popliteal fossa is inspected for a high posterior trim line, which could lead to vascular embarrassment. The short-leg cast is extended into a long-leg cast up to the groin with the knee flexed 90°. The cast material is trimmed away from around the toes.

Complications

Vascular

Vasospasm may occur following percutaneous tenotomy and forced dorsiflex-

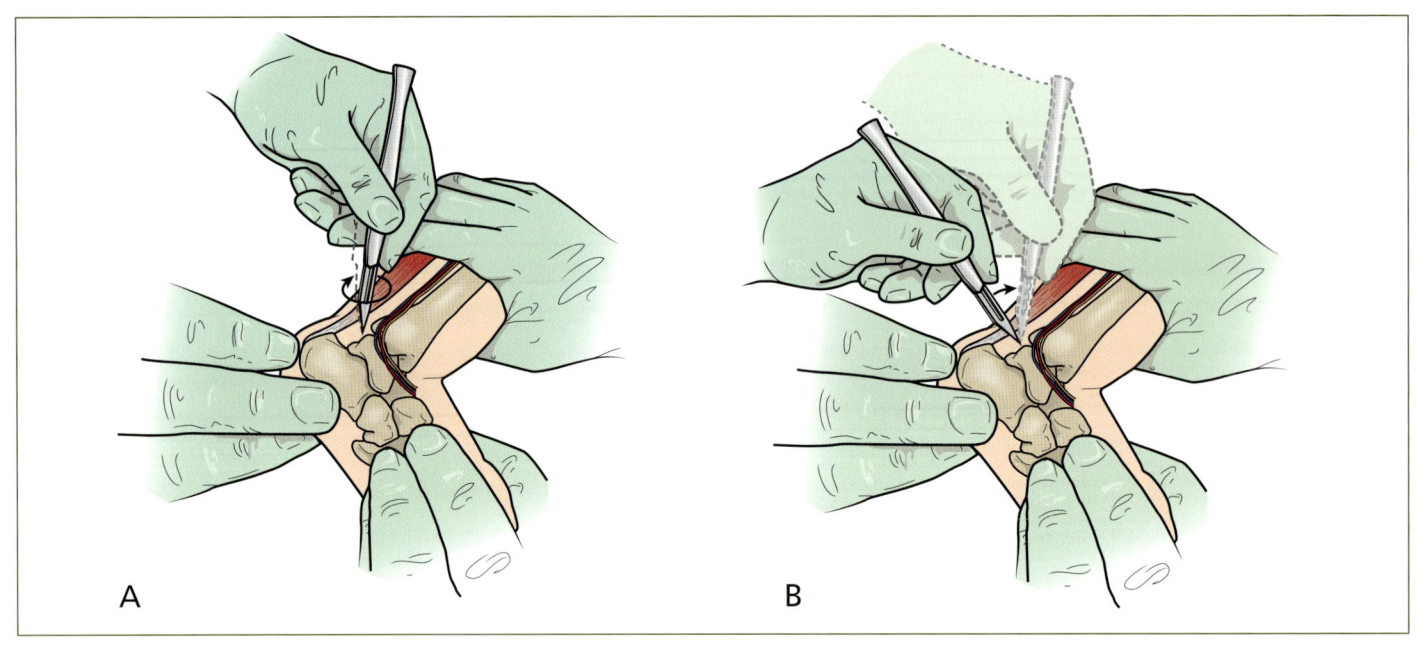

Figure 7 Illustrations demonstrate two techniques for percutaneous Achilles tenotomy in clubfoot deformity. **A,** In the first technique, the blade is inserted parallel to the tendon, followed by rotation of the blade to make contact with and transect the tendon. **B,** In an alternative technique, the blade is inserted at a 45° angle to the skin. The handle is then lifted anteriorly to bring the blade into contact with the tendon and perform the transection.

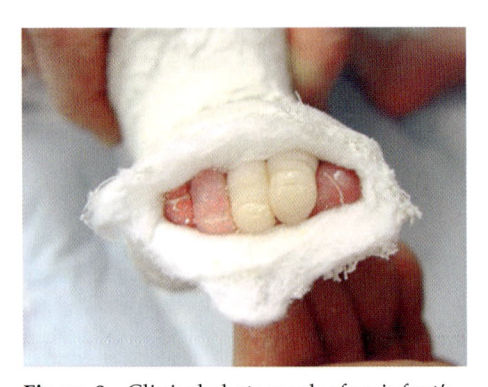

Figure 8 Clinical photograph of an infant's foot following release of dorsiflexion during casting after percutaneous Achilles tenotomy for clubfoot. Pallor of the second and third toes is seen; the first, fourth, and fifth toes demonstrate return of blood flow. Perfusion of the second and third toes returned within seconds.

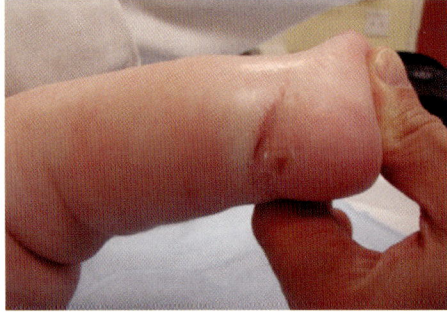

Figure 9 Clinical photograph shows a heel sore following cast removal in a patient with spina bifida who was undergoing Ponseti casting for clubfoot.

ion, resulting in pale digits (**Figure 8**). Typically, reperfusion will occur once the excessive dorsiflexion applied during casting is released and the cast relaxes slightly. If reperfusion does not occur, the cast should be removed and reapplied.

Parents should be advised to expect a small amount of blood spotting (no larger than 2 cm in diameter) on the posterior portion of the cast. Increased or prolonged bleeding should be evaluated because transection of the lateral vessels (lesser saphenous vein and/or peroneal artery) may have occurred.[9]

Pseudoaneurysm has been reported following percutaneous Achilles tenotomy.[11]

Cast Sores
Pulling back in the cast can result in pressure sores. Children with spina bifida may be especially susceptible because they typically have stiff feet with insensitive skin that predisposes to pressure sores (**Figure 9**).

Fractures
Tibial fractures may occur in children with spina bifida.[2]

Postoperative Care and Rehabilitation
The final cast, following percutaneous Achilles tenotomy, should be left in place for 3 weeks before removal to allow for healing of the tendon.[12] After removal of the final cast, the child is placed in a foot abduction brace. Multiple models of braces exist; some are specifically designed for use in children with clubfeet.

Shoes for clubfeet should be externally rotated on the bar as far as the maximum abduction obtained during cast correction—ideally, 70° for idiopathic clubfeet, 40° to 50° for complex clubfeet, and 40° to 70° for teratologic clubfeet. The heels of the shoes are placed at shoulder width. In unilateral cases, the unaffected foot is abducted 30° (**Figure 10**). Front-entry shoes should be used for complex clubfeet; ankle-foot orthoses attached to an articulated bar should be used for teratologic clubfeet.

The foot abduction brace is worn full time for 3 months, followed by nighttime and naptime wear until 4 years of age. Improved compliance with recommended brace wear has been demonstrated when close telephone and/or clinic follow-up is used to address problems with tolerance of brace wear.[13] Recurrence occurs in 80% of patients who do not wear the brace as recommended.

Intolerance of the bar and shoes may occur if the foot is incompletely corrected or the bar and shoes do not fit properly, or if the child excessively plantar flexes the foot, lifting the heel within the shoes.

Recurrences are addressed by repeat casting. Repeat tenotomy may be indicated if less than 15° of dorsiflexion is present after repeat casting (<5° for complex/teratologic clubfeet). Repeat percutaneous tenotomy, which is performed only if the tendon is discretely palpable, should be done in the operating room. If the tendon is scarred and diffi-

Chapter 105: Treatment of Clubfoot Using the Ponseti Method

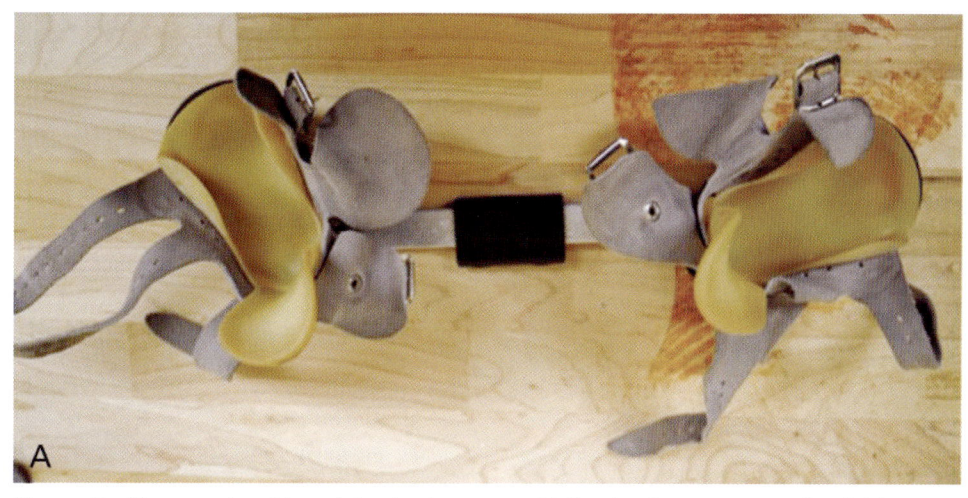

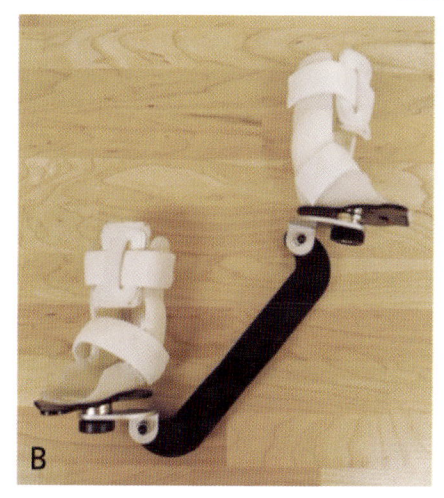

Figure 10 Photographs of foot abduction braces used following Ponseti casting for clubfoot. **A,** Positioning of the shoes on the bar. Affected feet are abducted to the degree of maximum correction. In this case, the right foot is abducted 70°; the unaffected (left) foot is abducted 30°. **B,** Foot abduction brace that uses an articulated bar to allow independent movement of the legs.

cult to palpate, an open tendon dissection and posterior release may be the more definitive approach. The use of a different brace construct (front-entry shoes, articulated bar, ankle-foot orthoses, or a combination of these) may prevent recurrence after recasting.

In instances of persistent recurrence refractory to repeated casting, limited soft-tissue surgery is indicated. Achilles tendon lengthening and posterior release is used for equinus that is refractory to repeat percutaneous tenotomy. Transfer of the anterior tibialis tendon to the third cuneiform corrects persistent varus and is performed once the first cuneiform has ossified, usually between 3 and 4 years of age; an Achilles tendon lengthening may be performed at the same time if indicated.

Pearls

- Pronation of the forefoot should be avoided during abduction; this will re-create the deformity.
- The foot should be assessed before cast removal to identify subtle pulling back within the cast.
- After cast removal, the foot is examined and casting is adapted to correct the deformities identified in accordance with the expected progression of correction, with an understanding that some feet correct slower (or faster) than others.
- The features of a complex clubfoot must be recognized early in the casting process, and the casting technique should be appropriately modified to correct the persistent cavus deformity and prevent further deformity associated with overabduction.
- Good education of caregivers and close follow-up improve compliance with the recommended use of the foot abduction brace.
- Recurrences should be treated early with repeat casting, using percutaneous Achilles tenotomy, Achilles tendon lengthening, posterior release, and/or anterior tibialis tendon transfer as necessary. A wide posterior and medial release should be avoided in patients with residual foot deformity because this can lead to overcorrection. Selectively releasing only those aspects involved in the recurrence will avoid this pitfall.

References

1. Janicki JA, Narayanan UG, Harvey B, Roy A, Ramseier LE, Wright JG: Treatment of neuromuscular and syndrome-associated (nonidiopathic) clubfeet using the Ponseti method. *J Pediatr Orthop* 2009;29(4): 393-397.
2. Gerlach DJ, Gurnett CA, Limpaphayom N, et al: Early results of the Ponseti method for the treatment of clubfoot associated with myelomeningocele. *J Bone Joint Surg Am* 2009;91(6):1350-1359.
3. Lourenço AF, Morcuende JA: Correction of neglected idiopathic club foot by the Ponseti method. *J Bone Joint Surg Br* 2007;89(3):378-381.
4. Garg S, Dobbs MB: Use of the Ponseti method for recurrent clubfoot following posteromedial release. *Indian J Orthop* 2008;42(1):68-72.
5. Mammen L, Benson CB: Outcome of fetuses with clubfeet diagnosed by prenatal sonography. *J Ultrasound Med* 2004;23(4):497-500.
6. Ponseti IV: *Congenital Clubfoot: Fundamentals of Treatment*. New York, NY, Oxford Medical Publications, 1996.
7. Ponseti IV, Zhivkov M, Davis N, Sinclair M, Dobbs MB, Morcuende JA: Treatment of the complex idiopathic clubfoot. *Clin Orthop Relat Res* 2006;451:171-176.
8. Morcuende JA, Abbasi D, Dolan LA, Ponseti IV: Results of an accelerated Ponseti protocol for clubfoot. *J Pediatr Orthop* 2005;25(5):623-626.
9. Dobbs MB, Gordon JE, Walton T, Schoenecker PL: Bleeding complications following percutaneous tendoachilles tenotomy in the treatment of clubfoot deformity. *J Pediatr Orthop* 2004;24(4): 353-357.
10. Greider TD, Siff SJ, Gerson P, Donovan MM: Arteriography in club foot. *J Bone Joint Surg Am* 1982;64(6):837-840.
11. Burghardt RD, Herzenberg JE, Ranade A: Pseudoaneurysm after Ponseti percutaneous Achilles tenotomy: A case report. *J Pediatr Orthop* 2008;28(3):366-369.
12. Mangat KS, Kanwar R, Johnson K, Korah G, Prem H: Ultrasonographic phases in gap healing following Ponseti-type Achilles tenotomy. *J Bone Joint Surg Am* 2010;92(6):1462-1467.
13. Dobbs MB, Rudzki JR, Purcell DB, Walton T, Porter KR, Gurnett CA: Factors predictive of outcome after use of the Ponseti method for the treatment of idiopathic clubfeet. *J Bone Joint Surg Am* 2004;86(1):22-27.

Video Reference

105.1 Ponseti IV: Video: *Treatment of Congenital Clubfoot*. Rosemont, IL, American Academy of Orthopaedic Surgeons, 2002.

© 2013 *American Academy of Orthopaedic Surgeons*

Chapter 106
Treatment of Tarsal Coalitions

Scott J. Mubarak, MD

Patient Selection

Patients who present with tarsal coalitions have myriad presenting symptoms, but the most common include foot pain, foot deformity, and a history of an injury or multiple injuries to the ankle or foot. The orthopaedic surgeon must always be suspicious of a tarsal coalition in a teenager with multiple ankle sprains.

The history should alert the orthopaedic surgeon to the possibility of a coalition, but the physical examination will all but confirm its presence. A stiff flatfoot is the hallmark of a foot with a tarsal coalition. This is especially dramatic in presentation when the pathology is unilateral (**Figure 1**). The findings for a calcaneonavicular coalition are restricted subtalar motion; a palpable, often tender, bony ridge in the sinus tarsi; and restricted plantar flexion of the affected foot compared with the unaffected side[1-3] (**Figure 1, B**). A patient with a talocalcaneal coalition may present with a tender bony prominence around the sustentaculum tali (just below the medial malleolus) and, of course, restricted subtalar motion. Any of these findings should prompt further diagnostic imaging, as discussed below.

In my opinion, nonsurgical treatment of a symptomatic tarsal coalition does not benefit the patient long term. Periods of immobilization may provide temporary relief but do not address the altered mechanics that can cause adjacent joint degeneration. I also believe that patients with coalitions are at risk for future foot/ankle injuries due to the coalitions. I recommend excision in all young patients.

Preoperative Imaging

Much has been written about diagnostic imaging of tarsal coalitions. Both the calcaneonavicular and talocalcaneal coalitions have radiographic signs named for them: the anteater sign (**Figure 2, A**) and the C-sign (**Figure 2, B**), respectively.[2] Plain radiographs can be helpful screening tools, but I believe that all patients going to the operating room for resection of a coalition should have a CT scan of both feet and, if at all possible, three-dimensional reconstructions of those images. These images are extremely useful not only to delineate the extent of the coalition in three dimensions but also to ensure that multiple coalitions are not present. MRI may be useful for a patient with stiff talar motion but no obvious evidence on a CT. Sometimes MRI will show fibrocartilaginous coalitions not seen on CT scan.

The spectrum of each type of coalition as seen on diagnostic imaging is detailed in two articles. Upasani et al[3] described calcaneonavicular coalitions (**Figure 3**), and Rozansky et al[4] described talocalcaneal coalitions (**Figure 4**).

Procedure

Room Setup/Patient Positioning

The patient's foot should be positioned near the end of the operating table in such a way that the surgical team can be seated for the procedure. The patient's entire limb is prepared and draped from the anterior superior iliac spine distally.

Special Instruments/Equipment/Implants

A C-arm should be available if needed to identify the subtalar joint with a talocalcaneal coalition and for complete removal of a calcaneonavicular coalition. Useful instruments include Kerrison rongeurs (3 or 4 mm), osteotomes, and a high-speed burr (3 or 4 mm), which is helpful for a large talocalcaneal coalition. Additional helpful instruments include Freer

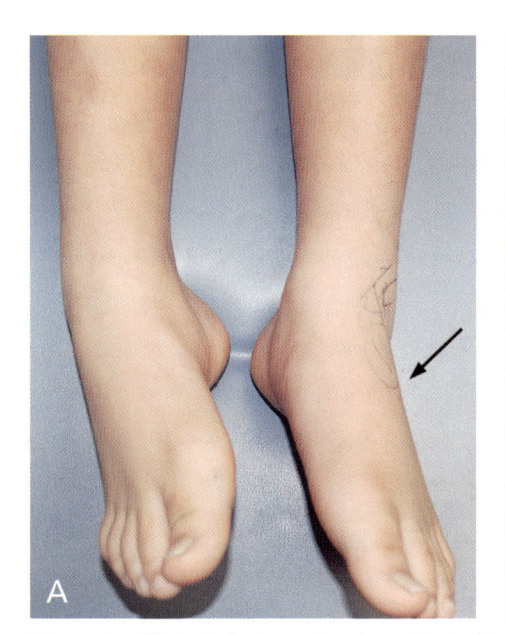

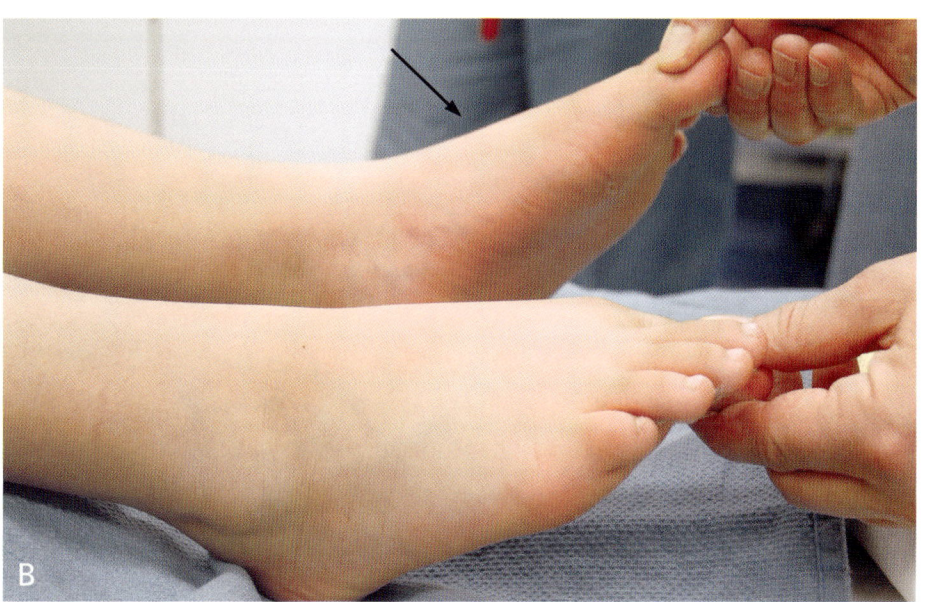

Figure 1 Clinical photographs of a patient with a unilateral calcaneonavicular coalition. In the supine position, the affected foot (arrows) fails to form an arch (**A**) and has diminished plantar flexion (**B**).

Dr. Mubarak or an immediate family member has stock or stock options held in Rhino Pediatric Orthopedic Designs.

Section 8: Pediatric Orthopaedics

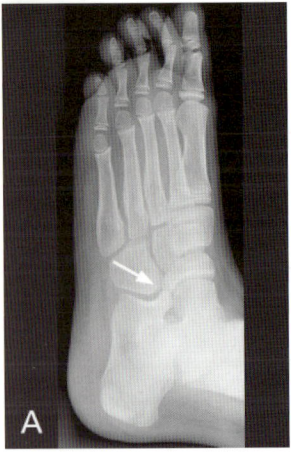

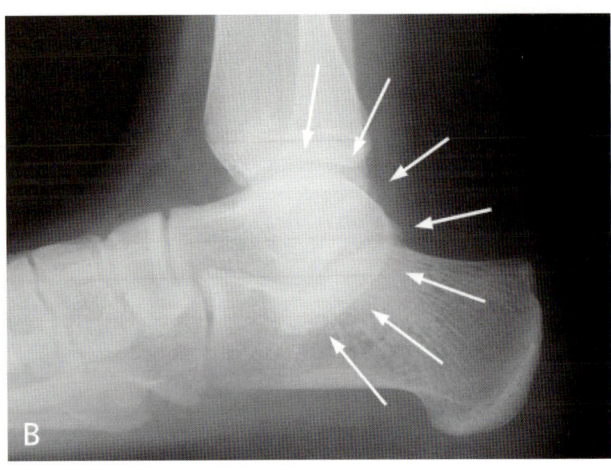

Figure 2 Radiographs demonstrate typical findings of a tarsal coalition. **A,** The calcaneonavicular coalition is demonstrated on the internal rotation oblique view (arrow). **B,** The C-sign, observed on a lateral view, indicates a talocalcaneal coalition. This sign is present when the posterior margin of the talus appears to be continuous with the sustentaculum tali (arrows). The C-sign can also be seen in flexible flatfoot.

Figure 3 Classification of calcaneonavicular coalition (circled) according to Upsani et al[3] based on three-dimensional CT reconstruction images.

Figure 4 Classification of talocalcaneal coalitions according to Rozansky et al[4] based on coronal and three-dimensional CT scans.

elevators, small Hohmann retractors, Bovie electrocautery, and an Allis clamp.

Surgical Technique

A sterile tourniquet is placed on the proximal thigh. After Esmarch exsanguination and tourniquet inflation, the initial foot incision is made.

Calcaneonavicular Coalition Resection

The approach for calcaneonavicular excision follows the technique described by Mubarak et al.[1] An oblique modified Ollier incision is made over the site of the coalition, along the Langer lines (**Figure 5, A**). The location of this incision is just distal to the sinus tarsi overlying the coalition. This incision is taken down to the level of the extensor digitorum brevis (EDB) fascia, with careful dissection to avoid the lateral branches of the superficial peroneal nerve. After releasing the origin, the EDB is elevated from proximal to distal. The coalition should be visible beneath the reflected EDB (**Figure 5, B**). The three-dimensional CT reconstructions obtained preoperatively should be available in the operating room to aid in delineating the appropriate plane of dissection (**Figure 5, C**).

Prior to resection, the surgeon should identify the synchondrosis junction between the calcaneus and the navicular. A curet or rongeur can be used to unroof the periosteum, revealing the cartilaginous interface (synchondrosis) (**Figure 6, A**). This line should mark the center of the resection. Next, the calcaneocuboid and talonavicular joints should be identified. Two Freer elevators used as retractors are placed around the coalition into these joints. With the joints protected, the resection can proceed. Initially, a 1-cm osteotome can be used to resect the coalition. As the depth of the bridge is approached, a 0.5-cm straight Lambotte osteotome is used (**Figure 6, B**). Care must be taken to not damage the underlying cuboid, which may be prominent, or the head of the talus. This normal cuboid prominence is present with a type I (forme fruste) coalition.[3] In more complete coalitions, the cuboid has a truly cuboid shape and therefore is less likely to be injured by the osteotome in the field of resection. Once the wedge is removed, subsequent dissection is performed with 3- or 4-mm Kerrison rongeurs until the resection is complete (**Figure 6, C**). A gap of about 1 cm × 1 cm is usually required before stopping. Fluoroscopic images should be obtained at this time. The most

Chapter 106: Treatment of Tarsal Coalitions

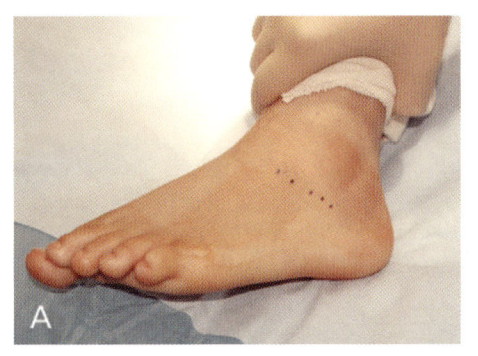

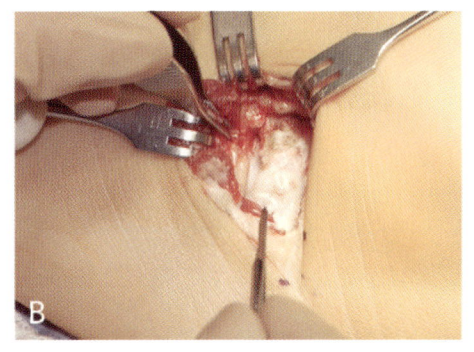

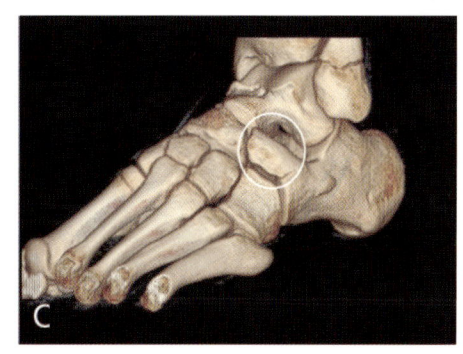

Figure 5 Calcaneonavicular coalition resection: approach and exposure. **A,** Clinical photograph shows a planned reverse Ollier incision, within the Langer lines. **B,** Intraoperative photograph shows the extensor digitorum brevis elevated off the coalition by proximal release at its origin. The coalition is visible directly beneath the elevated muscle. **C,** Example of a three-dimensional CT scan; such images are invaluable for ensuring that the intended plane of dissection is the correct one.

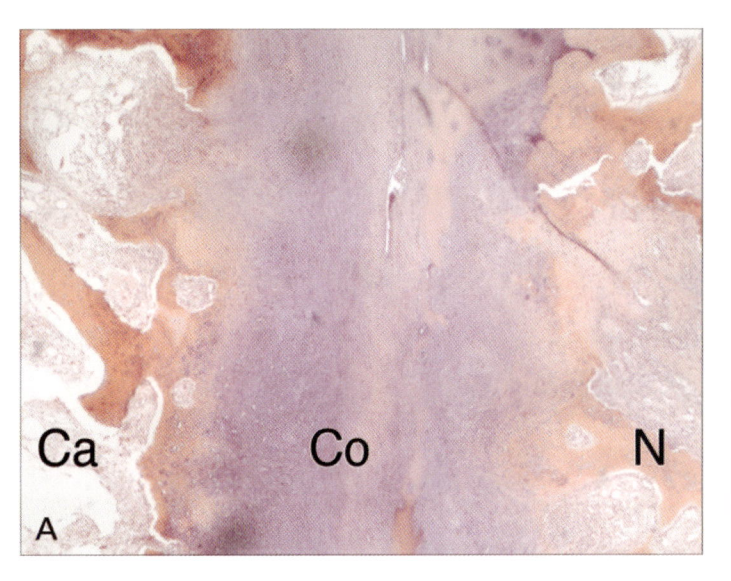

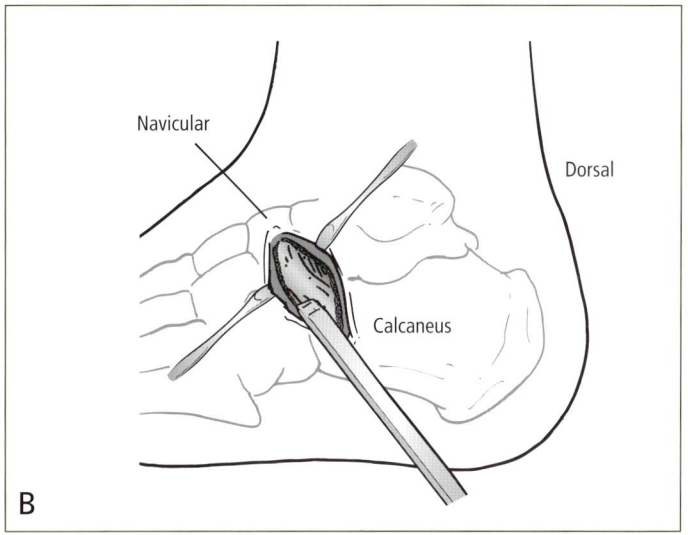

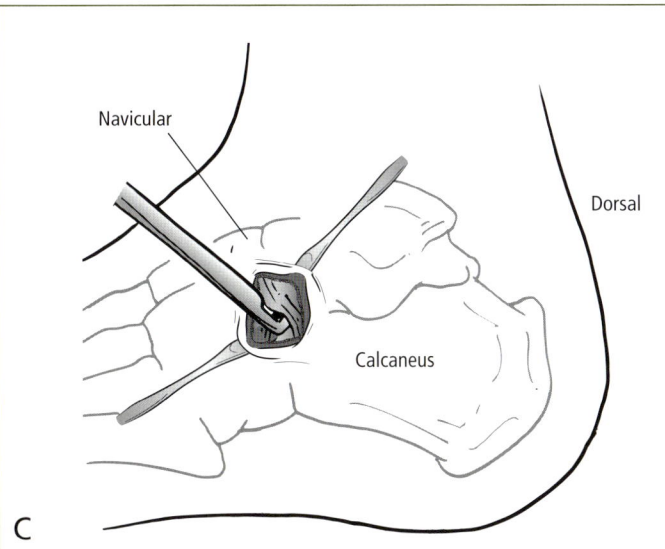

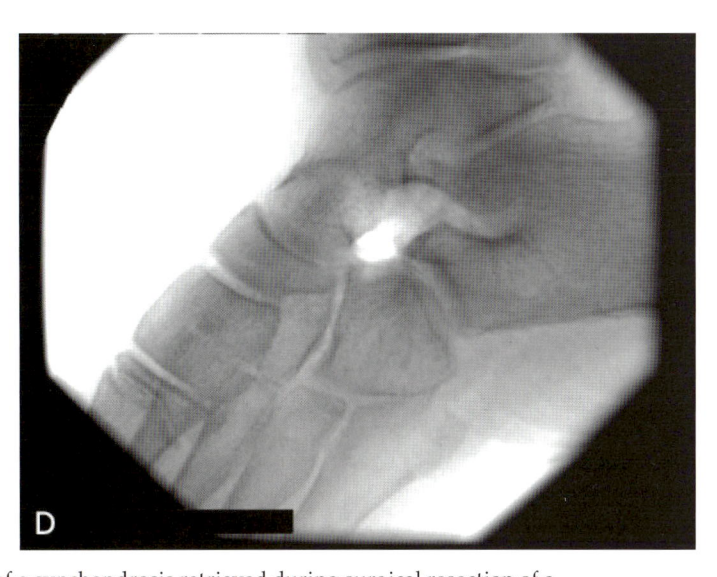

Figure 6 Calcaneonavicular coalition resection. **A,** Photomicrograph of a synchondrosis retrieved during surgical resection of a calcaneonavicular coalition (Ca = calcaneus, Co = coalition, N = navicular). **B,** A small Lambotte osteotome is used to remove the first wedge of bone. **C,** Final resection of the coalition is performed with Kerrison rongeurs. True excision is confirmed with a range-of-motion examination and an internal oblique fluoroscopic image (**D**).

helpful view is the internal oblique view (**Figure 6, D**).

The hindfoot range of motion is now examined and compared with the preoperative measurements. Near normal range-of-motion values should not be expected at this point, but the surgeon should be able to visualize that the calcaneus and navicular now move independently.

The fat graft is harvested (see below) and prepared for insertion. The fat should be tucked into the gap; there should be enough fat to fill the gap completely (**Figure 7, A**). The EDB fascia is then sutured back into its normal position with 0 Vicryl (Ethicon) absorbable sutures (**Figure 7, B**). The EDB fascia must be sutured

© 2013 American Academy of Orthopaedic Surgeons

691

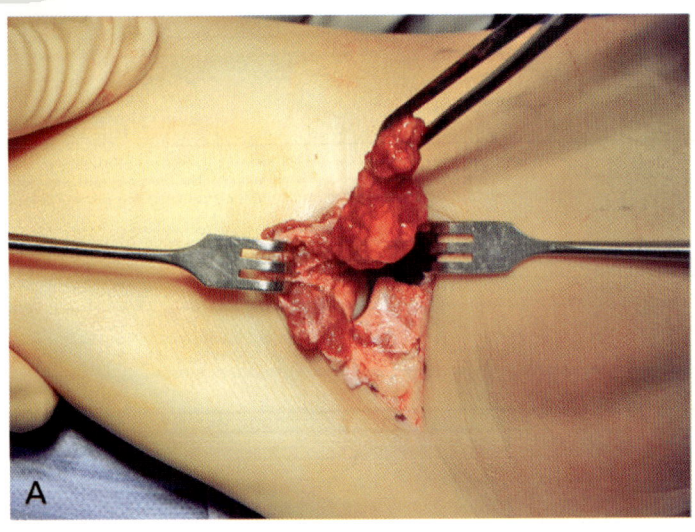

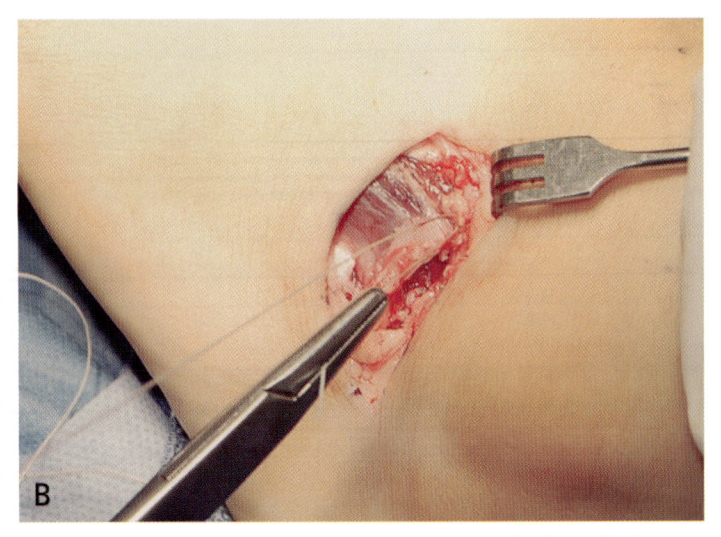

Section 8: Pediatric Orthopaedics

Figure 7 Intraoperative photographs demonstrate calcaneonavicular coalition excision: Fat graft. Intraoperative photographs show the fat graft placed within the cavity (**A**) and the extensor digitorum brevis repaired back to its origin (**B**).

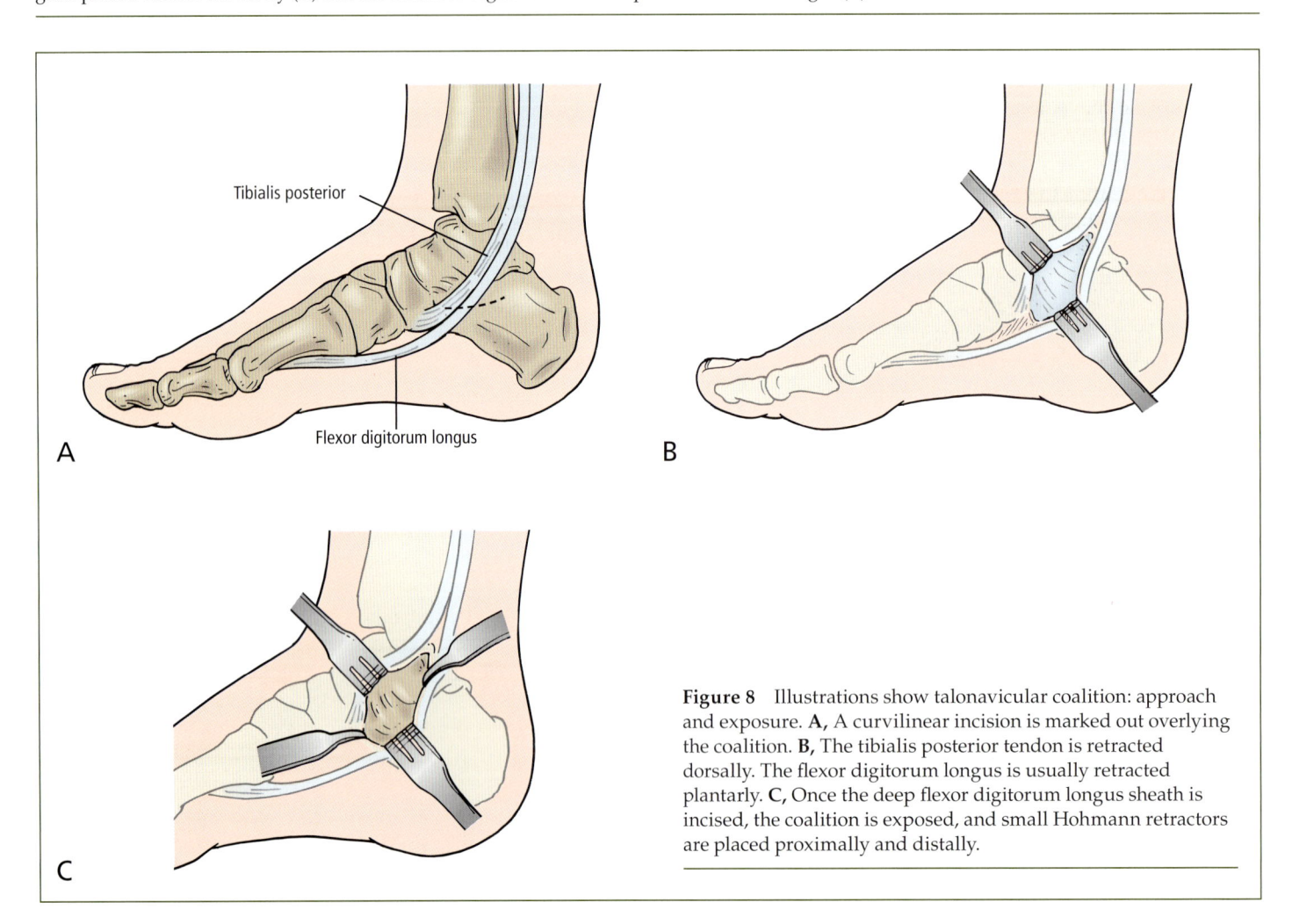

Figure 8 Illustrations show talonavicular coalition: approach and exposure. **A**, A curvilinear incision is marked out overlying the coalition. **B**, The tibialis posterior tendon is retracted dorsally. The flexor digitorum longus is usually retracted plantarly. **C**, Once the deep flexor digitorum longus sheath is incised, the coalition is exposed, and small Hohmann retractors are placed proximally and distally.

back down appropriately or the normal contours of the foot will be altered, leaving a less cosmetic result. The skin is approximated with a 3-0 Vicryl suture, followed by a running subcuticular skin closure with a 3-0 Monocryl (Ethicon) suture. Adhesive skin closure strips are then applied to the wound, followed by a sterile dressing. The patient is placed in a synthetic short-leg cast, which is split to allow for swelling. The tourniquet is deflated, and the graft site wound is closed as described in the Fat Graft Harvest section.

Talocalcaneal Coalition Resection

An incision is made over the sustentaculum tali about 1.5 to 2 cm distal to the medial malleolus (**Figure 8, A**). Often, a palpable prominence can be felt approximately 1.0 to 1.5 cm inferior to the medial malleolus. The incision should be long enough to expose the medial facet and often the entire subtalar joint. My preferred technique[5] is based on the technique first described by Olney and Asher.[6]

The incision is taken sharply through the skin. Where the path of the incision is inferior to the saphenous vein, the crossing branches of the vein should be identified and coagulated with a Bovie cautery. The tendons of the tarsal tunnel are then identified within their sheaths. The pos-

© 2013 American Academy of Orthopaedic Surgeons

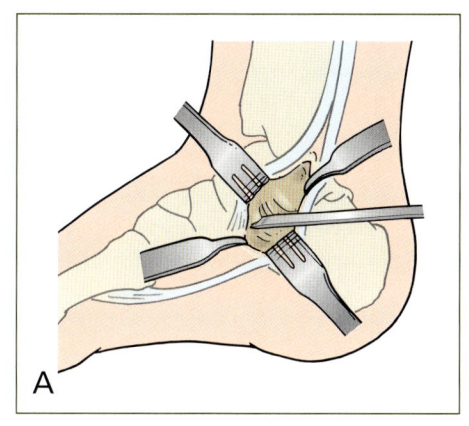

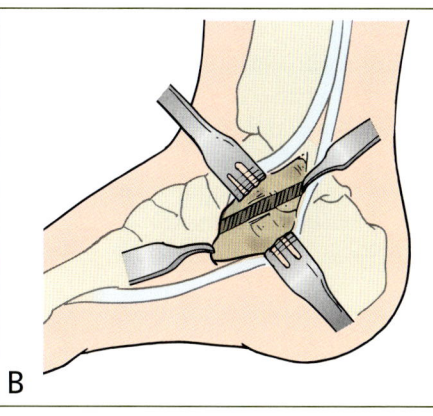

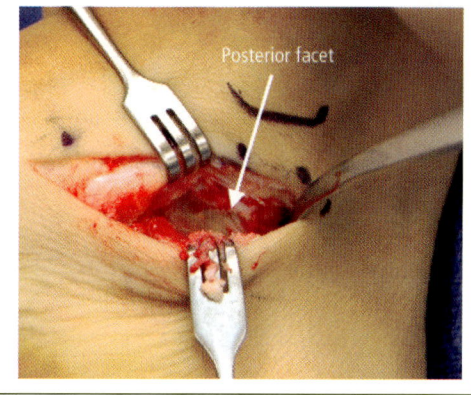

Figure 9 Images demonstrate talonavicular coalition: resection. **A,** Initial resection is performed with an osteotome. Illustration (**B**) and intraoperative photograph (**C**) show the completed resection. Resection is not complete until the posterior facet is visualized and motion can be seen to occur within the subtalar joint.

terior tibial tendon should be freed from its sheath and retracted dorsally. The flexor digitorum longus tendon is identified in its sheath by extending the toes and observing movement of the tendon within its sheath. The sheath is incised in line with its fibers, and the tendon can be retracted plantarly as needed for the exposure of the coalition (**Figure 8, B**). The deep sheath is then incised, exposing the middle facet coalition.

To completely view the coalition, further dissection posteriorly is necessary. The flexor hallucis longus lies just below the coalition and the neurovascular bundle just posterior. Small Hohmann retractors are then placed around the coalition (**Figure 8, C**). With good exposure, the surgeon should be able to identify the borders of the medial facet proximally and distally. In all coalitions except the completely osseous coalitions (type IV, representing 11% of talocalcaneal coalitions), a synchondrosis is visible.[6] Checking the preoperative three-dimensional CT scan is exceptionally helpful at this time. The surgeon can easily become "lost" during the resection if the relationship of the synchondrosis plane relative to the true subtalar joint is not well understood.

A combination of osteotomes, Kerrison rongeurs, and high-speed burrs are now used to remove the coalition. I prefer to start with osteotomes (**Figure 9, A**). The amount of bone resected and the plane in which it is resected depend on the type of coalition and the extent of involvement of the sustentaculum and talus. Some coalitions can be very large (up to 3 cm in length and 2 cm in depth). Once the coalition is identified, resection is continued until the articular cartilage of the joint is visualized anteriorly and posteriorly (**Figure 9, B and C**). This is especially crucial posteriorly. My experience is that if a small posterior hook is left unresected, it will continue to restrict subtalar motion. The advantage of being able to see the entire medial coalition cannot be overstated; a complete resection must be performed to ensure maximal benefit to the patient.

The range of motion of the hindfoot is assessed continually throughout the resection. A Freer elevator can be inserted around and through the middle facet defect into the posterior facet to liberate capsular adhesions and "free up" the joint. Great care is taken to not strip the interosseous ligament. Once range of motion is significantly improved and the entire posterior facet is visualized, the surgeon may stop the resection.

The fat graft is harvested as described below and prepared for insertion. The fat graft should fill the space of the resection (**Figure 10**). The graft is held in place with a Freer elevator while the overlying layer (the tendon sheath) is closed with a No. 1 Vicryl suture. The skin edges are approximated with a 3-0 Vicryl suture, and a running 3-0 Monocryl suture is placed in the subcutaneum. Adhesive skin closure strips cut to one-third length are placed over the foot. The tourniquet is deflated, and the graft site wound is closed as described below. The patient is placed in a synthetic short-leg cast, which is split to allow for swelling.

Fat Graft Harvest

After resection of the coalition, a fat graft is obtained. I prefer to harvest the fat graft from the gluteal crease on the ipsilateral side. This leaves a very cosmetic scar, and there is always enough fat in this region, even in the thinnest of patients. In obese patients, abdominal fat from the lower abdominal crease can be considered.

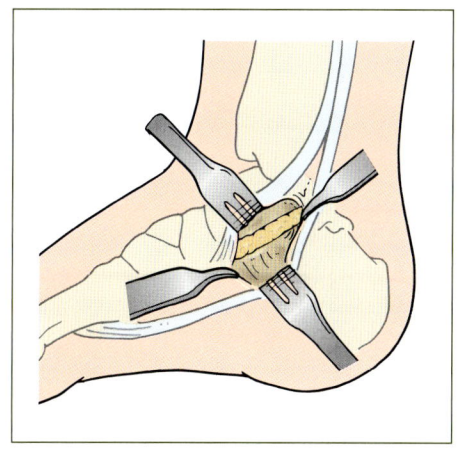

Figure 10 The harvested fat is placed within the space left following resection of the coalition.

This is an easier location for obtaining the fat, but the scar is more obvious to the patient. The size of the fat graft required is generally 3 cm × 1 cm × 1 cm for calcaneonavicular coalition resections and slightly smaller for talocalcaneal coalition resections.

A 4-cm incision is made in the gluteal crease and taken through the dermis only. Elevation of the dermis off the fat proximally in the buttock is then performed, with care taken to not buttonhole the skin. This dissection should be performed to approximately 1 cm on all sides of the wound. Once this has been done, an Allis clamp is clamped on the fat at one corner of the wound. With the help of traction on the fat, a 3-cm-long × 1-cm-wide × 1-cm-deep fat graft is resected. The fat is passed off in a moistened sponge. The wound is packed off until after the foot wound is closed. After closure of the foot wound and removal of the tourniquet, the buttock wound is closed subcutaneously with 0 and 3-0 Vicryl sutures, and a running subcuticular

© 2013 American Academy of Orthopaedic Surgeons

closure of the skin is performed with a 3-0 Monocryl suture. I usually also use several 0 Vicryl skin retention sutures to prevent dehiscence because of the stretch on this wound. Adhesive skin closure strips are placed over the wound, and a dressing is applied.

Complications

Early problems include occasional wound dehiscence from the buttocks if retention sutures are not used. Wound infections are extremely rare.

Possible long-term problems include continued pain, stiffness, and deformity (usually pes valgus). If the pain persists, further workup, including CT scans, may be necessary to rule out coalition recurrence or incomplete removal.

Postoperative Care and Rehabilitation

A below-knee synthetic cast is applied and univalved. All patients are admitted overnight for pain control and observation. The patient is made weight bearing as tolerated and is encouraged to walk on the cast. The patient returns at 1 week for cast closure and at around 2 to 3 weeks for cast removal, after which patients are encouraged to begin active ankle and subtalar motion. They are counseled to expect that the foot will not feel "normal" for up to 6 months. At 6-week follow-up, the patient is cleared for activities as tolerated. Some patients may require physical therapy if return of motion is slow. The patient is seen at 3 months, 6 months, and 1 and 2 years postoperatively for examination. Radiographs are obtained at approximately 1 year postoperatively.

Pearls

- For each type of resection, understanding the subtypes (as shown in **Figures 3** and **4**) will help avoid pitfalls.
- In type I calcaneonavicular coalitions, the cuboid prominence should not be excised; it is not pathologic.
- In talocalcaneal coalitions, three-dimensional CT reconstructions are invaluable to help avoid becoming lost and resecting too much normal talus or calcaneus.
- Type II and V talocalcaneal coalitions have a posterior component. The posterior facet must be visualized to ensure complete resection of the coalition.
- Type IV talocalcaneal coalitions do not have a visible physis to guide the resection. The anterior and posterior borders of the coalition should be identified and visualized and small Hohmann retractors inserted. The surgeon should begin with small rongeurs (eg, Kerrison) and proceed along the line connecting the Hohmann retractors. Intraoperative lateral fluoroscopic images may help. The normal subtalar joint will soon present itself.
- Severe preoperative pes valgus will not improve after resection. The family must be consulted on this important point before any surgery.
- When lateral ankle/foot pain or deformity is still present at 6 to 12 months postoperatively, I recommend correction. About 20% of calcaneonavicular coalitions need further corrective surgery because of deformity present preoperatively. My preferred method is the "triple C" (calcaneal-cuboid-cuneiform) osteotomy.[7]

References

1. Mubarak SJ, Patel PN, Upasani VV, Moor MA, Wenger DR: Calcaneonavicular coalition: Treatment by excision and fat graft. *J Pediatr Orthop* 2009;29(5):418-426.
2. Lateur LM, Van Hoe LR, Van Ghillewe KV, Gryspeerdt SS, Baert AL, Dereymaeker GE: Subtalar coalition: Diagnosis with the C sign on lateral radiographs of the ankle. *Radiology* 1994;193(3):847-851.
3. Upasani VV, Chambers RC, Mubarak SJ: Analysis of calcaneonavicular coalitions using multi-planar three-dimensional computed tomography. *J Child Orthop* 2008;2(4):301-307.
4. Rozansky A, Varley E, Moor M, Wenger DR, Mubarak SJ: A radiologic classification of talocalcaneal coalitions based on 3D reconstruction. *J Child Orthop* 2010;4(2):129-135.
5. Gantsoudes GD, Roocroft JH, Mubarak SJ: Treatment of talocalcaneal coalitions. *J Pediatr Orthop* 2012;32(3):301-307.
6. Olney BW, Asher MA: Excision of symptomatic coalition of the middle facet of the talocalcaneal joint. *J Bone Joint Surg Am* 1987;69(4):539-544.
7. Rathjen KE, Mubarak SJ: Calcaneal-cuboid-cuneiform osteotomy for the correction of valgus foot deformities in children. *J Pediatr Orthop* 1998;18(6):775-782.

Chapter 107
Lower Extremity Surgery in Children With Cerebral Palsy

Nirav K. Pandya, MD   Henry G. Chambers, MD

Introduction

Cerebral palsy (CP) is an abnormality of motor function that results from an insult to the brain during early development. The musculoskeletal manifestations of this disorder are progressive. Surgical management of the lower extremity in these patients requires a thorough understanding of the indications for these procedures and how the procedures will affect the functional status of these patients. Surgery should be delayed as long as possible (until the patient is older than 6 years), and spasticity management should be used as an adjunct to surgery. When multiple deformities exist, single-stage surgery is recommended to prevent decompensation from unbalanced correction.

Traditionally, the patient with CP is classified based on the Gross Motor Functional Classification System (GMFCS),[1] which assigns patients with CP to one of five functional groups based on self-initiated ambulatory function and postural control (**Figure 1**). The Functional Mobility Scale (FMS)[2] also rates ambulatory ability at 5 m, 50 m, and 500 m, giving a more dynamic assessment of a patient's mobility (**Figure 2**).

The combination of these two scales can help to define quickly and reproducibly the ambulatory status of patients with CP. This is important, because the type of surgery recommended for the patient with CP depends largely on whether the patient is ambulatory (GMFCS levels I through III) or nonambulatory (levels IV and V). Whereas the goals of surgery in the ambulatory patient are to improve or maintain the patient's ability to walk, nonambulatory surgery is performed to increase comfort, positioning, sitting balance, and posture. Using ambulatory procedures in a nonambulatory child (and vice versa) may lead to significant loss of function.

GMFCS E & R between 6th and 12th birthday: Descriptors and illustrations

GMFCS Level I
Children walk at home, school, outdoors and in the community. They can climb stairs without the use of a railing. Children perform gross motor skills such as running and jumping, but speed, balance and coordination are limited

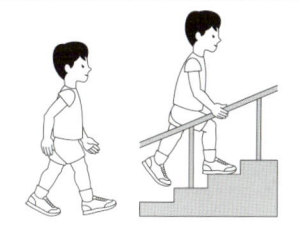

GMFCS Level II
Children walk in most settings and climb stairs holding onto a railing. They may experience difficulty walking long distances and balancing on uneven terrain, inclines, in crowded areas or confined spaces. Children may walk with physical assistance, a hand-held mobility device or used wheeled mobility over long distances. Children have only minimal ability to perform gross motor skills such as running and jumping.

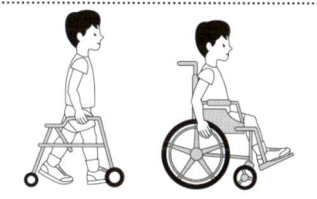

GMFCS Level III
Children walk using a hand-held mobility device in most indoor settings. They may climb stairs holding onto a railing with supervision or assistance. Children use wheeled mobility when traveling long distances and may self-propel for shorter distances.

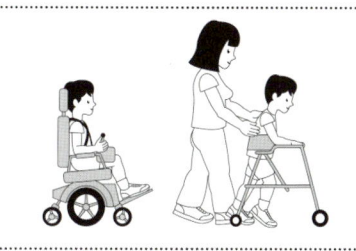

GMFCS Level IV
Children use methods or mobility that require physical assistance or powered mobility in most settings. They may walk for short distances at home with physical assistance or use powered mobility or a body support walker when positioned. At school, outdoors and in the community children are transported in a manual wheelchair or use powered mobility.

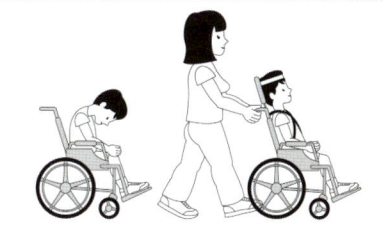

GMFCS Level V
Children are transported in a manual wheelchair in all settings. Children are limited in their ability to maintain antigravity head and trunk postures and control leg and arm movements.

Figure 1 The Gross Motor Function Classification System (GMFCS) for cerebral palsy. **A**, Levels I through III (ambulatory). **B**, Levels IV and V (nonambulatory). E & R = expanded and revised. (© Kerr Graham, Bill Reid and Adrienne Harvey, The Royal Children's Hospital, Melbourne, Australia. Data from Palisano R, Rosenbaum P, Walter S, Russell D, Wood E, Galuppi B: Development and reliability of a system to classify gross motor function in children with cerebral palsy 1997;39[4]:214-223 and data from CanChild Centre for Childhood Disability Research Institute for Applied Health Sciences, Ontario, Canada.)

Dr. Pandya or an immediate family member serves as a board member, owner, officer, or committee member of the Pediatric Orthopaedic Society of North America. Dr. Chambers or an immediate family member serves as a paid consultant to or is an employee of Allergan, Merz Pharmaceuticals, and Orthopediatrics, and serves as a board member, owner, officer, or committee member of the American Academy of Orthopaedic Surgeons, the American Academy for Cerebral Palsy and Developmental Medicine, and the Pediatric Orthopaedic Society of North America.

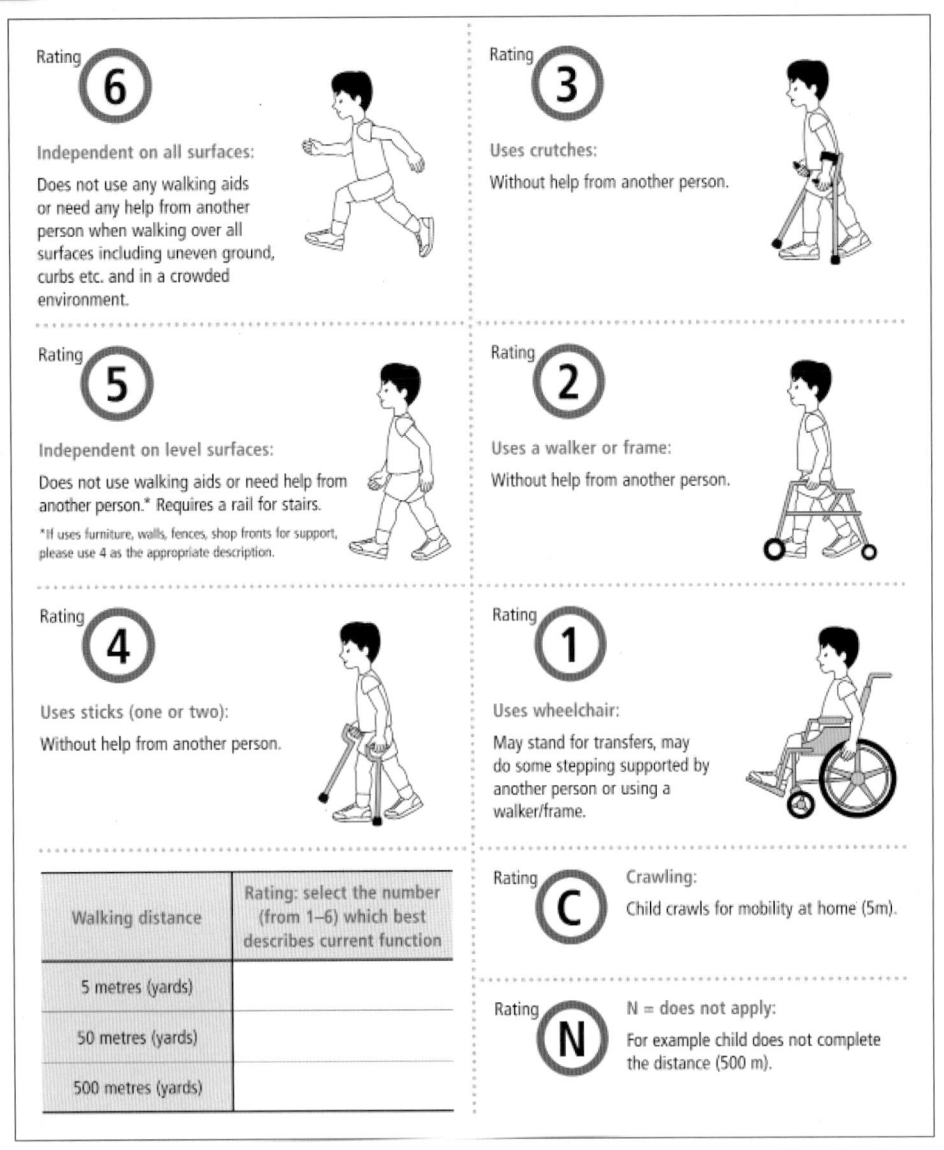

Figure 2 The Functional Mobility Scale for cerebral palsy. (© Kerr Graham, Bill Reid and Adrienne Harvey, The Royal Children's Hospital, Melbourne, Australia.)

Ambulatory Patients

The clinician must have a thorough understanding of gait analysis when evaluating the ambulatory patient with CP. Once the appropriate gait abnormality is identified, the correct surgical procedure can be chosen. Common gait abnormalities seen in the ambulatory patient with CP include scissoring gait (excessive hip adduction), crouch gait (excessive hip flexion, knee flexion, and ankle dorsiflexion), jump gait (excessive hip flexion, knee flexion, and ankle plantar flexion), stiff-knee gait (swing-phase knee stiffness due to an overactive rectus femoris muscle), and recurvatum gait (knee hyperextension due to equinus contracture).

At the level of the foot, ambulatory patients also may have a pure ankle equinus deformity (excessive ankle plantar flexion), equinovarus deformity (excessive ankle plantar flexion with an overactive tibialis posterior or tibialis anterior), or pes planovalgus deformity (overactive peroneals and/or bony deformity).

The surgical options for the components of the gait abnormalities mentioned above are shown in **Table 1**.

The ambulatory patient with CP also may have rotational abnormalities (lever-arm disease) at the level of the hip and knee (eg, increased femoral anteversion, internal/external tibial torsion) that may require corrective surgery. Unlike the typically developing patient, who may be able to compensate for these rotational abnormalities, the patient with CP requires correction via proximal or distal femoral osteotomies and/or tibial derotational osteotomies to preserve ambulatory function.

Therefore, before determining the appropriate surgical procedure in an ambulatory patient with CP, the clinician must consider the following: (1) the gait abnormality present, (2) the soft-tissue and bone components that may be causing the ambulatory dysfunction, (3) the appropriate procedures to correct the gait abnormalities based on the anatomic contractures/imbalances leading to them, and (4) that rotational abnormalities need to be corrected more aggressively in the patient with CP than in the nonneuromuscularly impaired patient.

Nonambulatory Patients

Nonambulatory patients with CP also can undergo procedures around the hip, knee, and ankle; however, the options are not as extensive as those for the ambulatory patient. In the hip, spastic subluxation or dislocation with severe acetabular dysplasia can be present. This can lead to difficulty in sitting and transfers and can exacerbate scoliosis. A combined adductor, psoas, and proximal hamstring lengthening, open reduction and capsulorrhaphy of the hip, pericapsular pelvic osteotomy, and femoral shortening varus derotation osteotomy (particularly in patients with increased valgus and femoral anteversion) can manage this problem. In the knee, severe flexion contractures that interfere with sitting and hygiene can be corrected with distal hamstring lengthening. Finally, deformities of the foot in nonambulatory patients can be corrected as in ambulatory patients (**Table 1**), resulting in a foot that can rest plantigrade on a wheelchair platform.

Soft-Tissue Lengthening Procedures
Adductor Lengthening
Indications

The indications for adductor tenotomy[3] are scissoring gait and spastic hip subluxation/dislocation.

Preoperative Imaging

No preoperative imaging is required unless the adductor tenotomy is part of a larger procedure for spastic hip subluxation/dislocation. In that case, imaging includes AP and frog-leg lateral views of the pelvis and bilateral hips and possibly CT with three-dimensional reconstructions.

Surgical Technique

For this procedure, the patient is positioned supine. The perineum is draped free. A transverse incision is made over the palpably tight adductor longus tendon, one fingerbreadth distal to the groin crease. The fascia overlying the adductor longus tendon should be opened (**Figure 3, A**), and a right-angle clamp should be used to isolate the adductor longus tendon, passing the clamp from medial to lateral. The tendon should be cut as proximal to its attachment to the pelvis as possible with an electrocautery. After the adductor longus tendon has been transected, the surgeon should encounter the anterior branch of the obturator nerve overlying the adductor brevis tendon inferiorly, the pectineus muscle superiorly, and the gracilis muscle medially (**Figure 3, B**). If an intraoperative test confirms that abduction of the leg is hindered more with the leg in extension than in flexion, the gracilis muscle also can be isolated with a right-angle clamp and transected (**Figure 3, C**). If further abduction is desired, the adductor brevis can be isolated with a right-angle clamp and transected as well. The goal should be to obtain 45° of abduction. Lying below the adductor brevis, the large adductor magnus and its overlying posterior branch of the obturator nerve must be preserved to maintain the ability to adduct. After all tenotomies are performed, hemostasis should be obtained to prevent hematoma formation. The wound should be closed in layers.

Complications
Complications include hematoma formation and inadvertent transection of the branches of the obturator nerve.

Postoperative Care and Rehabilitation
Postoperatively, the patient is placed in Petrie casts with a bar between the legs or into an abduction brace, which is worn full time for 4 weeks and then worn at night for 6 months.

Pearl
The initial incision should not extend too far laterally beyond the lateral border of the adductor longus tendon to avoid encountering the femoral neurovascular bundle.

Distal Hamstring Lengthening
Indications
Indications for distal hamstring lengthening[4] include crouch gait, jump gait, and knee flexion contracture. The surgeon must be cautious when performing hamstring lengthening in ambulatory patients. The patient should have a popliteal angle greater than 40° combined with a posterior pelvic tilt. If the patient has an anterior pelvic tilt, then there may be worsening of the gait after hamstring lengthening.

Surgical Technique
The patient is positioned supine if this procedure is performed with other surgeries or prone if performed as an isolated procedure. If the patient is supine, medial and lateral incisions can be made; if the patient is prone, a single midline incision is used. The incision(s) should begin 1 to 2 cm proximal to the knee joint and extend proximally for 5 to 7 cm (**Figure 4, A**). For the two-incision technique, the incisions should be placed slightly anterior to the hamstring tendons, which

Table 1 Typical Abnormalities and Potential Surgical Options in Ambulatory Patients with Cerebral Palsy

Abnormality	Potential Surgical Treatments
Hip adduction contracture	Adductor tenotomy
Hip flexion contracture	Psoas release at pelvic brim
Knee flexion contracture	Distal hamstring lengthening
	Distal femoral extension osteotomy with patellar tendon advancement
Knee recurvatum	Ankle plantar flexor lengthening
Stiff-knee gait	Rectus femoris transfer
Equinus contracture	Ankle plantar flexor lengthening
Equinovarus deformity of the foot	Posterior tibialis lengthening
	Split posterior tibial tendon transfer
	Split anterior tibialis transfer
	Ankle plantar flexor lengthening
Pes planovalgus deformity	Peroneus brevis lengthening
	Calcaneal lengthening osteotomy (± cuneiform osteotomy)
	Calcaneal sliding osteotomy (± cuboid and cuneiform osteotomy)
	Subtalar arthrodesis
	Triple arthrodesis

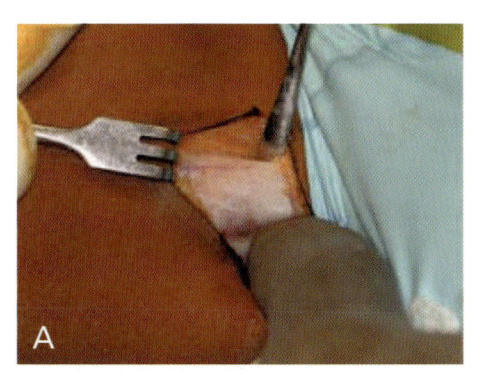

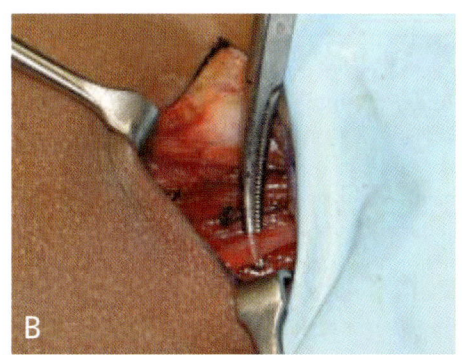

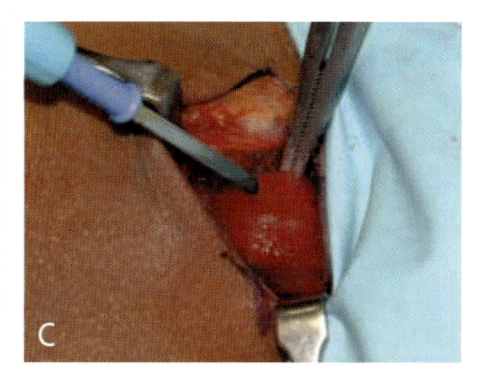

Figure 3 Intraoperative photographs demonstrate the surgical technique for adductor lengthening. **A,** The adductor longus tendon is shown with its overlying fascia identified before tenotomy. **B,** The anterior branch of the obturator nerve is identified with a hemostat. **C,** The gracilis tendon is identified before tenotomy. (Reproduced with permission from Sawyer JR: Cerebral palsy, in Canale ST, Beaty JH, eds: *Campbell's Operative Orthopaedics*, ed 11. Philadelphia, PA, Mosby/Elsevier, 2007, pp 1333-1399.)

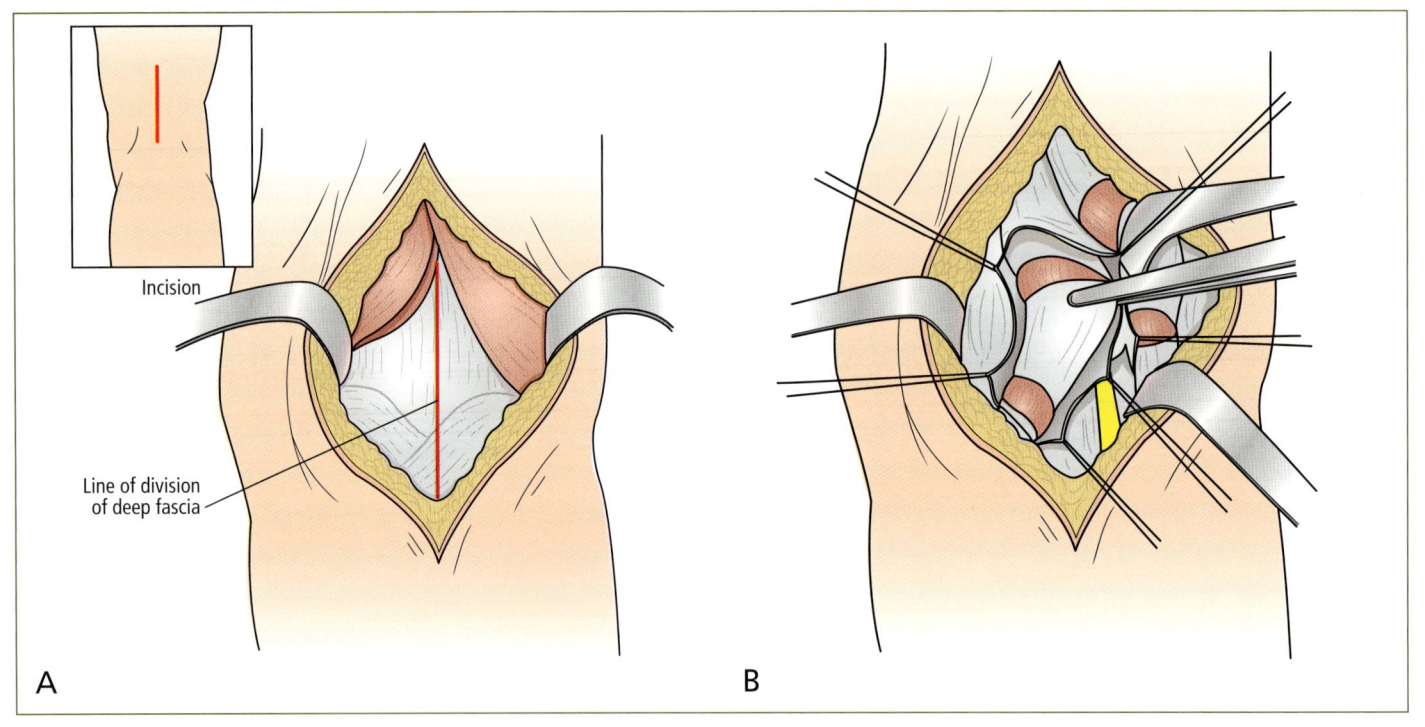

Figure 4 Illustrations demonstrate surgical technique for distal hamstring lengthening using a single midline incision. **A,** The approach. **B,** Transection of the tendon overlying the semimembranosus muscle belly (in forceps). Two cuts have been made in the muscle belly to gain additional length.

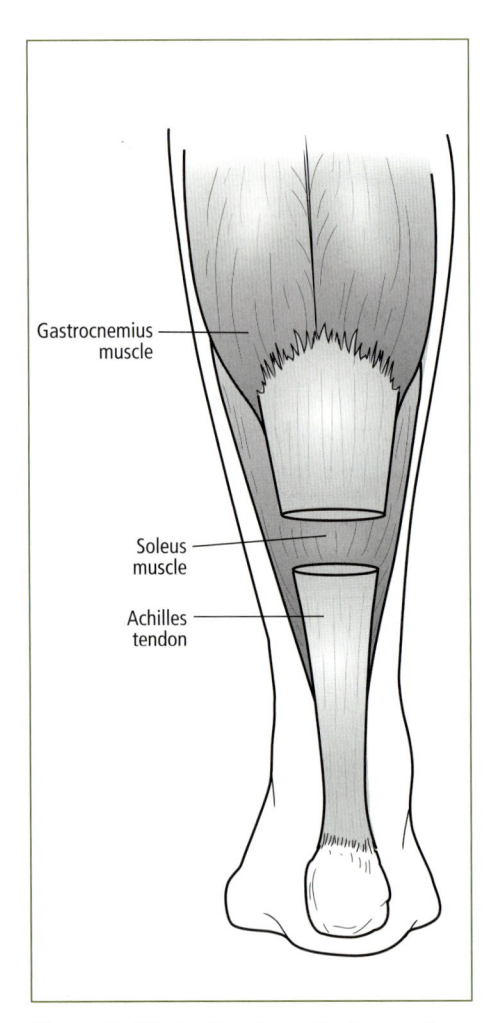

Figure 5 Illustration shows the transection of the tendon overlying the gastrocnemius and soleus muscle in gastrocnemius-soleus lengthening.

should be palpably tight with the leg extended. Dissection on the medial side of the leg should be taken posterior to the sartorius muscle (the most superficial muscle) to open the fascia overlying the gracilis muscle. The tendon overlying the gracilis muscle belly should be cut with a knife or electrocautery. Deep to the gracilis, the semitendinosus tendon should be encountered and the fascia over the muscle opened, followed by cutting of the tendon overlying the muscle belly or a Z-lengthening if additional length is required. The deepest, broadest muscle that will be encountered is the semimembranosus muscle; its fascia should be opened as well, followed by transection of the tendon overlying the muscle belly. Two cuts can be made in the tendon if necessary (**Figure 4, B**). After all tendons have been cut, straight-leg raising can be performed to provide an additional amount of lengthening. Forceful extension should not be performed, to avoid sciatic nerve damage.

Lengthening of the lateral hamstrings is rarely indicated; however, if necessary, attention is turned to the lateral incision, if a two-incision technique is used, or to the lateral aspect of the incision, if a single midline incision is used. For the two-incision approach, the incision is made anterior to the biceps tendon to avoid the peroneal nerve. Dissection is carried down to the level of the fascia overlying the biceps tendon that is opened, and the tendon overlying the muscle belly is transected. Both wounds can now be closed in a layered fashion.

Complications
Complications from this procedure include sciatic nerve transection and sciatic nerve palsy from excessive extension.

Postoperative Care and Rehabilitation
A knee immobilizer or knee range-of-motion brace should be placed in the amount of flexion that can be achieved comfortably without stretching the sciatic nerve. The patient is allowed to bear weight as tolerated with the cast. The immobilizer is kept in place for 4 weeks, and then the patient is allowed to return to a stretching program.

Pearl
The sciatic nerve should be monitored carefully postoperatively.

Lengthening of the Gastrocnemius-Soleus
Indications
Lengthening of the gastrocnemius-soleus[5] is indicated for equinus contracture, jump gait, and recurvatum gait secondary to gastrocnemius-soleus contracture. Generally, the gastrocnemius should be the only muscle lengthened in diplegia, whereas the gastrocnemius and

soleus should be lengthened in hemiplegia. Actual lengthening of the Achilles tendon by Z lengthening should be discouraged in ambulatory patients because of the risk of overlengthening and weakening of the muscles.

Surgical Technique
The patient is positioned supine. A posteromedial incision is made over the middle third of the leg, posterior to the calf muscles. Blunt dissection should be used to develop the plane above the gastrocnemius and soleus muscles. The fascia overlying the gastocnemius and soleus muscles is opened, and the tendons overlying these muscles are released from medial to lateral under direct visualization, with the foot held in maximal dorsiflexion (**Figure 5**). Care should be taken to preserve the muscle underlying the tendons. The sural nerve should be identified. Further dorsiflexion can be performed after the release, and spreading of the underlying muscle should be visualized. The wound is closed in a layered fashion.

Complications
Complications include Achilles tendon rupture and sural nerve injury.

Postoperative Care and Rehabilitation
Patients are placed in a short-leg weight-bearing cast with the foot in a neutral position for 4 to 6 weeks. The patients then may be transitioned to an ankle-foot orthosis for maintenance of correction, based on disease severity.

Pearls
- Overaggressive dorsiflexion of the foot after release should be avoided to prevent a complete tear of the Achilles tendon.
- If an associated peroneus brevis lengthening is being performed, the incision also can be made laterally.
- Posterior tibialis lengthening also can be performed through the medial incision.

Peroneus Brevis Lengthening
Indications
Peroneus brevis lengthening[6] is indicated for pes planovalgus.

Surgical Technique
The patient is positioned supine. A posterolateral incision is made over the distal one third of the leg. Care is taken to identify and protect the superficial peroneal nerve. The peroneus longus tendon is identified, and the fascia overlying the tendon is opened. The peroneus longus tendon is retracted inferiorly, and the fascia overlying the peroneus brevis tendon is opened. The tendon overlying the muscle belly is transected, and foot is placed in inversion to provide further lengthening. The wound is closed in a layered fashion.

Complications
The primary complication is superficial peroneal nerve injury.

Postoperative Care and Rehabilitation
Because this procedure rarely is performed in isolation, postoperative care should be dictated by the larger procedure that is performed.

Pearl
If gastrocnemius-soleus lengthening is performed concomitantly, it can be performed within the same incision before the peroneus brevis lengthening

Posterior Tibial Tendon Lengthening
Indications
Posterior tibial tendon lengthening[7] is indicated for equinovarus.

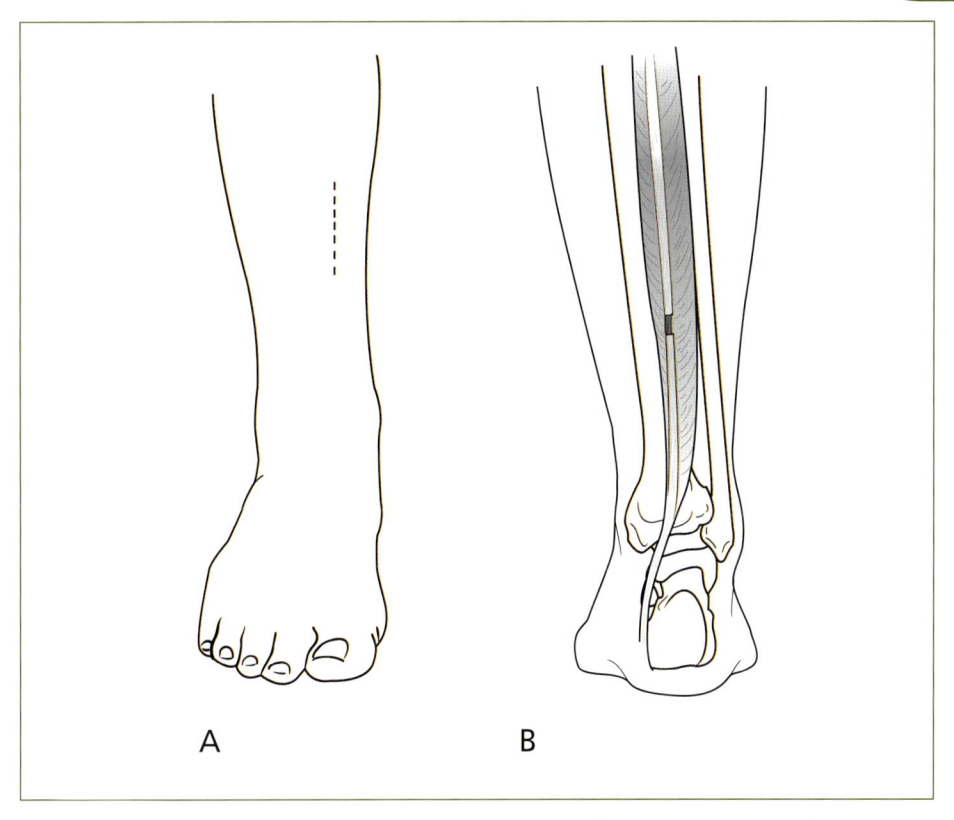

Figure 6 Illustrations demonstrate the surgical technique for posterior tibial tendon lengthening. **A**, The incision (dashed line). **B**, Transection of the tendon overlying the muscle belly.

Surgical Technique
The patient is positioned supine, with a bump under the hip. An approximately 3-cm incision over the medial border of the tibia at the junction of the middle and distal one third of the leg is made (**Figure 6, A**). The posterior border of the tibia is palpated, and dissection is carried down to the deep posterior compartment of the leg, the fascia of which is opened. The flexor digitorum longus muscle, which lies medial to the posterior tibialis tendon at this level, is encountered. The flexor digitorum longus tendon is retracted posteriorly, and the fascia overlying the posterior tibial tendon is encountered and opened. The tendon overlying the posterior tibial muscle belly should then be transected with a knife (**Figure 6, B**). The wound is closed in a layered fashion.

Complications
Complications of posterior tibial tendon lenthening include inadvertent lengthening of the flexor digitorum longus and injury to the posterior tibial artery and tibial nerve.

Postoperative Care and Rehabilitation
Because this procedure rarely is performed in isolation, postoperative care

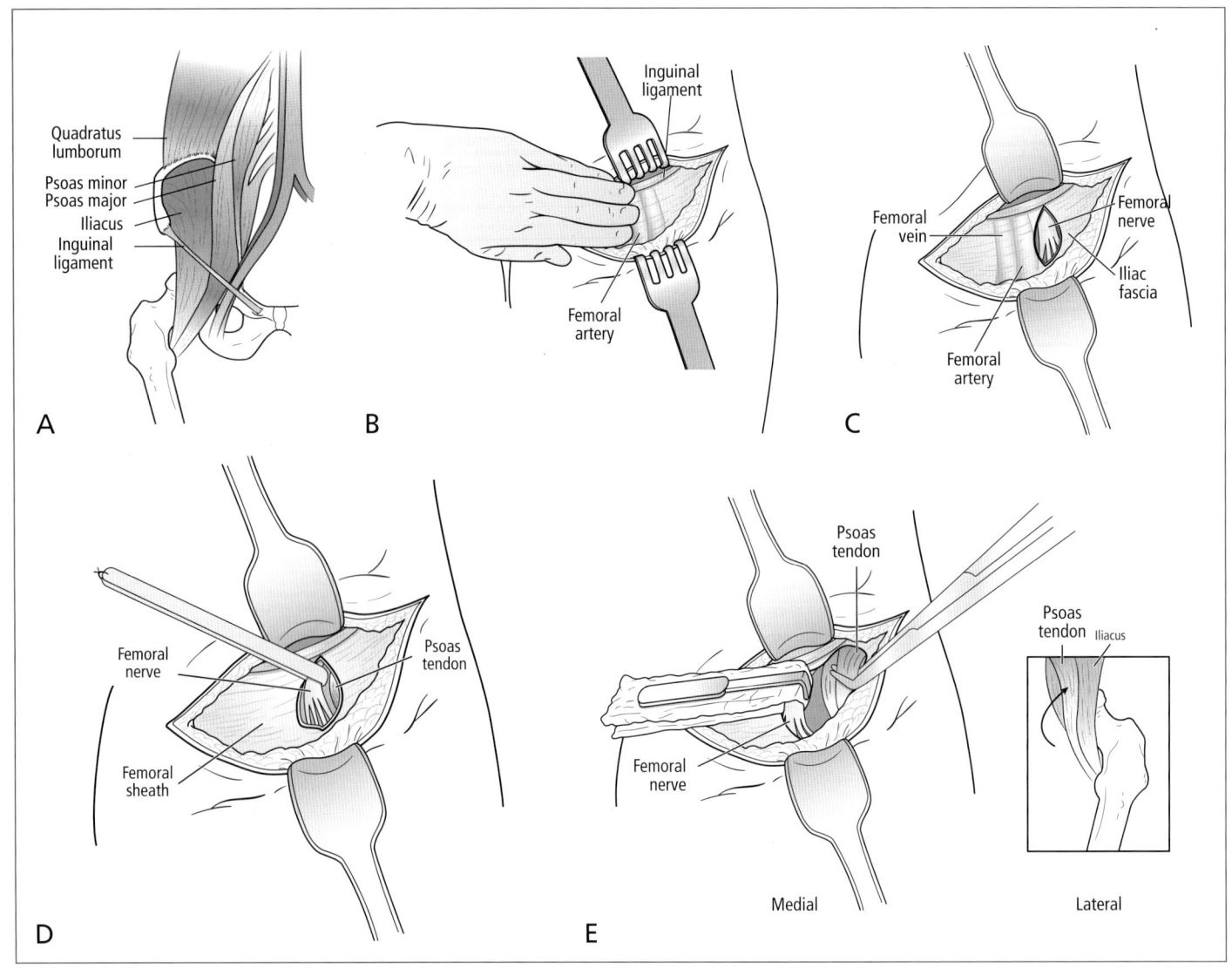

Figure 7 Illustrations demonstrate the surgical technique for psoas lengthening at the pelvic brim. **A,** The anatomy of the psoas and iliacus muscle at the pelvic brim. **B,** Palpation of the femoral artery during the superficial dissection. **C,** After division of the iliac fascia, the femoral nerve is encountered. **D,** The femoral nerve is retracted medially, revealing the psoas tendon. **E,** The psoas tendon is isolated, taking care to preserve the iliacus muscle, and transected at the pelvic brim.

should be dictated by the larger procedure that is performed.

Pearl
When opening the deep posterior compartment, the flexor digitorum longus muscle is first encountered. An error can be made if this muscle is assumed to be the posterior tibial tendon.

Psoas Release at the Pelvic Brim
Indications
Indications for psoas release at the pelvic brim[8] are hip flexion contracture and spastic hip subluxation/dislocation.

Preoperative Imaging
No imaging is required unless this is part of a larger procedure for spastic hip subluxation/dislocation, which calls for AP and frog-leg lateral views of the pelvis and bilateral hips and possibly CT with three-dimensional reconstructions.

Surgical Technique
The patient is positioned supine for this procedure. The lower extremity is draped completely free. The femoral artery is palpated and marked, and an oblique incision is made parallel and slightly distal to the anterior hip flexion crease (**Figure 7, A** and **B**). Dissection is taken down to the iliac fascia, which is divided vertically lateral to the femoral artery (**Figure 7, C**). The femoral nerve is encountered and retracted medially toward the femoral sheath with a Penrose drain (**Figure 7, D**). The iliopsoas muscle is encountered in the depth of the wound (**Figure 7, D**). The medial border of the muscle is identified and rolled laterally to expose the inner wall of the pelvis. Flexion and external rotation of the hip will relax the muscle and expose the psoas tendon (**Figure 7, E**). The tendon is isolated with a right-angle forceps and cut at the level of the pelvic brim, avoiding the transaction of any iliacus muscle fibers. The wound is closed in a standard layered fashion.

Complications
Complications include hematoma formation and damage to the femoral neurovascular bundle.

Postoperative Care and Rehabilitation
Because this procedure rarely is performed in isolation, postoperative care should be dictated by the larger procedure that is performed.

Pearl

It is of utmost importance to retract the inguinal ligament proximally and palpate the rim of the pelvis to make certain that the location for release of the psoas tendon is at the level of the pelvic brim. There are other approaches to lengthening above the pelvic brim, and the same considerations should be made.

Soft-Tissue Transfer Procedures

Rectus Femoris Transfer to the Hamstrings

Indications

Rectus femoris transfer to the hamstrings[9] is indicated for stiff-knee gait.

Surgical Technique

The patient is positioned supine. A longitudinal incision is made in the midthigh region from the superior pole of the patella extending proximally 10 cm (**Figure 8**). Dissection is carried down to the deep fascia over the rectus muscle, which is opened. The tendon of the rectus is isolated from the vastus intermedius, and its insertion on the superior pole of the patella is freed. Entering the knee joint should be avoided. A medial incision over the hamstrings is made distally, and dissection is taken down to the level of the semimembranosus and semitendinosus. The proximal aspect of the semitendinosus is sutured to the semimembranosus at its musculotendinous junction. The semitendinosus is transected distally.

A tunnel is prepared under the adipose tissue to allow the rectus tendon to be passed from the anterior to the medial incision, and any impediments to tendon gliding should be cut free. The rectus should be passed through the tunnel. The free end of the semitendinosus is passed through the rectus tendon using a Pulvertaft technique with heavy nonabsorbable suture securing the transfer. This transfer should be fixed in about 20° of flexion. The wound is closed in a standard fashion.

Complications

The primary complication is inadequate excursion of the rectus tendon from tethering of the tendon in the wound tunnel.

Postoperative Care and Rehabilitation

The patient is placed in a knee immobilizer for 3 weeks and is allowed to bear weight as tolerated. Range-of-motion exercises should be started as soon as tolerated.

Pearl

The gracilis and fascia lata also can be used as a potential transfer point for the rectus.

Split Posterior Tibial Tendon Transfer

Indications

Split posterior tibial tendon transfer[10] is indicated for dynamic equinovarus, particularly hindfoot varus.

Surgical Technique

The patient is positioned supine. Four incisions are used in this surgery. Attention is first turned to an incision directly over the medial border of the foot from the navicular to the tip of the medial malleolus (**Figure 9, A**). The posterior tibial tendon sheath is identified and opened in its entirety from its insertion on the navicular to the tip of the medial malleolus. Care should be taken to free the tendon within its sheath proximally beyond the incision with scissors. The inferior portion of the tendon is split and detached from its navicular insertion.

A second incision approximately 5 cm in length is made over the medial border of the tibia at the junction of the middle and

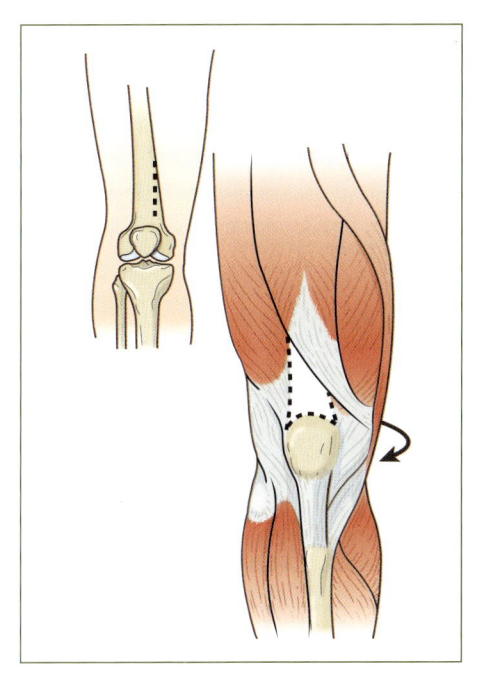

Figure 8 Illustration shows the incision used for rectus transfer and illustrates the new line of pull of the rectus tendon after transfer.

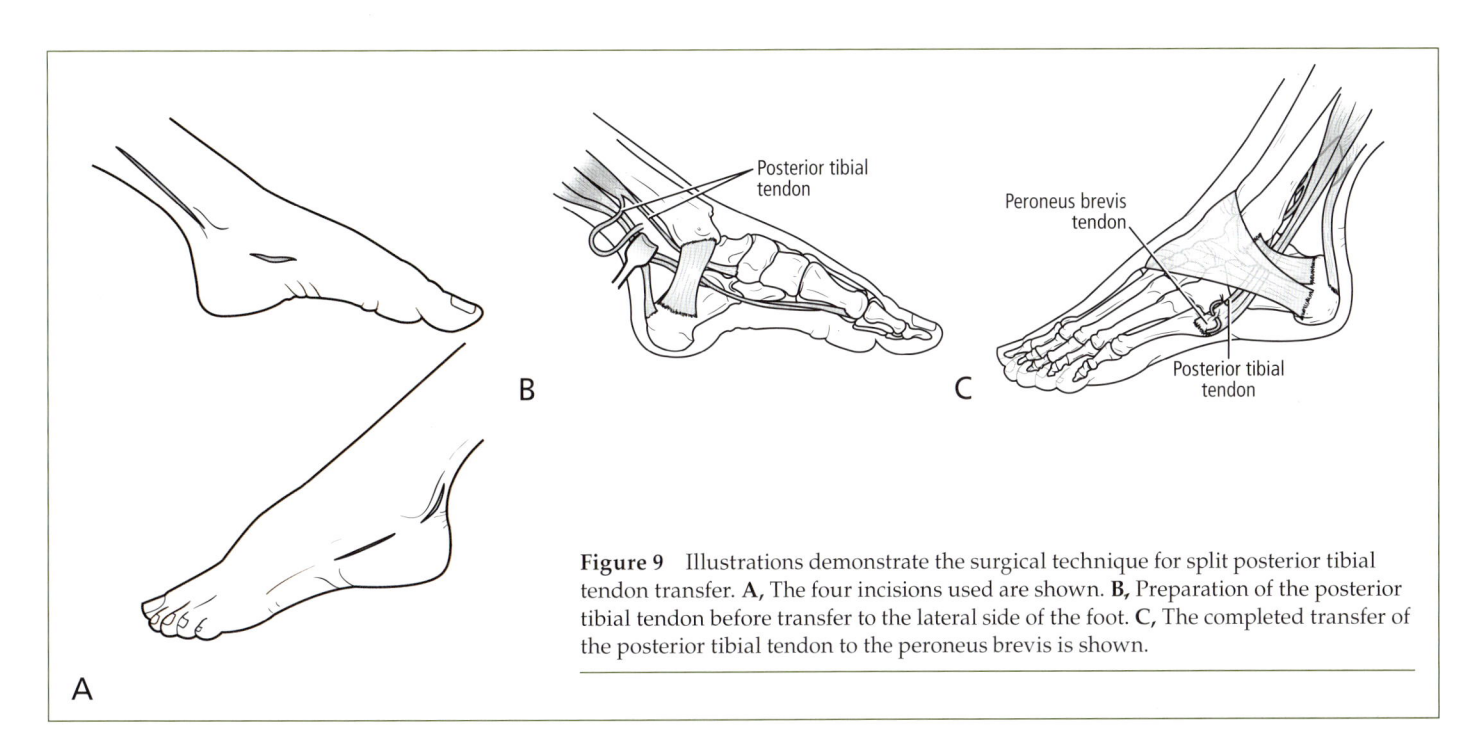

Figure 9 Illustrations demonstrate the surgical technique for split posterior tibial tendon transfer. **A**, The four incisions used are shown. **B**, Preparation of the posterior tibial tendon before transfer to the lateral side of the foot. **C**, The completed transfer of the posterior tibial tendon to the peroneus brevis is shown.

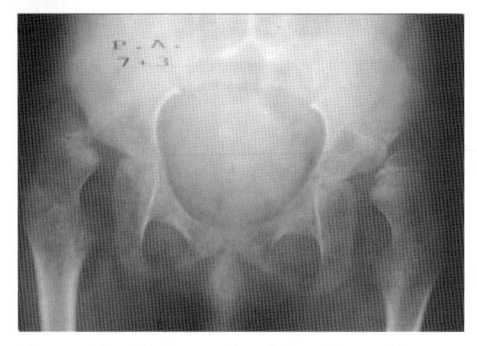

Figure 10 Preoperative AP radiograph of a patient with Gross Motor Functional Classification System level V cerebral palsy with spastic hip subluxation.

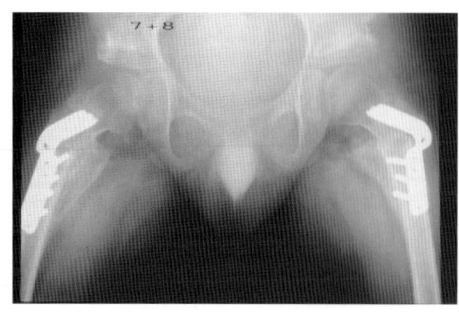

Figure 11 Postoperative AP radiograph of the patient in Figure 10 after proximal soft-tissue lengthening, varus derotational osteotomy, and acetabuloplasty for spastic hip subluxation.

distal one third of the leg (**Figure 9, A**). The posterior border of the tibia is palpated, and dissection is carried down to the deep posterior compartment of the leg. The fascia overlying the deep posterior compartment should be opened, and the flexor digitorum muscle should be retracted posteriorly. An umbilical tape can be placed between the two arms of the posterior tibialis muscle and retrieved with a tendon passer, which is placed within the posterior tibialis sheath and pulled into the posterior compartment. The tape can then be used to divide the tendon by pulling proximally. Alternatively, the fascia overlying the posterior tibial tendon should be opened longitudinally, and the split tendon pulled proximally into this wound. The split in the tendon is carried proximally with a scissors to the musculotendinous junction of the muscle (**Figure 9, B**).

A third incision is made behind the lateral malleolus (**Figure 9, A**). The incision should extend from the tip of the malleolus to a point 5 to 7 cm proximal. The peroneal tendon sheaths should be encountered and opened. A tendon passer is taken from the proximal medial wound into the wound. The tendon passer should be directly in contact with the posterior surface of the tibia to avoid the neurovascular bundle. The split posterior tibial tendon should be passed from the proximal medial wound to the lateral wound using the tendon passer (**Figure 9, B**). The tendon should be passed anterior to the peroneal tendons.

At this point, both medial wounds should be closed in a standard fashion to avoid manipulation of the foot after tendon transfer.

A fourth incision is made overlying the peroneus brevis tendon from the tip of the lateral malleolus to the base of the fifth metatarsal. The split portion of the posterior tibial tendon is passed from the third incision under the peroneal retinaculum into the sheath of the peroneus brevis tendon. With the foot held in the neutral position, the posterior tibial tendon is sutured to the peroneus brevis tendon using a heavy nonabsorbable suture (**Figure 9, C**). The lateral wounds are closed in a standard fashion.

Complications
Complications include neurovascular damage when passing the split tendon posterior to the tibia, and inadvertent transection of the posterior tibial tendon.

Postoperative Care and Rehabilitation
The patient is put in a short-leg weight-bearing cast for 4 to 6 weeks, followed by an ankle-foot orthosis.

Pearl
Preoperative gait analysis is helpful to ensure that the tibialis anterior is not the deforming force.

Bone Procedures
Combined Procedure for Spastic Hip Subluxation/Dislocation
The combined procedure[11,12] is indicated for spastic hip subluxation/dislocation. The combined procedure includes adductor tenotomy, psoas lengthening, proximal hamstring tenotomy, acetabuloplasty, varus derotational osteotomy of the femur, and hip open reduction and capsulorrhaphy.

Preoperative Imaging
AP and frog-leg lateral radiographs of the pelvis and bilateral hips are needed (**Figures 10 and 11**). Three-dimensional CT is optional.

Implants
Implants used in the combined procedure include the pediatric blade plate and the pediatric locking compression plate.

Surgical Technique
The patient is positioned supine, with a bump placed under the flank on the ipsilateral side. The leg is draped completely free, with care taken to include the iliac crest in the operative field. The first incision is made in the perineum to perform the adductor tenotomy as described previously.

A second anterior incision is made 1 cm lateral to the iliac crest and extending distally, ending medial to the anterior superior iliac spine. A standard Smith Petersen approach is performed, with the iliac apophysis elevated off the inner and outer table. The iliac wing is stripped subperiosteally down to the sciatic notch both medially and laterally. The lateral exposure allows full visualization of the sciatic notch, and the medial exposure allows full visualization of the anterior inferior iliac spine (AIIS). Attention is turned to the distal aspect of the wound, and the direct and indirect heads of the rectus muscle are released and reflected distally. The capsule is opened through a T-shaped incision for subsequent capsular repair. The ligamentum teres is removed, the transverse acetabular ligament is transected, and any other obstructions to reduction are removed, including lengthening the psoas tendon. Psoas lengthening also can be performed through this incision.

A third incision is made over the lateral aspect of the proximal thigh, from just below the tip of the greater trochanter and extending distally 6 cm. The femur should be subperiosteally exposed. The femoral neck anteversion should be palpated through the anterior incision. A Kirschner wire (K-wire) should be placed perpendicular to the femoral shaft in line with the femoral neck anteversion, and a second K-wire should be placed in the center of the femoral neck in relation to the perpendicular wire to obtain a neck-shaft angle of 110° post fixation, based on preoperative planning (**Figure 12, A**). The chisel for the blade plate should be seated toward its desired depth in the femoral neck, and care should be taken to not penetrate the calcar. Rotational K-wires are placed in the femur to aid in the planning of derotation. Three cuts are made with a saw: one perpendicular to the femoral shaft proximally, a second cut in line with the chisel to remove a medial wedge, and a third cut that bevels the lateral edge of the proximal fragment to allow for medialization. The blade plate is placed into the femoral neck, and the plate is reduced to the bone with a clamp.

Prior to securing the clamp, the appropriate rotation of the distal fragment should be set using the rotational K-wires. Screws are placed in a compression mode in the blade plate. Alternatively, the chisel can be kept in place until the pelvic osteotomy has been performed.

Attention is once again turned to the anterior incision. Five nonabsorbable sutures should be placed in the T-shaped capsulotomy but not tied. A K-wire is placed 0.5 to 1.0 cm above the lateral aspect of the acetabulum at the planned level of the acetabular osteotomy (**Figure 12, B**) and checked under fluoroscopy. This is a bending acetabuloplasty, so only the lateral cortex of the pelvis is cut except at the anterior (AIIS) and posterior (sciatic) corners of the osteotomy. With a straight osteotome approximately the size of the femoral head, an osteotomy is made through the lateral cortex (**Figure 13, A and B**). A Kerrison rongeur can be used to complete the cuts at the corners. At this point, a curved osteotome (1.9 to 2.5 cm wide) is directed toward the triradiate cartilage, just at the medial aspect of the triradiate cartilage. After confirming correct placement, a wider osteotome is used to widen the osteotomy site. A blunt laminar spreader is placed in the posterior portion of the osteotomy and opened 1.0 to 1.5 cm. The wedge that was removed from the proximal femur is then placed to keep the osteotomy open. Alternatively, wedges from the iliac crest can be used. Gentle pressure opens the osteotomy laterally 1.0 to 1.5 cm (**Figure 13, C**). No further fixation of these grafts is necessary (**Figure 13, D and E**).

The hip is reduced with abduction and internal rotation, and the capsule is repaired with the sutures placed previously. The iliac apophysis is repaired with a heavy absorbable suture. The vastus lateralis and tensor fascia lata also are repaired with a heavy absorbable suture through the lateral wound. Standard wound closure can be performed.

Complications
Complications include sciatic nerve palsy, osteonecrosis, iatrogenic fracture, and loss of hip reduction.

Postoperative Care and Rehabilitation
Although many authors suggest no immobilization is necessary, we place these patients in a one-and-one-half hip spica for 2 to 3 weeks postoperatively for pain relief while positioning the child in the immediate postoperative period.

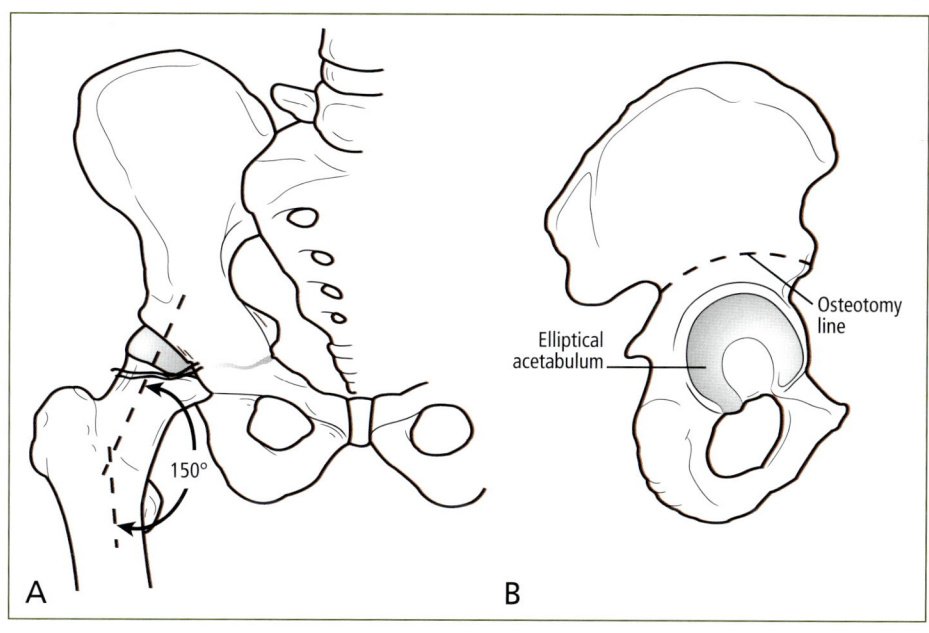

Figure 12 Illustrations show planning for the combined procedure for spastic hip subluxation/dislocation. **A,** The preoperative proximal femoral deformity noted in patients with spastic hip subluxation/dislocation with coxa valga is shown. **B,** The intended path of the acetabuloplasty, 0.5 to 1.0 cm above the acetabulum through the greater sciatic notch and the anterior inferior iliac spine is shown.

- When exposing the outer table of the pelvis, the surgeon should pay special attention to fully visualizing the sciatic notch posteriorly so that the osteotomy can be made easily.
- After the hip is reduced, an assistant should maintain the leg in abduction and internal rotation to prevent dislocation in the cast (if the surgeon chooses to use a spica cast).

Proximal Femoral Rotational Osteotomy
Indications
Indications for the proximal femoral rotational osteotomy[13,14] are increased femoral anteversion and lever-arm syndrome.

Preoperative Imaging
AP and frog-leg lateral radiographs of the pelvis and bilateral hips are taken. Three-dimensional CT with torsional profile is optional.

Implants
The implants required for proximal femoral rotational osteotomy include a pediatric blade plate and a pediatric locking compression plate.

Surgical Technique
The patient is positioned prone, with a bump under the hip. The prone position is used so that intraoperative internal and external rotation of the hips can be measured with the knees flexed 90°. A straight lateral incision is made over the lateral aspect of the proximal thigh from just below the tip of the greater trochanter and extending distally 6 cm. The vastus lateralis should be elevated, and the femur should be subperiosteally exposed and protected with retractors. A K-wire should be placed perpendicular to the femoral shaft in line with the femoral neck anteversion. Another K-wire is placed in the distal femur. This K-wire should be rotated the appropriate number of degrees away from the proximal pin, based on preoperative planning, to achieve 10° to 20° of femoral anteversion postoperatively. If a blade plate is the desired method of fixation at this point, the surgical technique described previously for the spastic/dislocated hip procedure is followed, starting with chisel placement. Of note, only a transverse osteotomy (at or below the level of the lesser trochanter) is necessary. The appropriate derotation is performed.

If a locking compression plate is used, a 6-hole plate generally is preferred. The proximal two or three holes of the plate are placed above the area of the intended transverse osteotomy (at or below the level of the lesser trochanter), and screws are drilled and measured. The transverse osteotomy is made, the distal fragment is derotated, the proximal portion of the plate is secured to the proximal frag-

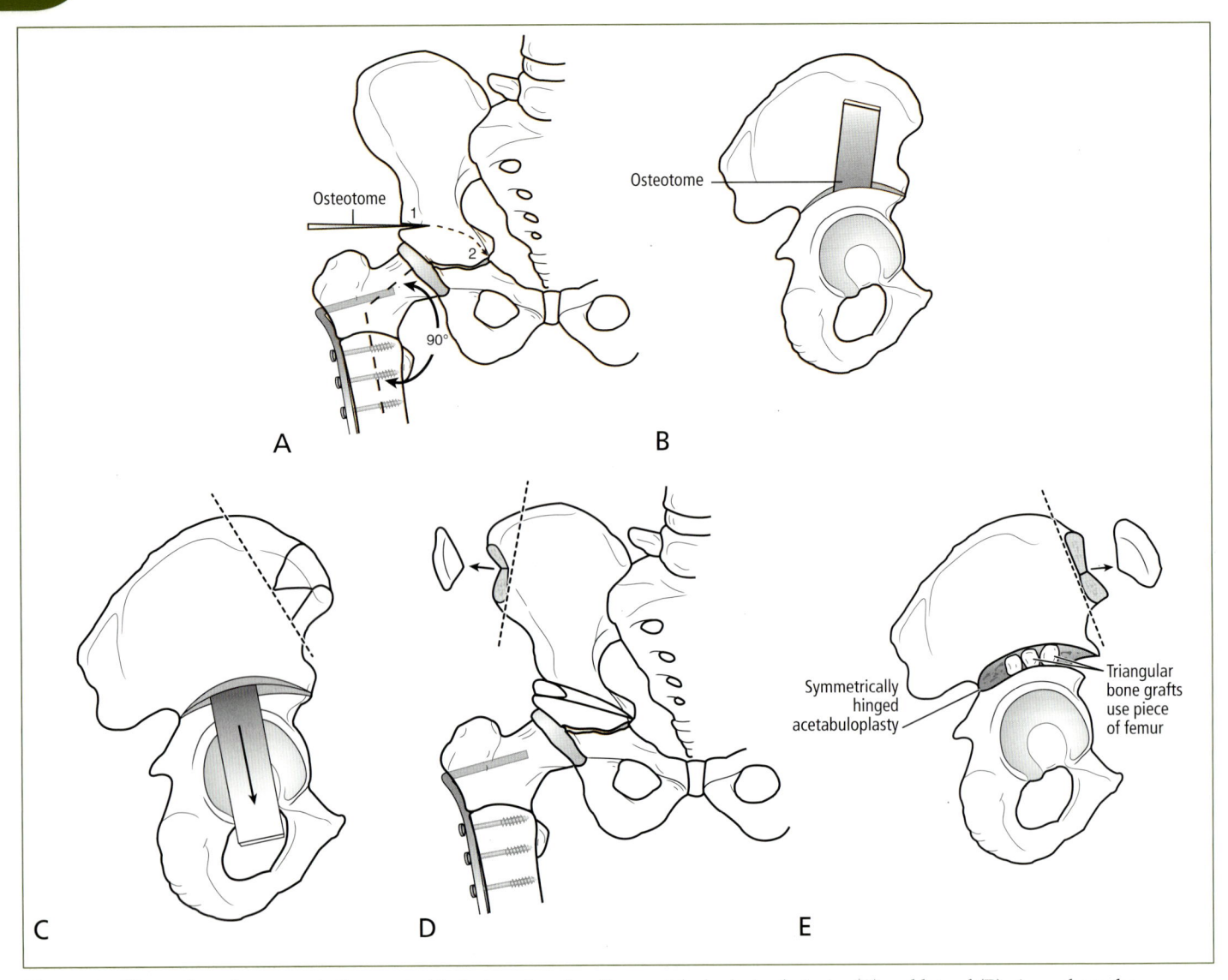

Figure 13 Illustrations demonstrate the surgical technique for a bending acetabuloplasty. Anterior (**A**) and lateral (**B**) views show the intended path of the acetabuloplasty. A straight No. 1 and curved No. 2 osteotome are used to perform the acetabuloplasty and correction of the coxa valga with a varus derotational osteotomy. **C,** Lateral view shows a curved osteotome directed toward the triradiate cartilage to perform the bending acetabuloplasty. Anterior (**D**) and lateral (**E**) views show the bicortical graft taken from the iliac crest and used to hold open the acetabuloplasty.

ment with the predrilled screws, and the distal fragment is finally secured to the distal three holes of the plate with a clamp. These locking or cortical screws are placed, and an intraoperative examination ensuring correction of the internal rotation (decreased) and external rotation (increased) of the hip is performed on the operating room table (**Figure 14**). Standard wound closure is performed after the vastus lateralis and tensor fascia lata are closed with a heavy absorbable suture.

Complications
Complications of this procedure include nonunion/malunion, overcorrection, and angular deformity.

Postoperative Care and Rehabilitation
A one-and-one-half hip spica cast is used for 4 to 6 weeks. If bone quality is deemed to be appropriate, several authors have suggested not using a spica cast.

Pearl
Care must be taken to fully expose the femur subperiosteally at the level of the osteotomy so that appropriate rotation can occur.

Tibial Derotational Osteotomy
Indications
Tibial derotational osteotomy[13,14] is indicated for tibial torsion and lever-arm syndrome.

Preoperative Imaging
AP and lateral radiographs of the knee, tibia, and ankle are taken. Three-dimensional CT with torsional profile is optional.

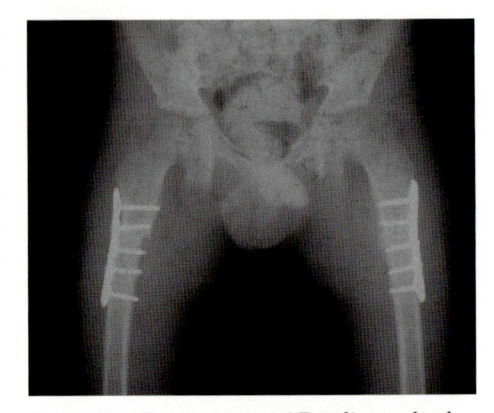

Figure 14 Postoperative AP radiograph of a patient after proximal femoral rotational osteotomy for increased femoral anteversion with plate fixation.

Implants
The implants required for this procedure are a 6-hole 3.5-mm compression plate and K-wires.

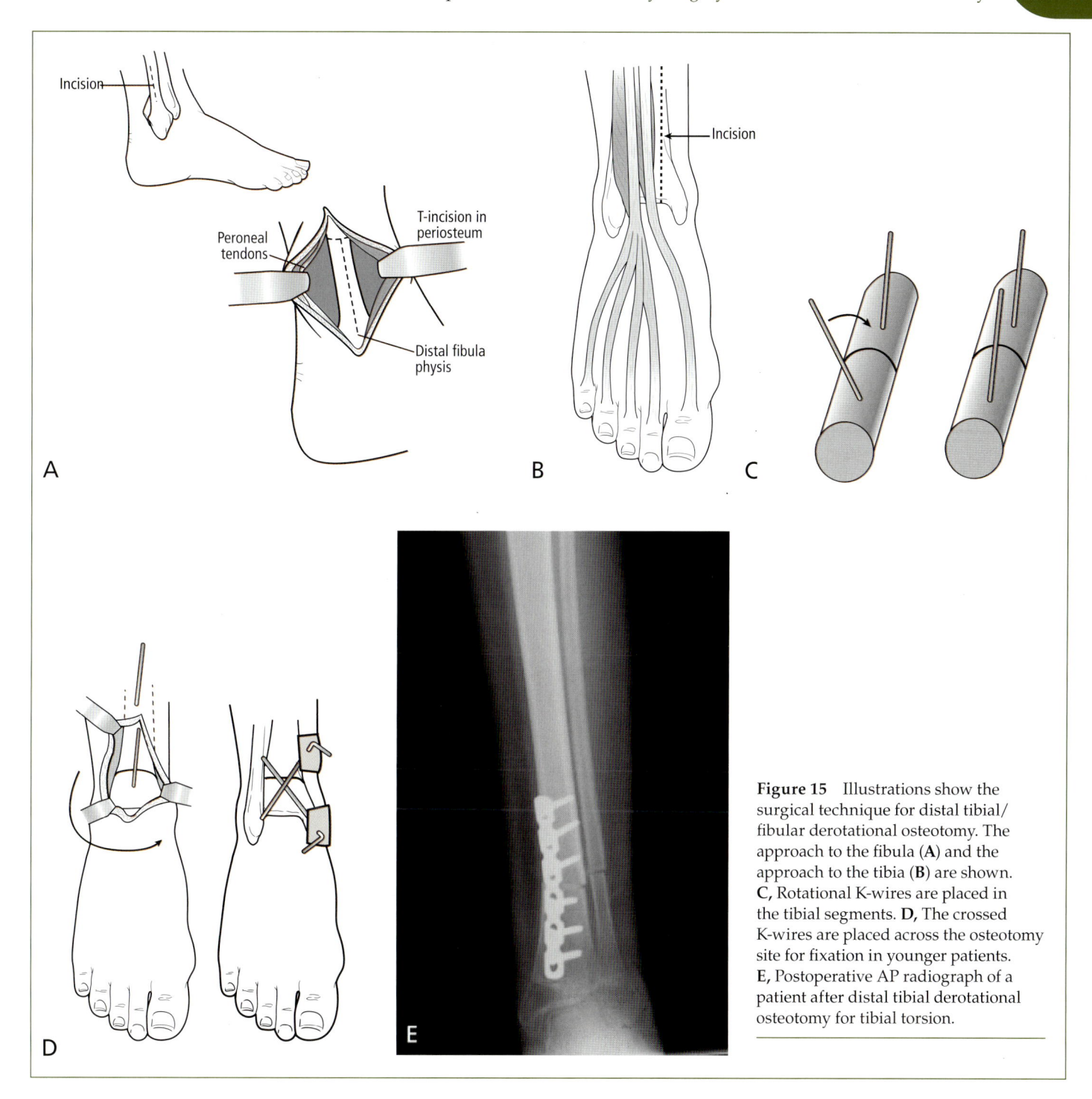

Chapter 107: Lower Extremity Surgery in Children With Cerebral Palsy

Figure 15 Illustrations show the surgical technique for distal tibial/fibular derotational osteotomy. The approach to the fibula (**A**) and the approach to the tibia (**B**) are shown. **C**, Rotational K-wires are placed in the tibial segments. **D**, The crossed K-wires are placed across the osteotomy site for fixation in younger patients. **E**, Postoperative AP radiograph of a patient after distal tibial derotational osteotomy for tibial torsion.

Surgical Technique

The patient is positioned supine, with a bump under the hip. If the surgeon is contemplating making more than a 20° to 30° derotation, a fibular osteotomy should be considered. An incision directly over the fibula is made first. The fibula is exposed subperiosteally, taking care to protect the superficial peroneal nerve. A transverse osteotomy is made in the fibula, 3 to 4 cm above the ankle joint (**Figure 15, A**).

Attention is turned to the anterior aspect of the tibia. An incision approximately 10 cm in length, if using a plate for fixation, or 5 cm in length, if using K-wires for fixation in a younger child, is made lateral to the anterior border of the tibia, extending from the ankle crease proximally (**Figure 15, B**). The tibialis anterior is reflected medially off the tibia. The tibia is exposed in a subperiosteal fashion at the level of the intended osteotomy. Two rotational K-wires, one placed distally just proximal to the physis and one placed proximally away from the osteotomy site, are placed in the tibia in a perpendicular fashion (**Figure 15, C**). The distal wire is rotated away from the proximal wire such that the intended degree of rotational correction based on preoperative templating can be visualized when the distal fragment is rotated (**Figure 15, D**).

If a compression plate is used, the proximal three holes above the osteotomy are drilled and measured. The plate is removed and the transverse osteotomy perpendicular to the tibia is made with an oscillating saw. The distal fragment is rotated. The proximal portion of the plate is secured to bone, the distal fragment is reduced to the plate, and the screws are placed in a compression fashion (**Figure 15, E**). If K-wire fixation is chosen in lieu of a compression plate (in young children with good bone quality), the crossed K-wires can be placed across the osteotomy (**Figure 15, D**). The pins are bent, cut, and placed out of the skin. A drain is placed. Standard wound closure follows in a layered fashion.

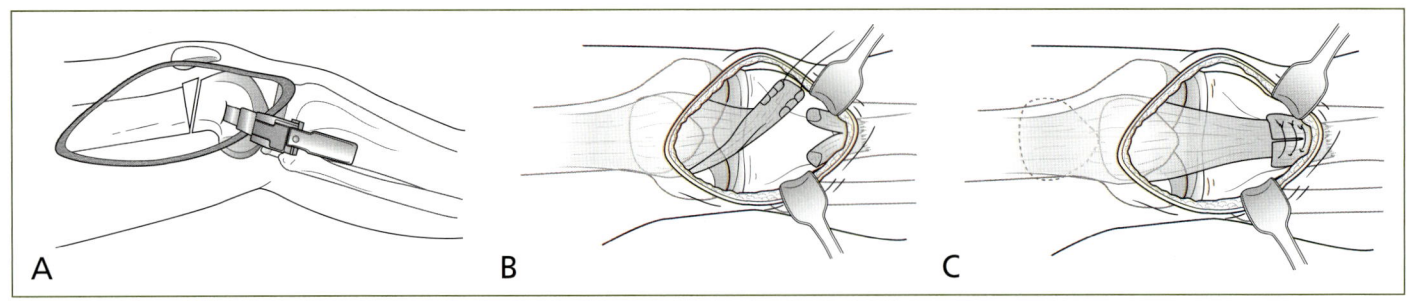

Figure 16 Illustrations demonstrate the surgical technique for a distal femoral extension osteotomy. **A**, A distal cut is made perpendicular to the blade plate chisel and the proximal cut is made perpendicular to the femur. **B**, Medial and lateral Krackow sutures are placed in the patellar tendon for advancement. **C**, The patellar tendon is advanced under the periosteal flaps, with the flaps repaired over the tendon.

Complications
Complications include nonunion/malunion, compartment syndrome, overcorrection or undercorrection, and hardware irritation (if a plate is used).

Postoperative Care and Rehabilitation
A short-leg non–weight-bearing cast is used for 4 weeks (if present, pins are pulled at 4 weeks), followed by a short-leg weight-bearing cast for an additional 4 weeks.

Pearl
Patients are at risk for compartment syndrome and should be monitored closely postoperatively.

Distal Femoral Extension Osteotomy With Patellar Tendon Advancement
Indications
This procedure[15] is indicated for knee flexion contracture and crouch gait.

Preoperative Imaging
AP and lateral radiographs of the knee are taken.

Implants
The implants required for this procedure include a pediatric blade plate (90°) or distal femoral locking plate and 3.5- or 4.5-mm screws.

Surgical Technique
The patient is positioned supine, with a bump under the hip. An incision is made over the lateral aspect of the distal femur, taking care to stay proximal to the knee joint and the distal femoral physis, if it still is open. This incision should be posterior to the vastus lateralis. The distal femur is exposed in a subperiosteal fashion, and a K-wire is placed perpendicular to the femur. This K-wire should be placed just proximal to the distal femoral physis. If a blade plate is being used, the chisel is impacted into the bone just proximal to the K-wire previously placed. This chisel should be perpendicular to the tibia at the knee joint to correct the flexion deformity of the osteotomy. At this point, the appropriate anterior wedge of bone based on preoperative planning should be cut from the distal femur (**Figure 16, A**). The chisel is removed, and the blade plate is impacted into the distal fragment. Bone that may be present posteriorly on the distal fragment is removed, and the blade plate is secured to the proximal fragment with screws placed in a compression mode.

A second anterior incision is made over the tibial tubercle and patella. Dissection is taken down to the level of the patellar tendon. The medial and lateral retinacula are divided to isolate the patellar tendon. The tendon is dissected free from its inferior attachment at the level of the tibial tubercle. The periosteum distal to the tubercle is divided in a T-shaped fashion to expose the tibia. The patellar tendon is advanced distally until the inferior pole of the patella is at the joint line (**Figure 16, B**). The tendon is repaired with a nonabsorbable, heavy suture under the periosteal flaps that were created (**Figure 16, C**). In a skeletally immature patient, patellar tendon advancement is achieved in this way. In a skeletally mature patient, a block of the tibial tubercle with the tendon attached is moved distally and secured with screws. Most patients who require this surgery are skeletally mature and will require this distalization of the tibial tubercle. The goal is to have the inferior pole of the patella at the level of the Blumensaat line on the lateral radiograph. The repair is reinforced with a tension band construct through the inferior aspect of the patella and the proximal tibia. The wound is closed in a layered fashion.

Complications
Complications include nonunion/malunion, anterior knee pain, tendon rupture, sciatic nerve palsy, compartment syndrome, and symptomatic hardware.

Postoperative Care and Rehabilitation
A knee range-of-motion brace is placed and kept in approximately 10° to 20° of flexion for 2 weeks. Motion is advanced gradually over the ensuing 4 to 6 weeks until the osteotomies have healed.

Pearls
- In a skeletally immature patient, the surgeon can imbricate the patellar tendon without cutting it or distalizing the tibial tubercle. This can be achieved by rotating the tendon over a clamp and suturing the tendon on top of itself, using nonabsorbable sutures.
- Keeping the knee slightly flexed until swelling has resolved will prevent stretching of the nerve.

Calcaneal Lengthening Osteotomy
Indications
Calcaneal lengthening osteotomy[16,17] is indicated for pes planovalgus foot.

Preoperative Imaging
AP, lateral, oblique, and Harris radiographs of the feet are taken. Three-dimensional CT scan is optional.

Surgical Technique
The patient is positioned supine, with a bump under the hip. An incision is made over the lateral border of the foot from the midportion of the calcaneus to the level of the calcaneocuboid joint. Dissection should proceed plantar to the sural nerve; the peroneus brevis tendon is identified and lengthened. A second incision is made medially over the talonavicular joint. The talonavicular joint capsule is exposed, and an elliptical portion of it is removed. Attention is turned again to the lateral incision. The calcaneus is subperiosteally exposed 2 to 2.5 cm proximal to the calcaneocuboid joint. The calcaneocu-

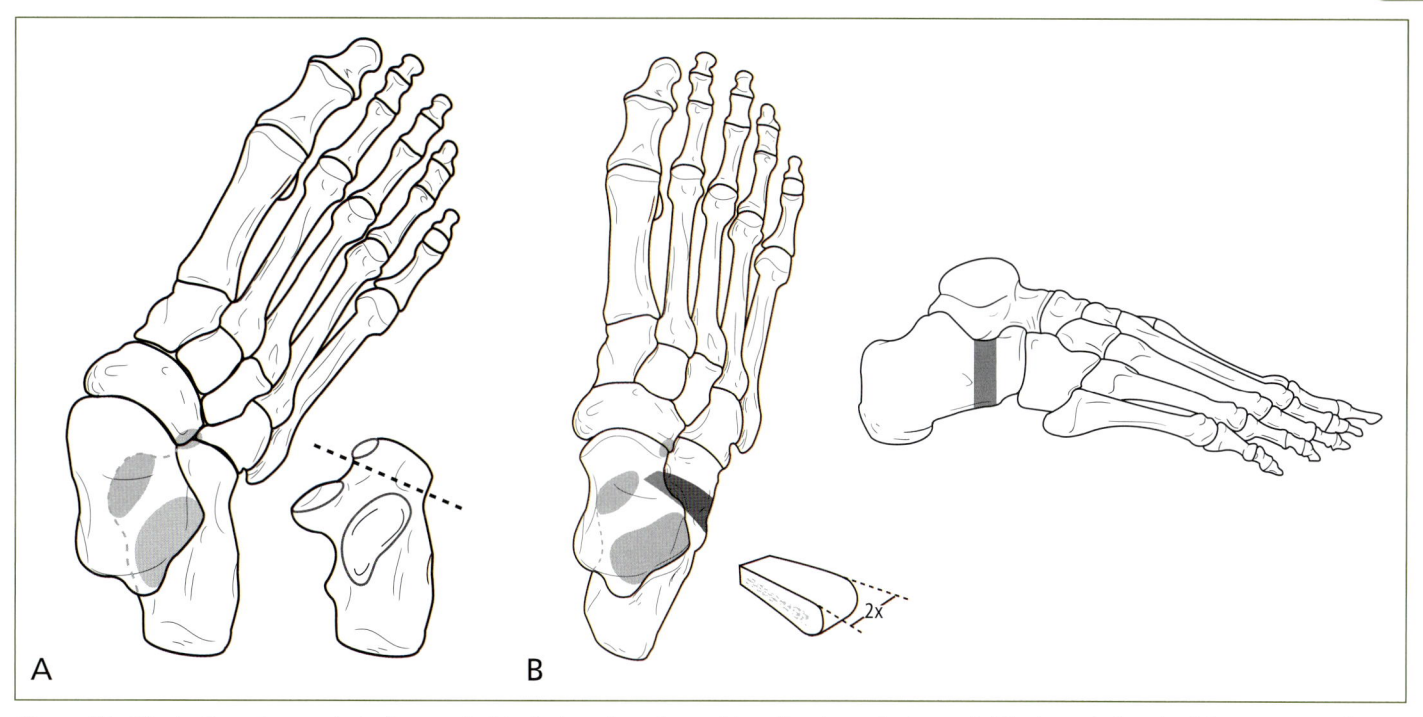

Figure 17 Illustrations demonstrate the surgical technique for calcaneal lengthening osteotomy. **A,** The intended path of the osteotomy for calcaneal lengthening is shown, exiting between the anterior and middle facets. **B,** The calcaneal lengthening osteotomy after placement of the graft.

boid joint is pinned in a reduced position prior to making the osteotomy. A transverse osteotomy is made in the calcaneus (**Figure 17, A**) after confirmation of the appropriate position with fluoroscopy. A laminar spreader is used to open the osteotomy site, and a trapezoidal piece of allograft or autograft is placed into the osteotomy (**Figure 17, B**). A K-wire can be passed across the osteotomy (if additional fixation is necessary), bent, and placed out of the skin.

Attention is returned to the medial incision, and the talonavicular joint capsule is imbricated with a nonabsorbable suture. The talonavicular capsulorrhaphy is not necessary in all cases. A closing-wedge osteotomy of the medial cuneiform is performed to plantar flex the medial column. Both wounds are closed in a layered fashion.

Complications
Complications include malunion/nonunion and inadvertent lengthening of the peroneus longus, leading to iatrogenic dorsal bunion.

Postoperative Care and Rehabilitation
A short-leg non–weight-bearing cast is used for 4 weeks (pins are pulled at 4 weeks), followed by a short-leg weight-bearing cast for an additional 4 weeks. An ankle-foot orthosis then may be used, depending on disease severity.

Pearls
- Because this osteotomy is inherently stable, no fixation generally is needed.
- Care should be taken to protect the calcaneus on its dorsal and plantar aspect with retractors when making the osteotomy.
- If residual forefoot supination is present, a plantar-based opening-wedge osteotomy of the medial cuneiform can be performed to plantar flex and pronate the foot.

Calcaneal Sliding Osteotomy
Indications
Calcaneal sliding osteotomy[16,17] is another procedure indicated for pes planovalgus foot.

Preoperative Imaging
AP, lateral, oblique, and Harris radiographs of the feet are taken. Three-dimensional CT is optional.

Surgical Technique
The patient is positioned supine, with a bump under the hip. An incision from the posterosuperior aspect of the calcaneus to its plantar-anterior surface is made. Dissection is taken plantar to the sural nerve from the distal plantar aspect of the calcaneus to the proximal-superior aspect near the tuberosity in an extraperiosteal fashion. A Key elevator is used to dissect the soft tissue between the calcaneus and the Achilles as well as between the calcaneus and peroneal tendons. Hohmann-type retractors are placed in these areas to protect the soft tissues. Subperiosteal dissection is performed in the path of the intended osteotomy, which should be parallel to the posterior facet and perpendicular to the calcaneus in a lateral-to-medial direction (**Figure 18, A**).

An oscillating saw is used to cut through the lateral cortex of the calcaneus. The osteotomy is completed with an osteotome (**Figure 18, B**). The distal fragment is slid medially approximately 1 cm. Correction of the hindfoot valgus should be noted. Two K-wires are placed from the dorsolateral foot to the medial-plantar portion of the osteotomy. The pins are cut and bent over the skin.

The incision is extended distally, and the lateral aspect of the cuboid bone is exposed. A Hohmann retractor is placed under the cuboid, protecting the peroneus longus tendon. A vertical osteotomy is performed in the cuboid.

Attention is turned to the medial aspect of the foot. The tibialis anterior tendon is identified and dissected off the medial cuneiform. A plantar-based closing-wedge osteotomy is performed and the resected bone is removed. A K-wire is placed from the lateral aspect of the foot to the level of the cuboid osteotomy. The resected bone is placed into the cuboid osteotomy site to perform an opening-wedge osteotomy,

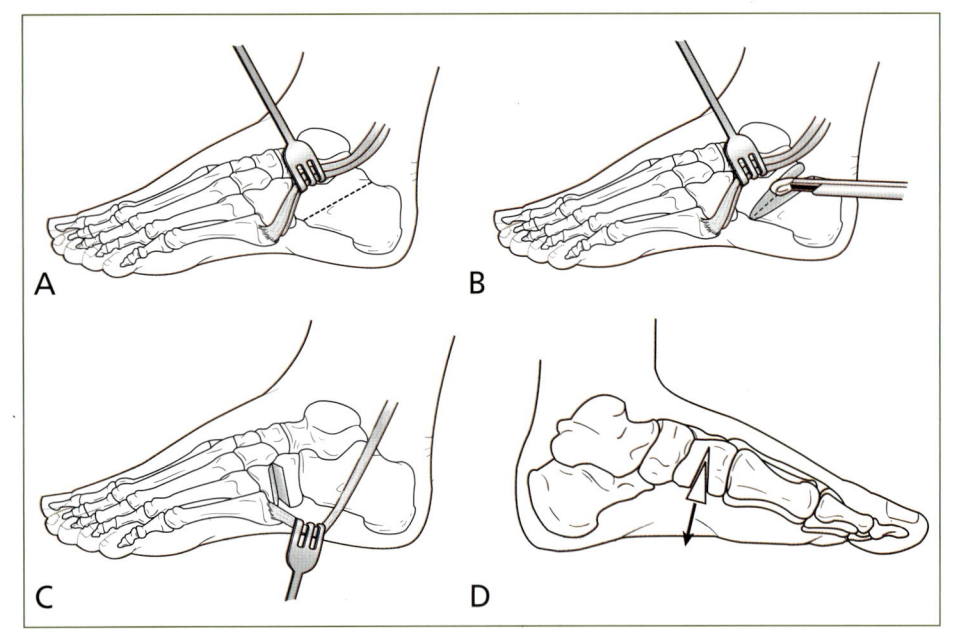

Figure 18 Illustrations demonstrate the surgical technique for calcaneal sliding osteotomy. **A,** The recommended location of the osteotomy in the calcaneus for sliding correction. **B,** Completion of the calcaneal osteotomy with an osteotome. **C,** An opening-wedge osteotomy of the cuboid can be performed for additional lateral column correction. **D,** Residual forefoot supination can be corrected with a plantar-based closing-wedge osteotomy of the medial cuneiform.

and the K-wire is advanced across the osteotomy. A K-wire is placed across the medial closing-wedge osteotomy, on the medial aspect of the foot.

Complications
Complications after calcaneal sliding osteotomy include lateral wound necrosis and nonunion/malunion.

Postoperative Care and Rehabilitation
The patient wears a short-leg non–weight-bearing cast for 4 weeks (pins are pulled at 4 weeks), followed by a short-leg weight-bearing cast for an additional 4 weeks. An ankle-foot orthosis then may be used, depending on disease severity.

Pearls
- Meticulous closure of the lateral wound must be performed to prevent wound complications.
- The calcaneal osteotomy must have two smooth surfaces for appropriate sliding to occur.
- An osteotome is used to complete the medial cut to prevent damage to neurovascular structures.
- A gastrocnemius-soleus recession and/or peroneus lengthening also may be necessary as an adjunct to this bony procedure.

- If additional lateral column lengthening is needed, an opening-wedge cuboid osteotomy can be performed (**Figure 18, C**).
- Residual forefoot supination can be corrected with a plantar-based closing-wedge osteotomy of the medial cuneiform (**Figure 18, D**).

References
1. Palisano R, Rosenbaum P, Walter S, Russell D, Wood E, Galuppi B: Development and reliability of a system to classify gross motor function in children with cerebral palsy. *Dev Med Child Neurol* 1997;39(4):214-223.
2. Graham HK, Harvey A, Rodda J, Nattrass GR, Pirpiris M: The Functional Mobility Scale (FMS). *J Pediatr Orthop* 2004;24(5):514-520.
3. Presedo A, Oh CW, Dabney KW, Miller F: Soft-tissue releases to treat spastic hip subluxation in children with cerebral palsy. *J Bone Joint Surg Am* 2005;87(4):832-841.
4. Chang WN, Tsirikos AI, Miller F, et al: Distal hamstring lengthening in ambulatory children with cerebral palsy: Primary versus revision procedures. *Gait Posture* 2004;19(3):298-304.
5. Javors JR, Klaaren HE: The Vulpius procedure for correction of equinus deformity in cerebral palsy. *J Pediatr Orthop* 1987;7(2):191-193.
6. Nather A, Fulford GE, Stewart K: Treatment of valgus hindfoot in cerebral palsy by peroneus brevis lengthening. *Dev Med Child Neurol* 1984;26(3):335-340.
7. Majestro TC, Ruda R, Frost HM: Intramuscular lengthening of the posterior tibialis muscle. *Clin Orthop Relat Res* 1971;79:59-60.
8. Sutherland DH, Zilberfarb JL, Kaufman KR, Wyatt MP, Chambers HG: Psoas release at the pelvic brim in ambulatory patients with cerebral palsy: Operative technique and functional outcome. *J Pediatr Orthop* 1997;17(5):563-570.
9. Sutherland DH, Santi M, Abel MF: Treatment of stiff-knee gait in cerebral palsy: A comparison by gait analysis of distal rectus femoris transfer versus proximal rectus release. *J Pediatr Orthop* 1990;10(4):433-441.
10. Green NE, Griffin PP, Shiavi R: Split posterior tibial-tendon transfer in spastic cerebral palsy. *J Bone Joint Surg Am* 1983;65(6):748-754.
11. Mubarak SJ, Valencia FG, Wenger DR: One-stage correction of the spastic dislocated hip: Use of pericapsular acetabuloplasty to improve coverage. *J Bone Joint Surg Am* 1992;74(9):1347-1357.
12. Elmer EB, Wenger DR, Mubarak SJ, Sutherland DH: Proximal hamstring lengthening in the sitting cerebral palsy patient. *J Pediatr Orthop* 1992;12(3):329-336.
13. Staheli LT, Corbett M, Wyss C, King H: Lower-extremity rotational problems in children: Normal values to guide management. *J Bone Joint Surg Am* 1985;67(1):39-47.
14. Gage JR, DeLuca PA, Renshaw TS: Gait analysis: Principle and applications with emphasis on its use in cerebral palsy. *Instr Course Lect* 1996;45:491-507.
15. Novacheck TF, Stout JL, Gage JR, Schwartz MH: Distal femoral extension osteotomy and patellar tendon advancement to treat persistent crouch gait in cerebral palsy: Surgical technique. *J Bone Joint Surg Am* 2009;91(Suppl 2):271-286.
16. Mosca VS: Calcaneal lengthening for valgus deformity of the hindfoot: Results in children who had severe, symptomatic flatfoot and skewfoot. *J Bone Joint Surg Am* 1995;77(4):500-512.
17. Rathjen KE, Mubarak SJ: Calcaneal-cuboid-cuneiform osteotomy for the correction of valgus foot deformities in children. *J Pediatr Orthop* 1998;18(6):775-782.

Index

A

Achilles tendon rupture repair
   acute, 505
   chronic/neglected, 506–507
   complications, 507–508
   pearls, 508
Acromioclavicular (AC) joint reconstruction
   complications, 34
   patient selection, 31
   pearls, 34
   postoperative care and rehabilitation, 34
   preoperative imaging, 31–32
   room setup/patient positioning, 32
   special instruments/equipment, 32
   surgical technique, 32–34
Amputations
   Chopart, 555
   Lisfranc, 554–555
   midfoot, 551–556
   transtibial, 545–549
Ankle arthroscopy
   complications, 487–488
   contraindications, 485
   indications, 485
   outcomes, 488
   patient selection, 485
   pearls, 488
   postoperative care and rehabilitation, 488
   preoperative imaging, 485
   room setup/patient positioning, 486
   special instruments/equipment, 486
   surgical technique, 486–487
Ankle fractures, surgical treatment of
   complications, 448
   instruments/equipment/implants, 445
   patient selection, 443–444
   pearls, 449
   postoperative care and rehabilitation, 448
   preoperative imaging, 444–445
   room setup/patient positioning, 445
   surgical technique, 445–448
Ankle ligament reconstruction
   anesthesia, 500
   closure, 503
   complications, 503
   contraindications, 499
   indications, 499
   patient positioning, 499–500
   patient selection, 499
   pearls, 503
   postoperative care, 503
   preoperative imaging, 499
   surgical technique, 500–503
Anterior cervical corpectomy and fusion (ACCF)
   approach, 565
   central decompression, 569–570
   closure, 572
   complications, 572
   contraindications, 563–564
   deep exposure, 566–567
   disk removal, 567–568
   end-plate preparation, 571
   foraminal decompression and uncinate resection, 570
   graft, 564, 571
   indications, 563
   initial corpectomy, 569
   patient positioning, 564
   patient selection, 563–564
   pearls, 572
   postoperative care and rehabilitation, 572
   preoperative imaging, 564
   screw sizing, 571
   special instruments/equipment/implants, 564
   surgical technique, 565–572
Anterior cervical diskectomy and fusion (ACDF)
   complications, 561
   contraindications, 559
   indications, 559
   patient selection, 559
   pearls, 561–562
   postoperative care and rehabilitation, 561
   preoperative imaging, 559
   room setup/patient positioning, 560
   special instruments/equipment/implants, 560
   surgical technique, 560–561
Anterior cruciate ligament reconstruction, double-bundle
   closure, 114
   complications, 114–115
   contraindications, 109
   femoral fixation, 114
   femoral tunnel, anteromedial, 113–114
   femoral tunnel, posterolateral, 113
   graft preparation, 112
   indications, 109
   patient selection, 109
   pearls, 115
   portals and diagnostic arthroscopy, 111–112
   postoperative care and rehabilitation, 115
   preoperative imaging, 109
   room setup/patient positioning, 111
   soft-tissue débridement, 112–113
   surgical technique, 111–114
   tibial fixation, 114
   tibial tunnels, 113
Anterior cruciate ligament reconstruction, pediatric
   complications, 122
   conclusions/results, 122–123
   distal fixation, 121
   graft preparation, 119
   knee balance, 119-120
   lateral approach, 120
   patient selection, 118
   pearls, 122
   postoperative care and rehabilitation, 122
   preoperative imaging, 118
   proximal fixation, 121
   room setup/patient positioning, 118
   surgical technique, 118–121
   tibial tunnel preparation, 120–121
Anterior cruciate ligament reconstruction, single-bundle transtibial technique
   closure, 99–100
   complications, 100
   contraindications, 95

diagnostic arthroscopy and notch preparation, 97–98
graft harvest, 96–97
graft passage and interference screw fixation, 99
graft preparation, 97
indications, 95
patient selection, 95
pearls, 101
postoperative care and rehabilitation, 100–101
preoperative imaging, 95
room setup/patient positioning, 96
special instruments/equipment/implants, 96
surgical technique, 96–100
tibial tunnel placement, 98–99
Anterior cruciate ligament reconstruction, two-tunnel technique
complications, 107
femoral and tibial insertion site preparation, 105
femoral tunnel placement, 106
graft choice, 103
graft harvest and preparation, 105
graft passage and fixation, 107
patient selection, 103
pearls, 107–108
portals and incisions, 104–105
postoperative care and rehabilitation, 107
preoperative imaging, 103–104
room setup/patient positioning, 104
special instruments/equipment/implants, 104
tibial tunnel placement, 106–107
Anterior lumbar interbody fusion
complications, 627–628
contraindications, 625
diagnosis, 625
indications, 625
patient selection, 625
pearls, 628–629
postoperative care and rehabilitation, 628
preoperative imaging, 625–626
room setup/patient positioning, 626
special instruments/equipment/implants, 626–627
surgical technique, 627
APL suspensionplasty, 296–298
Arthritis
basal joint of thumb, 295–304
septic arthritis of hip, pediatric 653
subtalar arthrodesis, 515–518
tibiotalar arthrodesis, 509–514
Arthroplasty. *See* specific procedure
Arthroscopy
ankle, 485-489
anterior cruciate ligament double-bundle reconstruction, 111–112
anterior cruciate ligament reconstruction, 97–98
Bankart repair, 10–12
elbow, 203–209
femoroacetabular impingement, 55–58
medial meniscal root tears, 73–78
meniscectomy, 61
patellofemoral arthritis, 132
pediatric anterior cruciate ligament reconstruction, 118–121
rotator cuff disorders, 159–168
rotator cuff tears, partial-thickness, 3–8
subacromial decompression and distal clavicle resection, 150
superior labrum anterior-to-posterior tears, 17–24

B

Ball-tipped guide rod, 432
Bankart lesions, arthroscopic and open repair of
complications, 14–15
contraindications, 9
indications, 9
patient selection, 9
pearls, 15
postoperative care and rehabilitation, 15
preoperative imaging, 9
special instruments/equipment/implants, 10
surgical technique for arthroscopic repair, 10–12
surgical technique for open repair, 12–14
Basal joint arthritis of the thumb, surgical treatment of
APL suspensionplasty, 296–298
complications, 303
LRTI arthroplasty, 298–301
patient selection, 295
pearls, 303
postoperative care and rehabilitation, 303
preoperative imaging, 295–296
surgical technique, 296–303
thumb TMC arthroscopy, 301–303
Biceps tenotomy and tenodesis
complications, 28
contraindications, 25
indications, 25
patient selection, 25
postoperative care and rehabilitation, 28
preoperative imaging, 25–26
room setup/patient positioning, 26
surgical decision making, 26
surgical technique, 26–28
Boyd and Anderson two-incision approach for distal biceps repair, 44
Bryan-Morrey triceps-reflecting approach for total elbow arthroplasty, 226–227

C

Calcaneal fractures, open reduction and internal fixation of
assessing the peroneal tendons, 463
complications, 464
contraindications, 459
definitive fixation, 463
delayed wound healing/wound dehiscence, 464
indications, 459
mobilization of the fragments, 462
pathoanatomy, 460
patient selection, 459
pearls, 464–465
postoperative care and rehabilitation, 464
posttraumatic subtalar arthritis, 464
preoperative imaging, 459-460
reduction of the anterior process, 462–463
reduction of the articular surface, 462
resolution of soft-tissue swelling, 460–461
room setup/patient positioning, 461
special instruments/equipment/implants, 461
split tongue–type variant patterns, 462
surgical technique, 461–464
wound closure, 463
Calcaneal lengthening osteotomy, 706–707
Calcaneal sliding osteotomy, 707–708
Calcaneonavicular coalition resection, 690–692
Carpal ganglionectomy, 290

Carpal tunnel release (CTR)
    approach, 236
    complications, 240
    electrodiagnostic testing, 235
    open, 236–237
    outcomes, 235
    patient positioning, 236
    patient selection, 235
    pearls, 240
    postoperative care and rehabilitation, 240
    revision, 239–240
    single-incision endoscopic (modified Agee technique), 237–238
    surgical technique, 236–240
    two-incision endoscopic (Chow technique), 239
Carpal tunnel syndrome (CTS), 235, 239–240
Cerebral palsy, lower extremity surgery in children with
    adductor lengthening, 696–697
    bone procedures, 702–708
    calcaneal lengthening osteotomy, 707
    calcaneal sliding osteotomy, 707–708
    combined procedure for spastic hip subluxation/dislocation, 702–703
    distal femoral extension osteotomy with patellar tendon advancement, 706–707
    distal hamstring lengthening, 697–698
    Functional Mobility Scale, 696
    Gross Motor Function Classification System, 695
    lengthening of the gastrocnemius-soleus, 698–699
    pearls, 708
    peroneus brevis lengthening, 699
    posterior tibial tendon lengthening, 699–700
    proximal femoral rotational osteotomy, 703–705
    proximal femoral rotational osteotomy with patellar tendon advancement, 706
    psoas release at the pelvic brim, 700–701
    rectus femoris transfer to the hamstrings, 701
    soft-tissue lengthening procedures, 696–701
    soft-tissue transfer procedures, 701–702
    split posterior tibial tendon transfer, 702
    tibial derotational osteotomy, 705–706
Cervical laminoplasty
    complications, 588–589
    contraindications, 585
    indications, 585
    laminar closure, 589
    patient selection, 585
    pearls, 589
    postoperative care and rehabilitation, 589
    preoperative imaging, 585–587
    room setup/patient positioning, 587
    special instruments/equipment/implants, 587
    surgical technique, 587–588
    types of laminoplasty, 585
Chondrolysis, complication of Bankart repair, 14
Chopart amputation, 555
Clavicle fractures, open reduction and internal fixation of
    complications, 37
    contraindications, 35
    indications, 35
    intramedullary nailing, 36–37
    patient selection, 35
    pearls, 38
    plate fixation, 35–36
    postoperative care and rehabilitation, 37–38
    preoperative imaging, 35
    room setup/patient positioning, 35
    surgical technique, 35–37
Clubfoot, treatment using Ponseti method
    complex clubfoot, 684
    complications, 685–686
    contraindications, 683
    evaluation, 683
    indications, 683
    patient selection, 683
    pearls, 687
    percutaneous Achilles tenotomy, 685
    postoperative care and rehabilitation, 686–687
    serial casting, 684
    special instruments/equipment/implants, 683
    surgical technique, 684–685
    teratologic clubfoot, 684
    vascular complications, 685–686
Compartment syndrome of the leg, fasciotomy for
    complications, 372
    patient selection, 371
    pearls, 373
    postoperative care and rehabilitation, 372–373
    surgical technique, 371–372
Complex regional pain syndrome (CRPS)
    distal radius fractures, 266–267
    partial palmar fasciectomy, 309
Cubital tunnel syndrome, surgical treatment of
    anterior submuscular transposition, 245
    complications, 246
    contraindications, 242
    electrodiagnostic testing, 241–242
    endoscopic decompression (Hoffmann technique), 242–243
    indications, 242
    intramuscular transposition, 245
    medial epicondylectomy, 245
    open decompression, 242
    patient selection, 241–242
    pearls, 246
    physical examination, 241
    postoperative care and rehabilitation, 243, 246
    preoperative imaging, 242
    room setup/patient positioning, 242
    in situ decompression, 242–243
    special instruments/equipment/implants, 242
    subcutaneous anterior transposition, 244–245
    transposition techniques and medial epicondylectomy, 243–246
Cuff tear arthropathy, reverse total shoulder arthroplasty for
    complications, 200–201
    contraindications, 197
    indications, 197
    patient selection, 197
    pearls, 201
    postoperative care and rehabilitation, 201
    preoperative imaging, 197–198
    room setup/patient positioning, 198
    surgical technique, 198–200

D

de Quervain syndrome. *See* First dorsal extensor compartment release
Deep venous thrombosis (DVT)
    meniscal repair, 72
    meniscectomy, 64
Diaphyseal femur fractures, intramedullary nailing of
    complications, 410

contraindications, 407
indications, 407
patient selection, 407
pearls, 410
postoperative care and rehabilitation, 410
preoperative imaging, 407
room setup/patient positioning, 407
special instruments/equipment/implants, 407
surgical technique, 407–410
Digital mucous cyst excision
   complications, 291, 294
   contraindications, 293
   indications, 293
   patient selection, 293
   pearls, 294
   postoperative care and rehabilitation, 294
   preoperative imaging, 293
   surgical technique, 294
Discoid meniscus, 64
Distal biceps repair
   complications, 46
   patient selection, 43
   pearls, 46
   postoperative care and rehabilitation, 46
   preoperative imaging, 43
   special instruments/equipment/implants, 43
   surgical technique, 43–46
Distal clavicle resection, 151
Distal femoral fractures, surgical fixation of
   approaches, 416–417
   complications, 420
   contraindications, 413
   indications, 413
   patient selection, 413
   pearls, 420
   plate insertion, 418–420
   postoperative care and rehabilitation, 420
   preoperative imaging, 413
   reduction techniques, 417–418
   room setup/patient positioning, 414–415
   special instruments/equipment/implants, 415
   surgical technique, 415–420
   timing, 413–414
Distal humerus fractures, open reduction and internal fixation of
   complications, 223
   contraindications, 219
   indications, 219
   olecranon osteotomy, 221
   paratricipital approach, 220–221
   patient selection, 219
   pearls, 224
   postoperative care and rehabilitation, 223–224
   preoperative imaging, 219
   reduction and fixation, 221–222
   surgical technique, 220–223
   triceps peel, 221
   triceps split, 221
Distal metatarsal osteotomy, 536–537
Distal radius fractures, external fixation of
   closed reduction and adjunctive procedures, 264–265
   complications, 266–267
   contraindications, 263
   indications, 263
   outcomes, 267–268
   patient positioning and setup, 264

patient selection, 263
pearls, 268
placement of distal fixator pins, 265–266
placement of proximal fixator pins, 265
postoperative care and rehabilitation, 267
preoperative imaging, 264
surgical technique, 264–266
Distal radius fractures, open reduction and internal fixation with volar locking plate
   complications, 261
   patient selection, 259
   pearls, 261
   postoperative care and rehabilitation, 261
   preoperative imaging, 259
   surgical technique, 259–261
Dupuytren disease, partial palmar fasciectomy for
   addressing joint contracture, 308
   complications, 308–309
   contraindications, 305
   fasciectomy types, 307
   incisions, 307
   indications, 305
   initial dissection, 307
   pearls, 309
   postoperative care and rehabilitation, 309
   preoperative imaging, 305
   preoperative planning, 306
   recurrence and extension of disease, 309
   room setup/patient positioning, 305–306
   special instruments/equipment, 306
   surgical technique, 306–307
   tissue excision, 307–308
   wound closure, 308

E

Elastic intramedullary nailing in pediatric femur fractures
   complications, 669
   pearls, 669
   special instruments/equipment/implants, 667–668
   surgical technique, 668–669
Elbow arthroplasty. *See* Total elbow arthroplasty (TEA)
Elbow arthroscopy
   accessory posterolateral portal, 207
   anatomy, 203–204
   anesthesia, 204
   anterolateral portal, 206
   anteromedial portal, 205
   arthroscopic synovectomy, 208–209
   complications, 209
   contraindications, 204
   diagnostic arthroscopy, 207
   direct lateral portal, 206
   equipment, 204
   indications, 204
   lateral decubitus position, 205
   loose bodies, 207–208
   patient positioning, 204–205
   patient selection, 204
   pearls, 209
   portal placement, 205–207
   posterior portal, 206
   posterolateral portal, 207
   prone position, 205
   proximal anterolateral portal, 206
   proximal anteromedial portal, 205–206

Electrodiagnostic testing
    carpal tunnel syndrome, 235–236
    cubital tunnel syndrome, 241–242
Electromyographic (EMG) studies, 235, 236
Ellman classification system, for partial thickness rotator cuff tears, 4
Endoscopic decompression (Hoffmann technique), 242–243
Extended trochanteric osteotomy, revision total hip arthroplasty via
    complications, 338
    contraindications, 334
    exposure, 335
    indications, 333–334
    osteotomy, 335–338
    patient selection, 333–334
    pearls, 338–339
    postoperative care and rehabilitation, 338
    preoperative imaging, 334
    preoperative planning, 334–335
    special instruments/equipment/implants, 335

F
Femoral derotation osteotomy
    complications, 674
    contraindications, 673
    indications, 673
    patient selection, 673
    pearls, 675
    postoperative care and rehabilitation, 674–675
    preoperative imaging, 673
    room setup/patient positioning, 673
    surgical technique, 673–674
Femoral neck fractures, open reduction and internal fixation of
    complications, 397
    fixation in the older patient, 397
    instruments/equipment/implants, 393–394
    patient selection, 393
    pearls, 398
    postoperative care and rehabilitation, 397
    preoperative imaging, 393
    surgical technique, 394–397
Femoroacetabular impingement (FAI), arthroscopic management of
    complications, 58
    contraindications, 55
    indications, 55
    patient selection, 55
    pearls, 58
    postoperative care and rehabilitation, 58
    preoperative imaging, 55
    room setup/patient positioning, 55–56
    special instruments/equipment/implants, 56
    surgical technique, 56–58
First dorsal extensor compartment release
    complications, 249–250
    patient selection, 247
    pearls, 251
    postoperative care and rehabilitation, 250–251
    preoperative imaging, 247
    room setup/patient positioning, 247
    special instruments/equipment/implants, 247
    surgical technique, 247–249
Forearm fractures, open reduction and internal fixation of
    approach for radial fixation, 378
    complications, 381–383
    evaluation, 376
    fixation of the radial fracture, 379–380
    fixation of the ulnar fracture, 380
    patient positioning/room setup, 376
    patient selection, 375–376
    pearls, 383
    postoperative care and rehabilitation, 383
    preoperative imaging, 376
    preoperative planning, 376
    provisional reduction of the radial fracture, 378–379
    surgical technique, 376–381
    wound closure, 380–381
Fracture-dislocation patterns, 460
Fractures
    flexion-type, 637–638
    forearm, 375–384
    lateral condyle fractures of the distal humerus, 641–646
    open, 638–639
    pediatric femur, 663–672
    pediatric radial and ulnar shaft, 647–652
    supracondylar humerus, 633–640
    type IV, 638
Frozen shoulder, arthroscopic management of
    complications, 156–157
    patient selection, 153
    pearls, 157
    postoperative care and rehabilitation, 157
    preoperative imaging, 153–154
    surgical technique, 154–156
Functional Mobility Scale for cerebral palsy, 696

G
Ganglion cysts of the wrist and hand, excision of
    arthroscopic ganglionectomy, 289
    carpal ganglionectomy, 290
    complications, 290–291
    contraindications, 288
    dorsal wrist ganglionectomy, 290
    indications, 287–288
    instruments/equipment, 288
    mucous cyst excision, 290
    open dorsal wrist ganglionectomy, 288–289
    open volar wrist ganglionectomy, 289
    patient presentation, 287
    patient selection, 287–288
    pearls, 291
    postoperative care and rehabilitation, 291
    preoperative imaging, 288
    radial-side ganglionectomy, 289
    retinacular cyst excision, 289–290
    room setup/patient positioning, 288
    surgical technique, 288–290
    ulnar-side ganglionectomy, 289
    wound closure, 289
Gastrocnemius-soleus lengthening, 698–699
Golfer's elbow. See Medial epicondylitis
Gross Motor Function Classification System, 695

H
Hallux valgus, osteotomies for
    complications, 538–539
    contraindications, 535
    distal metatarsal osteotomy, 536–537
    indications, 535
    patient selection, 535–536
    pearls, 539
    postoperative care and rehabilitation, 539

preoperative imaging, 536
proximal metatarsal osteotomy, 537–538
room setup/patient positioning, 536
special instruments/equipment/implants, 536
surgical technique, 536–538
Hemiarthroplasty, hip
direct anterior approach, 329–330
direct lateral approach, 321–322
Hip arthroplasty, direct anterior approach
contraindications, 325
indications, 325
patient selection, 325
pearls, 331
postoperative care and rehabilitation, 330–331
preoperative imaging, 325
room setup/patient positioning, 325–326
special instruments/equipment/implants, 326
surgical technique, 326–330
Hip arthroplasty, via a direct lateral approach
complications, 322
contraindications, 319
indications, 319
patient selection, 319
pearls, 323
postoperative care and rehabilitation, 322–323
preoperative imaging, 319
room setup/patient positioning, 319
special instruments/equipment, 319
surgical technique, 319–321
Hip arthroplasty, via small-incision enhanced posterior soft-tissue repair
complications, 317
contraindications, 313
hemiarthroplasty, surgical technique, 316–317
indications, 313
patient selection, 313
pearls, 317
postoperative care and rehabilitation, 317
preoperative imaging and planning, 313
room setup/patient positioning, 313
SIEPSTR approach, 316
special instruments/equipment, 313
surgical technique, 313–317

I

Infection
anterior cruciate ligament reconstruction, 100
Bankart repair, 14
cervical laminoplasty, 588
clavicle fractures, 37
cubital tunnel syndrome, 246
cuff tear arthropathy, 201
distal radius fractures, 261, 266
Dupuytren disease, 308
hip arthroplasty, 322
meniscal repair, 72
total elbow arthroplasty, 230
total shoulder arthroplasty for osteoarthritis, 196
transforaminal lumbar interbody fusion, 620
Instrumented lumbar fusion
complications, 614–615
contraindications, 611
indications, 611
patient selection, 611
pearls, 615
postoperative care and rehabilitation, 615

preoperative imaging, 611
room setup/patient positioning, 612
special instruments/equipment/implants, 612
surgical technique, 612–614
Intertrochanteric fracture fixation
complications, 404
contraindications, 401
indications, 401
patient selection, 401
pearls, 405–405
postoperative care and rehabilitation, 404
preoperative imaging, 401
room setup/patient positioning, 401–402
special instruments/equipment, 402
surgical technique for cephalomedullary nail, 402–403
surgical technique for sliding hip screw, 403–404
Intramedullary (IM) nailing, 36–37

K

Kyphosis line concept, 585–586

L

Laminoplasty, types of, 585
Lateral condyle fractures of the distal humerus, reduction and fixation of
complications, 644
patient selection, 641
pearls, 644
postoperative care and rehabilitation, 644
preoperative imaging, 641
special instruments/equipment/implants, 642
surgical technique, 642–644
Lateral epicondylitis, open treatment of
complications, 40
patient selection, 39
pearls, 41
postoperative care and rehabilitation, 40–41
preoperative imaging, 39
room setup/patient positioning, 39
special instruments/equipment/implants, 39
surgical technique, 39
Letournel classification system, 385
Ligament reconstruction tendon interposition (LRTI) arthroplasty, 295, 298–301
Lisfranc amputation, 554–555
Lobenhoffer approach, 424–429
Long head of the biceps tendon (LHBT), 25–29
Lumbar laminectomy
complications, 609–610
contraindications, 607
indications, 607
patient selection, 607
pearls, 610
postoperative care and rehabilitation, 610
preoperative imaging, 607
room setup/patient positioning, 607
surgical technique, 608–609
Lumbar microdiskectomy
complications, 605
contraindications, 601
indications, 601
patient selection, 601
pearls, 605
postoperative care and rehabilitation, 605
preoperative imaging, 601
room setup/patient positioning, 601–602

special instruments/equipment/implants, 601
surgical technique for, 602–604
surgical technique for far-lateral, 604–605

M

Mayo classification system, 215
Medial epicondylectomy, 245
Medial epicondylitis, open treatment of
    complications, 40
    patient selection, 39
    pearls, 41
    postoperative care and rehabilitation, 40–41
    preoperative imaging, 39
    room setup/patient positioning, 39
    special instruments/equipment/implants, 39
    surgical technique, 39–40
Medial meniscal root tears (MMRTs), repair of
    complications, 76
    diagnostic arthroscopy, 74–75
    patient selection, 73
    pearls, 77
    portals and incisions, 74
    posteromedial portal, 75
    postoperative care and rehabilitation, 76–77
    preoperative imaging, 73–74
    repair of, 73–78
    room setup/patient positioning, 74
    special instruments/equipment/implants, 74
    surgical technique, 74–76
Medial patellofemoral ligament reconstruction, for recurrent patellar instability
    complications, 128–129
    contraindications, 125
    indications, 125
    patient positioning/examination, 126
    patient selection, 125
    pearls, 129–130
    postoperative care and rehabilitation, 129
    preoperative imaging, 125
    surgical technique, 126–128
Meniscal repair
    complications, 71–72
    contraindications, 67
    indications, 67
    patient selection, 67
    pearls, 72
    postoperative care and rehabilitation, 72
    preoperative imaging, 67
    room setup/patient positioning, 68
    special instruments/equipment/implants, 68–69
    surgical technique, 69–71
Meniscal root tears, 63
Meniscectomy
    arthroscopy, 61
    complications, 64
    diagnosis, 60
    discoid meniscus, 64
    displaced bucket-handle tears, 63
    evaluation and tear morphology, 61–62
    horizontal cleavage tears, 62–63
    meniscal root tears, 63
    patient selection, 60
    pearls, 65
    preoperative imaging, 60–61
    radial tears, 62
    setup/equipment, 61
    surgical technique, 61–64
    vertical tears, 63
Metacarpal fractures, surgical fixation of
    metacarpal head fractures, 284–285
    metacarpal neck fractures, 282–283
    metacarpal shaft fractures, 283–284
    patient selection, 282
    pearls, 285
    postoperative care and rehabilitation, 285
    preoperative imaging, 282
Metatarsophalangeal (MTP) joint arthrodesis
    alternative treatments, 531
    complications, 533
    contraindications, 531
    indications, 531
    patient selection, 531
    pearls, 533
    postoperative care and rehabilitation, 533
    preoperative imaging, 531
    special equipment and implants, 531–532
    surgical technique, 532–533
Microfracture
    complications, 81
    contraindications, 79
    indications, 79
    patient selection, 79
    pearls, 82
    postoperative care and rehabilitation, 81–82
    preoperative imaging, 79
    surgical technique, 80–81
Midfoot amputations
    complications, 555
    contraindications, 551
    imaging, 552
    indications, 551
    laboratory and diagnostic tests, 551–552
    patient selection, 551
    pearls, 556
    postoperative care and rehabilitation, 555–556
    preoperative evaluation, 551–553
    room setup/patient positioning, 553
    surgical technique, 553–555
Milch classification system, 641
Motor root palsies, 589
Mucous cyst excision, 290
Multimodal pain management, 354
Myerson classification system, 468

N

Navicular stress fractures, surgical treatment of
    complications, 529–530
    patient positioning, 527–528
    patient selection, 527
    pearls, 530
    preoperative imaging, 527
    surgical technique, 528–529
Nerve conduction studies (NCS), 235, 236

O

Olecranon fractures, open treatment of
    complications, 217
    excision, 216
    open reduction and internal fixation, 216–217
    patient selection, 215–216
    pearls, 218
    postoperative care, 217–218

preoperative imaging, 216
room setup/patient positioning, 216
special instruments/equipment/implants, 216
surgical technique, 216–217
Olecranon osteotomy, 221
Osteoarthritis, total shoulder arthroplasty for
approach, 192–193
closure, 195–196
complications, 196–197
glenoid component placement, 194–195
glenoid exposure, 194
humeral preparation, 193–194
patient selection, 191
pearls, 196
postoperative care and rehabilitation, 196
preoperative imaging, 191
room setup/patient positioning, 191–192
special instruments/equipment/implants, 192
surgical technique, 192–196
Osteochondral lesions of the talus (OLTs), arthroscopic treatment of
classification of, 491–493
complications, 496
diagnostic imaging, 491
equipment, 493
pearls, 496
postoperative care, 496
setup/patient positioning, 493
surgical technique, 493–496
treatment options/indications, 492–493
Osteochondritis dissecans (OCD) lesions, surgical treatment of
comorbidities, 93
patient selection, 85–86
pearls, 93
preoperative imaging, 86–87
reparative procedures, 88–90
restorative procedures, 90–93
room setup/patient positioning, 87
surgical technique, 87–93
treatment decisions, 85

P

Patellar tendon injuries, surgical treatment of
acute patellar tendon repair, 140–141
complications, 143–144
extensor mechanism disruptions after total knee arthroplasty, 143–144
patient selection, 138
pearls, 145
postoperative care and rehabilitation, 144–145
preoperative imaging, 138–139
Patellofemoral arthritis, realignment for
complications, 133
diagnostic arthroscopy, 132
examination under anesthesia, 132
patient selection, 131
pearls, 134
postoperative care and rehabilitation, 133–134
preoperative imaging, 131
room setup/patient positioning, 132
special instruments/equipment/implants, 132
surgical technique, 132–133
Pediatric femur fractures, fixation of
complications, 666–667
elastic intramedullary nailing, 667–669
indications, 663

patient selection, 663
pearls, 667, 669, 670
postoperative care and rehabilitation, 667
preoperative imaging, 663
submuscular plating, 663
surgical technique, 664–666, 668–670
trochanteric intramedullary fixation, 669–670
Peroneus brevis lengthening, 699
Phalangeal fractures, open reduction and internal fixation of
complications, 276–278, 280
patient selection, 275
pearls, 278
phalangeal condylar fractures, 275–278
phalangeal shaft fractures, 278–280
postoperative care and rehabilitation, 276
surgical technique, 275–276, 279-280
Ponseti method, 683–687
Posterior cervical foraminotomy
complications, 577
contraindications, 575
indications, 575
patient selection, 575
pearls, 577
postoperative care and rehabilitation, 577
preoperative imaging, 575
room setup/patient positioning, 575
surgical technique, 575–577
Posterior cervical laminectomy and fusion
complications, 582–583
dural injury, 583
lateral mass instrumentation, 583
neurologic complications, 582–583
patient selection, 579
pearls, 583
postlaminectomy kyphosis, 583
postoperative care and rehabilitation, 583
preoperative imaging, 579
room setup/patient positioning, 579–581
special instruments/equipment/implants, 581
surgical technique, 581–582
vascular complications, 582
Posterior tibial tendon lengthening, 699–700
Posterior wall acetabular fractures, open reduction and internal fixation of
associated injuries, 385–386
classification of, 385
complications, 390
early management of dislocation, 386
equipment/implants, 386
exposure, 386–387
implant selection, 388
intra-articular fragments, 387
marginal impaction, 387
pearls, 390
postoperative care and rehabilitation, 390
preoperative imaging, 386
preoperative planning and patient positioning, 386
provisional fixation, 388
surgical technique, 386–390
wound management, 388–390
Posttraumatic osteoarthritis, 37
Posttraumatic subtalar arthritis, 464
Propionibacterium acnes, 14
Proximal femoral rotational osteotomy, 703–705
Proximal femoral rotational osteotomy with patellar tendon advancement, 706

Proximal fifth metatarsal fractures, open reduction and internal fixation of
  approach, 473–474
  complications, 478
  contraindications, 473
  guide pin positioning and drilling, 474–476
  indications, 473
  patient selection, 473
  pearls, 479–480
  postoperative care and rehabilitation, 478–479
  preoperative imaging, 473
  room setup/patient positioning, 473
  screws, 477–478
  special instruments/equipment/implants, 473
  surgical technique, 473–478
Proximal humerus fractures, hemiarthroplasty for
  complications, 187–188
  contraindications, 183
  history and physical examination, 183
  humeral prosthesis positioning, 185–186
  indications, 183
  patient selection, 183
  pearls, 188
  postoperative care and rehabilitation, 188
  preoperative imaging, 183–184
  room setup/patient positioning, 184
  special instruments/equipment/implants, 184
  surgical technique, 184–187
  tuberosity handling, 184–185
  tuberosity reduction and fixation, 186–187
Proximal humerus fractures, fixation of
  assessment of reduction, 180
  complications, 180–181
  contraindications, 175
  definitive fixation, 180
  exposure, 177–178
  extensile maneuvers, 178
  humeral head support, 179
  indications, 175
  patient selection, 175
  pearls, 181–182
  postoperative care and rehabilitation, 181
  preoperative imaging, 175
  provisional fixation, 179
  reduction maneuvers, 178–179
  room setup for fluoroscopic imaging/patient positioning, 175–176
  special instruments/equipment/implants, 176–177
  surgical technique, 177–180
Proximal humerus fractures, percutaneous pinning of
  complications, 172
  contraindications, 169
  indications, 169
  patient selection, 169
  pearls, 173
  postoperative care and rehabilitation, 172–173
  preoperative imaging, 169
  room setup/patient positioning, 169–170
  special instruments/equipment/implants, 170
  surgical technique, 170–172
Proximal metatarsal osteotomy, 537–538
Psoas release at the pelvic brim, 700–701

Q
Quadriceps injuries, surgical treatment of
  chronic quadriceps repairs, 141–143
  complications, 143–144
  extensor mechanism disruptions after total knee arthroplasty, 143
  patient selection, 138
  pearls, 145
  postoperative care and rehabilitation, 144–145
  preoperative imaging, 138–139
  tendon repair, 139–140

R
Radial and ulnar shaft fractures, intramedullary fixation of in skeletally immature patients
  complications, 651–652
  contraindications, 648
  indications, 647–648
  patient selection, 647–648
  pearls, 652
  postoperative care and rehabilitation, 652
  preoperative imaging, 648
  room setup/patient positioning, 648
  special instruments/equipment/implants, 648–649
  surgical technique, 649–651
Radial head fractures, open treatment of
  complications, 214
  patient selection, 211
  pearls, 215
  postoperative care, 214–215
  preoperative imaging, 211
  room setup/patient positioning, 211
  special instruments/equipment/implants, 211–212
  surgical technique, 212–214
Rectus femoris transfer to the hamstrings, 701
Retinacular cyst excision, 289–290
Revision total knee arthroplasty, via quadriceps snip
  clinical results, 361
  complications, 361
  contraindications, 359
  indications, 359
  patient selection, 359
  pearls, 361
  postoperative care and rehabilitation, 361
  room setup/patient positioning, 359
  special instruments/equipment/implants, 359
  surgical technique, 359–360
Revision total knee arthroplasty, via tibial tubercle osteotomy
  complications, 365
  contraindications, 363
  indications, 363
  patient selection, 363
  pearls, 365–366
  postoperative care and rehabilitation, 365
  preoperative imaging, 363
  room setup/patient positioning, 363
  special instruments/equipment/implants, 364
  surgical technique, 364–365
Rockwood classification system, 31
Rotator cuff disorders, arthroscopic repair of
  anchor placement and suture passage, 164–165
  closure, 166
  complications, 166
  contraindications, 160
  indications, 160
  intra-articular arthroscopy and débridement, 162
  knot tying, 165
  lateral-row repair, 165–166
  marginal convergence sutures, 164

patient selection, 159–160
pearls, 167
postoperative care and rehabilitation, 166–167
preoperative imaging, 160
special instruments/equipment/implants, 161
subacromial bursectomy and acromioplasty, 162–163
surgical technique, 161–166
tear characterization and mobilization, 163
tips for portal placement, 162
tuberosity and tendon preparation, 163–164
Rotator cuff tears, arthroscopic repair of partial-thickness
bursal-side tears, 6
classification of, 4
complications, 6–7
contraindications, 3
diagnostic arthroscopy, 4
indications, 3
patient selection, 3
pearls, 7
postoperative care and rehabilitation, 7
preoperative imaging, 3
repair of, 4–6
room setup/patient positioning, 3
special instruments/equipment, 4
surgical technique, 4–6
transosseous-equivalent technique, 5–6

S

Scaphoid fractures, open reduction and internal fixation of
complications, 272–273
dorsal approach, 272–273
patient selection, 269–270
pearls, 273–274
postoperative care and rehabilitation, 273
preoperative imaging, 269
room setup/patient positioning, 270
special instruments/equipment/implants, 270
surgical technique, 270–272
volar approach, 270–272
Scapular notching, 200
Seebauer classification system, 198
Septic hip, incision and drainage of
complications, 655–656
patient selection, 653
pearls, 656
postoperative care and rehabilitation, 656
preoperative imaging, 653
room setup/patient positioning, 653
special instruments/equipment/implants, 653
surgical technique, 654–655
SIEPSTR approach, 316
Single-incision endoscopic CTR (modified Agee technique), 237–238
Slipped capital femoral epiphysis (SCFE), percutaneous in situ fixation of
complications, 660–661
patient selection, 657
pearls, 662
postoperative care and rehabilitation, 661–662
preoperative imaging, 657
room setup/patient positioning, 657–659
surgical technique, 659–660
Snyder classification system, 17
Spastic hip subluxation/dislocation, combined procedure for, 702–703
Split posterior tibial tendon transfer, 701–702

Stenosing tenosynovitis. *See* Trigger finger
Subacromial decompression, arthroscopic
acromioplasty and subacromial decompression, 150–151
complications, 152
diagnostic arthroscopy, 150
distal clavicle resection, 151
examination under anesthesia, 150
patient selection, 149
pearls, 152
postoperative care and rehabilitation, 152
preoperative imaging, 149
room setup/patient positioning, 149
special instruments/equipment/implants, 149
surgical technique, 150–152
Subtalar arthrodesis
complications, 517
contraindications, 515
deformity correction, 516–517
implants, 515
indications, 515
outcomes, 517–518
patient selection, 515
pearls, 518
postoperative care and rehabilitation, 517
preoperative imaging, 515
setup/patient positioning, 515
surgical technique, 515–517
Superior labrum anterior-to-posterior (SLAP) tears, arthroscopic repair of
alternative repair techniques and considerations, 21–22
cannula placement, 20
complications, 22–23
contraindications, 18
diagnostic arthroscopy, 20
indications, 18
patient selection, 18
pearls, 23
postoperative care and rehabilitation, 23
preoperative imaging, 18
range of motion goals following repair, 23
room setup/patient positioning, 19
special instruments/equipment/implants, 19–20
surgical considerations, 18–19
surgical technique, 20–22
suture anchor placement, 20–21
Supracondylar humerus fractures, closed and open reduction of
dressing and casting, 637
flexion-type fractures, 637–638
fracture fixation, 636–637
fracture reduction, 634–636
lateral-entry vs. medial-entry pins, 637
nonsurgical management, 634
open fractures, 638–639
patient evaluation, 633–634
pearls, 639
postoperative care and rehabilitation, 639
room setup/patient positioning, 634
surgical technique, 634–637
type IV fractures, 638
Surgical débridement, general principles of
postoperative care and rehabilitation, 369
surgical technique, 369

T

Talus fractures, surgical management of
  anatomy, 451
  classification of, 452
  complications, 455
  contraindications, 452
  indications, 452
  instruments/equipment/implants, 453–454
  mechanism of injury, 451–452
  patient positioning, 453
  patient selection, 452
  pearls, 455–456
  postoperative care and rehabilitation, 455
  preoperative imaging, 452–453
  surgical technique, 454–455
Tarsal coalitions, treatment of
  calcaneonavicular coalition resection, 690–692
  complications, 694
  fat graft harvest, 693–694
  patient selection, 689
  pearls, 694
  postoperative care and rehabilitation, 694
  preoperative imaging, 689
  room setup/patient positioning, 689
  special instruments/equipment/implants, 689–690
  surgical technique, 690–694
  talocalcaneal coalition resection, 692–693
Tarsometatarsal joint, arthrodesis of
  anatomy, 519
  complications, 523–524
  contraindications, 519
  indications, 519
  patient selection, 519
  pearls, 524
  postoperative care and rehabilitation, 524
  surgical technique, 519–523
Tarsometatarsal joint fracture-dislocations, open reduction and internal fixation of
  complications, 470
  patient selection, 467
  pearls, 470
  postoperative care and rehabilitation, 470
  preoperative (diagnostic) imaging, 467–468
  room setup/patient positioning, 468
  special instruments/equipment/implants, 468–489
  surgical technique, 469–470
Tennis elbow. *See* Lateral epicondylitis
Thoracic pedicle screws, placement of
  closure, 596–597
  complications, 597
  contraindications, 591
  gearshift probing, 594–595
  incision and exposure, 592–593
  indications, 591
  patient selection, 591
  pearls, 598
  pedicle sounding, 595–596
  postoperative care and rehabilitation, 598
  preoperative imaging, 591
  room setup/patient positioning, 591–592
  special instruments/equipment/implants, 592
  starting point and trajectory, 593–594
  surgical technique, 592–597
Thrower's elbow. *See* Medial epicondylitis
Tibial diaphyseal intramedullary nailing
  approach and start site, 430
  complications, 435
  contraindications, 429
  fracture reduction, 431
  incision closure, 434–435
  indications, 429
  interlocking screw enhancement, 434
  patient selection, 429
  pearls, 435
  postoperative care and rehabilitation, 435
  preoperative imaging, 429
  room setup/patient positioning, 429
  special instruments/equipment/implants, 429–430
  surgical technique, 430–435
Tibial plafond, open reduction and internal fixation of
  complications, 441–442
  contraindications, 437
  definitive surgery, 440–441
  implants, 441
  index surgery, 438–440
  indications, 437
  patient selection, 437
  pearls, 442
  postoperative care and rehabilitation, 442
  preoperative imaging, 437
  room setup/patient positioning, 438
  sequence of reduction, 441
  surgical technique, 438–441
Tibial plateau fractures, open reduction and internal fixation of
  alternative treatments, 421
  anterolateral approach, 423–424
  approaches, 422
  classification of, 421
  complications, 425–427
  contraindications, 421
  indications, 421
  Lobenhoffer approach, 424–425
  patient selection, 421
  pearls, 427
  postoperative care and rehabilitation, 427
  preoperative imaging, 421–422
  room setup/patient positioning, 422
  special instruments/equipment/implants, 422–423
  surgical technique, 423–425
Tibial spine fractures in children, surgical reduction and fixation of
  complications, 681
  contraindications, 677
  indications, 677
  patient selection, 677
  pearls, 681–682
  postoperative care and rehabilitation, 681
  preoperative imaging, 677
  room setup/patient positioning, 677–678
  special instruments/equipment/implants, 678
  surgical technique, 678–681
Tibiotalar arthrodesis
  contraindications, 509
  general principles of, 509–510
  indications, 509
  outcomes/complications, 512–514
  patient positioning, 510
  patient selection, 509
  pearls, 514
  postoperative care, 514
  preoperative imaging, 509

special instruments/equipment/implants, 510
surgical technique, 510–512
Total elbow arthroplasty (TEA)
bone preparation, 228–229
Bryan-Morrey triceps-reflecting approach, 226–227
complications, 230–231
contraindications, 225
indications, 225
patient selection, 225
pearls, 231
postoperative care and rehabilitation, 231
preoperative evaluation, 225
preoperative imaging, 225
preoperative planning, 225
room setup/patient positioning, 225–226
surgical technique, 226–229
triceps-sparing approach, 227–228
Total knee arthroplasty, via the medial parapatellar approach
arthrotomy, 342–343
bone resection, 343
complications, 344
contraindications, 341
implantation of components, 343–344
indications, 341
patellar eversion and additional exposure, 343
patient selection, 341
pearls, 344
posteromedial soft-tissue release, 343
postoperative care and rehabilitation, 344
preoperative evaluation, 341
room setup/patient positioning, 342
special instruments/equipment, 342
surgical technique, 342–343
Total knee arthroplasty, via the mini-subvastus approach
applicability, 355–356
complications, 356
concerns about minimally invasive, 355
contraindications, 351
femoral and tibial preparation, 352–354
incision and arthrotomy, 351–352
indications, 351
learning curve, 356
mobilization, 354–355
multimodal pain management, 354
patellar mobilization, 352
patient selection, 351
pearls, 355
postoperative care and rehabilitation, 354
room setup/patient positioning, 351
special instruments/equipment/implants, 351
surgical technique, 351–354
trialing, balancing, and final preparation, 354
Total knee arthroplasty, via small-incision midvastus approach
closure, 349
complications, 349
component insertion, 349
contraindications, 345
distal femoral resection, 346–347
exposure, 346
femoral sizing and anterior-posterior resection, 348
final preparation, 348–349
indications, 345
patellar preparation, 348
patient positioning, 345
patient selection, 345
pearls, 350

postoperative care and rehabilitation, 350
preoperative imaging, 345
special instruments, 345–346
surgical technique, 346–349
tibial preparation, 347–348
Total shoulder arthroplasty for osteoarthritis, 191–198
Transforaminal lumbar interbody fusion (TLIF)
complications, 620–622
contraindications, 617
indications, 617
infection, 620
patient selection, 617
pearls, 622
pedicle screw malposition, 621
postoperative care and rehabilitation, 622
postoperative radiculopathy, 621
preoperative imaging, 617
pseudarthrosis, 621
room setup/patient positioning, 617
special instruments/equipment/implants, 617
surgical technique, 618–620
Transtibial amputation
complications, 548
contraindications, 545
indications, 545
patient selection, 545
pearls, 549
postoperative care and rehabilitation, 548–549
preparation for a bone-bridge procedure, 547–548
room setup/patient positioning, 545–546
special instruments/equipment/implants, 546
surgical technique, 546–547
Triceps peel, 221
Triceps split, 221
Trigger finger release
anatomy, 254
complications, 256
contraindications, 254
indications, 253–254
patient selection, 253–254
patients with diabetes, 253
patients with distal triggering, 253
patients with PIP contracture, 253
patients with rheumatoid arthritis, 253
pearls, 256
postoperative care and rehabilitation, 256
preoperative imaging, 254
release of the central digits (ring or long finger), 254–256
special populations/situations, 253
trigger thumb release, 256
Two-incision endoscopic CTR (Chow technique), 238–239

U

Ulnar collateral ligament (UCL) reconstruction
complications, 52
contraindications, 50
indications, 49–50
patient positioning/special equipment, 50
patient selection, 49–50
pearls, 53
postoperative care and rehabilitation, 52–53
preoperative planning, 50
surgical technique, 50–52